Breast Cancer Screening and Diagnosis

Mahesh K. Shetty
Editor

Breast Cancer Screening and Diagnosis

A Synopsis

Springer

Editor
Mahesh K. Shetty, MD, FRCR, FACR, FAIUM
Department of Radiology
Baylor College of Medicine,
Houston, TX
USA

Woman's Center for Breast Care and MRI,
Woman's Hospital of Texas
Houston, TX
USA

ISBN 978-1-4939-1266-7 ISBN 978-1-4939-1267-4 (eBook)
DOI 10.1007/978-1-4939-1267-4
Springer New York Heidelberg Dordrecht London

Library of Congress Control Number: 2014949798

Printed on acid-free paper

Springer is part of Springer Science+Business Media (www.springer.com)

To women who have suffered the devastation of breast cancer and faced the disease with grit, to their loved ones who had to endure the agony of the suffering or loss of a beloved one.

To Dr. Al Watson, a mentor, a guide, and a friend, who has nurtured me throughout my career as a Breast Imager, for his unwavering and relentless support of my professional pursuits.

To my sister, Shobha, for her love and affection, to my mother, Sundari, and to my daughters, Ambika and Sarika, who inspire my life.

Mahesh K. Shetty, MD, FACR

Foreword

One of my favorite sayings is that "Times Change."

Over the past 40 years breast imaging has dramatically changed. The 1970s and 1980s we transitioned from xeromammography to film-screen mammography and from mostly diagnostic to screening and diagnostic mammography. Early mammographic screening trials, the HIP of New York and BCCDP and later the Swedish Trials, provided statistically significant data to support the reduction of breast cancer mortality through screening. As screening mammography was developed, there was a need for standardization of breast imaging which led to the development of ACR and MQSA standards. In the 1990s, breast ultrasound helped take some of the mystique out of the diagnosis of breast masses. Use of core needle biopsies and later vacuum assisted tissue sampling greatly reduced the need for open surgical biopsies. During this evolution of breast imaging, the care of breast diseases was transferred from the surgical specialties to radiology with the development of breast imaging specialization. Since 2000, digital mammography has nearly replaced film screen mammography. The use of breast MRI has further improved the diagnosis of benign vs. malignant breast diseases. Breast tomosynthesis, nuclear medicine (breast specific gamma imaging), and screening breast ultrasounds are also being used today to improve the diagnosis of early or subtle breast cancer findings.

Yes, "Times Change"! This text book, *Breast Cancer Screening and Diagnosis*, brings the reader up to date on changing times in breast imaging and provides a holistic approach to breast imaging. The authors are experts in all breast imaging modalities, screening and diagnostic mammography, breast ultrasound, breast MRI, tomosynthesis and breast interventional procedures. These are also authors whose expertise includes a multidisciplinary approach to breast cancer management.

The textbook carries an underlying theme: development of an interdisciplinary approach in the diagnosis, management and treatment of breast diseases. The targeted readers are not only breast imagers, general radiologists, and radiology residents, but also include breast oncologists, breast surgeons, radiation oncologists, pathologists, and the clinicians who refer their patients for breast imaging.

The chapter on multidisciplinary approach in breast cancer management provides the most concise synopsis of clinical trials that support the chemo-prevention, adjuvant, non-adjuvant, surgical, and radiation treatment of breast cancer. It provides all medical disciplines with the most recent evidence-based data to support different therapies in treating breast cancer.

Dr. Shetty has a life-long passion for decreasing breast cancer mortality through early diagnosis and appropriate treatment of breast cancer. He has spent the past 18 years as a dedicated breast imager who has lectured nationally and internationally, published peer-reviewed articles, formed organizations to promote early diagnosis of breast cancer, and taught radiology residents, clinicians, and technologists. This book further expands

Dr. Shetty's teaching and educational endeavors to those who promote breast imaging. He has been a part of the emerging breast imaging specialty and now provides an extremely well written and complete synopsis of breast cancer screening and diagnosis.

"Times Change": breast imaging is changing! Read, enjoy, and keep up to date.

Alfred B. Watson, Jr., MD, MPH, FACR, FACPM
Department of Radiology,
Baylor College of Medicine,
Houston, TX, USA

Preface

Breast cancer is now the leading cause of cancer in women worldwide and the most common cause of cancer-related deaths in women. Organized and opportunistic screening programs in the developed countries have resulted in a significant decrease in breast cancer mortality. Mammography, while not the perfect tool, is the best available and the only modality scientifically proven to be of value in reducing mortality from breast cancer based on data from multiple clinical trials. To obtain maximum benefit from mammography, highest quality is mandatory, and, rightly so, the quality of mammography is strictly overseen by a federal mandate in the USA. There is a need to further strengthen this mandate to optimize performance and interpretation of mammography. The ultimate goal of screening mammography is to find a high percentage of small, nonpalpable cancers while keeping the false positives at a minimally acceptable level. Technology of mammography has made steady progress, leading to improving sensitivity.

There has been an expanded role for sonography and MRI as supplemental tools in breast cancer screening and diagnosis. New technologies continue to emerge. Molecular imaging holds great promise in the imaging armamentarium, and, as our knowledge and understanding of tumor behavior and biology expand, this has particular relevance in being able to predict response to treatment.

This textbook is a synopsis of the current trends and practices in breast imaging. The chapters are organized and presented in a format that addresses the needs of residents in training, radiologists in practice, as well as physicians in the affiliated specialties of breast oncology and surgery. This book covers topics that include mammographic interpretation, postoperative breast, current and new technology in breast imaging, breast intervention with imaging pathological correlation, and the management of the symptomatic breast in young, pregnant, and lactating women. An excellent description of current and emerging technologies is provided by Drs. Svahn, Newell, and Holbrook in their respective chapters. The management of breast cancer is challenging and requires a multidisciplinary approach. This is discussed by Drs. Hunt and DeSnyder in their chapter on the multidisciplinary approach to breast cancer. Dr. Destounis and colleagues provide an overview of the operations and design of a comprehensive breast center. Each contributor is a recognized expert in the screening, diagnosis, and management of the breast cancer patient and has translated his/her experience and expertise into a well-written and informative chapter. The information provided in this text book will serve as a ready reference for Physicians involved in Breast cancer management.

Houston, TX, USA Mahesh K. Shetty, MD, FRCR, FACR, FAIUM

Contents

Contributors

Andrea Arieno, BS Elizabeth Wende Breast Care LLC, Rochester, NY, USA

Abigail S. Caudle, MD, MS Department of Surgical Oncology, University of Texas MD Anderson Cancer Center, Houston, TX, USA

Anu Chittenden, MS, CGC Department of Medical Oncology/Population Sciences, Dana-Farber Cancer Institute, Boston, MA, USA

Sarah M. DeSnyder, MD Department of Surgical Oncology, University of Texas MD Anderson Cancer Center, Houston, TX, USA

Stamatia Destounis, MD, FACR Elizabeth Wende Breast Care LLC, Rochester, NY, USA

Lilian O. Ebuoma, MD Department of Radiology, Baylor College of Medicine, Houston, TX, USA

Riham H. El Khouli, MD, PhD Department of Radiology and Radiological Sciences, The Johns Hopkins University School of Medicine, Baltimore, MD, USA

Nan M. Garrett, MD Department of Radiology, Woman's Hospital of Texas, Houston, TX, USA

Karen E. Gerlach, MD, MS Department of Radiology, Woman's Hospital of Texas, Houston, TX, USA

Anna I. Holbrook, MD Department of Radiology and Imaging Sciences, Emory University, Atlanta, GA, USA

Kelly K. Hunt, MD Department of Surgical Oncology, University of Texas MD Anderson Cancer Center, Houston, TX, USA

Michael A. Jacobs, PhD The Russell H. Morgan Department of Radiology and Radiological Sciences, Sidney Kimmel Comprehensive Cancer Center, The Johns Hopkins University School of Medicine, Baltimore, MD, USA

H. Carisa Le-Petross, MD, FRCPC Department of Radiology, University of Texas MD Anderson Cancer Center, Houston, TX, USA

Katarzyna J. Macura, MD, PhD The Russell H. Morgan Department of Radiology and Radiological Sciences, The Johns Hopkins University School of Medicine, Baltimore, MD, USA

Renee Morgan, RT Elizabeth Wende Breast Care LLC, Rochester, NY, USA

Mary S. Newell, MD Department of Radiology and Imaging Sciences, Emory University, Atlanta, GA, USA

Tamara Ortiz-Perez, MD Department of Radiology, Baylor College of Medicine, Houston, TX, USA

Candace E. Roberts, MD Department of Radiology,
Baylor College of Medicine, Houston, TX, USA

Department of Radiology, The Woman's Hospital of Texas, Houston, TX, USA

Karla Arabela Sepulveda, MD Department of Radiology,
Baylor College of Medicine, Houston, TX, USA

Kristen Mahoney Shannon, MS, CGC Cancer Center Genetics Program,
Center for Cancer Risk Assessment, Massachusetts General Hospital, Boston, MA, USA

Mahesh K. Shetty, MD, FRCR, FACR, FAIUM Department of Radiology,
Baylor College of Medicine, Houston, TX, USA

Woman's Center for Breast Care and MRI, Woman's Hospital of Texas, Houston, TX, USA

Tony Martin Svahn, PhD Department of Clinical Sciences,
Skåne University Hospital, Malmö, Lund University, Helsingborg, Sweden

Alfred B. Watson, Jr., MD, MPH, FACR, FACPM Department of Radiology,
Baylor College of Medicine, Houston, TX, USA

Breast Cancer Genetics and Risk Assessment

1

Kristen Mahoney Shannon and Anu Chittenden

Introduction

An accurate estimation of breast cancer risk is essential in guiding clinical management for women at all levels of risk. The goal of providing the appropriate clinical management is to increase survival in high-risk women and decrease cost and complications in low-risk women. Women can be at high risk of developing breast cancer based on benign disease (like ADH and LCIS) as well as family history of cancer. While the former is determined by the surgeon, the genetic counselor is essential in using the family history to distinguish those at high risk for breast cancer.

Recognizing Risk

It is essential to identify women who would benefit from genetic counseling and risk assessment and refer them to a provider who can assess risk using the aforementioned models and clinical judgment. Several health and professional organizations strongly encourage referral to a certified/credentialed cancer genetics professional for pretest counseling, prior to genetic testing. The National Comprehensive Cancer Network® (NCCN®) has established criteria for those individuals that need further genetics risk assessment (Box 1.1). If an individual meets these criteria, the NCCN® recommends that individual be referred to a cancer genetics professional for further work-up and potential genetic testing [1]. While these criteria are very helpful in identification, each individual practice/institution should establish a protocol so that the criteria are utilized.

The process of identifying and referring those needing further genetics assessment varies widely. Many practices will rely on physicians and other health-care providers to recognize and refer these individuals for further risk assessment [2]. The success of this strategy, however, relies on multiple factors – the strongest of which is patient inquiry about their need for genetic testing for cancer [3, 4]. Other programs implement a "pen and paper" family history questionnaire that is reviewed by a trained staff member to identify and refer for genetic counseling. Still others use a more complex approach, where a patient inputs his or her personal and family history into a computerized software program, and the software identifies those needing genetic counseling [5–7]. This software output must be reviewed systematically so as no woman identified as "high risk" is overlooked. The use of the Internet in the identification of at-risk women is a potentially powerful tool, and interest in this modality is high [8]. More research is needed to determine which of the strategies noted herewith are most efficient at identifying individuals at risk [9, 10].

Once an individual is recognized as being at increased risk, it is important that they are referred to a cancer genetics professional [1] as the importance of pretest and post-test genetic counseling for cancer susceptibility testing is widely recognized [11]. Referral to a cancer genetics professional is also important because the provider ordering the genetic testing must understand the complexities of genetic testing and the appropriate interpretation of the test results. One study reported that patients undergoing genetic testing for APC mutations often received inadequate counseling and would have been given incorrectly interpreted results [12]. The authors concluded that physicians should be prepared to offer

K.M. Shannon, MS, CGC (✉)
Cancer Center Genetics Program,
Center for Cancer Risk Assessment,
Massachusetts General Hospital, 55 Fruit Street,
YAW 10B, Boston, MA 01803, USA
e-mail: keshannon@partners.org

A. Chittenden, MS, CGC
Department of Medical Oncology/Population Sciences,
Dana-Farber Cancer Institute, 450 Brookline Avenue,
Boston, MA 02215, USA
e-mail: achittenden@partners.org

M.K. Shetty (ed.), *Breast Cancer Screening and Diagnosis: A Synopsis*,
DOI 10.1007/978-1-4939-1267-4_1, © Springer Science+Business Media New York 2015

Box 1.1 NCCN Criteria for Referral to Genetics Provider: Hereditary Breast and/or Ovarian Cancer Syndrome Testing Criteria [a,b,c] (V4.2013)

Individual from a family with a known deleterious BRCA1/BRCA2 mutation

Personal history of breast cancer[d] + one or more of the following:

- Diagnosed at age ≤45 years
- Two breast primaries[e] when first breast cancer diagnosis occurred ≤ age 50 years
- Diagnosed at age ≤50 years with ≥1 close blood relative with breast cancer at any age or with a limited family history
- Diagnosed at age ≤60 years with a triple-negative breast cancer
- Diagnosed at any age with ≥1 close blood relative[f] with breast cancer diagnosed ≤50 years
- Diagnosed at any age with ≥2 close blood relatives[f] with breast cancer at any age
- Diagnosed at any age with ≥1 close blood relative with epithelial ovarian cancer
- Diagnosed at any age with ≥2 close blood relatives[f] with pancreatic cancer or aggressive prostate cancer (Gleason score ≥7) at any age
- Close male blood relative[f] with breast cancer
- For an individual of ethnicity associated with higher mutation frequency (e.g., Ashkenazi Jewish), no additional family history may be required.[g]

Personal history of epithelial ovarian[h] cancer

Personal history of male breast cancer

Personal history of pancreatic cancer or aggressive prostate cancer (Gleason score ≥7) at any age with ≥2 close blood relatives[f] with breast and/or ovarian[h] and/or pancreatic or aggressive prostate cancer (Gleason score ≥7) at any age

Family history only (significant limitations of interpreting test results for an unaffected individual should be discussed):

- First- or second-degree blood relative meeting any of the above criteria
- Third-degree blood relative with breast cancer[d] and/or ovarian[h] cancer with ≥2 close blood relatives[f] with breast cancer (as least one with breast cancer ≤50 years) and/or ovarian[h] cancer
- Clinical judgment should be used to determine if the patient has reasonable likelihood of a mutation, considering the unaffected patient's current age and the age of the female unaffected relatives who link the patient with the affected relatives
- Testing of unaffected individuals should only be considered when an appropriate affected family member is unavailable for testing

HBOC testing criteria met, then see follow-up (HBOC-2)

HBOC testing criteria not met, then cancer screening as per NCCN screening guidelines

[a]One or more of these criteria are suggestive of hereditary breast/ovarian cancer syndrome that warrants further personalized risk assessment, genetic counseling, and often genetic testing and management. The maternal and paternal sides should be considered independently. Melanoma has been reported in some HBOC families

[b]Patients who have received an allogeneic bone marrow transplant should not have molecular genetic testing via blood or buccal samples due to unreliable test results from contamination by donor DNA. If available, DNA should be extracted from a fibroblast culture. If this source of DNA is not possible, buccal samples can be considered, subject to the risk of donor DNA contamination.

[c]Individuals with limited family history, such as fewer than 2 first- or second-degree female relatives or female relatives surviving beyond 45 years in either lineage, may have an underestimated probability of a familial mutation

[d]For the purposes of these guidelines, invasive and ductal carcinoma in situ breast cancers should be included

[e]Two breast primaries include bilateral (contralateral) disease or two or more clearly separate ipsilateral primary tumors either synchronously or asynchronously

[f]Close blood relatives include first-, second-, and third-degree relatives on the same side of family (see BR/OV-3)

[g]Testing for Ashkenazi Jewish founder-specific mutation(s) should be performed first. Full sequencing may be considered if ancestry also includes non-Ashkenazi Jewish relatives or other HBOC criteria are met. Founder mutations exist in other populations

[h]For the purposes of these guideline, fallopian tube and primary peritoneal cancers are included. Ovarian/fallopian tube/primary peritoneal cancers are component tumors of Lynch syndrome/hereditary nonpolyposis colorectal cancer; be attentive for clinical evidence of this syndrome. See NCCN guidelines for colorectal cancer screening

genetic counseling if they order genetic tests. Another study examining the genetic testing ordered at a large genetic testing company (including genetic testing for hereditary predisposition to cancer) showed that as high as 30 % of all ordered tests were inappropriately ordered [13]. Among frequently misordered tests in this study were requests for full gene sequencing when a familial mutation was known or when a screening panel would have been more appropriate. These studies suggest that if a physician is not adequately trained in the complexities of cancer genetic testing, a referral to cancer genetics professional should be made. The genetics professional will obtain a more detailed family history and determine who is appropriate for genetic testing. Practice guidelines exist to guide the genetic counselor in this process [14, 15].

Defining Risk

There exist various models which are used to estimate a woman's risk of breast cancer (Table 1.1). Most of these models can be classified into two groups: those that estimate the risk of developing breast cancer over time [16, 17] and those that estimate the probability of detecting a mutation in a cancer susceptibility gene [18, 19]. The most commonly used breast cancer risk assessment models are the Gail and Claus models. The model of Gail and colleagues [16] estimates breast cancer risk by taking into account a woman's age at menarche, age at first live birth, number of first-degree relatives with breast cancer, and previous biopsies, with specific focus on the presence of atypical hyperplasia. The Gail model will underestimate the risk of developing breast cancer in many women with a family history of cancer as it does not include breast cancer in non-first-degree relatives or a family history of ovarian cancer [20]. For this reason, the model is more appropriately used to determine breast cancer risk in individuals who do not have family histories suggestive of a hereditary breast cancer syndrome or who have tested negative for a known genetic mutation. The tables of Claus and colleagues [17] also determine the risk of breast cancer for unaffected women, taking into consideration the number and age at breast cancer diagnosis of first- and second-degree female

Table 1.1 Models used to predict the risk of breast cancer and the probability of a BRCA mutation

Model	Variables in model	Comments/limitations
Risk of breast cancer for unaffected women		
Gail et al. [16] Provides risk of breast cancer by a given age Available as an interactive tool at www.cancer.gov/bcrisktool	Age, FH of breast cancer, reproductive factors (age at menarche, menopause, and first childbirth and the number of live births), number of breast biopsies, personal history of atypia	Does not incorporate paternal FH of breast or ovarian cancer; does not include breast cancer in non-FDR; does not consider age of onset of breast cancer in relatives; derived from a population undergoing screening
Claus et al. [17] Provides 5-year and lifetime probability of breast cancer Available for download at www4.utsouthwestern.edu/breasthealth/cagene/default.asp	Age, FH of breast cancer (first- and second-degree relatives)	Limited to specific combinations of affected relatives; does not incorporate risk factors other than family history
Probability of detecting BRCA mutation (affected and unaffected women)		
Tyrer et al. [18] Also provides a 10-year and lifetime probability of breast cancer	Personal or family history of breast and ovarian cancer, Ashkenazi ethnic background	Incomplete validation, especially in nonwhite populations
Frank et al. [21] Provides empirical experience of one laboratory Available for download at www.myriadtests.com/provider/brca-mutation-prevalence.htm	Personal or family history of breast and ovarian cancer, Ashkenazi ethnic background	Empirical model with incomplete validation; does not include unaffected family members
BRCAPRO [19] Also provides age-specific probability of breast cancer Available for download at www4.utsouthwestern.edu/breasthealth/cagene/default.asp	Personal or family history of breast or ovarian cancer, Ashkenazi ethnic background	Requires information on all affected and unaffected family members; incorporates only FDR and SDR relatives and may need to change proband to best capture risk; uses high-penetrance estimates

Abbreviations: *FH* family history, *FDR* first-degree relative, *SDR* second-degree relative relatives. Despite this, the Claus model also underestimates the risk of a woman developing breast cancer if she has a hereditary predisposition to developing breast cancer because it does not take into consideration ethnicity or the presence of ovarian cancer in the family. This model, too, is more helpful in women without a family history suggestive of a known hereditary cancer syndrome.

For women with a family history of cancer, there exist models that help determine the likelihood of indentifying a mutation in a highly penetrant cancer susceptibility gene. There are a handful of models that are designed to estimate the likelihood of identifying a mutation in the *BRCA1* or *BRCA2* gene [18, 19, 21–23], for example. These models have both strengths and limitations that health-care providers must be familiar with to use and interpret them appropriately [24–26]. Probably the most widely used model is BRCAPRO which estimates the probability that an individual is a carrier of a *BRCA* mutation using family history and Bayes' theorem [19]. One limitation of the model is that it only incorporates relevant family history up to the second-degree relatives, potentially underestimating the probability of *BRCA* mutations in individuals with extended family history (e.g., early-onset breast cancer or ovarian cancer in cousins). On the other hand, the BRCAPRO model analysis is based primarily on large, high-penetrance families, thus this may lead to overestimation of risk in a more diverse risk assessment clinic.

A web-based model to predict the likelihood of identifying a mutation in the PTEN gene (which is responsible for Cowden syndrome) has been proposed by the researchers at Cleveland Clinic (http://www.lerner.ccf.org/gmi/ccscore/documents/adult_criteria.php). This model is based on a paper by Tan and colleagues [27] and proposes a clinical scoring system for selection of patients for PTEN mutation on the basis of a prospective study of 3,042 probands. The web-based model consists of a series of >20 clinical questions, with the output result of >3 % being the threshold for consideration of PTEN genetic testing. The major limitation of this model is that there is probable referral bias in the data it was based on, as the data were derived from two cohorts of patients representing patients recruited at two major cancer centers. While not a risk assessment model, the NCCN also has proposed criteria for when to offer PTEN testing. In these criteria, many of the clinical correlates present in the PTEN risk assessment model proposed by the Cleveland Clinic are removed. It remains unclear which of the previously mentioned is the most appropriate for determining those individuals at risk for PTEN mutations.

There are no statistical models that predict the likelihood of identifying mutations in the *TP53* or *CDH1* genes to date. Because there is no well-defined risk assessment model, it is important to be able to recognize other genetic syndromes based on personal and family history. (Please refer to full discussion of individual syndromes later in this chapter.)

It is important when using any risk assessment model to understand the limitations of these risk calculations and to place risk estimates into the appropriate context. It is important to note that risk estimates calculated by different models may vary—a factor that complicates the use of quantitative thresholds for making screening recommendations [28]. The health-care provider must use clinical judgment in addition to the estimates from models in order to provide the most precise risk assessment for an individual patient.

Genetic Counseling

The genetics professional will most often begin the assessment with collecting a detailed 3- generation family history in the form of a pedigree [29, 30]. It is important to gather information on both maternal and paternal lineages, with particular focus on individuals with malignancies (affected). Table 1.2 illustrates effective questions used by providers in obtaining this information [31]. It is imperative to include those family members without a personal history of cancer (unaffected) because the ratio and pattern of affected and unaffected influences the risk assessment. It is equally important to include the presence of nonmalignant findings in the proband and family members, as some inherited cancer syndromes have other physical characteristics associated with them (e.g., trichilemmomas with Cowden syndrome).

Table 1.2 Useful questions to use when obtaining a family history

Questions to ask all patients	Questions to ask patients who have had cancer or regarding relatives with cancer
Age	Organ in which tumor developed
Personal history of benign or malignant tumors	Age at time of diagnosis
Major illnesses	Number of tumors[a]
Hospitalizations	Pathology, stage, and grade of malignant tumors
Surgeries	Pathology of benign tumors
Biopsy history	Treatment regimen (surgery, chemotherapy, radiation)
Reproductive history[b]	Age at time of diagnosis
Cancer surveillance	
Environmental exposures	

Data from Trepanier et al. [31]

[a]For patients who have developed more than one tumor, it is important to discriminate whether the additional tumor(s) was a separate primary, recurrence, or the result of metastatic disease

[b]Especially important for women at increased risk of breast, ovarian, or endometrial cancer. Inquire about age at menarche, age at first live birth, history of oral contraceptive use, infertility medications, or hormone replacement therapy including dosage and duration, and age at menopause

When taking the family history, the accuracy of the information obtained from an individual patient should be considered. Sometimes individuals are even unclear about their own medical health history. One study reported that individuals who have had colonic polyps identified on colonoscopy do not recall key details about their own polyps (number, size, or pathology features) required to establish appropriate screening and surveillance intervals [32].

When talking about relatives, many factors can influence an individual's knowledge of their family history. A recent study indicates that individuals are often confident that a family member has had cancer but are typically unsure of the details surrounding that diagnosis [9, 33]. Reports of breast cancer tend to be accurate, while reports of ovarian cancer are less trustworthy [34, 35]. In a large study of 2,605 relatives that were sampled for confirmation of cancer reports on breast, colorectal, prostate, and lung cancer, sensitivity and positive predictive values were low to moderate and varied by cancer type: 60.2 and 40.0 %, respectively, for lung cancer reports, 27.3 and 53.5 % for colorectal cancer reports, 61.1 and 61.3 % for breast cancer reports, and 32.0 and 53.4 % for prostate cancer reports [36]. Studies have also found significant reporting differences between maternal and paternal family history of cancer, in addition to degree of relative [36, 37]. It is also important to note that family histories can change over time, with new diagnoses arising in family members as time passes [38]. See Box 1.2 [39].

All of these factors must be considered during the consultation, as the risk assessment and differential diagnosis is based primarily on this information. The primary purpose of the risk assessment process is to distinguish a hereditary form of cancer from familial clustering of cancer and sporadic forms of cancer. Features of a family history that are suggestive of a hereditary cancer syndrome include a preponderance of relatives with similar or related cancers; earlier age at onset of cancer; autosomal dominant pattern of cancer inheritance; the presence of rare cancers; the presence of multifocal, bilateral, or multiple primary cancers in one individual; and the absence of environmental risk factors. When a hereditary form of cancer is suspected, genetic testing should be entertained.

Box 1.2 Challenges in Collecting an Accurate Family History

Family history is incomplete
- Family members live far away
- Clients are not prepared to answer questions
- Cancer is not discussed in the family

Family history information is not available
- Lost contact with relatives
- Estrangement from the family
- Adoption

Reported history is false
- Mistaken about the cancer diagnosis
- Confused about the diagnosis
- Deliberately fabricating history

Adapted from Schneider [39]

Although some published guidelines for genetic testing exist, much of the time the decision to offer genetic testing is based on clinical judgment. The American Society of Clinical Oncology (ASCO) recommends that genetic testing be offered when (1) the individual has personal or family history features suggestive of a genetic cancer susceptibility condition, (2) the test can be adequately interpreted, and (3) the results will aid in diagnosis or influence the medical or surgical management of the patient or family members at hereditary risk of cancer [11]. The NCCN provides NCCN Clinical Practice Guidelines in Oncology (NCCN Guidelines®) for individuals that should be offered genetic testing for hereditary breast/ovarian cancer syndrome, Li-Fraumeni syndrome, and Cowden syndrome [1]. In the end, however, it is up to the individual provider's judgment as to whether or not genetic testing is indicated.

Genetic Testing Process

Once it has been determined that genetic testing is appropriate, the next step is to determine which individual in the family should be tested first. If there is not a known mutation in a family, testing should begin with a person that has the highest probability of finding a mutation. Typically, this is a person who has been diagnosed with cancer at an early age. If there is no such person available, the person with the highest a priori risk of carrying a mutation in the gene should be tested. If there is a known mutation in the family, testing should begin with those family members with the highest risk of carrying the familial mutation.

Testing Logistics

Finding the appropriate laboratory to perform the testing is also very important. Genetic testing for most cancer susceptibility genes is available at a variety of laboratories in a variety of settings. It is important to note that many genetic tests can be done in a research lab as well as in a clinical laboratory. Clinical certification via the Clinical Laboratory Improvement Amendments of 1988 (CLIA), however, is essential when using the DNA tests for clinical management of the individual. When choosing a laboratory, it is also important to consider the fact that laboratory techniques (as well as sensitivity of the technique) vary. Finally, cost of testing as well as insurance coverage issues need to be taken into account when choosing a laboratory to perform the genetic test.

The turnaround time for the genetic test will vary by gene and by laboratory. For most of the syndromes discussed in this chapter, genetic testing takes 4–12 weeks, and results are not available in enough time to impact the surgical management of a newly diagnosed breast cancer patient. There are two very important exceptions to this.

BRCA1/2 genetic test results are typically available within 14 days of the blood draw. The information gleaned from this has the potential to affect surgical decision-making if the results are available prior to definitive surgery. If a woman tests positive for a deleterious mutation, for example, she may choose mastectomy to treat her cancer and also undergo contralateral prophylactic mastectomy to reduce the risk of developing a second breast malignancy. Although women are interested in obtaining this genetics information at the time of diagnosis to help them plan their choice of surgery [40], women who report that they would not consider bilateral mastectomies even with a BRCA mutation are likely to proceed with breast-conserving surgery regardless of BRCA result [41].

Genetic testing for *TP53* mutations can take as little as 3 weeks if ordered as an "urgent" test. It is well known that *TP53* mutant cells are extremely sensitive to DNA damage [42, 43]. In vivo studies suggest that DNA damaging agents (e.g., chemotherapy and radiotherapy) used for treatment of a cancer in an individual with LFS can cause a second malignancy [44]. One study showed the risk of developing second cancer after radiotherapy treatment was as high as 57 % [45]. Although avoidance of chemotherapy in many situations is not plausible, radiotherapy can sometimes be avoided by different surgical techniques (e.g., mastectomy rather than lumpectomy for surgical treatment of breast cancer). It is important that oncologists realize that radiation should be avoided if possible (e.g., choosing mastectomy over lumpectomy). In many cases, however, radiation is needed for proper treatment of the current cancer, and in these cases, it should not be avoided. In these cases, it is imperative that the physicians and patient be aware of the risk of a second primary in the radiation field [44, 46].

For several reasons, it is important that the identification of women who are interested in and would use this genetic testing information in their surgical decision-making be done *prior to* any definitive treatment. First, when women undergo genetic counseling after definitive surgery, they are less likely to consider genetic testing pertinent to them [47]. Second, women may be subjected to additional surgical procedure and all of the associated risks. For example, one study showed that women who had *BRCA1/2* testing and who had initially undergone breast-conserving surgery chose to undergo subsequent bilateral mastectomies prior to receiving radiation therapy [48]. Finally, women with a family history of breast cancer may be advised to consider bilateral mastectomies for treatment of their newly diagnosed breast cancer. Most of these women if tested for BRCA mutations would find that they are not mutation carriers. Silva reported that in a group of such women, finding out that they are not mutation carriers *after* the prophylactic procedure leads many to question the decision to undergo prophylactic surgery. This, in turn, is often associated with complications and quality of life problems which they never envisioned [49].

Box 1.3 Components of Informed Consent

1. Purpose of the test and who to test
2. General information about the gene(s)
3. Possible test results
   Positive result
   Negative result: no mutation in the family (i.e., uninformative negative)
   Negative results: known mutation in the family (i.e., true negative)
   Variant of uncertain significance
4. Likelihood of positive result
5. Technical aspects and accuracy of the test
6. Economic considerations
7. Risks of genetic discrimination
8. Psychosocial aspects
   Anticipated reaction to results
   Timing and readiness for testing
   Family issues
   Preparing for results
9. Confidentiality issues
10. Utilization of test results
11. Alternatives to genetic testing
12. Storage and potential reuse of genetic material

Adapted from Trepanier et al. [31]

Informed Consent

Once a laboratory has been identified, it is necessary to obtain informed consent from the individual undergoing the test. The components and process of informed consent for cancer genetic testing have been described thoroughly [50–52] and are presented in Box 1.3. It is important to note that some US states have very specific laws that provide requirements as to what are the necessary components of the informed consent document itself.

Test Results and Follow-Up

Once the results are available, it is important to disclose the results to the patient in a timely fashion. The provider should review the significance of the results and quantify the patient's risk for developing cancer, the emotional impact of the test results on the individual, screening recommendations and how his/her medical management should proceed given the test results, and the importance of sharing the information with his/her relatives and resources if desired [31].

It is incredibly important for the health-care provider and patient to maintain communication [31]. For those individuals who are found to carry a mutation in a cancer predisposition gene, the follow-up can ensure that the patient is adhering to appropriate screening recommendations and also ensure that there is dissemination of the test result through family. For individuals who are found to be "true negative," the future contact can ensure that the patient understands the appropriate screening (i.e., not too much screening but not avoidance of appropriate, general population screening recommendations). Patients receiving a "variant of uncertain significance" should stay in touch with the ordering provider so that if the variant is reclassified, that new information can be communicated quickly to the patient and his/her family.

For patients receiving an uninformative negative (i.e., a negative result when no mutation has been previously identified in the family), it is crucial to remain in contact with their genetics health-care provider. As new genetic tests become available, for example, the provider can advise whether or not these newer techniques are appropriate for them. The most appropriate method for recontacting patients has yet to be determined, and interestingly, the uptake of the additional testing was quite low in one study [53]. Nonetheless, every attempt to communicate with individuals should be made to ensure that they receive the best care.

This issue has come up twice in recent history with genetic testing for *BRCA1/2*. In 2002, Myriad Genetics labs introduced a newer technique for detecting mutations in *BRCA1*. Again in 2006, Myriad Genetics added a technique called "rearrangement testing" or "BART" which brought the sensitivity of the *BRCA1/2* test up to nearly 99 %. For those women who had testing prior to these newer technologies, it was important to communicate the availability of these tests so that they could decide to proceed with the additional test or not.

More recently in 2013, laboratories started offering "breast cancer gene panel" testing for patients. These tests include mutational analysis for many genes that have been associated with an increased risk of breast cancer. (Please see sections later in this chapter for full discussion of each gene.) Genetic counseling and testing for gene panels is more complex than testing for single gene disorders because of the length of time to obtain results, the higher likelihood of variants of uncertain significance, and the number of syndromes and associated cancer risks that need to be reviewed and the potential difficulty in management recommendations.

With single gene analysis, genetic counselors can discuss the specific disorder in depth and can focus on the patient's questions related to the syndrome. In gene panel testing, counselors are faced with reviewing multiple syndromes in a short period of time and synthesizing pertinent information about each syndrome or associated cancer risk without overwhelming the patient. Currently, test reporting can take anywhere from 2 to 6 months, so this type of testing may not be feasible for decision-making regarding surgical intervention or oncology treatment.

In addition, testing for multiple genes means that there is a higher risk for finding unclear results. With BRCA testing, for example, the number of variants of uncertain significance has decreased dramatically over time, with a rate of 5 % or less for patients of most ancestries [54]. With panel testing, many of these genes on the panels are not well characterized in any population. This means that the likelihood of finding a variant of uncertain significance is quite high when testing multiple genes in this setting. One laboratory that has been doing gene panel testing notes that the rate of finding at least one uncertain variant is over 30 % for its breast cancer gene panel testing (personal communication, Ambry Genetics Laboratories).

Because of the large number of genes that are "new" and therefore not well studied, there are many questions about how to manage individuals with deleterious mutations in these genes. Even in the genes that are considered to have well-defined cancer risks, management issues can be controversial. With high-risk breast cancer genes, there are often clear or at least published guidelines on how to follow and treat women with mutations in these genes. Typically, if a woman is tested for a particular single gene, it is usually because her personal and family history is consistent with the syndrome. With the approach of testing for multiple genes simultaneously, alterations may be found in genes that are not consistent with the history in the family or the individual. Consider the following example:

BRCA testing was negative in a woman with an invasive ductal breast cancer diagnosed at 45 who has multiple first- and second-degree relatives with early breast cancer. She meets with a genetic counselor to consider additional genetic testing and goes forward with breast cancer gene panel testing, and 3 months later, analysis reveals that she has a deleterious *CDH1* mutation, which is associated with Hereditary Diffuse Gastric Cancer (HDGC) syndrome. Standard management recommendations include prophylactic gastrectomy. Do you recommend this to your patient, knowing that she does not have the typical type of breast cancer seen in HDGC and has no family history of gastric cancer?

With more moderate-penetrance genes, there are generally few if any published guidelines on how to manage individuals with these types of gene mutations. Management strategies are even harder to determine in the "unknown" category of genes on these panels, which often have few studies to provide clinicians with evidence-based research.

Inherited Breast Cancer Syndromes

The identification of individuals with cancer predisposition gene mutations affords the mutation carriers the ability to use the information in making medical management decisions. The most clearly described hereditary breast cancer syndromes for which genetic testing is available include hereditary breast and ovarian cancer syndrome (HBOC), Cowden syndrome (CS), Li-Fraumeni syndrome (LFS), Peutz–Jeghers syndrome (PJS), and hereditary diffuse gastric carcinoma syndrome (HDGC). All of these syndromes are inherited in an autosomal dominant pattern and are associated with other cancers and clinical features. As noted previously in this chapter, genetic testing for each of the genes associated with these syndromes is available through commercial and research laboratories, thus allowing for appropriate clinical care, genetic counseling, and testing for at-risk individuals. Newer "breast cancer panel tests" include testing for lesser known genes and are discussed at length next.

Hereditary Breast and Ovarian Cancer Syndrome

Hereditary breast and ovarian cancer syndrome is the most common form of hereditary breast cancer and hereditary ovarian cancer. The vast majority of cases of HBOC are due to mutations in the *BRCA1* and *BRCA2* genes [21, 55]. *BRCA1* and *BRCA2* mutations are found in approximately 1 of 400 individuals but found more commonly in the Ashkenazi Jewish population in which 1 of 40 individuals carries one of three main disease-causing mutations: two in *BRCA1* (187delAG and 5385insC, previously named 185delAG and 5382insC) and the 6174delT mutation in *BRCA2* [56, 57]. Other founder mutations have been identified in populations that tend to be isolated by culture or geography [58, 59].

BRCA-associated cancers have been studied extensively. *BRCA2*-associated breast cancers are similar in phenotype and clinical behavior to sporadic breast cancers [60, 61]. *BRCA1*-related breast cancers are often of higher histological grade, show an excess of medullary histopathology, and are more likely than sporadic tumors to be "triple negative" (i.e., estrogen receptor negative, progesterone receptor negative, and are less likely to demonstrate HER2/neu overexpression) [62]. Ovarian cancers found in women with *BRCA1* and *BRCA2* mutations tend to be serous papillary cancers. Endometrioid and clear-cell subtypes of ovarian cancer have been observed [63], but borderline and mucinous ovarian tumors do not seem to be a part of the phenotype [64]. Both primary tumors of the fallopian tubes and peritoneum occur with increased frequency in mutation carriers [65]. The prognosis of ovarian cancer in *BRCA1* and *BRCA2* carriers is better than age-matched controls [63, 66, 67].

Table 1.3 BRCA1/2 cancer risks (lifetime risks)

Cancer site	BRCA1 mutation (%)	BRCA2 mutation (%)
Female breast	50–80	40–70
Ovarian cancer	<40	<20
Prostate	<30	<39
Pancreatic	1.3–3.2	2.3–7

Adapted from Ford et al. [55], King et al. [69], Antoniou et al. [74], Risch et al. [75], The Breast Cancer Linkage Consortium [76], and Ozcelik et al. [70]

The penetrance associated with mutations in *BRCA1* and *BRCA2* remains an active area of research. The range of breast cancer risk is influenced by the population under study: higher-risk estimates have come from studies with affected families and somewhat lower-risk estimates from studies in populations. Also, the risk of ovarian cancer is not the same for all *BRCA2* mutations, with mutations in the central 'ovarian cancer cluster region', conferring a higher lifetime risk [68]. Other factors, such as birth cohort, oral contraceptive use, age at first pregnancy, and exercise, have all been shown to influence penetrance risk in populations [69]. There has been a report of increased risk of gallbladder and bile duct, stomach, and melanoma with *BRCA2* mutation, none of which seem to be clinically actionable [70, 71]. Pancreatic cancer risk is also increased in families with *BRCA1* and especially *BRCA2* alterations, although studies differ as to the magnitude of this risk [72, 73]. The risks of developing specific cancers can be found in Table 1.3 [55, 69, 70, 74–76].

The current NCCN screening recommendations for women are listed in Box 1.4. Risk-reducing mastectomies are an appropriate consideration for women at the highest hereditary risk for breast cancer. Studies have shown a 90–95 % reduction in breast cancer risk following prophylactic mastectomy [77–80]. The evidence for the use of tamoxifen or raloxifene as chemopreventive agents in *BRCA* carriers is limited; however, tamoxifen has been shown to reduce the risk of contralateral breast cancers in *BRCA* carriers [81–83]. Two fairly recent studies support the role of risk-reducing salpingo-oophorectomy: the hazard ratio for ovarian cancer for women who underwent prophylactic surgery compared to those who chose close surveillance was 0.15 and 0.04, respectively [84, 85]. Women should be informed about the potential for the subsequent development of peritoneal carcinomatosis, which has been reported up to 15 years following RRBSO [65, 86].

Male *BRCA* mutation carriers face an increased risk for breast cancer and prostate cancer. They are advised to undergo training in breast self-examination with regular monthly practice and semiannual clinical breast examinations, and work-up of any suspicious breast lesions is recommended. The NCCN Guidelines® also recommend that a baseline mammogram be considered, with an annual mammogram if gynecomastia or parenchymal/glandular breast density is identified

Box 1.4 NCCN Screening for Female BRCA Carriers

- Breast awareness[a] starting at age 18 years
- Clinical breast exam, every 6–12 months,[b] starting at age 25 years
- Annual mammogram and breast MRI[c] screening starting at age 25, or individualized based on earliest age of onset in family[d]
- Discuss option of risk-reducing mastectomy.
  - Counseling may include a discussion regarding degree of protection, reconstruction options, and risks.
- Recommend risk-reducing salpingo-oophorectomy,[e] ideally between 35 and 40 years, and upon completion of child bearing, or individualized based on earliest age of onset of ovarian cancer in the family.
  - Counseling includes a discussion of reproductive desires, extent of cancer risk, degree of protection for breast and ovarian cancer, management of menopausal symptoms, possible short-term hormone replacement therapy to a recommended maximum age of natural menopause, and related medical issues.
- Address psychosocial, social, and quality-of-life aspects of undergoing risk-reducing mastectomy and/or salpingo-oophorectomy.
- For those patients who have not elected risk-reducing salpingo-oophorectomy, consider concurrent transvaginal ultrasound (preferably days 1–10 of menstrual cycle in premenopausal women) + CA-125 (preferably after day 5 of menstrual cycle in premenopausal women)[f] every 6 months starting at age 30 years or 5–10 years before the earliest age of first diagnosis of ovarian cancer in the family.
- Consider chemoprevention options for breast and ovarian cancer, including discussing risks and benefits[g] (see NCCN guidelines for breast cancer risk reduction).
- Consider investigational imaging and screening studies, when available (e.g., novel imaging technologies, more frequent screening intervals), in the context of a clinical trial.

[a]Women should be familiar with their breasts and promptly report changes to their health-care provider. Periodic, consistent breast self-examination (BSE) may facilitate breast self-awareness. Premenopausal women may find BSE most informative when performed at the end of the menses

[b]Randomized trials comparing clinical breast exam versus no screening have not been performed. Rationale for recommending clinical breast exam every 6–12 months is the concern for interval breast cancers

[c]High-quality MRI limitations include having a need for a dedicated breast coil, the ability to perform biopsy under MRI guidance, experienced radiologists in breast MRI, and regional availability. Breast MRI is performed preferably days 7–15 of menstrual cycle for premenopausal women

[d]The best screening strategy for women age 25–30 is uncertain with some data suggesting that mammogram be added to MRI only after age 30. The appropriateness of imaging modalities and scheduling is still under study [225]

[e]Given the high rate of occult neoplasms, special attention should be given to sampling and pathologic review of the ovaries and fallopian tubes. (See discussion for details.) See the College of American Pathologists, Protocol for the Examination of Specimens from patients with Carcinoma of the Ovary

[f]There are data that show that annual transvaginal ultrasound and CA-125 are not effective strategies for screening for ovarian cancer in high-risk women. There are limited data regarding the effectiveness of a 6-month screening interval. Thus, until such data are available, it is reasonable to consider this approach in high-risk women, especially in the context of a clinical research setting

[g]Data suggest that oral contraceptives (OCs) reduce ovarian cancer risk in BRCA mutation carriers. The risk/benefit ratio is uncertain because of contradictory evidence about OC's increasing breast cancer risk; however, OC use for contraception is acceptable. Other chemoprevention options for breast cancer include tamoxifen and raloxifene; however, only very limited data with these agents are available in patients with BRCA mutations. (See discussion for details.)

on baseline study [1]. The guidelines also recommend that male BRCA mutation carriers should adhere to the current prostate cancer screening guidelines [1, 87].

Li-Fraumeni Syndrome [88]

Li-Fraumeni syndrome (LFS) is a rare cancer predisposition syndrome that is thought to be responsible for ~1 % of breast cancer [89]. LFS is often thought of as a hereditary predisposition to cancer in general, involving many tumor types and occurring at any point in an individual's lifetime, often early adult and childhood cancers. The majority of cases of LFS are due to mutations in the *TP53* gene [90–93]. The component tumors of LFS include bone sarcomas (primarily osteosarcomas and chondrosarcomas), soft-tissue sarcomas, breast cancer, brain tumors, leukemia, and adrenocortical carcinomas [94]. The classic component tumors are thought to account for 63–77 % of cancer diagnoses in individuals with Li Fraumeni syndrome [94–97]. Breast cancer is the most common tumor

Box 1.5 Other Tumors Associated with LFS

Wilms' tumor
Malignant phyllodes tumor
Lung cancer
Choroid plexus tumor
Colorectal cancer
Prostate cancer
Pancreatic cancer
Bladder cancer
Hepatoblastoma
Neuroblastoma
Lymphomas
Nasopharyngeal cancer
Teratomas
Ureteral tumors
Testicular cancer
Laryngeal cancer
Ovarian cancer
Melanoma
Gonadal germ cell tumors
Stomach cancer

Adapted from Gonzalez et al. [95], Nichols et al. [96], Hwang et al. [97], Kleihues et al. [98], Olivier et al. [99], Birch et al. [100], and Strong et al. [101]

in *TP53* mutation carriers (24–31.2 %), followed by soft tissue sarcomas (11.6–17.8 %), brain tumors (3.5–14 %), osteosarcomas (12.6–13.4 %), and adrenocortical tumors (6.5–9.9 %) [98, 99]. Other tumors that have been argued to be component tumors of LFS are listed in Box 1.5 [95–101].

There are some data regarding common histology of LFS component tumors. Breast cancers are most commonly invasive ductal carcinomas and may have a tendency toward being "triple positive" [94, 102]. Rhabdomyosarcomas account for 55 % of soft-tissue sarcomas, followed by fibrosarcomas (13 %), and then malignant fibrous histiocytomas [98]. For LFS-associated brain tumors, 69 % are astrocytic (astrocytoma or glioblastoma), followed by medulloblastoma/PNET tumors (17 %) [98].

Typically, LFS-associated tumors occur at significantly younger ages than when they occur sporadically. However, depending on tumor type, the mean age of diagnosis varies from childhood well into adulthood [98]. Understanding cancer risk for LFS is somewhat complicated as the ranges of risk vary greatly between studies and depend largely on study population. When pooling studies that examine overall cancer risk in *TP53* mutation carriers (both female and male), the risk of developing cancer by ages 15–20 is 12–42 %, by ages 40–45 is 52–66 %, by age 50 is 80 %, and by age 85 is 85 % [96, 97, 103, 104]. When separating out the sexes, it is apparent that female *TP53* mutation carriers have generally a higher lifetime cancer risk in comparison to males [97, 104, 105].

Individuals diagnosed with LFS are also at markedly increased risk to develop multiple primary tumors. Hisada et al. found that following a first cancer diagnosis, there is a 57 % risk for a second primary tumor within 30 years of the first diagnosis, followed by a 38 % risk for a third primary tumor within 10 years of the second cancer diagnosis [45]. In addition, it has been widely observed that second, third, etc. primary cancers commonly occur in the radiation field of previously treated cancers [45, 90, 94, 104].

Currently, NCCN management recommendations (Box 1.6) for individuals with LFS center around proven screening techniques such as mammography and MRI for the detection of breast cancer and early colonoscopy [88]. Because of the wide variety of tumors that can be seen in LFS, researchers have begun to consider whole-body imaging techniques such as MRI or PET scans for individuals who have *TP53* mutations. One study published in 2011 involved the use of whole-body MRI, in addition to certain targeted MRI screening and biochemical testing, to screen children and adults with LFS. Researchers were successful in detecting cancers presymptomatically and early [106]. While this cohort was relatively small, promising studies like these give hope to families with Li-Fraumeni syndrome for the possibility of screening and detecting cancers at an earlier, curable stage.

Cowden Syndrome

Cowden syndrome (CS) is a rare hereditary cancer syndrome that is characterized by overgrowth in different organ systems. The incidence of CS is thought to be about 1 in 200,000 but may be underdiagnosed. CS belongs to the set of syndromes known as the *PTEN* hamartoma tumor syndromes (PHTS) [107]. *PTEN* (phosphatase and tensin homolog) mutations are found in the vast majority of patients with Cowden syndrome, although mutations in other genes such as *BMPR1A* and the succinate dehydrogenase (SDH) genes have been reported in a small number of patients who have features of Cowden syndrome but do not meet diagnostic criteria (Cowden syndrome like) [108, 109].

Diagnostic criteria for Cowden syndrome are complicated [110]. The National Comprehensive Cancer Network's (NCCN) most recent NCCN guidelines (v.4.2013) for testing for Cowden syndrome are included in Box 1.7 [88].

Breast cancer is the most frequent cancer seen in Cowden syndrome. Reports of the risk of cancers associated with CS vary widely [111, 112]. It was initially felt that Cowden syndrome patients faced moderate increased risks for cancer; however, a paper published in 2012 by a group from the Cleveland Clinic reported much higher risks for cancer than previously thought. In 2013, the French Cowden disease network published similar high risks for cancer

Box 1.6. NCCN Screening for Li-Fraumeni Syndrome

Breast cancer risk, women

- Breast awareness[a] starting at age 18 years
- Clinical breast exam, every 6–12 months, starting at age 20–25 years or 5–10 years before the earliest known breast cancer in the family (whichever comes first).
- Annual mammogram and breast MRI screening starting at 20–25 years[b] or individualized based on earliest age of onset in family[c,d]
- Discuss risk-reducing mastectomy and counsel regarding degree of protection, degree of cancer risk, and reconstruction options.
- Address psychosocial, social, and quality-of-life aspects of undergoing risk-reducing mastectomy.

Other Cancer Risks

- Address limitations of screening for many cancers associated with LFS. Because of the remarkable risk of additional primary neoplasms, screening may be considered for cancer survivors with LFS and a good prognosis from their prior tumor(s).
- Annual comprehensive physical exam with high index of suspicion for rare cancers and second malignancies in cancer survivors includes careful skin and neurologic examinations.
- Therapeutic RT for cancer should be used with caution.
- Consider colonoscopy every 2–5 years starting no later than 25 years.
- Pediatricians should be apprised of the risk of childhood cancers in affected families.
- Discuss option to participate in novel screening approaches using technologies within clinical trials when possible, such as whole-body MRI, abdominal ultrasound, and brain MRI.[e]
- Additional surveillance based on individual family histories.
- Education regarding signs and symptoms of cancer.

Risk to Relatives

- Advise about possible inherited cancer risk to relatives, options for risk assessment, and management.
- Recommend genetic counseling and consideration of genetic testing for at-risk relatives.

Reproductive Options

- For patients of reproductive age, advise about options for prenatal diagnosis and assisted reproduction including preimplantation genetic diagnosis. Discussion should include known risks, limitations, and benefits of these technologies. See discussion for details.

[a]Women should be familiar with their breasts and promptly report changes to their health-care provider. Periodic, consistent breast self exam (BSE) may facilitate breast self awareness. Premenopausal women may find BSE most informative when performed at the end of the menses

[b]Given theoretical concerns with harmful effects of radiation exposure in LFS, for patients aged 20–30 years, annual MRI-only screening may be sufficient based on physician's discretion

[c]The appropriateness of imaging modalities and scheduling is still under study

[d]High-quality MRI limitations include having a need for a dedicated breast coil, the ability to perform biopsy under MRI guidance, experienced radiologists in breast MRI, and regional availability. Breast MRI is performed preferably days 7–15 of menstrual cycle for premenopausal women

[e]A surveillance study has been published that utilizes these screening approaches [106]

in carriers [113]. See Table 1.4. There is a possibility of ascertainment bias in these more recent papers because of recruitment strategies. The screening recommendations for individuals with Cowden synrome are seen in Box 1.8.

Peutz-Jeghers Syndrome

Peutz-Jeghers syndrome (PJS) is a rare autosomal dominant gastrointestinal polyposis syndrome. The incidence is not well known but is estimated at 1 in 25,000 to 1 in 300,000

Table 1.4 French Cowden disease network published high risks for cancer in carriers

	Pilarski (2009) [111]	Tan et al. (2012) [112]	Bubien et al. (2013) [113]
Breast cancer risk	25–50 %	85 %	77 %
Thyroid cancer	3–10 %	35 %	38 %
Endometrial cancer	5–10 %	28 %	NS
Renal cell cancer	Unknown	34 %	NS
Melanoma	Unknown	6 %	NS
Colorectal cancer	Unknown	9 %	NS

Adapted from Pilarski [111], Tan et al. [112], Bubien et al. [113]
NS not specified

Box 1.7 NCCN Guidelines for Testing for Cowden Syndrome (v.4.2013)

- Bannayan-Riley-Ruvalcaba syndrome (BRRS)
- Adult Lhermitte-Duclos disease (dysplastic gangliocytoma of the cerebellum)
- Autism spectrum disorder and macrocephaly or
- ≥2 biopsy-proven trichilemmomas
- ≥2 major criteria (one must be macrocephaly)
- ≥3 major criteria, without macrocephaly or
- 1 major and ≥3 minor criteria
- ≥4 minor criteria
- Fewer criteria are needed when an individual has a relative with a clinical diagnosis of Cowden syndrome (any one major criteria or two minor criteria)

Major criteria

- Breast cancer
- Endometrial cancer
- Follicular thyroid cancer
- Multiple GI hamartomas or ganglioneuromas
- Macrocephaly (≥97th percentile, 58 cm in adult women, 60 cm in adult men)
- Macular pigmentation of glans penis
- Mucocutaneous lesions
  - One biopsy-proven trichilemmoma
  - Multiple palmoplantar keratoses
  - Multifocal or extensive oral mucosal papillomatosis
  - Multiple cutaneous facial papules (often verrucous)

Minor criteria

- Autism spectrum disorder
- Colon cancer
- Esophageal glycogenic acanthosis (≥3)
- Lipomas
- Mental retardation (intelligence quotient ≤75)
- Papillary or follicular variant of papillary thyroid cancer
- Thyroid structural lesions (e.g., adenoma, nodule(s), goiter)
- Renal cell carcinoma
- Single GI hamartoma or ganglioneuroma
- Testicular lipomatosis
- Vascular anomalies (including multiple intracranial developmental venous anomalies)

Box 1.8 NCCN Guidelines for Cancer Screening and Prevention: Cowden Syndrome

Women

- Breast awareness starting at age 18 years
- Clinical breast exam, every 6–12 months, starting at age 25 years or 5–10 years before the earliest known breast cancer in the family.
- Annual mammography and breast MRI screening starting at age 30–35 years or 5–10 years before the earliest known breast cancer in the family (whichever comes first).
- For endometrial cancer screening, encourage patient education and prompt response to symptoms and participation in a clinical trial to determine the effectiveness and necessity of screening modalities.
- Discuss option of risk-reducing mastectomy and hysterectomy and counsel regarding degree of protection, extent of cancer risk, and reconstruction options.
- Address psychosocial, social, and quality-of-life aspects of undergoing risk-reducing mastectomy and hysterectomy and/or hysterectomy.

Men and women

- Annual comprehensive physical exam starting at age 18 or 5 years before the youngest age of diagnosis of a component cancer in the family (whichever comes first), with particular attention to breast and thyroid exams.
- Baseline thyroid ultrasound at age 18 years and consider annually thereafter.
- Consider colonoscopy starting at age 35 years, then every 5–10 years or more frequently if patient is symptomatic or polyps found.
- Consider annual dermatologic exam.
- Education regarding the signs and symptoms of cancer.

Risk to relatives

- Advise about possible inherited cancer risk to relatives, options for risk assessment, and management.
- Recommend genetic counseling and consideration of genetic testing for at-risk relatives.

Reproductive options

- For women of reproductive age, advise about options for prenatal diagnosis and assisted reproduction including preimplantation genetic diagnosis. Discussion should include known risks, limitations, and benefits of these technologies. See discussion for details.

live births by the National Institutes of Health [114]. Peutz-Jeghers is characterized by the development of Peutz-Jeghers polyps (a specific type of hamartoma) in the intestine in conjunction with pigmentation (brown or bluish spots) around and inside the mouth, nose and lips, perianal area, as well as other parts of the body. The mucocutaneous lesions are often most prominent in childhood and fade with age.

Most families with PJS have mutations in the *STK11* gene, although this gene does not explain all inherited cases of PJS as well as many simplex cases [115]. The lifetime risk of breast cancer in females with PJS is reported in a wide range, with the most consistent risks being in the 30–50 % range [116, 117]. Other cancers that can be seen in PJS include cancers of the colon, pancreas, stomach, ovary, small intestine, lung, cervix, testes, uterus, and esophagus [118]. Consensus diagnostic criteria were published in 2010 and are listed in Box 1.9 [118]. Screening and surveillance guidelines are also included in Table 1.5 [119].

Box 1.9 Clinical Diagnostic Criteria for Peutz-Jeghers

Any *ONE* of the following is present:

- Two or more histologically confirmed PJ polyps
- Any number of PJ polyps detected in one individual who has a family history of PJS in close relative(s)
- Characteristic mucocutaneous pigmentation in an individual who has a family history of PJS in close relative(s)
- Any number of PJ polyps in an individual who also has characteristic mucocutaneous pigmentation

Adapted from Beggs et al. [118]

Hereditary Diffuse Gastric Cancer Syndrome

Hereditary diffuse gastric cancer syndrome is a rare autosomal dominant hereditary cancer syndrome characterized by diffuse or signet ring cell pathology cancer of the stomach. The incidence of this syndrome is not well known. The lifetime risk of stomach cancer is thought to be approximately 80 % compared to less than 1 % in the general population [120, 121]. The second most common cancer in families with this syndrome is lobular breast cancer, with a lifetime risk of about 40 % in women [122–126]. Colorectal cancer and cleft lip and palate have also been reported in some families [123, 127]. The International Gastric Cancer Linkage Consortium (IGCLC) published clinical criteria in 2010 seen in Box 1.10 [128]. Screening and prevention adapted from consensus guidelines are included in Box 1.11 as well [129].

Box 1.10 Clinical Criteria for Hereditary Diffuse Gastric Cancer Syndrome

Any of the following:

- Two gastric cancer (GC) cases in a family, one individual under age 50 years with confirmed diffuse gastric cancer (DGC)
- Three confirmed DGC cases in first- or second-degree relatives independent of age
- Simplex case (i.e., a single occurrence in a family) of DGC occurring before age 40 years
- Personal or family history of DGC and lobular breast cancer, one diagnosed before age 50 years

Adapted from Fitzgerald et al. [128]

Table 1.5 NCCN screening and surveillance guidelines for Peutz-Jeghers syndrome

Site	Procedure	Onset (year)	Interval (year)
Stomach	Upper endoscopy[a]	8	2–3
Small intestine	Capsule endoscopy or MR enterography[b]	8	2–3
Large intestine	Colonoscopy	18	2–3
Breast	Breast examination	25[c]	Monthly
	Mammography or MRI	25[c]	1
Ovary	Transvaginal ultrasound and serum CA 125[c]	18	1
Cervix and uterus	Pelvic exam with Pap smear[d]	18	1
Pancreas	MRI-MRCP or endoscopic ultrasound and CA 19-9	25	1–2
Testes	Testicular exam; ultrasound if symptomatic or abnormality on exam	Birth	1

Adapted from the NCCN Clinical Practice Guidelines in Oncology (NCCN Guidelines®) for Genetic/Familial High-Risk Assessment: Breast and Ovarian V.4.2013.

[a]Extended upper endoscopy beginning at age 18 years

[b]CT enterography as alternative

[c]Discuss prophylactic mastectomy

[d]Discuss prophylactic hysterectomy and oophorectomy

Box 1.11 Consensus Screening and Prevention Guidelines for CDH1 + Patients

Consider prophylactic gastrectomy with close nutritional follow-up.

If refused, annual EGD with biopsy

If biopsy is positive for signet ring cells, recommend prophylactic gastrectomy and close nutritional follow-up.

Screening for lobular breast cancer from age 35 years

Consider colorectal cancer screening in families with CRC beginning at age 40 years or 10 years younger than the earliest case.

Adapted from Fitzgerald et al. [128]

Moderate- and Low-Penetrance Breast Cancer Genes

Besides the high-risk genes and syndromes listed previously, several familial forms of breast cancer have been reported. These include families with *CHEK2* and *ATM* mutations. The risk of breast cancer associated with alterations in these genes is thought to be lower than with traditional hereditary breast cancer syndromes; other factors are likely to interact with the effects of changes in these genes and result in a more moderate increase in risk for breast cancer.

Researchers at the University of Washington published a study on germline mutations in 12 genes linked to ovarian cancer that are also being analyzed in families with breast cancer [130–132]. Many laboratories are offering genetic testing for panels of genes that are important in DNA repair pathways. This grouping is adapted and expanded from categories presented by Pennington and Swisher in 2012 [133].

Group 1: Genes Functionally Related to BRCA1 and BRCA2 (ATM, BARD1, CHEK2, MRE11A, NBN, RAD50, FAM175A)

ATM (Ataxia Telangiectasia Mutated)

ATM is a serine threonine kinase that mediates checkpoint regulation and homologous repair [134]. *ATM*-deficient cells display increased chromosome breakage and abnormal cell cycle progression, especially in the presence of ionizing radiation. An increased risk for breast cancer was first observed in the mothers of patients with ataxia telangiectasia (a recessive condition characterized by cerebellar ataxia, telangiectasias, immune deficiency, and a high risk of cancer) more than 30 years ago [135]; breast cancer is also seen more often in A-T patients [136]. The relative risk of breast cancer for *ATM* mutation carriers is thought to be about 2.4-fold over that of noncarriers [137].

BARD1 (BRCA1-Associated RING Domain 1)

BARD1 helps to mediate the tumor suppressor function of *BRCA1* and has an independent role in tumor suppression as well. Initial studies on *BARD1* seemed to indicate a higher frequency of mutations in familial breast cancer or breast/ovarian cancer than in controls, although the significance of these mutations was unclear [138, 139]. Clearly deleterious mutations of *BARD1* have been reported in families with breast and/or ovarian cancer, but in a small percentage of cases [140]. Relative risks for breast cancer are not well known.

CHEK2 (Cell Cycle Checkpoint Kinase 2)

CHEK2 is a serine threonine kinase involved in double-strand DNA break repair. *CHEK2* was initially reported in a few families with a clinical diagnosis of Li-Fraumeni syndrome but does not play a major role in LFS [141, 142]. Several different mutations have been reported to be associated with increased breast cancer risk; one specific common mutation in *CHEK2*, 1100delC, appears to confer about a 2.4-fold increase in breast cancer risk [143]. The interaction of 1100delC with family history of breast cancer yields a relative risk of almost fivefold (approximately 37 % by age 70) [143]. Women who are homozygous for 1100delC seem to have an even higher risk for breast cancer and multiple primary tumors [144]. The carrier frequency of 110delC is higher in some European populations than in North America and, consequently, support for widespread testing of this mutation is more common in Europe than in the USA [131, 145].

MRE11A (Meiotic Recombination 11 Homolog A, S. Cerevisiae)

Recessively inherited mutations in *MRE11A* cause ataxia-telangiectasia-like disorder (ATLD), another chromosomal instability syndrome. *MRE*11A is part of an important complex along with Rad50 and Nbn/Nbs1, called MRN, which is critical for genomic integrity and tumor suppression. *MRE11A* germline mutations were found in a small number of women whose breast tumors showed loss or reduction of all three MRN complex proteins [146]. Few studies have analyzed the risk of breast cancer associated with mutations in this gene.

NBN (Nibrin aka NBS1)

Nijmegen breakage syndrome is a recessively inherited chromosomal instability syndrome characterized by microcephaly, growth retardation, immune deficiency, and cancer caused by alterations in *NBN* (OMIM #251260). Two common mutations, 657del5 and R215W, have been seen in Slavic cancer populations and at low frequency in controls [147, 148]. The relative risk of breast cancer in this population appears to be about threefold higher in carriers of the 657del5 mutation [149]. A germline missense mutation, Leu150Phe, has been reported in a small number of Northern European breast cancer families [150]. However, deleterious mutations have not been found in other populations [151, 152].

RAD50

One patient has been reported with Nijmegen breakage syndrome-like disorder (NBSLD), another recessively inherited chromosomal instability syndrome; she was found to be a compound heterozygote for mutations in *RAD50* (OMIM #613078 [151]). *RAD50* mutations have been reported in similar cohorts as *NBN* [150]. The significance of a previously reported mutation, 687delT, found in Finnish families, has been challenged [153]. *RAD50* mutations have not been seen consistently in other populations [151, 154, 155]. Therefore, the relative risk of breast cancer associated with carriers of *RAD50* mutations is unknown.

FAM175A (Family with Sequence Similarity 175, Member A aka ABRA1, CCDC98)

FAM175A produces a BRCA1-associated protein that links BRCA1 to a core complex dedicated to ubiquitin chain recognition and hydrolysis at DNA double-strand breaks. One study indicates that mutations in this gene may be linked with a rare form of hereditary breast cancer in Finnish families [156].

Group 2: Other Genes in the Fanconi Anemia Pathway That Increase Breast Cancer Risk (BRIP1, PALB2)

BRIP1(BRCA-Interacting Protein C-Terminal Helicase 1 or FANCJ)

BRIP1 is important in the double-strand DNA repair function of *BRCA1*. Seal and colleagues published a report in 2006 which showed truncating mutations in 9/1,212 women with breast cancer and 2/2,081 controls [157]. They calculated a relative risk of 2.0 associated with a truncating *BRIP1* mutation. Several studies have shown a low frequency of *BRIP1* mutation in various cohorts, but often the mutation does not segregate with cancer in the family [158–161]. Many studies have not observed a link between *BRIP1* and breast or ovarian cancer risk [162–167]. It is unclear whether the relative risk of 2 for breast cancer is accurate, but if there is an association, it is likely to be a small one for most populations. There are specific founder mutations which seem to confer a much higher risk for cancer; for example, an Icelandic *BRIP1* mutation, c.2040_2041insTT, confers an odds ration of ~8 for ovarian cancer [168].

PALB2 (Partner and Localizer of BRCA2 or FANCN)

PALB2 co-localizes with BRCA2 in the nucleus and helps to stabilize the protein, making it critical for homologous recombination [169]. *PALB2* mutations were first reported in breast cancer patients in 2007; a link between breast cancer and pancreatic cancer has also been seen. A UK group found a frequency of mutation of ~1 % in familial breast cancer cases (10/923 versus 0/1,084 controls); they estimated a two-fold increase in risk for breast cancer [170]. In Finland, a founder mutation, c.1592delT, was seen in ~1 % of unselected breast cancer cases and 2.7 % of familial breast cancer cases [171]. In greater than 20 studies, the frequency of *PALB2* mutations in breast cancer cohorts varies from 0 to 5 %, with most populations having a frequency of 0.5–1 % in cases [161, 172–197]. The Finnish mutation (c.1592delT) may be more highly penetrant than other mutations with an estimated lifetime risk of 40 % by age 70 with triple-negative tumors seen more often [190, 198]. There is a question of whether the location of the truncating mutation has differential effects on breast cancer risk [198].

Group 3: RAD51 Gene Family Members

RAD51 Paralogs

RAD51 is a critical part of DNA repair through homologous recombination [199]. Members of the *RAD51* gene family which share homology to *RAD51* and each other are also important in homologous recombination and have independent DNA repair functions; these *RAD51* paralogs include *RAD51B*, *RAD51C*, *RAD51D*, *XRCC2*, and *XRCC3* [200]. While RAD51 mutations have not been linked with hereditary cancer, associations have been made with several gene family members. *RAD51C* has been implicated in one family with Fanconi anemia-like phenotype and is likely to represent one of the Fanconi anemia complementation groups (FANCO) [201]. *RAD51C* and *RAD51D* mutations have been found in women with ovarian cancer [202–207]. While *RAD51C* and *RAD51D* mutations appear to be relatively rare, families with mutations in these genes (especially *RAD51D*) could represent a small but important fraction of hereditary ovarian cancer. The risk of breast cancer associated with *RAD51C* and *RAD51D* mutations is not well known, but they do not appear to be major contributors to risk. One study which analyzed 689 multiple breast cancer case families through whole exome sequencing reported two families with *XRCC2* mutations, one protein-truncating mutation and one missense [208]. However, a larger analysis of 3,548 familial breast cancer cases and 1,435 controls did not find any evidence of *XRCC2* mutations as causative in cases [209]. One particular SNP in *XRCC3*, T241M, found in about 10 % of Asian women has been associated with a moderate increase in risk for breast cancer [210, 211]. An SNP in *RAD51B* has been associated with a modest increase in risk for male breast cancer [212]. Yet, a larger study of *RAD51B* on multiple-case, non-BRCA families did not reveal any germline mutations [213].

Group 4: Hereditary Colorectal Cancer/ Polyposis Genes

Lynch Syndrome and MYH-Associated Polyposis

Lynch syndrome (LS) is the most common hereditary form of colorectal cancer accounting for about 2–3 % of colorectal cancer cases. It is caused by mutations in genes involved in DNA mismatch repair, including *MLH1*, *MSH2*, *MSH6*, *PMS2*, and, indirectly, *EPCAM*. LS is typically characterized by the development of relatively early onset colorectal and uterine cancer; increased risks for other cancers include stomach cancer, cancer of the small intestine, pancreatic cancer, sebaceous carcinomas, ovarian cancer, cancers of the urinary collecting tract, and rarely brain tumors [214]. Most studies have not shown a significant increase in breast cancer risk for MMR mutation carriers versus noncarriers [215], although a more recent paper studying a cohort of Lynch syndrome families prospectively did show a fourfold increase in breast cancer risk [216]. It is clear that defective mismatch repair can be seen in some breast cancers in women from Lynch syndrome families [217, 218]. Whether there is a true increase in risk (and the magnitude of this risk) is a matter of debate at this point.

MUTYH-associated polyposis (MAP) is a recessive form of adenomatous polyposis. *MUTYH* is involved in base excision repair; without MUTYH, oxidative DNA damage leads to the formation of 8-oxo-G which mispairs with adenine. This leads to an increase in G:C>T:A transversions in *APC* and other genes [219]. MAP is associated with an attenuated phenotype; adenomas typically number less than 100 and a mixture of polyp types (serrated adenomas, hyperplastic polyps) and duodenal polyps are often seen [220, 221]. Extraintestinal manifestations, including breast cancer, have been reported in MAP [222, 223]. However, *MUTYH* does not appear to be a common cause of breast cancer [224].

Summary

Cancer genetics has become an integral subspecialty of the practice of preventive medicine and oncology. Genetic counselors provide expertise in the attainment of the family history, cancer risk assessment, and guidance for individuals as they pursue genetic testing through the informed consent process. The identification of individuals who harbor mutations in cancer predisposition genes enables the utilization of appropriate screening and prevention techniques. Cancer genetic care begins with the identification of individuals at high risk, proceeds through the genetic counseling and testing process, and culminates in targeted and effective medical management for these individuals. As genetic testing becomes more routine, the hope is that information about hereditary and familial cancer predisposition will lead to the development of better screening techniques, earlier detection, less morbidity from preventive options, and longer disease-free survival.

References

1. NCCN guidelines: NCCN Clinical Practice Guidelines in Oncology (NCCN Guidelines) for Genetic/Familial High – Risk Assessment: Breast and Ovarian V.4.2013. http://www.nccn.org.
2. Pal T, Vadaparampil ST. Genetic risk assessments in individuals at high risk for inherited breast cancer in the breast oncology care setting. Cancer Control. 2012;19(4):255–66.
3. Sifri R, et al. Use of cancer susceptibility testing among primary care physicians. Clin Genet. 2003;64(4):355–60.
4. Wideroff L, et al. Physician use of genetic testing for cancer susceptibility: results of a national survey. Cancer Epidemiol Biomarkers Prev. 2003;12(4):295–303.
5. Acheson LS, et al. Validation of a self-administered, computerized tool for collecting and displaying the family history of cancer. J Clin Oncol. 2006;24(34):5395–402.
6. Sweet KM, Bradley TL, Westman JA. Identification and referral of families at high risk for cancer susceptibility. J Clin Oncol. 2002;20(2):528–37.
7. Drohan B, et al. Hereditary breast and ovarian cancer and other hereditary syndromes: using technology to identify carriers. Ann Surg Oncol. 2012;19(6):1732–7.
8. Simon C, et al. Patient interest in recording family histories of cancer via the internet. Genet Med. 2008;10(12):895–902.
9. Reid GT, et al. Family history questionnaires designed for clinical use: a systematic review. Public Health Genomics. 2009;12(2): 73–83.
10. Hilgart JS, Coles B, Iredale R. Cancer genetic risk assessment for individuals at risk of familial breast cancer. Cochrane Database Syst Rev. 2007;(2):CD003721.
11. ASCO. American Society of Clinical Oncology policy statement update: genetic testing for cancer susceptibility. J Clin Oncol. 2003;21(12):2397–406.
12. Giardiello FM, et al. The use and interpretation of commercial APC gene testing for familial adenomatous polyposis. N Engl J Med. 1997;336(12):823–7.
13. Miller C. The value of genetic counselors in the laboratory. ARUP Laboratories; Salt Lake City, UT, 2011.
14. Berliner JL, et al. NSGC practice guideline: risk assessment and genetic counseling for hereditary breast and ovarian cancer. J Genet Couns. 2013;22(2):155–63.
15. Riley BD, et al. Essential elements of genetic cancer risk assessment, counseling, and testing: updated recommendations of the National Society of Genetic Counselors. J Genet Couns. 2012; 21(2):151–61.
16. Gail MH, et al. Projecting individualized probabilities of developing breast cancer for white females who are being examined annually. J Natl Cancer Inst. 1989;81(24):1879–86.
17. Claus EB, Risch N, Thompson WD. Autosomal dominant inheritance of early-onset breast cancer. Implications for risk prediction. Cancer. 1994;73(3):643–51.

18. Tyrer J, Duffy SW, Cuzick J. A breast cancer prediction model incorporating familial and personal risk factors. Stat Med. 2004; 23(7):1111–30.
19. Berry DA, et al. BRCAPRO validation, sensitivity of genetic testing of BRCA1/BRCA2, and prevalence of other breast cancer susceptibility genes. J Clin Oncol. 2002;20(11):2701–12.
20. MacKarem G, Roche CA, Hughes KS. The effectiveness of the Gail model in estimating risk for development of breast cancer in women under 40 years of age. Breast J. 2001;7(1):34–9.
21. Frank TS, et al. Sequence analysis of BRCA1 and BRCA2: correlation of mutations with family history and ovarian cancer risk. J Clin Oncol. 1998;16(7):2417–25.
22. Couch FJ, et al. BRCA1 mutations in women attending clinics that evaluate the risk of breast cancer. N Engl J Med. 1997;336(20): 1409–15.
23. Shattuck-Eidens D, et al. BRCA1 sequence analysis in women at high risk for susceptibility mutations. Risk factor analysis and implications for genetic testing. JAMA. 1997;278(15):1242–50.
24. Kang HH, et al. Evaluation of models to predict BRCA germline mutations. Br J Cancer. 2006;95(7):914–20.
25. Barcenas CH, et al. Assessing BRCA carrier probabilities in extended families. J Clin Oncol. 2006;24(3):354–60.
26. James PA, et al. Optimal selection of individuals for BRCA mutation testing: a comparison of available methods. J Clin Oncol. 2006;24(4):707–15.
27. Tan MH, et al. A clinical scoring system for selection of patients for PTEN mutation testing is proposed on the basis of a prospective study of 3042 probands. Am J Hum Genet. 2011;88(1):42–56.
28. Saslow D, et al. American Cancer Society Guideline for human papillomavirus (HPV) vaccine use to prevent cervical cancer and its precursors. CA Cancer J Clin. 2007;57(1):7–28.
29. Bennett RL, et al. Standardized human pedigree nomenclature: update and assessment of the recommendations of the National Society of Genetic Counselors. J Genet Couns. 2008;17(5): 424–33.
30. Bennett RL, et al. Recommendations for standardized human pedigree nomenclature. Pedigree Standardization Task Force of the National Society of Genetic Counselors. Am J Hum Genet. 1995;56(3):745–52.
31. Trepanier A, et al. Genetic cancer risk assessment and counseling: recommendations of the national society of genetic counselors. J Genet Couns. 2004;13(2):83–114.
32. Kumaravel V, et al. Patients do not recall important details about polyps, required for colorectal cancer prevention. Clin Gastroenterol Hepatol. 2012;11(5):543–7 e1-2.
33. Jefferies S, Goldgar D, Eeles R. The accuracy of cancer diagnoses as reported in families with head and neck cancer: a case-control study. Clin Oncol (R Coll Radiol). 2008;20(4):309–14.
34. Murff HJ, Spigel DR, Syngal S. Does this patient have a family history of cancer? An evidence-based analysis of the accuracy of family cancer history. JAMA. 2004;292(12):1480–9.
35. Chang ET, et al. Reliability of self-reported family history of cancer in a large case-control study of lymphoma. J Natl Cancer Inst. 2006;98(1):61–8.
36. Mai PL, et al. Prevalence of family history of breast, colorectal, prostate, and lung cancer in a population-based study. Public Health Genomics. 2010;13(7–8):495–503.
37. Ozanne EM, et al. Bias in the reporting of family history: implications for clinical care. J Genet Couns. 2012;21(4):547–56.
38. Ziogas A, et al. Clinically relevant changes in family history of cancer over time. JAMA. 2011;306(2):172–8.
39. Schneider KA. Counseling about cancer: strategies for genetic counseling. 2nd ed. New York: Wiley-Liss; 2002. xviii, 333 p.
40. Schwartz MD, et al. Impact of BRCA1/BRCA2 counseling and testing on newly diagnosed breast cancer patients. J Clin Oncol. 2004;22(10):1823–9.
41. Ray JA, Loescher LJ, Brewer M. Risk-reduction surgery decisions in high-risk women seen for genetic counseling. J Genet Couns. 2005;14(6):473–84.
42. Liang L, et al. Radiation-induced genetic instability in vivo depends on p53 status. Mutat Res. 2002;502(1–2):69–80.
43. Shay JW, et al. Spontaneous in vitro immortalization of breast epithelial cells from a patient with Li-Fraumeni syndrome. Mol Cell Biol. 1995;15(1):425–32.
44. Heyn R, et al. Second malignant neoplasms in children treated for rhabdomyosarcoma. Intergroup Rhabdomyosarcoma Study Committee. J Clin Oncol. 1993;11(2):262–70.
45. Hisada M, et al. Multiple primary cancers in families with Li-Fraumeni syndrome. J Natl Cancer Inst. 1998;90(8):606–11.
46. Salmon A, et al. Rapid development of post-radiotherapy sarcoma and breast cancer in a patient with a novel germline "de-novo" TP53 mutation. Clin Oncol (R Coll Radiol). 2007;19(7): 490–3.
47. Vadaparampil ST, et al. Experiences of genetic counseling for BRCA1/2 among recently diagnosed breast cancer patients: a qualitative inquiry. J Psychosoc Oncol. 2008;26(4):33–52.
48. Stolier AJ, Corsetti RL. Newly diagnosed breast cancer patients choose bilateral mastectomy over breast-conserving surgery when testing positive for a BRCA1/2 mutation. Am Surg. 2005;71(12): 1031–3.
49. Silva E. Genetic counseling and clinical management of newly diagnosed breast cancer patients at genetic risk for BRCA germline mutations: perspective of a surgical oncologist. Fam Cancer. 2008;7(1):91–5.
50. Bernhardt BA, et al. Toward a model informed consent process for BRCA1 testing: a qualitative assessment of women's attitudes. J Genet Couns. 1997;6(2):207–22.
51. Geller G, et al. Genetic testing for susceptibility to adult-onset cancer. The process and content of informed consent. JAMA. 1997;277(18):1467–74.
52. Geller G, et al. "Decoding" informed consent. Insights from women regarding breast cancer susceptibility testing. Hastings Cent Rep. 1997;27(2):28–33.
53. Shannon KM, et al. Uptake of BRCA1 rearrangement panel testing: in individuals previously tested for BRCA1/2 mutations. Genet Med. 2006;8(12):740–5.
54. Eggington JM, Burbidge LA, Roa B, Pruss D, Bowles K, Rosenthal E, Esterling L, Wenstrup R. Current variant of uncertain significance rates in BRCA1/2 and lynch syndrome testing (MLH1, MSH2, MSH6, PMS2, EPCAM). American College of Medical Genetics and Genomics annual meeting, Charlotte, NC, Mar 2012.
55. Ford D, et al. Genetic heterogeneity and penetrance analysis of the BRCA1 and BRCA2 genes in breast cancer families. The Breast Cancer Linkage Consortium. Am J Hum Genet. 1998;62(3): 676–89.
56. Struewing JP, et al. The risk of cancer associated with specific mutations of BRCA1 and BRCA2 among Ashkenazi Jews. N Engl J Med. 1997;336(20):1401–8.
57. Kauff ND, et al. Incidence of non-founder BRCA1 and BRCA2 mutations in high risk Ashkenazi breast and ovarian cancer families. J Med Genet. 2002;39(8):611–4.
58. Thorlacius S, et al. A single BRCA2 mutation in male and female breast cancer families from Iceland with varied cancer phenotypes. Nat Genet. 1996;13(1):117–9.
59. Unger MA, et al. Screening for genomic rearrangements in families with breast and ovarian cancer identifies BRCA1 mutations previously missed by conformation-sensitive gel electrophoresis or sequencing. Am J Hum Genet. 2000;67(4):841–50.
60. Chappuis PO, Nethercot V, Foulkes WD. Clinico-pathological characteristics of BRCA1- and BRCA2-related breast cancer. Semin Surg Oncol. 2000;18(4):287–95.

61. Phillips KA, Andrulis IL, Goodwin PJ. Breast carcinomas arising in carriers of mutations in BRCA1 or BRCA2: are they prognostically different? J Clin Oncol. 1999;17(11):3653–63.
62. Rakha EA, Reis-Filho JS, Ellis IO. Basal-like breast cancer: a critical review. J Clin Oncol. 2008;26(15):2568–81.
63. Boyd J, et al. Clinicopathologic features of BRCA-linked and sporadic ovarian cancer. JAMA. 2000;283(17):2260–5.
64. Lakhani SR, et al. Pathology of ovarian cancers in BRCA1 and BRCA2 carriers. Clin Cancer Res. 2004;10(7):2473–81.
65. Levine DA, et al. Fallopian tube and primary peritoneal carcinomas associated with BRCA mutations. J Clin Oncol. 2003;21(22): 4222–7.
66. Cass I, et al. Improved survival in women with BRCA-associated ovarian carcinoma. Cancer. 2003;97(9):2187–95.
67. Arun B, et al. Response to neoadjuvant systemic therapy for breast cancer in BRCA mutation carriers and noncarriers: a single-institution experience. J Clin Oncol. 2011;29(28):3739–46.
68. Thompson D, Easton D. Variation in cancer risks, by mutation position, in BRCA2 mutation carriers. Am J Hum Genet. 2001; 68(2):410–9.
69. King MC, Marks JH, Mandell JB. Breast and ovarian cancer risks due to inherited mutations in BRCA1 and BRCA2. Science. 2003;302(5645):643–6.
70. Ozcelik H, et al. Germline BRCA2 6174delT mutations in Ashkenazi Jewish pancreatic cancer patients. Nat Genet. 1997;16(1):17–8.
71. van Asperen CJ, et al. Cancer risks in BRCA2 families: estimates for sites other than breast and ovary. J Med Genet. 2005;42(9): 711–9.
72. Mocci E, et al. Risk of pancreatic cancer in breast cancer families from the breast cancer family registry. Cancer Epidemiol Biomarkers Prev. 2013;22(5):803–11.
73. Iqbal J, et al. The incidence of pancreatic cancer in BRCA1 and BRCA2 mutation carriers. Br J Cancer. 2012;107(12): 2005–9.
74. Antoniou A, et al. Average risks of breast and ovarian cancer associated with BRCA1 or BRCA2 mutations detected in case series unselected for family history: a combined analysis of 22 studies. Am J Hum Genet. 2003;72(5):1117–30.
75. Risch HA, et al. Prevalence and penetrance of germline BRCA1 and BRCA2 mutations in a population series of 649 women with ovarian cancer. Am J Hum Genet. 2001;68(3):700–10.
76. The Breast Cancer Linkage Consortium. Cancer risks in BRCA2 mutation carriers. J Natl Cancer Inst. 1999;91(15):1310–6.
77. Hartmann LC, et al. Efficacy of bilateral prophylactic mastectomy in BRCA1 and BRCA2 gene mutation carriers. J Natl Cancer Inst. 2001;93(21):1633–7.
78. Rebbeck TR, et al. Bilateral prophylactic mastectomy reduces breast cancer risk in BRCA1 and BRCA2 mutation carriers: the PROSE Study Group. J Clin Oncol. 2004;22(6):1055–62.
79. Meijers-Heijboer H, et al. Breast cancer after prophylactic bilateral mastectomy in women with a BRCA1 or BRCA2 mutation. N Engl J Med. 2001;345(3):159–64.
80. Robson M, et al. Appropriateness of breast-conserving treatment of breast carcinoma in women with germline mutations in BRCA1 or BRCA2: a clinic-based series. Cancer. 2005;103(1):44–51.
81. Narod SA, et al. Tamoxifen and risk of contralateral breast cancer in BRCA1 and BRCA2 mutation carriers: a case-control study. Hereditary Breast Cancer Clinical Study Group. Lancet. 2000;356(9245):1876–81.
82. Gronwald J, et al. Tamoxifen and contralateral breast cancer in BRCA1 and BRCA2 carriers: an update. Int J Cancer. 2006;118(9): 2281–4.
83. Phillips KA, et al. Tamoxifen and Risk of Contralateral Breast Cancer for BRCA1 and BRCA2 Mutation Carriers. J Clin Oncol. 2013;21(35):3091–9.
84. Kauff ND, et al. Risk-reducing salpingo-oophorectomy in women with a BRCA1 or BRCA2 mutation. N Engl J Med. 2002;346(21): 1609–15.
85. Rebbeck TR, et al. Prophylactic oophorectomy in carriers of BRCA1 or BRCA2 mutations. N Engl J Med. 2002;346(21):1616–22.
86. Piver MS, et al. Primary peritoneal carcinoma after prophylactic oophorectomy in women with a family history of ovarian cancer. A report of the Gilda Radner Familial Ovarian Cancer Registry. Cancer. 1993;71(9):2751–5.
87. Liede A, Karlan BY, Narod SA. Cancer risks for male carriers of germline mutations in BRCA1 or BRCA2: a review of the literature. J Clin Oncol. 2004;22(4):735–42.
88. Daly MB, et al. NCCN Clinical Practice Guidelines in Oncology (NCCN Guidelines®): genetic/familial high-risk assessment: breast and ovarian V.4.2013. © 2013 National Comprehensive Cancer Network, Inc. Available at NCCN.org. Accessed 4 Dec 2013.
89. Sidransky D, et al. Inherited p53 gene mutations in breast cancer. Cancer Res. 1992;52(10):2984–6.
90. Malkin D, et al. Germ line p53 mutations in a familial syndrome of breast cancer, sarcomas, and other neoplasms. Science. 1990; 250(4985):1233–8.
91. Birch JM, et al. Prevalence and diversity of constitutional mutations in the p53 gene among 21 Li-Fraumeni families. Cancer Res. 1994;54(5):1298–304.
92. Srivastava S, et al. Germ-line transmission of a mutated p53 gene in a cancer-prone family with Li-Fraumeni syndrome. Nature. 1990;348(6303):747–9.
93. Varley JM, et al. Germ-line mutations of TP53 in Li-Fraumeni families: an extended study of 39 families. Cancer Res. 1997; 57(15):3245–52.
94. Li FP, et al. A cancer family syndrome in twenty-four kindreds. Cancer Res. 1988;48(18):5358–62.
95. Gonzalez KD, et al. Beyond Li Fraumeni syndrome: clinical characteristics of families with p53 germline mutations. J Clin Oncol. 2009;27(8):1250–6.
96. Nichols KE, et al. Germ-line p53 mutations predispose to a wide spectrum of early-onset cancers. Cancer Epidemiol Biomarkers Prev. 2001;10(2):83–7.
97. Hwang SJ, et al. Germline p53 mutations in a cohort with childhood sarcoma: sex differences in cancer risk. Am J Hum Genet. 2003;72(4):975–83.
98. Kleihues P, et al. Tumors associated with p53 germline mutations: a synopsis of 91 families. Am J Pathol. 1997;150(1):1–13.
99. Olivier M, et al. Li-Fraumeni and related syndromes: correlation between tumor type, family structure, and TP53 genotype. Cancer Res. 2003;63(20):6643–50.
100. Birch JM, et al. Relative frequency and morphology of cancers in carriers of germline TP53 mutations. Oncogene. 2001;20(34): 4621–8.
101. Strong LC, Williams WR, Tainsky MA. The Li-Fraumeni syndrome: from clinical epidemiology to molecular genetics. Am J Epidemiol. 1992;135(2):190–9.
102. Masciari S, et al. Breast cancer phenotype in women with TP53 germline mutations: a Li-Fraumeni syndrome consortium effort. Breast Cancer Res Treat. 2012;133(3):1125–30.
103. Le Bihan C, et al. ARCAD: a method for estimating age-dependent disease risk associated with mutation carrier status from family data. Genet Epidemiol. 1995;12(1):13–25.
104. Chompret A, et al. P53 germline mutations in childhood cancers and cancer risk for carrier individuals. Br J Cancer. 2000;82(12): 1932–7.
105. Wu CC, et al. Joint effects of germ-line p53 mutation and sex on cancer risk in Li-Fraumeni syndrome. Cancer Res. 2006;66(16): 8287–92.
106. Villani A, et al. Biochemical and imaging surveillance in germline TP53 mutation carriers with Li-Fraumeni syndrome: a prospective observational study. Lancet Oncol. 2011;12(6):559–67.
107. Eng C. PTEN Hamartoma Tumor Syndrome (PHTS). In: Pagon RA, Bird TD, Dolan CR, et al., editors. GeneReviews [Internet]. Seattle: University of Washington; 2001 Nov 29 [Updated 2011 Jul 21].

108. Zhou XP, et al. Germline mutations in BMPR1A/ALK3 cause a subset of cases of juvenile polyposis syndrome and of Cowden and Bannayan-Riley-Ruvalcaba syndromes. Am J Hum Genet. 2001;69(4):704–11.
109. Ni Y, et al. Germline mutations and variants in the succinate dehydrogenase genes in Cowden and Cowden-like syndromes. Am J Hum Genet. 2008;83(2):261–8.
110. Eng C. Will the real Cowden syndrome please stand up: revised diagnostic criteria. J Med Genet. 2000;37(11):828–30.
111. Pilarski R. Cowden syndrome: a critical review of the clinical literature. J Genet Couns. 2009;18(1):13–27.
112. Tan MH, et al. Lifetime cancer risks in individuals with germline PTEN mutations. Clin Cancer Res. 2012;18(2):400–7.
113. Bubien V, et al. High cumulative risks of cancer in patients with PTEN hamartoma tumour syndrome. J Med Genet. 2013;50(4):255–63.
114. Kutscher AH, et al. Incidence of Peutz-Jeghers syndrome. Am J Dig Dis. 1960;5:576–7.
115. Aretz S, et al. High proportion of large genomic STK11 deletions in Peutz-Jeghers syndrome. Hum Mutat. 2005;26(6):513–9.
116. Lim W, et al. Relative frequency and morphology of cancers in STK11 mutation carriers. Gastroenterology. 2004;126(7):1788–94.
117. Hearle N, et al. Frequency and spectrum of cancers in the Peutz-Jeghers syndrome. Clin Cancer Res. 2006;12(10):3209–15.
118. Beggs AD, et al. Peutz-Jeghers syndrome: a systematic review and recommendations for management. Gut. 2010;59(7):975–86.
119. Amos CI, et al. Peutz-Jeghers syndrome. In: Pagon RA, et al., editors. GeneReviews. Seattle: University of Washington; 1993.
120. Kluijt I, et al. Familial gastric cancer: guidelines for diagnosis, treatment and periodic surveillance. Fam Cancer. 2012;11(3):363–9.
121. Howlader N, Noone AM, Krapcho M, Neyman N, Aminou R, Waldron W, Altekruse SF, Kosary CL, Ruhl J, Tatalovich Z, Cho H, Mariotto A, Eisner MP, Lewis DR, Chen HS, Feuer EJ, Cronin KA, Edwards BK, editors. SEER Cancer Statistics Review, 1975–2008. Bethesda: National Cancer Institute; 2010. Posted to the SEER website 2011.
122. Kaurah P, et al. Founder and recurrent CDH1 mutations in families with hereditary diffuse gastric cancer. JAMA. 2007;297(21):2360–72.
123. Brooks-Wilson AR, et al. Germline E-cadherin mutations in hereditary diffuse gastric cancer: assessment of 42 new families and review of genetic screening criteria. J Med Genet. 2004;41(7):508–17.
124. Pharoah PD, et al. Incidence of gastric cancer and breast cancer in CDH1 (E-cadherin) mutation carriers from hereditary diffuse gastric cancer families. Gastroenterology. 2001;121(6):1348–53.
125. Keller G, et al. Diffuse type gastric and lobular breast carcinoma in a familial gastric cancer patient with an E-cadherin germline mutation. Am J Pathol. 1999;155(2):337–42.
126. Oliveira C, et al. Screening E-cadherin in gastric cancer families reveals germline mutations only in hereditary diffuse gastric cancer kindred. Hum Mutat. 2002;19(5):510–7.
127. Frebourg T, et al. Cleft lip/palate and CDH1/E-cadherin mutations in families with hereditary diffuse gastric cancer. J Med Genet. 2006;43(2):138–42.
128. Fitzgerald RC, et al. Hereditary diffuse gastric cancer: updated consensus guidelines for clinical management and directions for future research. J Med Genet. 2010;47(7):436–44.
129. Kaurah P, Huntsman DG. Hereditary diffuse gastric cancer. In: Pagon RA, et al., editors. GeneReviews. Seattle: University of Washington; 1993.
130. Walsh T, et al. Mutations in 12 genes for inherited ovarian, fallopian tube, and peritoneal carcinoma identified by massively parallel sequencing. Proc Natl Acad Sci U S A. 2011;108(44):18032–7.
131. Ripperger T, et al. Breast cancer susceptibility: current knowledge and implications for genetic counselling. Eur J Hum Genet. 2009;17(6):722–31.
132. Lalloo F, Evans DG. Familial breast cancer. Clin Genet. 2012;82(2):105–14.
133. Pennington KP, Swisher EM. Hereditary ovarian cancer: beyond the usual suspects. Gynecol Oncol. 2012;124(2):347–53.
134. Shuen AY, Foulkes WD. Inherited mutations in breast cancer genes–risk and response. J Mammary Gland Biol Neoplasia. 2011;16(1):3–15.
135. Swift M, et al. Malignant neoplasms in the families of patients with ataxia-telangiectasia. Cancer Res. 1976;36(1):209–15.
136. Reiman A, et al. Lymphoid tumours and breast cancer in ataxia telangiectasia; substantial protective effect of residual ATM kinase activity against childhood tumours. Br J Cancer. 2011;105(4):586–91.
137. Renwick A, et al. ATM mutations that cause ataxia-telangiectasia are breast cancer susceptibility alleles. Nat Genet. 2006;38(8):873–5.
138. Ghimenti C, et al. Germline mutations of the BRCA1-associated ring domain (BARD1) gene in breast and breast/ovarian families negative for BRCA1 and BRCA2 alterations. Genes Chromosomes Cancer. 2002;33(3):235–42.
139. Ishitobi M, et al. Mutational analysis of BARD1 in familial breast cancer patients in Japan. Cancer Lett. 2003;200(1):1–7.
140. Ratajska M, et al. Cancer predisposing BARD1 mutations in breast-ovarian cancer families. Breast Cancer Res Treat. 2012;131(1):89–97.
141. Bell DW, et al. Heterozygous germ line hCHK2 mutations in Li-Fraumeni syndrome. Science. 1999;286(5449):2528–31.
142. Ruijs MW, et al. The contribution of CHEK2 to the TP53-negative Li-Fraumeni phenotype. Hered Cancer Clin Pract. 2009;7(1):4.
143. Weischer M, et al. CHEK2*1100delC genotyping for clinical assessment of breast cancer risk: meta-analyses of 26,000 patient cases and 27,000 controls. J Clin Oncol. 2008;26(4):542–8.
144. Adank MA, et al. CHEK2*1100delC homozygosity is associated with a high breast cancer risk in women. J Med Genet. 2011;48(12):860–3.
145. Offit K, Garber JE. Time to check CHEK2 in families with breast cancer? J Clin Oncol. 2008;26(4):519–20.
146. Bartkova J, et al. Aberrations of the MRE11-RAD50-NBS1 DNA damage sensor complex in human breast cancer: MRE11 as a candidate familial cancer-predisposing gene. Mol Oncol. 2008;2(4):296–316.
147. Steffen J, et al. Increased cancer risk of heterozygotes with NBS1 germline mutations in Poland. Int J Cancer. 2004;111(1):67–71.
148. Buslov KG, et al. NBS1 657del5 mutation may contribute only to a limited fraction of breast cancer cases in Russia. Int J Cancer. 2005;114(4):585–9.
149. Steffen J, et al. Germline mutations 657del5 of the NBS1 gene contribute significantly to the incidence of breast cancer in Central Poland. Int J Cancer. 2006;119(2):472–5.
150. Heikkinen K, et al. RAD50 and NBS1 are breast cancer susceptibility genes associated with genomic instability. Carcinogenesis. 2006;27(8):1593–9.
151. Cao AY, et al. Some common mutations of RAD50 and NBS1 in western populations do not contribute significantly to Chinese non-BRCA1/2 hereditary breast cancer. Breast Cancer Res Treat. 2010;121(1):247–9.
152. He M, et al. RAD50 and NBS1 are not likely to be susceptibility genes in Chinese non-BRCA1/2 hereditary breast cancer. Breast Cancer Res Treat. 2012;133(1):111–6.
153. Tommiska J, et al. Evaluation of RAD50 in familial breast cancer predisposition. Int J Cancer. 2006;118(11):2911–6.
154. Mosor M, et al. RAD50 gene mutations are not likely a risk factor for breast cancer in Poland. Breast Cancer Res Treat. 2010;123(2):607–9.
155. Uhrhammer N, Delort L, Bignon YJ. Rad50 c.687delT does not contribute significantly to familial breast cancer in a French

population. Cancer Epidemiol Biomarkers Prev. 2009;18(2): 684–5.
156. Solyom S, et al. Breast cancer-associated Abraxas mutation disrupts nuclear localization and DNA damage response functions. Sci Transl Med. 2012;4(122):122ra23.
157. Seal S, et al. Truncating mutations in the Fanconi anemia J gene BRIP1 are low-penetrance breast cancer susceptibility alleles. Nat Genet. 2006;38(11):1239–41.
158. Lewis AG, et al. Mutation analysis of FANCD2, BRIP1/BACH1, LMO4 and SFN in familial breast cancer. Breast Cancer Res. 2005;7(6):R1005–16.
159. Rutter JL, et al. Mutational analysis of the BRCA1-interacting genes ZNF350/ZBRK1 and BRIP1/BACH1 among BRCA1 and BRCA2-negative probands from breast-ovarian cancer families and among early-onset breast cancer cases and reference individuals. Hum Mutat. 2003;22(2):121–8.
160. Luo L, et al. No mutations in the BACH1 gene in BRCA1 and BRCA2 negative breast-cancer families linked to 17q22. Int J Cancer. 2002;98(4):638–9.
161. McInerney NM, et al. Evaluation of variants in the CHEK2, BRIP1 and PALB2 genes in an Irish breast cancer cohort. Breast Cancer Res Treat. 2010;121(1):203–10.
162. Kuusisto KM, et al. Screening for BRCA1, BRCA2, CHEK2, PALB2, BRIP1, RAD50, and CDH1 mutations in high-risk Finnish BRCA1/2-founder mutation-negative breast and/or ovarian cancer individuals. Breast Cancer Res. 2011;13(1):R20.
163. Silvestri V, et al. Mutation analysis of BRIP1 in male breast cancer cases: a population-based study in Central Italy. Breast Cancer Res Treat. 2011;126(2):539–43.
164. Solyom S, Pylkas K, Winqvist R. Screening for large genomic rearrangements of the BRIP1 and CHK1 genes in Finnish breast cancer families. Fam Cancer. 2010;9(4):537–40.
165. Ameziane N, et al. Lack of large genomic deletions in BRIP1, PALB2, and FANCD2 genes in BRCA1/2 negative familial breast cancer. Breast Cancer Res Treat. 2009;118(3):651–3.
166. Cao AY, et al. Mutation analysis of BRIP1/BACH1 in BRCA1/BRCA2 negative Chinese women with early onset breast cancer or affected relatives. Breast Cancer Res Treat. 2009;115(1): 51–5.
167. Guenard F, et al. Mutational analysis of the breast cancer susceptibility gene BRIP1/BACH1/FANCJ in high-risk non-BRCA1/BRCA2 breast cancer families. J Hum Genet. 2008; 53(7):579–91.
168. Rafnar T, et al. Mutations in BRIP1 confer high risk of ovarian cancer. Nat Genet. 2011;43(11):1104–7.
169. Tischkowitz M, Xia B. PALB2/FANCN: recombining cancer and Fanconi anemia. Cancer Res. 2010;70(19):7353–9.
170. Rahman N, et al. PALB2, which encodes a BRCA2-interacting protein, is a breast cancer susceptibility gene. Nat Genet. 2007; 39(2):165–7.
171. Erkko H, et al. A recurrent mutation in PALB2 in Finnish cancer families. Nature. 2007;446(7133):316–9.
172. Harinck F, et al. Routine testing for PALB2 mutations in familial pancreatic cancer families and breast cancer families with pancreatic cancer is not indicated. Eur J Hum Genet. 2012;20(5): 577–9.
173. Blanco A, et al. Detection of a large rearrangement in PALB2 in Spanish breast cancer families with male breast cancer. Breast Cancer Res Treat. 2012;132(1):307–15.
174. Hellebrand H, et al. Germline mutations in the PALB2 gene are population specific and occur with low frequencies in familial breast cancer. Hum Mutat. 2011;32(6):E2176–88.
175. Stadler ZK, et al. Germline PALB2 mutation analysis in breast-pancreas cancer families. J Med Genet. 2011;48(8):523–5.
176. Hofstatter EW, et al. PALB2 mutations in familial breast and pancreatic cancer. Fam Cancer. 2011;10(2):225–31.
177. Casadei S, et al. Contribution of inherited mutations in the BRCA2-interacting protein PALB2 to familial breast cancer. Cancer Res. 2011;71(6):2222–9.
178. Peterlongo P, et al. PALB2 germline mutations in familial breast cancer cases with personal and family history of pancreatic cancer. Breast Cancer Res Treat. 2011;126(3):825–8.
179. Southey MC, et al. A PALB2 mutation associated with high risk of breast cancer. Breast Cancer Res. 2010;12(6):R109.
180. Bogdanova N, et al. PALB2 mutations in German and Russian patients with bilateral breast cancer. Breast Cancer Res Treat. 2011;126(2):545–50.
181. Ding YC, et al. Germline mutations in PALB2 in African-American breast cancer cases. Breast Cancer Res Treat. 2011;126(1):227–30.
182. Ding YC, et al. Mutations in BRCA2 and PALB2 in male breast cancer cases from the United States. Breast Cancer Res Treat. 2011;126(3):771–8.
183. Balia C, et al. PALB2: a novel inactivating mutation in a Italian breast cancer family. Fam Cancer. 2010;9(4):531–6.
184. Adank MA, et al. PALB2 analysis in BRCA2-like families. Breast Cancer Res Treat. 2011;127(2):357–62.
185. Kim JH, et al. PALB2 mutations 1592delT and 229delT are not present in Korean breast cancer patients negative for BRCA1 and BRCA2 mutations. Breast Cancer Res Treat. 2010;122(1):303–6.
186. Silvestri V, et al. PALB2 mutations in male breast cancer: a population-based study in Central Italy. Breast Cancer Res Treat. 2010;122(1):299–301.
187. Dansonka-Mieszkowska A, et al. A novel germline PALB2 deletion in Polish breast and ovarian cancer patients. BMC Med Genet. 2010;11:20.
188. Ghadirian P, et al. The contribution of founder mutations to early-onset breast cancer in French-Canadian women. Clin Genet. 2009;76(5):421–6.
189. Papi L, et al. A PALB2 germline mutation associated with hereditary breast cancer in Italy. Fam Cancer. 2010;9(2):181–5.
190. Heikkinen T, et al. The breast cancer susceptibility mutation PALB2 1592delT is associated with an aggressive tumor phenotype. Clin Cancer Res. 2009;15(9):3214–22.
191. Sluiter M, Mew S, van Rensburg EJ. PALB2 sequence variants in young South African breast cancer patients. Fam Cancer. 2009; 8(4):347–53.
192. Gunnarsson H, et al. Evidence against PALB2 involvement in Icelandic breast cancer susceptibility. J Negat Results Biomed. 2008;7:5.
193. Pylkas K, et al. Analysis of large deletions in BRCA1, BRCA2 and PALB2 genes in Finnish breast and ovarian cancer families. BMC Cancer. 2008;8:146.
194. Cao AY, et al. The prevalence of PALB2 germline mutations in BRCA1/BRCA2 negative Chinese women with early onset breast cancer or affected relatives. Breast Cancer Res Treat. 2009;114(3): 457–62.
195. Garcia MJ, et al. Analysis of FANCB and FANCN/PALB2 fanconi anemia genes in BRCA1/2-negative Spanish breast cancer families. Breast Cancer Res Treat. 2009;113(3):545–51.
196. Foulkes WD, et al. Identification of a novel truncating PALB2 mutation and analysis of its contribution to early-onset breast cancer in French-Canadian women. Breast Cancer Res. 2007;9(6):R83.
197. Tischkowitz M, et al. Analysis of PALB2/FANCN-associated breast cancer families. Proc Natl Acad Sci U S A. 2007;104(16): 6788–93.
198. Erkko H, et al. Penetrance analysis of the PALB2 c.1592delT founder mutation. Clin Cancer Res. 2008;14(14):4667–71.
199. Krejci L, et al. Homologous recombination and its regulation. Nucleic Acids Res. 2012;40(13):5795–818.
200. Suwaki N, Klare K, Tarsounas M. RAD51 paralogs: roles in DNA damage signalling, recombinational repair and tumorigenesis. Semin Cell Dev Biol. 2011;22(8):898–905.

201. Vaz F, et al. Mutation of the RAD51C gene in a Fanconi anemia-like disorder. Nat Genet. 2010;42(5):406–9.
202. Thompson ER, et al. Analysis of RAD51C germline mutations in high-risk breast and ovarian cancer families and ovarian cancer patients. Hum Mutat. 2012;33(1):95–9.
203. Vuorela M, et al. Further evidence for the contribution of the RAD51C gene in hereditary breast and ovarian cancer susceptibility. Breast Cancer Res Treat. 2011;130(3):1003–10.
204. Romero A, et al. A HRM-based screening method detects RAD51C germ-line deleterious mutations in Spanish breast and ovarian cancer families. Breast Cancer Res Treat. 2011;129(3):939–46.
205. Wickramanyake A, et al. Loss of function germline mutations in RAD51D in women with ovarian carcinoma. Gynecol Oncol. 2012;127(3):552–5.
206. Coulet F, et al. Germline RAD51C mutations in ovarian cancer susceptibility. Clin Genet. 2013;83(4):332–6.
207. Pelttari LM, et al. RAD51C is a susceptibility gene for ovarian cancer. Hum Mol Genet. 2011;20(16):3278–88.
208. Park DJ, et al. Rare mutations in XRCC2 increase the risk of breast cancer. Am J Hum Genet. 2012;90(4):734–9.
209. Hilbers FS, et al. Rare variants in XRCC2 as breast cancer susceptibility alleles. J Med Genet. 2012;49(10):618–20.
210. Lee SA, et al. Genetic polymorphism of XRCC3 Thr241Met and breast cancer risk: case-control study in Korean women and meta-analysis of 12 studies. Breast Cancer Res Treat. 2007;103(1):71–6.
211. Zhang B, et al. Genetic variants associated with breast-cancer risk: comprehensive research synopsis, meta-analysis, and epidemiological evidence. Lancet Oncol. 2011;12(5):477–88.
212. Orr N, et al. Genome-wide association study identifies a common variant in RAD51B associated with male breast cancer risk. Nat Genet. 2012;44(11):1182–4.
213. Johnson J, et al. Mutation analysis of RAD51L1 (RAD51B/REC2) in multiple-case, non-BRCA1/2 breast cancer families. Breast Cancer Res Treat. 2011;129(1):255–63.
214. Weissman SM, et al. Genetic counseling considerations in the evaluation of families for Lynch syndrome–a review. J Genet Couns. 2011;20(1):5–19.
215. Watson P, et al. The risk of extra-colonic, extra-endometrial cancer in the Lynch syndrome. Int J Cancer. 2008;123(2):444–9.
216. Win AK, et al. Colorectal and other cancer risks for carriers and noncarriers from families with a DNA mismatch repair gene mutation: a prospective cohort study. J Clin Oncol. 2012;30(9):958–64.
217. Walsh MD, et al. Lynch syndrome-associated breast cancers: clinicopathologic characteristics of a case series from the colon cancer family registry. Clin Cancer Res. 2010;16(7):2214–24.
218. Buerki N, et al. Evidence for breast cancer as an integral part of Lynch syndrome. Genes Chromosomes Cancer. 2012;51(1):83–91.
219. Lefevre JH, et al. MYH biallelic mutation can inactivate the two genetic pathways of colorectal cancer by APC or MLH1 transversions. Fam Cancer. 2010;9(4):589–94.
220. Sieber OM, et al. Multiple colorectal adenomas, classic adenomatous polyposis, and germ-line mutations in MYH. N Engl J Med. 2003;348(9):791–9.
221. Boparai KS, et al. Hyperplastic polyps and sessile serrated adenomas as a phenotypic expression of MYH-associated polyposis. Gastroenterology. 2008;135(6):2014–8.
222. Vogt S, et al. Expanded extracolonic tumor spectrum in MUTYH-associated polyposis. Gastroenterology. 2009;137(6):1976–85 e1-10.
223. Nielsen M, et al. Multiplicity in polyp count and extracolonic manifestations in 40 Dutch patients with MYH associated polyposis coli (MAP). J Med Genet. 2005;42(9):e54.
224. Beiner ME, et al. Mutations of the MYH gene do not substantially contribute to the risk of breast cancer. Breast Cancer Res Treat. 2009;114(3):575–8.
225. Lowry KP, et al. Annual screening strategies in BRCA1 and BRCA2 gene mutation carriers: a comparative effectiveness analysis. Cancer. 2012;118:2021–30.

Screening for Breast Cancer

2

Mahesh K. Shetty

Introduction

Screening is defined as the presumptive identification of unrecognized disease by means of tests, examinations, or other procedures that can be applied rapidly. The World Health Organization outlines a number of important prerequisites to justify implementation of an effective screening program [1]:

- Target cancer should have a high prevalence and be associated with a high mortality and morbidity.
- The screening test has to be safe, effective, and acceptable.
- The compliance of the target population in attending initial screening and diagnosis and in follow-up visits has to be high.
- Effective treatment should be available to be delivered to screen positive cases.

An ideal screening test is one which detects a high percentage of cancers [sensitivity] and has low false-positive rate so that disease-free women are not subjected to unnecessary diagnostic tests. A high prevalence of cancer in the target population being screened is an important prerequisite since even the best screening test will be ineffective when deployed in a population with a low prevalence of cancer. National and/or professional or regulatory body guidelines in individual countries for cancer screening should be based on cancer incidence and prevalence statistics. These need to address at what age and how frequent screening needs to be performed; additional influencing factors to be taken into consideration will also include cost-effectiveness of screening strategy. Quality control and assurance to ensure effectiveness, accuracy, and consistency has to be applied to and monitored for health-care personnel performing and interpreting these tests as well as for the equipment used for this purpose. A tested and a robust referral system for women testing positive for cancers needs to be in place. An information system that can send out invitations for initial screening, follow-up visits, and repeat screening at predetermined intervals is a must to ensure success [1].

Mammographic Screening for Breast Cancer

Randomized clinical trials study the efficacy of a screening methodology; efficacy is thus measured in experimental studies. The effectiveness of a screening modality on the other hand is defined as the extent to which a specific intervention when deployed in routine circumstances does what it is supposed to do in a specific population [2]. The role of mammography in reducing breast cancer mortality has been demonstrated in multiple randomized clinical trials as well as in organized mammography screening services. The first randomized controlled study to demonstrate a significant benefit of screening mammography was the Swedish Two-County trial. A total of 77,080 women aged 40–74 years were randomized in geographical clusters and invited to be screened, and 55,985 women were assigned to a no invitation group. A single view mammogram was performed every 33 months in women of age group 50–74 years and every 24 months in the age group 40–49 years. In this trial a 30 % mortality reduction was achieved when those women who were invited to be screened were compared to those who were not [3]. In the same study when those women who actually attended screening were compared to those who did not, a still higher mortality reduction of 42 % was observed [3].

A meta-analysis of all the randomized clinical trials [RCTs] testing the efficacy of screening mammography to date demonstrated a significant reduction in breast cancer mortality of 20–35 % in women of age group 50–69

M.K. Shetty, MD, FRCR, FACR, FAIUM
Department of Radiology, Baylor College of Medicine, Houston, TX, USA

Woman's Center for Breast Care and MRI, Woman's Hospital of Texas, Fannin 7600, Houston, TX 77054, USA
e-mail: mshettymd@womans-clinic.com

M.K. Shetty (ed.), *Breast Cancer Screening and Diagnosis: A Synopsis*, DOI 10.1007/978-1-4939-1267-4_2, © Springer Science+Business Media New York 2015 years [4]. How do the results of these RCTs translate to clinical practice, i.e., service screening, effectiveness versus efficacy. This has been studied by Tabar and others. In the age group of women between 20 and 69 years, there were 6,807 who were diagnosed with breast cancer over a 29-year period in two counties in Sweden and 1,863 breast cancer deaths [5]. These investigators reported a 63 % mortality reduction in mortality from incident breast carcinoma in women ages 40–69 years during the service screening period of 1988–1996 compared with breast cancer mortality during the time period when no screening was available (1968 1977). The reduction in mortality observed during the service screening period when adjusted for selection bias was 48 %. The reason for a more significant mortality reduction in service screening compared to RCTs can be attributed to a number of logical factors. These include significant improvements in mammographic techniques since the randomized trial era, and the inherent limitations of RCTs in quantifying mortality reduction due to compliance and contamination rates, and prevalence screen. The number of screening rounds, length of follow-up, and length of screening intervals which in the Swedish Two-County trial was 33 months for women aged 50–74 years are additional factors that lead to better results in service screening [5]. A review of seven population-based community screening programs in the USA that included 463,372 women, the sensitivity of mammography was 75 % and the specificity was 92.3 %. Sensitivity was similar to what was shown in RCTs. Breast density contributes to the overall sensitivity with only 63 % sensitivity noted in women with dense breasts and 87 % in women with entirely fatty breasts [6].

The literature supporting the benefits of screening mammography in reducing mortality from breast cancer is extensive, and the overwhelming body of evidence is strongly in favor of offering this service to women in countries with a high prevalence of breast cancer. The controversy regarding benefits of screening mammography and the debate as to when breast cancer screening should commence, how often to screen, and when to stop screening rages on. The council of the European Union and the International Agency for Research on Cancer expert working group has recommended the use of biannual mammography for women age 50–69 [7].

Recommendations for Screening for Breast Cancer with Imaging in the USA [8]

In the USA, the Society of Breast Imaging and the Breast Imaging Commission of the American College of Radiology recommends women at average risk to undergo annual screening mammography starting at age 40 [8]. The recommendations for screening women at average and elevated risk are outlined in Table 2.1. The recommendations are based on presence or absence of risk factors.

Table 2.1 The American College of Radiology and the Society of Breast Imaging recommendation for breast cancer screening with imaging

Population to be screened	Age to commence screening
Women at average risk	
Annual screening mammograms	40 years
Women at an elevated risk	
(a) Women with certain BRCA 1 or BRCA mutations or those who have not been tested but have first degree relatives[Mother, sisters, daughters] with such proven mutations	Yearly starting by 30 years of age but not before 25
(b) Women ≥ 20 % lifetime risk of breast cancer based on maternal or paternal family history	Yearly starting by 30 years of age but not before age 25 or 10 years before diagnosis of youngest affected relative whichever occurs later
(c) Women with mothers or sisters with premenopausal cancer	Yearly starting by 30 years of age but not before 25 or 10 years before diagnosis of youngest affected relative whichever occurs later
(d) Women with history of mantle radiation usually for Hodgkin's lymphoma received between 10 and 30 years	Yearly starting 8 years after therapy but not before age 25
(e) Women with biopsy proven lobular carcinoma in situ, atypical lobular hyperplasia, atypical ductal hyperplasia, ductal carcinoma in situ, invasive carcinoma, ovarian carcinoma	Yearly from the time of diagnosis regardless of age

Data from Lee et al. [8]

Annual screening mammography is recommended for women starting at the age of 40 years based on overwhelming evidence showing a benefit with significant mortality rate reduction. In those at risk screening at an earlier age is recommended [8]. There are no data from large clinical trials on the effectiveness of screening for breast cancer in the high-risk population. Screening is recommended in young women with an elevated risk based on the assumption that the risk for developing breast cancer is same or higher than women 40 and older therefore justified to offer screening. Women with personal history of breast cancer have a 5–10 % risk of developing a second cancer in the first 10 years after diagnosis, and those with ovarian cancer have a three- to fourfold increased risk for development of breast cancer; hence, it is reasonable to subject these women to annual mammographic surveillance from the time of diagnosis of breast or ovarian cancer. Those women who have received mantle radiation between the ages of 10 and 30 years have a significantly elevated risk of developing breast cancer; 35 % by the age of 40 years has been reported [8]. Histopathologies that indicate an increased risk for developing breast cancer include lobular

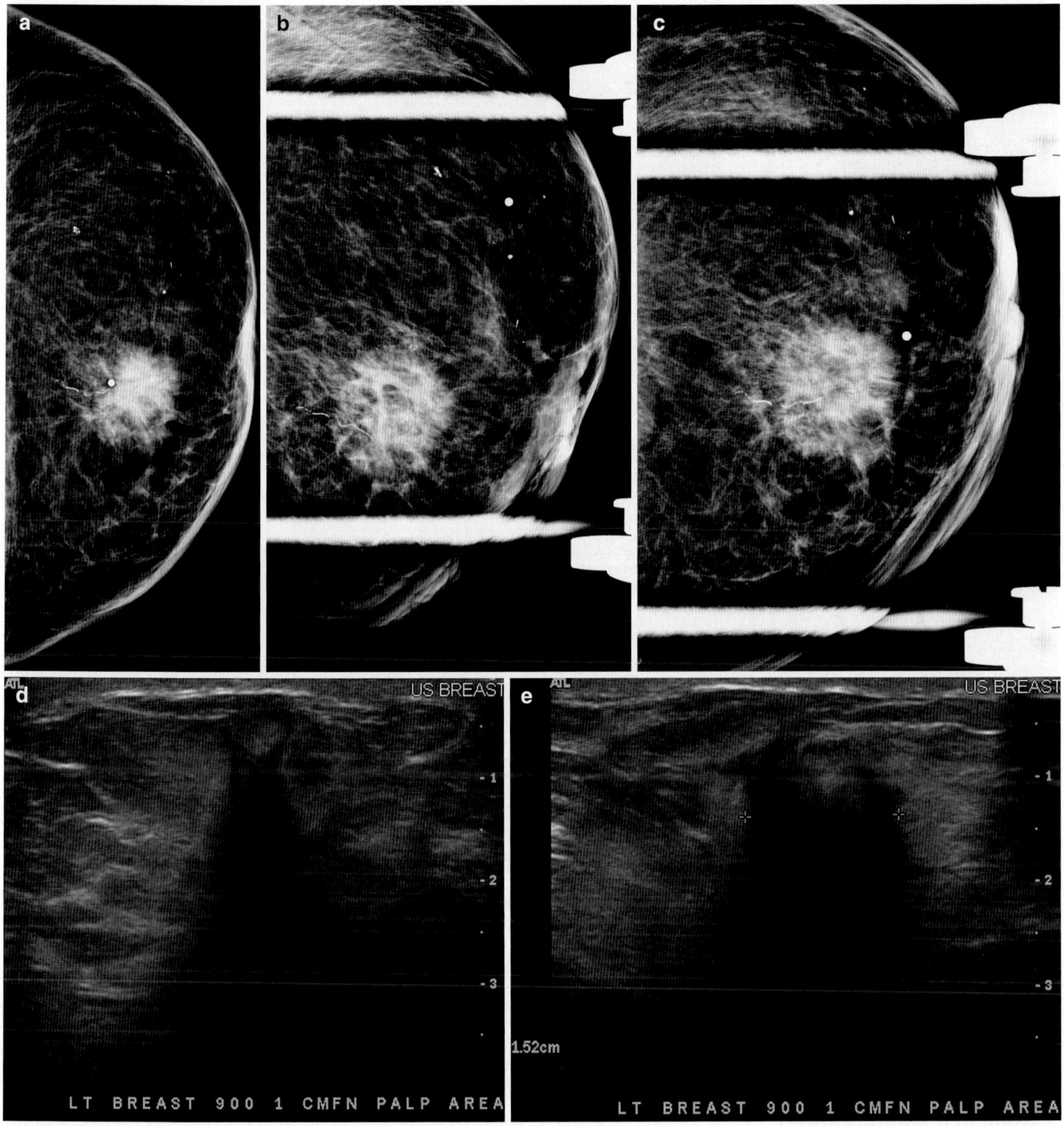

Fig. 2.1 (**a–e**) A 95-year-old with a palpable lump in left breast. (**a**) Left mediolateral view shows a 1.5 cm irregular mass. (**b, c**) Spot compression views show a spiculated mass. (**d, e**) Radial and antiradial ultrasound images demonstrate a 1.5 cm mass with malignant features. Histology showed an invasive ductal carcinoma

neoplasia, and atypical ductal hyperplasia is a justifiable indication to commence screening before the age of 40 years. Hereditary breast cancer is caused by several genetic mutations. BRCA 1 mutation carries a 19 % risk for breast cancer by the age of 40 years and a lifetime risk of 85 %, BRCA 2 mutation carries a similar lifetime risk, but cancer tends to occur at a later stage, and screening should start by 30 years of age [8]. Although there are no specific recommendations as to when screening should be stopped, it is generally desirable to offer screening mammograms until there is at least a 7 years of life expectancy remaining. In our practice occasionally we receive requests for screening in women in their 80s, and we had recently a case of an unsuspected cancer found on a screening mammogram in a 95-year-old woman (Fig. 2.1a–e). It is also not uncommon to find larger cancers in women who have skipped several years of undergoing screening mammograms (Figs. 2.2a–c and 2.3a–d).

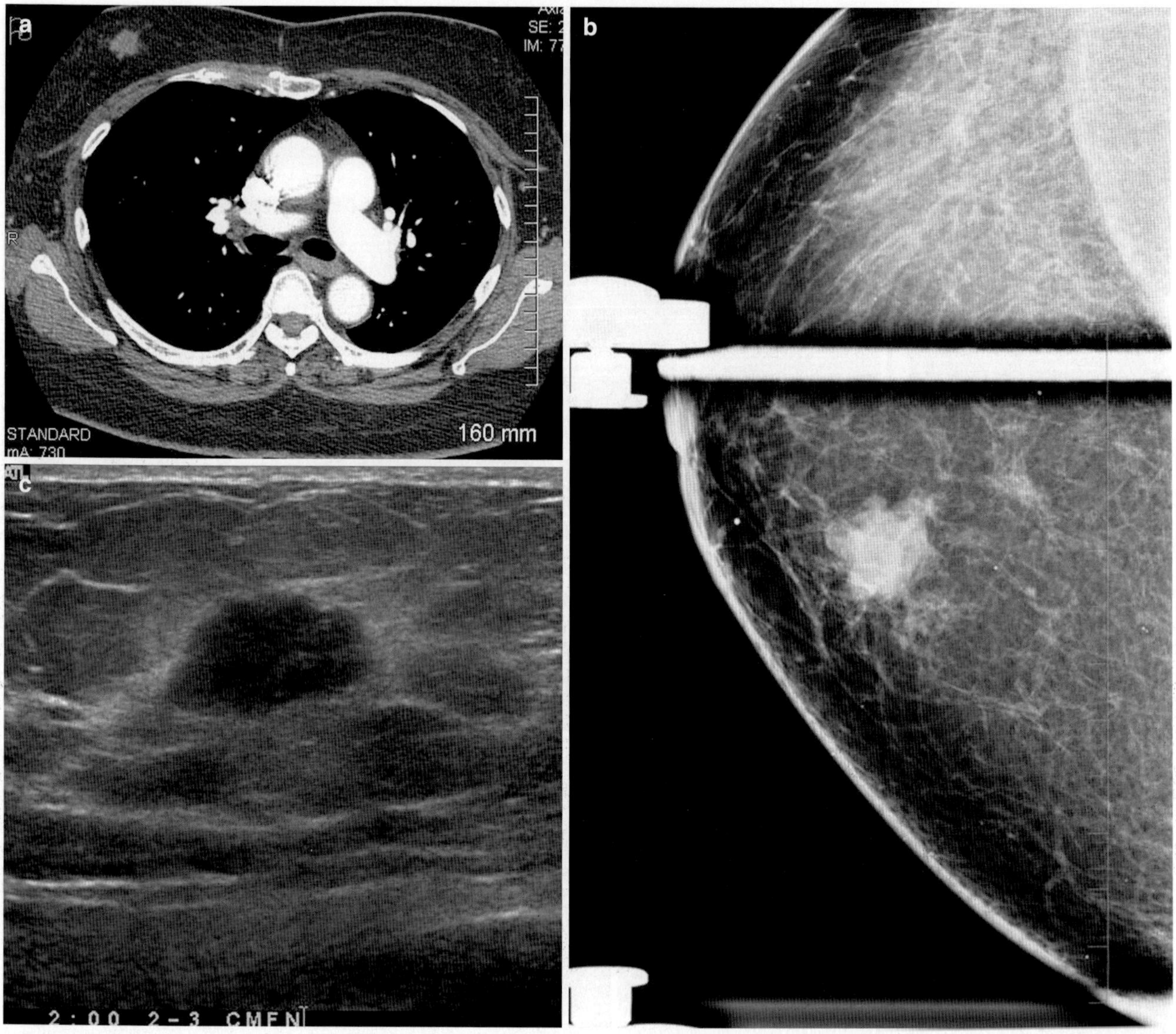

Fig. 2.2 (**a**–**c**) A 60-year-old who had not undergone screening mammogram in 4 years. (**a**) CT pulmonary angiogram performed for chest pain reveals a 2 cm mass in right breast. (**b**) Spot compression craniocaudad view of the right breast shows an irregular mass in the inner right breast. (**c**) Sonography reveals a 2 cm mass with irregular borders suggestive of malignancy. Histology showed an invasive ductal carcinoma

Limitations and Potential Harm from Screening Mammography

There are some who question the benefit of screening mammography. Controversies regarding the false positives resulting from mammography, the benefit of performing screening in women in their 40s, and whether mammography overdiagnoses cancer, leading to unneeded treatment interventions, are some of the issues. Approximately 95 % of women with abnormalities on the screening mammogram do not have breast cancer [9]. In a review commissioned by the US Preventive Services Task Force, the sensitivity of mammography for a 1-year screening interval was found to be 71–96 % and substantially lower for women in their 40s. The specificity was 94–97 %; it has to be borne in mind that false positive meant recall of the patient for additional views and resolution of the abnormality in most instances without the need for a biopsy or surgical intervention. The positive predictive value of one-time mammography ranged from 2 to 12 % for abnormal results requiring further evaluation and from 12 to 78 % for abnormal results requiring biopsy. There is continued increase in predictive value with age [10].

Screening Women in Their 40s

The mammographic sensitivity is lower in women in their 40s mostly due to increased prevalence of dense breast tissue in this age group. The incidence of cancer in this age group is lower about 140 per 100,000 compared to 500 per

100,000 in women older than 50 years. An evidence-based analysis from Canada concluded that there is Level 1 evidence that screening mammography in women aged 40–49 years at average risk for breast cancer is not effective in reducing mortality [11]. The Canadian Task Force of Preventive Services supports neither the inclusion nor the exclusion of screening mammography for women in their 40s. In the USA there is disagreement among nation organizations regarding the benefit of screening in their 40s. The National Institutes of Health, the American Association for

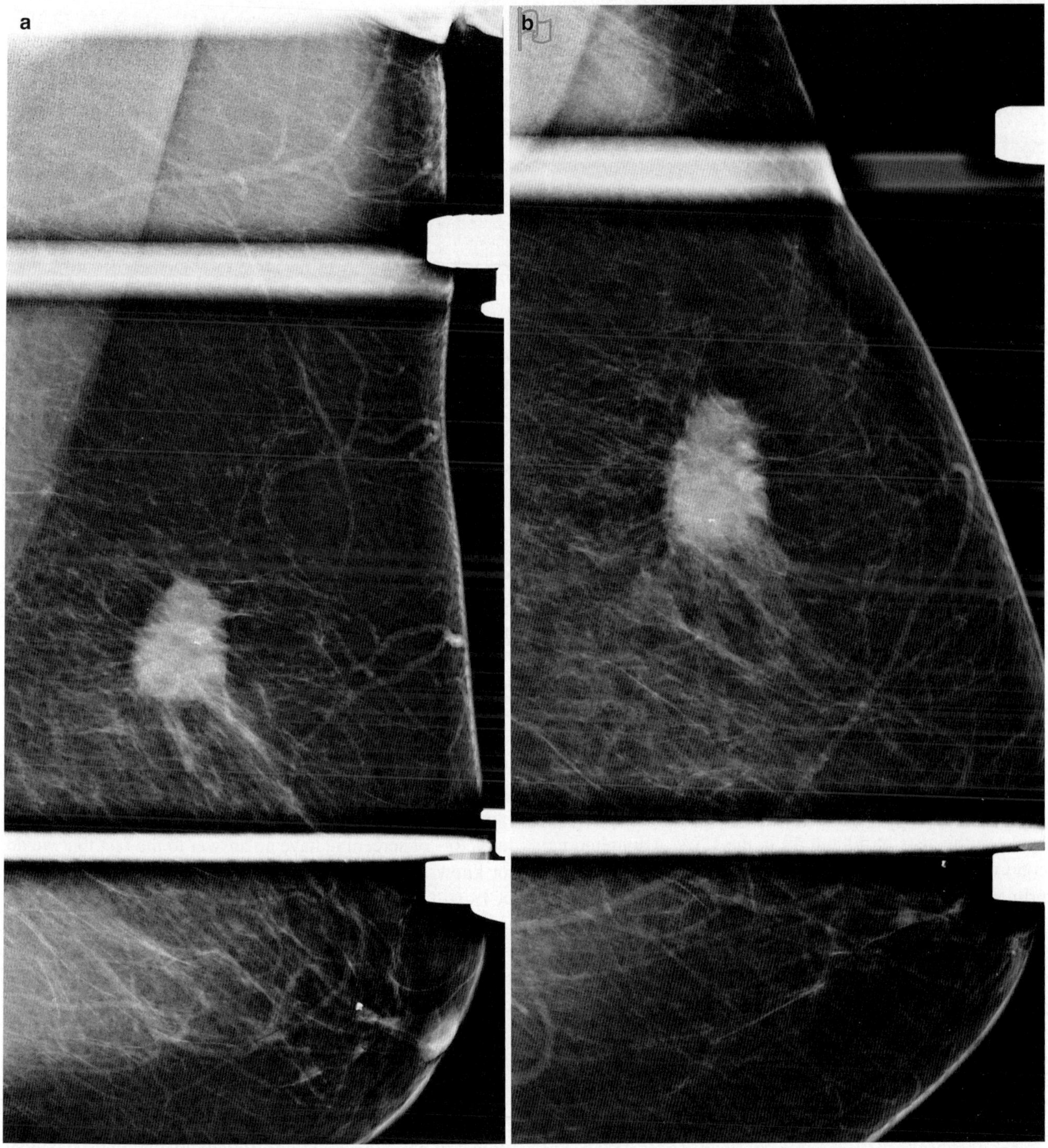

Fig. 2.3 (**a–d**) A 72-year-old woman not screened in 6 years. (**a**) Left breast mediolateral oblique view with spot compression demonstrates an irregular spiculated mass. (**b**) Left breast craniocaudad view with spot compression. (**c, d**) Left breast ultrasound shows a 3 cm mass with malignant features. Histology showed an invasive ductal carcinoma

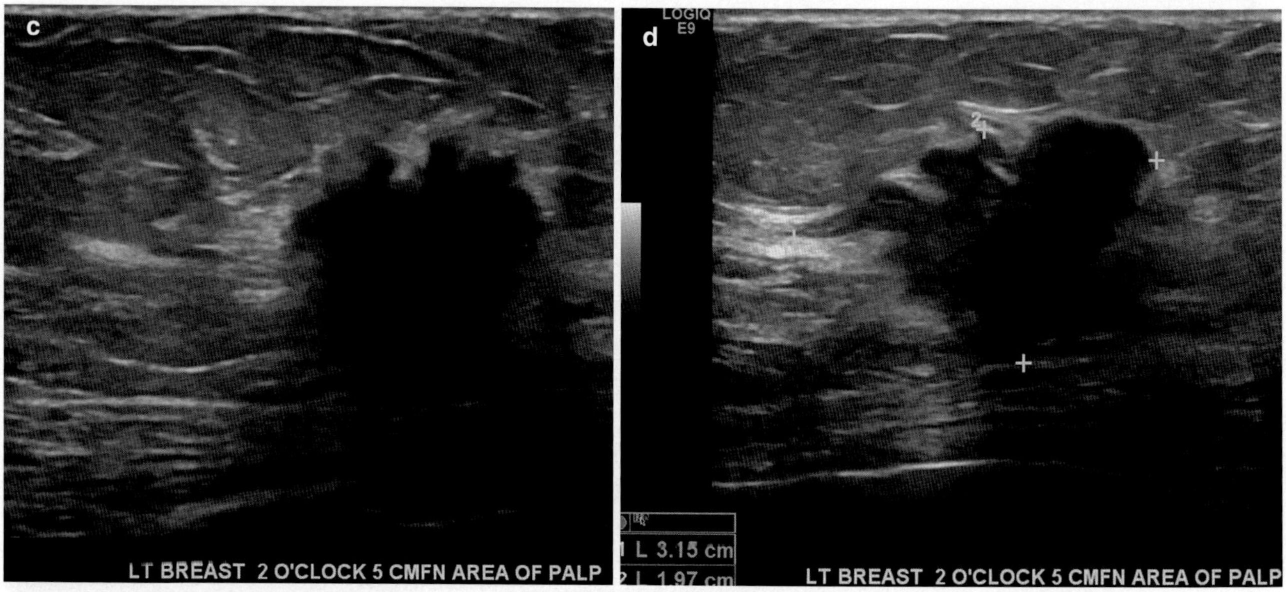

Fig. 2.3 (continued)

Cancer Research, and the American Academy of Family Physicians do not recommend screening women in their 40s, whereas the National Cancer Institute, the American Cancer Institute, the American Cancer Society, the American College of Radiology, and the American College of Obstetricians and Gynecologists do.

Although women in their 40s have denser breast and a lower incidence of breast cancer accounting for decreased sensitivity of mammography, in this age group, women tend to have faster growing cancers [9]. The evidence of reduction of mortality for women between 40 and 49 years is lower yet significant. A study that looked at the data from all four Swedish trials for women in this age group reported a 23 % mortality reduction at randomization achieved from a median trial time of 7 years, a median follow-up of 12.8 years, and a screening interval of 18–24 months [12]. About 18 % of cancers both in situ and malignant are reported in women between the ages of 40 and 49 in the USA. A longitudinal cohort study of 1977 women in this age group who had primary breast cancer was undertaken over an 18-year period. A significant increase in the percentage of mammography-detected cancer was seen over time (28–58 %), and a concurrent decline in patient- and physician-detected breast cancer (73–42 %), with a consequent increase in lower stage disease detection and decrease in higher stage disease [13]. A study of 31,814 average-risk women found that the positive predictive value for further evaluation was 1–4 % for women aged 40–49 years, 4–9 % for women aged 50–59 years, 10–19 % for women aged 60–69 years, and 18–20 % for women aged 70 years or older [14].

Harms of Mammography Screening

Overdiagnosis refers to diagnosis of cancers particularly DCIS [ductal carcinoma in situ] which may have never progressed to an invasive stage and resulted in death. Such patients would have undergone surgery, chemotherapy, and/or radiotherapy with consequent harm to women [15]. The presumptive evidence for "overdiagnosis" is suggested by the fact that breast cancer diagnosis in the screened group remained persistently higher even after many years when compared to the control group of non-screened women in large randomized clinical trials. This assertion is contentious because diagnosing more breast cancer cannot be somehow construed to be a bad thing, and mortality rate reduction which has been shown beyond question should be the one and only benchmark of success of screening mammography. Despite the criticism that mammography may find DCIS that may never become invasive is a moot point since the same detractors of screening have no answer to the fact that we do not know or have a means of determining which cases of DCIS will progress on to the invasive stage and which ones do not.

On the other hand two observational studies among women who underwent the current standard technique of a two view mammography and included millions of person years of observation reported a much stronger mortality reduction than what has been shown in RCTs of 30–40 % for women in their 40s. In fact RCTs tend to underestimate the benefit from screening mammography because it includes all women in the screened group who are invited to be screened including those who do not actually end up getting a mammogram and do not exclude women in the control group who may end up getting a mammogram outside the trial. As has been previously pointed out, in several RCTs, the mammographic quality was not comparable to the current standards, and one-view mammogram only was obtained which limits the cancer detection rate [16].

Interpretive accuracy varies among radiologists, especially in mammography. A study that examined the relationship between radiologists' confidence in their assessments and their accuracy in interpreting mammograms found that confidence in mammography assessments was associated with better accuracy, especially for low-volume readers. Asking for a second opinion when confidence in an assessment is low may increase accuracy [17]. The other significant potential harm resulting from screening mammography is from false-positive results that lead to unnecessary patient anxiety and unneeded breast biopsies. Although this is a shortcoming of mammography, it is a given that any screening modality is bound to have some false positive as no test is perfect. However, much can be done to minimize the false positives, and the following section addresses ways of achieving this objective.

The most recent review of the benefits and potential harms of breast cancer screening was performed by an independent panel in the UK [18].The review was performed based on the UK screening program which offers screening for women 50 years or older once every 3 years. The review included assessment of the relative mortality benefit in women who were invited to be screened and looked at 11 randomized clinical trials with a 13-year follow-up, a mortality rate reduction of 20 % was noted, and the benefit is higher among women who underwent screening as opposed to those who were invited to and did not undergo screening. This increased benefit is difficult to ascertain. This panel looked only at RCTs that were conducted 20–30 years ago, and since then there has been significant improvement in both the quality of mammographic technique and interpretive accuracy. More recently published studies have been observational studies, namely, ecological studies, case control studies, and incidence-based mortality studies that showed a greater benefit but were not included in the review. The absolute mortality benefit is variable but was estimated to be one breast cancer death prevented for 180 women screened [18].

The overdiagnosis rate is hard to quantify and varied from 0 to 36 %. Of more importance is the fact that neither the woman nor her physician has any means of knowing which of the screen detected DCIS or invasive cancer is an "overdiagnosed case." If it was somehow possible to distinguish at screening those cancers that would not lead to death if left untreated from those cancers that would, the overdiagnosis problem would be solved. Even DCIS that is often diagnosed on screening does not inevitably equate to overdiagnosis since 10 % of DCIS leads to subsequent development of invasive cancer even when treated with wide local excision [18]. The sources of data for overdiagnosis are few, and data are mostly based on indirect estimates. Data from three RCTs that did not screen the control group and followed them for several more years showed an estimated rate of overdiagnosis in order of 11 % from a population perspective and about 19 % from the perspective of a woman invited to screening. It has been estimated that for every 10,000 women invited to screening from 50 years onward for 20 years, there will be 681 cancers, estimated overdiagnosis rate is 129 cases, but 43 deaths from breast cancer will be prevented. An expert opinion panel after an exhaustive review of data opined that benefits of screening and benefits of better treatment are independent. Uncertainty as to whether some of the benefits in mortality rate reduction are due to better treatment is not a justification to stop screening [18].

The benefits of screening mammography have been questioned, and it has been suggested that RCTs were fundamentally flawed in design and that the results are not scientifically valid [19, 20]. An opposing view on the benefits of screening mammography that was recently published claimed that a review of clinical trials with adequate randomization did not show a statistically significant mortality rate reduction at 13 years [20]. The total rate of lumpectomies, mastectomies, and radiation therapy was increased in the screened group. When seven trials including 600,000 women were reviewed, the mortality rate reduction was seen to be only 15 % with a significant overdiagnosis and overtreatment which was estimated to be at 30 %. These authors concluded that for every 2,000 women invited for screening throughout 10 years, one breast cancer death will be prevented and ten healthy women will be treated unnecessarily. About 200 women will be subjected to anxiety and distress due to false-positive findings [20].

Nonmammographic Screening for Breast Cancer

Mammography is still the gold standard for breast cancer screening of the general population [2–5].

Breast MRI and whole breast ultrasound survey have been shown to be of greater sensitivity than mammography in the early detection of breast cancers [9, 21–39]. However, unlike mammography, these two modalities have not been proved to reduce breast cancer mortality. Proof of mortality rate reduction will require a randomized controlled clinical trial involving a large number of women receiving screening with the new modality, who will then have to be followed for at least 15 years and be matched with a control group of women who receive the current standard care. The new modality being tested would have to show mortality rate reduction over and above what has been achieved with screening mammography; this is unlikely to be the case anytime in the near future [9]. At the present time, ultrasound and MRI are being used to supplement mammography for breast cancer screening in women with an elevated risk for cancer. The role of ultrasound for this reason is discussed next; the role of MRI in breast cancer screening is discussed in the chapters on breast MRI (Chaps. 8 and 9). A brief discussion on two additional examinations that have been used as supplemental tools or primary means for screening, namely, breast self-examination and clinical breast examination, follows.

Supplemental Screening with Ultrasound in Women with an Elevated Risk for Breast Cancer

In North America, breast ultrasound has been predominantly used as a targeted examination for a clinical or mammographic problem, whereas in Europe whole-breast ultrasound survey has been more prevalent [26]. It is not uncommon to identify incidental nonpalpable cancers during diagnostic sonographic evaluation of a mammographic or physical finding [26]. Mammography is known to have a limited sensitivity in women with dense breast tissue. The use of breast ultrasound as a supplemental modality for breast cancer screening has been studied in women with dense breast tissue and in those with an elevated risk for breast cancer. Dense breast tissue is by itself considered a risk factor for breast cancer [27]. It has been suggested that in women with a threefold relative risk compared with women without any known risk factors, it is enough to be categorized in the high-risk group [29]. To date, none of the major professional societies in the USA or elsewhere recommend the use of screening ultrasound for breast cancer.

A systematic search and review of studies involving mammography and ultrasound performed for screening of breast cancer found 6 cohort studies, of which only two had follow-up on patients with negative or benign findings. Screening ultrasound performed in women with American College of Radiology breast density types 2–4 identified primarily invasive cancers in 0.32 % of women. The mean tumor size was 9.9 mm, and 90 % of the cancers were node negative. Biopsy rate was high at 2.3–4.7 %, with positive predictive value of 8.4–13.7 % for those biopsied because of an abnormal finding on the ultrasound examination. The added benefit of using ultrasound to screen for breast cancers in women with a negative mammogram might be lower in women aged 50–69 years [23].

The most notable and the largest clinical trial of screening ultrasound to date is the American College of Radiology Imaging Network trial 35 (ACRIN 6666). This study was a prospective multicenter trial randomized to a group receiving ultrasound and mammographic screening and one to mammographic screening alone to compare the diagnostic yield of performance of breast ultrasound and mammography versus mammography alone in women with elevated risk of cancer [22].The criteria used in this study to determine an elevated risk for breast cancer included a personal history of breast cancer, prior atypical biopsy, and elevated risk based on the Gail or Claus model or both. A standard protocol and interpretive criteria were used. Mammography and ultrasound were performed and read independently, allowing for reducing potential biases in patient recruitment and interpretation. Data were analyzed from 2,637 patients who underwent imaging. Thirty-one cancers were detected in the study group, 11.8 per 1,000 women; the increase in the cancer detection rate because of addition of ultrasound was 4.2 per 1,000 women. The diagnostic accuracy for mammography was 0.78, for ultrasound was 0.80, and for combined mammography and ultrasound was 0.91. Ultrasound hence proved a useful supplemental modality, identifying additional small node-negative invasive cancers in this cohort of women at an elevated risk for breast cancer [22].

Breast sonography has never been studied or been advocated to be used as the only modality to screen for breast cancer. The rationale against such an approach is sound; not the least is the low yield of ultrasound alone detected breast cancers. There is, however, some data from a study in Japan that demonstrate the value of sonography when used as the only modality for screening of breast cancer in women less than 40 years of age [29]. This study was undertaken in the Ibaraki prefecture of Japan where the breast cancer screening recommendations include performing annual screening ultrasound and CBE in women of ages 30 through 56 and biannual mammography in women of ages 40 through 65. There were 12,359 women in the age group of 30–39 years who received annual screening breast ultrasound and did not undergo mammographic screening. Of these, 4,501 women also received annual CBE in addition to whole breast screening ultrasound. In young women, i.e., younger than the age of 40 years, as expected, the cancer yield was low, with a cancer detection rate of 0.04–0.07 % [34]. In those women between the ages of 40–56 years in whom both mammography and ultrasound were used, the cancer detection rate ranged from 0.13 to 0.16 % for sonography and 0.1–0.22 % for mammography. Overall, 41,653 women underwent mammography, and 48,294 women underwent CBE and breast ultrasound. The rate of detection of stage I cancers was 72 % by ultrasound, 66 % by mammography, and 42 % by CBE. Cancer detection by mammography and ultrasound was complementary. Approximately one-third of cancers would have been missed if only one of these modalities were used, which once again proves the value of supplementing ultrasound with mammography, as has been shown in the ACRIN 6666 trial [29]. There have been other studies conducted in Japan, where a significant proportion of women tend to have small breasts with dense parenchyma and are better suited for whole breast ultrasound survey. These studies have also validated use of ultrasound in the detection of small cancers in women with dense breasts [30, 31].

Breast Ultrasound: Pros and Cons (Table 2.2)

The benefits of ultrasound as a screening modality are that it does not use ionizing radiation, is well-tolerated, does not require intravenous contrast administration, and is optimally amenable for percutaneous biopsy guidance. Ultrasound is able to identify small nonpalpable masses while undeterred by presence of dense breast tissue, which is an inherent limitation of mammography. More than 90 % of cancers identified at sonography are in women with >50 % of dense breast tissue [32, 33]. In addition ultrasound is a useful supplemental tool in identifying small cancers with subtle findings on a mammogram (Fig. 2.4a–e).

Due to its ability to detect intraductal calcifications associated with DCIS, mammography is able to identify intraductal cancers with a high degree of accuracy (Fig. 2.5). However, unlike mammography, the vast majorities of cancers that are seen on ultrasound are invasive cancers; DCIS is not usually identified by sonography [23]. On the other hand, MRI has been shown to readily identify DCIS [33]. Nevertheless, it is debatable whether a screening examination that identifies small node-negative cancers is adequate or whether detection of DCIS is a more critical requirement of a screening test. There are limitations for the use of ultrasound in screening for breast cancer. Ultrasound has never been proven to reduce mortality from breast cancer. Because the incidence of cancers seen on ultrasound is low, to prove mortality rate reduction, a large cohort will have to be studied in a randomized blinded controlled clinical trial [9]. These studies are unlikely to be conducted anytime in the near future, leaving this important question of whether ultrasound screening will lead to breast cancer mortality rate reduction unanswered. Ultrasound is an operator-dependent examination; standardization of the examination and having a skilled, adequately trained sonologist are critical for performance of a whole breast ultrasound [26]. This is compounded by intraobserver and interobserver variability when follow-up for probably benign lesions is recommended. Perhaps one of the most significant drawbacks for the use of ultrasound is the time that is takes to perform a high-quality bilateral breast ultrasound, which was reported to be a median of 19 min [26]. That compares very poorly with mammographic interpretation time. A breast radiologist might read up to 50 mammograms in the time taken to perform three breast ultrasounds [21]. Another limitation of ultrasound is the high rate of false-positive studies; the positive predictive value in those cases in which biopsy was performed was 8.8–8.9 %, compared with 23 % with mammography [22]. In this context it is worthwhile keeping in mind that a false-positive ultrasound might not have the same consequence as that of a false-positive mammogram. As Kuhl points out in an editorial, a suspicious finding on a mammogram requires a much more expensive and time-consuming biopsy procedure than an ultrasound-guided core biopsy or a fine-needle aspiration biopsy that can be performed often immediately after the ultrasound examination [21].

Table 2.2 Screening breast ultrasound: Pros and cons

Advantages	Disadvantages
Identifies small node-negative cancers that are missed by screening mammography	Operator dependent
Better tolerated by the patient, no ionizing radiation, no patient discomfort	Requires longer physician time compared to interpreting mammograms
May be beneficial as a supplemental modality in women with an elevated risk for breast cancer and/or in women with a dense breast	High false-positive rate
Biopsy of a suspicious abnormality is easier to perform than for mammographically identified abnormalities	Mortality rate reduction has not been proven in a randomized clinical trial as has been shown with mammography
	Lower sensitivity in identifying DCIS compared with mammography

Supplemental Screening with Ultrasound in Women with Dense Breasts

In the USA, there has been a movement that aims to make it a requirement to notify patients of their breast density on a mammogram when it is heterogeneously dense or very dense so their physicians could offer them supplemental screening with breast ultrasound and/or MRI depending on their risk factors [http://www.areyoudense.org/]. A handful of states like Texas, California, and Connecticut have passed such laws. In Connecticut, insurers are required to pay for supplemental screening with breast ultrasound. Connecticut Public Act 09–41 requires that radiologists inform patients with heterogeneous or extremely dense breasts at mammography that they may benefit from supplemental ultrasound or breast MRI [34]. In a report of 935 such women undergoing supplemental screening ultrasound, majority of whom were at low risk [65 %], 5 % were categorized as BI-RADS 4, and 63 interventions lead to a malignant diagnosis of three, all of which were small less than 1 cm cancer. There was one cancer each in the low-, intermediate-, and high-risk groups. As shown in multiple studies, the yield of cancer in a screening ultrasound is expected to be higher in women at elevated risk for breast cancer. Cancer detection rate was 3.2 per 1,000, and the positive predictive value was only 6.5 %. Another

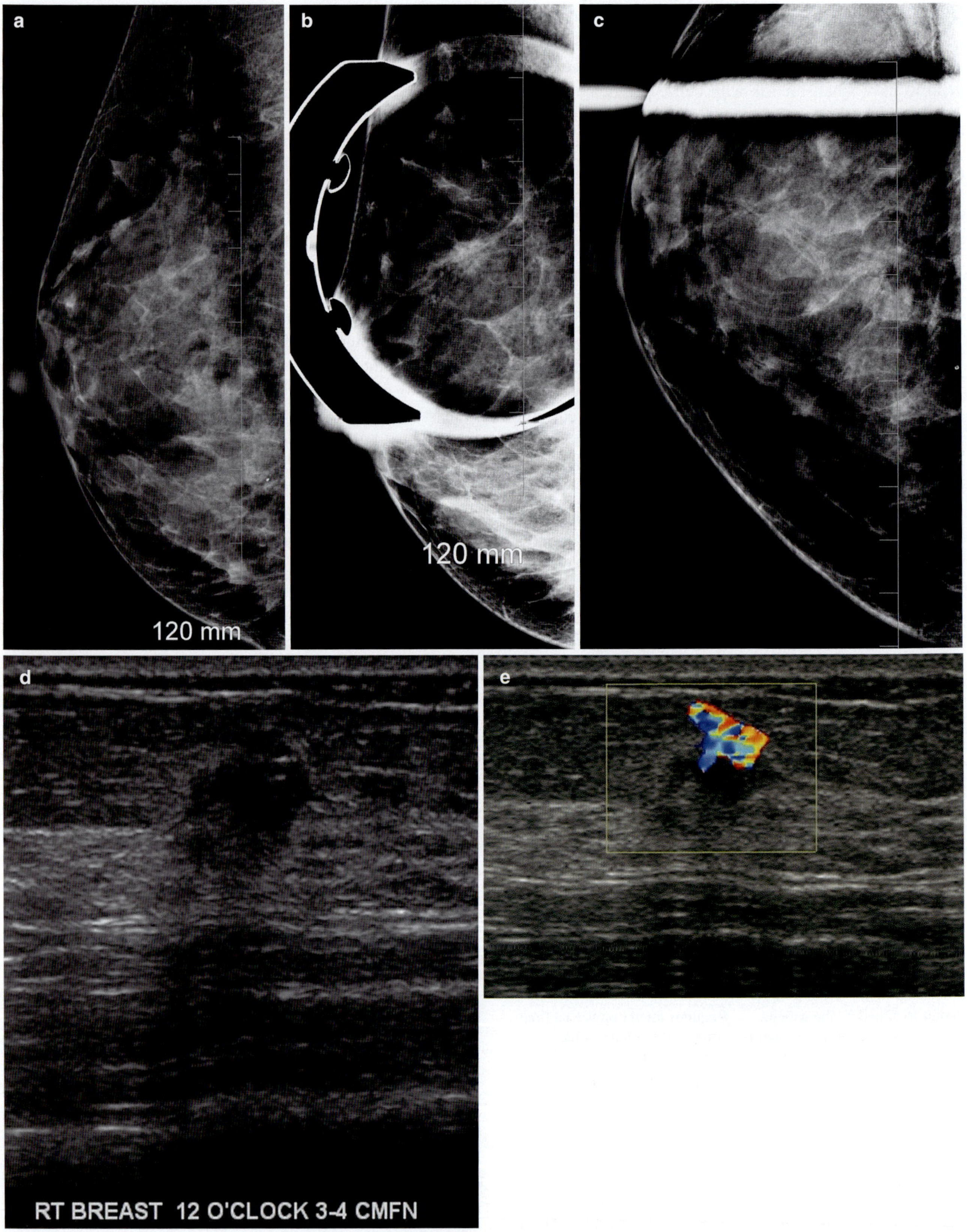

Fig. 2.4 (**a**–**e**) Mammographically subtle invasive ductal cancer in a 45-year-old female. (**a**) Mediolateral oblique view demonstrates a small focal asymmetry in the upper breast. (**b**) Spot compression mediolateral oblique view shows an irregular focal asymmetry. (**c**) Abnormality is barely visible on spot compression view in the craniocaudad projection. (**d**) Ultrasound demonstrates an irregular small mass with malignant features. (**e**) Color Doppler imaging demonstrates the mass to have prominent vascularity

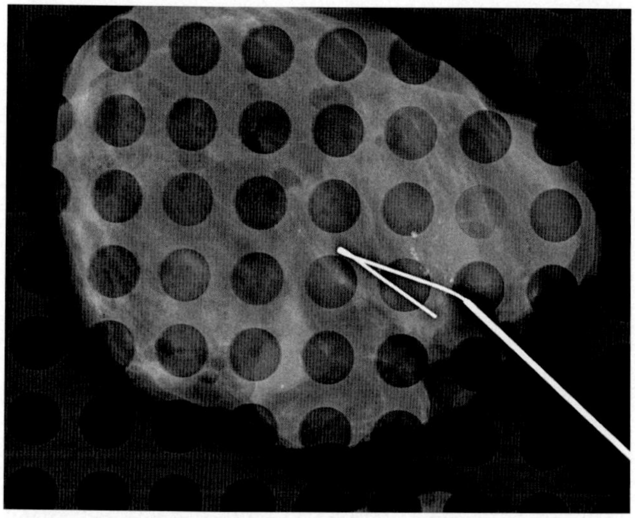

Fig. 2.5 Ductal carcinoma in situ appearing as clustered crushed stone type of pleomorphic microcalcifications in a specimen radiograph from an excisional biopsy. Localizing wire is seen within the specimen

study undertaken in Connecticut which included 8,647 screening breast ultrasound exams, 5 % were BI-RADS 4 or 5. There were 28 cancers in 418 of 429 in the BI-RADS 4/5 group for a positive predictive value of 6.7 %. The additional yield of cancers in women without an elevated risk was 3.25 per 1,000 [35].

A cancer detection rate of 4.4 per 1,000 has been reported in women with dense breasts in a study from Europe in women with average risk [36]. A systematic review of studies performed between 1995 and 2012 was undertaken to study the benefit of mammography supplemented with ultrasound as compared to mammography alone. There were no controlled studies undertaken to date. Extrapolation of results from women with an elevated risk for breast cancer suggested that the false-positive sonography could exceed 98 %. There is no sound evidence for routine use of ultrasound as a supplement to mammography. In clinical practice the use of supplemental ultrasound should be limited to women with dense breasts and/or in those with an elevated risk of breast cancer with a stronger justification for its use when both criteria exist [35, 38]. The role of ultrasound and/or MRI will remain debatable until controlled clinical trials are conducted to examine their efficacy as a supplemental tool particularly in women at average risk. Mammography will remain the gold standard methodology for screening for breast cancer [39].

Screening by Clinical Breast Exam

Most professional societies that issue recommendations for screening mammography also recommend that physician or health-care worker perform periodic clinical breast examination. Clinical breast examination in such a setting plays a complementary role. The number of women in the USA undergoing mammography has increased steadily since 1990, especially in women with limited access to health care [40]; In 1997, 71 % of women in the USA older than 41 years reported having undergone mammography in the previous 2 years compared to 54 % in 1989. Women and their physicians are making decisions about screening, and they need information about the underlying risk of the condition being screened for, the effectiveness of the procedure in preventing an untoward outcome such as death, and the potential ill effects of screening, such as false-positive tests. For policy makers and payers, cost-effectiveness is an important factor in decisions about the allocation of finite resources [2].

Clinical breast examination [CBE] has been studied as a low-cost alternative to mammographic surveillance to reduce mortality by early detection of breast cancer. CBE identifies about 60 % of cancers that are detected by mammography and a few that are not seen at mammography. There has been no randomized clinical trial undertaken to evaluate the efficacy of CBE in the early diagnosis of breast cancer by comparing women who received CBE and those who did not. An estimate based on all randomized clinical trials reported sensitivity of CBE for detection of breast cancer at 54 % and specificity at 94 %. Indirect evidence of its value comes from the Canadian National Breast Screening Study, where women were divided into two groups, one that received screening with physician-performed CBE alone and a second group that received both CBE and screening mammography. There were 39,405 women enrolled in this clinical trial. These investigators found that in the two groups, breast cancer mortality and nodal involvement was similar [2, 9, 41–43]. The sensitivity of CBE in clinical practice has been reported to be considerably lower compared to the Canadian National Breast Cancer Screening Study [CNBCSS]. A sensitivity of 28–36 % only in clinical practice compared to 63 % achieved with CNBCSS [42].

A cost-effectiveness analysis of screening mammography and clinical breast examination in India reported that a single CBE at age 50 leads to a 2 % decrease in breast cancer mortality rate and had an estimated cost-effectiveness ratio of Int.$793 per life year gained, a 16.3 % mortality rate reduction was possible with biennial CBE at a cost-effectiveness ratio of Int.$1341, and CBE performed annually from ages of 40–60 years was estimated to be as effective as screening mammography for reducing breast cancer mortality at a fraction of the cost [44]. It has been pointed out that health policy makers are critical of BSE and CBE and more tolerant toward inconsistent and negative findings of mammographic screening [44]. Clinical breast examination may find tumors that are not seen on mammography or in breast tissue that is not imaged at mammography, such as in the axilla or the chest wall above the breast an area that may not show up well or get excluded on routine mammographic views. The value of CBE which requires no special equipment should not be discredited particularly in developing countries. Failure to demonstrate efficacy in controlled clinical trials may not mean that an intervention is not effective particularly when can be implemented at a low cost. It is, however, imperative that primary care providers and health-care workers be well versed in the method of clinical breast examination, so that women who present with a complaint or in whom a lump is discovered are then offered appropriate further imaging with ultrasound.

Screening by Breast Self-Examination [BSE]

Breast self-examination has the advantage of being patient centered noninvasive and can be carried out by women in the comfort of their home. If the challenge of educating women on breast self-awareness, training to perform structured BSE, is overcome, it makes sense to implement it as part of a breast cancer screening strategy. Compliance is the greatest challenge, and even in the USA, only one-third of women perform regular BSE, and the reported sensitivity is also low [20–30 %]; the prospects in developing countries may be even more challenging [45]. A large randomized controlled trial in Shanghai, China, that included 266,064 women who worked in textile factories provided half of the women with intensive initial instruction that included practice with breast models, regular reminders, and practice examinations under supervision biannually for 5 years [46]. There was no change in breast cancer mortality in the intervention group at 10 years of follow-up. There was a significantly higher rate of biopsy due to false-positive findings [1.8 % in the instruction group compared to 1 % in the control group]. However, these findings have to be interpreted with caution, since the study group had a high percentage of young women [40 % in their 30s]; in this age group, no method of screening has ever been shown to be effective in reducing mortality, and also a higher false-positive rate is to be expected due to the hormonally induced cyclical changes in the breast tissue. The time to measure mortality change in this large clinical trial may have been too short [47]. The first large-scale clinical trial conducted in Russia also did not show any benefit in reducing breast cancer mortality in women undergoing BSE [48]. This trial has been criticized for not having practiced BSE well and the lack of critical analysis of data of cluster randomization [49, 50]. A case–control study within the CNBSS women showed that in those with a higher score, there was a lower score of being diagnosed with advanced breast cancer and thereby lower odds of death from breast cancer [51]. A similar benefit was seen in a cohort of nearly 30,000 women in Finland, where a relative risk of 0.75 for breast cancer mortality relative to that expected from the general population was found [47]. This study suggested that a well-performed BSE combined with a physician visit to act on the findings of BSE was critical in providing this benefit [47].

Conclusion

Screening mammography has proven benefits in reducing mortality from breast cancer, and this is independent of the benefits of improved therapy. The controversy regarding whether screening for breast cancer is justified, if it is when to start screening and how often to screen are controversies that will continue to rage on. The number of women needed to be screened to prevent one breast cancer death using the cancer intervention and surveillance modeling network [CISNET] is lower than the model based on RCTs that was used by the US Preventive Services Task Force [USPSTF]. For instance, for women between the ages of 40 and 49, the number of women to be screened to avoid one breast cancer death was 746 based on the CISNET model, whereas if the model based on RCTs was utilized, it is 1,904. The difference is attributed to two factors because RCTs do not account for nonattendance among women invited to be screened or for crossover of uninvited control group who end up being screened [52–55]. Only 67–68 % of women invited to be screened actually attended screening in the first year, and this number progressively decreased during subsequent years. In the control group as 20–30 % of women can undergo at least one round of screening [54]. The second confounding factor is that most of the large RCTs were performed in the 1970s and 1980s and therefore do not reflect current mammography technology, screening practice, or interpretation skills and therefore are likely to underestimate the current benefit of screening mammography. A recent publication reported that only 84 women needed to be screened annually between 40 and 84 years to save one life from breast cancer, and 5.3 need to be screened annually to gain one life-year from breast cancer [55]. The evidence in favor of mammographic screening is overwhelming. While there is a need to define and set benchmarks of performance for interpreting physicians to avoid unnecessary biopsy and optimize false positive, the rationale for screening women annually from 40 years of age is sound and scientifically validated.

It is generally recommended that screening mammography should be continued until that age where life expectancy is at least 7 years on the basis of age or comorbid conditions or when abnormal results would not result in intervention because of age or comorbid conditions. All the RCTs included women under the age of 74 years; however, it is known that mammographic sensitivity and specificity increases with age, and a study of 690,000 women aged 66–79 years showed a significant reduction [43 %] in the incidence of metastatic cancer in the screened versus the non-screened group [56]. These findings justify continuing screening beyond 74 years in otherwise healthy women.

In women with an elevated risk, there is proven benefit for supplementing screening with breast ultrasound and breast MRI particularly in women with dense breasts where mammographic screening may be compromised. Ultimately reduction in breast cancer mortality will require a multipronged approach, effective use of screening, and optimal treatment, and reduction of risk factors such as obesity would be the best approach [57]. The benefits of screening mammography in clinical practice has been also validated in a study just published that showed that 71 % of deaths from breast cancer occurred in women who were not screened for breast cancer and the median age of diagnosis of these fatal cancers was 49 years [58].

References

1. World Health Organization. Screening for various cancers. http://www.who.int/cancer/detection/variouscancer/en/index.html.
2. Fletcher SW, Elmore JG. Clinical practice: mammographic screening for breast cancer. N Engl J Med. 2003;348:1672–80.
3. Tabár L, Fagerberg CJG, Gad A, et al. Reduction in mortality from breast cancer after mass screening with mammography: randomized trial from the breast cancer screening working group of the Swedish national board of health and welfare. Lancet. 1985;1:829–32.
4. Tabar L, Fagerberg G, Chen HH, et al. Efficacy of breast cancer screening by age. New results from the Swedish two county trials. Cancer. 1995;75:2507–17.
5. Tabar L, Vitak B, Chen H-H, Yen MF, Duffy SW, Smith RA. Beyond randomized controlled trials: organized mammographic screening substantially reduces breast carcinoma mortality. Cancer. 2001;91(9):1724–31.
6. Carney PA, Miglioretti DL, Yankaskas BC, et al. Individual and combined effects of age, breast density, and hormone replacement therapy use on the accuracy of mammography. Ann Intern Med. 2003;138:168–75.
7. Perry N, Broeders M, Wolf CD, Tornberg S, Holland R, Karsa LV. European guidelines for quality assurance in breast cancer screening and diagnosis. Fourth edition-summary document. Ann Oncol. 2008;19:614–22.
8. Lee CH, Dershaw DD, Kopans D, Evans P, Monsees B, Monticello D, et al. Breast cancer screening with imaging: recommendations from the society of breast imaging and the ACR on the use of mammography, breast MRI, breast ultrasound, and other technologies for the detection of clinically occult breast cancer. J Am Coll Radiol. 2010;7:18–27.
9. Elmore JG, Armstrong K, Lehman CD, Fletcher SW. Screening for breast cancer. JAMA. 2005;293(10):1245–56.
10. Humphrey LL, Helfand M, Chan BKS, Woolf SH. Breast cancer screening: a summary of the evidence. Ann Intern Med. 2002;137:347–60.
11. Medical Advisory secretariat. Screening mammography for women aged 40 to 49 years at average risk for breast cancer: an evidence-based analysis. Ont Health Technol Assess Ser. 2007;7(1):1–32.
12. Larsson LG, Andersson I, Bjurstam N, Fagerberg G, Frisell J, Tabár L, Nyström L. Updated overview of the Swedish randomized trials on breast cancer screening with mammography: age group 40–49 at randomization. J Natl Cancer Inst Monogr. 1997;22:57–61.
13. Malmgren J, Parikh JA, Atwood MK, Kaplan HJ. Impact of mammography detection on the course of breast cancer in women aged 40–49 years. Radiology. 2012;262(3):797–806.
14. Kerlikowske K, Grady D, Barclay J, Sickles EA, Eaton A, Ernster V. Positive predictive value of screening mammography by age and family history of breast cancer. JAMA. 1993;270(20):2444–50.
15. Woloshin S, Schwartz LM. The benefits and harms of mammography screening. Understanding the trade-offs. JAMA. 2010;303(2):164–5.
16. Berg WA. Benefits of screening mammography. JAMA. 2010;303(2):168–9.
17. Geller BM, Bogart A, Carney PA, Elmore JG, Monsees BS, Miglioretti DL. Is confidence of mammographic assessment a good predictor of accuracy? AJR Am J Roentgenol. 2012;199(1):W134–41.
18. Marmot MG, Altman DG, Cameron DA, Dewar JA, Thompson SG, Wilcox M. The benefits and harms of breast cancer screening: an independent review. Br J Cancer. 2013;108(11):2205–40.
19. Bleyer A, Welch HG. Effect of three decades of screening mammography on breast-cancer incidence. N Engl J Med. 2012;367(21):1998–2005.
20. Gøtzsche PC, Jørgensen KJ. Screening for breast cancer with mammography. Cochrane Database Syst Rev. 2013;(6):CD001877.
21. Kuhl CK. The "coming of age" of nonmammographic screening for breast cancer. JAMA. 2008;299:2203–5.
22. Berg WA, Blume JD, Cormack JB, et al. Combined screening with ultrasound and mammography vs mammography alone in women with elevated risk of breast cancer. JAMA. 2008;299:2151–63.
23. Nothacker M, Duda V, Hahn M, et al. Early detection of breast cancer: benefits and risks of supplemental breast ultrasound in asymptomatic women with mammographically dense breast tissue: a systematic review. BMC Cancer. 2009;9:1–9.
24. Le-Petross HT, Shetty MK. Magnetic resonance imaging and breast ultrasonography as an adjunct to mammographic screening in high-risk patients. Semin Ultrasound CT MR. 2011;32(4):266–72.
25. Berg WA. Beyond standard mammographic screening: mammography at age extremes, ultrasound, and MR imaging. Radiol Clin North Am. 2007;45:895–906.
26. Gordan PB. Ultrasound for breast cancer screening and staging. Radiol Clin North Am. 2002;40:431–41.
27. Boyd NF, Guo H, Martin LJ, et al. Mammographic density and the risk and detection of breast cancer. N Engl J Med. 2007;356:227–36.
28. Berg WA. Supplemental screening sonography in dense breasts. Radiol Clin North Am. 2004;42:845–51.
29. Tohno E, Ueno E, Watanabe H. Ultrasound screening of breast cancer. Breast Cancer. 2009;16:18–22.
30. Tunoda H, Tohno E, Ueno E, et al. Examination of effectiveness of breast cancer detection by modalities and age groups. J Jpn Ass Breast Cancer Screen. 1998;7:281–5.
31. Osako T, Takahashi K, Iwase T, et al. Diagnostic ultrasonography and mammography for invasive and noninvasive breast cancer in women aged 30 to 39 years. Breast Cancer. 2007;14:229–33.
32. Corsetti V, Ferrari A, Ghirardi M, et al. Role of ultrasonography in detecting mammographically occult breast carcinoma in women with dense breasts. Radiol Med (Torino). 2006;111:440–8.
33. Menell JH, Morris EA, Dershaw DD, et al. Determination of the presence and extent of pure ductal carcinoma in situ by mammography and magnetic resonance imaging. Breast J. 2005;11:382–90.
34. Hooley RJ, et al. Screening US in patients with mammographically dense breasts: initial experience with Connecticut Public Act 09–41. Radiology. 2012;265(1):59–69.

35. Weigert J, Steenbergen S. The Connecticut experiment: the role of ultrasound in the screening of women with dense breasts. Breast J. 2012;18(6):517–22.
36. Corsetti V. Evidence of the effect of adjunct ultrasound screening in women with mammography-negative dense breasts: interval breast cancers at 1 year follow-up. Eur J Cancer. 2011;47(7):1021–6.
37. Gartlehner G, et al. Adjunct ultrasonography for breast cancer screening in women at average risk: a systematic review. Int J Evid Based Health. 2013;11(2):87–93.
38. Gartlehner G. Mammography in combination with breast ultrasonography versus mammography for breast cancer screening in women at average risk. Cochrane Database Syst Rev. 2013;(4):CD009632.
39. D'Orsi CJ, Newell MS. On the frontline of screening for breast cancer. Semin Oncol. 2011;38(1):119–27.
40. Meissner HI, Breen N, Yabroff KR. Whatever happened to clinical breast examination. Am J Prev Med. 2003;25(3):259–63.
41. Weiss NS. Breast cancer mortality in relation to clinical breast examination and breast self examination. Breast J. 2003;9 suppl 2:S86–9.
42. Barton MB, Harris R, Fletcher SW. Does this patient have breast cancer? The screening clinical breast examination: should it be done? How? JAMA. 1999;282:1270–80.
43. Miller AB, To T, Baines CJ, Wall C. Canadian National Breast Screening Study-2: 13-year results of a randomized trial in women aged 50–59 years. Natl Cancer Inst. 2000;92:1490–9.
44. Okonkwo QL, Draisma G, Kinderen AD, et al. Breast cancer screening policies in developing countries: a cost effectiveness analysis for India. J Natl Cancer Inst. 2008;100:1290–300.
45. Kearney AJ, Murray M. Breast cancer screening recommendations: is mammography the only answer? J Midwifery Womens Health. 2009;54:393–400.
46. Thomas DB, Gao DL, Ray RM, et al. Randomized trial of breast self-examination in Shanghai: final results. J Natl Cancer Inst. 2002;94:1445–57.
47. Gastrin G, et al. Incidence and mortality from breast cancer in the Mama program for breast screening in Finland, 1973–1986. Cancer. 1994;73:2168–74, c J. 157, 1205–1212.
48. Semiglazov VF, et al. Study of the role of breast self-examination in the reduction of mortality from breast cancer. Eur J Cancer. 1993;29A:2039–46.
49. O'Malley MS, Fletcher SW, US Preventive Services Task Force. Screening for breast cancer with breast self-examination: a critical review. JAMA. 1987;257:2196–203.
50. Miller AB, Bianes CJ. The role of clinical breast examination and breast self-examination. Prev Med. 2011;53:118–20.
51. Harvey BJ, et al. Effect of breast self-examination techniques on the risk of death from breast cancer. Can Med Assoc. 1997;157(9):1205–12.
52. Hendrick RE. Helvie mammography screening: a new estimate of number needed to screen to prevent one breast cancer death. AJR. 2012;198:723–8.
53. Demissie K, Mills OF, Rhoads GG. Empirical comparison of the results of randomized controlled trials and case–control studies in evaluating the effectiveness of screening mammography. J Clin Epidemiol. 1998;51:81–91.
54. Moss SM, Cuckle H, Evans A, et al. Effect of mammographic screening from age 40 years on breast cancer mortality at 10 years' follow-up: a randomized controlled trial. Lancet. 2006;368:2053–60.
55. Hendrick RE. Mammography screening: a new estimate of number needed to screen to prevent one breast cancer death. AJR Am J Roentgenol. 2012;198(3):723–8.
56. Smith-Bindman R, Kerlikowske K, Gebretsadik T. Is screening mammography effective in elderly women? Am J Med. 2000;108:112–9.
57. Mandelblatt J, et al. Which strategies reduce breast cancer mortality most? Collaborative modeling of optimal screening, treatment, and obesity prevention. Cancer. 2013;119(14):2541–8.
58. Webb ML, Cady B, Michaelson JS, Bush DM, Calvillo KZ, Kopans DB, Smith BL. A failure analysis of invasive breast cancer. Cancer. 2013. doi:10.1002/cncr.28199 [Epub ahead of print].

Mammography Techniques, Positioning, and Optimizing Image Quality

3

Tamara Ortiz-Perez and Alfred B. Watson Jr.

Introduction

Mammography is the gold standard screening examination for early breast cancer detection. For women in the United States of America, breast cancer is the most commonly diagnosed type of cancer and the second most common cause of cancer-related mortality after lung cancer [1]. The American Cancer Society (ACS) estimates that in 2011, the expected number of new cases of female breast cancer cases will be 288,130 (57,650 in situ cases and 230,480 invasive cases) and the expected number of breast cancer-related deaths in females will be 39,520 [2]. The ACS estimates that in 2011, about 2,140 new cases of breast cancer are expected to be diagnosed in men (accounting for less than 1 % of all breast cancer cases) and the expected number of breast cancer-related deaths in males will be 450 [2].

Based on the most recent data from the Surveillance, Epidemiology, and End Results (SEER) program, the relative survival rates for all women diagnosed with breast cancer are 89 % at 5 years after diagnosis, 82 % after 10 years, and 77 % after 15 years [2]. Since these data are based on women treated with past therapies and do not reflect recent improvements in early detection or advances in treatment, long-term survival rates may be even higher than these figures. It is known that 5-year relative survival is lower among women with a more advanced stage at diagnosis, with 98.4 % with localized stage at diagnosis (stages 0 and I) versus 83.9 % with regional disease and 23.8 % with distant disease [3]. Larger tumor size at diagnosis is also associated with decreased survival, with the 5-year survival rate being 95 % for tumors less than or equal to 2 cm, 82 % for tumors between 2.1 and 5 cm, and 63 % for tumors greater than 5 cm [2].

Accreditation of Mammography Programs: Historical Overview

The Mammography Quality Standards Act (MQSA) was enacted by the US Congress to regulate the quality of care in mammography. It requires mammography facilities in the United States to meet uniform quality standards. MQSA was signed into law on October 27, 1992, to establish national quality standards for mammography. In order to provide mammography services after October 1, 1994, all facilities (except facilities of the Department of Veterans Affairs) must be (1) accredited by an accreditation body approved by the Food and Drug Administration (FDA), (2) be certified by the FDA or its State, (3) go through an annual MQSA inspection, and (4) display the certificate of inspection issued by the agency that conveyed said inspection. These regulations were last updated in October 2002. The ACR is one of four FDA-approved accreditation bodies.

In 1987, the American College of Radiology (ACR) Task Force on Breast Cancer developed and initiated the National Mammography Accreditation Program (MAP) as a voluntary program. This program provided facilities with peer review and feedback on the following topics: staff qualifications, equipment, quality control (QC), quality assurance (QA), image quality, and radiation dose. This was the United States first and the largest program of this kind for mammography and was directed by radiologists and medical physicists on the Committee on Mammography Accreditation of the ACR Commission on Quality and Safety [4]. The success of the ACR program in improving the quality of mammography motivated the US Congress to develop the Mammography Quality Standards Act (MQSA) in 1992 after the provisions

T. Ortiz-Perez, MD (✉)
Department of Radiology, Baylor College of Medicine, One Baylor Plaza, Mail Stop BCM 360, Houston, TX 77030, USA
e-mail: toperez@bcm.edu

A.B. Watson Jr., MD, MPH, FACR, FACPM
Department of Radiology, Baylor College of Medicine, One Baylor Plaza, Mail Stop BCM 360, Houston, TX 77030, USA

Smith Clinic, Harris Health System, Houston, TX, USA
e-mail: alfredw@bcm.edu

M.K. Shetty (ed.), *Breast Cancer Screening and Diagnosis: A Synopsis*,
DOI 10.1007/978-1-4939-1267-4_3, © Springer Science+Business Media New York 2015

established by the ACR's Mammography Accreditation Program. After the enactment of the Mammography Quality Standards Act (MQSA) by the US Congress and its subsequent execution by the Food and Drug Administration (FDA), both quality assurance (QA) and quality control (QC) in mammography are a mandatory component of the practice of mammography.

Mammographic Techniques: An Overview

Annual screening mammography is the only method shown to decrease mortality for breast cancer, as breast cancers are being detected at an earlier and more treatable stage. The importance of adequate mammographic technique is paramount to achieving this goal. In order to do this, one needs to take advantage and maximize the intrinsic tissue contrast between normal and abnormal breast tissue.

Optimal mammographic technique is one of the cornerstones of breast cancer detection and diagnosis. Both mammographic positioning and technique are essential in order to achieve the goal of early detection of breast cancer. The radiologist that interprets the study is only as good as the images submitted for interpretation. Therefore, it is of utmost importance that both the radiologists and the technologists work closely and continuously in order to achieve the overall goal: obtaining the best images possible for each patient.

Mammography has its own and unique challenges, which are closely related to the anatomy of the breast. There are several considerations that one has to keep in mind when performing and interpreting a mammogram. The volume of breast tissue is larger as one moves more posterior and closer to the chest wall. It is extremely important that the breast is imaged in its entirety to evaluate all the breast tissue and to avoid missing significant pathology, including breast cancer. Both a skilled technologist and a cooperative patient are needed so that the highest-quality imaging can be obtained. From the technologist's end, this includes performing the technical maneuvers needed to make the patient as comfortable as possible while obtaining the high-quality images in a time-efficient fashion. From the patient's end, this includes cooperating with the technologist to achieve adequate positioning and compression.

As previously stated, the goal of mammography is to image the breast tissue in its entirety with both high contrast and high resolution while minimizing the radiation dose and artifacts and maximizing cost-effectiveness, allowing for the early detection and diagnosis of breast cancer. Many pieces are needed to complete this puzzle: appropriate equipment, appropriate technique (including positioning and exposure), and engaged, committed patients. Without these, the quality of the mammographic study suffers, which compromises the interpretation accuracy. The screening mammogram may be the sole opportunity to effectively alter the natural progression of this disease. Therefore, every effort should be made to ensure that every mammogram is of the highest quality possible.

There are many components to the imaging chain that must be carefully monitored to assure that the end result is an optimal mammogram for the radiologist to read. It all starts with testing of the equipment by the medical physicist with participation from the radiologist. Elements included in this chain include the mammography unit assembly, the focal spot size measurements, the collimation, the beam quality, the accuracy and reproducibility of the x-rays generated, the use of automated exposure control, the compression mechanics, the role of the mammography phantom image and dose measurements, among others.

Some basic considerations should be taken into account when performing the mammogram, regardless if it is a screening or diagnostic study. Ideally, the nipple should be imaged in profile (i.e., projected in a tangential fashion to the x-ray beam) on all the images obtained. This allows the nipple to be used as a landmark when performing other imaging studies (breast ultrasound or magnetic resonance imaging) as well as minimizing the possibilities of mistaking the nipple for a true retroareolar mass, often termed "pseudomass" (Fig. 3.1a, b). The appropriate labeling of mammography films is illustrated in Box 3.1.

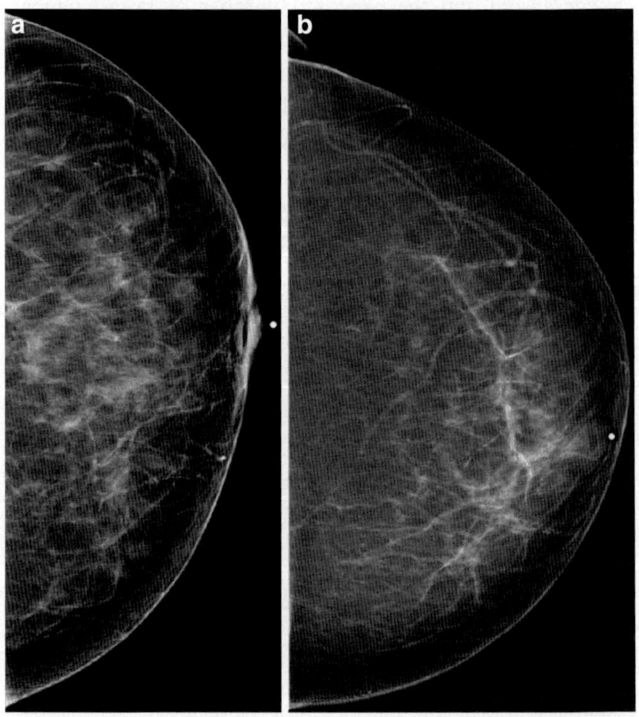

Fig. 3.1 (**a**, **b**) Comparison of two craniocaudal (CC) views: nipple in profile (**a**) versus nipple not in profile, with the nipple mimicking a retroareolar mass (**b**)

Box 3.1 Mammography Film Labeling

Patient's full name
Unique patient identification number
Name and address of facility
Mammography unit
Date of examination
Laterality and view
Technologist's initials

Screening Mammography

Screening mammograms are performed on asymptomatic women who have periodic mammograms to detect early breast cancer. The American College of Radiology (ACR) and other organizations recommend screening mammography for asymptomatic women 40 years of age and to continue annually. Screening mammography can be started before age 40 for high-risk women [5, 6]. However, there is controversy concerning the start of screening mammography as well as its frequency, which is discussed in other chapters. The screening mammogram is generally a two-view study. These standard views are described next.

Standard Mammographic Projections

Two projections are the basic components of the standard routine mammogram: the craniocaudal (CC) and the mediolateral oblique (MLO) views (Fig. 3.2a–d). This allows for maximum visualization of the breast tissues while obtaining the information required in order to gain a three-dimensional understanding of the visualized structures. This three-dimensional understanding is paramount to accomplish two objectives: (1) minimize the patient recall that would result from normal overlapping structures if only a single projection was obtained and (2) improved breast cancer detection by increasing the amount of breast tissues being imaged [5]. Additional views may be necessary for evaluation of women with breast implants (standard views as well as implant displaced or pushback views).

Craniocaudal (CC) View

An adequately positioned CC view maximizes the amount of tissue imaged (Fig. 3.3). Every effort should be made

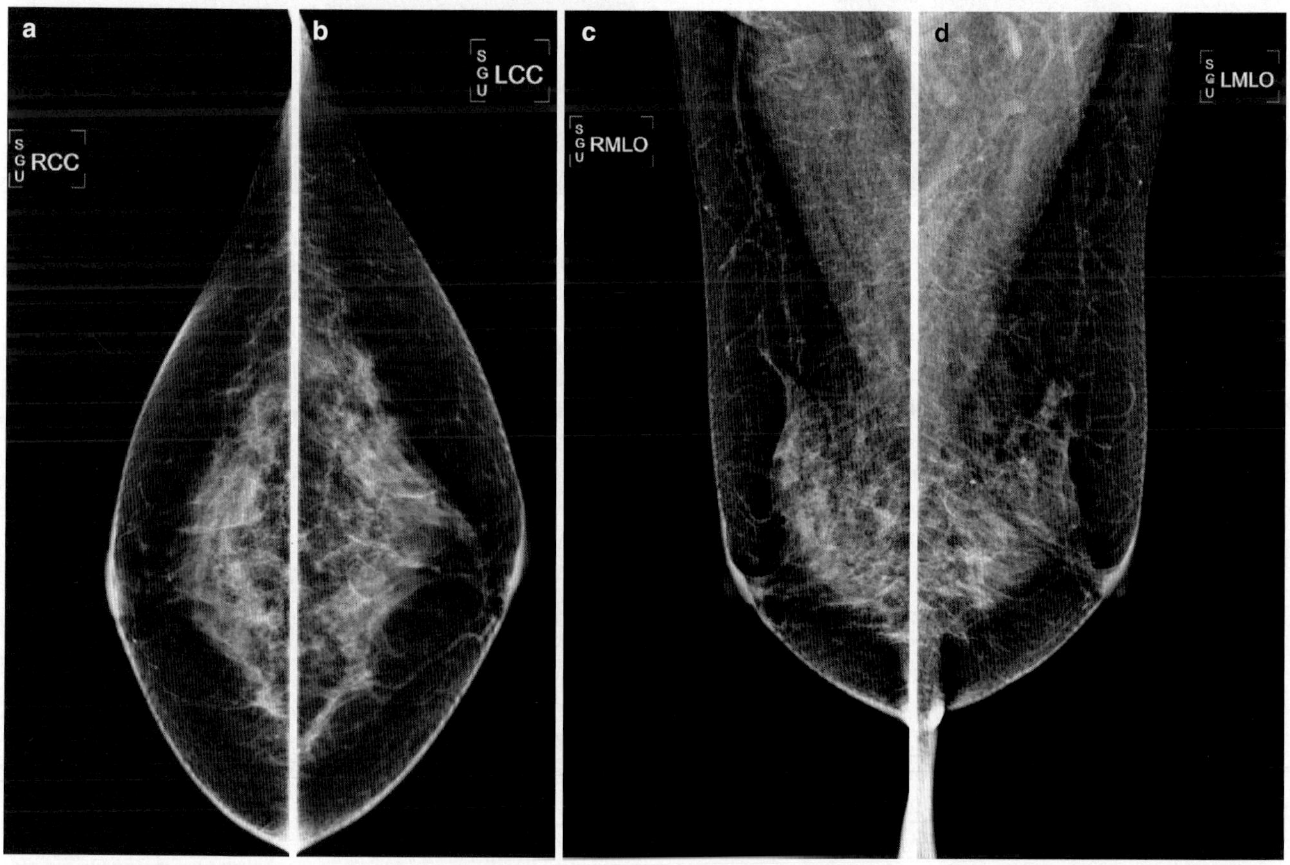

Fig. 3.2 (a–d) Standard images obtained for screening mammography

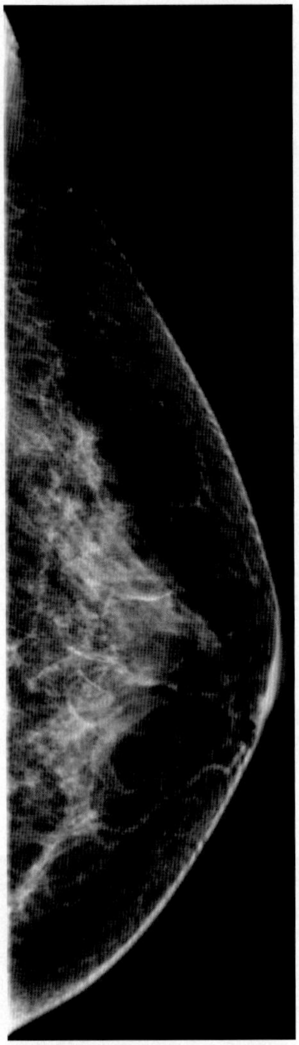

Fig. 3.3 Technically adequate craniocaudal (CC) view of both breasts

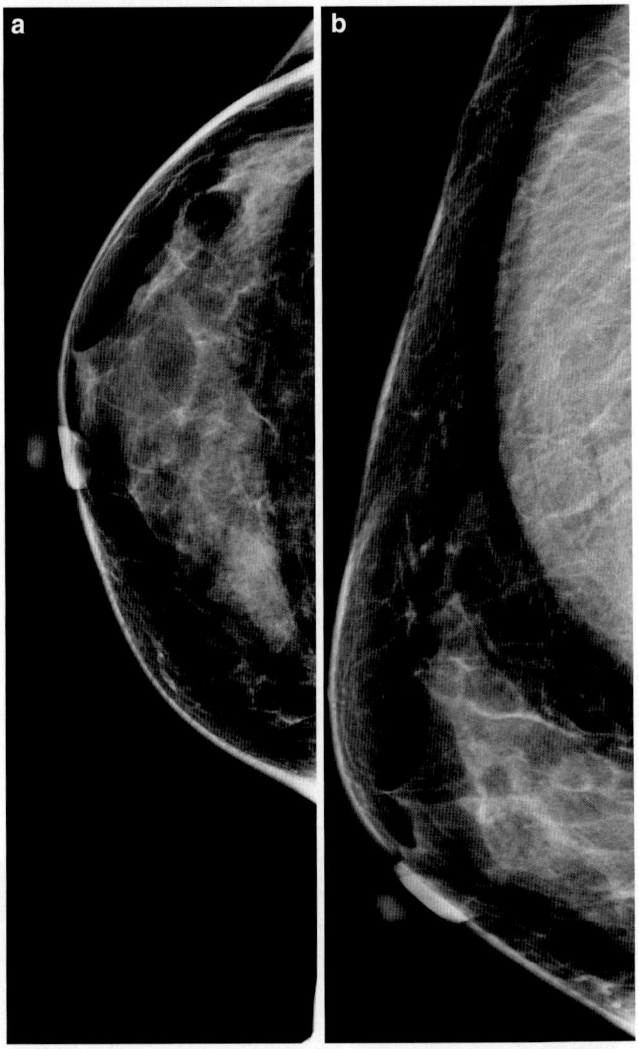

Fig. 3.4 (**a**, **b**) Example of standard craniocaudal (CC) view and exaggerated craniocaudal view laterally (XCCL) images, respectively. Note the increased amount of lateral breast tissues imaged

by the technologist in order to include all the medial and lateral breast tissues on the CC view. This is a more challenging task than on the MLO view since more breast tissue can be included in the latter as a result of the normal chest wall anatomy. The distance from the mid-nipple to the most medial and lateral skin line should be about equal. Every effort should be made by the technologist so that the medial tissues are included on the CC view. This may result in limited visualization of the lateral tissues. Additional imaging occasionally may be necessary as determined by the mammography technologist to ensure adequate visualization of all the breast tissues. The most frequent additional imaging needed is an exaggerated laterally CC view (also known as XCCL) so that there is visualization of fat behind the lateral portion of the fibroglandular tissues (Fig. 3.4a, b).

To determine the adequacy of the amount of breast tissue seen on the craniocaudal (CC) view, one should measure the distance starting from just underneath the nipple to the posterior edge of the image or the anterior edge of the pectoralis muscle in this projection. This distance is also known as the posterior nipple line (PNL). This distance should not differ by more than one centimeter when compared to the distance from just underneath the nipple to the pectoralis muscle at the level of the nipple on the mediolateral oblique (MLO) projection (Fig. 3.5a, b).

Mediolateral Oblique (MLO) View

An adequately positioned MLO view allows visualization of the tissues from the inframammary fold (IMF) in the upper abdominal wall to the axillary tail. The pectoralis muscle should extend in a convex curve obliquely in the upper half of the image and extend inferiorly to or below

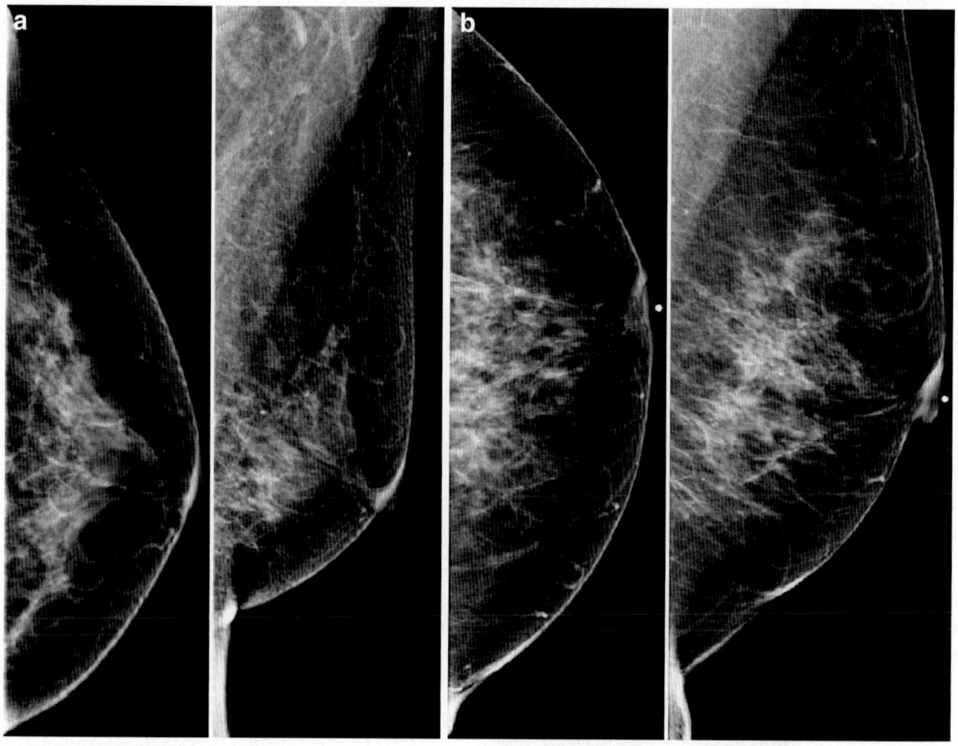

Fig. 3.5 (**a**) Adequate posterior nipple line (PNL) measurement differences between the craniocaudal (CC) and mediolateral oblique (MLO) views. The difference in this distance between the two views is less or equal to 1 cm. (**b**) Inadequate posterior nipple line (PNL) measurement differences between the craniocaudal (CC) and mediolateral oblique (MLO) views. The difference in this distance between the two views is greater than 1 cm. Nipple markers are present in these images

the level of the nipple while tapering during this course. This maximizes the amount of breast tissue that is imaged resulting in improved visualization and resultant cancer detection. The x-ray tube should be moved so that the detector plane is directly paralleling the muscle fibers. This way, pulling the breast away from the chest wall and achieving effective compression is easier for the imaging technologist and more comfortable for the patient. The degree of x-ray tube rotation will vary as appropriately from patient to patient depending on the different body habitus of the individual imaged. As mentioned earlier, the inframammary fold (IMF) should be included on the image. In particular, the inferior aspect of the breast and the upper abdomen do not overlap, opening up this area (Fig. 3.6).

One can measure the length of the posterior nipple line (PNL) from underneath the nipple to the pectoralis muscle. This line should be perpendicular to the pectoralis muscle line. The length of the PNL can be utilized, and the adequacy of the amount of breast tissue included in the craniocaudal (CC) projection (Fig. 3.7a, b).

Additional Views

Since every individual has a different anatomy, there will likely be breast tissues that are not included in the standard projections, particularly the more mobile upper inner quadrant. Additional projections can be performed on a case-by-case basis according to the different anatomy of the patients being imaged. Additional views can be obtained to maximize visualization of a region of interest. Some examples include:

- Lateral tissues: Exaggerated craniocaudal view laterally (XCCL) or the axillary tail (AT) view (Fig. 3.8a, b)
- Medial tissues: Exaggerated craniocaudal view medially (XCCM), cleavage (CV) view, or mediolateral (ML) view (Fig. 3.9a, b)
- Superior tissues: Caudocranial view

These will be discussed in more detail in the section later in this chapter titled "Additional views."

Diagnostic Mammography

Overview

There are numerous indications to perform diagnostic mammograms. These include:

1. Signs and/or symptoms indicated by the patient and/or the health care provider. Examples include palpable complaints, nipple or skin changes (retraction, induration), nipple discharge, or axillary adenopathy. The ACR guidelines also include persistent focal areas of pain or tenderness. In the author's (ABW) 35 years of practice in mammography, this symptom is rarely secondary to breast cancer.

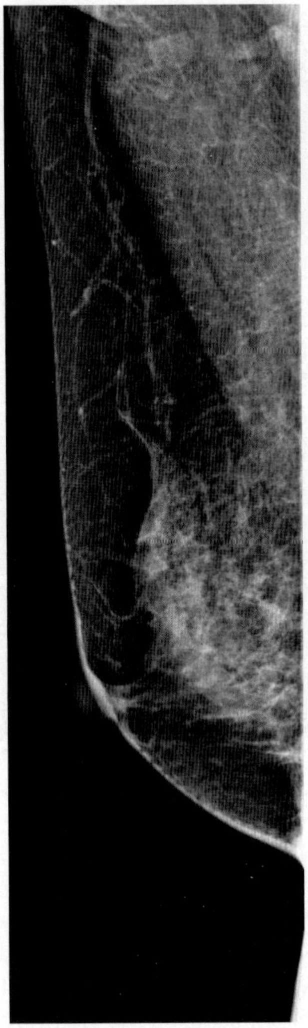

Fig. 3.6 Technically adequate right mediolateral oblique (MLO) view

2. Further evaluation of a finding noted on screening mammography.
3. Short-interval follow-up of a probably benign mammographic finding as described by the ACR Breast Imaging Reporting and Data System (BI-RADS®) to assess stability [7].
4. Patients treated for breast cancer. These patients, if asymptomatic, can undergo screening or diagnostic mammography [8].
5. Examinations requiring direct supervision by the radiologist such as consultation, direct breast examination, or directed additional views.

Additional Views

Spot Compression Views

Another technique that is employed in the work-up of breast lesions is obtaining spot views. The effective pressure generated in standard imaging is less than on spot imaging, as the pressure generated on standard imaging covers a larger area by using a larger paddle. When a smaller compression paddle is used, the pressure is then applied over a smaller area. This serves a dual purpose: (1) it spreads overlapping structures that may form a "pseudomass" on the original images, and (2) it helps to better define the morphological features of the lesion of interest.

The preferred compression device is the round spot compression paddle. This device is utilized for mid to large masses and small area of asymmetries (Fig. 3.10a). The larger square spot compression devices are best utilized for mid to large areas of asymmetry and very large masses (Fig. 3.10b). The smaller round spot compression device provides better compression with better resolution of the area of interest.

Magnification Views

Magnification mammography is most used for the analysis of morphology and distribution of microcalcifications. However, it can also be used in the analysis of the margins and internal architecture of masses.

The breast is elevated off the normal platform to obtain 1.5–2x magnification of the area of concern. Standard mammography uses a small focal spot size (traditionally, a nominal 0.4 mm focal spot). By using a smaller focal spot size (specifically, a 0.2 mm for 1.5× magnification and smaller) and elevating the breast above the receptor, magnification mammography can be performed. This allows for improved resolution due to a reduction in scatter and noise. This improved resolution comes at a cost, which are a higher patient dose as well as the exposure time. This can result in increased motion blur, which degrades the examination. Therefore, magnification views should be used appropriately realizing that what is obtained in increased resolution may be nullified by motion artifact from the longer exposure time.

Both small round (Fig. 3.11a, b) and larger square (Fig. 3.11c, d) magnification devices can be used. Again, the smaller round spot device provides better resolution of the area of interest, as seen in the corresponding figures.

Mediolateral (ML) and Lateromedial (LM) Views

The mediolateral (ML) or lateromedial (LM) views are utilized to better evaluate the morphology of lesions and assist in localizing lesions (Fig. 3.12a, b). The decision as to which view to use is mainly based on the medial or lateral location of a finding on the CC view so the abnormality is placed closest to the image receptor. If the area of concern is located in the lateral aspect of the breast, then a mediolateral (ML) view is obtained, and if it is located in the medial aspect, then a lateromedial (LM) view is obtained.

There is better compression on the ML or LM views than the MLO view because the pectoralis muscle is not included

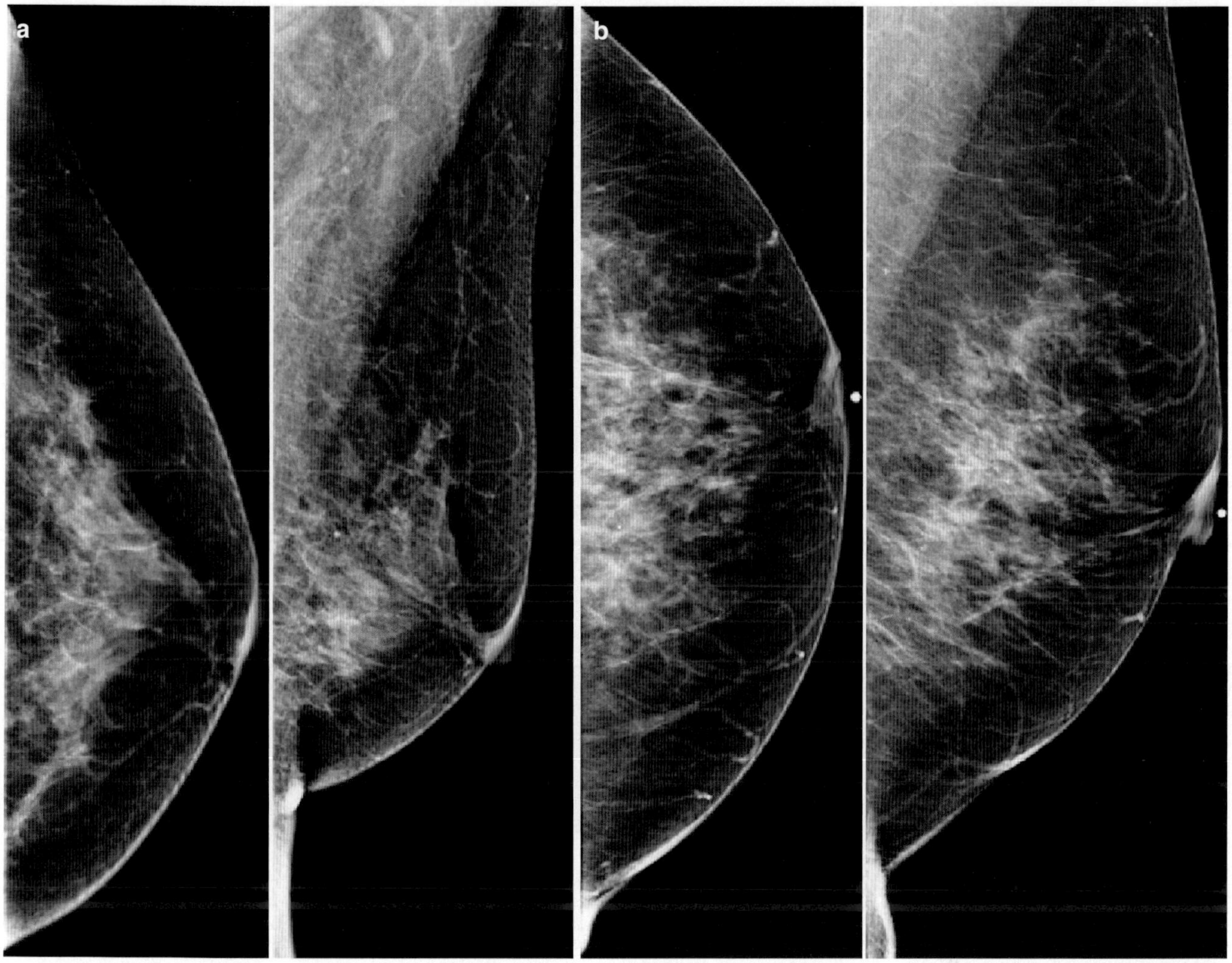

Fig. 3.7 (**a**) Adequate posterior nipple line (PNL) measurement differences between the craniocaudal (CC) and mediolateral oblique (MLO) views. The difference in this distance between the two views is less or equal to 1 cm. (**b**) Inadequate posterior nipple line (PNL) measurement differences between the craniocaudal (CC) and mediolateral oblique (MLO) views. The difference in this distance between the two views is greater than 1 cm. Nipple markers are present in these images

in the image. The ML or LM views also allow for more accurate prediction of the location of a mass or calcifications in the superior or inferior aspect of the breast by measuring its distance from the nipple. This is particularly beneficial when one is correlating a mammography finding to perform a focused breast ultrasound examination or when performing a second-look ultrasound in anticipation of biopsy of a breast magnetic resonance imaging (MRI) finding.

Another use of the ML or LM views is in the evaluation of microcalcifications. These are particularly useful for making the diagnosis of milk of calcium (MOC), which have a distinctive appearance in the lateral views versus on the CC view and constitute a benign process. This entity is discussed in more detail in other chapters in this book.

In addition, if a lesion is seen on the MLO view and not on the CC view, one can further help localize the lesion by performing an ML or LM view. This concept is discussed in more detail under the section "Localization Techniques" found later in this chapter.

Exaggerated Craniocaudal View Laterally (XCCL View)

This view is to further evaluate lesions that are in the extreme lateral/axillary part of the breast that are not seen or partially seen on the routine CC view. On the XCCL view, the nipple is off center and located in the medial aspect of the view with extra tissue visualized in the lateral aspect of the breast (Fig. 3.13a, b). This view is commonly utilized as it better visualizes lesions where cancer occurs more frequently, the upper outer quadrant of the breast. One can also utilize this view with magnification techniques to better evaluate small masses and calcifications.

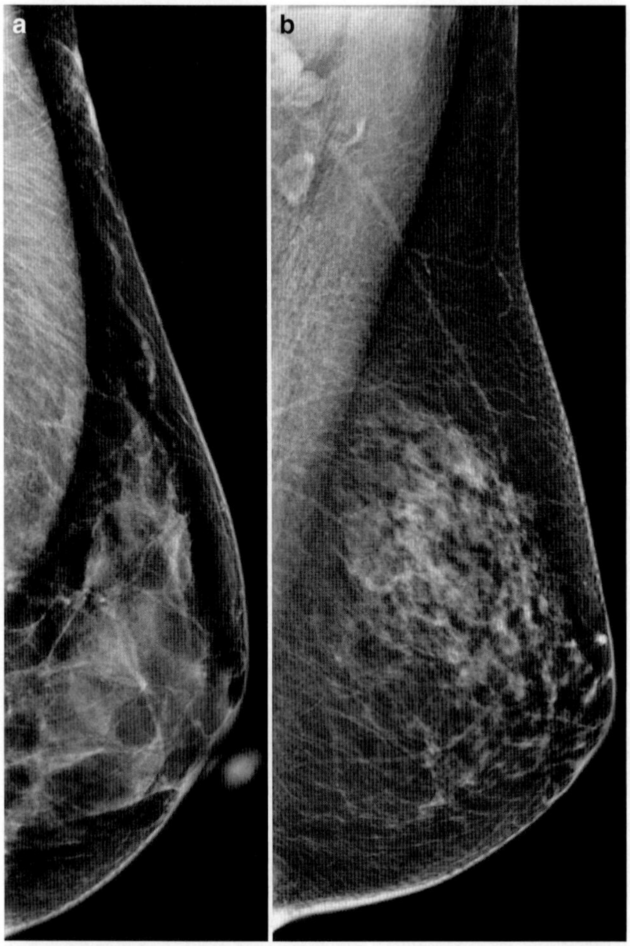

Fig. 3.8 (**a**) Example of improved visualization of the lateral tissues using an exaggerated craniocaudal view laterally (XCCL). (**b**) Example of improved visualization of the lateral tissues using an axillary tail view

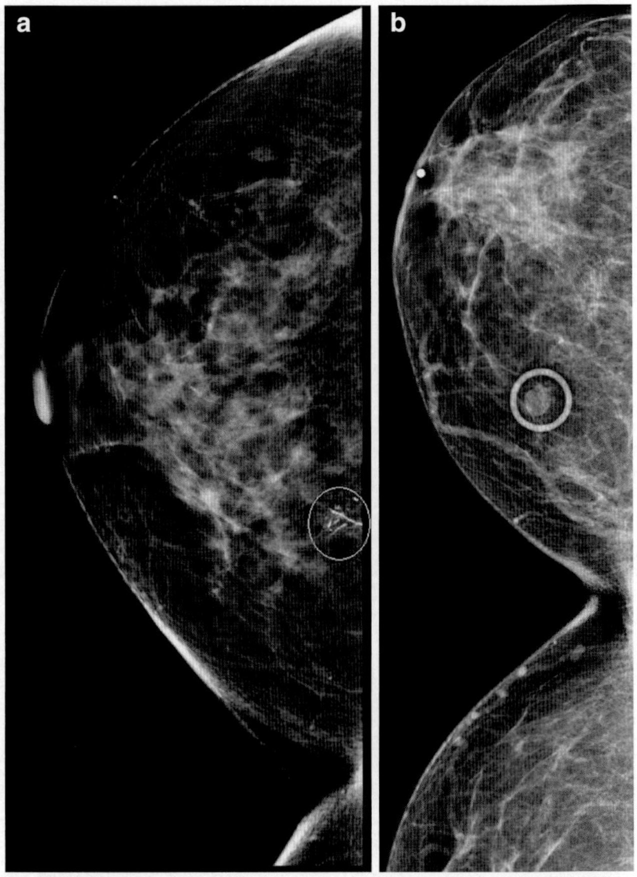

Fig. 3.9 (**a**) Example of improved visualization of the medial tissues using an exaggerated craniocaudal view medially (XCCM). In this example, the circled highly suspicious calcifications are biopsy-proven ductal carcinoma in situ (DCIS). (**b**) Example of improved visualization of the medial tissues using a cleavage view

Exaggerated Craniocaudal View Medially (XCCM View)

This view is used to further evaluate lesions that are located in the extreme medial part of the breast and therefore not seen or partially seen on the routine CC view. On the XCCM view, the nipple is off center and located in the lateral aspect of the view with extra tissue visualized in the medial aspect of the breast (Fig. 3.14).

Cleavage View

The cleavage (CV) view is an alternate method to the XCCM view for imaging the most medial aspect of both breasts (Fig. 3.15).

Rolled Medial and Rolled Lateral Views

The rolled medial CC and/or rolled lateral CC views (also known as RM or RL views) are utilized to further evaluate a finding seen only on the CC view (Fig. 3.16a) and not the MLO or lateral views (Fig. 3.16b, c). The finding may represent a "pseudomass" from overlapping tissue or a real mass that is not visualized on the MLO or lateral views. If the finding is secondary to a "pseudomass" from overlapping tissue, the process of rolling the breast medially (Fig. 3.16d) and laterally (Fig. 3.16e) will separate the overlapping tissue and the mass disappears. One can add spot compression views to the full rolled views to further evaluate the questionable finding (Fig. 3.16f).

The rolled views can also help localize a lesion if it persists on these views and is still not seen on the MLO view. This concept is discussed in more detail under the section "Localization Techniques" found later in this chapter.

Another technique instead of rolling the breast medially and laterally on the 0° plane is to rotate the imaging receptor 15–20° off the 0° plane (usual CC plane). This technique is more reproducible and is tolerated better by the patient than rolling the breast medially and laterally.

Tangential Views

The tangential views of the breast are utilized to determine if a lesion, usually calcifications, are dermal or intraparenchymal

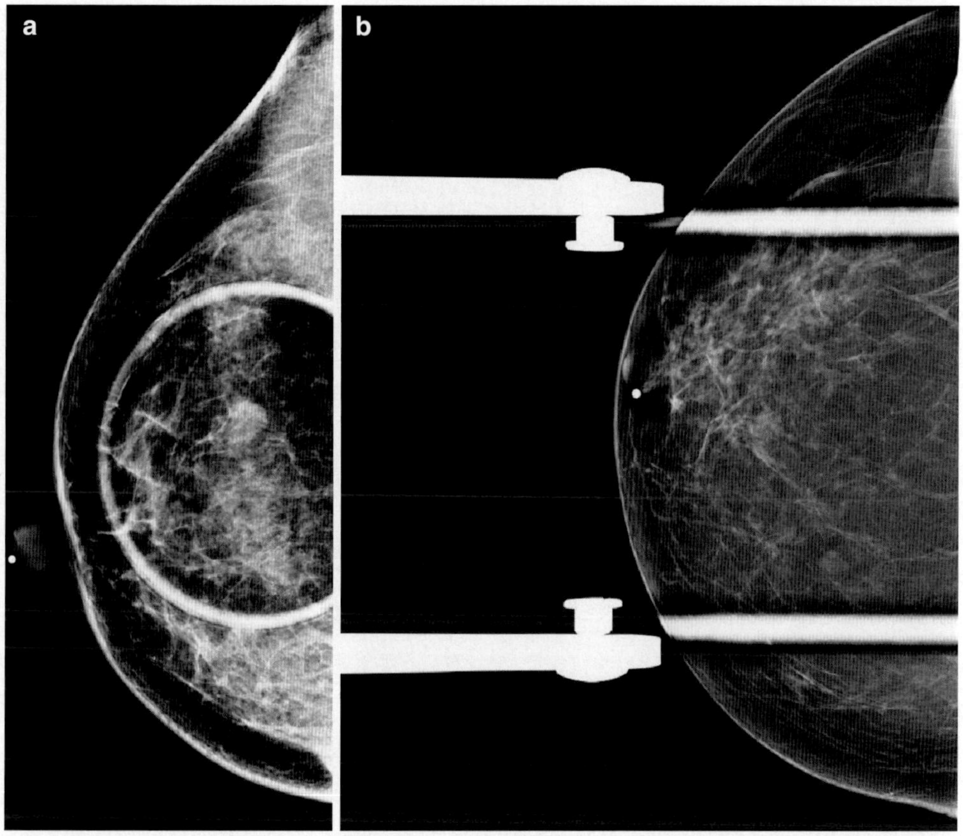

Fig. 3.10 (**a**, **b**) The round spot compression paddle (**a**) provides better characterization of the morphological features of the lesion of interest when compared to the larger square compression paddle (**b**). Images correspond to different cases, as in our institution we do not routinely use the larger square paddle

in location. It is important to make this determination prior to scheduling a patient for stereotactic biopsy for suspicious calcifications. These additional views are discussed in more detail under the section "Localization Techniques" found next.

Localization Techniques

For increased diagnostic accuracy, any suspicious lesion should be seen on at least two views so that its true three-dimensional location can be established. One way to determine the location of the lesion of interest is by employing the triangulation technique. The craniocaudal (CC), mediolateral oblique (MLO), and true lateral views (either mediolateral (ML) or lateromedial (LM) views) should be placed with the nipples at the same level and the mediolateral oblique view put in the middle. A straight line drawn passing the lesion of interest on the true lateral view and the mediolateral oblique view will point to the location on the breast in the craniocaudal view. The opposite is also true, as a straight line drawn passing the lesion of interest on the craniocaudal view and the lateral view will point to the location on the breast in the true lateral view. If the lesion "falls" closer to or below the nipple on the ML or LM view as compared to the MLO view, the lesion is located in the lateral aspect of the breast. An easy way to remember is "lead falls," i.e., if the lesion falls on the ML or LM view, it is lateral in location (Fig. 3.17a–c). Likewise, if the lesion rises closer or is above the nipple on the ML or LM view as compared to the MLO view, the lesion is located in the medial aspect of the breast. The way to easily remember this is the saying "muffins rise," i.e., if the lesion rises on the ML or LM view, it is medial in location (Fig. 3.17d–f). These steps assist in directing additional imaging to the appropriate quadrant of the breast for spot compression views and/or focused breast ultrasound examination.

Another technique that can be employed to further determine the location of a lesion seen on one view only is the use of rolled views. When a lesion is only seen on the craniocaudal view, we only know its location in regard to the medial versus the lateral aspect of the breast (Fig. 3.18a, b). Rolling the breast in both medial (Fig. 3.18c) and lateral (Fig. 3.18d) directions can provide information on the location of this lesion with regard to the upper versus the lower aspect of the breast based on how it moves in these additional images (Fig. 3.18e). If the lesion moves in the same direction as the breast is being rolled in (moves laterally in the rolled lateral view or medially in the rolled medial view), then the lesion

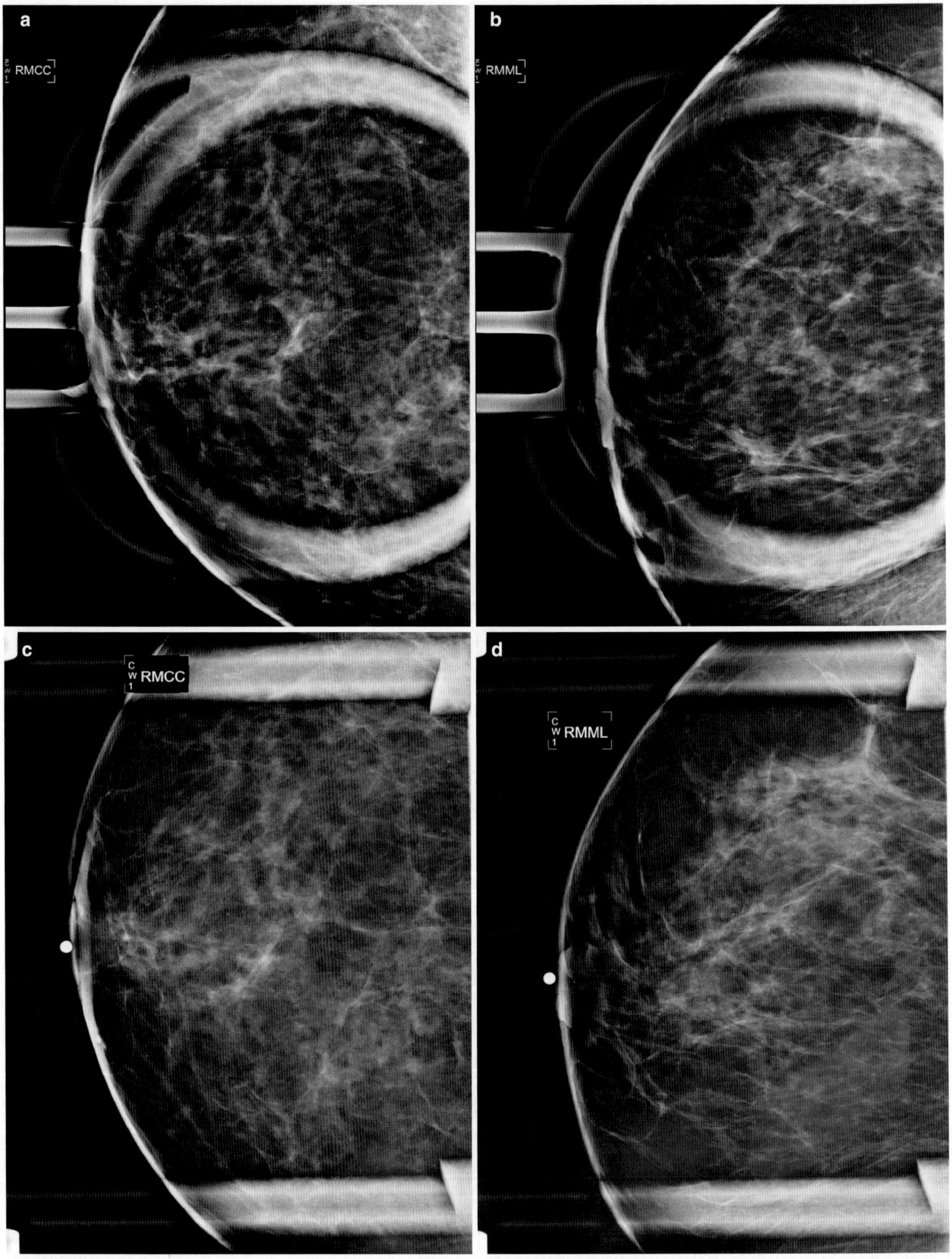

Fig. 3.11 (**a–d**) The small round magnification paddle (**a**, **b**) provides better visualization of the microcalcifications versus the larger square paddle (**c**, **d**). The use of the smaller magnification paddle aids in improved characterization of their morphology and distribution

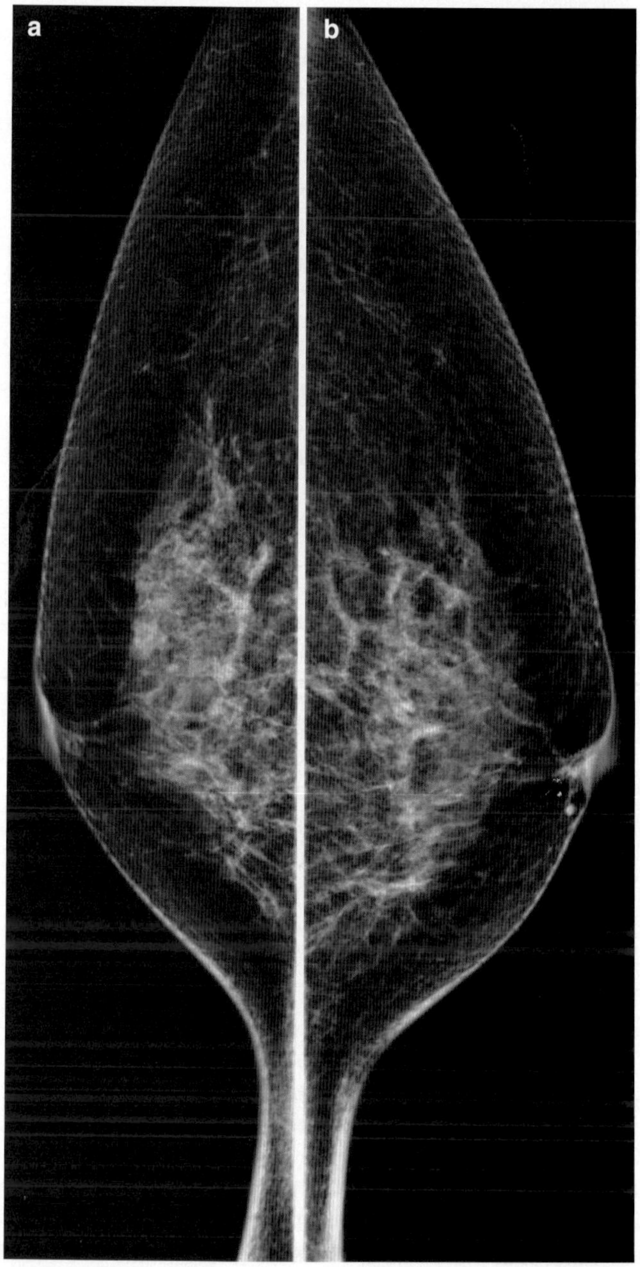

Fig. 3.12 (**a**, **b**) Technically adequate bilateral mediolateral (ML) views

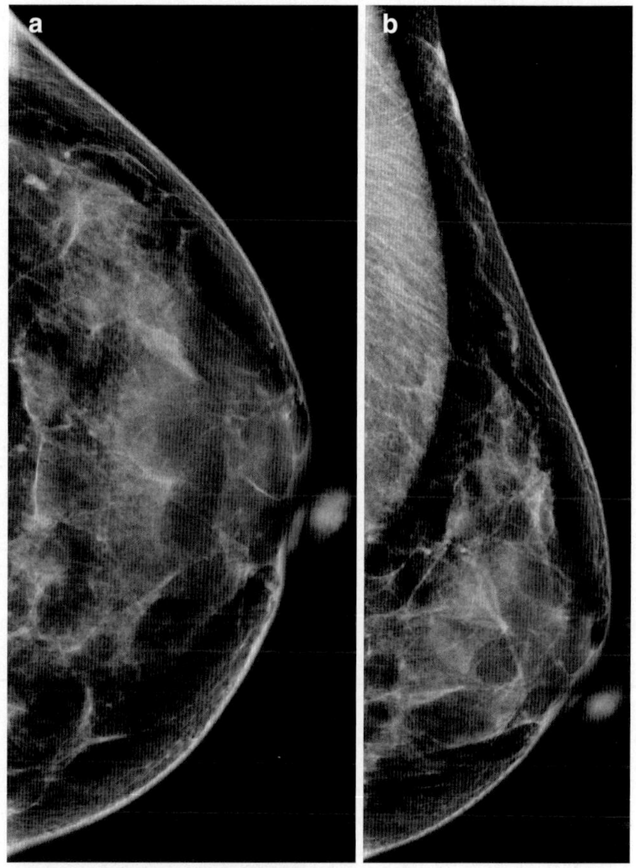

Fig. 3.13 (**a**, **b**) Example of exaggerated craniocaudal view laterally (XCCL). Note the increased amount of lateral breast tissues imaged on the XCCL view (**b**) compared to the CC view (**a**)

is located in the upper aspect of the breast. If the lesion moves in the opposite direction as the breast is being rolled in (moves laterally in the rolled medial view or medially in the rolled lateral view), then the lesion is located in the lower aspect of the breast. This process assists in further evaluation of the area of interest by focused breast ultrasound as it identifies the quadrant of the breast in which the lesion is expected to be found.

Several other parallax techniques can be employed to determine the expected location of a lesion of interest seen only on one view on additional views, such as the nipple-arc

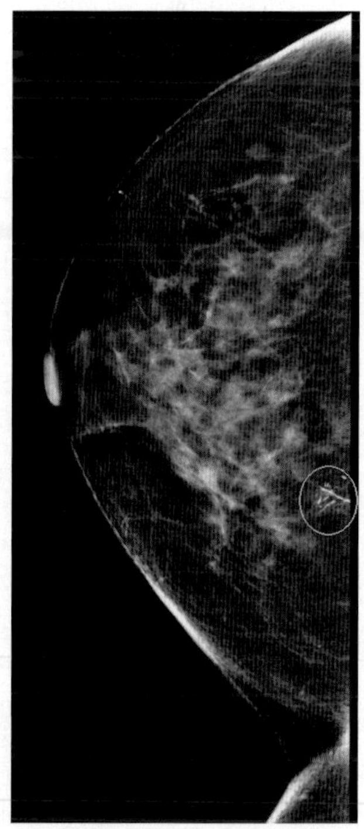

Fig. 3.14 Example of exaggerated craniocaudal view medially (XCCM). Note the increased amount of medial breast tissues imaged. In this example, the *circled* highly suspicious calcifica tions are biopsy-proven ductal carcinoma in situ (DCIS)

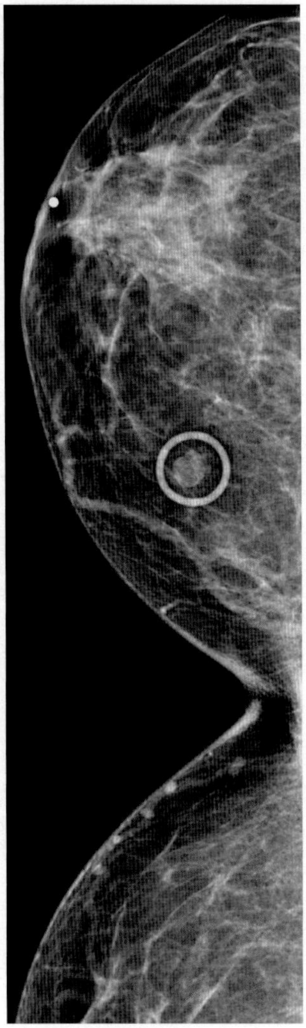

Fig. 3.15 Example of cleavage view. This is an alternate method to the XCCM view for imaging the most medial aspect of both breasts

method versus the parallel perpendicular parallel (P^3) method described next:

- Nipple-arc method: Martin [9] was the first to refer to a method for correlating an abnormality on one view with the corresponding abnormality on the complimentary view, known as the "nipple-arc method." The nipple-arc technique identifies the abnormality of the view and determines the length of the nipple as the reference point to the edge or epicenter of the abnormality. On the other view, where the location of the abnormality is not positively identified, one draws a line the same length, from the nipple reference point into the breast parenchyma in the form of an arc. The abnormality should be located on or near the arc line (Fig. 3.19).
- Parallel perpendicular parallel (P^3) method: Watson [10] first reported this method in 1995. For the P^3 method, one draws a line labeled "A" parallel to the posterior plane of the nipple on the view where the lesion is seen. A line labeled "B" is then drawn perpendicular to the nipple, i.e., "A" line, to the edge or epicenter of the visualized abnormality. On the other view where the abnormality is not positively identified, the same process is accomplished, assuring the "A" line is parallel to the back of the nipple and the perpendicular "B" line is the same length as the "B" line on the visualized lesion. Then one draws a line labeled "C" perpendicular to the "B" line and parallel to the "A" line through the breast tissue. The abnormality should be located on or near the "C" line (Fig. 3.20).

Identifying the dermal location of findings that project as intramammary lesions is a very important task. The use of skin markers (best known as "mole markers") cannot be stressed enough in order to avoid mistaking a true dermal lesion that is imaged on a mammogram as a true breast lesion. All skin lesions that are raised and therefore have an air/soft tissue interface, this confirms their true location at the time of imaging.

Dermal calcifications can also be identified by their classic morphology, as they can be lucent centered. When this classic morphology is absent, you can mark the calcifications with a BB marker while using an alphanumeric grid and subsequently obtain a tangential view to the skin to determine if they are dermal versus intraparenchymal in location (Figs. 3.22a–d and 3.23a–d). There are six steps in performing tangential views, which are outlined herewith:

1. Determine if the calcifications are in the superior versus inferior or medial versus lateral aspect of the breast.
2. Place the breast in an alphanumeric grid with the calcifications of interest visualized within the dimensions of the grid.
3. Identify the calcifications of interest and place the crosshairs so they intersect over the calcifications.
4. Place a BB marker on the skin where the crosshairs intersect.
5. Take the breast out of the alphanumeric grid and position the breast so the BB marker is tangential to the x-ray beam.
6. If the calcifications are dermal in location, they will be immediately under the BB marker on the image. If the calcifications are intraparenchymal, they will be deep in the tissue and not immediately under the BB marker.

Tangential views are also useful to determine if a mass seen on the routine views is dermal/subdermal or parenchymal. If the mass is palpable, then a BB can be placed over the mass, and the BB marker is placed in a tangential view to the x-ray beam. If dermal or subdermal in location, the mass will be noted immediately under the BB marker.

Mammographic Evaluation After Breast Augmentation

Breast Implants

Breast implants obscure and displace a significant amount of the breast tissue, therefore limiting evaluation for breast cancer screening. The Mammography Quality Standards Act (MQSA) recommends four mammographic views of each

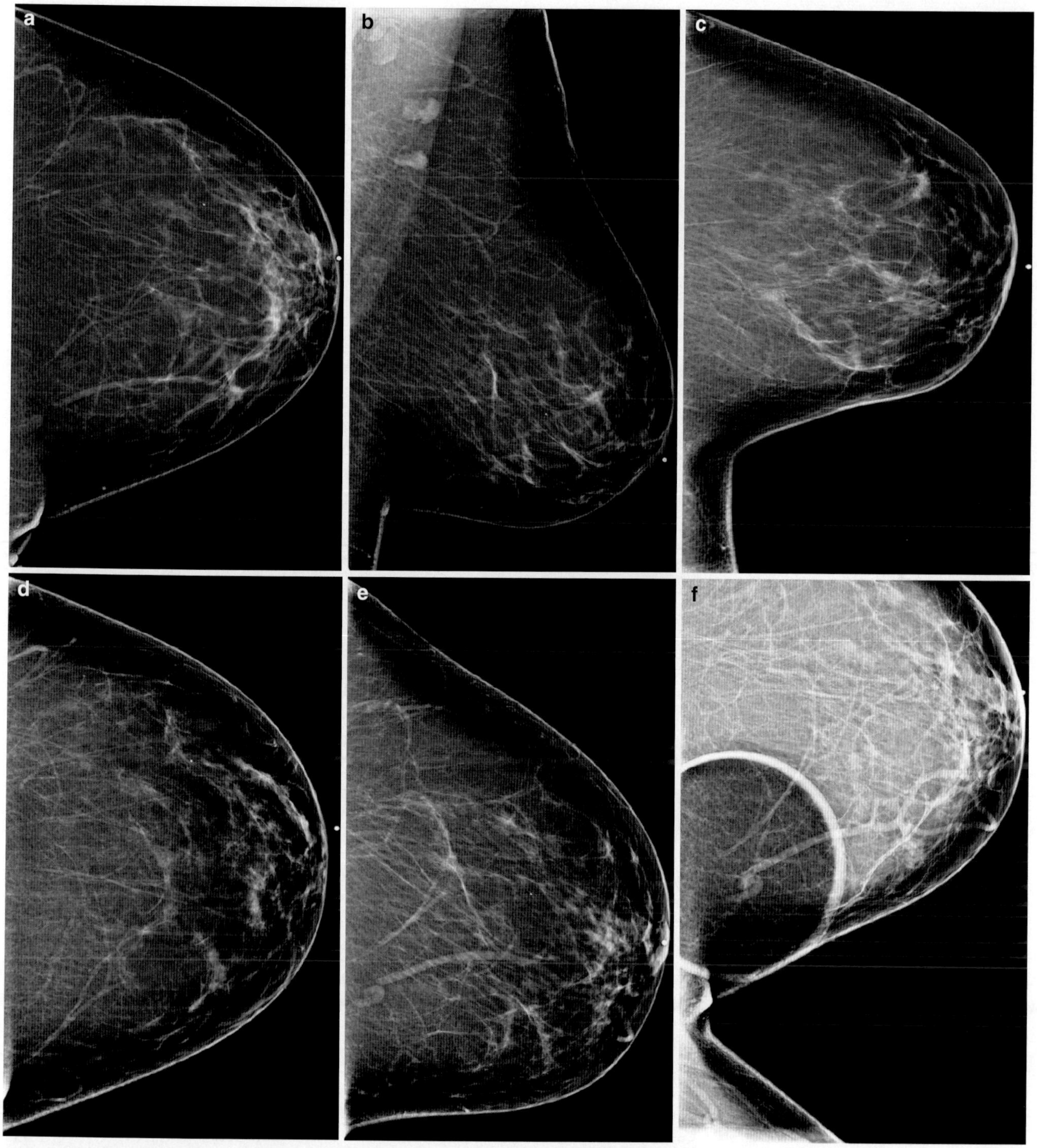

Fig. 3.16 (**a**–**f**) Use of rolled views to differentiate between a "pseudomass" from overlapping tissue (**a**) and a real mass that is not visualized on the MLO (**b**) or lateral (**c**) view. In this example, the finding is secondary to a "pseudomass" from overlapping tissue (**a**). The process of rolling the breast medially (**d**) and laterally (**e**) separates the overlapping tissue and the mass disappears. Spot compression view (**f**) was added to the rolled views to further evaluate the questionable finding

breast in this situation. Two views are included, where the breast implant is left in place (Fig. 3.24a) so that its integrity can be evaluated. These views are performed using limited compression to avoid the possibility of implant rupture. Two additional views are performed excluding as much of the breast implant as possible (also known as implant displaced views) in order to adequately visualize the surrounding breast tissues (Fig. 3.24b). These views are performed with normal compression. Additional views can be performed (e.g., lateral, magnification, or spot views) if deemed

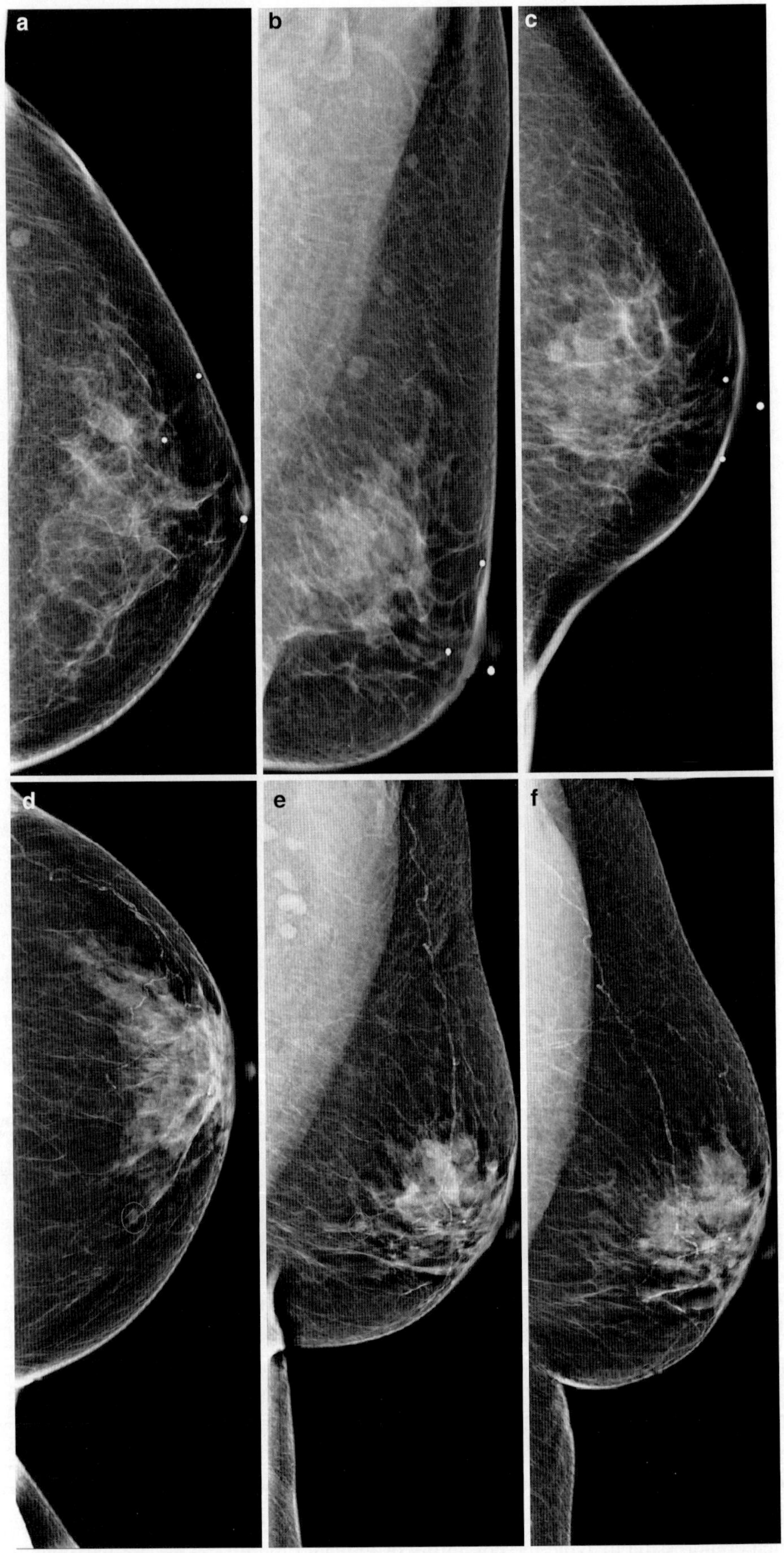

Fig. 3.17 (**a–c**) Triangulation techniques. To determine the location of a lesion seen in only one view, the CC (**a**), MLO (**b**), and true lateral (**c**) (either mediolateral or lateromedial) views should be placed with the nipples at the same level, and the MLO view is put in the middle. If the lesion "falls" closer to or below the nipple on the ML or LM view as compared to the MLO view, the lesion is located in the lateral aspect of the breast ("lead falls" = lateral location). (**d–f**) Triangulation techniques. To determine the location of a lesion seen in only one view, the CC (**d**), MLO (**e**), and true lateral (**f**) (either mediolateral or lateromedial) views should be placed with the nipples at the same level, and the MLO view is put in the middle. If the lesion "rises" closer to or below the nipple on the ML or LM view as compared to the MLO view, the lesion is located in the medial aspect of the breast ("muffins rise" = medial location)

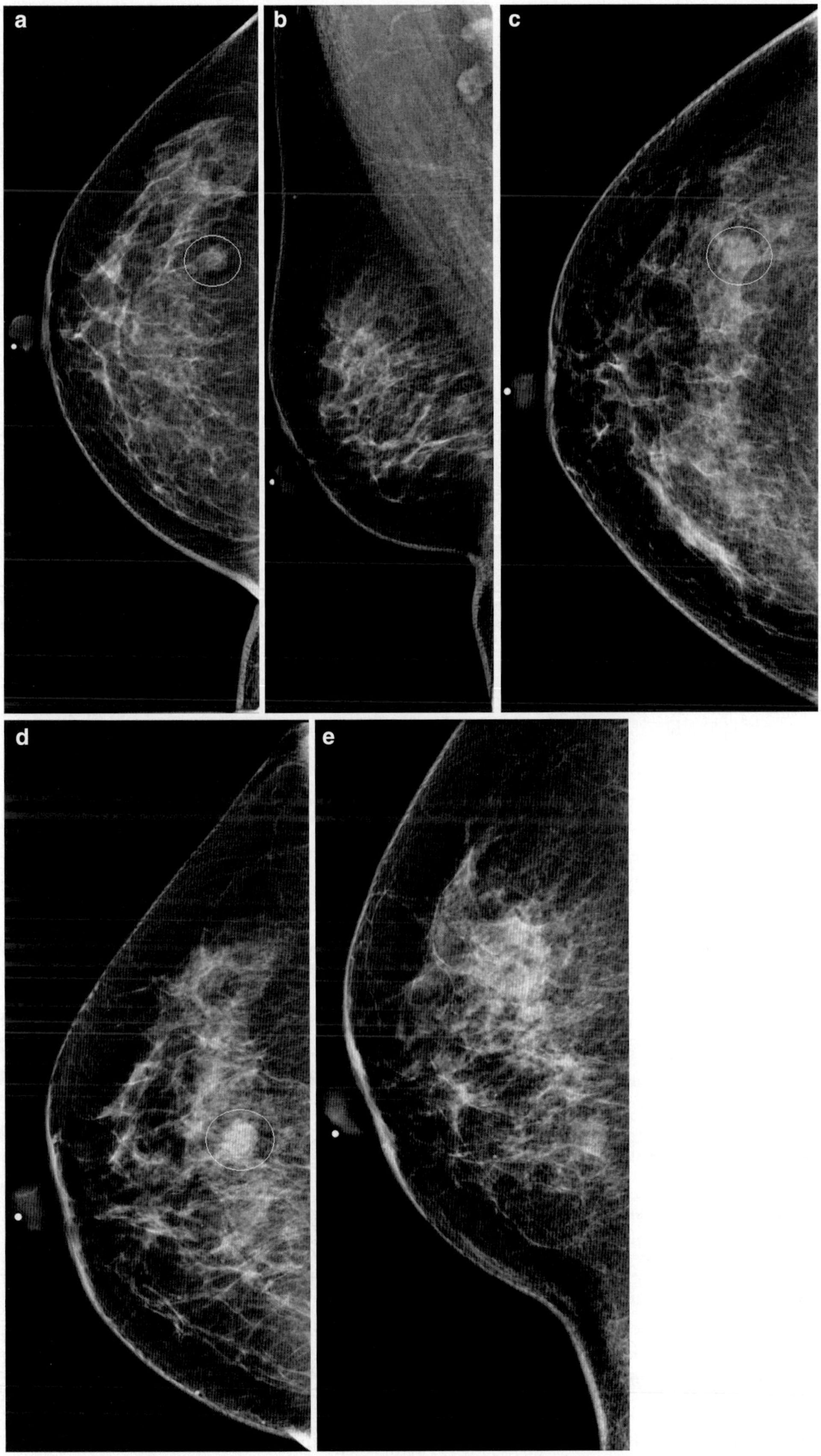

Fig. 3.18 (**a**–**e**) Localization techniques. To determine the location of a lesion seen only on the CC view (**a**, **b**), the breast can be rolled in both medial (**c**) and lateral (**d**) directions to determine the location of this lesion with regard to the upper versus the lower aspect of the breast (**e**). If the lesion moves in the same direction as the breast is being rolled in (moves laterally in the rolled lateral view or medially in the rolled medial view), then the lesion is located in the upper aspect of the breast. If the lesion moves in the opposite direction as the breast is being rolled in (moves laterally in the rolled medial view or medially in the rolled lateral view), then the lesion is located in the lower aspect of the breast. In this case, the lesion is located to the lower aspect of the breast

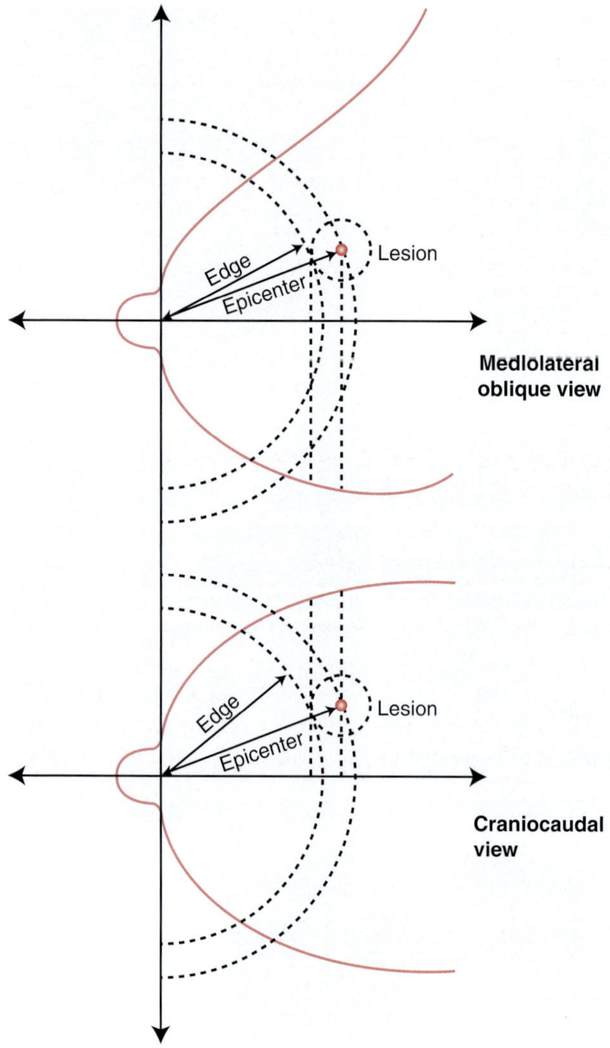

Fig. 3.19 Parallax techniques: Nipple-arc method

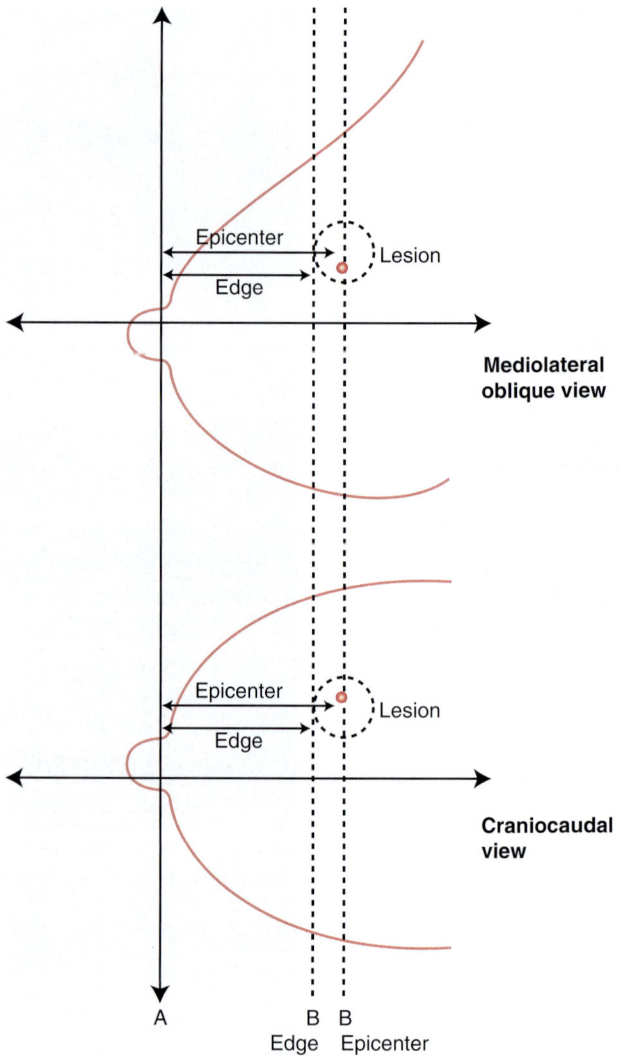

Fig. 3.20 Parallax techniques: Parallel perpendicular parallel (P^3) method

necessary. More detailed information regarding the different types and locations of breast implants will be discussed in another chapter.

Silicone Injections

Direct silicone or paraffin injections result in granulomas (round eggshell calcifications) that obscure the underlying breast parenchyma and therefore limiting evaluation for breast cancer detection (Fig. 3.25).

Mammography Artifacts

Artifacts are defined as any density difference in an image that is not the result of a true attenuation difference. These can have several sources or causes along the imaging chain. Artifacts can be related to the cleanliness as well as image processing (including chemical residues roller marks among others). Artifacts can also be equipment related (e.g., the presence of grid lines and inadequate selection, alignment or use of the compression devices). Finally, artifacts can be patient related (such as motion, projection of objects or structures located outside the breast on the images obtained, deodorant, and hair, among others). Some of these artifacts are discussed in this section.

Motion

Adequate compression prevents motion unsharpness. This is most commonly seen on the mediolateral (MLO) view than on the craniocaudal (CC) view, as the breast is supported by the imaging receptor on the CC view (Fig. 3.26a, b). The blurred appearance of calcifications and skin/nipple markers aids in noticing the unsharpness.

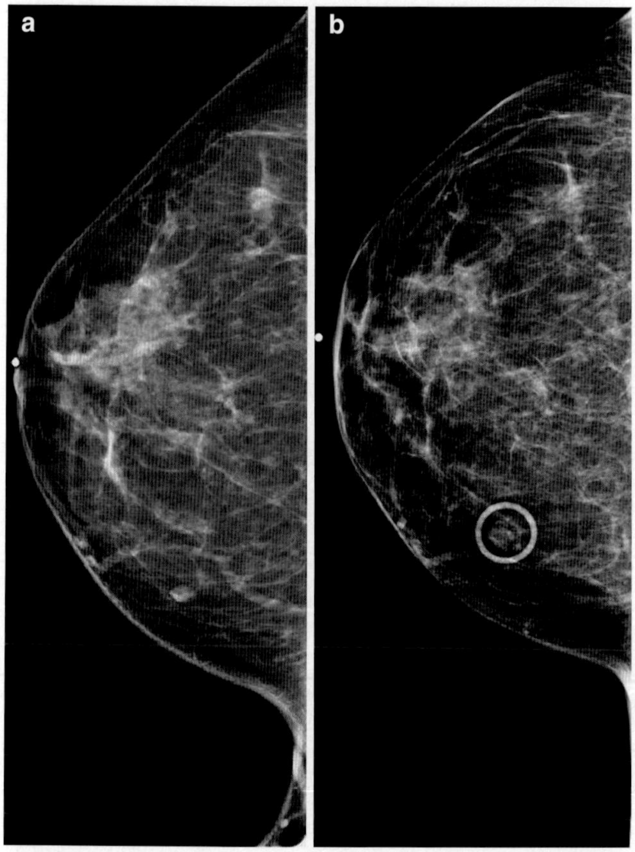

Fig. 3.21 (**a**, **b**) Dermal location of finding that projects as an intramammary lesion (**a**). The use of skin markers (commonly known as "mole markers") helps to avoid mistaking a true dermal lesion that is imaged on a mammogram as a true breast lesion (**b**)

Grid Lines

When utilizing a moving grid, the grid lines should not be visible on the images obtained. When they are, the drive mechanism for the moving grid needs to be repaired or replaced (Fig. 3.27a, b).

Deodorant/Antiperspirant

Radiopaque materials on the skin such as deodorant and antiperspirant may simulate breast calcifications. The location of these radiopacities over the axilla is characteristic and suggests this artifact (Fig. 3.28a, b). These should disappear on repeat images performed after the axilla has been washed.

Hair Artifact

This artifact consists of thin, strand-like opacities that are usually located close to the chest wall, particularly in patients with long hair that overlaps into the field of view (Fig. 3.29a). This artifact disappears when the patient's hair is pulled away on a repeat image (Fig. 3.29b).

Other Artifacts

Structures such as the chin or the knuckles can overlap the field of view (Fig. 3.30a, b). The chin can be seen overlying the axillary regions on the mediolateral oblique (MLO) view or the medial breast on the craniocaudal (CC) view.

Quality Assurance (QA) and Quality Control (QC)

After October 1, 1994, a certificate issued by the Food and Drugs Administration (FDA) is mandatory for lawful operation of all facilities under the regulatory jurisdiction of the United States that provide mammography services (except for the Department of Veteran Affairs). In order to obtain this mandatory certification, these facilities are required to meet the quality standards as designated by this agency as well as accreditation by an approved accreditation body or another entity as designated by the FDA. More details regarding the application as well as the reinstatement policy for this certification can be found on the web under the FDA web page dedicated to the discussion of the Mammography Quality and Standards Act (MQSA) regulations [6].

Quality Standards

Requirements have been established for all personnel involved in any facet of mammography (such as production, processing, and interpretation of mammograms as well as the associated quality assurance (QA) activities). Excerpts of Section 900.12 of the Mammography Quality Standards Act (MQSA) regulations applicable to interpreting physicians, radiology technologists, and medical physicists are included next [6]. The requirements for initial qualifications for interpreting physicians may be changed or modified with the upcoming changes in the initial certification process by the American Board of Radiology (ABR).

Interpreting Physicians

1. Initial qualifications
   (a) Licensed to practice medicine in a state.
   (b) Certified by a body determined by the FDA in an appropriate specialty area in order to ensure that they are competent to interpret radiological procedures, including mammography.

Fig. 3.22 (**a–d**) Use of an alphanumeric grid with a BB marker (**b**, **c**) and subsequent tangential view (**d**) to the skin to determine if calcifications are dermal versus intraparenchymal in location. In the illustrated case, the calcifications are located in the skin

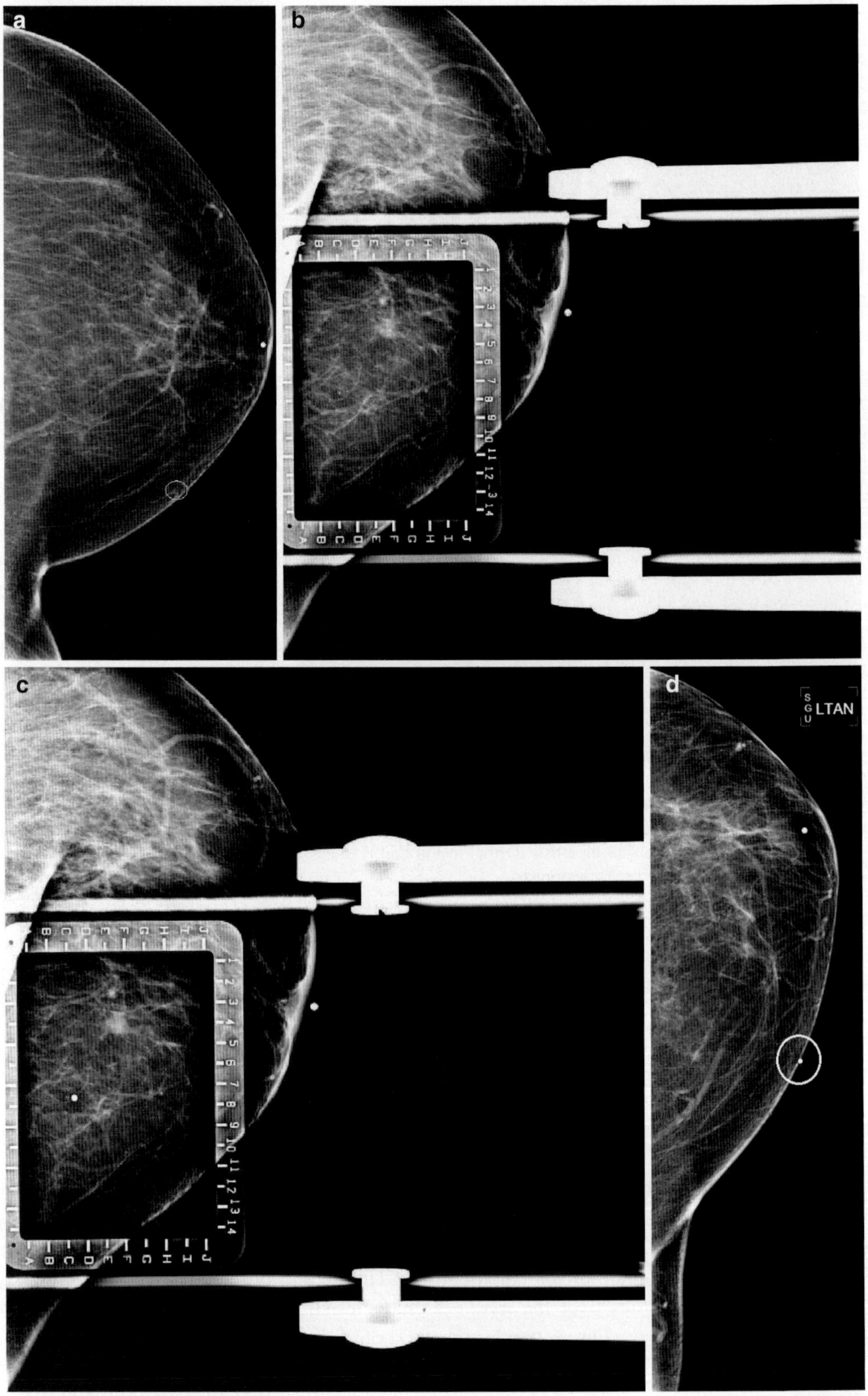

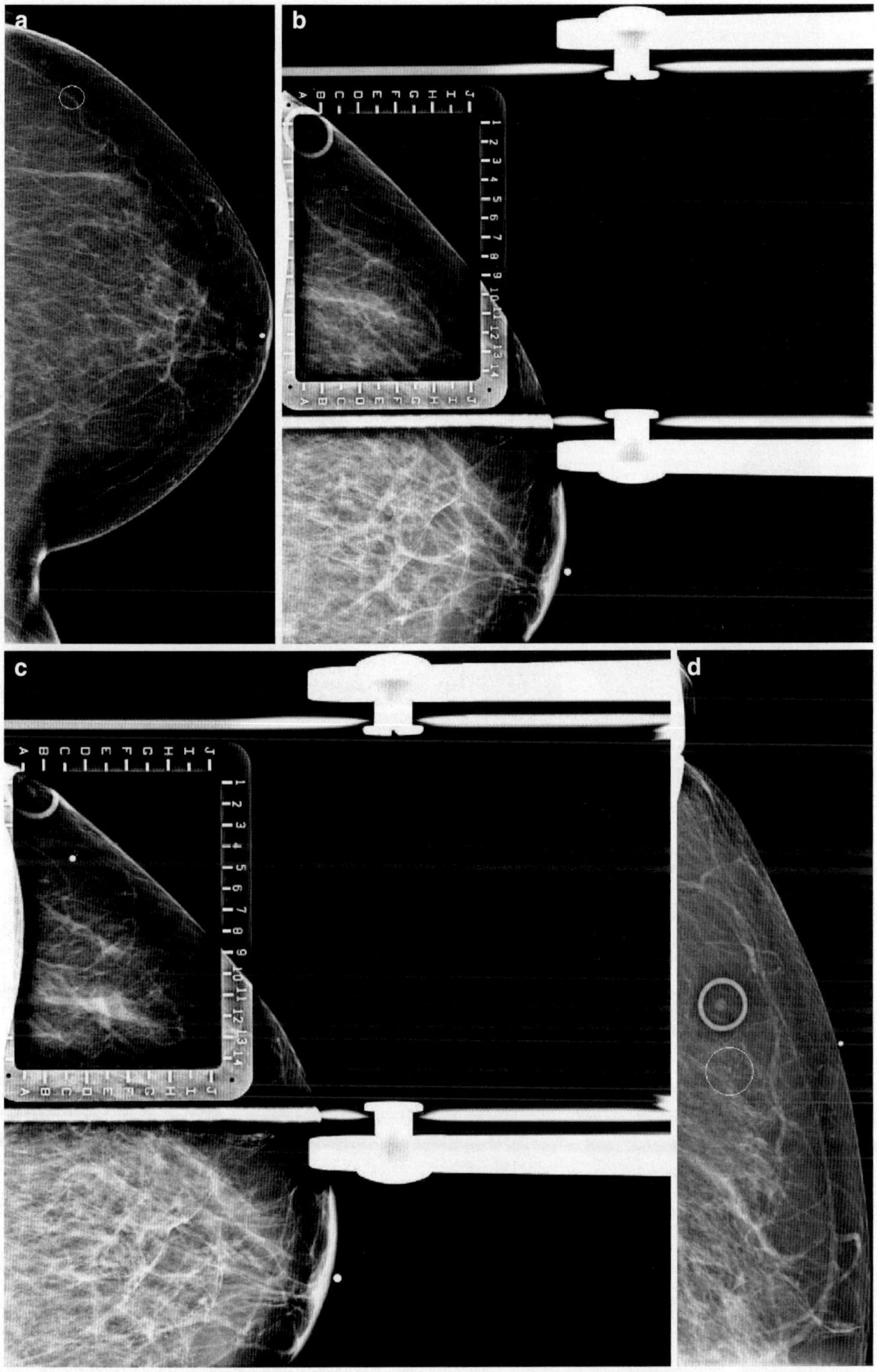

Fig. 3.23 (**a**–**d**) Use of an alphanumeric grid with a BB marker (**b**, **c**) and subsequent tangential view (**d**) to the skin to determine if calcifications are dermal versus intraparenchymal in location. In the illustrated case, the calcifications are intraparenchymal in location

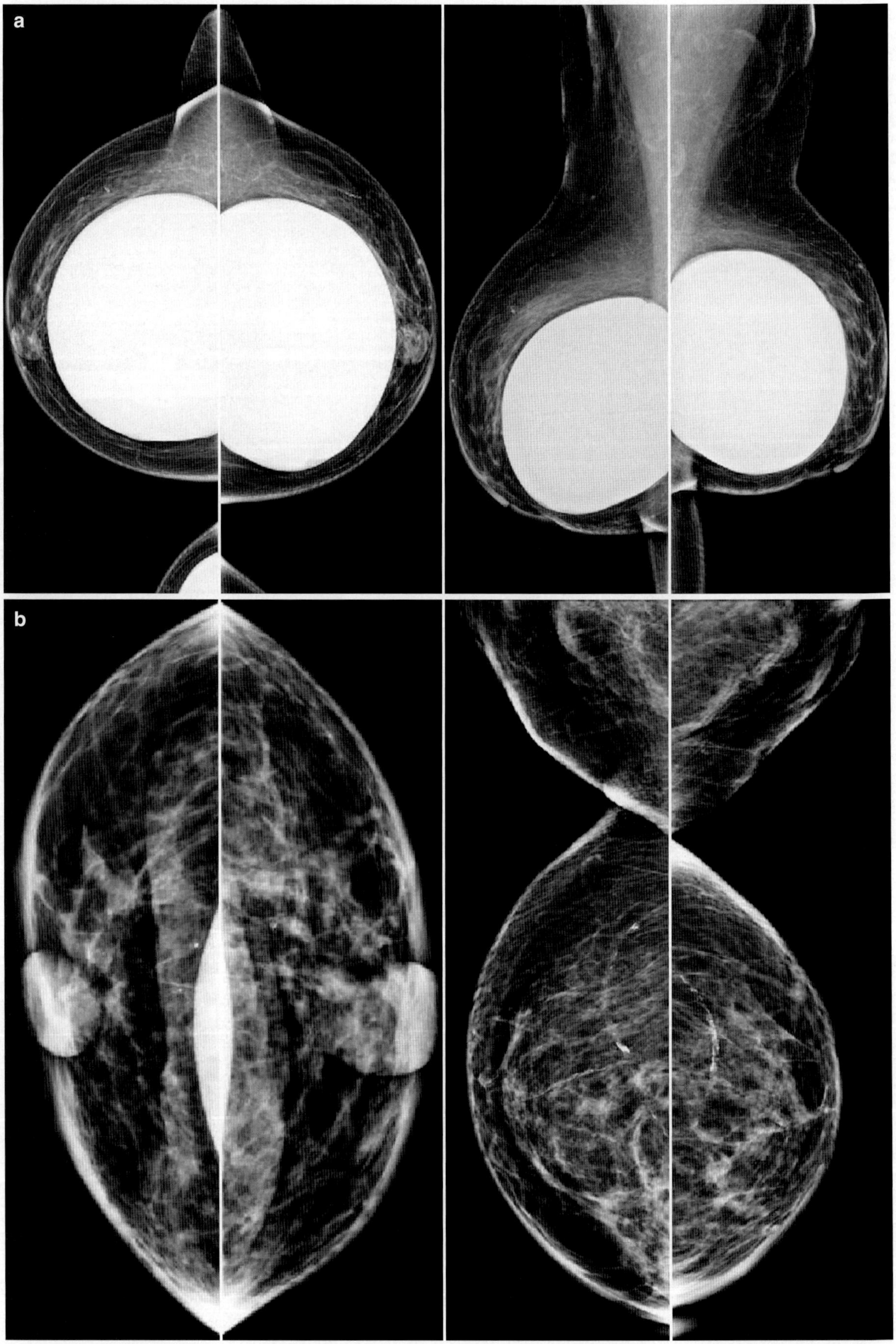

Fig. 3.24 (**a**, **b**) Mammographic evaluation with breast implants. Four views of each breast are acquired. Two views are obtained where the breast implant is left in place, and its integrity can be evaluated (**a**). Two additional views are performed excluding as much of the breast implant as possible (also known as implant displaced views) in order to adequately visualize the surrounding breast tissues (**b**)

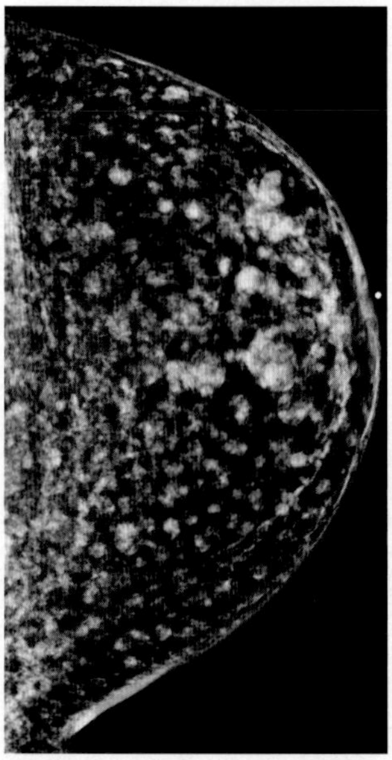

Fig. 3.25 Left CC view with multiple silicone granulomas in a patient status post breast augmentation. Note that the granulomas obscure the underlying breast parenchyma and therefore limiting evaluation for breast cancer detection

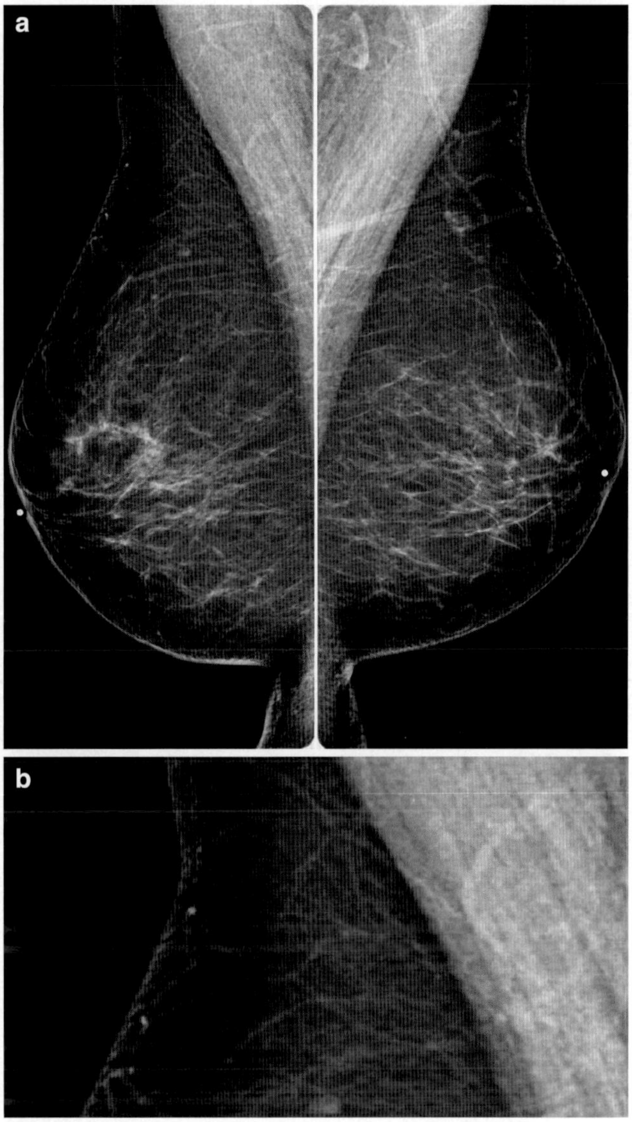

Fig. 3.27 (**a**, **b**) Example of grid lines visible on the right MLO view (**a**). Left MLO view is normal and provided for comparison. Closeup image of the right MLO view (**b**) shows grid lines in more detail

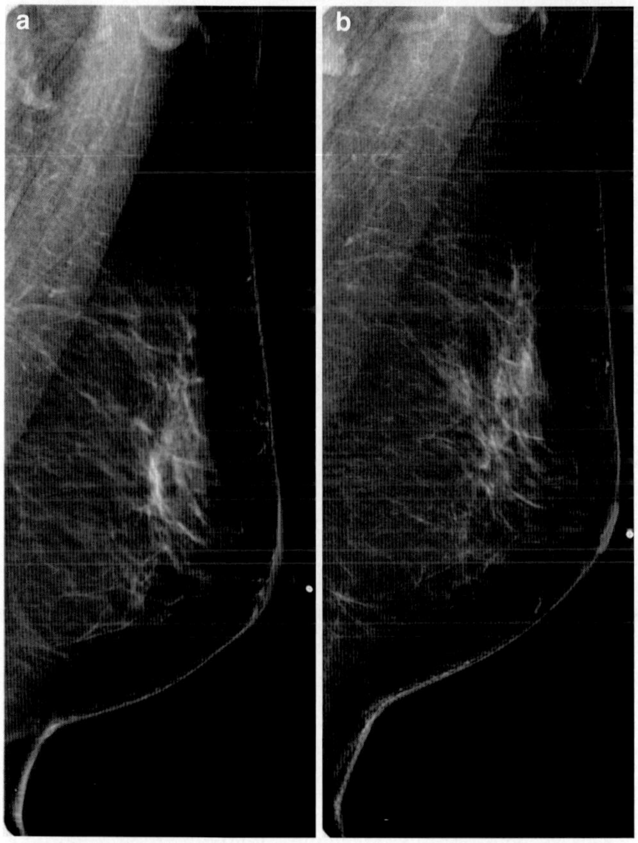

Fig. 3.26 Example of motion unsharpness on a left MLO view (**a**). Note the blurred appearance of the nipple marker. Repeat imaging (**b**) does not exhibit motion unsharpness

(i) Have had at least 3 months of documented formal training in the interpretation of mammograms and topics related to mammography (including radiation physics, radiation effects, and radiation protection specific to mammography). The component of mammographic interpretation will be performed under the direct supervision of a physician meeting the requirements specified previously.

(c) Minimum of 60 hours of documented medical education in mammography, including the following: instruction in the interpretation of mammograms and education in basic breast anatomy, pathology, physiology, technical aspects of mammography, and quality assurance and quality control in mammography.

(i) All of these hours shall be category I, and at least 15 of the category I hours must have been acquired within the 3 years immediately prior to the date that the physician qualifies as an interpreting physician.

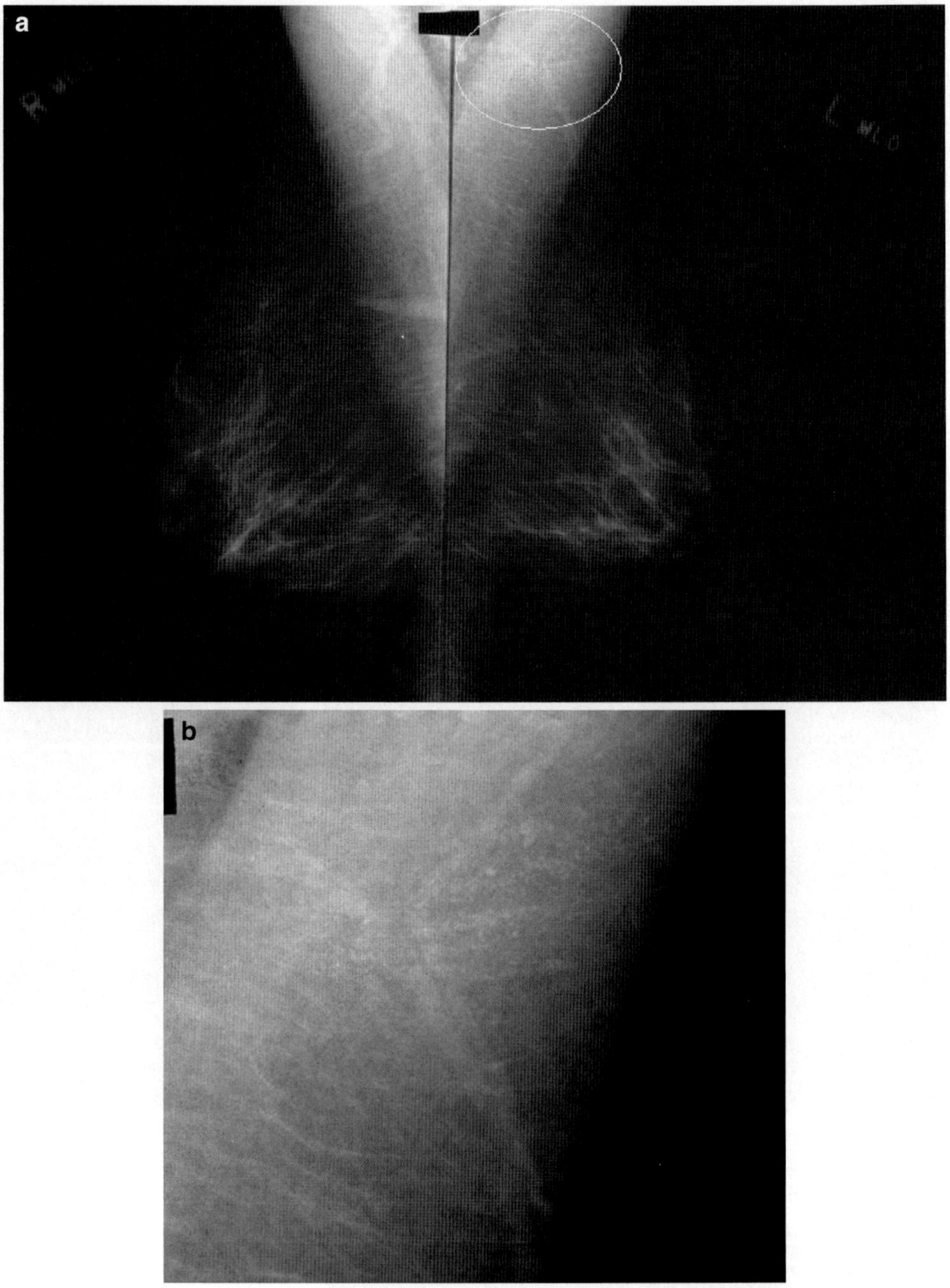

Fig. 3.28 (**a**, **b**) Example of deodorant/antiperspirant artifact simulating breast calcifications on a right MLO view (*circled* on **a**) and closeup view (**b**). These radiopacities should disappear on repeat images performed after the axilla has been washed

(ii) Hours spent in residency specifically devoted to mammography will be considered as equivalent to category I continuing medical education credits and will be accepted with written documentation by the appropriate representative of the training institution.

(iii) Unless the exemptions indicated in Section 900.12 of the original document apply, the interpreting physicians must have interpreted or multi-read at least 240 mammographic examinations within the 6-month period immediately prior to the date that the physician qualifies as an interpreting physician. This has to be performed under the direct supervision of an interpreting physician.

2. Continuing experience and education:

   All interpreting physicians maintain their qualifications by meeting the requirements as stipulated on the Mammography Quality and Standards Act (MQSA) regulations original document [6].

3. Exemptions

   (a) Physicians qualified as interpreting physicians prior to April 28, 1999, are considered to have met the initial requirements as detailed previously. They may continue to interpret mammograms provided they

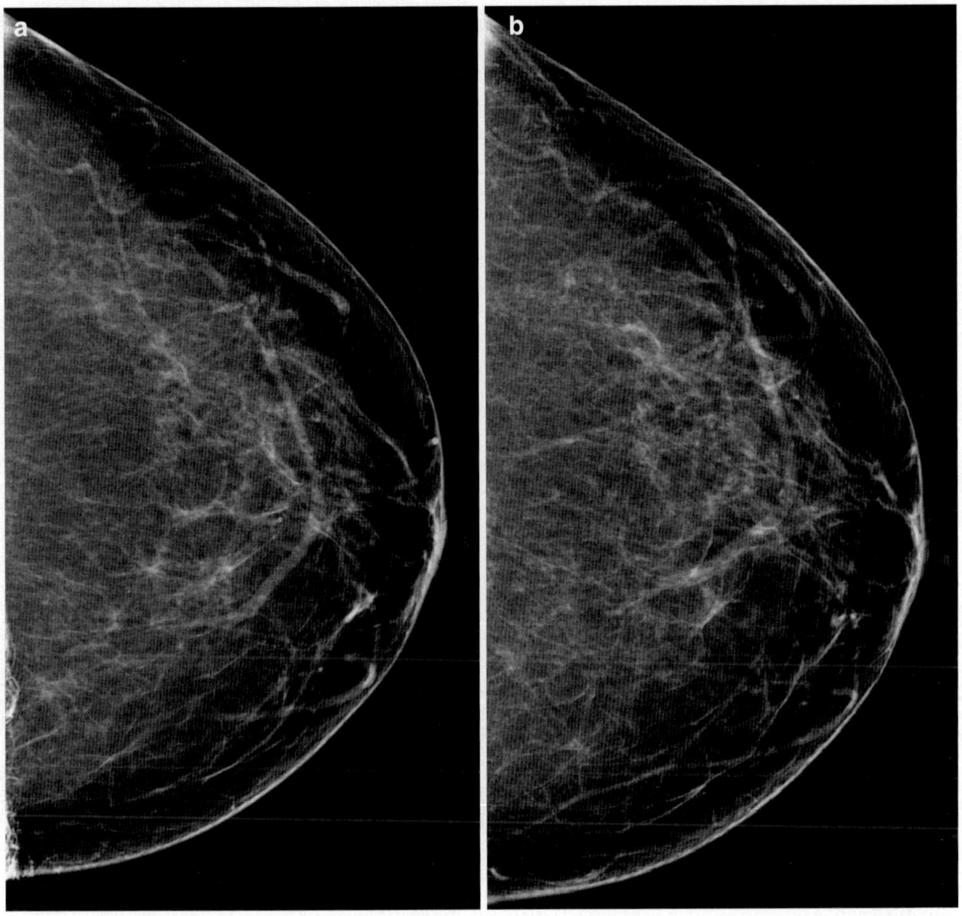

Fig. 3.29 (**a**, **b**) Example of hair artifact. Thin, strand-like opacities located close to the chest wall in this patient with long hair that overlaps into the field of view (**a**). This artifact disappears when the patient's hair is pulled away on a repeat image (**b**)

continue to meet the licensure requirements as established in this section.

(b) Physicians who have interpreted or multi-read at least 240 mammographic examinations under the direct supervision of an interpreting physician in any 6-month period during the last 2 years of a diagnostic radiology residency and who become appropriately board certified at the first allowable time, as defined by an eligible certifying body.

Radiology Technologists

1. General requirements
   (a) Licensed to perform general radiographic procedures in a state.
   (b) General certification from one of the bodies determined by FDA to have procedures and requirements adequate to ensure that technologists certified by the body are competent to perform radiologic examinations.
2. Mammography requirements:
   Have prior to April 28, 1999, qualified as a radiologic technologist under the requirements delineated in this section or completed at least 40 contact hours of documented training specific to mammography under the supervision of a qualified instructor. These hours will include, but are not necessarily limited to:
   (a) Training in breast anatomy and physiology, positioning and compression, quality assurance/quality control techniques, and imaging of patients with breast implants.
   (b) Performance of a minimum of 25 examinations under the direct supervision of an individual qualified under the requirements established by this section.
   (c) At least 8 h of training in each mammography modality to be used by the technologist in performing mammography exams.
3. Continuing education and continuing experience requirements: All radiology technologists maintain their qualifications by meeting the requirements as stipulated on the Mammography Quality and Standards Act (MQSA) regulations original document [6].

Medical Physicists

Applicable to all medical physicists conducting surveys of mammography facilities and providing oversight of the facility quality assurance programs:

1. Initial qualifications
   (a) State licensure or approval/certification in an appropriate specialty area by one of the bodies determined by

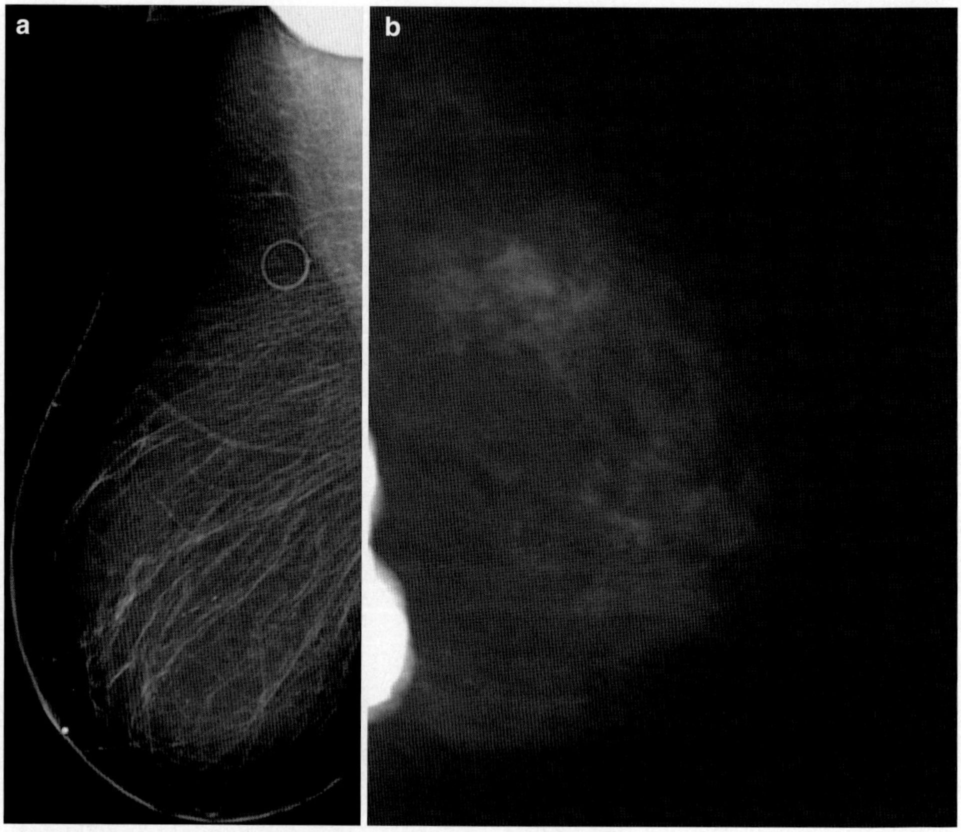

Fig. 3.30 (**a**, **b**) Examples of chin and knuckle artifacts. Structures such as the chin (**a**) or the knuckles (**b**) can overlap the field of view on the mammographic images

the FDA to have procedures and requirements to ensure that they are competent to perform physics survey.

(i) Have a masters degree or higher in a physical science from an accredited institution, with no less than 20 semester hours or equivalent [e.g., 30 quarter hours] of college undergraduate- or graduate-level physics.

(ii) Have 20 contact hours of documented specialized training in conducting surveys of mammography facilities.

(iii) Have the experience of conducting surveys of at least one mammography facility and a total of at least ten mammography units. No more than one survey of a specific unit within a period of 60 days can be counted toward the total mammography unit survey requirement. After April 38, 1999, experience conducting surveys must be acquired under the direct supervision of a medical physicist who meets all the requirements established in this section.

2. Alternative initial qualifications

(a) Have qualified as a medical physicist under the interim regulations specified in this section and retained that qualification by maintenance of the active status of any licensure, approval, or certification required under the interim regulations.

(b) Prior to April 28, 1999, have:

(i) A bachelor's degree or higher in a physical science form an accredited institution with no less than 10 semester hours or equivalent of college undergraduate- or graduate-level physics.

(ii) Forty contact hours of documented specialized training in conducting surveys of mammography facilities.

(iii) Have the experience of conducting surveys of at least one mammography facility and a total of at least 20 mammography units. No more than one survey of a specific unit within a period of 60 days can be counted toward the total mammography unit survey requirement. The training and experience requirements must be met after fulfilling the degree requirement.

3. Continuing qualifications: All medical physicists maintain their qualifications by meeting the requirements as stipulated on the Mammography Quality and Standards Act (MQSA) regulations original document [6].

Additional regulations and requirements regarding equipment, medical records and mammography reports, and the quality assurance programs are detailed under Section 900.12 of the MQSA Regulations original document [6].

Quality Assurance (QA) Program

Each facility has to establish and maintain a quality assurance program in order to ensure the safety, reliability, clarity, and accuracy of all of the mammography services performed. All of the mammography imaging facilities must designate a person in charge of establishing, implementing, administering, and documenting the quality assurance (QA) program. His or her responsibility includes establishing a quality assurance (QA)/quality control (QC) committee consisting of the radiologist, technologist, radiation safety officer (RSO), and medical physicist. The goal of this committee is to institute guidelines and testing mechanisms in order to comply with both the state and federal requirements established.

Part of the responsibilities of the lead interpreting physician, quality control technologist, and medical physicist is to ensure that the records concerning mammography technique and procedures, quality control (including monitoring data, problems detected as a result of data analysis, remedial actions, and the effectiveness of these actions), safety, protection, and employee qualifications to meet assigned quality assurance tasks are properly maintained and updated. These quality control records shall be kept for each test specified in this section until the next annual inspection is completed and the FDA has determined that the facility is in compliance with the quality assurance requirements or until the test has been performed two additional times at the required frequency, whichever is longer.

Quality Control (QC) Tests (Tables 3.1 and 3.2)

In order to perform high-quality imaging, a skilled, committed team is needed as the work is never done. The quality control (QC) tests for the QC mammography technologist and the medical physicist go hand in hand with the everyday work that the interpreting radiologist(s) does to achieve this goal. The scheduling of the QC tests should be based on the minimum frequencies mandated by the

Table 3.1 Technologist tests

Test	Minimum frequency
Daily checklist	Daily
Laser printer density consistency	Daily (wet)/monthly (dry)
Phantom image quality	Weekly
Display monitor QC	Weekly
Viewboxes/monitors and viewing conditions	Weekly
Full-field artifacts	Monthly
Monthly checklist	Monthly
Laser printer artifacts	Monthly
Resolution/modulation transfer function (MTF)	Quarterly
Repeat analysis	Quarterly
Printed image quality	Quarterly
Analysis of fixer retention	Quarterly
Compression force	Semiannually

Table 3.2 Medical physicist tests

Test	Minimum frequency
Mammographic unit assembly evaluation	Mammography equipment evaluation + annually
Phantom image quality	Mammography equipment evaluation + annually
Missed tissue	Mammography equipment evaluation + annually
Technique chart/AEC evaluation (SDNR)	Mammography equipment evaluation + annually
Viewboxes/monitors and viewing conditions	Mammography equipment evaluation + annually
Artifact evaluation	Mammography equipment evaluation + annually
kVp accuracy	Mammography equipment evaluation
Beam quality assessment (half-value layer)	Mammography equipment evaluation + annually
Breast entrance exposure and average glandular dose (AGD)	Mammography equipment evaluation + annually
Ghost image evaluation	Mammography equipment evaluation + annually
Collimation assessment	Mammography equipment evaluation + annually
Resolution/modulation transfer function (MTF)	Mammography equipment evaluation + annually
Noise	Mammography equipment evaluation + annually
Spatial linearity and geometric distortion of the detector	All – mammography equipment evaluation All with moving parts (slot scan and CR) – mammography equipment evaluation + annually
Monitor display, quality and baseline values (all soft copy)	Mammography equipment evaluation + annually
Monitor luminance, response, and viewing conditions (all soft copy)	Mammography equipment evaluation + annually
Viewbox luminance and room illuminance (if screen-film comparison films viewed/printed images interpreted)	Mammography equipment evaluation + annually
Laser printer evaluation and baseline values	Mammography equipment evaluation + annually
Evaluation of site tech QC	Annually

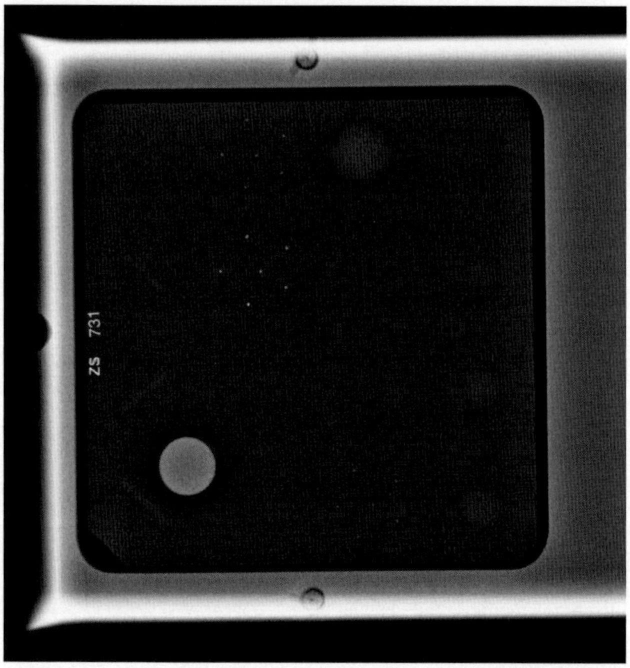

Fig. 3.31 Phantom image. Score phantom image contains six fibers, five speck groups, and five masses. For the minimum score, at least the four largest fibers, the three largest speck groups, and the three largest masses are visible

American College of Radiology (ACR) as part of their accreditation program. The objectives of the QC tests are to ensure that all the required equipment is functioning as it is needed so that the facility can meet all the performance criteria as indicated and if indicated, the appropriate corrective actions can be taken. A list of the quality control tests for screen-film mammography can be found next. More detailed information can be found in Section 900.12 of the Mammography Quality Standards Act (MQSA) Regulations [6].

A listing of quality control tests for screen-film mammography [6] follows:

1. Daily – Film processor performance test
   (a) Base plus fog density
   (b) Mid-density
   (c) Density difference
2. Weekly – Image quality evaluation test using an FDA-approved phantom (minimum frequency)
   (i) Background optical density
   (ii) Optical density difference from the established operating level
      1. Score phantom image contains six fibers, five speck groups, and five masses.
      2. Minimum score: At least the four largest fibers, the three largest speck groups, and the three largest masses are visible (Fig. 3.31).
3. Quarterly
   (a) Fixer retention in film
   (b) Repeat analysis
4. Semiannual
   (a) Darkroom fog
   (b) Screen-film contact
   (c) Compression device performance
5. Annual
   (a) Automatic exposure control (AEC) performance
   (b) Kilovoltage peak (kVp) accuracy and reproducibility
   (c) Focal spot condition
      (i) System resolution
      (ii) Focal spot dimensions
      (iii) Beam quality and half-value layer (HVL)
      (iv) Breast entrance air kerma and AEC reproducibility
      (v) Dosimetry
      (vi) X-ray field/light field/image receptor/compression paddle alignment
      (vii) Uniformity of screen speed
      (viii) System artifacts
      (ix) Radiation output
      (x) Decompression

Quality Control (QC) for Full-Field Digital Mammography Units

Full-field digital mammography (FFDM) differs from screen-film mammography in various ways, and the quality control tests are no exception. The FDA mandates that the facility's QC technologist and medical physicist abide by the quality control tests stipulated by the unit manufacturer. Not only some of the quality control tests may differ between the various units but also the frequencies and performance criteria specified by the different manufacturers. Therefore, the FDA mandate is for the facilities with full-field digital mammography units to follow the requirements stipulated by the manufacturer's quality assurance program. The American College of Radiology recommendations for FFDM quality control include the following tests, described in more detail in the Food and Drugs Administration (FDA) website dedicated to this topic [11].

Quality Control (QC) Tests: Other Modalities

For systems with image receptor modalities other than screen film, the quality assurance (QA) program is to a large extent similar to the program recommended by the image receptor manufacturer, except that the maximum allowable dose should not exceed the maximum allowable dose for screen-film systems outlined in this section.

Mobile Units

It is the main facility's responsibility to verify that the mobile mammography units meet the requirements outlined in this section. At each location, the main facility has the obligation to verify satisfactory performance of these units before any exams are performed.

References

1. Society AC. Cancer facts and figures 2012 Atlanta. 2012 [cited 22 Jan 2013]. Available from: http://www.cancer.org/acs/groups/content/@epidemiologysurveilance/documents/document/acspc-031941.pdf.
2. Society AC. Breast cancer facts and figures 2011–2012 Atlanta. 2012 [cited 22 Jan, 2013]. Available from: http://www.cancer.org/Research/CancerFactsFigures/BreastCancerFactsFigures/ACSPC-030975.
3. Howlader N, Noone A, Krapcho M, Neyman N, Aminou R, Altekruse SF, Kosary CL, Ruhl J, Tatalovich Z, Cho H, Mariotto A, Eisner MP, Lewis DR, Chen HS, Feuer EJ, Cronin KA, editors. SEER Cancer Statistics Review, 1975–2009. Bethesda. 2009 [cited 2012]. Available from: http://seer.cancer.gov/csr/1975_2009_pops09/.
4. Radiology ACO. American College of Radiology Mammography Accreditation Program requirements, Reston [updated 2 May 2012, cited 26 January 2013]. Available from: http://www.acr.org/~/media/ACR/Documents/Accreditation/Mammography/Requirements.pdf.
5. Sickles EA, Weber WN, Galvin HB, Ominsky SH, Sollitto RA. Baseline screening mammography: one vs two views per breast. AJR Am J Roentgenol. 1986;147(6):1149–53.
6. Administration USFaD. Mammography Quality Standards Act Regulations. Silver Spring [updated 4 Mar 2009; cited 8 June 2013]. Available from: http://www.fda.gov/Radiation-EmittingProducts/MammographyQualityStandardsActandProgram/Regulations/ucm110906.htm.
7. D'Orsi C, Berg WBL, et al. ACR breast imaging reporting and data system (BI-RADS atlas). 4th ed. Reston: American College of Radiology; 2003.
8. Kopans DB, Moore R, McCarthy KA, et al. Should women with implants or a history of treatment for breast cancer be excluded from mammography screening programs? AJR Am J Roentgenol. 1997;168:29–31.
9. Meyer JE. Atlas of mammography; histologic and mammographic correlation. Baltimore: Williams & Wilkins; 1982.
10. Watson AB, Lamki N, Michael E, Athey PA, Contant C. Geometric localization of breast lesions in two view mammography. Society of Breast Imaging 2nd Postgraduate Course; Orlando; 1995.
11. Radiology ACo. American College of Radiology Recommendations for full-field digital mammography quality control [updated 25 Sep 2006; cited 24 June 2013]. Available from: http://www.fda.gov/ohrms/dockets/ac/06/briefing/2006-4236b2-05-acr-table.pdf.

Digital Mammography and Digital Breast Tomosynthesis

4

Tony Martin Svahn

Introduction

In Western countries, about one in eight to ten women develops breast cancer during their lifetime [1]. Well-confirmed risk factors for breast cancer are reproductive factors (e.g., non-parity, late first birth, early menarche, and late menopause) [2], hormone replacement therapy (HRT) [2], genetic factors [3], ionizing radiation [4], and high breast density on mammography [5]. There is also evidence that lifestyle factors can increase the risk, such as high alcohol consumption [6] and low physical activity [7]. Mammography plays a central role in early detection, since it can show changes in the breast before the patient or a physician can feel them. Because of its clinical effectiveness, the technique has been used for detection of breast cancer for more than half a century [8], and since several decades also for screening of asymptomatic women. Screening mammography is one of the largest public health efforts to promote women's health, starting with pilot studies and proceeding with larger randomized controlled trials (RCTs) to determine the potential benefits [9–16]. In randomized controlled trials (RCTs), mammography screening was shown to reduce the breast cancer mortality by approximately 20–30 % [17, 18], which has led to today's population-based mammography screening programs. Screen-film mammography (SFM) has since long been the standard technique in breast cancer screening but advances in the digital detector technology and computers have paved the way for digital mammography (DM), and since the US Food and Drug Administration's (FDA) approval of the first commercial systems in the year 2000, two-dimensional (2D) DM became the accepted standard of care in breast cancer screening and diagnosis in North America as well as in Europe and in a majority of other developed countries. The use of DM has increased rapidly since it offers many advantages compared to SFM, such as higher image quality and/or lower radiation dose to the breast, omitting recalls due to technical failure, increased patient throughput, more efficient image management, and telemammography. However, despite the improvements, the mammographic accuracy has shown to be imperfect, and reader variability that may be influenced by various factors such as radiologist experience, case difficulty, and varying practices at different mammography centers has remained a great challenge. Sensitivities have been estimated from 68 % (as low as 48 % for very dense breasts) to 88 % at specificities from 82 to 98 %, suggesting that further improvements can be made [19, 20]. A major problem lies in the nature of the two-dimensional (2D) technique. Because a conventional mammogram is a 2D projection of the breast onto the detector plane, over-projected normal tissue (anatomical noise) can restrain the accuracy of mammography. In the clinical practice, cancer detection may be limited, particularly in younger women and in those with a high parenchymal density since the mammographic evidence of the tumor may be completely or partially concealed. Difficulty in characterizing breast lesions may be further emphasized, particularly in dense fibroglandular tissue, when they differ only marginally from normal glandular tissue or are diffusely infiltrating without forming a mass, such as lobular carcinoma. Conversely, overlying normal structures may produce an appearance in 2D mammography, which is suspicious for cancer, prompting false-positive recalls following routine screening. Hence, if the overlapping tissue effect is reduced, sensitivity as well as specificity could be improved. Digital breast tomosynthesis (DBT) is a three-dimensional (3D) imaging modality that resolves the tissue overlap by collecting 2D projection views over a limited angular range and permits image reconstruction of thin slices of the breast volume. In computed tomography (CT) hundreds of projection images are acquired covering 360° and subsequently the tissue overlap might be suppressed further but it is more

T.M. Svahn, PhD
Department of Clinical Sciences,
Skåne University Hospital, Malmö, Lund University,
Gustavlundsvägen 318, Helsingborg 25655, Sweden
e-mail: tony.svahn@med.lu.se

M.K. Shetty (ed.), *Breast Cancer Screening and Diagnosis: A Synopsis*,
DOI 10.1007/978-1-4939-1267-4_4, © Springer Science+Business Media New York 2015

difficult to image the entire breast volume, particularly close to the chest wall, and the spatial resolution has not been sufficiently high for adequate visualization of microcalcifications. Moreover, the average glandular dose has up to now been higher with CT, as have been imaging time and cost of the device. While there is ongoing research that has solved some of these issues [21–23], DBT has a number of potential advantages and there are commercialized FDA-approved units available [24]. DBT is increasingly being used as a diagnostic tool, though it is not yet considered the standard of care for breast cancer screening. Because it is relatively new, it is only available at a limited number of hospitals and research facilities. In order to appreciate the use and advantages of tomosynthesis, an understanding of mammography and its limitations is necessary. In this chapter, fundamental aspects of mammography are described, from the transition to the digital technology to the evolvement of tomosynthesis. Recent clinical tomosynthesis trials provide evidence of the effectiveness of tomosynthesis. A review of these and their results is summarized.

Fundamentals of Two-Dimensional Digital Mammography

Practical and Clinical Considerations

Digital mammography (DM) offers a range of benefits over traditional screen-film technology. Among the practical implications is the more reliable and efficient image management, which includes simplified archival, retrieval and transmission of images, higher throughput of patients, and possibilities for telemammography. Other advantages are related to image quality, for instance, the higher signal-to-noise ratio, detective quantum efficiency[1] (DQE), and contrast sensitivity.[2] In contrast to SFM where the image acquisition, storage, and display are all integrated in the film, these are decoupled in DM, which facilitates optimization of the components individually and adjustments in image characteristics (processing). This translates into more possibilities in improving image quality. The efficient use of incident X-rays in digital detector systems permits a considerable reduction of radiation dose to breast when compared to SFM. This is achieved with no excessive loss in spatial resolution and without sacrificing image quality [25]. The applied compression force to the breast does not differ substantially in between the systems [26]. However, the amount of compression force is important from a pain perspective as well as ensuring that optimal image quality is achieved so that small breast cancers will be visualized. Compression in mammography fixates the breast to eliminate motion blur and reduces the patient dose and amount of scattered radiation, which in general is a major source of image degradation. However, the pain from the breast compression might discourage women from attending (e.g., attendant anxiety) the screening program [27]. It has been recommended that compression force only should be applied until the minimum breast thickness has been reached; e.g., if breast compression is increased further from this point, it does not affect image quality or dose but rather increases the patient discomfort [28]. The use of soft copy (electronic) displays and readings is necessary to employ the advantages and flexibility of DM. The inherent advantages include features to enhance and aid the clinical evaluation such as windowing and leveling, pan[3] and zoom[4] functions, and edge-enhancement and customized algorithms to equalize tissue thickness. Before DM became the accepted standard, there was concern about whether the mammographic performance would be adversely affected by the use of soft-copy displays and readings. However, experimental clinical studies showed a similar or even better performance in their readings compared to that of hard-copy readings [29–32]. Because of the image quality-related improvements in DM, it has been expected to improve the clinical performance over SFM. However, as with trials performed in North America, the DM trials in Europe yielded mixed results. Although the sensitivity has been higher in DM than in SFM in a majority of the trials, the recall rates were usually higher as well.[5] As a consequence, only a few studies performed significantly better in overall performance in favor of DM [19]. One of them, e.g., the ACRIN trial, involved a subset of dense breasts including only women below 50 years of age [33]. With regard to specific lesion types, there was apprehension in how the detection of calcifications would be affected by the lower spatial resolution of DM (SFM (~15 line pairs/mm) vs. DM (~6–7 line pairs/mm)) [34]. Most studies have, however, shown a higher detection rate in DM for ductal carcinoma in situ (DCIS; usually presented as calcifications) [33, 35–39]. These results are in accordance with those obtained at experimental clinical studies [35–40] and might be explained by the higher contrast resolution and lesion conspicuity of DM [19, 41].

[1]Detective quantum efficiency (DQE) describes how effectively an x-ray imaging system can produce an image with a high signal-to-noise ratio (SNR) relative to an ideal detector.

[2]Contrast sensitivity refers to the ability of the visual system to distinguish between an object and its background.

[3]Pan = to move an image arbitrarily in a magnified view setting.

[4]Zoom in = magnification of an image to see more details.

[5]Overall performance = when changes in both sensitivity and specificity are considered. An increase in sensitivity (increased detection of cancer) may be associated with a decrease in specificity and does not necessarily indicate that a medical imaging device offers improved depiction of cancer.

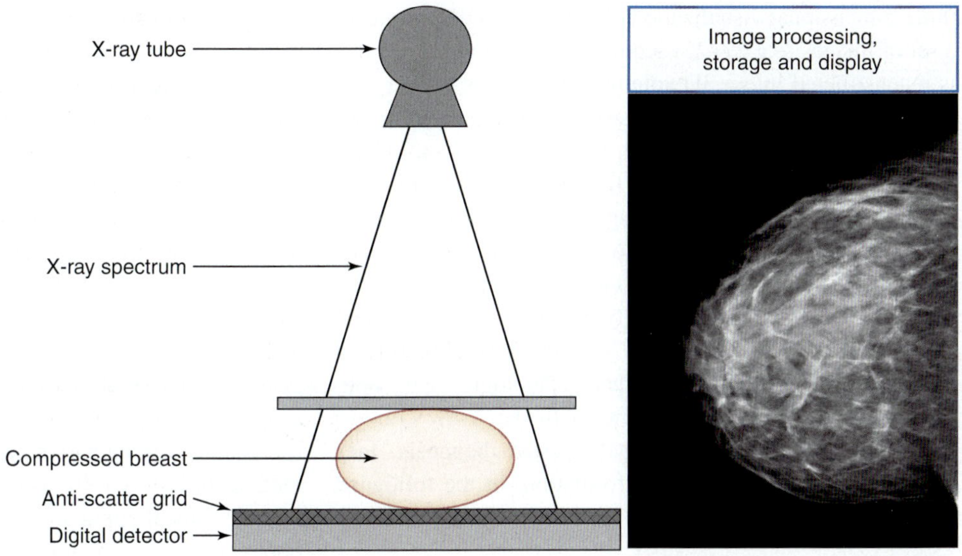

Fig. 4.1 Schematic description of the main components in digital mammography, from X-ray tube to image display. The image acquisition, display, and storage can be optimized separately in digital mammography, unlike screen-film mammography where they are integrated in the film

Imaging Procedure

The objective in mammography is to produce images that provide sufficient image quality with regard to visualization of breast anatomy and signs of disease without subjecting the patient to unnecessary radiation. Based on attenuation differences of the internal structures of the breasts, mammography utilizes low-energetic X-rays (typically around 24–32 kVp) to produce the image (radiograph or mammogram). During examination, the breast is compressed between the breast support and a paddle (Fig. 4.1). The compression is followed by exposure of the breast and the subsequent transmission and scattering of X-rays through the tissue. The attenuated X-ray photon beam passing through the grid is absorbed in the digital detector and transferred as a spatial electrical charge distribution in the form of pixels (i.e., picture elements). Unlike the film in screen-film mammography (SFM) that is nonlinear in sensitivity to X-ray photon flux with a narrow range in which small contrast differences can be detected (S-shaped, commonly referred to as the Hurter-Driffield curve), the digital detector elements provide a signal that is proportional (or linear) to detector exposure [25]. The high requirements of proper exposure in the film often result in suboptimal images (over- and underexposure), in particular in high- and low-density regions and occasionally for the entire imaged breast, which lead to repeated imaging and increased radiation dose to the patient. The large dynamic range in digital detectors permits visualization of all regions in the breast and hence eliminates the need for repeated imaging. With regard to the absorption process of X-rays, digital detector systems can be based on either an indirect or a direct capture process. Indirect capture uses a two-step process in which a scintillator such as cesium iodide (CsI) absorbs the X-rays and generates a scintillation, which is then detected by an array of photodiodes or charge-coupled devices [25]. The structure of the needlelike CsI crystals causes less side scattering of light and provides a high spatial resolution of the imaging system. The thickness of the crystal can be adjusted to desired sensitivity of the system, providing the appropriate level of absorption of X-rays, while maintaining a high spatial resolution [25]. In the direct capture process, the X-ray photons are captured by a photoconductor such as amorphous selenium (*a*-Se), which converts absorbed X-rays directly to a digital signal [42]. Some of the advantages of these systems are that there is no degradation of resolution due to light spread and spatial resolution is limited to pixel size and not to the thickness of the photoconductor [43]. Research and development in this area involves search for new X-ray-absorbing material with better qualities and improvements in the flat-panel array itself. The electrical charge that is generated by the detector is sent to an analog-to-digital (A/D) converter [43]. The magnitude of the charge depends on how much X-rays have passed through the breast at a particular point, which in turn depends on the attenuation properties of the tissues. Dense tissue involves more attenuation of X-rays (i.e., less charge to the A/D) in relation to fatty tissue. Based on the magnitude of the charge, a digital value is assigned by the A/D converter. This is done for each pixel in the mammogram. Prior to presentation, DM images are usually processed for gray-level equalization as well as edge and contrast enhancement [44] (Fig. 4.1).

Although, DM is superior to SFM in many aspects, its clinical performance is still less than perfect. The digital technology provides a platform that allows development of different technologies to facilitate early-stage detection of breast carcinoma. As such, in recent years digital breast tomosynthesis (DBT) has been developed for three-dimensional visualization of the breast. DBT produces a set of images (e.g., 9–25) acquired along a limited arc that is reconstructed into a 3D volume. The images have a high in-plane spatial resolution as determined by the detector system, while the depth resolution, which depends on system geometry, acquisition technique (number of views and angular range), and reconstruction algorithms, is lower but substantially increased in relation to 2D mammography. Aside from this, advantages of DBT include that it is integrated on units that have a dual functionality in that both DBT and DM can be performed on the same system. A combination of tomosynthesis and complementary technologies, e.g., optical procedures, nuclear medicine methods, X-ray contrast media, ultrasound, and computer-assisted diagnosis, may further increase the imaging information. In the following text section, technical aspects in DBT imaging are described.

Advancement of Digital Breast Tomosynthesis

History of DBT Imaging

Based on a sequence of projection views acquired during a single X-ray scan, tomosynthesis (a combination of two Greek words "tomos"—a section, slice, or a cutting—and "synthesis"—a process, resulting in formation of something new) permits any plane to be visualized in the imaged object. The principles of tomosynthesis were proposed by Ziedses des Plantes in the early 1930s who also built a tomography-based unit (i.e., the *planigraph*) [45, 46]. Three decades later the first tomosynthesis images were produced in an experiment performed by Garrison et al. [47] and reconstruction methods were presented [48]. From that point tomosynthesis underwent development in various periods of time. During the 1970s and 1980s, much of the research aimed at improving image quality and optimizing examination times, making tomosynthesis a potential candidate for a wide range of clinical applications. Various systems evolved in experimental settings using screen film, computed radiography detectors, and image intensifiers, but the need for acquiring multiple images made the procedure in these systems too time-consuming with a film change in between each exposure or nonoptimal in image quality for most clinical applications [49]. In addition, the possibilities for post-processing of the images were limited. Although these early systems have provided essential proof of concept, tomosynthesis imaging for clinical use is dependent on a digital detector with rapid readout capabilities, high-dose efficiency (detector quantum efficiency[6]; DQE), and low noise, allowing low-dose projections to be acquired under geometric stability. Because of lack of such detectors and since the popularity of computed tomography (CT) was rising, there was a marked reduction in research and development of tomosynthesis in the later 1980s. The situation changed substantially in the late 1990s, due to the development in flat-panel radiographic digital detectors with the appropriate qualities. The improvements in computers with regard to graphic cards, processing speed, random-access memory[7] (RAM), storage capacity, etc. have further enabled the rational use of the technique during the late 1990s. Initially, prototype tomosynthesis units with flat-panel detectors were developed for research and optimization purposes with a large degree of freedom in varying parameters, which was followed by commercialized units [50]. Tomosynthesis has been applied to several clinical applications over the years, including chest, bones, angiography, and dental imaging, and has emerged as a highly promising method in breast imaging.

Technical Aspects

Basic Imaging Procedure

As shown in Fig. 4.2, the basic equipment for digital breast tomosynthesis (DBT) image acquisition geometry is the same as that of 2D mammography but differs primarily in the rotation of the gantry and in acquisition of multiple images at various angles.

While the breast is being compressed and the detector is held in a fixed position, the X-ray tube translates over a limited angular range that can vary from 11° to 60° (manufacture dependent) and a low-dose exposure is made at every few degrees [51, 52]. Since DBT is a 3D imaging device, it might be desirable to use lower breast compression force than in 2D digital mammography. In 3D imaging, a lower compression force could be useful since it allows a greater depth within the breast volume (e.g., larger separation of the structures in the z-direction), which potentially can help to visualize obscured or partially obscured structures further. A couple of studies have addressed this question. Still, the lesser compression force needs to be weighted properly against the potential increase in average glandular dose (AGD) to the breast and possible degradation in image quality that originate from the increase of scattered radiation. The detector can be stationary or rotate with the tube during exposure; a moving detector results in a larger field of view, which might help to ensure that tissues located in the periphery of the breast are included. The fast readout employed in the detector permits the information from each

[6]Detective quantum efficiency (DQE) describes how effectively an X-ray imaging system can produce an image with a high signal-to-noise ratio (SNR) relative to an ideal detector.

[7]Random-access memory (RAM) is a type of computer data storage. Additional RAM offers increased computer speed, performance, and numbers of applications that can be run momentarily and ability to handle larger files.

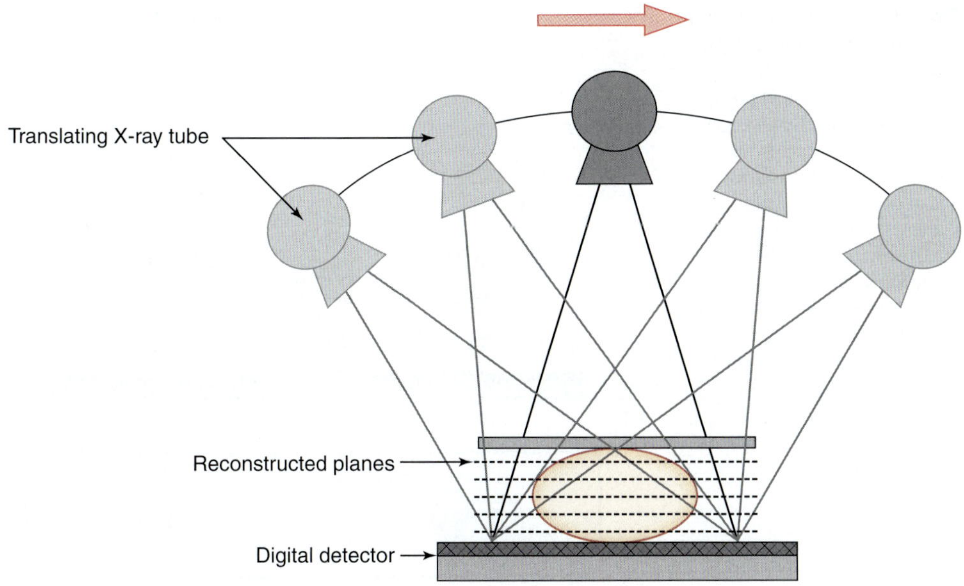

Fig. 4.2 Schematic geometry for digital breast tomosynthesis (DBT) acquisition. The X-ray tube moves (*arrow*) in an arc and information from multiple projection views are collected by a single digital flat-panel detector that can be static or rotating. The detector can be based on selenium alone, on cesium iodide crystals, on a silicon layer, or on photon-counting linear detectors. The latter provide low scatter signal with no electrical noise and may inherent energy resolution that is used in contrast-enhanced imaging to produce images at different energies. See Ref. [50] for further discussion on this

exposure to be extracted and stored prior to next exposure. In this way, a series of low-dose images are obtained, usually 9–25, that differ individually in depth information throughout the breast volume [51]. Many of the DBT parameters can be varied, which include the number of projection images and angular range. To a certain extent, a wider angular range offers increased separation of the breast tissues in depth and allows thinner slices to be reconstructed, while a larger number of images provide a better image quality [53]. The total radiation dose from the low-dose projection images is usually within the range of that from one to two standard mammograms. Low-dose imaging in DBT is possible because the image information in the reconstruction is additive, but as with other X-ray techniques, there is a trade-off (quantum mottle) where the appearance of image noise is noticeable and image quality degraded. With regard to the movement of the X-ray tube during DBT acquisition, different manufacturers have adopted one of two principles, based either on continuous movement or on step-and-shot movement in which the tube stops prior to each individual exposure [52]. Important considerations in the system design for continuous movement are that sufficiently short X-ray pulses are used and that the X-ray tube translates at an appropriate speed. If these two parameters are nonsynchronized, it could cause lack of sharpness in the images. Conversely, if the step-and-shot acquisition is applied, it is important that the gantry is stationary prior to the following exposure. If not, vibrations induced by the prompt stop could cause blur in the images. In general, short exposure times are necessary to obtain sharp images and since data acquisition using the step-and-shot method typically is longer, there is also a greater risk of more image artifacts induced by patient motion [54]. There is ongoing research and development on alternatives to the previously described acquisition methods. One proposed solution that avoids the problems in gantry movement and potential unsharpness in the images is a system based on a stationary array of X-ray sources [55], with the multiple X-ray sources already located in the various exposure angles. Qian et al. [55] have shown that this geometry yields higher modulation transfer function (MTF) over rotation-based systems and increases the sharpness of microcalcifications.

Image Reconstruction

The basic concept of DBT reconstruction is illustrated in Fig. 4.3. A set of projection images is acquired of the breast (in practice, typically 9–25). A DBT slice is created by summing information from the individual projection images about the same tissues (synthesized information). In the DBT slice of the lesion, the lesion contrast is enhanced, while the normal tissue is smeared out (Fig. 4.3). The same principle applies when the focus plane (slice) of the normal tissue is reconstructed. Shifting and adding the projection images repeatedly form a complete set of slices that describes the entire breast volume. The thickness of the reconstructed slices may vary, but typically, images are reconstructed with a slice separation of 1 mm. As such, a 40 mm thick compressed breast will be presented to the breast imager as a stack of at least 40 reconstructed images (slices).

There are two main benefits in the reduction of tissue overlap. First, in women with parenchymal densities that lie above or below a breast cancer, it yields a better differentiation of the lesion and benign or normal tissue, as illustrated in the schematics (Fig. 4.4a) and in a clinical case (Fig. 4.4b).

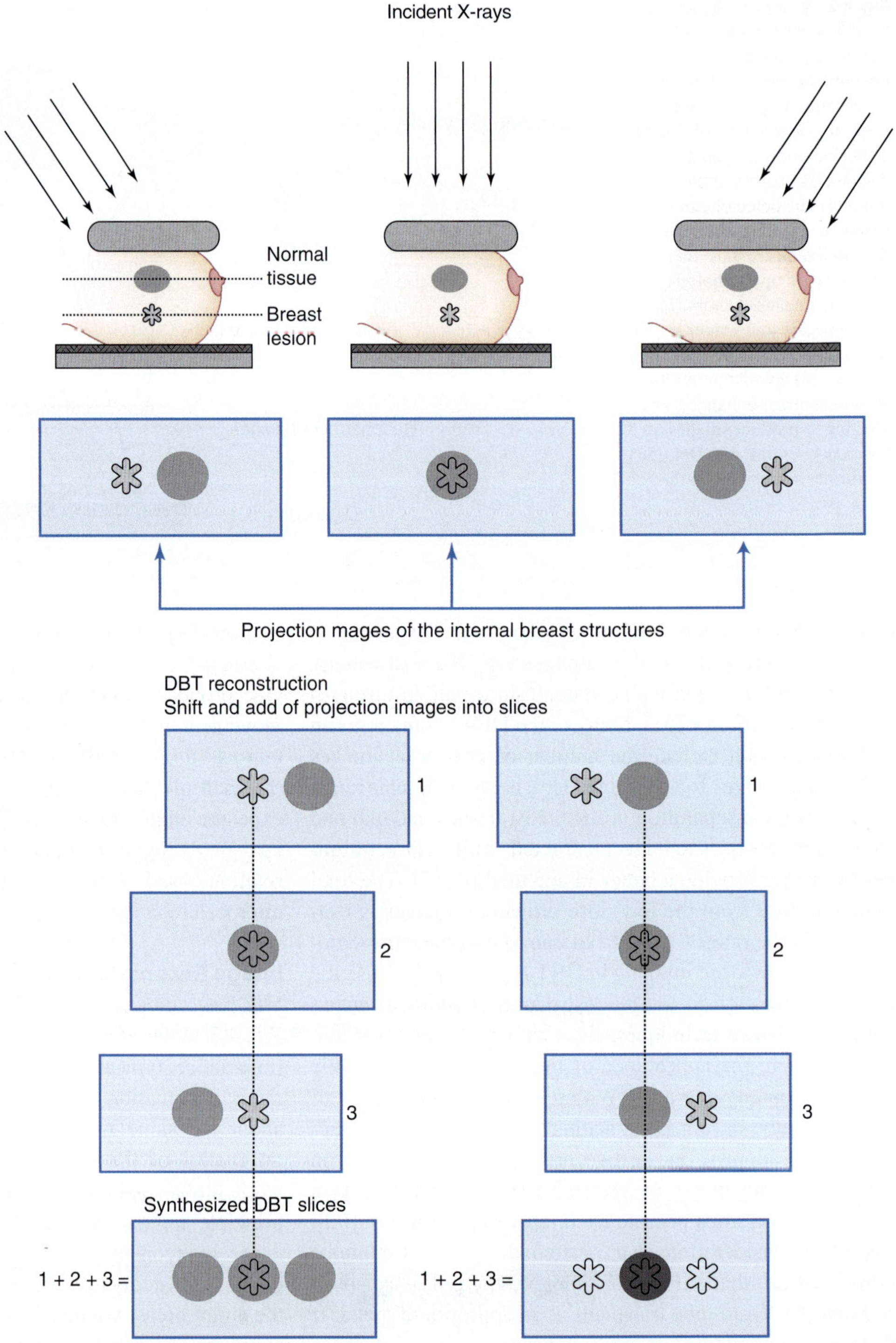

Fig. 4.3 Illustration of the basic image reconstruction in digital breast tomosynthesis. Images are acquired at different exposure angles and projection images collected. In the reconstruction, the projection images are shifted and added, which yields increased information of the breast structures. In the schematics, two slices are reconstructed: the in-focus plane of the lesion (*left*) and the in-focus plane of the normal tissue (*right*), which are enhanced in each DBT slice, respectively. (1–3) Number of projection images

Second, overlying normal structures that yield an appearance in 2D mammography that is suspicious for cancer may be resolved as superimposed glandular tissue in DBT (schematics and case; Fig. 4.5a, b).

Grant developed one of the first reconstruction algorithms for tomosynthesis imaging in 1972, e.g., the shift-and-add method (Fig. 4.3) [56]. Based on his work, several variants of the method followed. Multiple variants of reconstruction techniques have been tested or used in DBT imaging that estimate the 3D distribution of the tissues in the breast additively [51]. The two most common types of methods in commercially available DBT systems and prototype units are the filtered back projection (FBP) technique, which is an analytical method, and algebraic iterative reconstruction methods

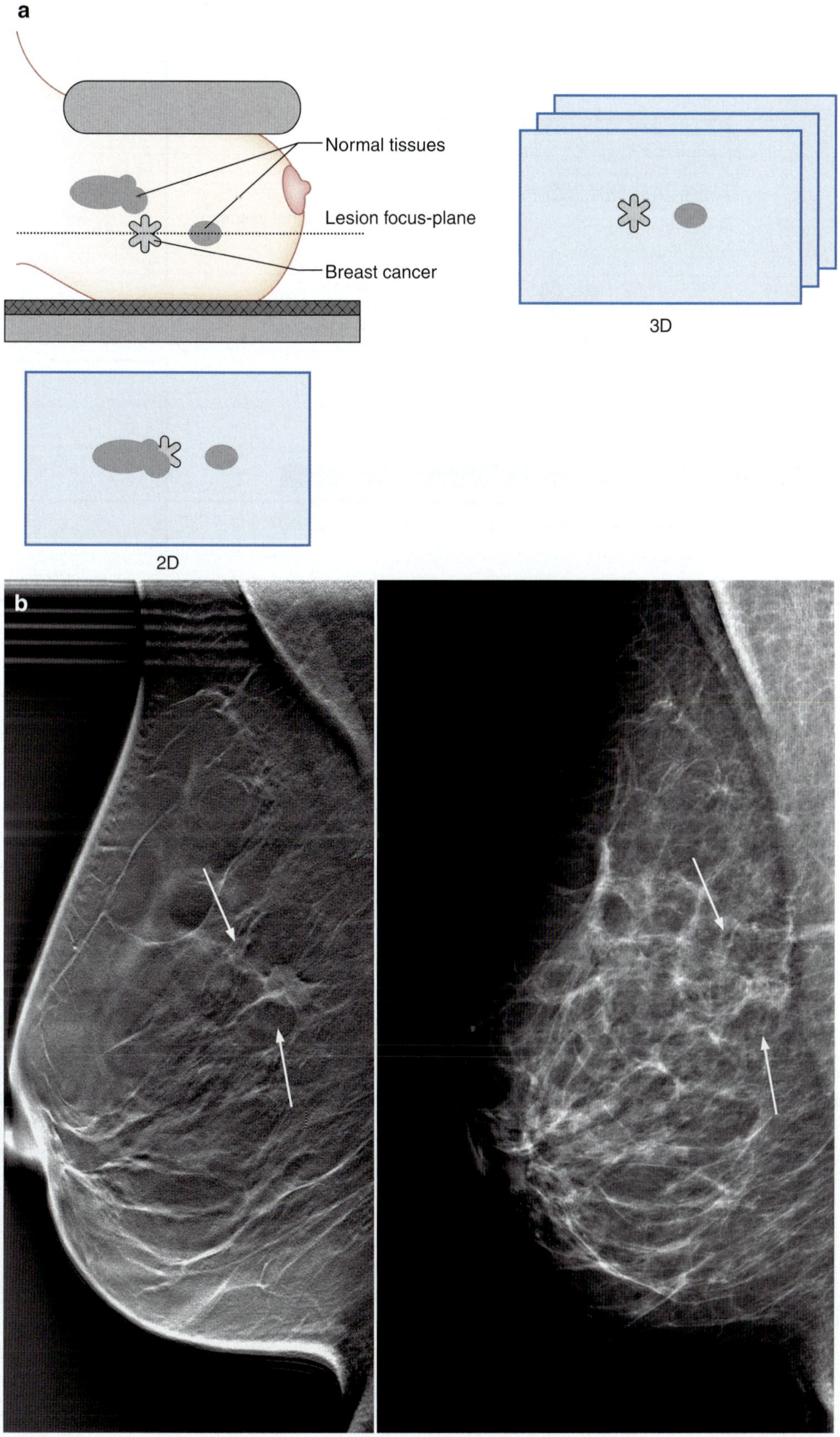

Fig. 4.4 (**a**) A breast cancer partially concealed by normal tissues in 2D mammography has a greater chance of becoming visible with 3D digital breast tomosynthesis (DBT). (**b**) A 62-year-old female with a 15 mm spiculated invasive lobular carcinoma (indicated by the *arrows*) imaged by digital breast tomosynthesis (*left*) and 2D digital mammography (*right*). The breast lesion is conspicuous in DBT, but lacks in contrast and edge characteristics in DM. The individual DBT slice contains less fibroglandular tissue than DM

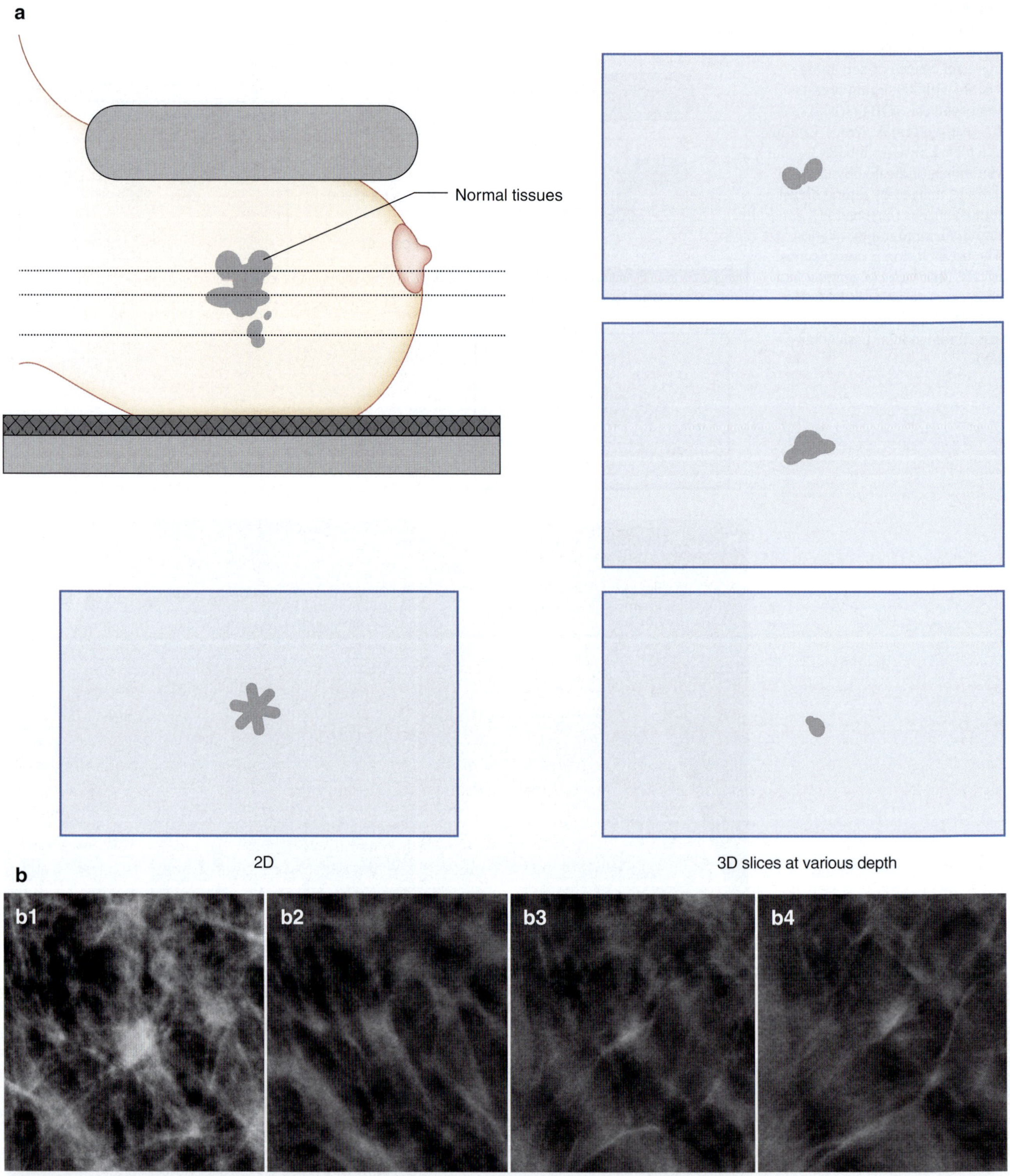

Fig. 4.5 (**a**) Normal tissues that are superimposed onto the 2D plane in 2D mammography may appear as an asymmetry that can result in an unnecessary recall of patient. In 3D imaging, the normal tissues can be better depicted to the radiologist by viewing them at different depths. (**b**) (1–4). Superimposition of normal tissues can lead to an asymmetry in 2D (**b1**) that is resolved as overlapping glandular tissue in 3D (**b2–b4**) (**b2–b4**: Images courtesy of Dr. Liane Philpotts and Dr. Brian Haas, Yale University, New Haven, USA)

[51]. Unlike the one-step operation in FBP, an iterative algorithm performs the reconstruction in a recursive fashion, e.g., repeatedly updated until it converges to a solution. Both types of algorithms have their own pros and cons. In general, FBP offers speed and ease of implementation, while iterative algorithms have potential to yield a better image quality by

yielding lower image noise and reduced artifacts, but it also requires more computational power or time. If DBT is to be used in the screening, it is essential to keep the time required for this post-acquisition processing step as low as possible. In recent years, the increase in computer processing speed and GPU-based image reconstruction has reduced the reconstruction time considerably, which is noticeable for iterative methods, in particular. However, more progress is underway [57, 58]. Most algorithms have a number of refinements (filters) implemented to remove image artifacts and improve image quality for presentation purposes, which can affect the quality of the reconstructed slices substantially. A general difficulty in the development of algorithms is to optimize them for all structures in the breast. For example, some methods visualize soft tissue components of low contrast better, such as masses, while other algorithms do a better job on smaller structures of high frequency, e.g., calcifications. Wu et al. [59] compared the standard back projection (BP), FBP, and the iterative maximum likelihood expectation maximization (MLEM) reconstruction methods in phantoms and in patient images and found that the BP algorithm resulted in the best in-plane image quality for low-contrast masses but resulted in more out-of-plane artifacts. The FBP algorithm performed better than BP for calcifications, while the iterative MLEM algorithm provided a high image quality with regard to both masses and calcifications. The development of tomosynthesis reconstruction algorithms is challenging, since data of only a limited number of low-dose projections are available. This type of data is where iterative methods could be useful the most; however, improvements in faster analytical methods have also been done. Since the clinical application of tomosynthesis is relatively new, continued work is needed.

Reconstruction Artifacts

One common phenomenon associated with digital breast tomosynthesis (DBT) is that the reconstructed images contain a certain degree of artifacts, mainly caused by the incomplete sampling during DBT image acquisition. Some of the artifacts can potentially obscure the breast tissue details and interfere with radiologist visual interpretation of subtle mammographic features. In-plane artifacts refer to falsely reconstructed signals arising from an object, e.g., a mass or calcification, contained within the same image plane as the object itself and can appear as either darker than the object from which they arise (Figs. 4.6 and 4.7a–c) or brighter, which depends on whether it is more or less attenuating than the surrounding tissue. Out-of-plane artifacts refer to falsely reconstructed signals arising from an object and contained within planes other than the object itself. They typically appear as multiple repeated ghost images, which gradually are smeared out (Fig. 4.7a–c). Both types of artifacts appear along the scan direction of the DBT system and are more pronounced for structures of higher contrasts, particularly large benign calcifications.

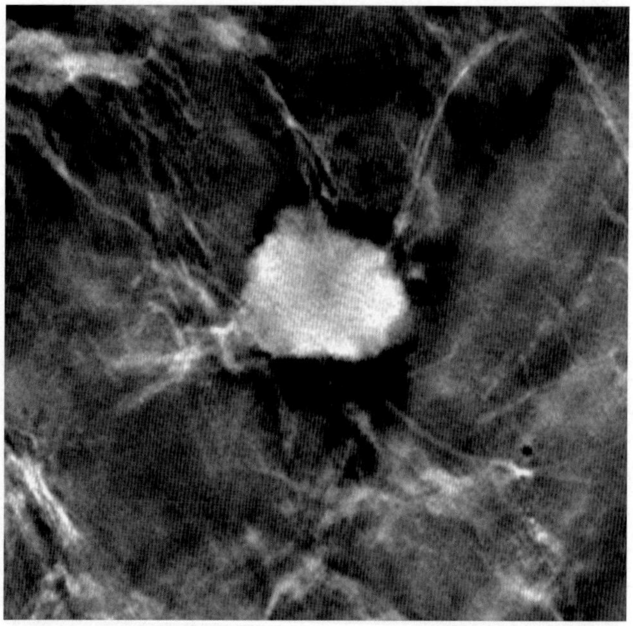

Fig. 4.6 In-plane artifacts surrounding an invasive lesion within a mastectomy specimen in DBT. The artifacts appear as dark rims in the scan direction

Several investigators have demonstrated that the nature of the artifacts is dependent both on the parameters used for image acquisition (e.g., angular range, number of images acquired during a scan, etc.) and on the image reconstruction method used. Iterative methods such as simultaneous algebraic reconstruction technique and maximum likelihood expectation maximization have in some studies shown to reduce the artifacts more than the filtered back projection technique [59–61], and integrated methods have been proposed (Fig. 4.8a, b). Alternatively, the artifacts can be suppressed by displaying thicker slices of the breast. It should be noted, though, that the use of thicker slices might suppress other relevant information in the images.

On one hand, these artifacts represent erroneously reconstructed signals, and the general aim is to attempt to minimize them, but on the other hand, since the peak values of the in-plane artifacts are situated at the edge of the breast lesion (Figs. 4.6 and 4.7a–c), they serve to some degree as edge enhancers, which may in turn increase the detection of some lesion types. The true effect of the artifacts on visualization of breast cancers remains to be studied.

Image Interpretation

As in 2D digital mammography, the digital breast tomosynthesis (DBT) image volume is interpreted in soft-copy format, using high-resolution monitors. It can be displayed in dynamic cine mode, which sequentially displays the slices

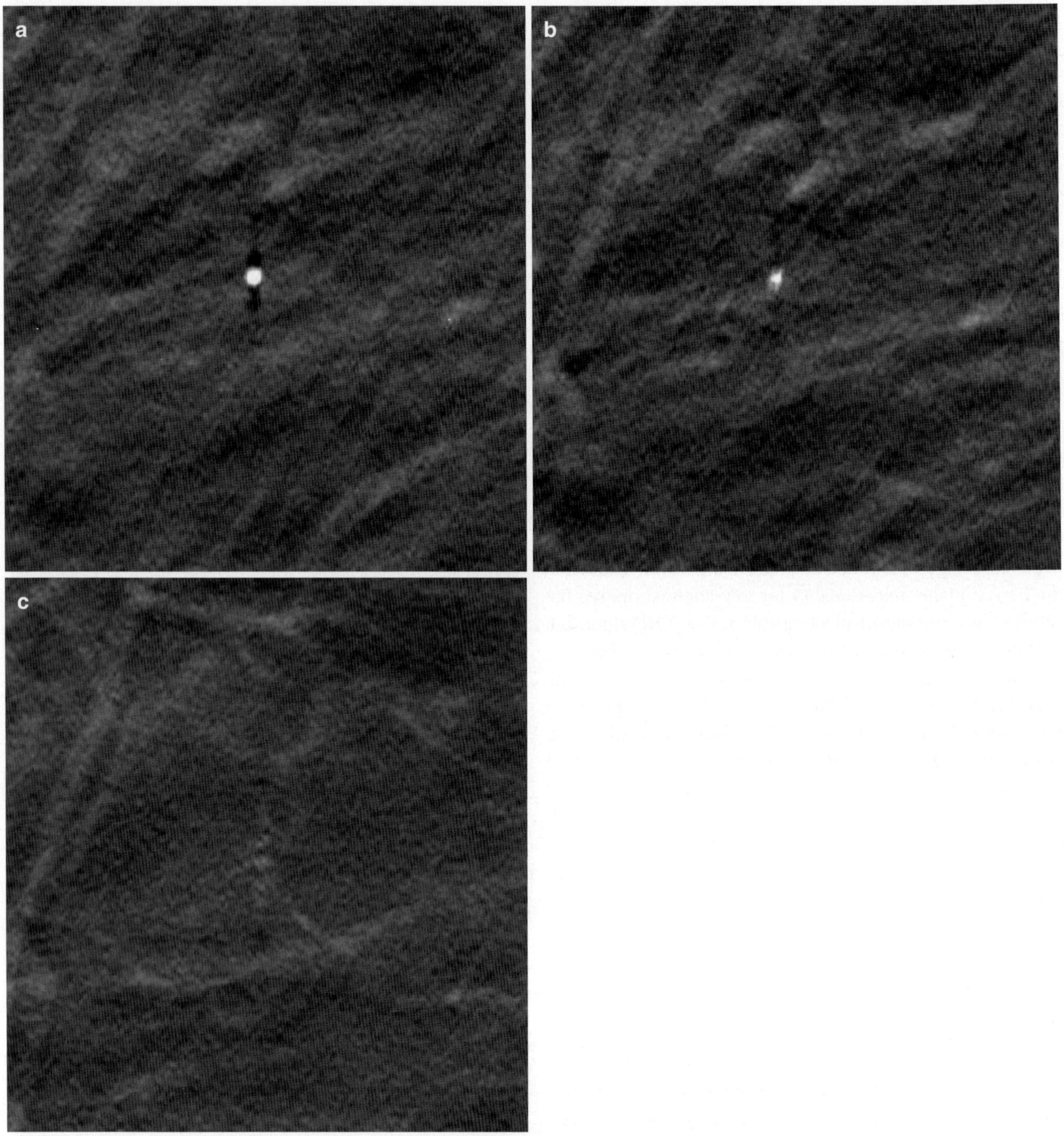

Fig. 4.7 (**a**) A calcification in its focus plane (**a**), (**b**) the slice 3 mm below and (**c**) 7 mm below the focus slice. The calcification is surrounded by in-plane artifacts (*dark shadows*) in (**a**) and out-of-plane artifacts can be seen in (**b**, **c**) as ghosting images that are gradually smeared out

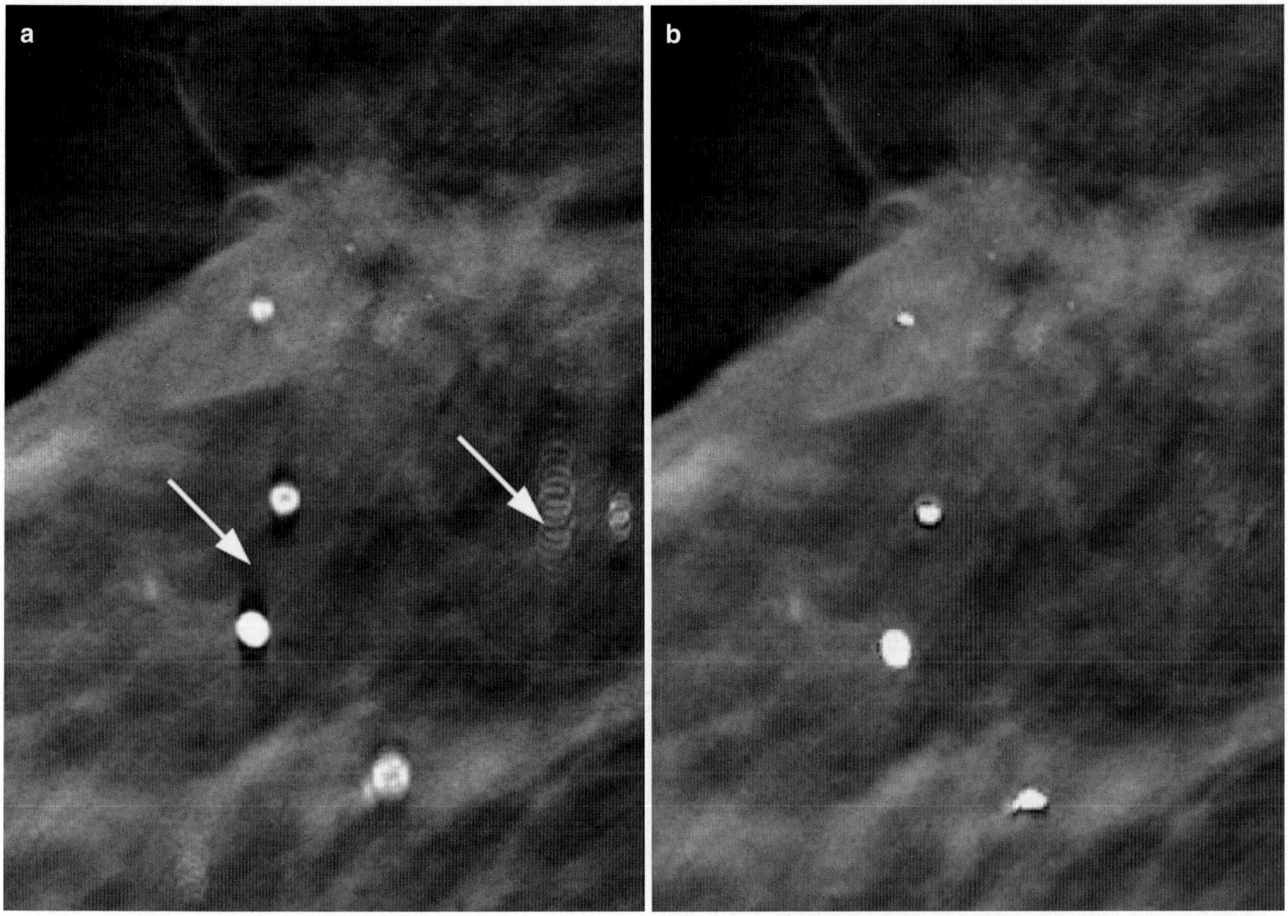

Fig. 4.8 Tomosynthesis reconstruction artifacts found in large benign calcifications (**a**: indicated by the *arrows*). The correction method developed by Wu et al. [62] eliminates the artifacts (**b**) (Reprinted with permission from Wu et al. [62])

automatically in a movie-like fashion, or they might be rendered through manually, slice by slice. The radiologist can scroll back and forth in the breast volume and, as in DM, use tools of pan, windowing and leveling, and zoom. These tools may also be altered in the dynamic mode. Alternatively, the tomosynthesis image volume can be reviewed at various slice thicknesses, also called slabs. A lesion is usually contained within multiple slices. A single tomosynthesis slice, however, describes only a cross section of the lesion. Hence, if several consecutive slices with a finding are added together, it may be enhanced further. The desired slice thickness can be reconstructed instantly at the workstation. Using thicker slices produces fewer images of the breast volume and allows faster image rendering. While thinner slices may be helpful for visualization of details such as morphology, thicker slices may increase lesion contrast or facilitate an overview of calcifications that are spread out at various depths (Fig. 4.9a–c). The slabs can be produced in different ways. Two common algorithms are the maximum intensity of projections (MIP) and simple averaging. The MIP provides high contrast, but results in an elevated noise level. On the contrary, the average algorithm results in lower contrast at a lower noise level. In a comparative study, the MIP provided best visualization of calcifications, while averaging was found to best visualize well-circumscribed or spiculated masses [63].

Synthesized 2D Images

It is possible to reconstruct 2D images from the 3D DBT image set. The concept is founded on the usefulness of reviewing 2D images in combination with DBT. A hybrid of the imaging modalities may speed up the assessment of calcifications and yield a more immediate overview of the breast. The synthesized 2D would be helpful in decreasing the radiation dose to the breast up to 50 % for two-view imaging, compared to if a set of 2D mammography images would be acquired. Gur et al. [64] found a lower sensitivity at a comparable specificity in an early study evaluating the performance of the synthesized 2D images in relation to standard 2D mammography images. However, the algorithm generating the 2D images has been developed since then and was recently used in screening trials [65, 66] (Fig. 4.10).

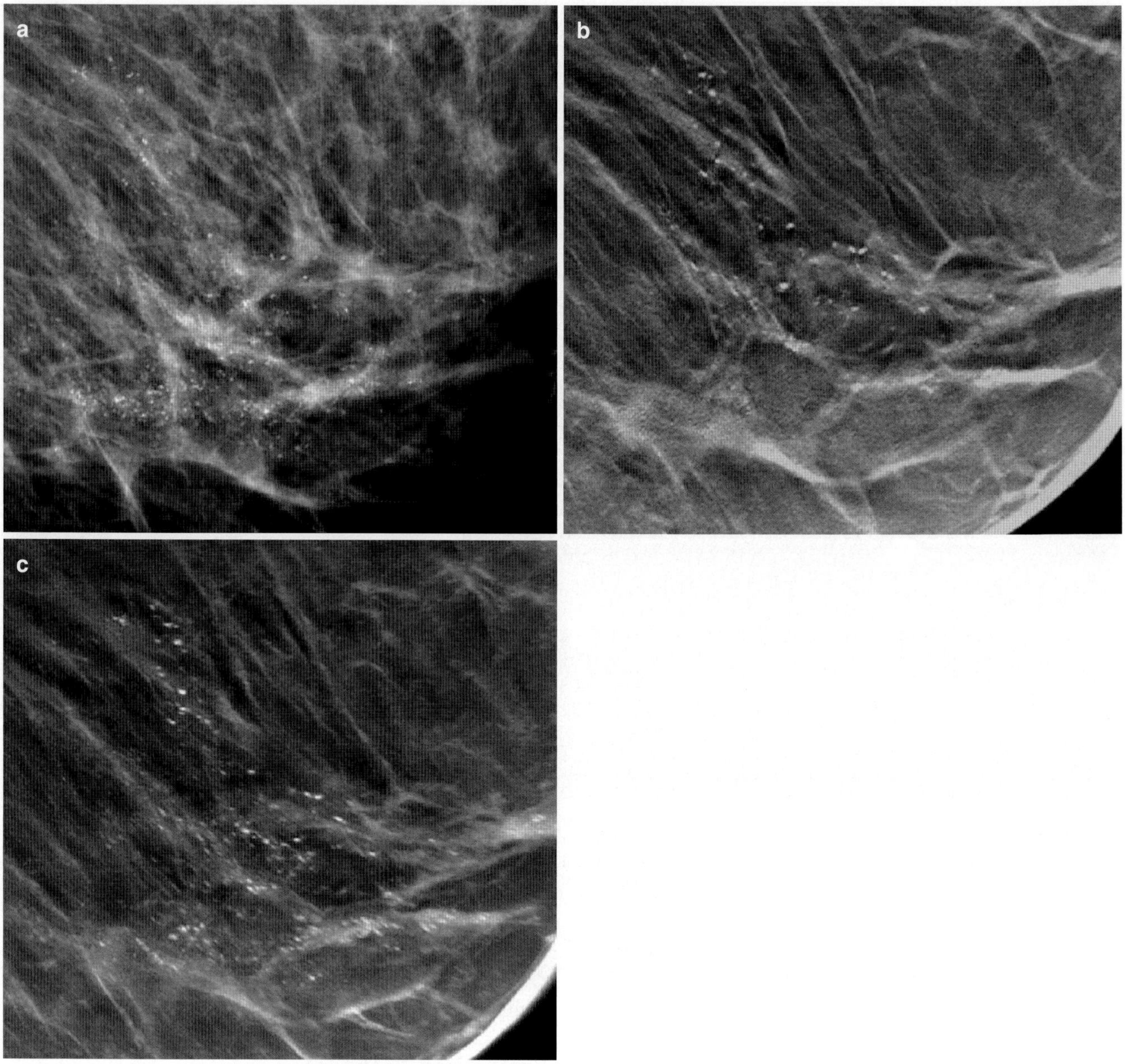

Fig. 4.9 (**a**) A 60-year-old female with a 40 mm DCIS indicated by microcalcifications located in the lower medial quadrant of the breast, imaged by DM (**a**) and DBT (**b**, **c**). (**b**) A central DBT slice has been extracted within the cluster of calcifications. (**c**) Slices have been added together using the maximum intensity of the projections. The most characteristic calcifications are seen with the comedo type of DCIS, which vary in size, form, and density and are clustered with partly ductal (linear) orientation

Clinical Studies of Breast Cancer Detection, Efficiency, and Aspects of Imaging Protocol

Introduction

Poplack et al. [67] performed one of the first clinical studies on patients that compared digital breast tomosynthesis (DBT) and conventional two-dimensional (2D) mammography. Image quality and recall rates were compared in images of 98 patients. The patients were selected consecutively from the screening program when the mammogram was interpreted as being abnormal. DBT and screen-film mammography (SFM) were compared in image quality, which included lesion conspicuity and feature analysis. The need for recall was assessed when DBT was combined with digital screening mammograms (DM). Image quality of DBT was similar ($n=51$) or superior ($n=37$) to SFM in 89 % of the cases. The numbers of recalls were reduced by 40 % when DM was supplemented with DBT. It was concluded that DBT has similar or superior image quality compared to SFM in a diagnostic setting and has potential to reduce screening recall rates when used in combination with digital screening mammograms. A number of retrospective studies on breast cancer detection have

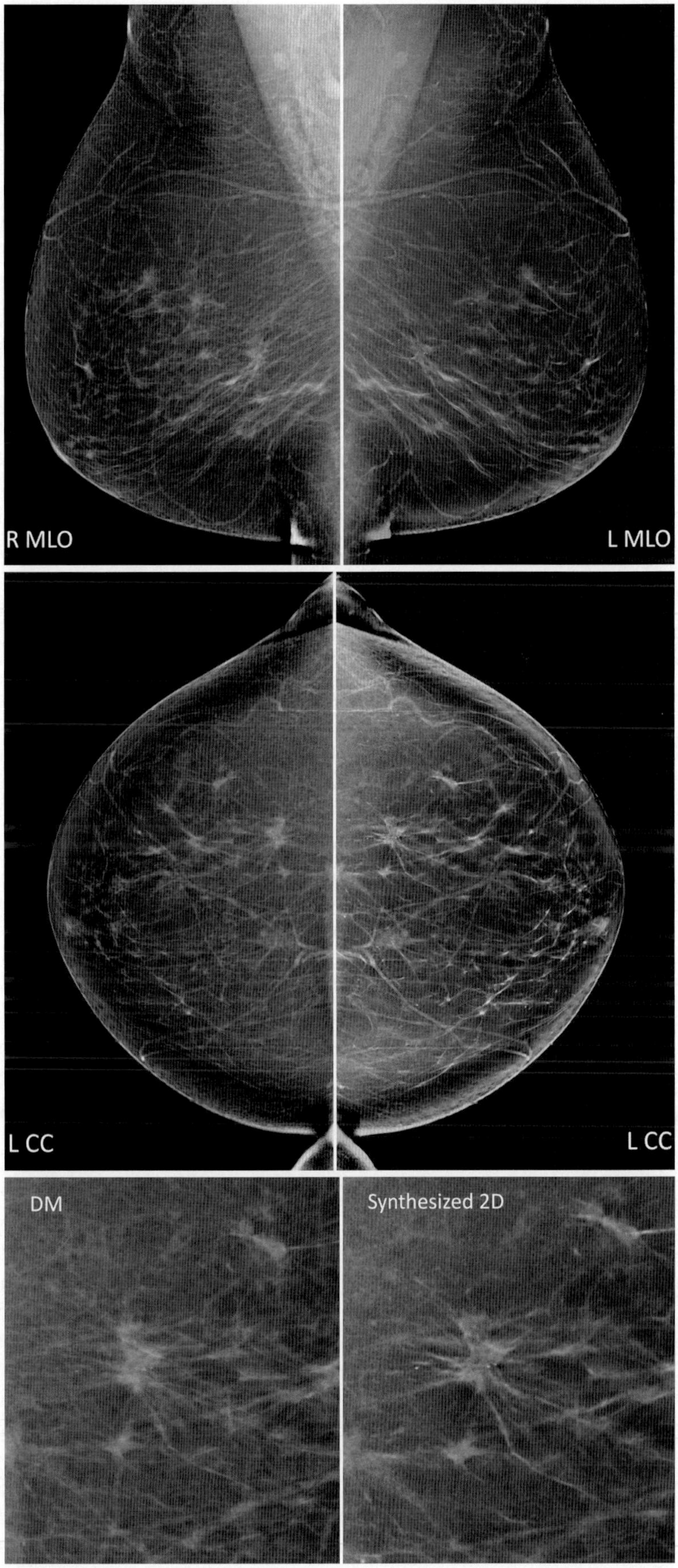

Fig. 4.10 Digital mammography (*left*) and synthesized 2D (*right*) mirrored in mediolateral oblique (MLO, *top*) and craniocaudal (*CC*, *middle*) views. The synthesized 2D images have been reconstructed from the series of tomosynthesis projection images. Close-ups (*bottom*) of the CC images show a spiculated invasive tumor with calcifications (Images courtesy of Professor Fiona Gilbert, University of Cambridge, Cambridge, UK)

followed that compares the diagnostic tests of tomosynthesis and mammography. Interpretation is done in a blinded fashion, usually by multiple radiologists independently to account for reader variability.

Reported Studies in 2008–2013

Table 4.1a, b show results of studies reported in 2008–2013 comparing DBT and conventional DM in breast cancer detection. The studies have been stratified according to (1) those that evaluated tomosynthesis alone, performed in one or in two views (Table 4.1a), and (2) those that evaluated tomosynthesis in adjunct to mammography (Table 4.1b). When the same populations of cases and readers have been used on several imaging modalities (paired study design), it allows for a matched comparison. Hence, if studies are listed in both tables by the same authors, the order of imaging modality in performance may be of interest. The tables show the results in increase (+) or in decrease (−) in performance measures using DBT in relation to conventional DM. The most common measures that have been used are presented: diagnostic accuracy (i.e., the radiologist's ability to discriminate between abnormal and normal/benign cases, fourth column), sensitivity and specificity (fifth column), and recall rate for assessment (sixth column). When statistical significance ($p<0.05$) has been achieved, the value is indicated with an asterisk*. As the sensitivity and specificity measures are correlated and depend on the individual threshold of the radiologist, it is valuable to use combined performance measures (denoted as diagnostic accuracy). Diagnostic accuracy has been estimated by the area under the ROC curve or by area under the alternative free-response ROC curve (applied in JAFROC analysis). The main difference in between the methods is that the ROC method considers the cases as a whole (e.g., if they are abnormal or normal/benign), while the free-response method also considers the locations of individual breast cancers, e.g., the radiologist needs to indicate the location of the finding [84]. By considering individual breast cancers, the free response method assesses a higher statistical strength and makes the evaluation more realistic [85, 86]. These and other observer performance methods have been described in more detail elsewhere [84, 85, 87]. Recall rate is defined as the percentage of screening studies in which further work-up was recommended by the radiologist. Reduced recall rate results in less anxiety, inconvenience, and cost for patients with false-positive findings. These numbers are known to vary widely, especially in between countries. Commonly reported recall rates ranges from around 5 % for mammography screening in northern Europe to 15 % for screening in North America [88]. However, the presented values (Table 4.1a, b) are based on enriched reader studies and are relative, in contrast to absolute performance values, which are being evaluated in clinical studies based on screening populations [89].

Although, diagnostic accuracy tends to increase (+) for tomosynthesis as a single imaging modality compared to mammography (Table 4.1a), there are few studies with significant improvements (31 %, 5 out of 16 comparisons). In studies comparing several different tomosynthesis imaging protocols, a trend of increased performance can be seen as the image information increases, by the addition of either tomosynthesis views or mammography views. A majority of studies evaluating DBT combined with DM (Table 4.1b) have found significant improvements (e.g., 78 %, in 7 out of 9 studies). When counting solely with the studies using a full set of two-view images from both imaging modalities, e.g., two-view tomosynthesis reviewed in adjunct to two-view mammography, they all showed significant improvements (Table 4.1b; 100 %, in 5 out of 5 studies). This image protocol has also resulted in the largest improvements [68, 75, 82]. Several of the studies did not show significant improvements using tomosynthesis, but resulted in rather similar performance values compared to conventional DM (Table 4.1a and a couple of studies in Table 4.1b). In one of these studies [69], six radiologists interpreted images of 376 subjects (63 abnormal). Subjective analysis found abnormal and benign lesions to be more conspicuous in one-view tomosynthesis than in mammography in substantially more cases. However, no significance was achieved in terms of improved breast cancer detection. In a follow-up study [83], tomosynthesis images were reviewed with the complementary DM view. Although the improvement was still statistically nonsignificant, the clinical performance increased, compared with tomosynthesis alone, as seen by the narrower confidence intervals, which were close to the limit of superiority. The same trend was seen in separate analyses of sensitivity and specificity. Besides the influence of image protocol used, there are several possible explanations for different results in studies. As discussed by Houssami and Skaane [89], it may depend on differences in readers or in research methods. Another aspect is the case difficulty. If only cases are included that are easy to detect and identify on both imaging modalities, any performance difference may be diluted or likewise is true if the cases are too difficult to detect on both imaging modalities [90]. Cases of borderline detection are essential to show differences in between medical imaging devices. The clinical occurrence of such cases can be registered in the data sampling of reader studies or naturally be assessed in population-based trials. At this stage, the fact that so many reader studies have found increase in accuracy should be regarded as very promising. Additionally, these studies have been performed in controlled environments and usually regard reader variability in a large extent. However, in many of the presented studies, readers are only included from the same mammography centers, which may result in smaller reader variability than using readers from different centers. In the same way, the use of mainly experienced

Table 4.1 Clinical studies reported in 2008–2013 on breast cancer detection using digital breast tomosynthesis alone (DBT; a), in one and in two views, and in adjunct to two-view digital mammography (DM; b) in comparison to standard two-view DM

4.1a: Studies comparing DBT only versus DM

Study		Subjects (anormal)	Radiologists	Diagnostic accuracy	Sensitivity/specificity	Recall rate (%)	
						Benign/normals	Cancer cases
One-view DBT	Svahn et al. [68]	50 (25)	5	+6.6			
	Gennaro et al. [69]	376 (63)	6	+1.5	−4.5/+4.1		
	Michell et al. [70]	501 (111)	8	+4.5*			
	Svane et al. [71]	144 (76)	2	−0.7	−3.9/+5.1		
	Svahn et al. [72]	185 (89)	5	+10.3*	+10.8*/+0.8		
	Wallis et al. [73]	130 (40)	10	+0.1		−11.2	−10.5
	Zanca et al. [74]						
	Exp. readers	130 (40)	5	+1		−12.5	−1.2
	Inexp. readers	130 (40)	5	−1		−10.7	−19.3
	Waldherr et al. [75]	144 (86)	2		+16.7*/+0.3	−69.7*	−52.5*
	Thibault et al. [76]	131 (55)	7	+2.27	−7/+11		
Two-view DBT	Good et al. [77]	30 (25)	9	+2		−2.6	+3.3
	Gur et al. [78]	125 (35)	6		+5/+4	−10	+5.7
	Teertstra et al. [79]	501 (111)	1	+1.5	0/−1.7		
	Wallis et al. [73]	130 (40)	10	+7.9*		−11.2	0
	Zanca et al. [74]						
	Exp. readers	130 (40)	5	+4.7		−17.5*	−1.2
	Inexp. readers	130 (40)	5	+11.0*		−5	−1.2

4.1b: Studies comparing DBT in adjunct to DM versus DM

Study[a]	Subjects (anormal)	Radiologists	Diagnostic accuracy	Sensitivity/specificity	Recall rate (%)	
					Benign/normals	Cancer cases
Smith et al. [80]	316 (48)	12	+7.1*		−42.6*	
Gur ct al. [78]	125 (30)	8		+5/+12	−30*	+5.7
Svahn et al. [68]	50 (25)	5	+11.3*			
Michell et al. [81][b]	738 (204)	6	+7.2*			
Waldherr et al. [75]	144 (86)	2		+21.1*/+2.2	−72.7*	−68.3*
Rafferty et al. I [82]	312 (48)	12	+7.2*	+10.7/+5.1	−69.7*	−7.8
Rafferty et al. II [82]	312 (51)	15	+7.1*	+16/−1.7	−38.3*	+1.1
Gennaro et al. [83]	469 (68)	6	+2.1	+3.4/−1.9		
Thibault et al. [76]	131 (55)	7	+2.39	−5/+11		

The results of the studies are presented in reader-averaged increase (+) or decrease (−) in tomosynthesis performance in relation to DM. Statistical significance is indicated by an asterisk (*)

[a]The studies by Svahn et al. [68], Gennaro et al. [83], Thibault et al. [76], and Waldherr et al. [75] are evaluating a single DBT MLO view combined with DM in comparison to conventional two-view DM (i.e., not a full set of 2-view images from both imaging modalities), while the other studies evaluated two-view DBT in adjunct to two-view DM

[b]Screen-film mammography (SFM) was also included in this comparison. The readers read SFM immediately followed by DM and DBT. The results are thus presented from when the readers had read SFM and DM, in comparison to those from when they had read SFM, DM, and DBT

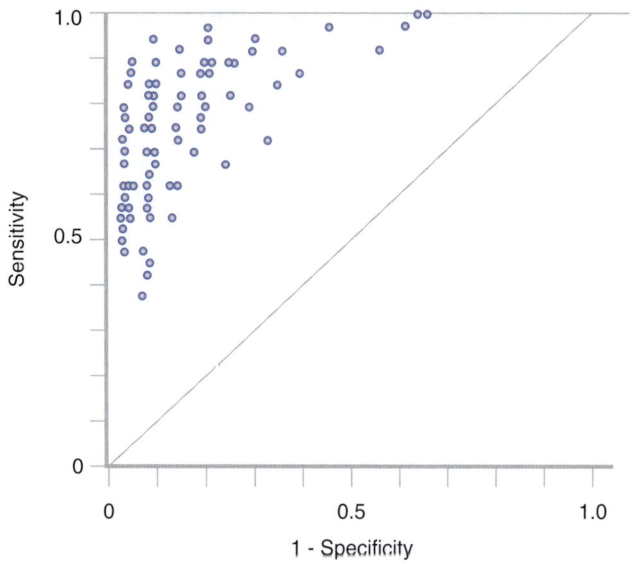

Fig. 4.11 Reader variability in 108 radiologists interpreting the same studies. A substantial variability is present in sensitivity (40 %) and in specificity (45 %) as described by the spread of reader data. The diagonal illustrates the performance associated with pure chance. When fitting ROC curves to the points and estimating the area under the curve, the reader variability was largely reduced (to 11 %) (Reprinted with permission from Chakraborty [85])

readers in a study might require a smaller number of readers, compared to using inexperienced, e.g., to obtain an acceptable level of uncertainty in the study results. To investigate the potential of DBT utmost, it is important to consider variability in different mammography centers that is described more in the following text section.

Multicenter, Multi-reader Trials

In a study by Beam et al. [91], the effectiveness of screening mammography was evaluated by randomly selecting fifty accredited mammography centers across the USA. A total of 108 radiologists at the centers interpreted the same set of 79 2D screening mammograms. The gold standard (state of truth) of the mammograms was obtained by either biopsy or follow-up during 2 years. The spread (dispersion) in radiologists' performance was large in sensitivity, at least 40 %, and in specificity, at least 45 %, but largely reduced (to 11 %) when estimating variability in the area under the curve (AUC) on the same reader data (Fig. 4.11). The study results demonstrate that a large part of the variability in sensitivity and specificity is due to the variable thresholds for reporting disease. Diagnostic accuracy considers individual shifts that might exist in sensitivity and specificity, for example, in between readers or for a specific reader interpreting cases obtained from different imaging modalities, and consequently, two radiologists may have identical AUC representing a similar skill in discriminating between abnormal and normal/benign findings but in practice perform at rather different values of sensitivity and specificity.

Variability has since long been noted in many areas of clinical medicine [92, 93]. The Breast Imaging Reporting and Data System (BIRADS) was initially introduced by the American College of Radiology in 1992 [94] as a tool designed to standardize breast imaging terminology and to help radiologists reduce false-positive screening mammograms. However, despite of this and many other improvements in mammography, the level of agreement among radiologists interpreting the same sets of mammograms has shown to be relatively low [93], which in practice can result in delayed detection of breast cancer and be both alarming for the patient and expensive. When comparing two medical imaging devices, large variability may compromise the aim of obtaining a value that represents radiologists in general and thus the reliability of the results. In worst case, the results of a study might be an effect of reader variability and subsequently it is essential to account for. Rafferty et al. [82] compared DBT in adjunct to DM with DM in two separate reader studies with a total of 27 radiologists participating from five different mammography centers (Table 4.1b). In both studies, the DBT modality was superior to digital mammography in diagnostic accuracy and in reduced recall rates. Other studies have included readers with various expertise in mammography from different countries and found benefits in breast cancer detection with tomosynthesis [73, 74].

Reading Time

Reading time is a crucial and important aspect if tomosynthesis is going to be used in population-based screening programs. Because there is more image information involved, tomosynthesis reading is at the current time more time-consuming, but it also depends on image protocol used (Table 4.2). Typically, reading time increases with additional image information. Screening trial results have found that the reading time for DBT in adjunct to DM was approximately double that for DM alone (91 s vs. 45 s), which may be acceptable when considering the substantial increase in diagnostic accuracy. In an optimized imaging protocol, the gain in accuracy needs to be balanced with radiologist time to interpret, radiation dose, and examination costs. Visualization tools, such as the slab function, synthesized 2D, and others, are under development for maximized reading efficiency [95, 96].

Tomosynthesis has shown to be able to improve breast cancer detection, but questions remain unanswered about what clinical uses are optimal. Should its primary application be in diagnostic imaging in selected high-risk groups of patients with specific types of abnormalities or as a screening tool in general? If so, should it be applied in one or two views alone or in adjunct to DM?

Table 4.2 Reported reading times (seconds and standard deviations) for digital mammography (DM) and different digital breast tomosynthesis (DBT) image protocols

Study	Two-view DM	One-view DBT	Two-view DBT	Two-view DM plus Two-view DBT
Gur et al. [78]	73±69		123±88 (68)	143±99 (96)
Zanca et al. [74]	79±10		134±15 (70)	
H/T 10 years of experience	74±22	99±19 (34)		
Zanca et al. [74]	56±9		115±17 (105)	
L/T 10 years of experience	74±10	94±24 (27)		
Average:	71±24	97±21 (37)	124±40 (76)	143±99 (96)

The numbers in the parentheses describe the percentage increase in reading time compared to that of DM

Two-View Imaging in Digital Mammography

When two-view imaging is used, which in many countries is the screening standard, a mediolateral oblique (MLO) view is acquired with the central X-ray beam passing the breast obliquely in a medial to lateral direction and a craniocaudal (CC) view with the central beam passing the breast in a vertical direction. In a randomized 2D mammography screening trial, a two-view setting was found to detect 24 % more women with breast cancer at a reduced recall rate by 15 % when compared to a one-view setting [97]. The use of several projection views in 2D mammography partially compensates for the overlapping effect of the normal tissue but to a limited extent since the 3D information is still overprojected onto the 2D plane in each individual projection view, hence the need for 3D imaging.

One- or Two-View Imaging in Digital Breast Tomosynthesis?

As in 2D mammography, a DBT examination can consist of either one or several images (projection views) of each breast. The use of a single MLO projection view in DBT has previously been suggested as the only view required [54, 98] as a substitute to two-view mammography. The use of the DBT MLO view is essential since it includes a larger amount of the breast, while the extra value of the CC view has been more uncertain. DBT can also be combined with DM, which in some publications is referred to as a "combo" mode. Because DBT is a 3D imaging modality, it has been hypothesized that additional views would not be needed. However, several reader studies have shown that breast cancer detection increases with the use of additional views, as indicated early on by Rafferty et al. [99]. In that study, a group of 34 patients undergoing biopsy were imaged with DBT and classified in breast cancer visibility. In a majority of the cases, the breast cancer was more clearly seen in the DBT CC view than in the DBT MLO view, e.g., in 67 % of the cases in study population. It was concluded that it might be desirable to use DBT in both views to optimally visualize lesions. Figure 4.12 shows a plot of performance in different image protocols, based on a study with subtle cases [68]. The performance was about 5 % higher for DBT with the complementary DM view compared to one-view DBT, and about 12 % higher when compared to DM. A sample-size prediction of the reader data, using the Hillis-Berbaum approach, estimates that statistical significance would be possible to achieve in between the tomosynthesis modalities, if the size of the study population would have been doubled (×2.34; $n=117$; most researchers seek a power at 80 % at $\alpha=0.05$, which was applied in the estimation). In the aspect of obtaining highest performance, the majority of studies with clear improvements (*) support two-view tomosynthesis imaging in combination with mammography (Table 4.1b). A recent trial found that the addition of one-view tomosynthesis to mammography improved the diagnostic accuracy

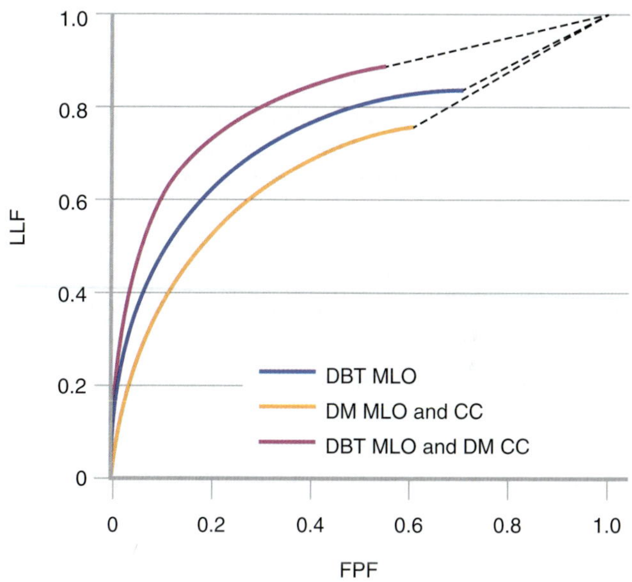

Fig. 4.12 Clinical performance of different DBT imaging protocols: conventional DM, one-view DBT, and DBT combined with DM estimated by the area under the alternative free-response ROC (AFROC). The performance was highest for DBT combined with DM, 5 % higher than one-view DBT, and 12 % higher than DM. The end points of the curves describe the numbers of breast cancers localized and identified (*LLF*) and the false-positive fraction (*FPF*). The combined modality found more breast cancers detected at fewer false positives. *DBT* Digital breast tomosynthesis, *MLO* Mediolateral oblique, *DM* Digital mammogram, *CC* Craniocaudal

and reduced the recall rate significantly, but the addition of two-view tomosynthesis to digital mammography yielded twice the performance gain at the same time further reducing the recall rate [100].

There are several possible explanations for the additional increase in performance when DBT is used in two views for each breast or in adjunct to DM. DBT images are collected within a limited angular range and reconstructed into a quasi-3D volume, and hence the anatomical noise is suppressed but not eliminated. A cancer can be missed because of incomplete elimination of anatomical noise. Moreover, the breast is compressed and the tissue lies in different positions in the breast in each view and breast cancers such as spiculated tumors might be preferentially oriented in one plane and difficult to identify in other planes. Some advantages in using one DBT view only would be a lower patient dose and examination time, faster post-processing, and decreased reading time for the radiologist, e.g., a more time-efficient process but with the disadvantage of not detecting some breast cancers. In the same manner, the choice of imaging protocol in DBT might affect the radiologists' ability to identify normal/benign cases (e.g., the specificity). Another aspect is the detection of calcifications. Two-dimensional mammography is the current reference standard for detection of microcalcifications, and early studies have reported lower image quality on calcifications or lower detection of them with DBT [67, 72, 101]. This might depend on motion artifacts in DBT that are caused by the longer DBT acquisition time than 2D mammography, or it can depend on the reconstruction algorithms used. Tomosynthesis reduces tissue overlap and thus structural noise, a quality that helps it better show breast masses. Microcalcifications are on the other hand not affected by it to the same degree and are in that way more amenable to viewing by 2D scans. Continued evolvement in DBT technology and developments in image post-processing can improve the detection of calcifications in DBT, as shown in more recent studies [55, 102]. In a reader study by Wallis et al., DBT and DM were compared using a photon-counting DBT unit employing iterative reconstruction methods. DBT images were reviewed, as a substitute to DM. Diagnostic accuracy of DBT applied in two views was found superior to conventional DM, while no clear improvement was found for DBT in one view versus DM. Masses and calcifications were also analyzed separately. The detection of both lesion types increased significantly in two-view tomosynthesis.

A majority of studies today show clear improvements when DBT and DM are used in a combined setting (Table 4.1b), whereas only a handful of studies have found similar results when tomosynthesis has been evaluated as a stand-alone imaging modality (Table 4.1a), and these have often included a limited number of abnormal DCIS cases in the study material, if any [63, 66] (Waldherr C, 2013, personal communication). There are some potential advantages of using DBT in adjunct to DM. First, it may offer increased sharpness with regard to the morphology of calcifications, but this depends on the reconstruction algorithm used. DM yields an overview of calcifications, which may speed up the assessment of them. Second, it may be more difficult or require more effort to mentally combine the information of two DBT views displayed side by side when rendering the image volumes than in DBT combined with DM, e.g., having at least one of the images "fixed." Breasts with a high amount of fat tissue (breast density of BIRADS 1 or 2) that involve a low probability of malignancy might be reviewed more time-efficiently with DM with little or no loss in performance. If a case contain no tissue that could obscure abnormalities, the DM interpretation might be sufficient. Third, the combined modality might involve lower learning curve effects for the radiologists since they are accustomed to 2D mammography. There are likely large effects on training involved since the appearance of the images by the different techniques is different (2D vs. 3D). During a possible transition, 2D mammography would also be useful for comparison with 2D priors. Computer-aided diagnosis (CAD) has since long been developed for 2D mammography, while research and development in CAD for tomosynthesis is relatively new. Using 2D mammography in a combined setting with DBT allows continued use of developed CAD systems. A situation where it was essential to apply tomosynthesis in two views is shown (Figs. 4.13, 4.14, 4.15, and 4.16). A 74-year-old female underwent 2D DM screening mammography that indicated no signs for malignancy when compared to 2D priors (Fig. 4.13).

A DBT mammogram (Fig. 4.14a–c) showed an area of architectural distortion in the lateral aspect of the left breast, seen on the DBT CC view and estimated location at the 3 o'clock position in the current slice of the reconstructed DBT volume.

The patient was asked to return for additional mammographic spot-compression views and ultrasonography examination. The finding detected in DBT was not seen on the mammography spot compression (Fig. 4.15). It was, however, seen on the target-based ultrasonography (Fig. 4.16) where a 5.5 mm spiculated tumor was located.

Architectural distortions are among the most commonly missed abnormalities in false-negative findings of screening mammography [104]. Pathology showed an infiltrating and in situ carcinoma. The case illustrates the potential of tomosynthesis in dense fibroglandular tissue but also stresses the importance of two-view imaging, as the cancer was detected in the craniocaudal tomosynthesis view only.

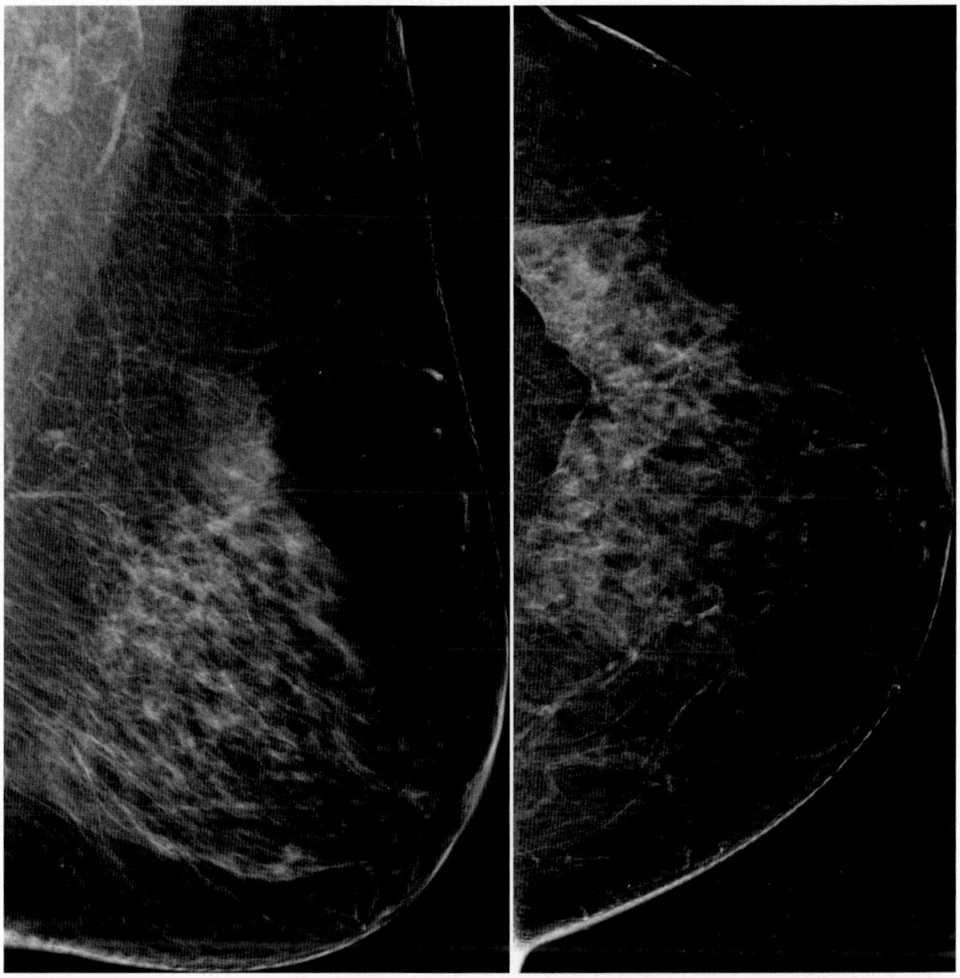

Fig. 4.13 The left 2D DM screening examination performed in DM MLO and CC view (*left* and *right* image, respectively) showed dense breast tissue, but no abnormality was detected (All used with permission from Andrejeva et al. [103])

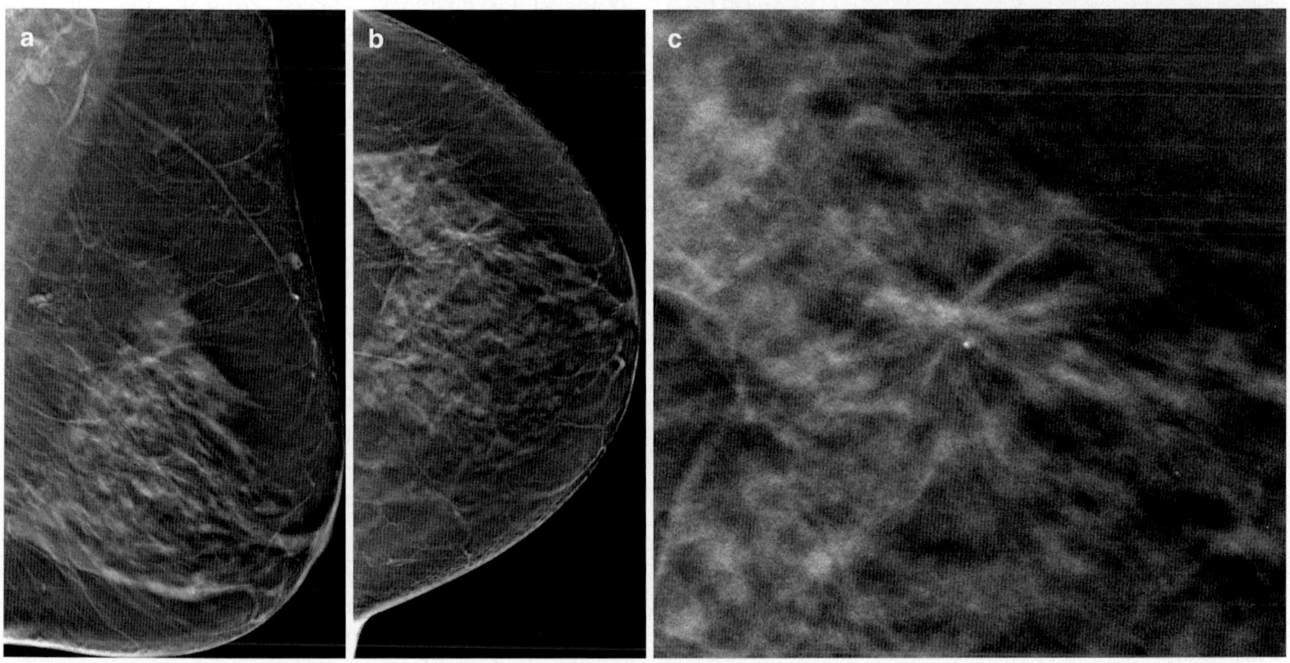

Fig. 4.14 The left DBT (**a**) MLO view showed no definite abnormality, but in the left DBT CC view (**b**), an architectural distortion (AD) was detected. (**c**) A close-up of the AD in the CC view (All used with permission from Andrejeva et al. [103])

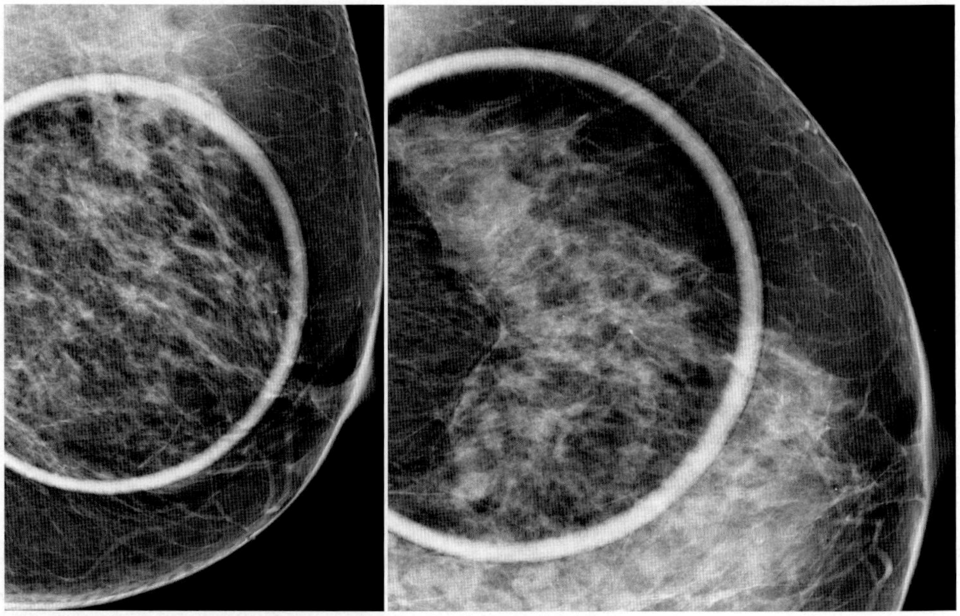

Fig. 4.15 The breast cancer was not visible in the spot compression in MLO or CC view (All used with permission from Andrejeva et al. [103])

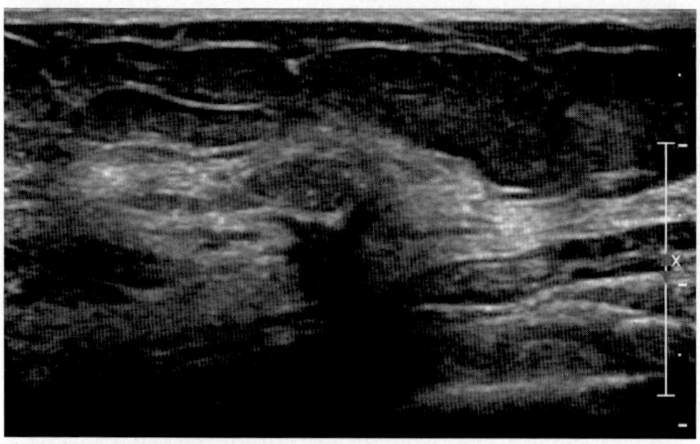

Fig. 4.16 Ultrasonography targeted at 3 o'clock in the breast revealed a hypoechoic lesion (Used with permission from Andrejeva et al. [103])

Key Points from Reader Studies on Breast Cancer Detection

DBT has shown to increase breast cancer detection in a variety of image protocols. However:

- Relatively few studies have found any clear improvements when using tomosynthesis [68, 70, 72, 75] alone (Table 4.1a, b).
- Accuracy of tomosynthesis has increased with the use of additional views (MLO plus CC) and when used as an adjunct to mammography [68, 73–75, 78, 81]
- A majority of studies using tomosynthesis combined with mammography in two-view imaging have found significant improvements. This image protocol has resulted in the largest improvements
- The potential of tomosynthesis has been validated accounting for reader variability, within and in between different mammography centers
- The interpretation time has increased in relation to mammography with 36–85 %, depending on the image protocol used for tomosynthesis

Population-Based Screening Trials

Introduction

As a medical imaging device, digital breast tomosynthesis is still undergoing large developments and is currently primarily used for symptomatic women. However, the long-term vision is to apply the technique for asymptomatic women in screening programs. Therefore, large population-based trials are currently ongoing that integrate tomosynthesis in the screening. In this section, trials and results are presented (Table 4.3).

Norwegian Trial

The Oslo tomosynthesis screening trial (OTST) evaluates tomosynthesis as a part of the screening program. The aim is to recruit 18,000 women in the age range 50–69. The trial comprises four arms with different reading strategies: mammography alone, mammography with computer-aided diagnosis, tomosynthesis with mammography, and tomosynthesis with synthesized 2D images. There have been two papers published on the first 12,600 women. In the first analysis, OTST I, the two primary modes of tomosynthesis plus mammography versus mammography alone were compared [105]. There were 27 % more breast cancers detected by the tomosynthesis modality (invasive and in situ cancers combined) and a 40 % increased detection of invasive breast cancers. These were associated with a decrease in false-positive rates with 13 %. For the whole study population, there were

Table 4.3 The results of screening trials in breast cancer detection rate, recall rate, or false-positive rate

		2D mammography (DM)			DBT		
Study[a]	Subjects (DM/DBT)	Detection per 1,000 women	Recall rate	False-positive rate	Detection per 1,000 women	Recall rate	False-positive rate
Oslo (OTST) I [105]	12,631	6.1		6.1	8.0 (+27*)		5.3 (−13.1*)
Oslo (OTST) II [106]	12,501	7.1	3.7	10.3	9.4 (+30*)	2.9 (−21.6*)	8.5 (−17.5*)
Yale I [107]	1,799 (1,475/324)		11.9			4.9 (−58.8*)	
Yale II [108]	13,174 (7,058/6,116)	5.2	11.7		5.7 (+9.6)	8.4 (−28.2*)	
Houston Breast Center	23,355 (13,856/9,499)	4	8.7		5.4 (+35)	5.5 (−37.5*)	
Trento/Verona (STORM) [109]	7,292	5.3	4.4		8.1 (+52.8*)	3.5 (−20*)	
Malmö (MBTST)	7,500	6.3	2.2		8.5 (+35)	3.3 (+50)	

All screening trials to date show statistically significant benefits in using DBT together with DM in comparison to conventional DM in either increased breast cancer detection or reduced recall rates/false-positive rates or both. The numbers in the parentheses show the percentage increase or decrease in performance measure. Statistical significance is indicated with an asterisk (*)

[a]The trials performed at Yale University and at Houston Breast Center uses non-paired retrospective study designs with single independent reading, while the other trials are prospective using paired image sampling with double reading. The Malmö (MBTST) trial compares one-view tomosynthesis (DBT) alone versus mammography (DM). The other trials investigate the efficacy of two-view DBT combined with DM. The OTST and the MBTST have incorporated arbitration management in their study designs

25 additional breast cancers detected in the tomosynthesis reading arm. A majority of them were small high-grade tumors (88 % were smaller than 15 mm, 36 % smaller than 10 mm) depicted as either spiculated tumors or architectural distortions (68 %). They were distributed in breasts of various densities, but most of them (84 %) were found in scattered fibroglandular or heterogeneously dense breasts. The mean interpretation time was about twice as large for the tomosynthesis modality and the radiation dose doubled compared to that of mammography alone.

The second analysis, OTST II, evaluated the performance of double reading with digital mammography, with double reading of tomosynthesis [106]. Double reading can improve the sensitivity, but may also result in an increase in recall rates. To reduce the recall rate, double reading with arbitration management (e.g., consensus decision) has been implemented in several European organized mammography screening programs. Double tomosynthesis reading was found to increase breast cancer detection rate by 30 % at a reduced recall rate by 22 %, in relation to double reading with mammography. The false-positive interpretations were reduced by 18 %. Double reading using tomosynthesis detected 27 additional invasive breast cancers with similar distributions as the prior analysis (OTST I). Synthesized 2D images were partially used in adjunct to tomosynthesis, as a substitute to mammography (Fig. 4.10), which reduced the average fibroglandular doses with 45 % (to 1.95 mGy ± 0.58).

US Trials

Two screening trials have recently been conducted at Yale, New Haven, USA. The first trial, Yale I, reported recall rates examining screening mammography in women undergoing tomosynthesis with mammography compared to those undergoing mammography alone, reviewed in different screening facilities [107]. Dedicated breast imagers interpreted screening mammograms of 1,799 women: 324 cases at tomosynthesis in adjunct to mammography and 1,475 cases at mammography only. The recall rates were also analyzed with regard to type of mammographic abnormality. The overall recall rate for DBT and 2D mammography decreased with 59 % for the tomosynthesis modality. When subdividing recall rates into type of mammographic abnormality, the largest reduction was found for asymmetries (1.8 % vs. 8.2 %, $p < 0.0001$).

The second trial, Yale II [108], compared cancer detection and recall rates for the same imaging modalities with a substantially larger population of women screened ($n = 13{,}174$). Recall rates were stratified by breast density and age. The overall recall rate for patients in the tomosynthesis group was 8.4 % compared to 11.7 % for conventional imaging ($p < 0.01$). Addition of tomosynthesis reduced recall rates for all breast density and patient age groups, with significant differences ($p < 0.05$) found for scattered fibroglandular, heterogeneously dense, and extremely dense breast density and for patients younger than 40 years and aged 40–49, 50–59, and 60–69. In patients receiving tomosynthesis, the cancer detection rate was 5.7 versus 5.2 per 1,000 in patients receiving 2D imaging alone ($p = 0.80$). Patients undergoing 2D+3D mammography had substantially lower screening recall rates. The largest reductions were for women under 50 years of age and for women with dense breasts.

Rose et al. [110] evaluated the efficacy of tomosynthesis in an observational screening study at Houston Breast Center, TX, USA. Recall rates, biopsy rates, and cancer detection rates were compared for six radiologists who interpreted mammography cases with ($n = 9{,}499$) and without ($n = 13{,}856$) tomosynthesis, accounting for reader variability. The introduction of tomosynthesis resulted in significant reduction in recall rates, from 8.7 to 5.5 %, and nonsignificant reductions in biopsy rates, e.g., from 15.2 to 13.5 % per

1,000 women screened. The cancer detection rate increased from 4 to 5.4 % per 1,000 screening examinations, while the invasive cancer detection rates increased from 2.8 to 4.3 % per 1,000 screening examinations.

Italian Trial

The Italian screening trial termed STORM [89] (Screening with Tomosynthesis OR standard Mammography) evaluated tomosynthesis in two-sequential reading phases, starting with interpretation of mammography alone, followed by interpretation of tomosynthesis with mammography. A total of 7,292 women aged 48–71 was recruited in the trial at the Trento and Verona screening facilities, Italy. Cancer detection rate was improved with 53 % for the tomosynthesis modality; 20 additional breast cancers were detected in the entire screening population. The recall rate was reduced with 20 % (Table 4.3). The incremental cancer detection rate in tomosynthesis was evident in both age stratifications (e.g., above and below 60 years of age) and in various breast density types (2.5 in denser breasts vs. 2.8 in less dense breasts, per 1,000 women). The findings in reduced recall rates were similar for different age intervals and breast density types.

Swedish Trial

The Malmö breast tomosynthesis screening trial (MBTST) is currently in progress. Women 40 years of age and older are randomly selected from the screening program to participate in the trial. The study evaluates the efficacy of one-view DBT alone in comparison to two-view imaging with DM. The aim is to recruit 15,000 patients who undergo both DM and DBT examinations. A follow-up period of 2 years after the intervention period will be used to establish the ground truth on the actual numbers of breast cancers and benign or normal cases. The number of breast cancers detected by the different techniques will be compared. A cost-effective analysis will be performed including potential benefits and acceptability to women undergoing screening. Results from an interim analysis showed improved breast cancer detection for DBT with 35 % at an increase in recall rate by 50 %; however, the recall rates were relatively low (3.3 % for one-view DBT and 2.2 % for DM) [111].

UK Trial

The TOMosynthesis with digital MammographY (TOMMY) trial is a retrospective multicenter multireader trial in the UK's breast cancer screening program that evaluates sensitivity and specificity of tomosynthesis in adjunct to mammography versus mammography alone. Twenty-five radiologists from different mammography centers participate in the trial, which have had extensive training in tomosynthesis by interpreting 500 image sets prior to the study. As a whole, the trial includes 7,000 women within 47–73 years of age, recalled after a positive DM screen. There are more than 1,000 verified cancers included in the population. A sub analysis will be made on small subtle masses and calcifications and in breast density. In addition, the radiologists interpret a test set before and after the study to evaluate effects of reader experience. Initial findings showed a small but borderline significant ($p = 0.05$) improvement in sensitivity for tomosynthesis combined with mammography over mammography alone, 88 % (955/1,087) versus 85 % (929/1,087). This was associated with a significantly ($p < 0.001$) greater specificity for tomosynthesis and DM compared to DM alone, 67 % (3,045/4,514) versus 55 % (2,474/4,514) [66].

Key Points from Tomosynthesis Screening Trials

Screening studies of tomosynthesis used in adjunct to DM or synthesized 2D compared to conventional 2D imaging show:

- A 27 % increase in detection of all cancers (invasive and in situ cancers combined).
- A 40 % increase in invasive breast cancers.
- A 13 % decrease in false-positive rates.
- Double reading of tomosynthesis-based examinations significantly increased the breast cancer detection with 30 %, while it significantly reduced the false-positive interpretations with 18 %.
- Reduction in overall recall rates with as much as 59 %. A stratification showed:
  - Large reduction of recalls in asymmetries
  - Significant improvements in a variety of breast densities and age groups, but particularly in women with dense breasts and in women below 50 years of age
- Increase in breast cancer detection with 53 %, associated with a 20 % reduction in false-positive rate

Complementary Applications

Several diagnostic procedures are being evaluated today in adjunct to tomosynthesis that provide additional image information to the radiologist. These can be divided into methods based on multimodality imaging and into advanced applications of tomosynthesis imaging. In difficult cases, the use of nuclear medicine [112], contrast media, or optical procedures [113] can be exploited to reduce false-positive rates and avoid unnecessary biopsies. Other applications may improve the actual biopsy procedure.

Contrast media is a well-known approach to characterize abnormalities. As the breast cancer grows, it is accompanied by development of new blood vessels (angiogenesis) with increased permeability [114]. The difference in absorption in vascular contrast agents in malignant breast tissue and in normal/benign tissues is used in the imaging process. Currently, contrast-enhanced MRI (CE-MRI) is the standard for vascular imaging of breast cancers,

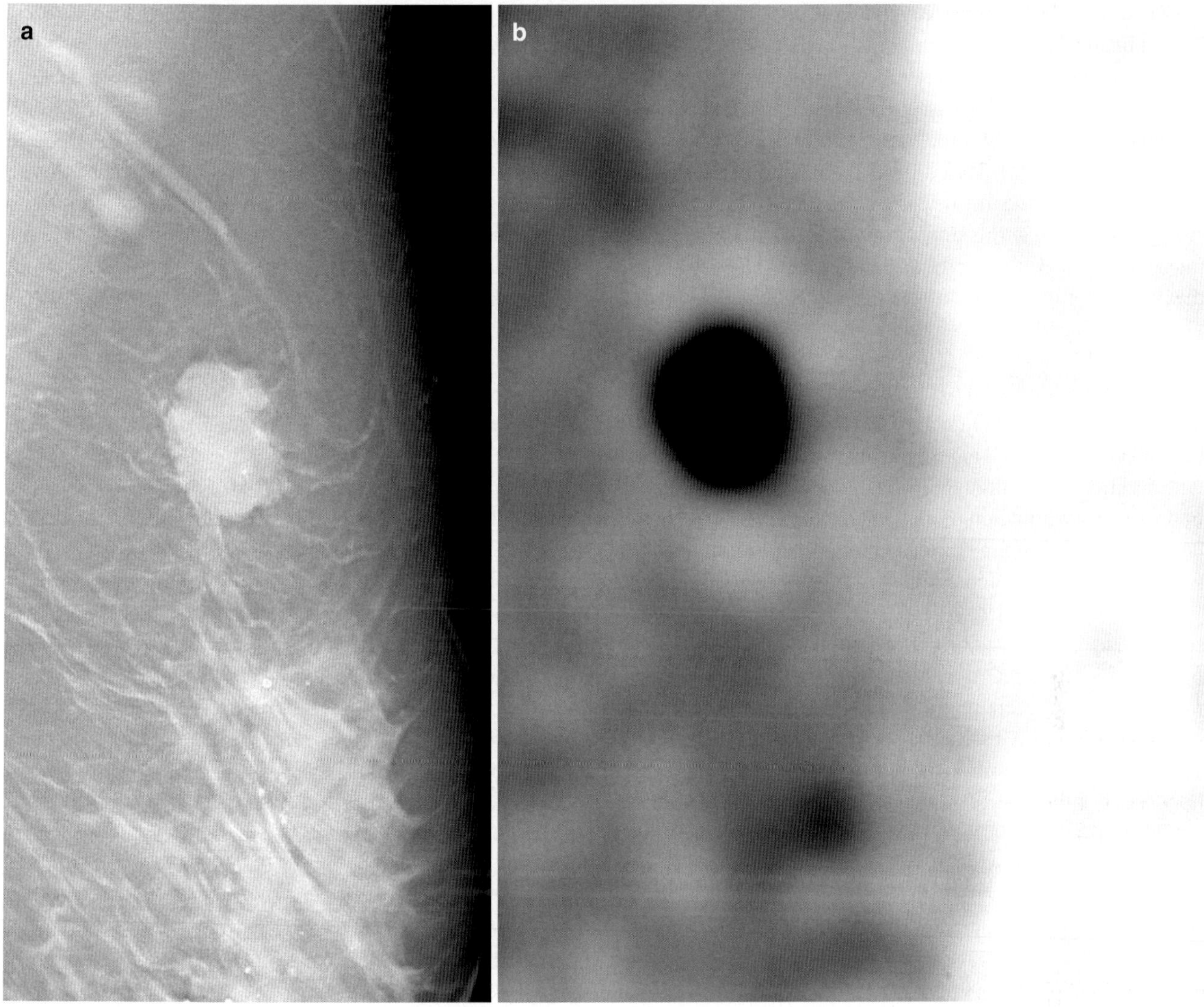

Fig. 4.17 An invasive ductal carcinoma, grade 2, can be seen in the upper quadrant of the breast in the tomosynthesis slice (**a**) and strong focal tracer uptake is present at the corresponding location in the gamma slice (**b**). A second smaller area of focal tracer uptake can be seen in the lower region of the gamma image, which corresponds to a region of radiodense tissue as seen on the X-ray slice (Images courtesy of Professor Mark B. Williams, University of Virginia, Charlottesville, USA)

which uses a gadolinium-based contrast substance as a contrast agent [115]. As a substitute, tomosynthesis could be performed after administrating intravenous-iodinated contrast material (e.g., CE-DBT). This would be less costly and more widely applicable than CE-MRI. In feasibility study, Carton et al. [116] found CE-DBT to provide morphology and kinetic information about malignancies that was qualitatively equivalent with the information obtained from CE-MRI.

Methods based on nuclear medicine return functional information, which is co-registered with the anatomical information obtained at X-ray imaging. A hybrid scanner (e.g., gamma camera and digital X-ray detector) that uses X-ray and gamma emission tomosynthesis conjoint has been developed and evaluated [112]. During the procedure, the patient is injected with a tracer (^{99m}Tc sestamibi), which accumulates preferentially in breast cancers. Absorbed dose to the breast is around 2 mGy (4.8 mGy to the whole body) and the imaging procedure takes around 12 min per breast. The dual-modality tomosynthesis (DMT) procedure may be particularly advantageous for women with radiographically dense breasts. In a small study among patients scheduled for biopsy, the system yielded high sensitivity and a perfect (100 %) specificity. Figure 4.17a, b shows a paired X-ray tomosynthesis and gamma emission tomosynthesis slices obtained by the DMT scanner.

Optical tomography has been evaluated with regard to the saturation state of hemoglobin and oxygen in adjunct to tomosynthesis [113]. The optical characteristic was found to differ substantially in between malignant lesions and benign lesions or normal tissues, which was found to be useful in characterizing lesions.

Vacuum-assisted biopsy (VAB) based on tomosynthesis, as a substitute for VAB with conventional 2D mammography, can increase the accuracy in targeting the lesion. VAB uses computer technology to pinpoint small masses or calcifications for biopsy. Multiple tissue samples are collected in the indicated area(s). Based on the obtained histology, the radiologist recommends the patient for surgery or other decision. Using DBT in this application may yield a more accurate placement of the target in depth. Other advantages are that it is faster and more dose efficient than the conventional procedure since it requires fewer image views to target the lesion [117].

Two recent studies have been published evaluating with ultrasound (US) as an adjunct to DBT [76, 118]. None of these have, however, showed any significance performance increase with addition of US, though in one of them a trend was seen in improved discrimination of malignancy [118]. As in the other described applications, there are limited clinical studies and further research is required to identify their specific roles.

Computer-aided detection (CAD) is used as an assisting supplement to the radiologist's own interpretation of the image, to highlight structures that are suspicious for malignancy. In screening programs, CAD has shown to have a positive effect on breast cancer detection [119, 120], but occasionally it has suffered from low specificity. There is hope in that the use of tomosynthesis data could increase CAD performance further. Several studies have been performed evaluating CAD for tomosynthesis for breast cancer detection. Singh et al. [121] have developed a CAD program specifically for mass detection, which performed at a sensitivity of 85 % with 2.4 false positives per case, while Reiser et al. [95] developed a calcification detection program that performed at a sensitivity of 86 % at 1.3 false positives per image volume. Mazurowski et al. [122] investigated the possibilities in translating the knowledge of detection problems from 2D CAD system directly to 3D DBT. The computational aid for a new medical imaging device is usually a time-consuming process, and it could speed up the development process of 3D CAD system if inter-modality information could be used. In the Mazurowski study, similar performance levels were found in tomosynthesis and mammography, hence showing that the use of mutual information can be beneficial. The results and progress in CAD systems for DBT are encouraging, taking into account that the studies until now have been comprised by limited sets of patient images.

Summary

As shown in reported trials, digital breast tomosynthesis can help to reduce one major problem in conventional mammography, namely, the effect of tissue overlap, which is substantial in breasts with dense parenchyma. Screening trial results are largely in agreement with those obtained from clinical reader trials and show promising findings. One of them found an increase in breast cancer detection rate with as much as 53 %, obtained at a reduced false-positive rate. Another trial showed significant benefits using DBT in reduced recall rate, which were primarily associated with asymmetries. When the results were stratified according to age (patients younger than 40 years and aged 40–49, 50–59, and 60–69), significant benefits were found for all age groups but were particularly large for women below 50 years of age. A third trial showed a significant increase in breast cancer detection rate, and a majority of the incremental breast cancers were found to be invasive node-negative carcinomas, depicted as spiculated masses or architectural distortions. Double reading with tomosynthesis-based examinations plus arbitration management significantly reduced the false-positive interpretations, while increasing the breast cancer detection rate.

A majority of the clinical studies show clear improvements when DBT has been used in a two-view imaging setting as an adjunct to DM. There are, however, both advantages and disadvantages in such an image protocol. While the performance is higher, the radiation dose is increased and the review time is typically longer. The increased performance of additional views must be considered in relation to the extra radiation dose, time to review the cases, and examination costs, which increases accordingly. Reading time is an important consideration, and visualization tools, such as the slab function, synthesized 2D (contributes with a dose reduction by ~50 %), and others, are currently in use and under continued development for maximized reading and dose efficiency [95, 96].

Like in 2D digital mammography, the components in the DBT imaging process, e.g., image acquisition, storage, and display, can be optimized and manipulated separately. Future work is needed to continue the development and validation of image reconstruction algorithms with better image quality, to optimize the digital breast tomosynthesis design, and to develop the imaging system and display further. Retrospective trials have shown that DBT can improve the mammographic accuracy significantly, but it does not achieve a perfect performance. A problem that still may occur is the lack of lesion contrast (e.g., minimal attenuation differences between the lesion and surrounding tissue), which can hamper breast cancer detection also in 3D imaging. In these and other difficult cases, the use of procedures that combines tomosynthesis with methods from nuclear medicine, contrast media, ultrasonography, and others may become valuable. The evolvement and use of these in adjunct to tomosynthesis depends on forthcoming study results.

Acknowledgments The author is grateful for valuable comments and helpful insights from Prof. Sören Mattsson and Dr. Dev Chakraborty.

The author also acknowledges the help from Dr. Federica Zanca and Dr. Christian Waldherr, who contributed with datasets, analyses, and other relevant information. The author was supported by the Franke and Margareta Bergqvist Foundation.

References

1. Sasieni PD, Shelton J, Ormiston-Smith N, Thomson CS, Silcocks PB. What is the lifetime risk of developing cancer?: the effect of adjusting for multiple primaries. Br J Cancer. 2011;105:460–5.
2. Veronesi U, Boyle P, Goldhirsch A, Orecchia R, Viale G. Breast cancer. Lancet. 2005;365:1727–41.
3. Tavtigian SV, et al. The complete BRCA2 gene and mutations in chromosome 13q-linked kindreds. Nat Genet. 1996;12:333–7.
4. ICRP (International Commission on Radiological Protection) Publication 103. Recommendation of the International Commission on Radiological Protection. Ann ICRP.
5. Boyd NF, et al. Quantitative classification of mammographic densities and breast cancer risk: results from the Canadian National Breast Screening Study. J Natl Cancer Inst. 1995;87:670–5.
6. Lash TL, Aschengrau A. Alcohol drinking and risk of breast cancer. Breast J. 2000;6:396–9.
7. Donville S, Brien R. Exercising to reduce breast cancer risk. Nurs Manag. 2000;36–7.
8. Leborgne R. Diagnosis of tumors of the breast by simple roentgenography; calcifications in carcinomas. Am J Roentgenol Radium Ther. 1951;65:1–11.
9. Tabar L, et al. Reduction in mortality from breast cancer after mass screening with mammography. Randomised trial from the Breast Cancer Screening Working Group of the Swedish National Board of Health and Welfare. Lancet. 1985;1:829–32.
10. Andersson I, et al. Mammographic screening and mortality from breast cancer: the Malmo mammographic screening trial. BMJ. 1988;297:943–8.
11. Frisell J, et al. Randomized study of mammography screening–preliminary report on mortality in the Stockholm trial. Breast Cancer Res Treat. 1991;18:49–56.
12. Bjurstam N, et al. The Gothenburg breast cancer screening trial: preliminary results on breast cancer mortality for women aged 39-49. J Natl Cancer Inst Monogr. 1997;53–5.
13. Shapiro S, Strax P, Venet L. Periodic breast cancer screening in reducing mortality from breast cancer. JAMA. 1971;215:1777–85.
14. Roberts MM, et al. Edinburgh trial of screening for breast cancer: mortality at seven years. Lancet. 1990;335:241–6.
15. Miller AB, Baines CJ, To T, Wall C. Canadian National Breast Screening Study: 1. Breast cancer detection and death rates among women aged 40 to 49 years. CMAJ. 1992;147:1459–76.
16. Miller AB, Baines CJ, To T, Wall C. Canadian National Breast Screening Study: 2. Breast cancer detection and death rates among women aged 50 to 59 years. CMAJ. 1992;147:1477–88.
17. Pisano ED, et al. Diagnostic performance of digital versus film mammography for breast-cancer screening. N Engl J Med. 2005; 353:1773–83. doi:10.1056/NEJMoa052911.
18. Holland R, Mravunac M, Hendriks JH, Bekker BV. So-called interval cancers of the breast. Pathologic and radiologic analysis of sixty-four cases. Cancer. 1982;49:2527–33.
19. Skaane P. Studies comparing screen-film mammography and full-field digital mammography in breast cancer screening: updated review. Acta Radiol. 2009;50:3–14.
20. Kolb TM, Lichy J, Newhouse JH. Comparison of the performance of screening mammography, physical examination, and breast US and evaluation of factors that influence them: an analysis of 27,825 patient evaluations. Radiology. 2002;225:165–75.
21. Kalender WA, et al. High-resolution spiral CT of the breast at very low dose: concept and feasibility considerations. Eur Radiol. 2012; 22:1–8.
22. Boone JM, et al. Computed tomography for imaging the breast. J Mammary Gland Biol Neoplasia. 2006;11:103–11.
23. Lindfors KK, et al. Dedicated breast CT: initial clinical experience. Radiology. 2008;246:725–33.
24. FDA U.S. Food and Drug Administration. Medical devices. Selenia Dimensions 3D System (P080003).
25. Pisano ED, Yaffe MJ. Digital mammography. Radiology. 2005;234: 353–62.
26. Saunders Jr RS, Samei E. The effect of breast compression on mass conspicuity in digital mammography. Med Phys. 2008;35:4464–73.
27. Miller D, Livingstone V, Herbison P. Interventions for relieving the pain and discomfort of screening mammography. Cochrane Database Syst Rev. 2008;(1):CD002942.
28. Poulos A, McLean D, Rickard M, Heard R. Breast compression in mammography: how much is enough? Australas Radiol. 2003;47: 121–6.
29. Venta LA, et al. Rates and causes of disagreement in interpretation of full-field digital mammography and film-screen mammography in a diagnostic setting. AJR Am J Roentgenol. 2001;176: 1241–8.
30. Pisano ED, et al. Interpretation of digital mammograms: comparison of speed and accuracy of soft-copy versus printed-film display. Radiology. 2002;223:483–8.
31. Obenauer S, et al. Soft copy versus hard copy reading in digital mammography. J Digit Imaging. 2003;16:341–4.
32. Skaane P, et al. Breast lesion detection and classification: comparison of screen-film mammography and full-field digital mammography with soft-copy reading–observer performance study. Radiology. 2005;237:37–44.
33. Pisano ED, et al. American College of Radiology Imaging Network digital mammographic imaging screening trial: objectives and methodology. Radiology. 2005;236:404–12.
34. Bartella L, Perry N, Young KC, Lawinski CP, Evans D. Assessment of full field digital mammography (FFDM) detected microcalcification is not hindered by low spatial resolution. Breast Cancer Res. 2002;4 Suppl 1:21.
35. Chan HP, et al. Digital mammography: observer performance study of the effects of pixel size on the characterization of malignant and benign microcalcifications. Acad Radiol. 2001;8:454–66.
36. Fischer U, et al. Comparative study in patients with microcalcifications: full-field digital mammography vs screen-film mammography. Eur Radiol. 2002;12:2679–83.
37. Obenauer S, et al. Screen film vs full-field digital mammography: image quality, detectability and characterization of lesions. Eur Radiol. 2002;12:1697–702.
38. Kim HH, et al. Comparison of calcification specificity in digital mammography using soft-copy display versus screen-film mammography. AJR Am J Roentgenol. 2006;187:47–50.
39. Suryanarayanan S, Karellas A, Vedantham S, Sechopoulos I, D'Orsi CJ. Detection of simulated microcalcifications in a phantom with digital mammography: effect of pixel size. Radiology. 2007;244: 130–7.
40. Krug KB, et al. Image quality of digital direct flat-panel mammography versus an analog screen-film technique using a phantom model. AJR Am J Roentgenol. 2007;188:399–407.
41. Skaane P. Screening of breast cancer. In: Kahán Z, Tot T, editors. Breast cancer, a heterogeneous disease entity the very early stages. Dordrecht/New York: Springer; 2011. p. 23–44.
42. Rowlands JA, Hunter DM, Araj N. X-ray imaging using amorphous selenium: a photoinduced discharge readout method for digital mammography. Med Phys. 1991;18:421–31.
43. Mahesh M. AAPM/RSNA physics tutorial for residents: digital mammography: an overview. Radiographics. 2004;24:1747–60.

44. Vuylsteke P, Schoeters E, Mortsel B. Computerized tomography for industrial applications and image processing in radiology. In: DGZfP proceedings BB 67-CD. Berlin; 1999. p. 87–101 .
45. Ziedses des Plantes BG. Eine neue methode zur di erenzierung in der roentgenographie. Acta Radiol. 1932;13:182–92.
46. Goodsitt MM. Introduction: In: Reiser I, Glick S, editors. Tomosynthesis imaging. London: Taylor & Francis; 2014.
47. Garrison JB, Grant DG, Guier WH, Johns RJ. Three dimensional roentgenography. Am J Roentgenol Radium Ther Nucl Med. 1969;105:903–8.
48. Grant DG. Tomosynthesis: a three-dimensional radiographic imaging technique. IEEE Trans Biomed Eng. 1972;19:20–8.
49. Dobbins 3rd JT, Godfrey DJ. Digital x-ray tomosynthesis: current state of the art and clinical potential. Phys Med Biol. 2003;48: R65–106.
50. Lewin JM, Niklason L. Advanced applications of digital mammography: tomosynthesis and contrast-enhanced digital mammography. Semin Roentgenol. 2007;42:243–52.
51. Sechopoulos I. A review of breast tomosynthesis. Part II. Image reconstruction, processing and analysis, and advanced applications. Med Phys. 2013;40:014302.
52. Matos Monteiro J, Santos Ribeiro A, Lacerda L. Review on digital breast tomosynthesis patents. Recent Patents Biomed Eng. 2012;5: 175–82.
53. Bissonette M, et al. Digital breast tomosynthesis using an amorphous selenium flat panel detector. Proc SPIE. 2005;5745:529–40.
54. Park JM, Franken Jr EA, Garg M, Fajardo LL, Niklason LT. Breast tomosynthesis: present considerations and future applications. Radiographics. 2007;27 Suppl 1:S231–40.
55. Qian X, et al. High resolution stationary digital breast tomosynthesis using distributed carbon nanotube x-ray source array. Med Phys. 2012;39:2090–9.
56. Dobbins 3rd JT. Tomosynthesis imaging: at a translational crossroads. Med Phys. 2009;36:1956–67.
57. Park JC, et al. Ultra-fast digital tomosynthesis reconstruction using general-purpose GPU programming for image-guided radiation therapy. Technol Cancer Res Treat. 2011;10:295–306.
58. Sidky EY. Introduction: In: Reiser I, Glick S, editors. Tomosynthesis imaging. London: Taylor & Francis; 2014.
59. Wu T, Moore RH, Rafferty EA, Kopans DB. A comparison of reconstruction algorithms for breast tomosynthesis. Med Phys. 2004;31:2636–47.
60. Sidky EY, et al. Enhanced imaging of microcalcifications in digital breast tomosynthesis through improved image-reconstruction algorithms. Med Phys. 2009;36:4920–32.
61. Zhang Y, et al. A comparative study of limited-angle cone-beam reconstruction methods for breast tomosynthesis. Med Phys. 2006; 33:3781–95.
62. Wu T, Moore RH, Kopans DB. Voting strategy for artifact reduction in digital breast tomosynthesis. Med Phys. 2006;33(7):2461–71.
63. Diekmann F, et al. Thick slices from tomosynthesis data sets: phantom study for the evaluation of different algorithms. J Digit Imaging. 2009;22:519–26.
64. Gur D, et al. Dose reduction in digital breast tomosynthesis (DBT) screening using synthetically reconstructed projection images: an observer performance study. Acad Radiol. 2012;19:166–71.
65. Skaane P, et al. In: RSNA 2013, VSBR31-07 Breast Series: Emerging technologies in breast imaging. Radiological Society of North America, Chicago, IL.
66. Gilbert FJ, Tucker L, Nagarajan S, Willsher P, Astley S, Young KC, Duffy S. Comparison of FFDM with DBT in a UK retrospective reading study. Vienna: European Congress of Radiology; 2014.
67. Poplack SP, Tosteson TD, Kogel CA, Nagy HM. Digital breast tomosynthesis: initial experience in 98 women with abnormal digital screening mammography. AJR Am J Roentgenol. 2007;189: 616–23.
68. Svahn T, et al. The diagnostic accuracy of dual-view digital mammography, single-view breast tomosynthesis and a dual-view combination of breast tomosynthesis and digital mammography in a free-response observer performance study. Radiat Prot Dosimetry. 2010;139:113–7.
69. Gennaro G, et al. Digital breast tomosynthesis versus digital mammography: a clinical performance study. Eur Radiol. 2010;20:1545–53.
70. Michell M, et al. Two-view 2D digital mammography versus one-view digital breast tomosynthesis. Breast Cancer Res. 2010;12(Suppl 3).
71. Svane G, et al. Clinical experience of photon counting breast tomosynthesis: comparison with traditional mammography. Acta Radiol. 2011;52:134–42.
72. Svahn TM, et al. Breast tomosynthesis and digital mammography: a comparison of diagnostic accuracy. Br J Radiol. 2012;85:e1074–82.
73. Wallis MG, Moa E, Zanca F, Leifland K, Danielsson M. Two-view and single-view tomosynthesis versus full-field digital mammography: high-resolution X-ray imaging observer study. Radiology. 2012;262:788–96.
74. Zanca F, et al. Diagnostic accuracy of digital mammography versus tomosynthesis: effect of radiologists' experience. In: Proceedings of SPIE 8318, Medical Imaging 2012: Image Perception, Observer Performance, and Technology Assessment, 83180W (23 Feb 2012). San Deigo, CA; 2012.
75. Waldherr C, et al. Value of one-view breast tomosynthesis versus two-view mammography in diagnostic workup of women with clinical signs and symptoms and in women recalled from screening. AJR Am J Roentgenol. 2013;200:226–31.
76. Thibault F, et al. Digital breast tomosynthesis versus mammography and breast ultrasound: a multireader performance study. Eur Radiol. 2013;23(9):2441–9.
77. Good WF, et al. Digital breast tomosynthesis: a pilot observer study. AJR Am J Roentgenol. 2008;190:865–9.
78. Gur D, et al. Digital breast tomosynthesis: observer performance study. AJR Am J Roentgenol. 2009;193:586–91.
79. Teertstra HJ, et al. Breast tomosynthesis in clinical practice: initial results. Eur Radiol. 2010;20:16–24.
80. Smith AP, Rafferty EA, Niklason LT. Clinical performance of breast tomosynthesis as a function of radiologist experience level. Lect Notes Comput Sci. 2008;5116:61–6.
81. Michell MJ, et al. A comparison of the accuracy of film-screen mammography, full-field digital mammography, and digital breast tomosynthesis. Clin Radiol. 2012;67:976–81.
82. Rafferty EA, et al. Assessing radiologist performance using combined digital mammography and breast tomosynthesis compared with digital mammography alone: results of a multicenter, multireader trial. Radiology. 2013;266:104–13.
83. Gennaro G, et al. Performance comparison of single-view digital breast tomosynthesis plus single-view digital mammography with two-view digital mammography. Eur Radiol. 2013;23:664–72.
84. Thompson JD, Manning DJ, Hogg P. The value of observer performance studies in dose optimization: a focus on free-response receiver operating characteristic methods. J Nucl Med Technol. 2013;41:57–64.
85. Chakraborty DP. New developments in observer performance methodology in medical imaging. Semin Nucl Med. 2011;41:401–18.
86. Chakraborty DP, Berbaum KS. Observer studies involving detection and localization: modeling, analysis, and validation. Med Phys. 2004;31:2313–30.
87. Svahn TM, Tingberg A. Observer experiments with tomosynthesis. In: Reiser I, Glick S, editors. Tomosynthesis imaging. Boca Raton: Taylor & Francis; 2014.
88. Smith-Bindman R, et al. Comparison of screening mammography in the United States and the United Kingdom. JAMA. 2003;290: 2129–37.
89. Houssami N, Skaane P. Overview of the evidence on digital breast tomosynthesis in breast cancer detection. Breast. 2013;22:101–8.

90. Metz CE. Some practical issues of experimental design and data analysis in radiological ROC studies. Invest Radiol. 1989;24: 234–45.
91. Beam CA, Layde PM, Sullivan DC. Variability in the interpretation of screening mammograms by US radiologists. Findings from a national sample. Arch Intern Med. 1996;156:209–13.
92. Feinstein AR. A bibliography of publications on observer variability. J Chronic Dis. 1985;38:619–32.
93. Elmore JG, Feinstein AR. A bibliography of publications on observer variability (final installment). J Clin Epidemiol. 1992;45: 567–80.
94. The Breast Imaging-Reporting and Data System (BIRADS). Reston: American College of Radiology. Reston, VA; 1992.
95. Reiser I, et al. Automated detection of microcalcification clusters for digital breast tomosynthesis using projection data only: a preliminary study. Med Phys. 2008;35:1486–93.
96. Chen Y, Lo JY, Dobbins 3rd JT. Importance of point-by-point back projection correction for isocentric motion in digital breast tomosynthesis: relevance to morphology of structures such as microcalcifications. Med Phys. 2007;34:3885–92.
97. Wald NJ, et al. UKCCCR multicentre randomised controlled trial of one and two view mammography in breast cancer screening. BMJ. 1995;311:1189–93.
98. Rafferty E, Kopans D, Wu T, Moore R. Breast tomosynthesis: will a single view do? Chicago: Radiological society of North America; 2004. http://rsna2004.rsna.rsna.org/rsna2004/V2004/search/search.cvn?ACTION=SEARCH&starttab=4. Accessed 1 Aug 2009.
99. Rafferty EA, Niklason L, Jameson-Meehan L. Breast tomosynthesis: one view or two? Presented at the Radiological Society of North America (RSNA), Session SSG01-04 Breast Imaging: digital tomosynthesis. Chicago, IL; 2006.
100. Rafferty EA, et al. Diagnostic accuracy and recall rates for digital mammography and digital mammography combined with one-view and two-view tomosynthesis: results of an enriched reader study. AJR Am J Roentgenol. 2014;202:273–81.
101. Spangler ML, et al. Detection and classification of calcifications on digital breast tomosynthesis and 2D digital mammography: a comparison. AJR Am J Roentgenol. 2011;196:320–4.
102. Kopans D, Gavenonis S, Halpern E, Moore R. Calcifications in the breast and digital breast tomosynthesis. Breast J. 2011;17:638–44.
103. Andrejeva L, et al. Stage 1 breast cancer diagnosed by tomosynthesis in dense breasts. Appl Radiol. 2012;41(12):27–9.
104. Uematsu T. The emerging role of breast tomosynthesis. Breast Cancer. 2013;20:204–12.
105. Skaane P, et al. Comparison of digital mammography alone and digital mammography plus tomosynthesis in a population-based screening program. Radiology. 2013;267:47–56.
106. Skaane P, et al. Prospective trial comparing full-field digital mammography (FFDM) versus combined FFDM and tomosynthesis in a population-based screening programme using independent double reading with arbitration. Eur Radiol. 2013;23(8):2061–71.
107. Philpotts L. Breastimaging: screening/emergingtechnologies (Initial experience with digital breast tomosynthesis in screening mammography). AJR Am J Roentgenol. 2012;198(Suppl).
108. Haas BM, et al. Comparison of tomosynthesis plus digital mammography and digital mammography alone for breast cancer screening. Radiology. 2013;269(3):694–700.
109. Ciatto S, et al. Integration of 3D digital mammography with tomosynthesis for population breast-cancer screening (STORM): a prospective comparison study. Lancet Oncol. 2013;14:583–9.
110. Rose SL, et al. Implementation of breast tomosynthesis in a routine screening practice: an observational study. AJR Am J Roentgenol. 2013;200:1401–8.
111. Zackrisson S, Lång K, Timberg P, Andersson I. Performance of one-view breast tomosynthesis versus two-view mammography in breast cancer screening: first results from the Malmö breast tomosynthesis screening trial. In: European College of Radiology. Vienna; 2014.
112. Williams MB, Judy PG, Gunn S, Majewski S. Dual-modality breast tomosynthesis. Radiology. 2010;255:191–8.
113. Fang Q, et al. Combined optical and X-ray tomosynthesis breast imaging. Radiology. 2011;258:89–97.
114. Weidner N, Semple JP, Welch WR, Folkman J. Tumor angiogenesis and metastasis–correlation in invasive breast carcinoma. -N Engl J Med. 1991;324:1–8.
115. Schnall MD, et al. Diagnostic architectural and dynamic features at breast MR imaging: multicenter study. Radiology. 2006;238: 42–53.
116. Carton AK, et al. Dual-energy contrast-enhanced digital breast tomosynthesis–a feasibility study. Br J Radiol. 2010;83:344–50.
117. Viala J, et al. Stereotactic vacuum-assisted biopsies on a digital breast 3D-tomosynthesis system. Breast J. 2013;19:4–9.
118. Padilla F, et al. Breast mass characterization using 3-dimensional automated ultrasound as an adjunct to digital breast tomosynthesis: a pilot study. J Ultrasound Med. 2013;32:93–104.
119. Skaane P, Kshirsagar A, Stapleton S, Young K, Castellino RA. Effect of computer-aided detection on independent double reading of paired screen-film and full-field digital screening mammograms. AJR Am J Roentgenol. 2007;188:377–84.
120. Gilbert FJ, et al. Single reading with computer-aided detection for screening mammography. N Engl J Med. 2008;359:1675–84.
121. Singh S, Tourassi GD, Baker JA, Samei E, Lo JY. Automated breast mass detection in 3D reconstructed tomosynthesis volumes: a featureless approach. Med Phys. 2008;35:3626–36.
122. Mazurowski MA, Lo JY, Harrawood BP, Tourassi GD. Mutual information-based template matching scheme for detection of breast masses: from mammography to digital breast tomosynthesis. J Biomed Inform. 2011;44:815–23.

5 Mammographic Signs of Breast Cancer

Mahesh K. Shetty

Introduction

The effectiveness of screening mammography in reducing mortality from breast cancer has been well documented in several randomized clinical trials. Mammographic signs of breast cancer cover a wide spectrum including the commonly encountered irregular spiculated masses, pleomorphic microcalcifications, as well as asymmetry and architectural distortion. There are certain mammographic signs that are subtle, and these account for a significant number of missed cancers. Such subtle signs include small developing densities or findings that are obscured by dense glandular tissue. The mammographic signs of breast cancer and the differential diagnosis are discussed in this chapter.

On a mammogram there are four signs that are commonly associated with breast cancer, and there are additional signs that are less commonly seen and represent subtle signs of breast cancer (Box 5.1). The two most common mammographic appearances of breast cancer on a mammogram are masses and calcifications. Masses have been reported in a higher percentage of cancers in those series that include a larger number of invasive cancers, and microcalcifications are reported in a higher percentage of cancers in series that have a larger proportion of ductal carcinoma in situ [DCIS]. Asymmetry and architectural distortion are other commonly seen signs of breast cancer although less frequently associated with breast cancer than are masses and calcifications. In a series of 1,552 breast cancers of which 1,287 were invasive, 56 % of cancers appeared mostly as masses, 29 % appeared as calcifications, with asymmetry (12 %) and architectural distortion (4 %) accounting for the remainder of the cases [1]. In a series of 543 cases of breast cancer where a larger proportion of cases were made of DCIS (36 %), microcalcifications (47 %) were seen more commonly than masses (41 %) [2]. A majority of breast cancers presenting as masses were invasive cancers [95 %], and a majority of calcifications (68 %) were associated with DCIS. Architectural distortion was seen as a sign of breast cancer in 4 % of cases in this series [2].

Box 5.1 Mammographic Signs of Breast Cancer

Classic signs of breast cancer
1. Mass
2. Architectural distortion
3. Malignant-appearing microcalcifications
4. Focal asymmetry

Subtle signs of breast cancer
1. Developing densities
2. Subtle asymmetries
3. Partially visualized abnormalities
4. One-view-only finding

The positive predictive value on a screening examination for masses and calcifications is similar and is slightly lower for developing asymmetry and least for focal asymmetry [1]. Although architectural distortion is the least common of the four frequent signs of breast cancer, its reported positive predictive value for breast cancer on a screening examination (10.2 %) is similar to masses (9.7 %) and calcifications (12.7 %) and higher than for developing asymmetry (7.4 %). Focal asymmetry has a relatively low PPV for breast cancer at 3.7 %. A mass with spiculated margins (PPV = 81 %) and linear calcifications (PPV = 81 %) had the highest predictive value among 225 cancers in a series of 492 cases undergoing surgical biopsy. Other mammographic features that also show a high positive predictive value for cancer include masses with an irregular shape (73 %) and calcifications in a segmental (74 %) or linear distribution (68 %) [3].

M.K. Shetty, MD, FRCR, FACR, FAIUM
Department of Radiology, Baylor College of Medicine, Houston, TX, USA

Woman's Center for Breast Care and MRI, Woman's Hospital of Texas, Fannin 7600, Houston, TX 77054, USA
e-mail: mshettymd@womans-clinic.com

M.K. Shetty (ed.), *Breast Cancer Screening and Diagnosis: A Synopsis*,
DOI 10.1007/978-1-4939-1267-4_5, © Springer Science+Business Media New York 2015

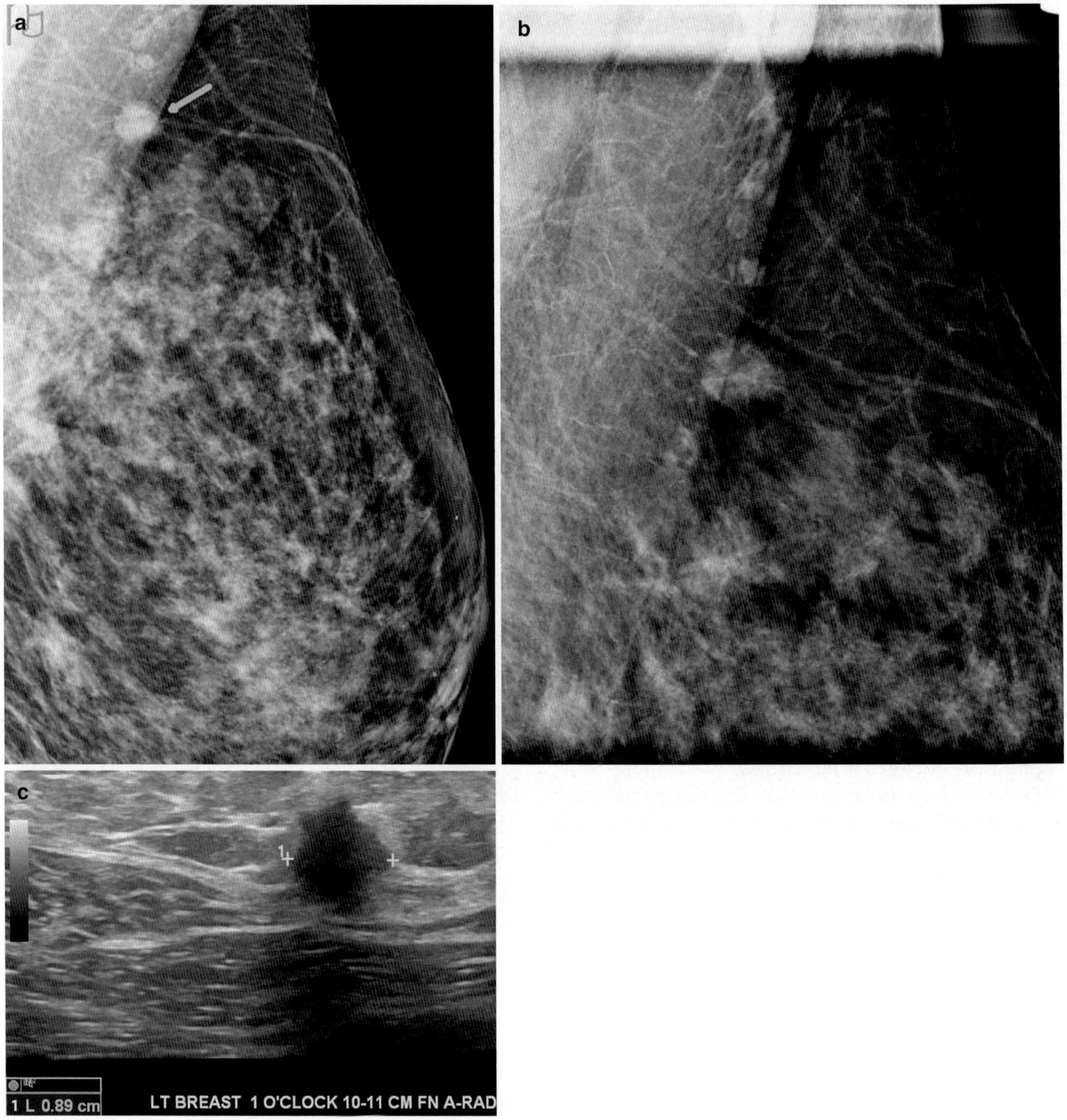

Fig. 5.1 (**a**–**c**) A 47-year-old with a 9 mm mass histologically proven to be a DCIS. (**a**) Mediolateral oblique view of a screening mammogram demonstrates a dense mass in the axillary tail (*arrow*). (**b**) Spot compression view in the mediolateral oblique projection reveals a mass with fine spiculated borders suspicious for a malignant mass. (**c**) Ultrasound demonstrates a 9 mm irregular mass with malignant features

Mass

A mass is a space-occupying lesion that is seen in two different mammographic projections. It has an outwardly convex border, is seen on two views, and is at least as dense centrally as in the periphery. Summation shadows on the other hand are produced by fortuitous superimposition of fibroglandular tissue and are not visualized in more than one projection [4]. When a mass is identified on a screening mammogram, an analysis of its features is done as follows: The shape of the mass is described as being round, oval, or lobular when a mass has an undulating contour. If a mass cannot be described as one of these, it is described as having an irregular shape (Fig. 5.1a–c). Once the primary features are ascertained, recall for a diagnostic assessment is often initiated. Spot compression views help define the margin characteristics of a mass. A margin that is sharply demarcated and well defined in at least 75 % of its extent and remainder is obscured is considered circumscribed with an abrupt transition from the mass to the surrounding tissue. Small undulations of the

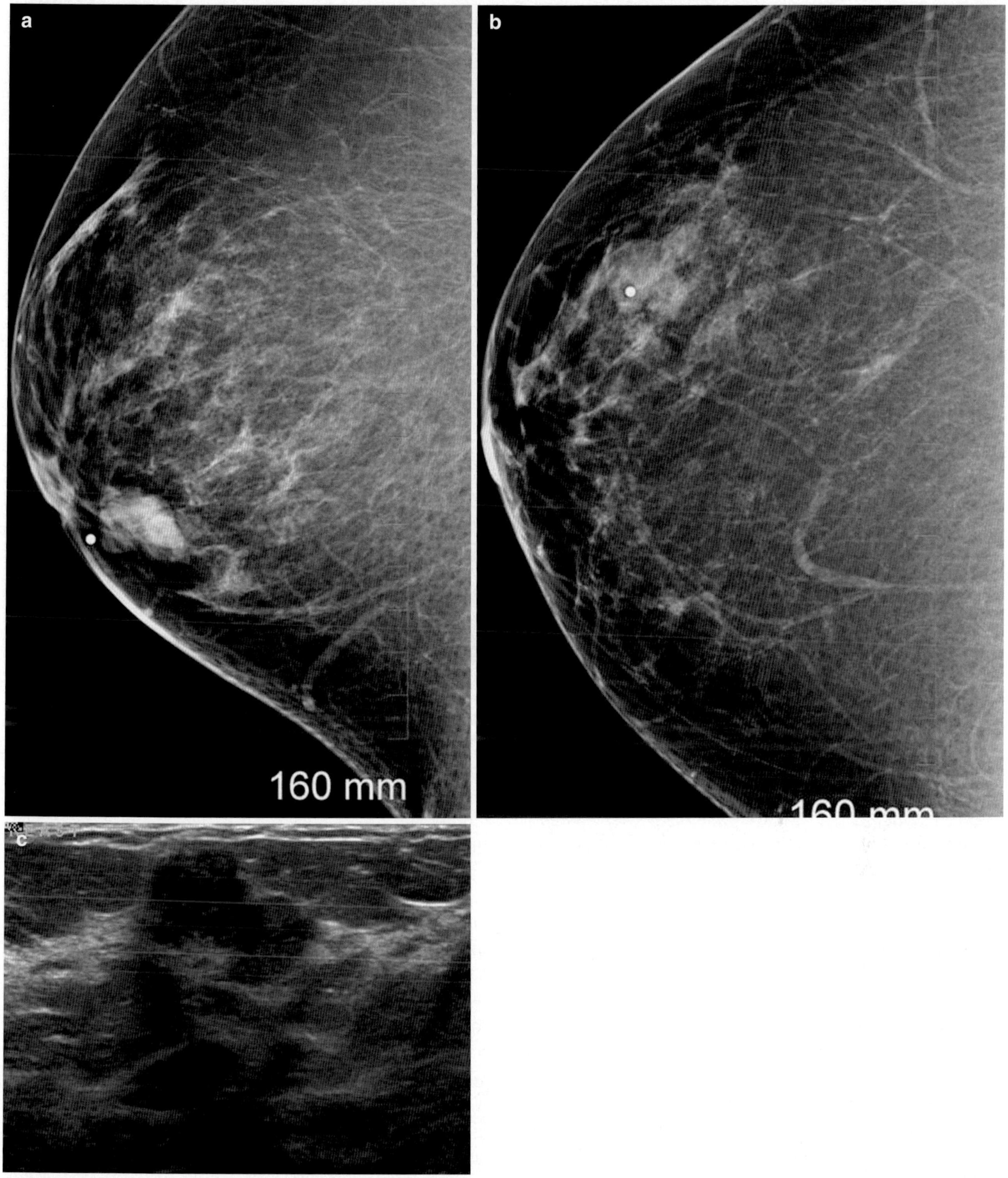

Fig. 5.2 (**a–c**) A 31-year-old with a palpable mass histologically proven to be invasive ductal cancer. (**a**) Mediolateral oblique view demonstrates a hyperdense mass with a circumscribed margin. (**b**) Craniocaudal projection reveals the mass with obscured borders. (**c**) Ultrasound shows a hypoechoic lobulated solid mass with ill-defined margins

border of a mass are defined as a macrolobulated border. A poor definition of the margin is suspicious for infiltration, a finding suggestive of malignancy. When lines radiate from the edge of a mass, the margin is described as being spiculated [5]. A mass with a density higher than of the surrounding fibroglandular parenchyma is more likely to be malignant than a low-density mass (Fig. 5.2a–c). In a retrospective study of 348 breast masses with biopsy confirmation, 70.2 % of the high-density masses were malignant, and 22.3 % of the iso- or low-density masses were malignant [6]. Similar

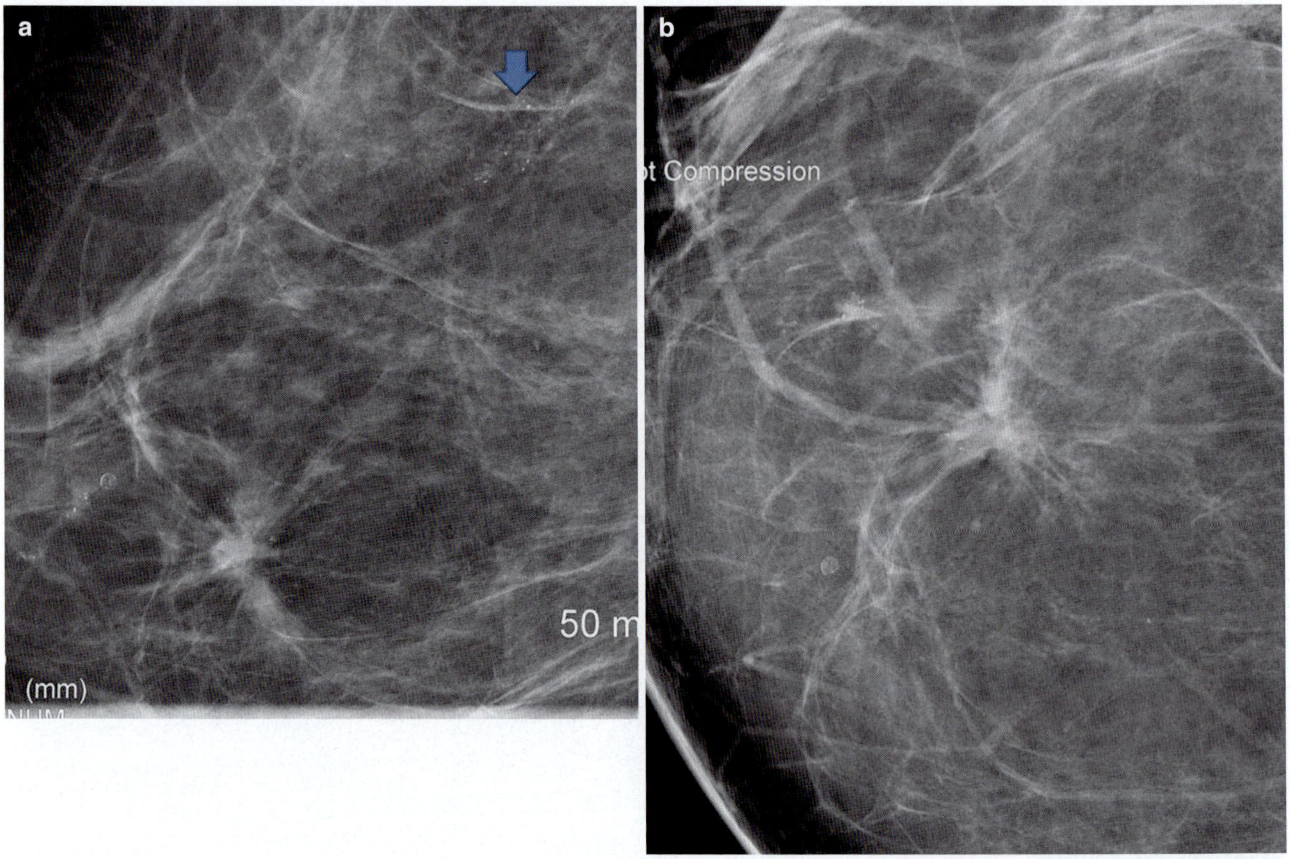

Fig. 5.3 (**a**, **b**) A 48-year-old with a screen-detected small spiculated mass histologically proven to be an invasive ductal cancer. (**a**) Spot compression magnification mediolateral view demonstrates a spiculated mass with microcalcifications and a second area of pleomorphic microcalcifications superiorly (*arrow*) that was proven to be DCIS. (**b**) Spot compression magnification craniocaudal view demonstrates a spiculated mass with microcalcifications

results have been reported using inductive logic programming and conditional probabilities and validating this association in an independent dataset [7].

There is a reported association between morphologic features and tumor stage and prognosis. Masses with spiculated margins are known to be associated with lower-grade tumors and hence have a better prognosis (Fig. 5.3a, b). On the other hand triple-negative breast cancers have been found to be associated with circumscribed masses and masses with microlobulations and with ill-defined borders. Lymphovascular invasion has been reported to be seen more often in breast cancers associated with architectural distortion rather than those with spiculated mass. The reason behind this association is unknown [8]. Lymphovascular invasion is also more common in masses with calcifications. In invasive cancers, the presence of calcifications is often associated with extensive intraductal component and necrosis. In one series breast cancers presenting as architectural distortion were reported to have positive margins in 65 % of cases. These investigators, however, did not find a significant correlate between mammographic features and tumor differentiation or ER (estrogen receptor)/PR (progesterone receptor) status [8].

It is known that the proportion of invasive cancers tends to be higher in younger women (Fig. 5.4a–c). The ratio of invasive to noninvasive cancers increased from 1:1 in those younger than 50 years of age to 3:1 in those over 70 years. Breast cancers presenting with calcifications are also decreased from 63 % in women younger than 50 years to 26 % in older than 70 years [2]. Generally calcifications that are malignant are associated with DCIS in 63 % of cases, whereas a spiculated mass is associated with invasive cancer in as high as 95 % of cases [9]. In a small percentage of cases, spiculated masses may represent pure DCIS or DCIS associated with a radial scar, 8 % of a series of 86 lesions with predominant DCIS in one series [10]. The prognosis is best and 8-year survival was the longest for small spiculated masses [95 %] that are 1–9 mm and good for rounded masses [91 %] compared to those presenting with calcifications [77 %]. Patients with casting or pleomorphic calcifications had significantly worst prognosis [11].

Architectural Distortion

Architectural distortion refers to a localized disruption of the breast architecture which can include spiculations or thin lines that radiate from a focal point or a localized retraction of the edge of the parenchyma at its interface with fat. It is a normal finding to see lines randomly crossing within the breast parenchyma; what is abnormal is when one sees these lines converging to a focal area. Not uncommonly overlapping crisscrossing tissue lines may simulate architectural distortion on a screening mammogram. Careful inspection alone with use of a magnifying lens may suffice to make this assertion; when unclear, recall for spot compression and rolled views of the breast in the projection where it is best seen will help to exclude an area of true architectural distortion (Fig. 5.5a, b). Architectural distortion when unassociated with other findings such as masses or clustered calcifications can be often subtle and accounts for a significant number of missed breast cancers; a discussion on missed cancers appears later. Architectural distortion is less common than a mass as a mammographic sign of breast cancer but is highly predictive of breast cancer both at screening and diagnostic mammography [1]. Architectural distortion is a sign of invasive ductal and invasive lobular cancer and results from the fibrosis in a scirrhous carcinoma. Ductal carcinoma in situ most commonly manifests as indeterminate or malignant-appearing microcalcifications. However, a small percentage of DCIS can appear as areas of distortion, 2.1 % [4/190] in one series [12]. Architectural distortion in an area of DCIS is often attributed to associated sclerosing adenosis rather

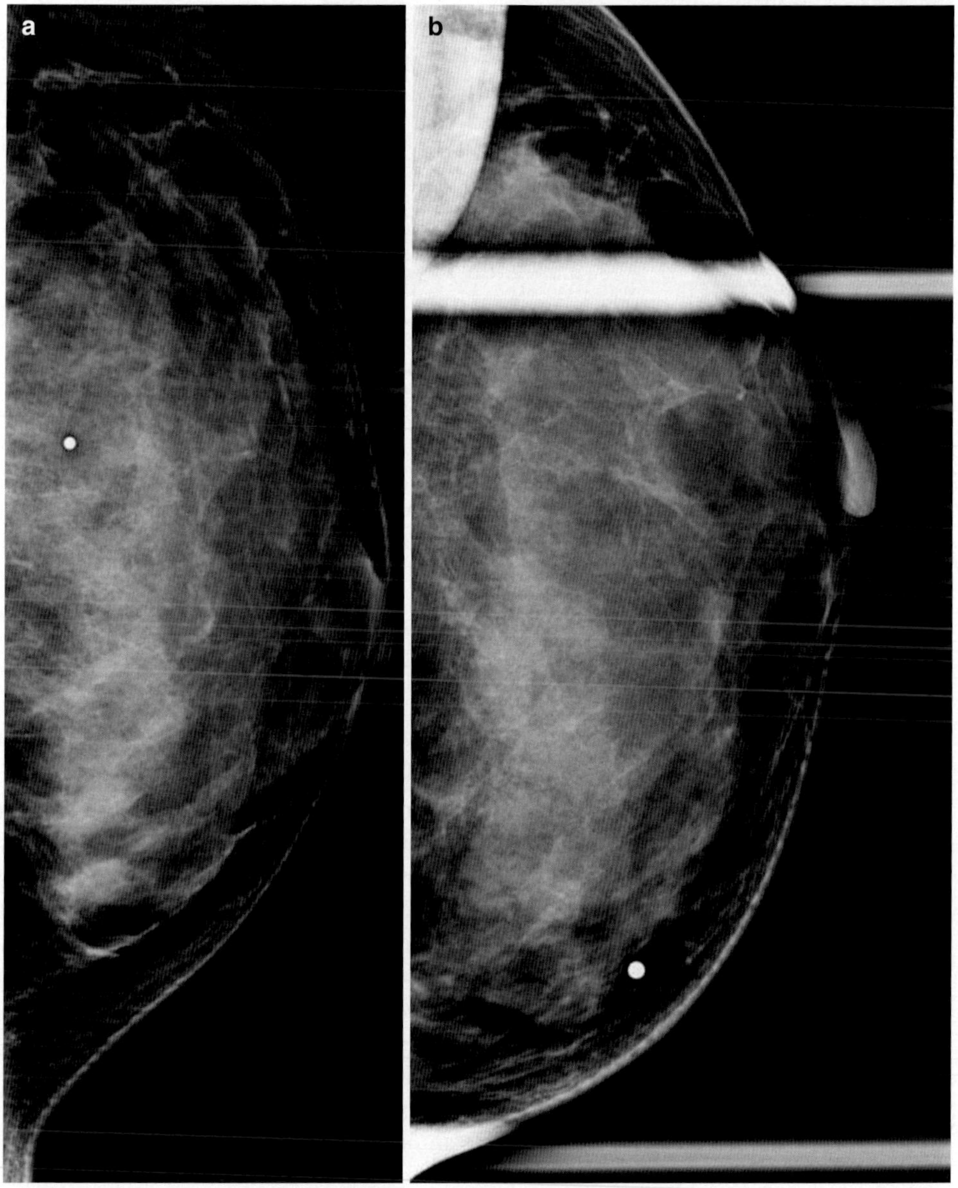

Fig. 5.4 (**a**–**c**) A 35-year-old with a palpable lump in left breast histologically proven to be invasive ductal cancer. (**a**) Mediolateral oblique view reveals no abnormality. (**b**) Craniocaudal view with spot compression demonstrates dense tissue but no mass. (**c**) Ultrasound demonstrates a solid hypoechoic mass with ill-defined and microlobulated borders suggestive of malignancy

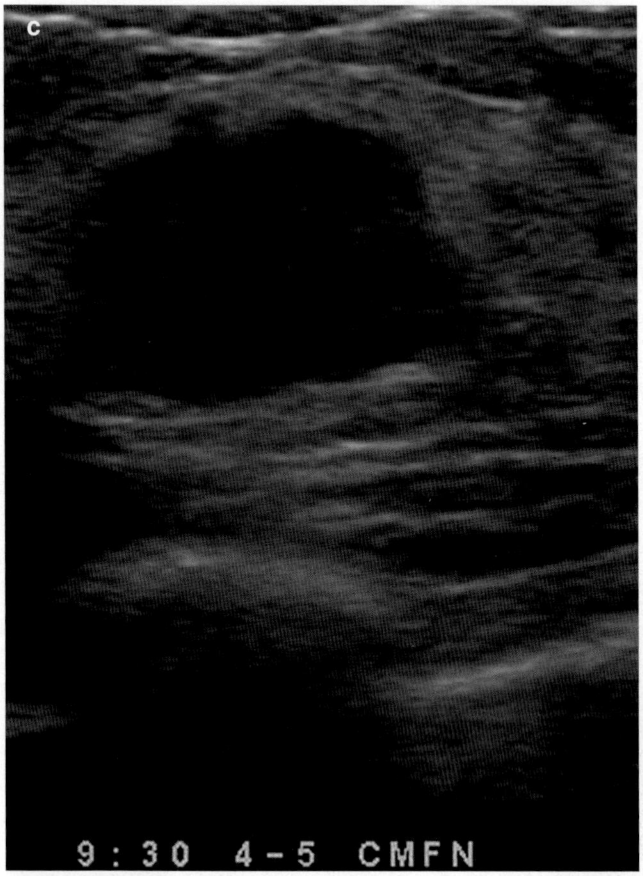

Fig. 5.4 (continued)

than due to the in situ cancer itself. In one series, 5 of 54 cases of DCIS [10.8 %] appeared as an area of architectural distortion. Histopathological correlation in this series showed that the AD in 4 of 5 cases correlated with sclerosis in the interstitium around DCIS, and DCIS in Cooper's ligament accounted for the appearance of AD on the mammogram [13].

It is also known that in patients with architectural distortion on mammography, there is more likely to be positive margins than those with masses or calcifications [2]. Breast cancer presenting as AD is also reported to be significantly larger than that seen on mammography compared to other mammographic abnormalities. It is therefore recommended that in those patients with nonpalpable architectural distortions, a wider excision be undertaken to minimize the risk of having positive margins. Although most series of invasive breast cancers have found architectural distortion a less common mammographic presentation, architectural distortion has been reported to be more frequently seen in invasive lobular cancer. Architectural distortion was found to be the second most common appearance after a mass, in some studies ranging from 10 to 34 % of cases of invasive lobular cancer [14]. The differential diagnosis of an area of architectural distortion appears in Box 5.2. A finding of an

Box 5.2 Differential Diagnosis of Architectural Distortion on a Mammogram

1. Invasive ductal and invasive lobular cancer
2. Radial scar
3. Sclerosing adenosis
4. Postsurgical or post biopsy
5. Post breast trauma

architectural distortion on a mammogram except for those that can definitively be attributed to prior surgery, biopsy, or trauma is an indication for excisional biopsy in most instances. Known mimics of cancers that can appear as areas of architectural distortion include a radial scar and sclerosing adenosis.

Differential Diagnosis of Architectural Distortion

Radial Scars

A radial scar is a known mammographic mimic of breast cancer. When these lesions are smaller than 1 cm, they are referred to as a radial scar and when larger than 1 cm are called complex sclerosing lesions (Fig. 5.6a–d). Mammographic features that are typical of radial scars include the presence of a central lucency from which thin long spicules radiate. The abnormality has a characteristic varying appearance on different projections and radiolucent linear structures parallel the spicules. Such a mammographic appearance has been called the black star in contradistinction to cancer where the central area of architectural distortion is dense and hence is referred as a white star. Radial scars are not typically palpable and not associated with microcalcifications [15, 16]. The mammographically described radial scar is distinct from those that are incidentally reported in histology specimens in about 28 % of cases [17]. These latter radial scars are small lesions, mammographically occult, and do not carry an increased risk of associated cancer.

The reported incidence of radial scars on screening mammograms is about 3 per 1,000 [18]. Although benign, when suspected on a mammogram, excisional biopsy is generally recommended due to the known association with invasive cancer and the difficulty in distinguishing tubular cancer from radial scar on core biopsy specimens [19]. Sonography is generally not performed when a radial scar is identified on the mammogram; however, sonographic appearance of radial scars has been described. Ultrasound is useful when the area of distortion is seen on one view only and if seen may then be used for presurgical localization [20–22].

Sclerosing Adenosis

Sclerosing adenosis is a proliferative benign abnormality characterized by proliferation of stromal and myoepithelial

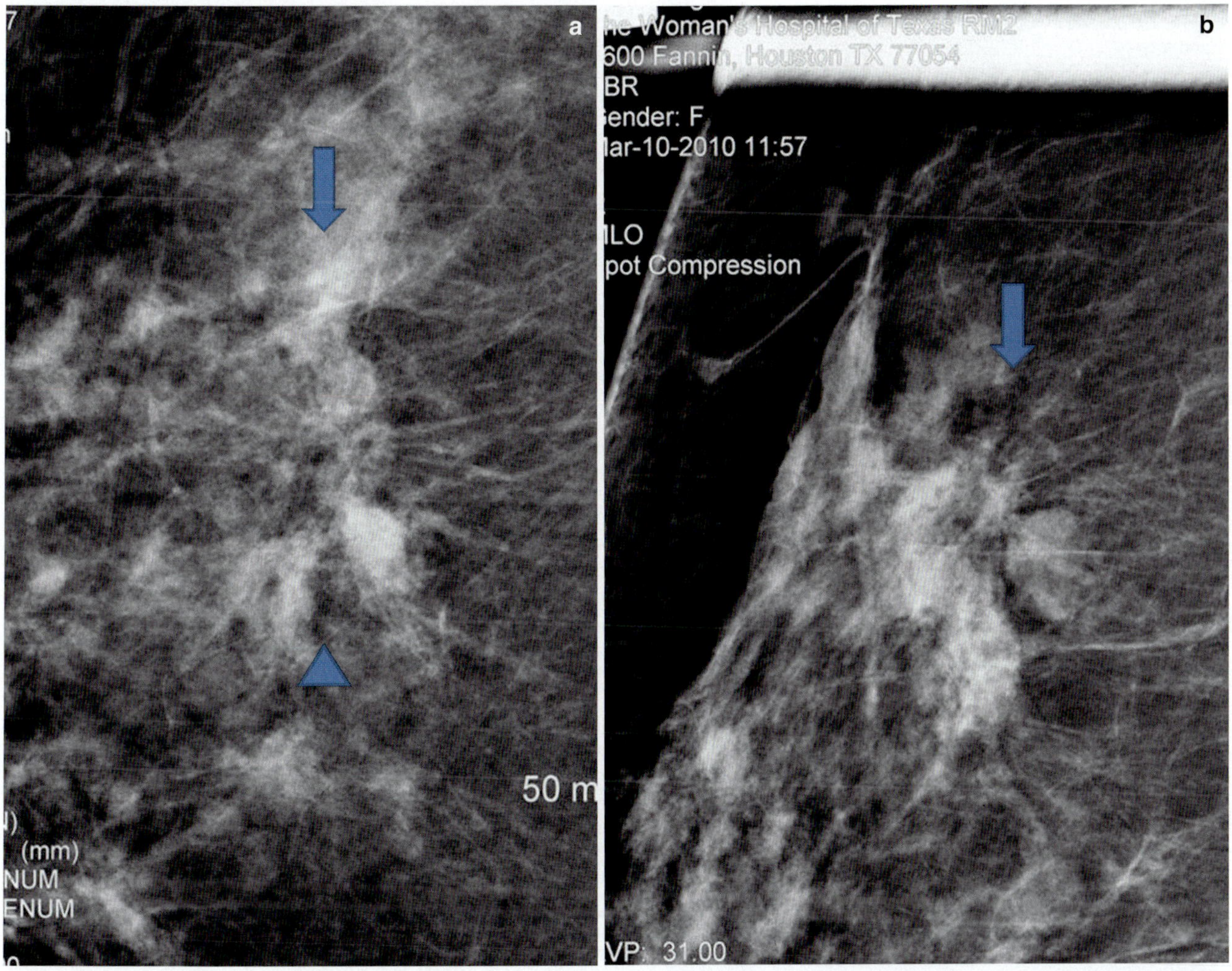

Fig. 5.5 (**a**, **b**) An invasive ductal cancer appearing as an area of architectural distortion. (**a**) Spot compression magnification views in the CC projection demonstrates an area of subtle architectural distortion (*between arrow and arrowhead*). (**b**) Spot compression magnification views in the MLO projection demonstrate an area of subtle architectural distortion (*arrow*)

cells leading to distortion of the acini. It is often associated with other benign and malignant abnormalities. When sclerosing adenosis exists as a dominant component, it may appear as a localized area of calcifications, mass, focal asymmetry, or an area of architectural distortion [23]. In one series of 69/76 cases of histologically proven sclerosing adenosis that were mammographically detectable, 12 % appeared as areas of localized architectural distortion [24]. In another series of 43 cases, 6.9 % [3/43] of sclerosing adenosis appeared on the mammogram as an area of architectural distortion [25].

Breast Trauma

Trauma to the breast may lead to mammographic findings that mimic cancer; however, appropriate history and evolution of changes in the appearance are helpful in the differential diagnosis (Fig. 5.7a, b). The spectrum of trauma encompasses blunt trauma such as in a seat belt injury, all types of breast biopsy, lumpectomy, as well as mammoplasty. Fat necrosis that can result from any insult to the breast parenchyma may also present diagnostic dilemma particularly when a reliable history is not present. A description of the postoperative breast appears in a separate chapter (Chap. 16).

Fat necrosis is a clinical and imaging mimic of breast cancer. The mammographic spectrum of findings includes a lipid cyst with or without calcification of the wall, clustered microcalcifications, spiculated mass, and nonlucent focal mass. Fat necrosis may result from accidental breast trauma or any of the previously listed causes of iatrogenic breast trauma, surgery, and biopsy [26]. Seat belt injuries cause appearance of areas of fat density necrosis and areas of increased density in a band-shaped distribution. In the short term the increased density may decrease in size, and the line of fibrosis is evident. These changes evolve over a period of time with development of calcifications and resultant architectural distortion [27].

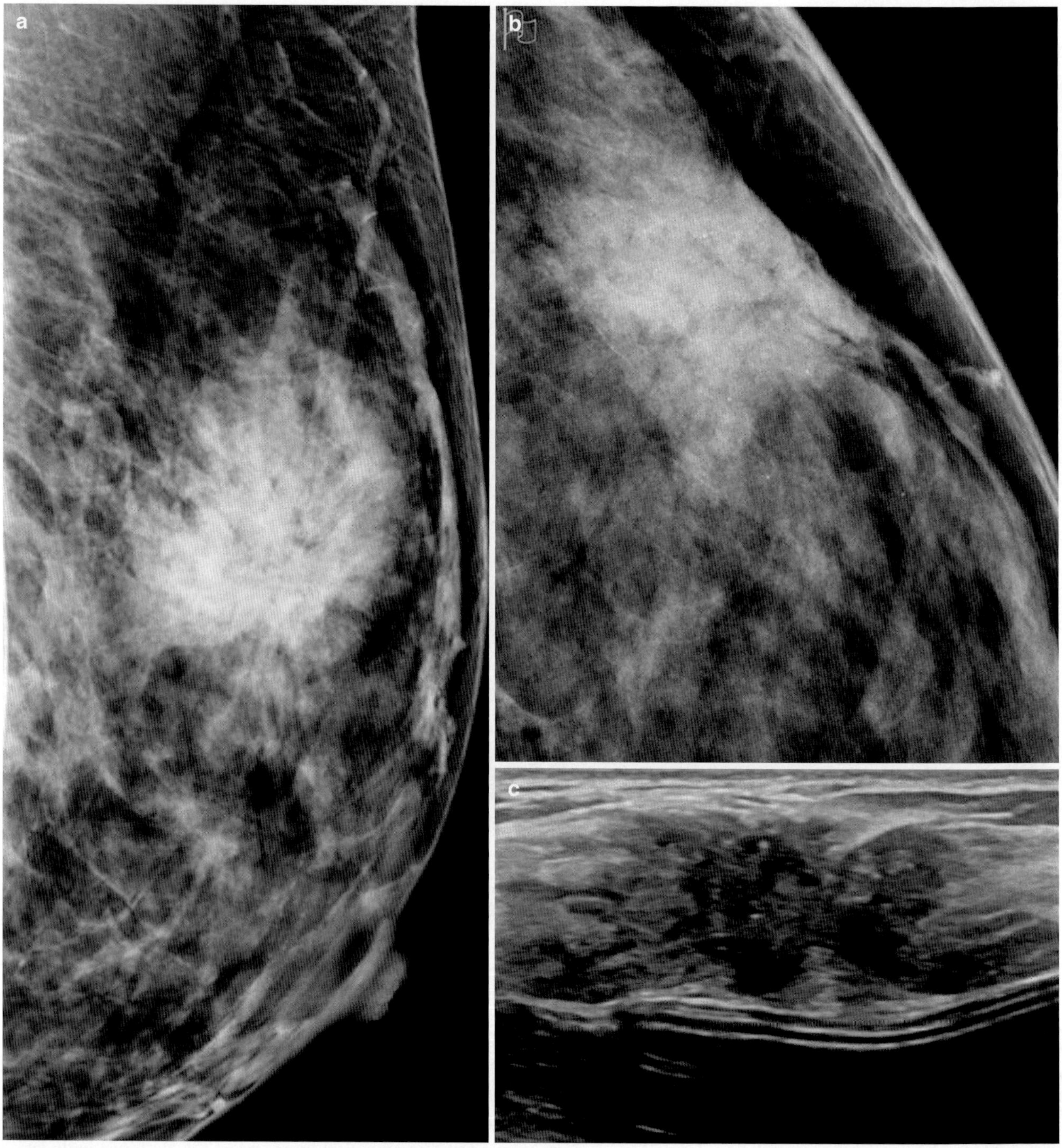

Fig. 5.6 (**a**–**d**) A 35-year-old with a family history of cancer and a palpable lump histologically proven to be a complex sclerosing lesion. (**a**) Mediolateral oblique view demonstrates a large irregular focal asymmetry with architectural distortion. (**b**) Craniocaudal view demonstrates a large irregular focal asymmetry with architectural distortion. (**c**, **d**) Ultrasound demonstrates an irregular mass that was considered probably malignant

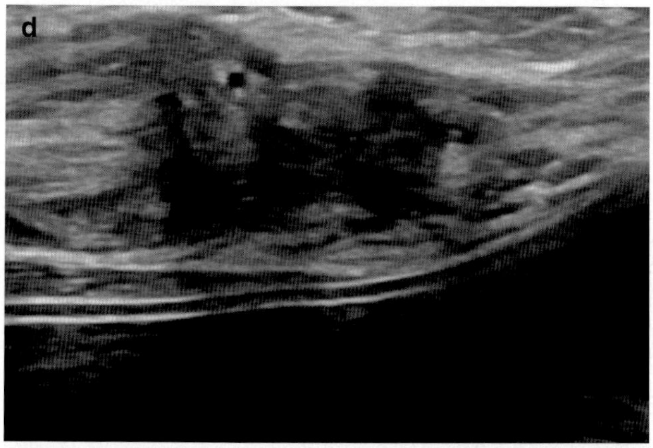

Fig. 5.6 (continued)

Microcalcifications

Calcifications that are identified on a screening mammogram and that do not exhibit the established criteria of benign calcifications are recalled to undergo a diagnostic mammogram. Spot compression magnification views in the mediolateral and craniocaudal projections are routinely obtained. The rationale for obtaining magnification views is to study the morphology and the distribution pattern of the calcifications. Magnification mammography decreases noise and improves image sharpness allowing for optimal evaluation of the morphology and distribution of calcifications. A description of mammographically identified calcifications should include the morphologic features and the distribution of the calcifications. Macrocalcifications are typically larger than 2 mm and are associated with benign

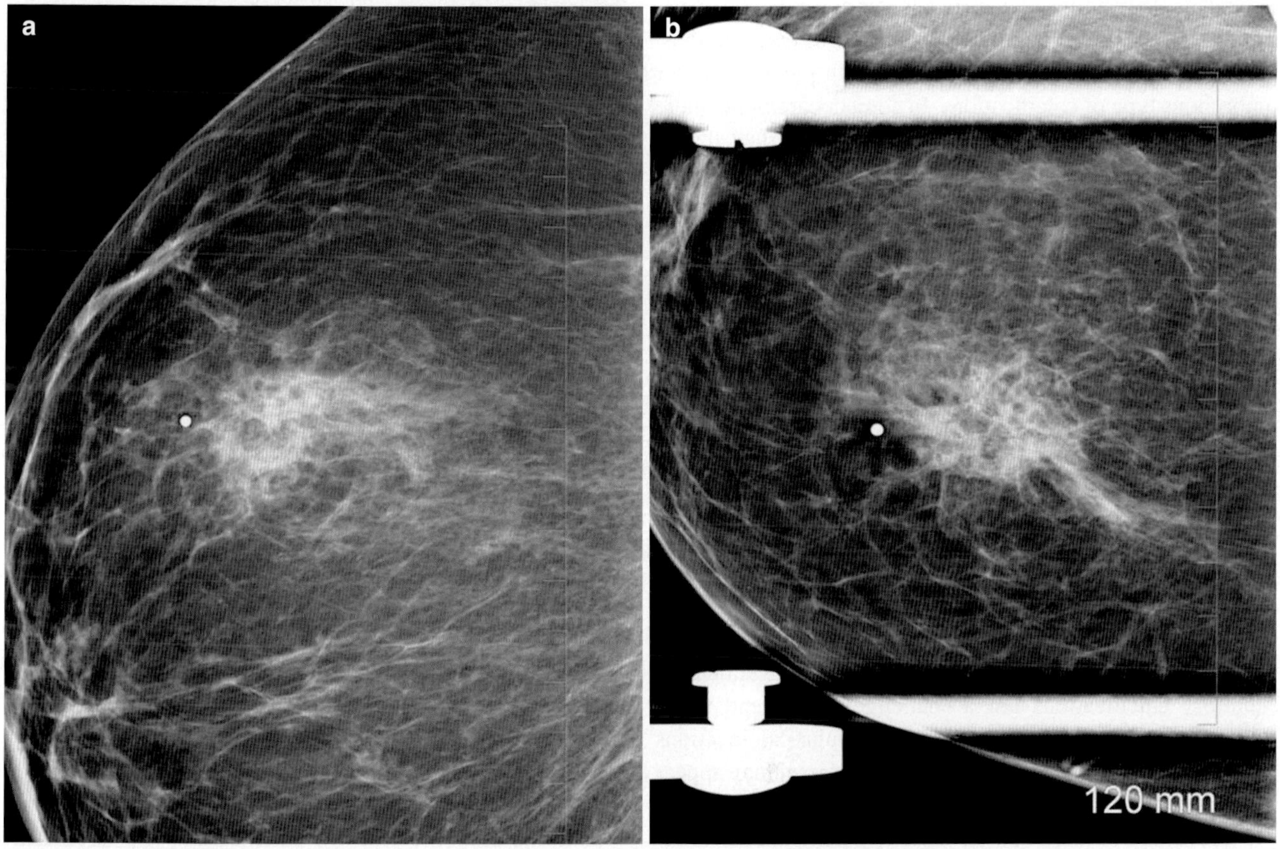

Fig. 5.7 (**a**, **b**) A 44-year-old with a history of a seat belt injury 3 months prior to a screening mammogram. (**a**) Mediolateral oblique view demonstrates an area of asymmetry and distortion in upper breast. (**b**) Spot compress view in the craniocaudal projection shows the area of distortion

processes; microcalcifications are smaller than 0.5 mm and can be associated with ductal carcinoma in situ or invasive cancer [28]. In DCIS the tumor grows within the duct, distending it but remaining within the basement membrane.

Malignancies presenting as calcifications on mammography are most commonly associated with DCIS and have been reported in up to 68 % of cases of ductal carcinoma in situ [2]. About 29–47 % of breast cancers appear as microcalcifications without a mass [1]. About 24 % of the suspicious calcifications are associated with DCIS. Microcalcifications in DCIS are most commonly linear, linear branching, and fine pleomorphic, in a linear distribution. Other forms described in DCIS include the dot-dash pattern, consisting of round and needle-shaped calcifications.

The histological high-grade carcinoma or comedocarcinoma tends to be associated with linear, branching, and irregular calcifications that are in a linear or segmental distribution, formerly referred to as casting type of calcifications. These cancers may also be associated with pleomorphic or amorphous type of calcifications. In comedocarcinoma there is significant necrosis within the lumen of the duct that is involved with cancer. About 90 % of high-grade DCIS is associated with microcalcifications. The lower-grade or non-comedo DCIS is associated more often with clustered calcifications of amorphous or coarse heterogeneous morphology calcifications. Overall unlike the high-grade DCIS, the low-grade DCIS is less frequently associated with microcalcifications and reported in about 50 % of cases. Sometimes in DCIS one sees clustered fine pleomorphic or coarse heterogeneous calcifications, and these are often associated with necrotic tumors of the cribriform or micropapillary type [28]. The differential diagnosis for linear calcifications includes two important benign causes, secretory calcifications and vascular calcifications. Linear calcifications can be associated with benign secretory disease of the breast; these calcifications are often bilateral, regional, and seen in older women. When confined to a smaller region and unilateral, secretory calcifications are a challenge, these tend to be dense and have smooth margins [29]. Vascular calcifications when patchy and confined to one wall of a vessel may appear as a linear calcification. Magnification views help to identify the true nature of these benign vascular calcifications.

There have been reports attempting to correlate the appearance of microcalcifications with likelihood of invasive cancers [30]. In malignant calcifications without a focal mass, invasive foci are more likely when calcifications were larger than 11 mm and with linear calcifications than with granular calcifications [30]. Invasive cancers presenting as calcifications are often associated with high-grade DCIS and are also more likely to be Her2/Neu [human epidermal growth factor receptor 2]-negative cancers [2]. Invasive ductal cancers may also be associated with fine pleomorphic calcifications (Fig. 5.8). Invasive lobular cancer on the other hand is rarely associated with microcalcifications.

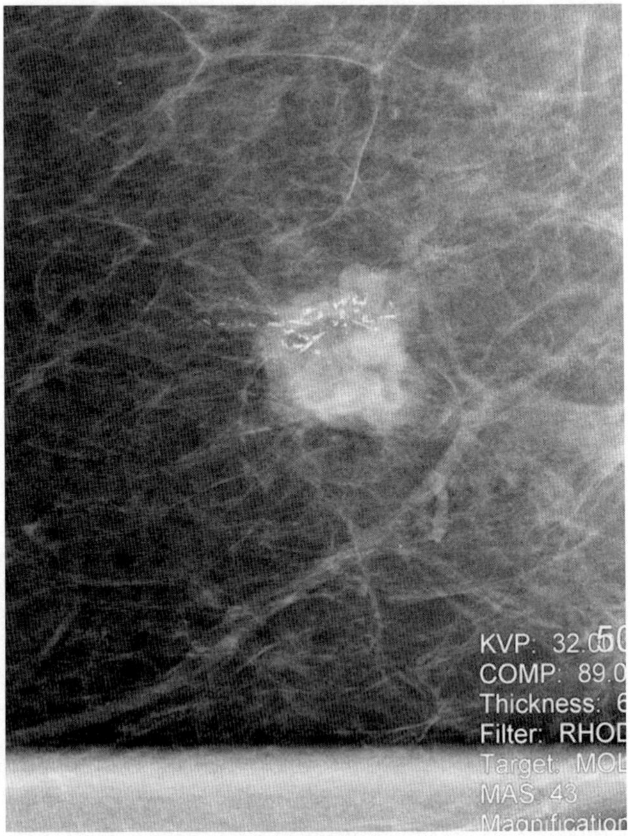

Fig. 5.8 A 67-year-old with histologically proven invasive ductal cancer in the right breast. Spot compression magnification view demonstrates linear branching pleomorphic calcifications associated with an irregular mass

Table 5.1 Morphology and distribution of calcifications and degree of concern

Benign	Intermediate concern	High probability for cancer
Diffuse, regional distribution	Grouped distribution	Linear, segmental distribution
Dystrophic, eggshell	Amorphous	Linear
Secretory, vascular	Granular	Linear branching
Vascular, sutural	Coarse heterogeneous	Pleomorphic

The morphologic types of calcifications that are suspicious for malignancy can be categorized as those with intermediate concern for cancer and those that have a higher probability of being associated with breast cancer [5] (Table 5.1).

Intermediate Concern for Malignancy

1. Amorphous or indistinct calcifications are small and hazy in appearance; a specific morphologic classification cannot be given. The distribution of such calcifications determines degree of suspicion, when diffuse and scattered are

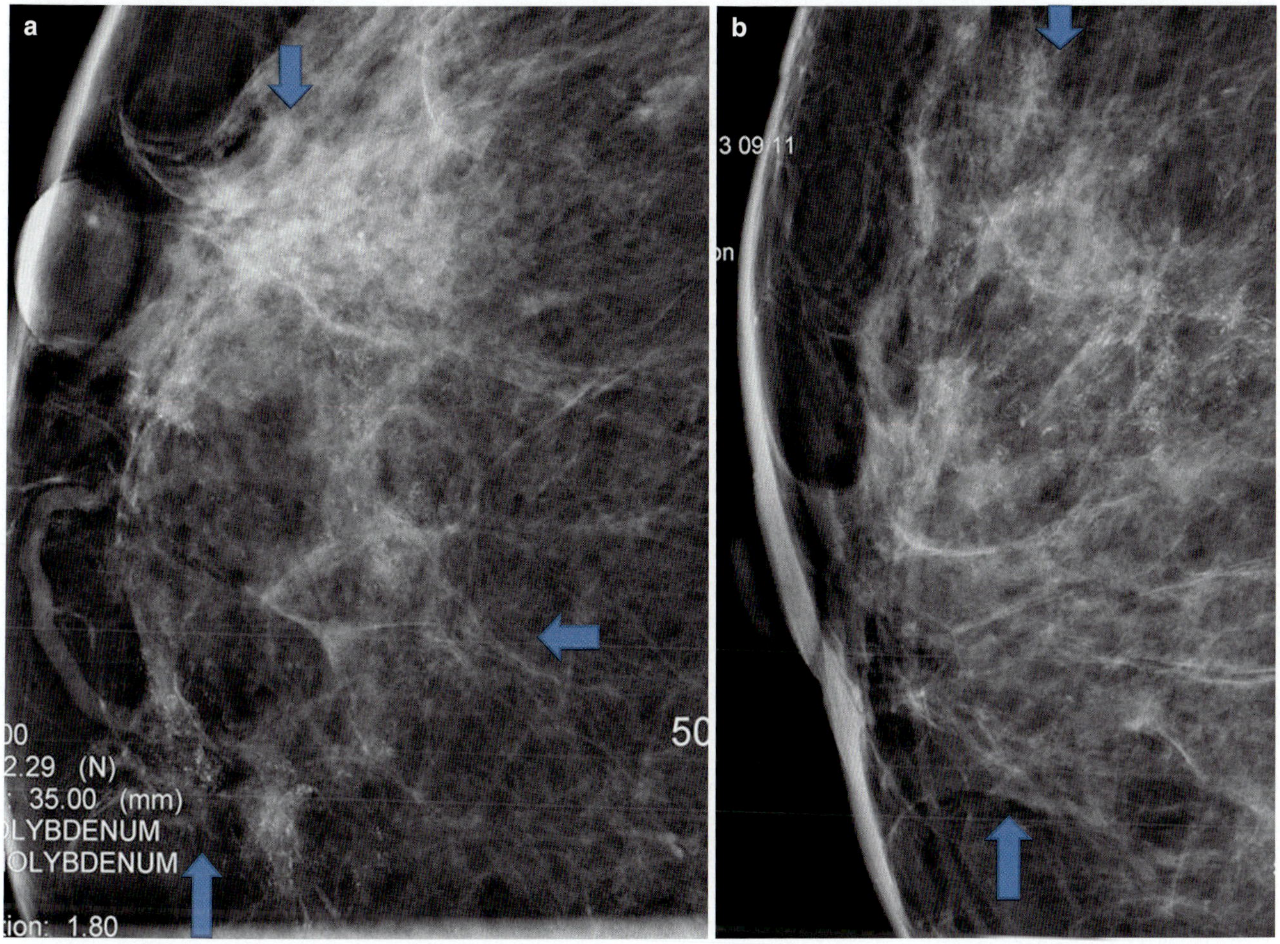

Fig. 5.9 (**a**, **b**) A 53-year-old with extensive calcifications identified on a screening mammogram histologically proven to be DCIS. (**a**) Spot compression magnification views in the craniocaudal projection demonstrate linearly arranged clusters of microcalcifications in a segmental distribution extending to the nipple. (**b**) Spot compression magnification views in the mediolateral projection demonstrate linearly arranged clusters of microcalcifications in a segmental distribution extending to the nipple. Area of microcalcifications is outlined by *arrows*

benign, however when seen on a baseline mammogram magnification views are generally obtained. When these types of calcifications have a regional, linear, or segmental distribution, they are considered suspicious and an indication for biopsy.

2. Coarse heterogeneous calcifications are irregular and larger than 0.5 mm and tend to be clustered. Such calcifications may be associated with malignancy and are also seen in benign lesions such as fibroadenomas, fibrosis, and trauma and in dystrophic calcifications.

Higher Probability of Malignancy

1. Fine pleomorphic: These are calcifications smaller than 0.5 mm and are more clearly defined than the amorphous type and are irregular with varying sizes and shapes.
2. Fine linear or fine-linear branching calcifications: These are thin linear or curvilinear irregular calcifications which may be discontinuous and smaller than 0.5 mm. This is suggestive of filling of the lumen of a duct by cancer cells (Fig. 5.9a, b).

Distribution of Calcifications

The distribution of calcifications is also an additional indicator of the likelihood of calcifications being associated with breast cancers:

1. Diffuse and scattered calcifications are usually benign particularly when bilateral. Such a distribution is often seen with punctuate and amorphous calcifications.
2. Regional calcifications may involve most of a quadrant or more than a single quadrant and do not conform to a duct distribution. Such a distribution is generally indicative of a benign etiology although careful assessment of the morphology may modify final assessment and the need for biopsy. Intermediate and high probability morphology even in such a distribution should prompt biopsy.

3. Grouped or clustered calcifications are when five or more calcifications are seen in a small volume of breast tissue. These are generally considered suspicious.
4. Linear distribution is when calcifications are arrayed in a line; such a distribution is highly suspicious for cancer and suggests that calcifications are intraductal.
5. Segmental distribution of calcifications implies calcifications in ducts and their branches and may imply extensive or multifocal breast cancer in a lobe or segment of the breast. Except in the case of coarse rodlike calcifications in older women associated with secretory calcifications, segmental distribution is worrisome and should prompt a biopsy.

Focal Asymmetry

Focal asymmetry is a localized area of increased density that is visible as a confined asymmetry with similar shape in two views, but does not fit the criteria of a mass and lacks defined borders. In majority of cases it represents an island of normal breast tissue especially when there is interspersed fat. Focal asymmetry that is associated with a palpable finding, architectural distortion, or microcalcifications is worrisome for malignancy [5, 31]. Breast asymmetry is generally a result of localized distribution of fibroglandular parenchyma and unlike a mass tends to have concave borders and is interspersed with fat and not dense centrally like one sees in a mass. To appreciate breast asymmetry views of each breast are inspected side by side as is standard practice of viewing mammograms. There are four types of breast asymmetry described [32]:

- Asymmetry of the breast is seen in one of two standard mammographic views, formerly referred to as a density. The likelihood of malignancy is slightly less than 2 %; nevertheless, Sickles rightly points out that it is not appropriate to categorize such findings as probably benign since 80 % of these asymmetries can be identified as summation artifact at screening or on additional evaluation and do not require short interval follow-up. The likelihood of malignancy for the remainder lesions is significantly higher [10.3 %], and thereby short interval follow-up is not justified [32, 33].
- Global asymmetry is when there is substantially more tissue in one breast compared to the other and occupies at least one quadrant of the breast. When not associated with a palpable abnormality, this finding is benign, and when associated with a palpable finding, a small percentage (3 %) may be associated with breast cancer [34].
- Focal asymmetry lacks convex borders of a mass and occupies less than one quadrant of the breast. The likelihood of malignancy for such a finding that is not associated with a mass, palpable finding, architectural distortion, calcifications, and sonographic correlate and with no prior mammograms to assess stability is less than 1 %.
- A developing asymmetry is a focal asymmetry that is new or enlarging or denser when compared to prior mammogram (Fig. 5.10a–g). Unlike such developing focal asymmetry, hormone-induced developing asymmetry is bilateral and global. Infection, trauma, and surgery are other nonsuspicious causes of a developing asymmetry that can be excluded by clinical history [31]. Developing asymmetry is an uncommon finding and reported in 0.16 % of 180,801 screening mammograms and 0.11 % of 27,330 diagnostic mammograms. On a screening examination, the incidence of cancer in a developing asymmetry has been reported to be 12.8 %, and in those that are persistent after a diagnostic work-up, irrespective of the presence of a correlative physical finding, the reported cancer rate is as high as 26.7 % [35]. Therefore, an uncomplicated developing asymmetry that is persistent after a diagnostic work-up unless proven to be due to benign finding such as a cyst by ultrasound should be categorized as a BI-RADS 4 with a recommendation for biopsy. A normal ultrasound does not preclude recommendation for a biopsy. In one series of 300 nonpalpable cancers, 6 % were manifest as developing asymmetry [36].

Sonography is an appropriate work-up for a focal asymmetry that is persistent mainly to exclude an underlying mass. In one series sonography had a negative predictive value for breast cancer of 89.4 % (7/9 cancers detected). One palpable focal asymmetry without a sonographic correlate proved to be an invasive ductal cancer as did one without a palpable correlate. A negative sonography should not preclude biopsy in those with a palpable focal asymmetry. However, the presence of localized hyperechoic tissue matching an area of focal asymmetry is suggestive of a benign process [37]. See Fig. 5.11a–d.

In summary, most cases of asymmetry are due to a summation artifact and appropriately categorized as benign with a recommendation for routine follow-up. Those that are determined not to be a summation artifact after a diagnostic work-up and if new or enlarging or palpable following either a negative ultrasound examination or an ultrasound finding of an indeterminate mass get a category 4 assessment with a recommendation for a biopsy. Uncomplicated focal asymmetry seen on a baseline screening mammogram or when there are no prior mammograms available for comparison need to be worked up with diagnostic mammography and if persistent assessed by sonography; if there is no benign finding accounting for the focal asymmetry, the finding is considered probably benign with a recommendation for a short interval follow-up in 6 months. Uncomplicated global asymmetry does not require a diagnostic work-up and is assigned a BI-RADS 2 category with a recommendation for

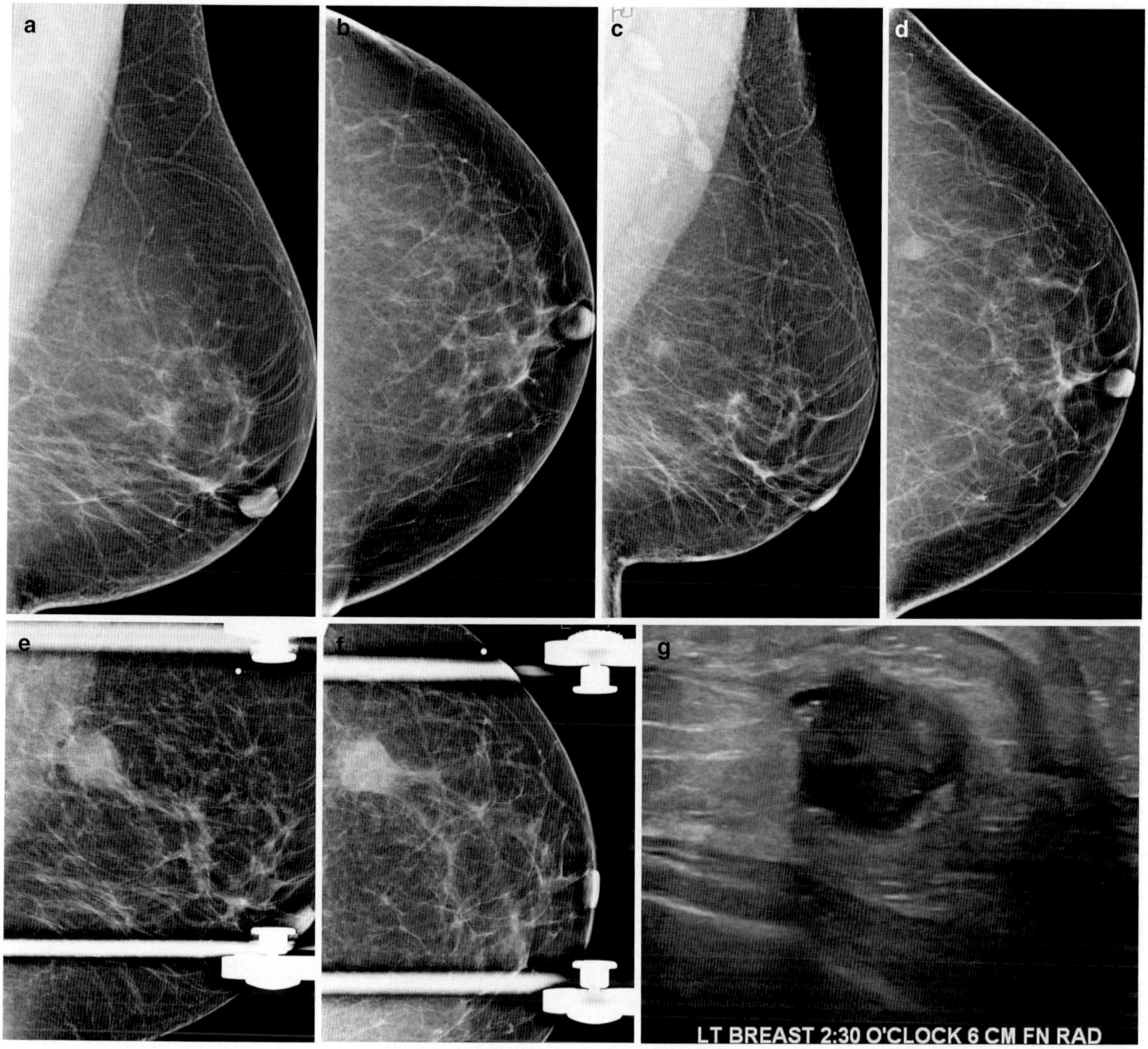

Fig. 5.10 (**a–g**) A 55-year-old with a new developing asymmetry that was subsequently proven to be invasive ductal carcinoma. (**a**) Left breast mediolateral oblique view obtained in August 2011 demonstrates a fat-replaced breast parenchymal pattern with no abnormal findings. (**b**) Left breast craniocaudal view obtained in August 2011 demonstrates no abnormal findings. (**c**) Left breast mediolateral oblique view obtained in August 2012 demonstrates a developing asymmetry in the posterior outer central breast. (**d**) Left breast craniocaudal view obtained in August 2012 demonstrates a developing asymmetry in the posterior outer central breast. (**e**) Spot compression mediolateral oblique view obtained in February 2013 demonstrates a high-density irregular mass in the posterior outer central breast. Patient had failed to return for a recommended diagnostic mammogram in August 2012. (**f**) Spot compression craniocaudal view obtained in February 2013 demonstrates a high-density irregular mass in the posterior outer central breast. (**g**) Ultrasound shows a solid mass with malignant features

routine screening. Uncomplicated developing asymmetry is always recalled and if determined not to be due to summation or a sonographic benign correlate is categorized as a BI-RADS 4, with a recommendation for a biopsy. Asymmetry, global asymmetry, or a focal asymmetry associated with a palpable finding, architectural distortion, or suspicious microcalcifications is always an indication for biopsy.

One-View Density

Density that is visible on one view and defined as asymmetry is often due to summation artifact. Women are recalled for a diagnostic mammogram where supplemental views are obtained to exclude summation artifact as well as to identify a corresponding area on the orthogonal view. Two methods have been described to triangulate a lesion in two

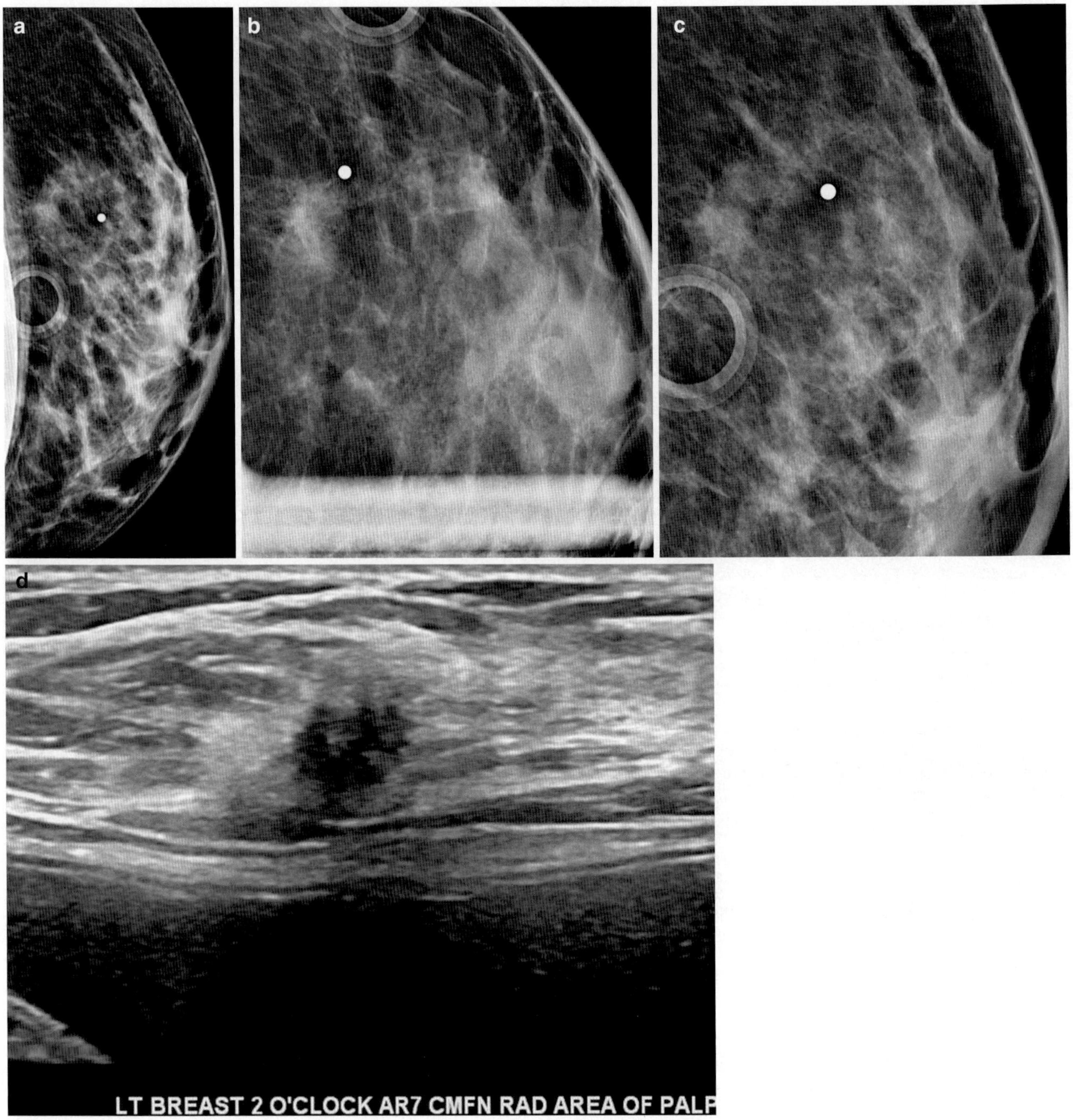

Fig. 5.11 (**a–d**) Small palpable invasive ductal cancer with subtle visibility on a screening mammogram. (**a**) Mediolateral view of left breast shows a questionable area of increased density in a breast with dense fibroglandular parenchyma. (**b**) Spot compression view in the craniocaudal projection reveals a small focal asymmetry. (**c**) Spot compression view in the mediolateral projection reveals a small focal asymmetry. (**d**) Ultrasound reveals a small solid mass with microlobulated borders and malignant features

projections [38]. First is the arc method where the distance from the nipple to the density is used to form the radius of an arc with the nipple at its center. In the straight line method, the distance from the nipple to a perpendicular line passing through the density is measured. A corresponding density is sought in the orthogonal plane along the arc or the line; if none is found the finding is considered as an asymmetry. One-view asymmetry if not a summation artifact may be caused by an abnormality that is not included on the second view due to technical difficulties in including that area of the breast, such as lesions in the axillary fold, very medial in the chest, very posterior, or in the inframammary fold [38]. When a lesion is apparent only on the mediolateral oblique view, a straight mediolateral view has to be obtained to determine if the finding persists and its location in the breast. Lesions that are in the medial breast will move superiorly and those in the lateral breast will move inferiorly on the straight mediolateral views. Rolled views are obtained for lesions that are seen only in the craniocaudal view, to confirm that it is a real finding or not [39].

A new area of focal asymmetry is sometimes related to initiation of hormone replacement therapy [HRT]. In such cases repeat mammogram after cessation of HRT may demonstrate a resolution of the focal asymmetry. A developing asymmetry that may appear less prominent but persists following cessation of therapy could at least in theory represent an estrogen-sensitive breast cancer [31]. Short-term cessation of hormone replacement prior to performance of screening mammography has been suggested although patient compliance may be an issue; one study reported that a majority of women [54 %] were unwilling to stop HRT for 1–2 months prior to undergoing a screening mammogram [40]. There is no proven benefit in stopping HRT in all patients prior to screening mammography. No significant reduction in recall rate was seen in those in whom HRT was suspended for 1–2 months prior to screening mammography [41].

Subtle Cancers/Missed Cancers

The sensitivity of mammography, i.e., the percentage of cancers with a positive interpretation, was 83.5 % based on 1,960,150 screening examinations performed between 2002 and 2006 [42]. Mammography misses 10–30 % of breast cancers [43]. Some of these cancers are truly occult, while others are missed due to perceptual error, interpretive error, or to limitation of the modality and/or technique such as dense breast parenchyma obscuring a lesion and poor positioning or technique [43]. Known pitfalls cited for missing a potential breast cancer on a screening mammogram include edge of the film findings, findings that are suspicious but stable, slowly developing asymmetry, architectural distortion, a finding seen on one-view only, benign-appearing nodule, presumed intramammary lymph node, shrinking breast, and scar carcinoma [44].

An edge of the image finding may also be due to lack of inclusion of the entire breast and should prompt recall and work-up to identify the lesion in orthogonal plane and if determined to be a true finding will need supplemental imaging with ultrasound. Another reason for failure to diagnose a breast cancer results from equating lesion stability with a benign process. Stable findings do not confirm benignity when morphological features are worrisome such as a mass with ill-defined borders or calcifications that have a suspicious distribution and/or morphology. A biopsy recommendation is appropriate after a diagnostic work-up for such lesions even if stability has been shown for 2–3 years. Architectural distortion when not associated with a mass particularly in a heterogeneously dense breast may be subtle and difficult to perceive or simulate the crisscrossing lines of normal breast parenchyma. Computer-aided detection [CAD] used to assist in lesion detection also tends to have low sensitivity for areas of architectural distortion. Certain cancers such as medullary, mucinous, and papillary cancers may appear as circumscribed masses that may appear benign and hence incorrectly categorized as benign and/or probably benign; such masses often reveal ill-defined borders on supplemental compression and magnification views. Close inspection of margin characteristics on ultrasound will often reveal suspicious morphology.

On occasion a small low-density nodule with a shallow notch may be presumed to be a lymph node and not be worked up. It is important to ensure that a fatty hilum is seen and that this finding is in the upper outer quadrant of the breast; multiplicity and bilaterality of such findings is also suggestive of intramammary lymph nodes. When masses appearing like lymph nodes are seen in locations that are not typical for lymph nodes such as in the inner breast, recall for a mammographic work-up, and identification of the sonographic correlate of a hyperechoic hilum is warranted to confirm the diagnosis of a benign intramammary lymph node. Although quite rare to develop at the site of a benign biopsy, it is not uncommon for recurrence of breast cancer to occur at the site of scar; careful analysis to look for increasing density, size, increasing convexity, or architectural distortion is required [44].

Findings seen in one view can also be problematic and a frequent reason for missing a breast cancer at screening mammography (Fig. 5.12a–c). About 3.3 % of such one-view findings have been reported in a series of 61,273 screening studies. A majority of these [82.7 %] are due to summation artifacts without a need for recall. There were 36 cancers, with a finding that was visible on one view only. An unusually large percentage of such missed cancers [33 %] were invasive lobular cancers; the remainder were DCIS [6 %] and invasive ductal cancers [18 %]. A large majority of these findings were density [84.8 %]; others included architectural distortion [10.7 %], calcifications [4.1 %], and combination [0.3 %]. Most one-view findings are seen on the MLO view since it includes more fibroglandular tissue than the CC view, with the exception of ILC which is often best seen on the CC view [33].

Poor mammographic technique and/or positioning can be an important cause of missing a breast cancer on a screening study. On occasion cancer may not be included on the mammographic views due to its location; this may happen particularly for those in the far medial breast or along the inframammary fold (Fig. 5.13a–d). Motion blurring, for instance, can mask out calcifications, small densities, and small areas of architectural distortion. Up to 62 % of breast cancers that presented as

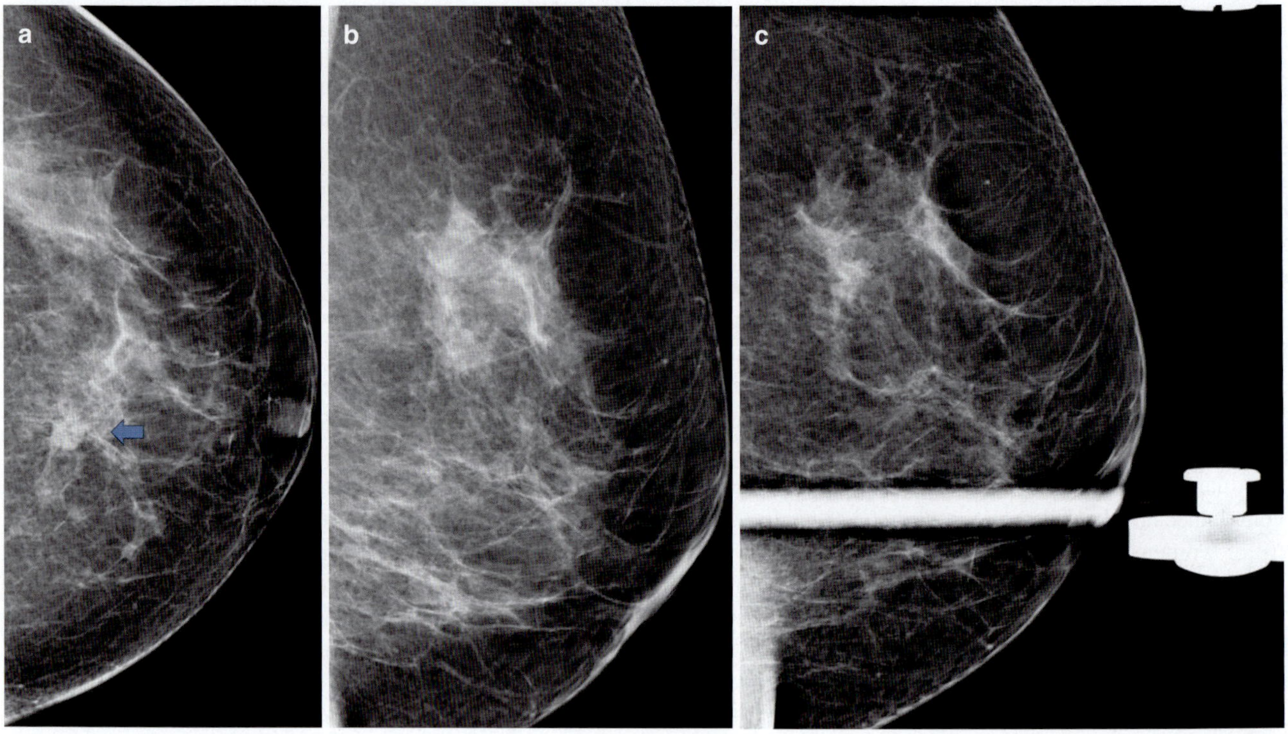

Fig. 5.12 (**a–c**) Small invasive ductal cancer visible on one view. Ultrasound (not shown) confirmed a 7 mm solid mass in the upper inner left breast. (**a**) Craniocaudal view shows a small round irregular density in the inner left breast (*arrow*). (**b**) Mediolateral view does not show a corresponding finding. (**c**) Mediolateral oblique view of the upper breast fails to demonstrate the cancer

microcalcifications were not biopsied and were attributed to blurring on magnification views [43]. A detailed description of and the importance of optimal technique and positioning is discussed elsewhere in this textbook.

Incorrect interpretation of a mammographic finding may be attributed to a lack of experience as in the case of general radiologist who may read a low number of mammograms or may be due to fatigue. Slow growing lesions or the absence of prior mammograms for comparison also increases the likelihood of misinterpreting subtle signs of a breast cancer [43]. Failure to adequately work up findings such as margin evaluation by spot compression views leads to erroneous interpretation of a mass with fine irregular margins as having a circumscribed border. In order to ensure that small cancers or cancers with subtle findings are not missed, careful and methodical inspection of mammograms comparing similar views of the right and left breast, looking for subtle asymmetry and changes from priors, and use of magnifying device to carefully evaluate the entire mammogram are needed. This will minimize the chances of missing subtle potential signs of breast cancer.

Meticulous attention to quality assurance and quality control to ensure proper positioning to include the entire breast, optimizing mammographic technical factors, and above all repeating mammograms that are blurred are also critical to avoid missing cancers with subtle signs.

A multi-institutional retrospective study examined the nonspecific findings on prior mammograms at locations where breast cancer subsequently developed. One unblinded radiologist determined that 286 findings of 493 examinations were deemed to be visible in retrospect at sites where cancer later developed. However, among a group of five blinded radiologists who reviewed these mammograms, none or only one or two of the radiologists recommended recall from screening [45]. The most frequent findings among interpretation factors were benign-appearing tissues, benign appearing calcifications, or too few calcifications. Among detection errors the most common were findings seen only on one view, overlooked calcifications, or findings at the edge of the glandular tissue. This study showed that a proportion of breast cancers display nonspecific mammographic findings that may not warrant recall and failure to act on such perceptible but nonspecific findings do not constitute interpretation below the standard of care. Berlin points out that during disposition of a malpractice claim, it is the testimony of individual experts that matters and majority votes of groups of expert witnesses are not considered in determining whether a defendant radiologist has or has not breached the standard of care [46]. In a comparison of retrospective versus blinded review of mammograms obtained prior to a diagnosis of impalpable breast cancers, in 30 patients [41 % of cancers] evidence of cancer was shown by blinded reviewers; however, in the remaining

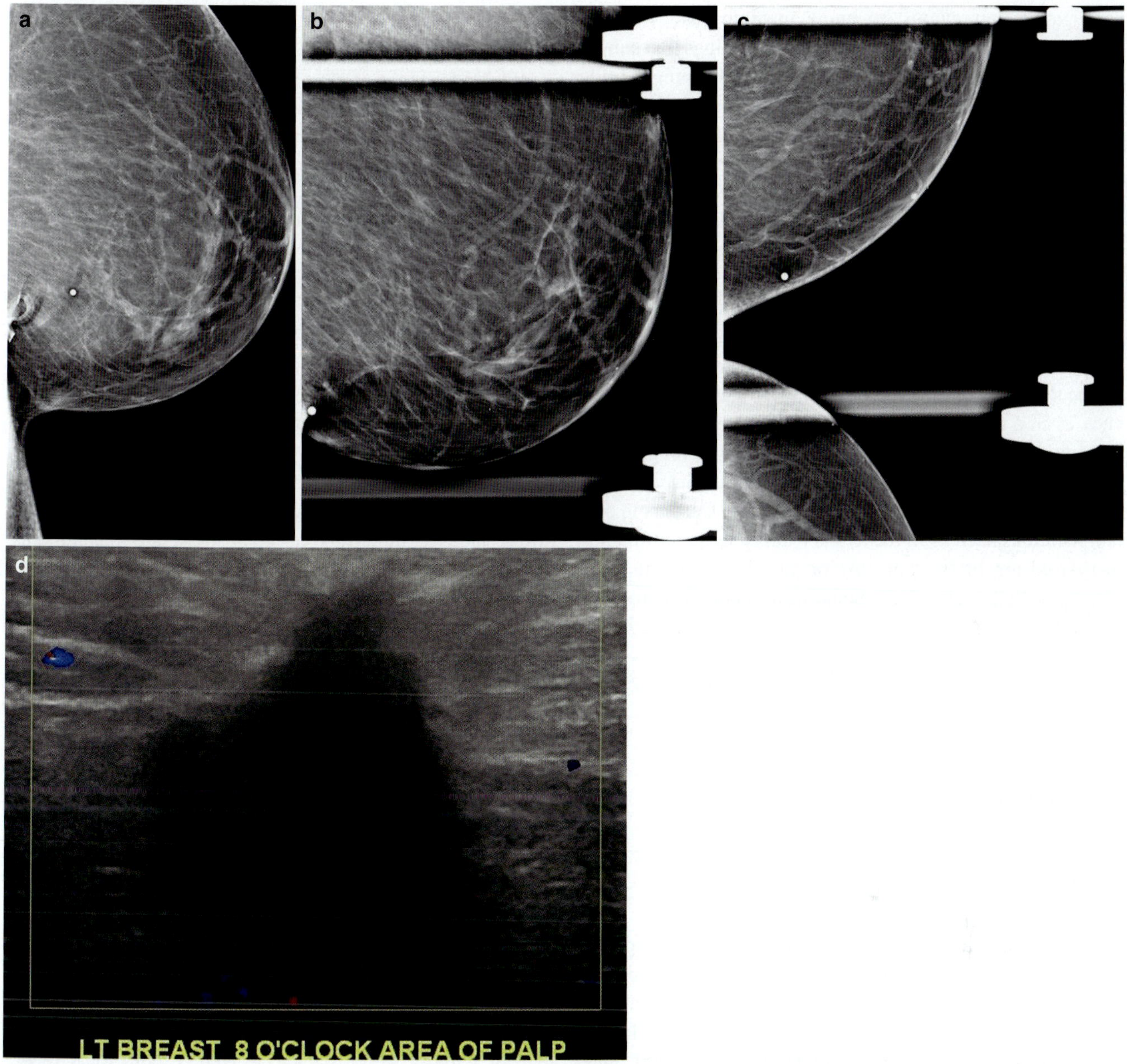

Fig. 5.13 (**a–d**) A palpable invasive ductal cancer mammographically occult in a fatty breast with failure to image the cancer due to its location. (**a**) Mediolateral oblique view does not show the palpable mass. (**b**) Spot compression view in the mediolateral view of the palpable finding fails to show the mass. (**c**) Spot compression view of the medial breast in the area of the palpable finding fails to show the mass. (**d**) Ultrasound demonstrates a large malignant-appearing mass close to the chest wall

43 patients [59 %] of those with cancers, the prior mammograms were read as negative or benign [47]. However, the retrospective reviewers thought that there was evidence of cancer in 25 of these patients. The majority of these findings that were called abnormal on a retrospective review were focal asymmetries. These authors concluded that impalpable cancers are frequently visible in retrospect on prior mammograms; however, since most are visible as an asymmetric density, these are not true radiologic errors. In a medical malpractice case of missed breast cancer, most experts testifying against a defendant radiologist are in essence performing a retrospective review having the benefit of knowing the diagnosis and location of the missed cancer. Retrospective reviews of this nature do not actually reflect the everyday practice of screening mammography; failure to detect or act upon a retrospectively evident finding should therefore not be considered as necessarily negligent [47].

The use of computer-aided detection (CAD) has been shown to decrease false-negative rate of mammography [48, 49]. In one study CAD decreased the false-negative rate at double reading by more than a third [31–19 %]. CAD system correctly marked 37 of 52 actionable findings that were read as negative in previous screening mammograms [48]. In another study CAD marked 42 % of 172 findings that subsequently developed cancer. Although CAD seemingly finds cancers that are subtle and missed, it can also lead to increased recall and biopsies [49]. A meta-analysis of studies looking at the value of CAD as a supplement to screening mammography showed that CAD yielded an additional 50 cancers in 100,000 women screened, but also led to recalls in 1,190 healthy women and 80 biopsies in healthy women. Ninety-six percent of women recalled based upon CAD and 65.1 % of women biopsied based upon CAD were healthy [50].

Missed cancers can be attributed to reader factors as well as due to subtle signs. The former may be a perceptual difference as in a cancer with subtle signs or interpretive errors. Suboptimal technique such as improper positioning and/or technical factors can also lead to decreased conspicuity of the cancer leading to a missed diagnosis [51]. Cancers in certain locations such as in the axillary tail or in the inframammary fold are often seen only on one view making their diagnosis challenging [52]. Some have reported that a significant number of missed cancers, up to a third, are in the retroglandular region of the breast [53], while others have found no statistically significant t difference in the location of missed cancers [54].

Uncommon Mammographic Signs of Breast Cancer

Solitary Dilated Duct

In the BI-RADS atlas, a solitary duct is described as a special case. Ducts are usually seen as tubular densities in a subareolar location; when prominent and bilateral, it is a benign finding indicative of duct ectasia. Wolfe has described a unilateral dilated duct as a possible sign of breast cancer [55]. One series looked at all cases of asymmetrically dilated ducts in a nonsubareolar location and found cancers in 11 [24 %] of 46 cases. Six [54 %] of these 11 cases had suspicious microcalcifications. They concluded that asymmetrically dilated ducts in a nonsubareolar location when associated with suspicious microcalcifications and/or interval change warrant biopsy [56].

Nevertheless the finding of a solitary dilated duct that is not associated with a mass, calcifications, or architectural distortion is exceedingly rare [57]. Only 21 [0.0079 %] cases were recorded for 264,476 consecutive mammography examinations. Ten were stable on follow-up for 2 years and presumed benign; 11 underwent biopsy. Among these there were two cancers, both DCIS [57]. Since the likelihood of malignancy is greater than 2 %, a BI-RADS 4 assessment may be warranted for this rare finding on mammography [57].

Box 5.3. Differential Diagnosis of Diffuse Skin Thickening of the Breast

1. Mastitis
2. Lymphatic obstruction
3. Lymphoma
4. Postradiation
5. Inflammatory breast cancer
6. Nephritic syndrome [bilateral]
7. Congestive heart failure [bilateral]

Diffuse Skin Thickening

Breast infection can demonstrate mammographic signs that mimic inflammatory breast cancer, namely, skin thickening, diffuse increase in density, irregular mass, and uncommonly architectural distortion. Mammography shows an abnormality in a significant number of patients with breast infection with sonography depicting an abscess in most cases when present [58]. The presence of diffuse breast thickening and of dense lymph nodes is suggestive of an underlying carcinoma. Diffuse skin thickening is rarely seen in unusual breast infections [58].

Breast skin thickening and edema may be caused by a variety of causes including mastitis, inflammatory breast cancer, lymphatic obstruction, lymphoma, postradiation changes, congestive heart failure, or nephritic syndrome [59] (Box 5.3). Granulomatous mastitis is a rare inflammatory disease of unknown origin that can mimic cancer. There is an association with oral contraceptive use. Pathologically it is characterized by granulomatous inflammation of the lobules with noncaseating granulomas. Mammographically peripheral areas of focal asymmetry are seen. Sonography demonstrated clustered tubular hypoechoic areas. Excisional biopsy with or without steroids may be needed, with local recurrence following excision having been reported [60, 61].

Inflammatory Breast Cancer

Inflammatory breast cancer is a rare but highly aggressive form of breast cancer and accounts for 1–6 % of breast cancer cases [62–64]. Prognosis is often poor due to the fact that micrometastasis is present at the time of diagnosis. Distant metastasis is present in 20 % of cases at the time of diagnosis, and the mean 5-year survival rate with modern multidisciplinary therapy is 20–40 %. Patients present with rapid onset of swelling and enlargement of the breast with skin erythema. A peau d'orange texture of the skin is caused by dermal edema resulting from lymphatic obstruction by tumor emboli. Tenderness, induration, and warmth are clinically apparent, and a palpable mass may or may not be present. IBC usually represents a poorly differentiated invasive ductal cancer.

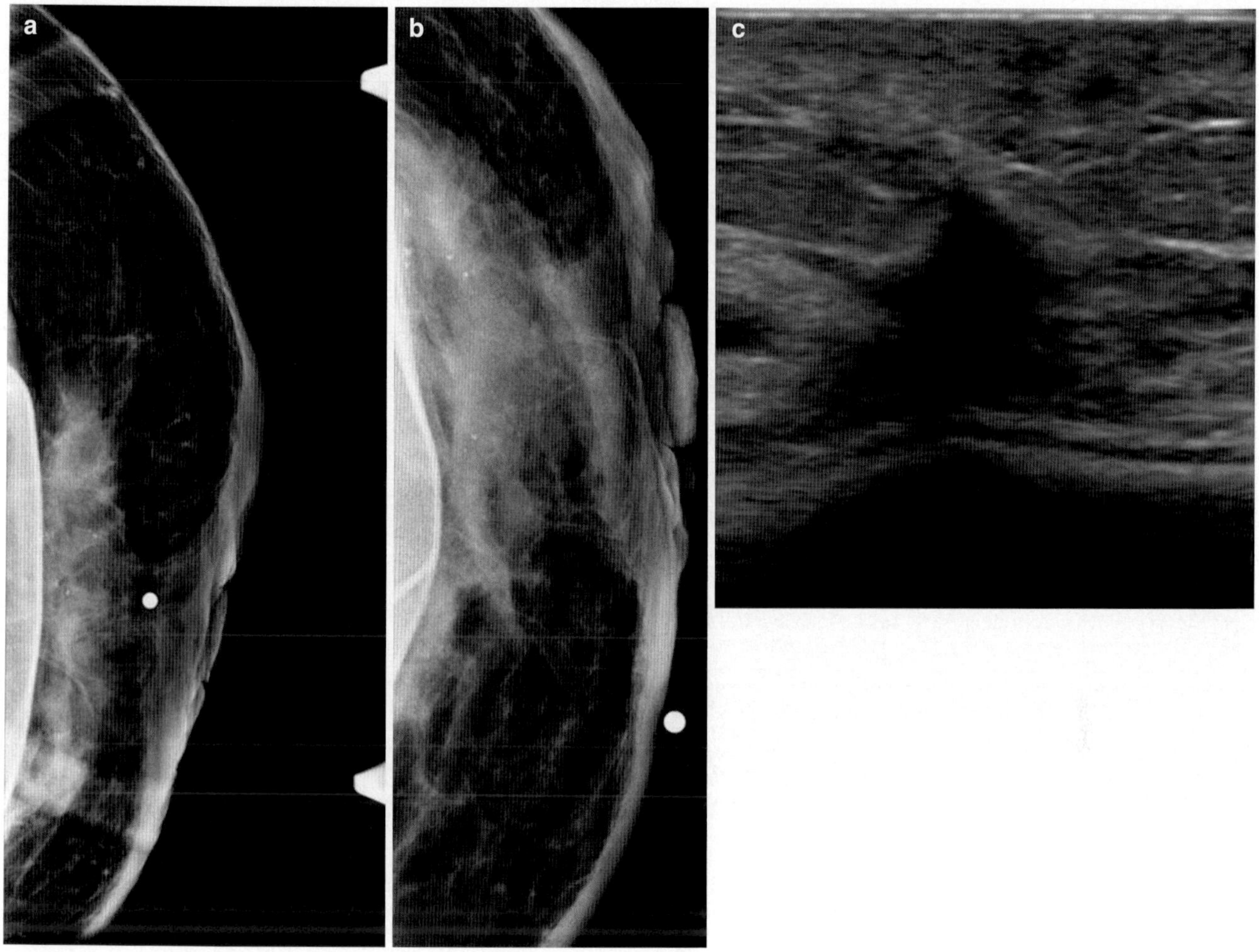

Fig. 5.14 (**a–c**) Inflammatory breast cancer in a 54-year-old woman. (**a**) Left mediolateral oblique view shows a large irregular focal asymmetry associated with suspicious-appearing microcalcifications. (**b**) Left craniocaudal view shows a large irregular focal asymmetry associated with suspicious-appearing microcalcifications and diffuse skin thickening. (**c**) Ultrasound demonstrates a large irregular malignant-appearing mass

Mammographic findings are seen in a majority of patients and include diffuse skin thickening, trabecular thickening, increased density, a mass, architectural distortion, and or calcifications [65–73]. Mammographic findings of a mass or calcifications are seen in 80–95 % of cases (Fig. 5.14a–c) [65, 66]. MRI has been reported to be the most accurate technique in detecting a breast parenchymal lesion in IBC patients [65]. The differential diagnosis of IBC is locally advanced breast cancer, primary breast lymphoma, and nonpuerperal mastitis, all of which are characterized by diffuse skin thickening, breast enlargement, and increased breast density [64].

Isolated Enlarged Lymph Nodes

In the BI-RADS™ atlas axillary adenopathy is included under associated findings with a guidance statement that reads "enlarged non fatty replaced axillary lymph nodes can be commented upon, mammographic assessment of these nodes is unreliable" [5]. The criteria to classify a lymph node as abnormal include a rounded shape, size > 2 cm, increased density, and absence of fatty hilum [74]. Unilaterally enlarged lymph nodes may be due to an underlying malignancy most commonly breast cancer, other malignancies, or non-neoplastic causes [74–80]. These may include those patients in whom enlarged lymph nodes are not associated with an underlying mammographic abnormality and represent an isolated finding. The malignancy rate reported in such instances varies from 33.3 to 52.3 %; sonographic evaluation of such abnormal lymph nodes identified at screening mammography has been shown to be useful in reducing false-positive and improving positive predictive value for biopsy [74]. The most common cause would be an occult breast primary; other causes would include lymphoma, metastasis from malignant melanoma, and lung, stomach, or ovarian carcinoma. Benign causes would include systemic inflammatory diseases such as

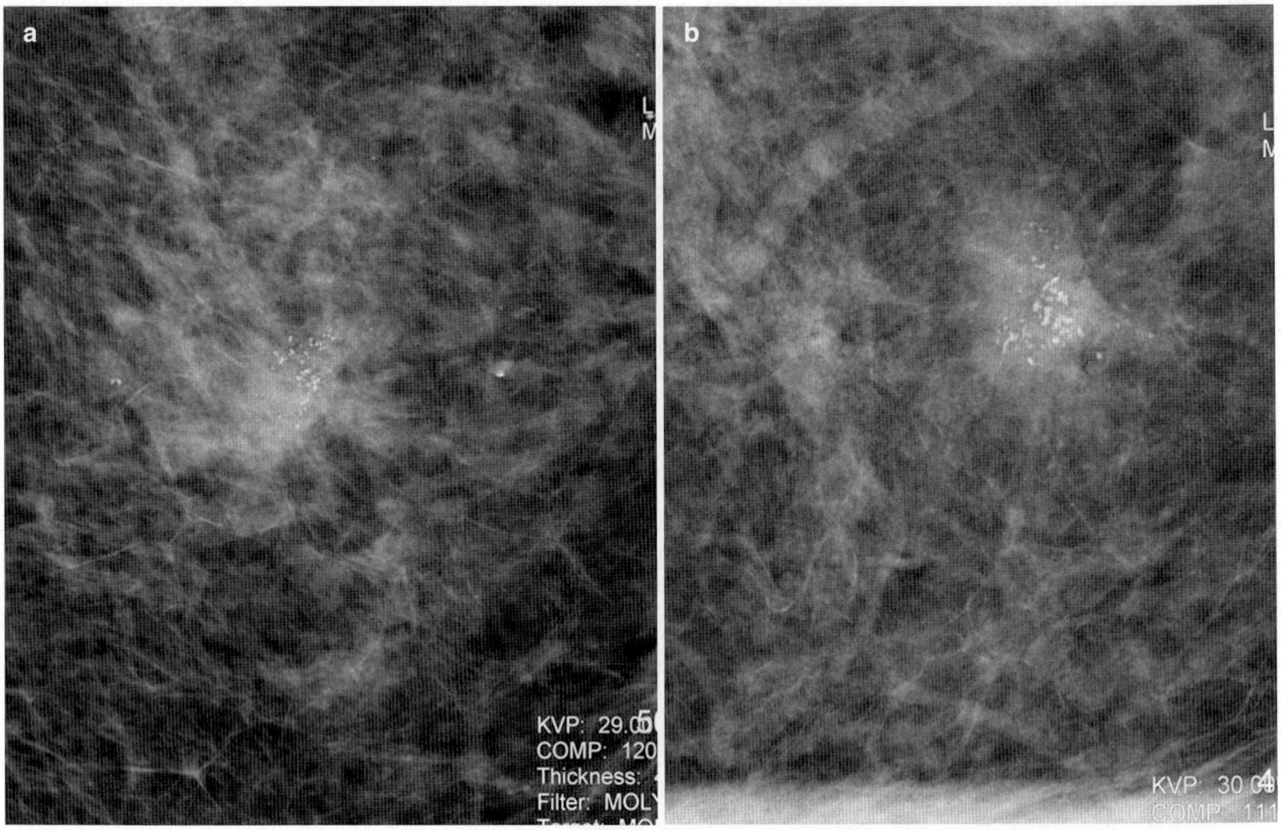

Fig. 5.15 (**a**, **b**) A 47-year-old woman with a triple-negative ductal carcinoma in situ with an invasive component. (**a**) Spot magnification view in the mediolateral projection shows a small irregular mass with clustered pleomorphic calcifications. (**b**) Spot magnification view in the craniocaudal projection shows a small irregular mass with clustered pleomorphic calcifications

sarcoidosis, infectious diseases such as tuberculosis, collagen vascular diseases, and miscellaneous causes such as silicone granulomas [74–78]. MRI is recommended in patients with isolated enlarged lymph nodes and a mammographically occult primary [81–83].

Triple-Negative Breast Cancers

Triple-negative breast cancers are a subgroup of breast cancers that do not express estrogen receptors (ER), progesterone receptors (PR), or human epidermal growth factor receptor 2 (HER 2). This particular phenotype of breast cancer has aggressive tumor biology and a higher degree of association with suppression of BRCA 1 function and a consequent poor prognosis. Triple-negative breast cancer (estrogen receptor-negative, progesterone receptor-negative, and HER2-negative) is a high-risk breast cancer that cannot be treated with drugs that target these proteins. Triple-negative breast cancers accounts for 11–20 % of all subtypes of breast cancer and accounts for 23–38 % of locally advanced disease [84]. Women with triple-negative tumors tend to be younger, more likely African-American, and overweight. Triple-negative cancers and HER 2+ cancers are less likely to be detected by screening mammography and less likely to be present as TI [46.5 %] or diagnosed as Stage 1 [32.6 %]. TN tumors are often high grade [83 %] and invasive [93 %] [84]. Despite the large size at the time of diagnosis, up to 28.9 % of TNBC may be mammographically occult. The most common presentation on a mammography is as a mass which is circumscribed in 20–24 % of cases and with absence of calcifications in 49–100 % of cases [84–88].

Triple-negative breast cancers may lack the common and typical features on mammography that are encountered with breast cancer such as irregular masses, spiculation, or malignant-appearing calcifications. Mammography may hence be of limited value in screening women who are at risk to develop TNBC. Ultrasound has a higher sensitivity than mammography; however, in a substantial number of cases masses may exhibit benign features (21–41 % of cases). MRI has a higher sensitivity than either mammography or ultrasound and has been proposed as a modality of choice for establishing baseline prior to neoadjuvant chemotherapy [85–87]. In one series ultrasound found all 88 of TN cancers, most frequently as masses [92.5 %]; posterior acoustic enhancement was seen in 41.6 % of TN tumors, and posterior acoustic attenuation was seen in only in 8.7 % of cases. An elasticity score of 4 or 5 was noted on elastography in

87.5 % of tumors [88]. Triple-negative DCIS present mammographically as calcifications less commonly than non-TN DCIS, 22 % in one series. They more commonly appeared as masses or focal asymmetry. Triple-negative DCIS are rare, reported in 3.6 % in one series of 494 cases [89] (Fig. 5.15a, b).

Invasive Lobular Cancer

Invasive lobular cancer accounts for 10–15 % of invasive breast cancers. ILC has a higher rate of multiplicity and bilaterality, despite which tends to have a better prognosis than invasive ductal cancers [14]. These cancers can be difficult to detect at mammography due to the fact that the opacity may be equal to or lower than normal fibroglandular tissue due to lack of incitement of a desmoplastic reaction. Mammographically they are often seen only on one view, often on the craniocaudal projection. These cancers often fail to form discrete palpable masses and hence may also remain occult to clinical examination [14]. Up to 19 % of false-negative rates are reported for ILC at mammography because of difficulty in mammographic detection [90, 91]. Ultrasound is superior to mammography in detecting multifocality and multicentricity of ILC. The size of tumor is more accurately assessed by sonography. The sensitivity of US for detection of ILC ranges from 68 to 98 %. Ultrasound is also a valuable adjunct to mammography to biopsy and preoperatively localizes ILC particularly when seen only on one view [14, 92].

Mammographic Features of ILC

The reported sensitivity of mammography is 57–81 % [14, 90, 93, 94]. ILC is most commonly seen on a mammogram as a mass [44–65 %] usually with spiculated margins. Architectural distortion is the next most common mammographic pattern [10–34 % of cases] followed by focal asymmetry [1–14 % of cases]. Calcifications are less commonly associated with a reported association in 0–24 % of cases [14, 90, 93, 94]. Round and circumscribed masses are uncommon and seen only in 1–3 % of cases [14, 95]. In a series of 49 patients with ILC, masses were seen in 43 % of cases, architectural distortion in 20 %, and asymmetries in 18 %. Surprisingly in 16 % of patients ILC was associated with microcalcifications. Normal or benign findings were seen in 10 % of cases [14]. The most common US manifestation of ILC is solid hypoechoic and heterogeneous mass with irregular or angular or spiculated borders and posterior acoustic shadowing seen in 54–61 % of cases [92, 95–97]. ILC can also appear on ultrasound as a circumscribed mass, an area of focal shadowing without a discreet mass, or be sonographically occult [95] (Fig. 5.16a–i).

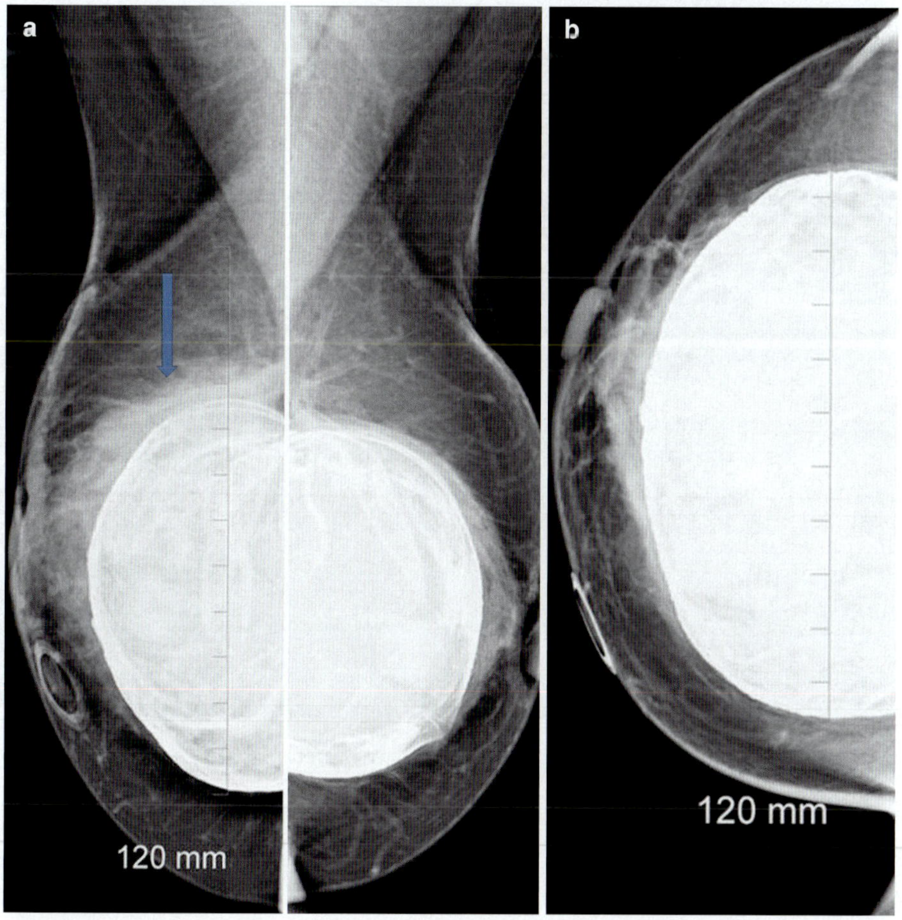

Fig. 5.16 (**a**–**i**) A 56-year-old woman with a palpable lump in right breast histologically proven to be infiltrating lobular cancer. (**a**) Mediolateral oblique view demonstrates an area focal asymmetry (*arrow*) in the upper right breast adjacent to the implant corresponding to the palpable finding. (**b**) Craniocaudal view of the right breast demonstrates no abnormal finding. (**c**) Ultrasound shows a large irregular malignant-appearing mass adjacent to the implant. (**d**) Ultrasound shows a large irregular malignant-appearing mass adjacent to the implant. (**e**) Mediolateral oblique view obtained at the end of 3 months of chemotherapy reveals near-complete resolution of the focal asymmetry. A post biopsy clip is visible. (**f**) Ultrasound obtained at the end of 3 months of chemotherapy reveals near-complete resolution of the focal asymmetry. A post biopsy clip is visible. (**g**) Post gadolinium sagittal T1-weighted fat-suppressed MRI image of the right breast demonstrates an enhancing cancer superior to the implant. (**h**) Subtracted image reveals the enhancing cancer in right breast. (**i**) Axial MRI CAD image demonstrates the enhancing tumor in the right breast

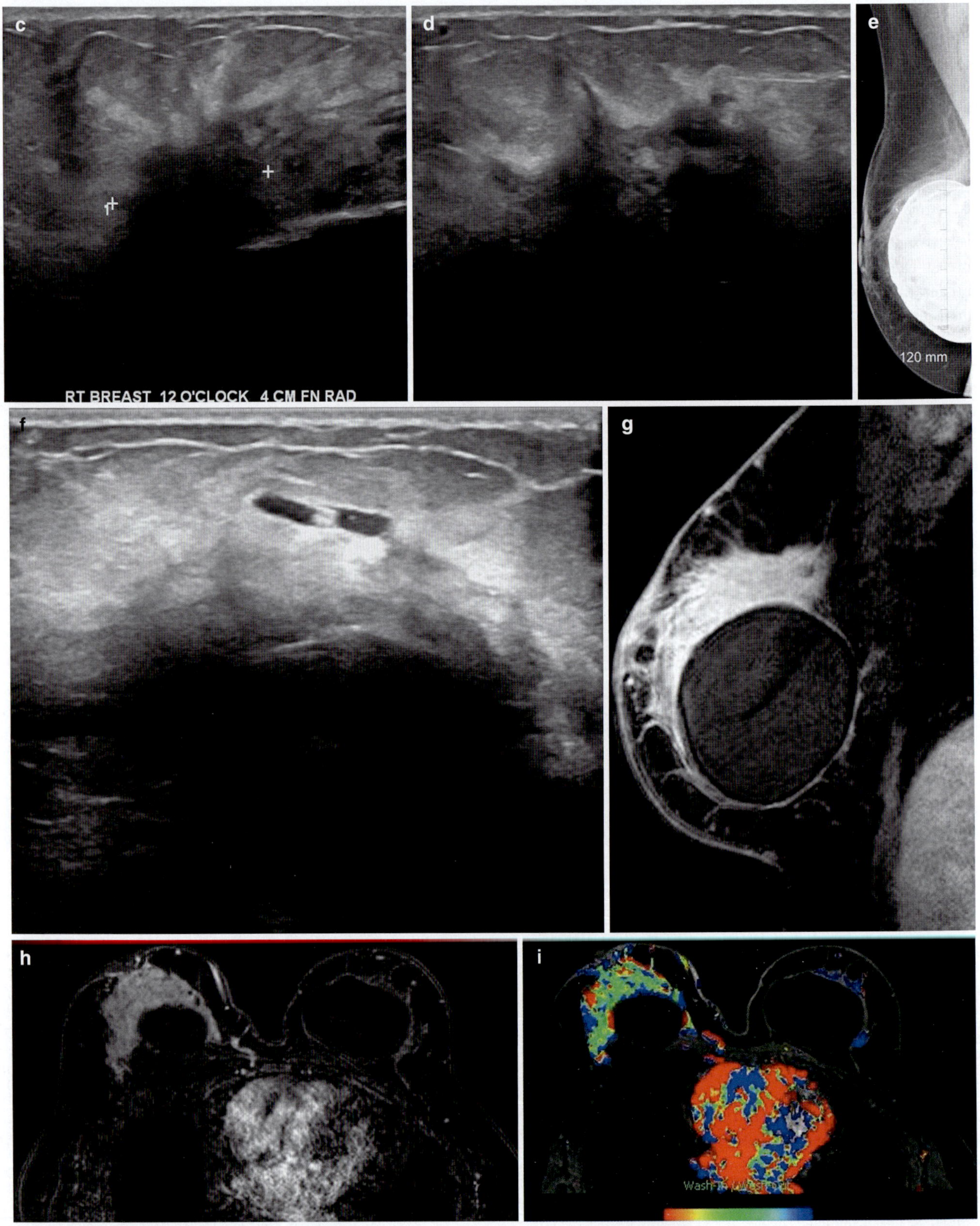

Fig. 5.16 (continued)

References

1. Venkatesan A, Chu P, Kerlikowske K, Sickles E, Smith-Bindman R. Positive predictive value of specific mammographic findings according to reader and patient variables. Radiology. 2009;250(3): 648–57.
2. Gajdos C, Tartler PI, Bleiweiss IJ. Mammographic appearance of nonpalpable breast cancer reflects pathologic characteristics. Ann Surg. 2002;235(2):246–51.
3. Liberman L, Abramson AF, Squires FB, Glassman JR, Morris EA, Dershaw DD. The breast imaging reporting and data system: positive predictive value of mammographic features and final assessment categories. AJR Am J Roentgenol. 1998;171(1):35–40.
4. Sickles EA. Breast masses: mammographic evaluation. Radiology. 1989;173(2):297–303.
5. American College of Radiology. Breast imaging reporting and data system (BI-RADS). 4th ed. Reston: American College of Radiology; 2003.
6. Woods RW, Sisney GS, Salkowski LR, Shinki K, Lin Y, Burnside ES. The mammographic density of a mass is a significant predictor of breast cancer. Radiology. 2011;258(2):417–25.
7. Woods RW, Oliphant L, Shinki K, Page D, Shavlik J, Burnside E. Validation of results from knowledge discovery: mass density as a predictor of breast cancer. J Digit Imaging. 2010;23(5):554–61.
8. Tamaki K, Ishida T, Miyashita M, Amari M, Ohuchi N, Tamaki N, Sasano H. Correlation between mammographic findings and corresponding histopathology: potential predictors for biological characteristics of breast diseases. Cancer Sci. 2011;102(12):2179–85.
9. Thurfjell MG, Lindgren A, Thurfjell E. Nonpalpable breast cancer: mammographic appearance as predictor of histologic type. Radiology. 2002;222(1):165–70.
10. Reiff DB, Cooke J, Griffin M, Given-Wilson R. Ductal carcinoma in situ presenting as a stellate lesion on mammography. Clin Radiol. 1994;49:396–9.
11. Thurfjell E, Thurfjell MG, Lindgren A. Mammographic finding as predictor of survival in 1–9 mm invasive breast cancers. Worse prognosis for cases presenting as calcifications alone. Breast Cancer Res Treat. 2001;67(2):177–80.
12. Ikeda DM, Anderson I. Ductal carcinoma in situ: atypical mammographic appearances. Radiology. 1989;172:661–9.
13. Sekine K, et al. DCIS showing architectural distortion on screening mammogram – comparison of mammographic and pathological findings. Breast Cancer. 2007;14(3):281–4.
14. Lopez JK, Bassett LW. Invasive lobular carcinoma of the breast: spectrum of mammographic, US, and MR imaging findings. Radiographics. 2009;29:165–76.
15. Tabar L, Dean PB. Stellate lesions. In: Tabar L, Dean PB, editors. Teaching atlas of mammography. Second revised. New York: Georg Thieme Verlag; 1985. p. 87–136.
16. Kennedy M, Masterson AV, Kerin M, Flanagan F. Pathology and clinical relevance of radial scars: a review. J Clin Pathol. 2003;56(10):721–4.
17. Neilsen M, Christensen L, Anderson J. Radial scars in women with breast cancer. Cancer. 1987;59:1019–25.
18. Ciatto S, Morrone D, Catarzi S, et al. Radial scars of the breast: review of 38 consecutive mammographic diagnoses. Radiology. 1993;187:757–60.
19. King TA, Scharfenberg JC, Smetherman DH, et al. A better understanding of the term radial scar. Am J Surg. 2000;180(6):428–32.
20. Cohen MA, Sferlazza SJ. Role of sonography in evaluation of radial scars of the breast. AJR Am J Roentgenol. 2000;174:1075–8.
21. Shetty MK. Radial scars of the breast: sonographic findings. Ultrasound Q. 2002;18(3):203–7.
22. Finlay ME, Liston JE, Lunt LG, et al. Assessment of the role of ultrasound in the differentiation of radial scars and stellate carcinomas of the breast. Clin Radiol. 1994;49:52–5.
23. Shaheen R, Schimmelpenninck CA, Stoddart L, Raymond H, Slanetz PJ. Spectrum of diseases presenting as architectural distortion on mammography: multimodality radiologic imaging with pathologic correlation. Semin Ultrasound CT MR. 2011;32(4):351–62.
24. Taşkin F, Köseoğlu K, Unsal A, Erkuş M, Ozbaş S, Karaman C. Sclerosing adenosis of the breast: radiologic appearance and efficiency of core needle biopsy. Diagn Interv Radiol. 2011;17(4):311–6.
25. Günhan-Bilgen I, Memiş A, Ustün EE, Ozdemir N, Erhan Y. Sclerosing adenosis: mammographic and ultrasonographic findings with clinical and histopathological correlation. Eur J Radiol. 2002;44(3):232–8.
26. Hogge JP, Robinson RE, Magnant CM, Zuurbier RA. The mammographic spectrum of fat necrosis of the breast. Radiographics. 1995;15(6):1347–56.
27. DiPiro PJ, Meyer JE, Frenna TH, Denison CM. Seat belt injuries of the breast: findings on mammography and sonography. AJR Am J Roentgenol. 1995;164(2):317–20.
28. Demitri-Lewis A, Slaentz PJ, Eisneberg RL. Breast calcifications: the focal group. AJR Am J Roentgenol. 2012;198:W325–43.
29. Bird RE. Critical pathways in analyzing breast microcalcifications. Radiographics. 1995;15:928–34.
30. Stomper PC, Geradts J, Edge SB, Levine EG. Mammographic predictors of the presence and size of invasive carcinomas associated with malignant microcalcifications lesions without a mass. AJR Am J Roentgenol. 2003;181:1679–84.
31. Samardar P, Shaw de Paredes E, Grimes MM, Wilson JD. Focal asymmetric densities seen at mammography: US and pathologic correlation. Radiographics. 2002;22:19–33.
32. Sickles EA. The spectrum of breast asymmetries: imaging features, work-up, management. Radiol Clin North Am. 2007;45(5): 765–71.
33. Sickles EA. Findings at mammographic screening on only one standard projection: outcomes analysis. Radiology. 1998;208(2): 471–5.
34. Kopans DB, Swan CA, White G, et al. Asymmetric breast tissue. Radiology. 1989;171(3):639–43.
35. Leung JWT, Sickles EA. Developing asymmetry identified on mammography: correlation with imaging outcome and pathologic findings. AJR Am J Roentgenol. 2007;188(3):667–75.
36. Sickles EA. Mammographic features of 300 consecutive nonpalpable breast cancers. AJR Am J Roentgenol. 1986;146:661–3.
37. Shetty MK, Watson AB. Sonographic evaluation of focal asymmetric density of the breast. Ultrasound Q. 2002;18(2):115–21.
38. Youk JH, Kim E, Ko KH, et al. Asymmetric mammographic findings based on the fourth edition of BI-RADS: types, evaluation, and management. Radiographics. 2009;29(1):1–48.
39. Brenner RJ. Strategies in the evaluation of breast asymmetries. Appl Radiol. 1998;27:15–20.
40. Reed SD, Buist DS, Anderson ML, Bowles EJ, Fitzgibbons D, Seger D, Newton KM. Short-term (1–2 mo) hormone therapy cessation before mammography. Menopause. 2009;16(6):1125–31.
41. Buist DS, Anderson ML, Reed SD, Aiello Bowles EJ, Fitzgibbons ED, Gandara JC, Seger D, Newton KM. Short-term hormone therapy suspension and mammography recall: a randomized trial. Ann Intern Med. 2009;150(11):752–65.
42. Performance measures for 1,960,150 screening mammography examinations from 2002 to 2006 by age – based on BCSC data as of 2009 NCI-funded Breast Cancer Surveillance Consortium co-operative agreement (U01CA63740, U01CA86076, U01CA86082, U01CA63736, U01CA70013, U01CA69976, U01CA63731, U01CA70040). Downloaded from the Breast Cancer Surveillance Consortium Web site. http://breastscreening.cancer.gov/data/performance/screening/2009/perf_age.html.

43. Majid AS, Parades ES, Doherty RD, Sharma NR, Salvador X. Missed breast carcinoma: pitfalls and pearls. Radiographics. 2003;23:881–95.
44. Roberts-Klein S, Iuanow E, Slaentz PJ. Avoiding pitfalls in mammographic interpretation. Can Assoc Radiol J. 2011;62:50–9.
45. Ikeda DM, Birdwell RL, O'Shaughnessy KF, Brenner RJ, Sickles EA. Analysis of 172 subtle findings on prior normal mammograms in women with breast cancer detected at follow-up screening. Radiology. 2003;226:494–503.
46. Berlin L. Missed mammographic abnormalities, malpractice, and expert witnesses: does majority rule in the courtroom? [letter]. Radiology. 2003;229:288–9.
47. Harvey JA, Fajardo LL, Innis CA. Previous mammograms in patients with impalpable breast carcinoma: retrospective vs blinded interpretation. 1993 ARRS President's Award. Am J Roentgenol. 1993;161:1167–72.
48. Destounis SV, DiNitto P, Logan-Young W, Bonaccio E, Zuley ML, Willison KM. Can computer-aided detection with double reading of screening mammograms help decrease the false-negative rate? Initial experience. Radiology. 2004;232(2):578–84.
49. Ikeda DM, Birdwell RL, O'Shaughnessy KF, Sickles EA, Brenner RJ. Computer-aided detection output on 172 subtle findings on normal mammograms previously obtained in women with breast cancer detected at follow-up screening mammography. Radiology. 2004;230(3):811–9.
50. Noble M, Bruening W, Uhl S, Schoelles K. Computer aided detection mammography for breast cancer screening: systematic review and meta-analysis. Arch Gynecol Obstet. 2009;279(6):881–90.
51. Giess CS, Frost EP, Birdwell RL. Difficulties and errors in diagnosis of breast neoplasms. Semin Ultrasound CT MR. 2012;33: 288–99.
52. Brenner RJ. False-negative mammograms: medical, legal, and risk management implications. Radiol Clin North Am. 2000;38: 741–57.
53. Bird RE, Wallace TW, Yankaskas BC. Analysis of cancers missed at screening mammography. Radiology. 1992;184:613–7.
54. Goergen SK, Evans J, Cohen GP, et al. Characteristics of breast carcinomas missed by screening radiologists. Radiology. 1997;204: 131–5.
55. Wolfe JN. Mammography: ducts as a sole indicator of breast carcinoma. Radiology. 1967;89:206–10.
56. Huynh PT, Parellada JA, de Paredes ES, et al. Dilated duct pattern at mammography. Radiology. 1997;204:137–41.
57. Chang CB, Lvoff NM, Leung JW, et al. Solitary dilated duct identified at mammography: outcomes analysis. AJR Am J Roentgenol. 2010;194:378–82.
58. Crowe DJ, Helvie MA, Wilson TE, Crowe DJ. Breast infection. Mammographic and sonographic findings with clinical correlation. Invest Radiol. 1995;30(10):582–7.
59. Kwak JY, Kim EK, Chung SY, You JK, Oh KK, Lee YH, et al. Unilateral breast edema: spectrum of etiologies and imaging appearances. Yonsei Med J. 2005;46:1–7.
60. An YY, Kim SH, Cha ES, et al. Diffuse infiltrative lesion of the breast: clinical and radiologic features. Korean J Radiol. 2011;12(1):113–21.
61. Han BK, Choe YH, Park JM, Moon WK, Ko YH, Yang JH, et al. Granulomatous mastitis: mammographic and sonographic appearances. AJR Am J Roentgenol. 1999;173:317–20.
62. Levine PH, Steinhorn SC, Ries LG, Aron JL. Inflammatory breast cancer: the experience of the surveillance, epidemiology, and end results (SEER) program. J Natl Cancer Inst. 1985;74:291–7.
63. Chang S, Parker SL, Pham T, Buzdar AU, Hursting SD. Inflammatory breast carcinoma incidence and survival: the surveillance, epidemiology, and end results program of the National Cancer Institute, 1975–1992. Cancer. 1998;82:2366–72.
64. Hance KW, Anderson WF, Devesa SS, Young HA, Levine PH. Trends in inflammatory breast carcinoma incidence and survival: the surveillance, epidemiology, and end results program at the National Cancer Institute. J Natl Cancer Inst. 2005;97: 966–75.
65. Yang WT, Le-Petross HT, Macapinlac H, et al. Inflammatory breast cancer: PET/CT, MRI, mammography, and sonography findings. Breast Cancer Res Treat. 2008;109(3):417–26.
66. Dershaw DD, Moore MP, Liberman L, et al. Inflammatory breast carcinoma: mammographic findings. Radiology. 1994;190:831–4.
67. Lee B, Tannenbaum N. Inflammatory carcinoma of the breast: a report of twenty-eight cases from the breast clinic of memorial hospital. Surg Gynecol Obstet. 1924;39:580–5.
68. Droulias CA, Sewell CW, McSweeney MB, et al. Inflammatory carcinoma of the breast: a correlation of clinical, radiologic and pathologic findings. Ann Surg. 1976;184:217–22.
69. Gunhan-Bilgen I, Ustun EE, Memis A. Inflammatory breast carcinoma: mammographic, ultrasonographic, clinical, and pathologic findings in 142 cases. Radiology. 2002;223:829–38.
70. Kushwaha AC, Whitman GJ, Stelling CB, et al. Primary inflammatory carcinoma of the breast: retrospective review of mammographic findings. AJR Am J Roentgenol. 2000;174:535–8.
71. Caumo F, Gaioni MB, Bonetti F, et al. Occult inflammatory breast cancer: review of clinical, mammographic, US and pathologic signs. Radiol Med (Torino). 2005;109:308–20.
72. Tardivon AA, Viala J, CorvellecRudelli A, et al. Mammographic patterns of inflammatory breast carcinoma: a retrospective study of 92 cases. Eur J Radiol. 1997;24:124–30.
73. Lee KW, Chung SY, Yang I, et al. Inflammatory breast cancer: imaging findings. Clin Imaging. 2005;29(22–250):1014–24.
74. Shetty MK, Carpenter WS. Sonographic evaluation of isolated abnormal axillary lymph nodes identified on mammograms. J Ultrasound Med. 2004;23(1):63–71.
75. Given-Wilson RM, Murray ME. The clinical importance of axillary lymphadenopathy detected on screening mammography. Clin Radiol. 1997;52:458–61.
76. Bergvist L, Frodis E, Hedborg-Mellander C, Hansen J. Management of accidentally found pathological lymph nodes on routine screening mammography. Eur J Surg Oncol. 1996;22:250–3.
77. Lee LH, Giurescu ME, Philpotts LE, Horvath LJ, Tocino I. Clinical importance of unilaterally enlarging lymph nodes on otherwise normal mammograms. Radiology. 1997;203:329–34.
78. Görkem SB, O'Connell AM. Abnormal axillary lymph nodes on negative mammograms: causes other than breast cancer. Diagn Interv Radiol. 2012;18(5):473–9.
79. Walsh R, Kornuguth PJ, Soo MS, Bentley R, Delong DM. Axillary lymph nodes: mammographic, pathologic and clinical correlation. AJR Am J Roentgenol. 1997;168:33–8.
80. Rahbar H, Partridge SC, Javid SH, Lehman CD. Imaging axillary lymph nodes in patients with newly diagnosed breast cancer. Curr Probl Diagn Radiol. 2012;41(5):149–58.
81. Morris EA, Schwartz LH, Dershaw DD, Van Zee KJ, Abramson AF, Liberman L. MR imaging of the breast in patients with occult primary breast carcinoma. Radiology. 1997;205:437–40.
82. Tilanus-Linthorst MM, Obdeijn AI, Bontenbal M, Oudkerk M. MRI in patients with axillary metastases of occult breast carcinoma. Breast Cancer Res Treat. 1997;44:179–82.
83. Obdeijn IM, Brouwers-Kuyper EM, Tilanus-Linthorst MM, Wiggers T, Oudkerk M. MR imaging-guided sonography followed by fine-needle aspiration cytology in occult carcinoma of the breast. AJR Am J Roentgenol. 2000;174:1079–84.
84. Lin NU, Vanderplas A, Hughes ME, et al. Clinicopathological features and sites of recurrence according to breast cancer subtype in the National Comprehensive Cancer Network (NCCN). J Clin Oncol. 2009;27(15s):Abstr 543.

85. Yang WT, Dryden M, Broglio K, et al. Mammographic features of triple receptor negative primary breast cancers in young premenopausal women. Breast Cancer Res Treat. 2008;111:405–10.
86. Wang Y, Ikeda DM, Narasimhan B, et al. Estrogen receptor-negative invasive breast cancer: imaging features of tumors with and without human epidermal growth factor receptor type 2 over expression. Radiology. 2008;246:367–75.
87. Dogan BE, Gonzalez-Angulo AM, Gilcrease M, et al. Multimodality imaging of triple receptor-negative tumors with mammography, ultrasound, and MRI. AJR Am J Roentgenol. 2010;194:1160–6.
88. Kojima Y, Tsunoda H. Mammography and ultrasound feature of triple-negative breast cancer. Breast Cancer. 2011;18:146–51.
89. Kojima Y, Tsunoda H, Honda S, Kikuchi M, Kawauchi N, Yoshida A, Yagata H, Yamauchi H, Suzuki K. Radiographic features for triple negative ductal carcinoma in situ of the breast. Breast Cancer. 2011;18(3):213–20.
90. Krecke KN, Gisvold JJ. Invasive lobular carcinoma of the breast: mammographic findings and extent of disease at diagnosis in 184 patients. AJR Am J Roentgenol. 1993;161(5):957–60.
91. Berg WA, Gutierrez L, NessAiver MS, et al. Diagnostic accuracy of mammography, clinical examination, US, and MR imaging in preoperative assessment of breast cancer. Radiology. 2004;233(3): 830–49.
92. Selinko VL, Middleton LP, Dempsey PJ. Role of sonography in diagnosing and staging invasive lobular carcinoma. J Clin Ultrasound. 2004;32(7):323–32.
93. Hilleren DJ, Andersson IT, Lindholm K, Linnell FS. Invasive lobular carcinoma: mammographic findings in a 10-year experience. Radiology. 1991;178(1):149–54.
94. Le Gal M, Ollivier L, Asselain B, et al. Mammographic features of 455 invasive lobular carcinomas. Radiology. 1992;185(3): 705–8.
95. Butler RS, Venta LA, Wiley EL, Ellis RL, Dempsey PJ, Rubin E. Sonographic evaluation of infiltrating lobular carcinoma. AJR Am J Roentgenol. 1999;172(2):325–30.
96. Paramagul CP, Helvie MA, Adler DD. Invasive lobular carcinoma: sonographic appearance and role of sonography in improving diagnostic sensitivity. Radiology. 1995;195(1):231–4.
97. Evans WP, Warren Burhenne LJ, Laurie L, O'Shaughnessy KF, Castellino RA. Invasive lobular carcinoma of the breast: mammographic characteristics and computer- computer-aided detection. Radiology. 2002;225(1):182–9.

Probably Benign Abnormalities of the Breast

6

Mahesh K. Shetty

Probably Benign Findings on Mammography

Screening mammography has been well established and is the modality of choice for screening for breast cancer in women who are at an average risk for cancer. False-positive mammographic findings are often cited as one of the limitations of mammographic screening. There is a clear need to reduce the number of biopsies of benign lesions. Some of the findings that lead to a biopsy recommendation are those with a low probability of cancer. A prospective study was undertaken by Sickles and others to evaluate mammographic findings that have a low likelihood for malignancy. The findings of that landmark study have been the basis of a probably benign assessment category. Mammographic findings with a low probability of representing breast cancer should not prompt a recommendation for a biopsy and should instead be subjected to short-interval surveillance. The rationale being that these findings have a less than 2 % likelihood of being representative of breast cancer and when so are identified by interval change at a stage with a favorable prognosis [1–6]. Decreasing the number of biopsies clearly is needed to reduce morbidity resulting from unnecessary biopsies and decrease the cost of the breast cancer screening program.

Criteria for categorizing findings on a mammogram as probably benign are summarized in Box 6.1 [2]. Mammographic findings that are clearly benign (Box 6.2) should not be placed in the probably benign category and do not need short-term surveillance. A clear understanding of the criteria is important to place an abnormality in the short-term follow-up category. It is also important to note that mammographic findings can be placed under short-interval surveillance only after a diagnostic workup of the findings that are initially identified on a screening mammogram. Probably benign assessment category should not be inappropriately used without a proper diagnostic workup. Benign abnormalities such as multiple similar-

Box 6.1. Mammographic Findings That Are Appropriate for Short-Interval Surveillance

1. Localized
   - Clusters of round or oval calcifications [38.8 %][a]
   - Noncalcified nonpalpable masses with well-defined margins and round, oval, or gently lobulated [18.5 %]
   - Focal asymmetry [14.1 %]
   - Miscellaneous: single dilated duct, architectural distortion at biopsy sites [1.3 %]
2. Generalized
   - Multiple tiny calcifications randomly distributed throughout both breast [16.4 %]
   - Multiple clusters of calcifications [3 %]
   - Multiple masses with similar appearance distributed throughout both breast [7.9 %]

Data from Sickles et al. [2]

[a]Percentages of abnormalities in the study group [2]

Box 6.2. Mammographic Findings That Are Clearly Benign and Requiring No Follow-Up

1. Dermal calcifications
2. Vascular calcifications
3. Mass with milk of calcium
4. Characteristic calcified fibroadenoma
5. Sutural calcifications
6. Rodlike calcifications often bilateral associated with duct ectasia
7. Fat density masses
8. Lymph nodes
9. Multiple bilateral similar appearing masses

M.K. Shetty, MD, FRCR, FACR, FAIUM
Department of Radiology, Baylor College of Medicine, Houston, TX, USA

Woman's Center for Breast Care and MRI, Woman's Hospital of Texas, Fannin 7600, Houston, TX 77054, USA
e-mail: mshettymd@womans-clinic.com

M.K. Shetty (ed.), *Breast Cancer Screening and Diagnosis: A Synopsis*,
DOI 10.1007/978-1-4939-1267-4_6, © Springer Science+Business Media New York 2015

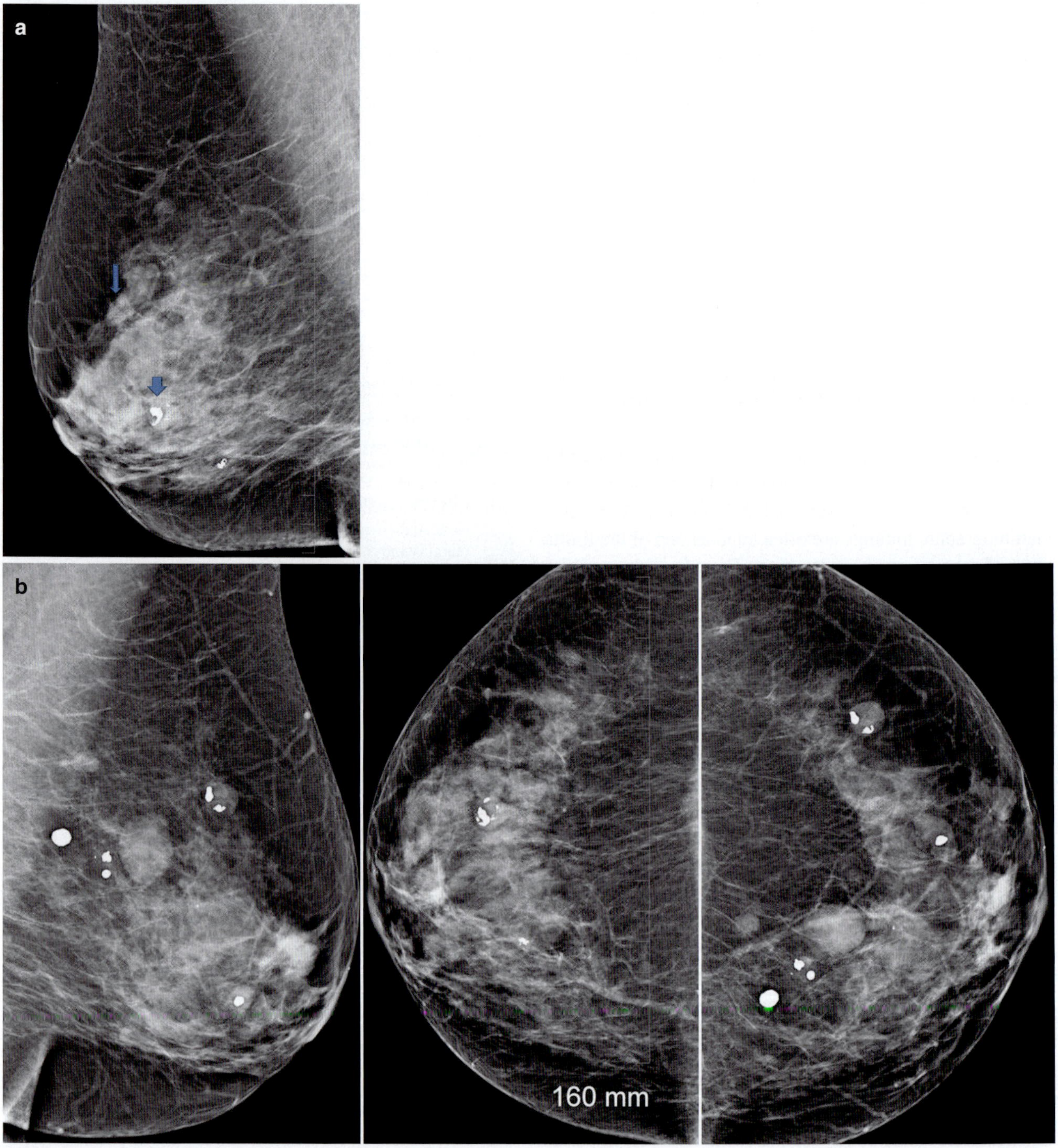

Fig. 6.1 Multiple bilateral masses in a 54-year-old woman categorized as benign findings. (**a**) Mediolateral oblique view demonstrates multiple masses of varying size (*arrows*) with a similar appearance some which demonstrate the classic appearance of coarse popcorn calcifications characteristic of calcified benign fibroadenomas. (**b**) Craniocaudal views demonstrate multiple masses of varying size with a similar appearance some which demonstrate the classic appearance of coarse popcorn calcifications characteristic of calcified benign fibroadenomas

appearing masses each breast do not need further workup and should not be categorized as probably benign. Multiple similar appearing masses with benign morphology represent benign process such as cysts or multiple fibroadenomas the latter may also show classic dystrophic popcorn type of calcifications (Fig. 6.1a, b). Such findings are appropriately classified as benign instead of probably benign and should instead undergo annual screening mammograms. Another example is global asymmetry that is characterized by increased tissue density or greater volume of tissue in one breast (Fig. 6.2a, b). This is a

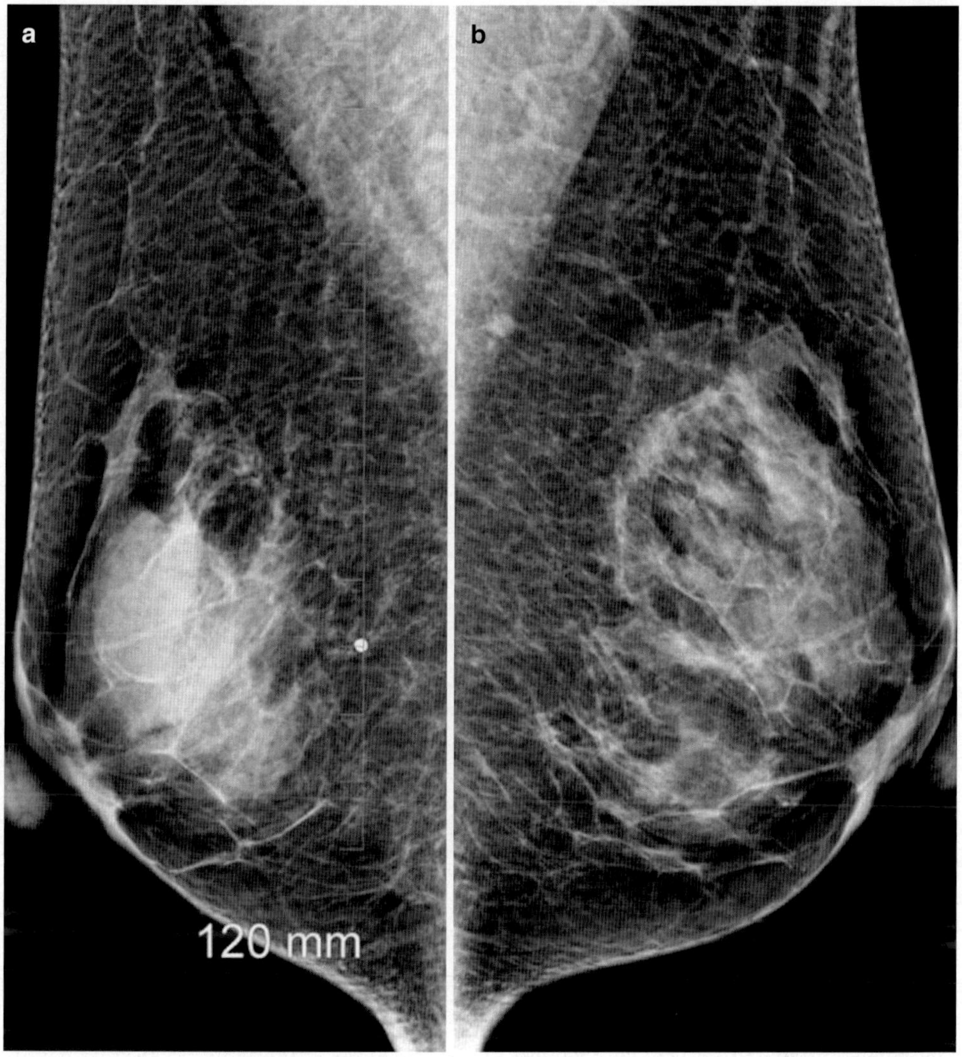

Fig. 6.2 Global asymmetry. (**a**) Right breast MLO view demonstrates greater volume of tissue in the central breast. (**b**) Left breast MLO view demonstrates lesser volume of tissue in the breast compared to the right

benign finding when not associated with a symptom or clinical finding and should be categorized as benign; there is no justification for a short-interval follow-up for such a finding.

Diagnostic workup for findings that are believed to have a low probability of malignancy may include spot compression views with or without magnification. It is important to note that palpable abnormities are excluded in the probably benign category and so are findings that demonstrate interval change. The mammographic signs that are appropriately assigned as being probably benign with a low likelihood for malignancy after additional workup can be grouped under two headings, one that includes findings that are focally distributed and confined to one segment and a second group that includes diffusely distributed findings.

The focal group includes a cluster of five or more calcifications that on magnification views are round or oval. Calcifications that are dense distributed in a regional or diffuse manner (Fig. 6.3a, b).Non-calcified masses with a round oval or gently lobulated shape, and margins that are seen clearly and are well defined [2]. Focal asymmetries that are non-palpable, clearly seen on two views and with concave margins and interspersed with fat (Fig. 6.4a, b). Also included in the focal group are several miscellaneous findings such a single dilated duct without a history of a nipple discharge, subtle areas of architectural distortions occurring at known biopsy sites and unassociated with central area of increased density. When two such clustered calcifications or nodules are seen, they are to be reported as one case.

The second group of probably benign abnormalities includes abnormalities that are diffusely distributed and consist of findings of multiple more than three lesions either tiny calcifications or nodules randomly distributed throughout both breasts. These findings are characterized by being of similar appearance. The calcifications may consist of diffusely scattered types or multiple clusters of calcifications. Again any abnormality that is associated with a palpable finding is excluded, as are those findings that demonstrate interval change whenever prior mammograms are available for comparison. An initial study of 90 such low suspicion lesions that were followed for at least 20 months or biopsied,

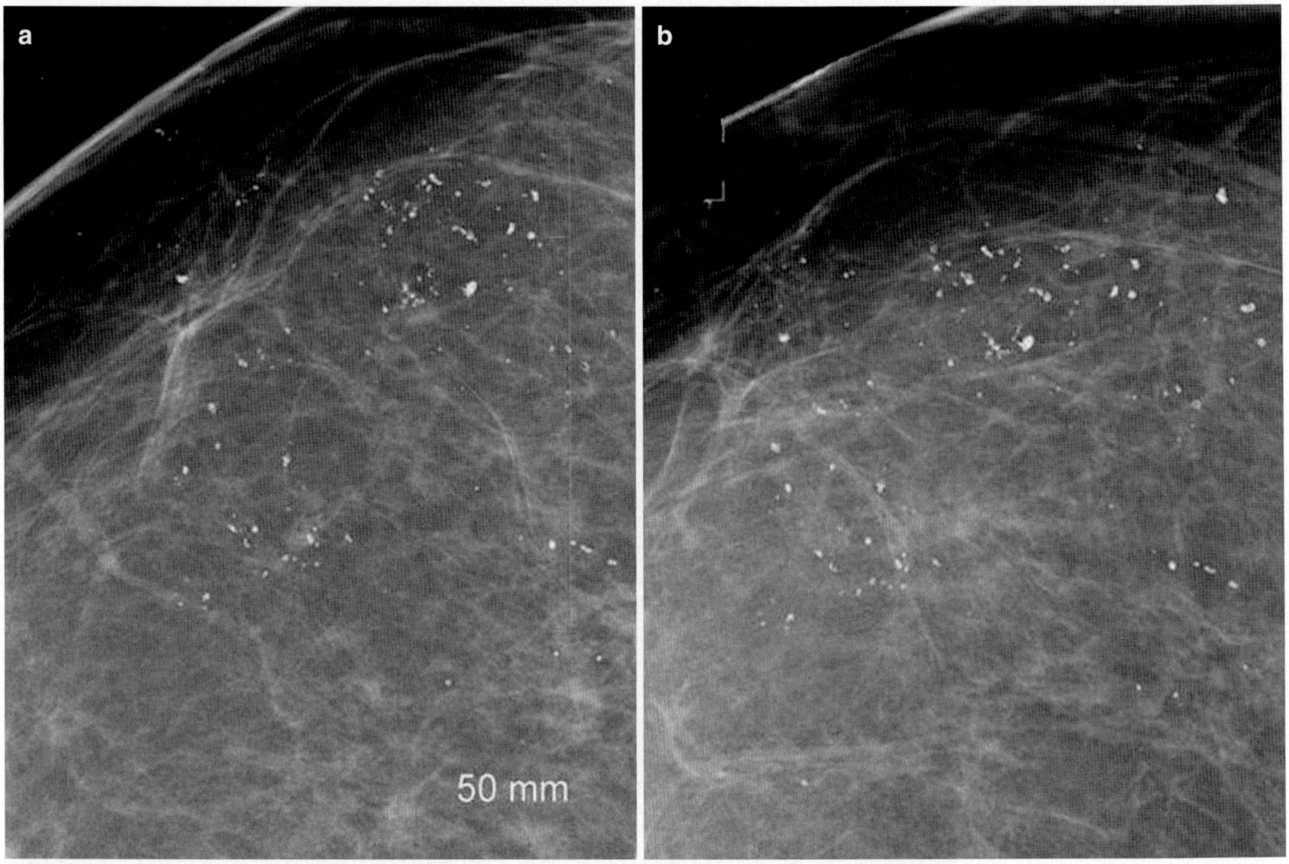

Fig. 6.3 A 45-year-old recalled for calcifications and categorized as probably benign. (**a**) Spot compression magnification views in the craniocaudal projection demonstrate dense macrocalcifications in a regional distribution appropriately classified as probably benign with short-interval follow-up recommendation. (**b**) Spot compression magnification views in the mediolateral projection demonstrate dense macrocalcifications in a regional distribution

one cancer was reported [1]. The validity of short-interval follow-up was for the first time proven by Sickles [2]. In a study of 3,184 cases that fulfilled these criteria to be assigned into a short-interval follow-up group, there were 17 cancers. 3,184 cases represented 11.2 % of the screening mammograms during the study period of 8.5 years. Tiny calcifications were the most frequently encountered findings [58.2 %] followed by well-defined nodules [26.4 %] [2]. Seventeen cancers were detected at follow-up corresponding to a malignancy rate of only 0.5 % in the study group. Fifteen of these 17 were biopsied based on interval growth during follow-up surveillance. None of the lesions that were biopsied despite displaying a stable appearance demonstrated a malignant histology. The majority of cancers were solitary circumscribed noncalcified masses (12/17). For noncalcified circumscribed masses, the malignancy rate was hence 2 %, higher than for the entire group although still within the acceptable range for short-interval follow-up [2]. Two circumscribed masses became palpable and hence biopsied with a malignant diagnosis. Two of the 17 cancers had metastasis to one node and none had systemic metastasis.

Similar results have been shown by others who have undertaken such studies to test the validity of short-interval follow-up for lesions with low probability for breast cancer [3–5]. In a study of 21,885 mammograms, 558 [2.5 %] abnormalities were categorized as probably benign with a malignancy rate of only 0.47 % [3]. In another study of 795 probably benign lesions representing 5.8 % of screening mammograms, the malignancy rate was 0.3 %. The probably benign abnormalities were followed for 2 years. Two cancers were seen in the low-suspicion group: one was a ductal carcinoma in situ and another 7 mm invasive cancer [4].

The value of a consensus opinion among two breast imagers in categorizing calcifications as being probably benign or suspicious enough to biopsy was studied prospectively using standard criteria. This study included for short-interval follow-up, 490 cases with clustered calcifications, 411 of which were single clusters and 81 had multiple clusters were subjected to a short-interval surveillance [6]. The malignancy rate was 0.5 % and both cases were DCIS that was diagnosed at 12 months. Among the calcifications that were deemed suspicious with a recommendation for biopsy, positive biopsy rate was 29 % [6]. The authors concluded that consensus review using standardized criteria by two breast imagers is a safe follow-up option.

In a study of 544 lesions that represented 3 % of screening mammograms, the malignancy rate was 0.4 %. The cancer

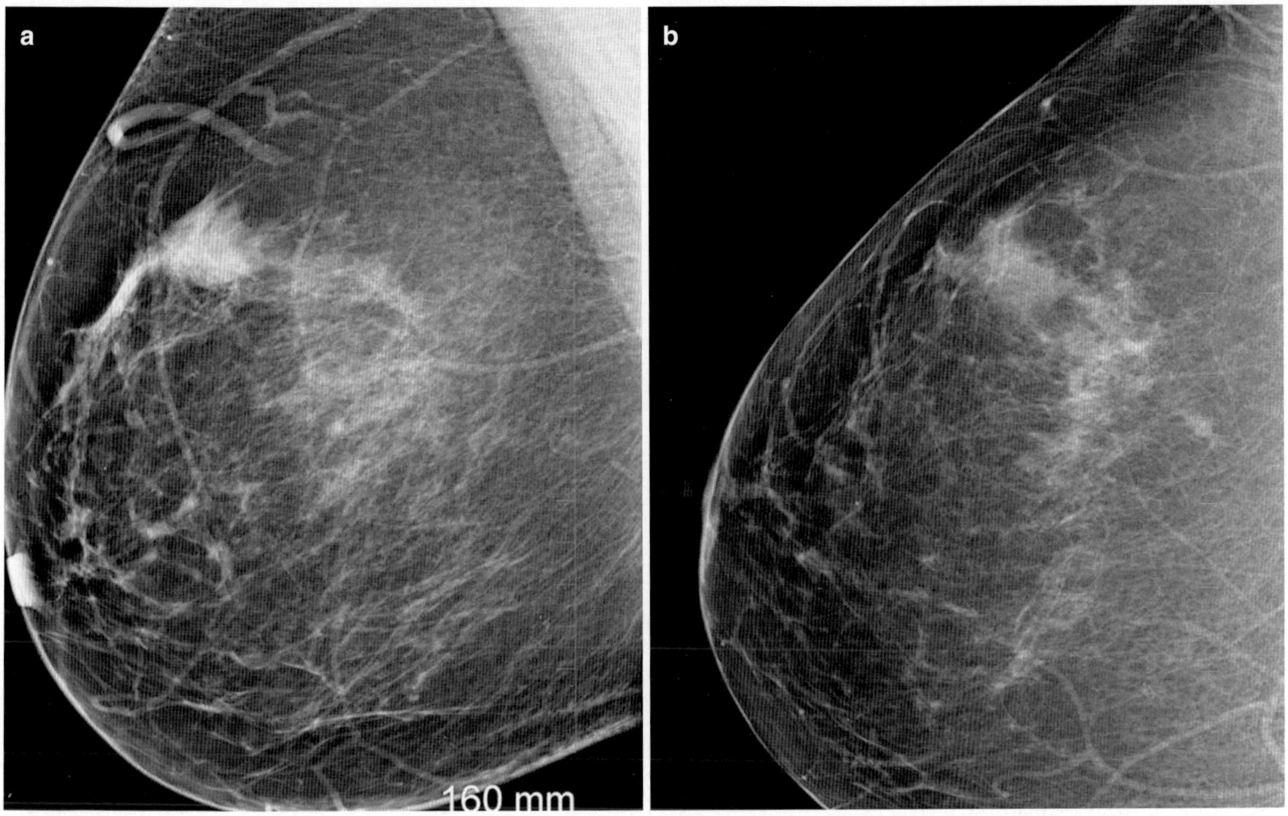

Fig. 6.4 Focal asymmetry seen on a baseline mammogram in an asymptomatic 43-year-old. Sonogram (not shown) did not demonstrate an abnormal finding. A probably benign finding assessment was given with a recommendation for a short-interval follow-up. (**a**) Mediolateral oblique view demonstrates a focal asymmetry in the upper breast. (**b**) Craniocaudal view demonstrates a focal asymmetry in the outer breast not associated with calcifications, distortion, or a mass

rate among those cases undergoing biopsy due to interval progression at two-year follow-up was 14 % [5].In this study masses formed the most common finding [40 %] followed by focal asymmetry [26 %] and calcifications [17 %].

Short-Interval Surveillance Follow-Up Protocol and Rate of Compliance

In the study by Sickles, initial follow-up was with a unilateral mammogram at 6 months which was then followed by a bilateral mammogram at 6–12 months depending on age appropriate screening protocol, followed by two more annual follow-ups for a total of four follow-up examinations spanning up to 3.5 years. In his study the compliance rate decreased at each of the follow-up exam with compliance dropping to 66 % for the fourth follow-up exam [2]. Others have reported a compliance rate of 94.5–96 % [3–5].

Notwithstanding the extremely low incidence of malignancy among probably benign lesions that underwent surveillance based on these studies, one does encounter a higher incidence of cancers in some practices among those lesions that are categorized as probably benign. This is often due to failure to use the criteria for placing abnormalities in the probably benign category. In one reported series there were 51 malignancies identified in a group of 178 biopsies performed in patients who were assigned a probably benign assessment. On review of these findings, it was noted none of the findings fulfilled strict criteria needed to be placed in a short-interval surveillance group [7]. Calcifications were the most frequent findings in those abnormalities that proved malignant and were seen in 45 % of these cases, followed by noncalcified masses and focal asymmetry in 24 % of cases.

Probably Benign Findings on Breast Ultrasound

Stavros and others in a prospective study were able to predict benignity of a solid mass with a high degree of accuracy using morphologic criteria based on a retrospective analysis [8] (Fig. 6.5). In their series the negative predictive value for benignity was 99.5 % and was high enough to avoid biopsy. In practice these strict criteria may not be strictly adhered to while assigning solid masses to the probably benign category [9–12]. Also to note that unlike with mammography, the prospective study on probably benign category for ultrasound

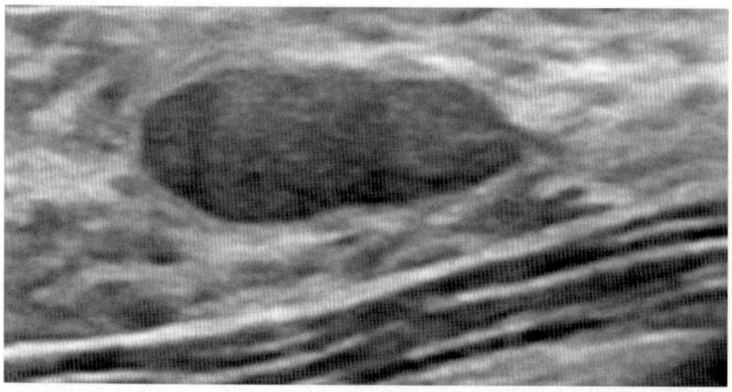

Fig. 6.5 Ultrasound demonstrates a non-palpable ovoid mass with circumscribed borders and a thin echogenic capsule considered probably benign with a recommendation for a short-interval follow-up in a 44-year-old woman seen as an incidental finding during evaluation for breast pain

abnormalities was studied in a group of patients who had both palpable and nonpalpable abnormalities [8].

The validity of the use of probably benign assignment for ultrasound-detected solid masses was studied in a series of 920 solid nodules assigned to the probably benign category based on established criteria. In this series 40.9 % of the solid masses did not fulfill the strict criteria needed for categorizing a mass as being benign. All 14 cancers that were diagnosed in the probably benign group in this study belonged to the group that subsequently was categorized as suspicious [9]. Nevertheless the malignancy rate among these 920 solid nodules was still an acceptable 1.5 % and also to be noted, 8 of the 14 cancers were palpable [9]. For ultrasound-detected masses the criteria for biopsy of a lesion placed in the probably benign finding group are either an increase in diameter beyond 10 % or change in margin characteristics on a follow-up examination [9]. Stable appearance at 2 years leads to a downgrade in final assessment category to a BI-RADS 2 [9]. The cost-effectiveness of follow-up of solid masses with benign features as an alternate to biopsy has been studied and reported to lead a reduction of cost by a third [13]. Recent studies have validated the use of probably benign assessment category for ultrasound-detected solid masses [14, 15]. The malignancy rate for lesions categorized as probably benign is still low and well below the accepted 2 % rate. A series of 4,000 women reported a malignancy rate of 0.8 %. As reported by others on retrospective analysis of the features, 29/32 [90.6 %] were incorrectly classified as benign and the error was mostly due to lack of appreciation of suspicious margin characteristics [14]. The malignancy rate among the probably benign lesions was higher among the lesions that were palpable, 2.4 % [21 of 859] compared to 0.4 % [11 of 3141] among nonpalpable lesions. In a study of 288 probably benign lesions that underwent immediate histological diagnosis, only three cancers were found for a malignancy rate of 1 % which was again within the acceptable range of 2 %. Two of these three cancers was ductal carcinoma in situ and one was an invasive ductal cancer. There were 195 masses in the study group [15]. Sonographic criteria for classifying a solid mass as benign were presence of circumscribed margins, round, oval, or slightly lobulated shape, wider than tall with parallel orientation to the skin surface, internal echotexture that was iso- or slightly hypoechoic to subcutaneous fat and with normal through transmission of sound. As in the study published by Stavros and others, size of the solid mass was considered a criterion for exclusion [8, 15]. Also included in the follow-up category were sonographic findings of hypoechoic masslike abnormalities with low-level internal echoes consistent with complicated and clustered microcysts. It is, however, important to follow these criteria strictly when categorizing as probably benign. Analysis of the margin characteristics is critical and dependency only on presence of an ovoid shape may lead to misdiagnosis (Fig. 6.6a–d).

The Case Against Short-Interval Follow-Up of Abnormalities in the Breast

Unnecessary patient anxiety has been cited as a potential deterrent for short-interval follow-up resulting from not knowing the possible outcome and living with the possibility of a very small albeit real risk of having a malignant lesion in the breast [16]. However, a study that assessed the level of anxiety among women who underwent biopsy and compared it to women who had a follow-up found that the women in the biopsy group experienced a higher level of anxiety than those in the follow-up group [17]. Hall points out that the number of screening mammograms that were assigned to the BI-RADS 3 category is declining [18]. In Sickles' original paper validating the low likelihood of malignancy in the probably benign lesions, 11.6 % of mammograms were placed in the short-interval follow-up group, and this percentage decreased to 1.2 % [2, 19]. The relatively more frequent use of this category in the USA compared to Europe may also be in part because of the heightened risk of a malpractice lawsuit in this country [18]. An additional consideration is masses versus calcifications. It has been suggested that it is more prudent to follow nonpalpable nodules than calcifications since growth of low-grade cancers among nodules is more predictable and easier to identify at follow-up compared to microcalcifications related to low-grade DCIS which may remain unchanged for years [18].

Screening mammography has a conflicting challenge of having to detect as high percentage of early-stage breast cancers as possible while causing as little harm as possible to the vast number of women that are screened and do not have breast cancer [20]. Rubin questions the need for short-interval surveillance and whether the follow-up should be 12 months instead of 6 months. She points out that unlike as

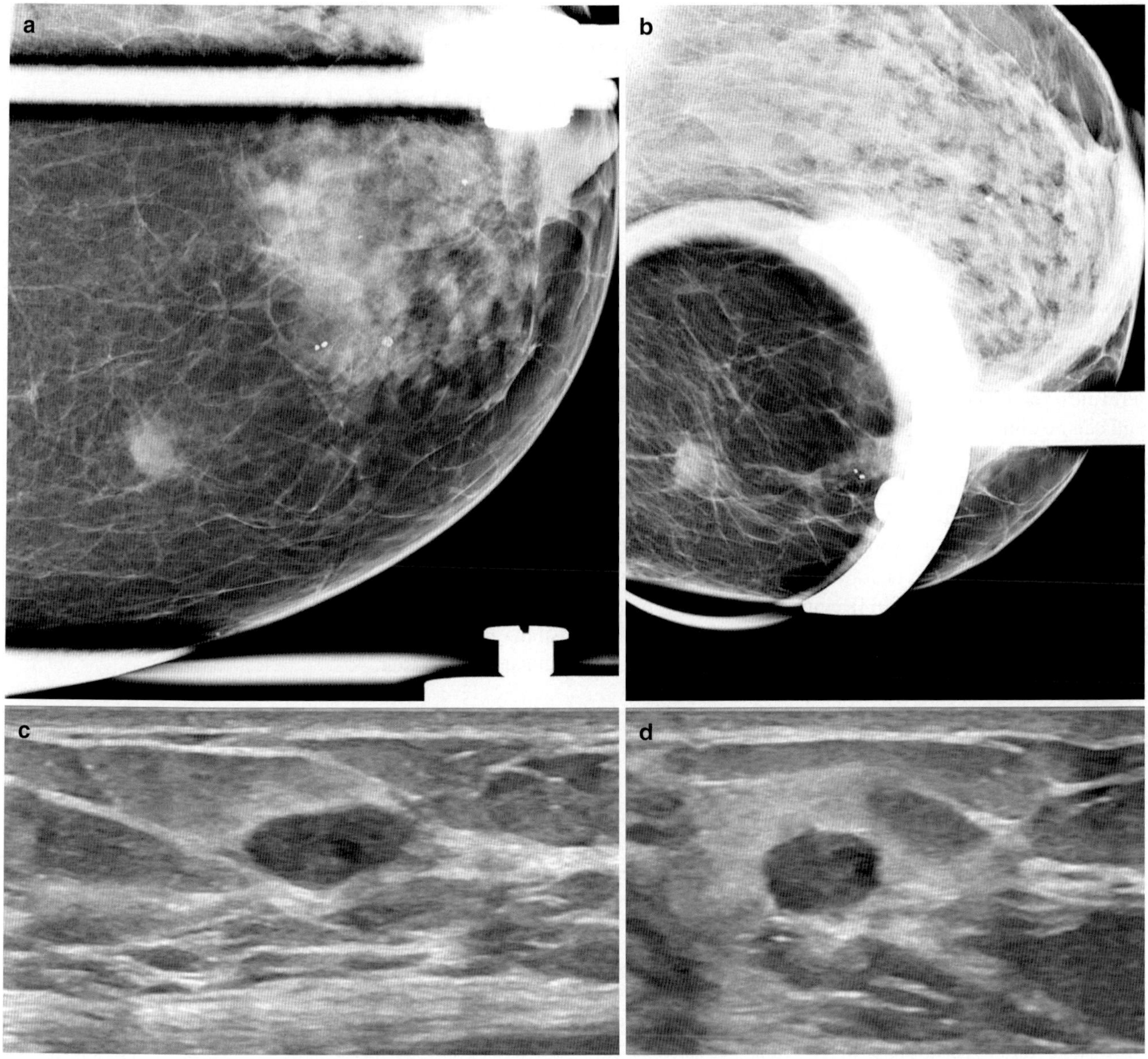

Fig. 6.6 A 44-year-old with a non-palpable solid mass incorrectly characterized as probably benign solid mass based on sonographic features histologically proven to be an invasive ductal cancer at follow-up. (**c**) Ultrasound in the radial plane demonstrates an ovoid circumscribed solid mass. (**d**) Ultrasound in the antiradial plane demonstrates irregular and ill-defined borders on close inspection. (**a**) Spot compression magnification views demonstrate a focal asymmetry with ill-defined borders. (**b**) Spot compression magnification views demonstrate a focal asymmetry with ill-defined borders

was proposed by Sickles, many radiologists perform 6-month follow-up for the entire course of 3 and sometimes up to 5 years [2, 20]. Although the rate of immediate biopsy resulting from a probably benign assessment in Sickles study was only 0.4 % in most practices, it is considerably higher [2, 20]. There is always a problem with who discusses the results with the patient; clinicians are often uncomfortable with the probably benign assessment and not able to explain the findings to the patient and depending on level of patient anxiety may prompt referral to a surgeon for a biopsy. Probably benign assessment can also trigger a desire to seek a second opinion [20]. The guidelines from the European Society of Breast Imaging for Diagnostic Interventional Breast Procedures recommend biopsy as an option to short-interval follow-up [21]. Studies conducted in the UK have shown that early recall is considered more stressful than biopsy both in the short and long term [22, 23].

Data from the recently published paper from the ACRIN6666 trial showed that BI-RADS category 3 lesions have a low malignancy rate of 0.8 %. Six malignancies were seen in 5 of 514 women. Only one of the six was node positive; three were biopsied because of interval change at follow-up. Based on these findings it may be appropriate to follow up by a diagnostic study at 1 year instead of at 6 months for probably benign lesions identified at screening ultrasound, thereby reducing anxiety, costs, and unnecessary biopsies [24].

Computer-Aided Diagnosis of Breast Masses on Ultrasound

Computer-aided diagnostic system has been studied to aid in the characterization of masses on ultrasound [25–31]. Distinction of benign from malignant tumors based on textural information alone has been found to be satisfactory and can be clinically useful as a second opinion tool to aid in the characterization of masses [25]. Others have used a combination of features such as speckle and shape in addition to texture [26]. Texture and speckle features in a solid mass on ultrasound are easy to extract but are affected by the region of interest that is drawn by the examining physician, based on where the ROI [Region of Interest] is placed the texture and speckle features can be different [26]. Shape features also called morphologic features are also effective tools to assess breast tumors by CAD. However, this is more cumbersome a process and involves extensive computation and training a CAD system can take a long time. A study of 210 breast tumors, 120 benign and 90 malignant, looked at shape and texture features and found an accuracy of 92.8 %, sensitivity of 94.4 % and specificity of 91.6 %, positive predictive value of 89.4 %, and a negative predictive value of 95.6 % [26]. A study of using a computer-aided classification system on lesions that were category 3 by two of four radiologists showed that CAC system correctly upgraded 38 of 42 malignant lesions [90 %] assigned to the probably benign group [27]. Others have used the CAD system to classify masses into the BI-RADS assessment categories of 3, 4, and 5 based on sonographic features of shape, orientation, margin, lesion boundary, echo pattern, and posterior acoustic features. These eight computerized features are quantified to characterize the mass in the CAD system. The classification results of the radiologists are used to train a basic system by the multinomial logistic regression. The diagnostic accuracy of such a system is strengthened by using a weighting strategy based on pathologic diagnosis to help in the CAD system training. Using such a system the authors were able to achieve an accuracy of 73 % [457/626], sensitivity of 98.1 % [215/219], specificity of 59.4 % [242 of 407], positive predictive value of 56.5 %[215 of 380], and a negative predictive value of 98.3 % [242 of 246] [30]. A computer-aided analysis with qualitative information from radiologists showed a promising result for breast tumor classification [31].

Special Types of Benign Abnormalities of the Breast

Superficial Lesions of the Breast

These include lesions that arise in the dermis, hypodermis (subcutaneous fat), or superficial breast tissue. Lesions that arise in the dermis are benign and do not require intervention or imaging follow-up. Lesions that arise in the subcutaneous fat are usually benign but may uncommonly represent breast cancer arising from the superficial terminal ductal lobular unit [32]. These include lesions that originate in the subcutaneous fat like fat necrosis, lipomas, and vascular lesions, lesions of lymphatic origin, or neurogenic tumors.

Dermal lesions include sebaceous cyst, epidermal inclusion cyst, and dermal calcifications.

Sebaceous Cyst

On mammography these may appear as superficially located low density, mixed density, or fat density mass. On ultrasound they are circumscribed and cystic with low-level echoes or solid like and may extend from the dermis into the subcutaneous tissue.

Epidermal Inclusion Cyst

Epidermal cysts may arise spontaneously or result from trauma. Mammographically these appear as iso- or hyperdense superficially located circumscribed masses that are palpable. The internal contents of an epidermal cyst determine the sonographic appearance which can consequently vary from being cystic to hypoechoic or heterogeneously hypoechoic. The abnormality is seen to be predominantly in the dermis and when inflamed may exhibit ill-defined margins and may exhibit a track leading into the subcutaneous fat.

Dermal Calcifications

These are superficially located calcifications, typically have a lucent center and result from inspissated material in sebaceous glands or due to chronic folliculitis. They are most commonly seen in the lower inner breast. When lucent centers are absent or when morphology appears irregular or pleomorphic, these can present diagnostic challenges; tangential views prove their dermal locations. Dermal calcifications need to be ascertained during a diagnostic workup to avoid the spectacle of identifying this fact during a failed stereotactic or presurgical localization biopsy.

Large Rodlike Calcifications

Calcifications that form solid or discontinuous smooth linear rods with a diameter of 1 mm or more and show a ductal distribution extending to the nipple are typically benign;

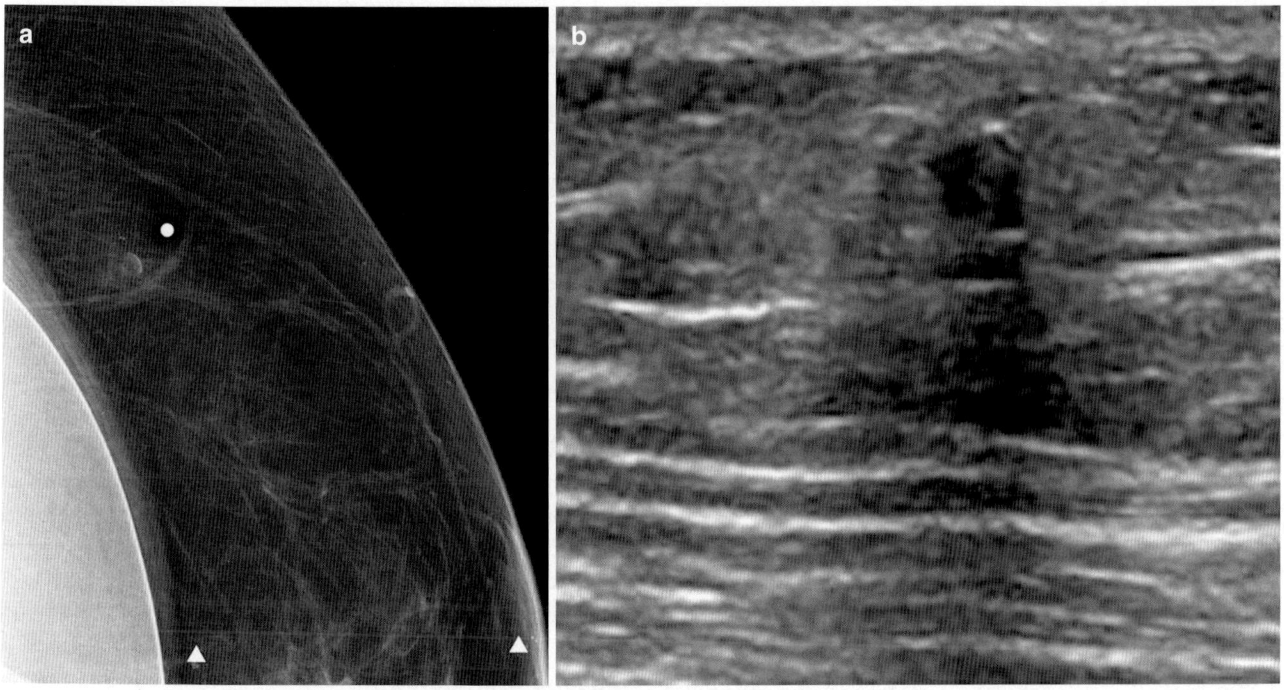

Fig. 6.7 A 56-year-old with a small palpable lump. (**a**) Mammogram reveals a small radiolucent mass with peripheral rim calcification suggestive of benign fat necrosis. (**b**) Ultrasound reveals a small solid mass with heterogeneous echotexture and an indeterminate appearance. Biopsy was deferred due to the benign mammographic appearance

these are associated with duct ectasia. They are solid when secretions in the lumen calcify or show lucent centers if calcium accumulates in the wall of the duct. These secretory calcifications are typically bilateral and seen in women older than 60 years. Bilaterality is seen in up to 80 % of women, and in about 10 % these calcifications are branching [33].

Fat Necrosis

Fat necrosis can have a wide spectrum of imaging appearance with findings that overlap with known mammographic signs of breast cancer [34–38]. Fat necrosis of the breast is fairly commonly encountered and results from breast trauma or surgery. It is a nonsuppurative inflammatory process [34]. Fat necrosis starts off as hemorrhage in fat. The area becomes well demarcated over several weeks. Cystic degeneration leads to a formation of a cavity that contains oily fluid representing necrotic fat. Calcifications can form along the cyst wall [35] (Fig. 6.7a, b). It frequently presents as a palpable lump. A clear understanding and knowledge of the findings is essential to avoid unnecessary biopsy. Generally the sonographic appearance may appear more worrisome and prompt intervention which may be avoided by correlating sonographic appearance with the mammographic findings and with underlying clinical history. While mammographic findings are frequently characteristic and predominantly benign, in some instances particularly when the sole manifestation is an irregular focal asymmetry or suspicious calcifications, biopsy is indicated to exclude a breast malignancy. The spectrum of the mammographic findings appears in Box 6.3 [34]. Lipid cysts appear as circumscribed radiolucent masses with a thin rim that may partially calcify. Lipoma also appears as radiolucent mass but generally does not calcify and the rim is less well defined; a lipoma is also frequently larger than fat necrosis. Microcalcifications when

Box 6.3. Mammographic and Sonographic Signs in Fat Necrosis

A. Mammographic signs
- Occult, clinically palpable
- Lipid cyst
- Microcalcifications
- Coarse calcifications
- Spiculated mass or focal asymmetry

B. Sonographic signs
- Hyperechoic solid mass
- Cystic mass with a mural nodule [D/D: intracystic carcinoma, papilloma, blood clot in a cyst]
- Cystic mass with echogenic bands
- An anechoic mass without posterior acoustic enhancement or with posterior acoustic shadowing
- Isoechoic mass

Data from Graf et al. [33]; and from Bilgen et al. [35]

seen may appear pleomorphic and particularly in the setting of lumpectomy for breast cancer will necessitate biopsy to exclude malignancy. Coarse calcifications are readily recognized as benign when there is underlying trauma, surgery, or biopsy. Spiculated masses or irregular focal asymmetry will require tissue diagnosis. Sonographically fat necrosis may appear as an isoechoic or hyperechoic circumscribed mass, complex cystic mass, or as a cyst without posterior acoustic enhancement or with posterior acoustic shadowing. A mass with echogenic internal bands that can shift in position with changes in patient position is a specific sign of fat necrosis. This results from interface between lipid and hemorrhagic components of fat necrosis [38]. Fat necrosis can have ill-defined or irregular margins on ultrasound prompting a recommendation for a biopsy.

Echogenic Masses on Us

A mass that is uniformly hyperechoic is rarely encountered and are almost always benign [8, 38–40]. There were no cancers in 42 such masses in the series reported by Stavros [8]. In a large series of 4,511 consecutive breast biopsies, only 0.6 % were hyperechoic, representing only 0.4 % of malignancies. The two features most distinguishing between benign and malignant masses were lesion margins and orientation of the mass; those with noncircumscribed margins or nonparallel orientation are more likely to be malignant [40]. There is some nonuniformity in the description of hyperechoic masses; some compare the echogenicity to fibroglandular tissue, although the proper description should compare it to subcutaneous fat [40]. Hyperechoic cancers are not associated with a specific histological type of breast cancer. Commonly encountered histology in hyperechoic masses are discussed next. See Box 6.4 for differential diagnoses for hyperechoic masses.

Lipoma

A lipoma is circumscribed often unilateral and solitary and radiolucent on a mammogram. A palpable lump is often associated. Ultrasound features are variable and may include a circumscribed hypoechoic, hyperechoic, or isoechoic mass without internal vascularity [40].

Box 6.4. Differential Diagnoses of Hyperechoic Masses

- Lipoma [lucent on a mammogram]
- Hematoma
- Silicone granuloma
- Abscess
- Galactocele
- Fat necrosis
- Hemangioma
- Pseudoangiomatous stromal hyperplasia [PASH]
- Metastasis
- Angiolipoma or liposarcoma [rare]

Angiolipoma

These are rarely encountered in the breast and may be associated with overlying skin discoloration. The noninfiltrative type is more commonly seen in the breast. A circumscribed mass that is iso- or hyperechoic is identified with internal vascularity necessitating biopsy. These are not malignant lesions and at pathology are characterized by microthrombi in small vessels. At mammography these appear as a mixed density or isodense mass.

Hematoma

A hematoma is a sequela of trauma or surgery and appears as an area of focal asymmetry which can have an irregular appearance. On ultrasound appearance depends on the age of the hematoma and may vary from being hypoechoic to heterogeneously hyperechoic.

Silicone Granuloma

Silicone granuloma represents a granulomatous reaction surrounding free silicone in the soft tissues and is most commonly encountered at the edge of the implants or in the axilla. These represent a consequence of an extra capsular rupture of the silicone implant or in those cases where silicone has been injected into the breast tissue as a breast augmentation procedure.

On ultrasound these granulomas have a hyperechoic appearance with fine internal echoes, described as a "snow storm" appearance caused by acoustic scattering by silicone. Mammographically these masses are iso- to hyperdense.

Hemangioma

These are uncommon benign tumors of the breast. Hemangiomas are typically superficial with circumscribed borders and oval or lobular shape with most of the tumors appearing heterogeneous or hypoechoic [41, 42]. Some of these tumors may be hyperechoic and when so tend to have less well-defined borders [42] (Fig. 6.8a, b).

The differential diagnosis of hyperechoic solid masses does include rare nonbreast malignant lesions.

Metastasis

Metastasis to the breast can appear as a hyperechoic mass on ultrasound. Lung cancer, ovarian cancer, melanoma, and lymphoma are the most common type of metastasis reported. A hyperechoic mass with internal vascularity may represent a lymphoma or a melanoma metastasis [43].

Angiosarcoma

Angiosarcoma of the breast is a very rare but highly aggressive tumor of the breast with a known association with

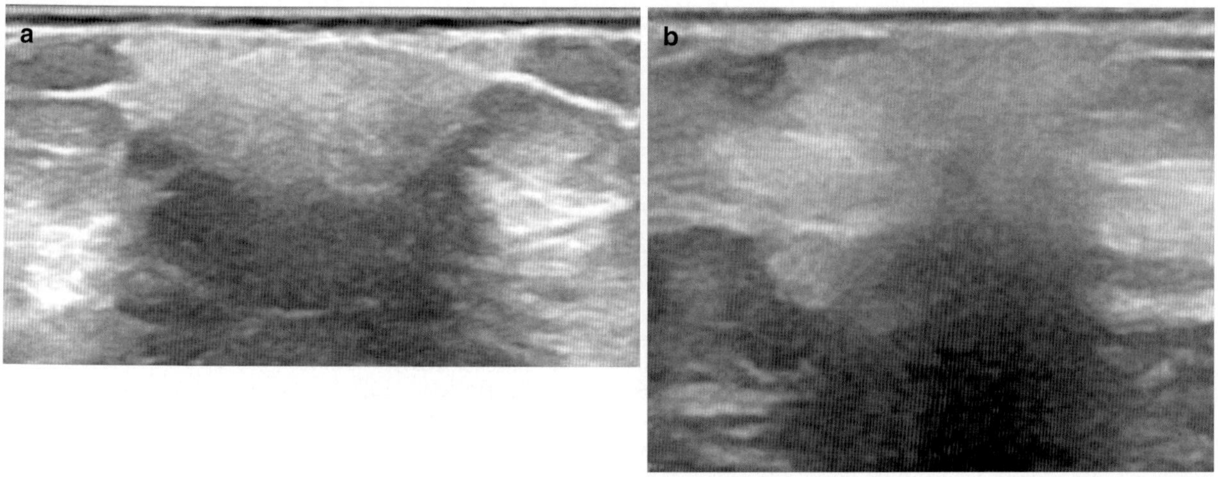

Fig. 6.8 A palpable mass in a 54-year-old woman histologically proven to be a hemangioma. (**a**) Radial sonographic image reveals a superficially located hyperechoic mass without circumscribed borders and posterior acoustic shadowing. (**b**) Sonographic image in an antiradial plane reveals a superficially located hyperechoic mass without circumscribed borders and posterior acoustic shadowing

radiation therapy occurring typically 5–10 years after irradiation. They arise from connective tissues of the breast and include angiosarcoma, fibrosarcoma, and malignant fibrous histiocytoma. These masses are irregular or circumscribed, hypervascular, heterogeneously hyperechoic, or less commonly uniformly hyperechoic [43].

References

1. Helvie MA, Pennes DR, Rebner M, Adler DD. Mammographic follow-up of low-suspicion lesions: compliance rate and diagnostic yield. Radiology. 1991;178(1):155–8.
2. Sickles EA. Periodic mammographic follow-up of probably benign lesions: results in 3,184 consecutive cases. Radiology. 1991;179:463–8.
3. Varas X, Leborgne F, Leborgne JH. Nonpalpable, probably benign lesions: role of follow-up mammography. Radiology. 1992;184:409–14.
4. Vizcaino I, Gadea L, Andreo L, et al. Short-term follow-up results in 795 nonpalpable probably benign lesions detected at screening mammography. Radiology. 2001;219:475–83.
5. Varas X, et al. Revisiting the mammographic follow-up of BI-RADS category 3 lesions. AJR. 2002;179:691–5.
6. Kuzmiak CM, Dancel R, Pisano E, Zeng D, Cole E, Koomen MA, McLelland R. Consensus review: a method of assessment of calcifications that appropriately undergo a six-month follow-up. Acad Radiol. 2006;13(5):621–9.
7. Rosen EL, Baker JA, Soo MS. Malignant lesions initially subject to short-term mammographic follow-up. Radiology. 2002;223:221–3.
8. Stavros AT, Thickman D, Rapp CL, Dennis MA, Parker SH, Sisney GA. Solid breast nodules: use of sonography to distinguish between benign and malignant lesions. Radiology. 1995;196:123–34.
9. Moon HJ, Kim MJ, Kwak JY, Kim EK. Probably benign breast lesions on ultrasonography: a retrospective review of ultrasonographic features and clinical factors affecting the BI-RADS categorization. Acta Radiol. 2010;51(4):375–82.
10. Kim EK, Ko KH, Oh KK, Kwak JY, You JK, Kim MJ, et al. Clinical application of the BI-RADS final assessment to breast sonography in conjunction with mammography. Am J Roentgenol. 2008;190:1209–15.
11. Park YM, Kim EK, Lee JH, Ryu JH, Han SS, Choi SJ, et al. Palpable breast masses with probably benign morphology at sonography: can biopsy be deferred? Acta Radiol. 2008;49:1104–11.
12. Raza S, Chikarmane SA, Neilsen SS, Zorn LM, Birdwell RL. BI-RADS 3, 4, and 5 lesions: value of US in management–follow-up and outcome. Radiology. 2008;248:773–81.
13. Lee CI, Wells CJ, Bassett LW. Cost minimization analysis of ultrasound-guided diagnostic evaluation of probably benign breast lesions. Breast J. 2013;19(1):41–8.
14. Moon HJ, et al. Malignant lesions initially categorized as probably benign breast lesions: retrospective review of ultrasonographic, clinical and pathologic characteristics. Ultrasound Med Biol. 2010;36(4):551–9.
15. Gruber R, et al. Histologic work-up of non-palpable breast lesions classified as probably benign at initial mammography and/or ultrasound (BI-RADS category 3). Eur J Radiol. 2013;82(3):398–403.
16. Jackson FI. Acceptability of periodic follow-up as an alternative to biopsy for mammographically detected lesions interpreted as probably benign. Radiology. 1989;173:580–1.
17. Lindfors KK, O'Connor J, Acredolo CR, Liston SE. Short-interval follow-up mammography versus immediate core biopsy of benign breast lesions: assessment of patient stress. AJR Am J Roentgenol. 1998;171(1):55–8.
18. Hall FM. Follow-up of probably benign breast lesions. Radiology. 2000;217(1):303–5.
19. Sickles EA. Commentary on Dr Rubin's viewpoint. Radiology. 1999;213:19–20.
20. Rubin E. Six-month follow-up: an alternative view. Radiology. 1999;213:15–8.
21. Wallis M, Tardivon A, Helbich T, Schreer I. Guidelines from the European Society of Breast Imaging for diagnostic interventional breast procedures. Eur Radiol. 2007;17:581–8.
22. Brett J, Austoker J, Ong G. Do women who undergo further investigation for breast screening suffer adverse psychological consequences? A multicentre follow-up study comparing different breast screening result groups five months after their last breast screening appointment. J Public Health Med. 1998;20:396–403.
23. Brett J, Austoker J. Women who are recalled for further investigations for breast screening: psychological consequences 3 years after

recall and factors affecting re-attendance. J Public Health Med. 2001;23:292–300.
24. Barr RG, Zhang Z, Cormack JB, Mendelson EB, Berg WA. Probably benign lesions at screening breast US in a population with elevated risk: prevalence and rate of malignancy in the ACRIN 6666 trial. Radiology. 2013;269(3):700–12.
25. Chen DR, Huang YL, Lin SH. Computer-aided diagnosis with textural features for breast lesions in sonograms. Comput Med Imaging Graph. 2011;35(3):220–6.
26. Wu WJ, Moon WK. Ultrasound breast tumor image computer-aided diagnosis with texture and morphological features. Acta Radiol. 2008;15(7):873–80.
27. Buchbinder SS, Leichter IS, Lederman RB, Novak B, Bamberger PN, Sklair-Levy M, Yarmish G, Fields SI. Computer-aided classification of BI-RADS category 3 breast lesions. Radiology. 2004;230(3):820–3.
28. Shen WC, Chang RF, Moon MK. Computed aided classification system for breast ultrasound based on Breast Imaging Reporting and Data System (BI-RADS). Ultrasound Med Biol. 2007;33(11):1688–98.
29. Kim KG, Cho SW, Min SJ, Kim JH, Min BG, Bae KT. Computerized scheme for assessing ultrasonographic features of breast masses. Acad Radiol. 2005;12:58–66.
30. Moon WK, Lo CM, Chang JM, Huang CS, Chen JH, Chang RF. Quantitative ultrasound analysis for classification of BI-RADS category 3 breast masses. J Digit Imaging. 2013;111(1):84–92.
31. Moon WK, Lo CM, Cho N, Chang JM, Huang CS, Chen JH, Chang RF. Computer-aided diagnosis of breast masses using quantified BI-RADS findings. Comput Methods Programs Biomed. 2013;111(1):84–92.
32. Giess CS, Raza S, Birdwell RL. Distinguishing breast skin lesions from superficial breast parenchymal lesions: diagnostic criteria, imaging characteristics, and pitfalls. Radiographics. 2011;31(7):1959–72.
33. Graf O, Berg WA, Sickles EA. Large rodlike calcifications at mammography: analysis of morphologic features. AJR Am J Roentgenol. 2013;200(2):299–303.
34. Hogge JP, Robinson RE, Magnant CM, Zuurbier RA. The mammographic spectrum of fat necrosis of the breast. Radiographics. 1995;15(6):1347–56.
35. Bilgen IG, Ustun EE, Memis A. Fat necrosis of the breast: clinical, mammographic and sonographic features. Eur J Radiol. 2001;39(2):92–9.
36. Taboada JL, Stephens TW, Krishnamurthy S, Brandt KR, Whitman GJ. The many faces of fat necrosis in the breast. AJR Am J Roentgenol. 2009;192(3):815–25.
37. Brenin DR. Management of the palpable breast mass. In: Harris JR, Lippman ME, Morrow M, Osborne CK, editors. Diseases of the breast. 3rd ed. Philadelphia: Lippincott Williams & Wilkins; 2004. p. 33–46.
38. Soo MS, Kornguth PJ, Hertzberg BS. Fat necrosis in the breast: sonographic features. Radiology. 1998;206:261–9.
39. Rahbar G, Sie AC, Hansen GC, et al. Benign versus malignant solid breast masses: US differentiation. Radiology. 1999;213(3):889–94.
40. Linda A, Zuiani C, Lorenzon M, et al. Hyperechoic lesions of the breast: not always benign. AJR Am J Roentgenol. 2011;196(5):1219–24.
41. Tilve A, Mallo R, Pérez A, Santiago P. Breast hemangiomas: correlation between imaging and pathologic findings. J Clin Ultrasound. 2012;40(8):512–7.
42. Mesurolle B. Sonographic and mammographic appearances of breast hemangioma. AJR Am J Roentgenol. 2008;191(1):W17–22.
43. Gao Y, Slanetz PJ, Eisenberg RL. Echogenic breast masses at US: to biopsy or not to biopsy? Radiographics. 2013;33(2):419–34.

Breast Ultrasound

7

Mahesh K. Shetty

Introduction

This chapter provides an overview of the role of ultrasound in breast imaging. Ultrasound plays a critical role in the evaluation of the asymptomatic and symptomatic breast. Ultrasound has an important role as a supplemental modality to mammography in screening for breast cancer in women with an elevated risk for breast cancer, for workup of screen-detected abnormalities, and in the evaluation of the symptomatic breast. The breast ultrasound BI-RADS lexicon is discussed. The technical aspects of the breast ultrasound examination are outlined. The spectrum of abnormal findings seen on workup of a screen-detected abnormality and those seen in a symptomatic breast are described. A brief review of the current status of supplemental methods such as Doppler ultrasound and elastography is presented.

Breast Ultrasound BI-RADS Lexicon

The just released American College of Radiology 2014 BI-RADS™ Atlas has updated descriptors for breast ultrasound lexicon (Table 7.1). Newly added and/or updated features include tissue composition and descriptors for calcifications.

There are a total of six descriptors in the BI-RADS-US lexicon for a mass that is visible in two projections (Table 7.1). The shape of a mass is described as being oval, round, or when neither as irregular. The orientation of the lesion is noted as being parallel to the skin surface indicating a horizontal orientation or as being not parallel, meaning in a vertical orientation or being round. The margin of the lesion is described as being circumscribed or not. When not circumscribed, the appearance is noted as being indistinct where no clear demarcation exists (Fig. 7.1), angular when sharp corners or borders forming acute angles is observed, microlobulated when the margin has a scalloped appearance, or spiculated when sharp lines project from the mass. Mass margins are especially important descriptors, and the distinction between circumscribed and noncircumscribed margin is critical since this distinction determines whether biopsy is required or if a mass can be followed up.

The echo pattern of the mass is either anechoic when no internal echoes are visible, hyperechoic when internal echoes are greater than that of fat or equal to fibroglandular tissue, complex when a combination of anechoic and echogenic components are seen, hypoechoic relative to fat indicating presence of low-level echoes, or isoechoic meaning having an echogenicity similar to fat. Fibroadenomas and complicated cysts typically are hypoechoic or isoechoic. Posterior acoustic features are described as being absent, enhanced, shadowing, or a combination of the latter two. Lesion boundary and surrounding tissue are also suggested although not commonly used.

Appropriate Indications for the Use of Breast Ultrasound [1–15]

Breast ultrasound is an established modality in the evaluation of the breast and is broadly used for two major indications, one as a supplemental method to assess abnormalities that are identified on a screening mammogram or in the evaluation of a breast symptom, most important of which is a patient with a palpable abnormality of the breast. There are guidelines suggested for the use of breast ultrasound by the American College of Radiology and the American Institute of Ultrasound in Medicine [1, 2]. Use of ultrasound as a screening modality is somewhat controversial and is discussed elsewhere in this textbook. The American College of

M.K. Shetty, MD, FRCR, FACR, FAIUM
Department of Radiology, Baylor College of Medicine, Houston, TX, USA

Woman's Center for Breast Care and MRI, Woman's Hospital of Texas, Fannin 7600, Houston, TX 77054, USA
e-mail: mshettymd@womans-clinic.com

M.K. Shetty (ed.), *Breast Cancer Screening and Diagnosis: A Synopsis*,
DOI 10.1007/978-1-4939-1267-4_7, © Springer Science+Business Media New York 2015

Radiology appropriateness criteria provide guidance for appropriate triaging of women depending on the age of the patient and specific indication (Tables 7.2 and 7.3) [14, 15]. Detailed descriptions of the appropriateness criteria can be found in Appendix 7A and Appendix 7B at the end of this chapter.

Indications [1, 3–13]

1. Evaluation and characterization of palpable breast masses and other breast related signs and symptoms.
2. Additional evaluation of abnormal findings seen on a mammogram or a breast MRI.

Table 7.1. ACR BI-RADS® — Ultrasound Lexicon Classification Form

For each of the following categories, select the term that best describes the dominant lesion feature. Whenever possible, definitions and descriptions used in BI-RADS® for mammography should be applied to ultrasound.

BREAST TISSUE		
A. Tissue composition (screening only): Heterogeneous background echotexture of the breast may affect the sensitivity of breast sonograms for lesion detection. *(select one)*		
☐ 1. a. Homogeneous background echotexture — fat		
☐ 2. b. Homogeneous background echotexture — fibroglandular		
☐ 3. c. Heterogeneous background echotexture		
FINDINGS		
B. Masses: A mass is three dimensional and occupies space. In 2-D US, it should be seen in two different planes; with volumetric acquisitions, in three planes.		
1. **Shape** *(select one)*	☐ a. Oval	Elliptical or egg-shaped (may include two or three undulations, i.e. gently lobulated or macrolobulated)
	☐ b. Round	Spherical, ball-shaped, circular, or globular
	☐ c. Irregular	Neither round nor oval
2. **Orientation** *(select one)*	☐ a. Parallel	Long axis of lesion parallels the skin line (wider than tall or horizontal)
	☐ b. Not parallel	Long axis not oriented along the skin line (taller than wide or vertical) — includes round
3. **Margin** *(select all that apply)*	☐ a. Circumscribed	Entire margin is well defined or sharp, with an abrupt transition between the lesion and surrounding tissue
	b. Not circumscribed	The mass has one or more of the following features: indistinct, angular, microlobulated, or spiculated in any portion of the margin
	☐ i. Indistinct	No clear demarcation between a mass and the surrounding tissue anywhere on the margin
	☐ ii. Angular	Some or all of the margin has sharp corners, often forming acute angles
	☐ iii. Microlobulated	Margin is characterized by short-cycle undulations
	☐ iv. Spiculated	Margin is characterized by sharp lines radiating from the mass
4. **Echo pattern** *(select one)*	☐ a. Anechoic	Without internal echoes
	☐ b. Hyperechoic	Having increased echogenicity relative to fat or equal to fibroglandular tissue
	☐ c. Complex cystic and solid	Contains both anechoic (cystic or fluid) and echogenic (solid) components
	☐ d. Hypoechoic	Defined relative to subcutaneous fat; less echogenic than fat; characterized by low-level echoes throughout (e.g., complicated cysts or fibroadenomas)
	☐ e. Isoechoic	Having the same echogenicity as subcutaneous fat
	☐ f. Heterogeneous	A mixture of echogenic patterns within a solid mass

Table 7.1 ACR BI-RADS® – ultrasound lexicon classification form Reprinted with permission of the American College of Radiology 2014. No other representation of this material is authorized without expressed, written permission from the American College of Radiology. Refer to the ACR website at www.acr.org/ac for the most current and complete version of the ACR Appropriate Criteria® This US lexicon classification form is for data collection and does not constitute a written US report

Table 7.1 (continued)

5. **Posterior features** *(select one)*	☐ a. No posterior features	No shadowing or enhancement deep to the mass
	☐ b. Enhancement	Appears as a column that is more echogenic (whiter) deep to the mass
	☐ c. Shadowing	The area posterior to the mass appears darker; (refractive edge shadowing is of no significance)
	☐ d. Combined pattern	More than one pattern of posterior attenuation, both shadowing and enhancement
C. Calcifications: Calcifications are poorly characterized with US but can be recognized as echogenic foci, particularly when in a mass. *(if present, select all that apply)*		
☐ 1. **Calcifications in a mass**		Small hyperechoic foci will be more conspicuous in a hypoechoic mass than within a volume of fibroglandular tissue (unless grouped very closely or individually coarse, they will not attenuate the US beam)
☐ 2. **Calcifications outside of a mass**		Calcifications situated in fat or fibroglandular tissue are less conspicuous than when present within a mass
☐ 3. **Intraductal calcifications**		
D. Associated features *(select all that apply)*		
☐ 1. **Architectural distortion**		
☐ 2. **Duct changes**		Manifested by cystic dilation of a duct or ducts involving irregularities in caliber and/or arborization, extension of duct(s) to or from a malignant mass, or the presence of an intraductal mass, thrombus, or detritus
3. **Skin changes** *(select all that apply)*	☐ a. Skin thickening	May be focal or diffuse, > 2 mm in thickness (in the periareolar area and inframammary folds up to 4 mm)
	☐ b. Skin retraction	Skin surface is concave or ill-defined, and appears pulled in
☐ 4. **Edema**		Increased echogenicity of surrounding tissue and reticulated (angular network of hypoechoic lines)
5. **Vascularity** *(select one)*		Must reference a contralateral normal area or unaffected site in the same breast as the basis for comparison
	☐ a. Absent	
	☐ b. Internal vascularity	Blood vessels present within the mass
	☐ c. Vessels in rim	Blood vessels may be marginal, occupying part or all of the rim of the mass
6. **Elasticity assessment** *(select one)*		Stiffness as a feature of malignant masses may be considered along with their much more important morphologic characteristics
	☐ a. Soft	
	☐ b. Intermediate	
	☐ c. Hard	

Table 7.1 (continued)

E. Special cases: These are cases with a unique diagnosis or finding. *(select all that apply)*		
☐ 1. **Simple cyst**		Circumscribed, round or oval, anechoic, shows posterior enhancement
☐ 2. **Clustered microcysts**		A cluster of anechoic masses, each < 2–3 mm in diameter with thin (< 0.5 mm) intervening septations and no discrete solid component
☐ 3. **Complicated cyst**		Cysts that contain debris; characterized by homogeneous, low-level internal echoes without a discrete solid component, and with an imperceptible wall: may have layered appearance which may shift slowly with changes in the patient's position; may also contain echogenic foci that appear to scintillate as they shift
☐ 4. **Mass in or on skin**		These masses are clinically apparent and may include sebaceous or epidermal inclusion cysts, keloids, moles, pimples, neurofibromas, and accessory nipples
☐ 5. **Foreign body including implants**		May include marker clips, coils, wires, catheter sleeves, injected or leaked silicone, metal or glass related to trauma, and implants
☐ 6. **Lymph nodes — intramammary**		Circumscribed, oval masses with hypoechoic cortices and echogenic fatty hila, often reniform and containing hilar fat; most commonly seen in the upper outer quadrant (especially the axillary tail); usually 3 mm to 1 cm
☐ 7. **Lymph nodes — axillary**		
8. **Vascular abnormalities** *(select one)*	☐ a. AVMs (arteriovenous malformations/ pseudoaneurysms)	
	☐ b. Mondor disease	
☐ 9. **Postsurgical fluid collection**		
☐ 10. **Fat necrosis**		

ASSESSMENT CATEGORIES *(select one)*		
Incomplete Assessment	**Management**	**Likelihood of Cancer**
☐ Category 0: Incomplete — Need Additional Imaging Evaluation	Recall for additional imaging	N/A
Final Assessment	**Management**	**Likelihood of Cancer**
☐ Category 1: Negative	Routine screening	Essentially 0% likelihood of malignancy
☐ Category 2: Benign	Routine screening	Essentially 0% likelihood of malignancy
☐ Category 3: Probably Benign	Short-interval (6-month) follow-up or continued surveillance	> 0% but ≤ 2% likelihood of malignancy
☐ Category 4: Suspicious	Tissue diagnosis	> 2% but < 95% likelihood of malignancy
☐ Category 4A: *Low suspicion for malignancy*		> 2% to ≤ 10% likelihood of malignancy
☐ Category 4B: *Moderate suspicion for malignancy*		> 10% to ≤ 50% likelihood of malignancy
☐ Category 4C: *High suspicion for malignancy*		> 50% to < 95% likelihood of malignancy
☐ Category 5: Highly Suggestive of Malignancy	Tissue diagnosis	≥ 95% likelihood of malignancy
☐ Category 6: Known Biopsy-Proven Malignancy	Surgical excision when clinically appropriate	N/A

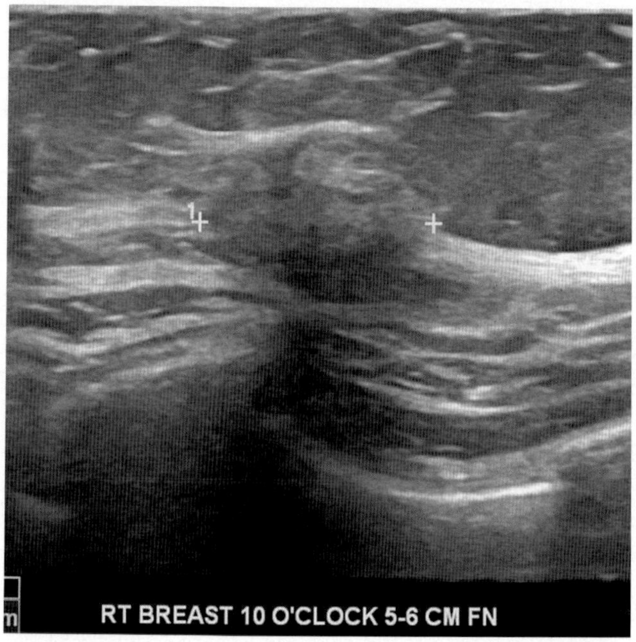

Fig. 7.1 A solid mass whose margins are indistinct. Histological diagnosis: invasive lobular cancer

Table 7.2 Appropriateness of use of ultrasound following a nonpalpable finding on a screening mammogram

Indication	Procedure rating for next exam to perform
Architectural distortion: no history of surgery or trauma	1
Architectural distortion: history of surgery or trauma at area of distortion	1
Mass seen on a mammogram indistinct, microlobulated, or spiculated margins	1
Mass seen on a mammogram, circumscribed margins with no suspicious features, new, enlarging, or no priors to compare	9
Multiple bilateral masses with no mass demonstrating suspicious features, no priors available or baseline	1
Multiple bilateral masses with one dominant mass or one or more demonstrating suspicious features	5
Focal asymmetry or symmetry seen on one view, no priors	1
Focal asymmetry or symmetry seen on one view, new or enlarging	1

Adapted from the American College of Radiology Appropriateness Criteria [14]

Rating scale: 1, 2, 3 usually not appropriate; 4, 5, 6 may be appropriate; 7, 8, 9 usually appropriate

Table 7.3 Appropriateness of use of ultrasound following a palpable finding on a screening mammogram

Indication	Procedure rating for next exam to perform
Woman 40 years or older, initial evaluation	4
Woman 40 years or older, initial evaluation, mammographic finding is suspicious	9
Woman 40 years or older, initial evaluation, mammographic finding is probably benign	8
Woman 40 years of age or older, mammography findings benign (like lipoma) at site of palpable mass.	2
Woman 40 years of age or older, mammography findings negative	9
Woman 30 years or younger, initial evaluation	9
Woman 30 years or younger, ultrasound findings probably benign: US short interval follow-up	9
Woman aged 30–39 years, initial evaluation	8
Ultrasound	8
Diagnostic mammogram	

Adapted from the American College of Radiology Appropriateness Criteria [15]

Rating scale: 1, 2, 3 usually not appropriate; 4, 5, 6 may be appropriate; 7, 8, 9 usually appropriate

3. Imaging modality of choice in women under the age of 30 years or those who are pregnant or lactating. Given the low incidence of breast cancer and to minimize exposure of the breast glandular tissue to diagnostic radiation.
4. Evaluation of breast implants.
5. For guidance of breast interventional procedures.
6. Treatment planning for radiotherapy.
7. Supplemental screening for occult breast cancer in defined population of women in whom MRI is not an option due to a contraindication or lack of access. These include women who are newly diagnosed with breast cancer or those who have a dense breast and are in addition at an elevated risk for breast cancer.
8. To detect a mass associated with architectural distortion or suspicious microcalcifications when surrounded by dense glandular tissue.
9. Assessment and biopsy guidance of abnormal axillary nodes such as in patients diagnosed with breast cancer.

The AIUM [American Institute of Ultrasound] practice and the American College of Radiology [ACR] guidelines have similar indications for the use of breast ultrasound with few notable exceptions. The AIUM does not recommend the use of breast ultrasound for breast cancer screening. The efficacy of sonography as a screening study for occult masses is an area for research; at this time, sonography is not considered a primary screening modality for breast cancer [1]. The ACR recommends supplemental use of ultrasound for breast cancer in a defined set of women who are at an elevated risk for breast cancer and in whom MRI is not an option [2, 10, 11].

Technical Aspects of Breast Ultrasound

Breast sonography is performed with a high-frequency linear array transducer operating at a center frequency of at least 10 MHz, with electronic adjustment of the focal zone. The highest frequency that is capable of satisfactory penetration to the depth of interest is desirable to obtain the best resolution; for very superficial lesions or lesions suspected to be in the dermis, standoff gel pad or a blob of gel and/or use of small hockey stick transducers is helpful. In special circumstances such as in deep lesions in large breasts or when a large abnormality is being assessed, lower-frequency transducers that allow better penetration can be used. The patient is positioned to minimize thickness of the portion of the breast being evaluated and to bring the area of interest within the optimal focal zone of the transducer [1, 2].

Breast ultrasound examination should be appropriately correlated with the indication for imaging be it a physical finding or a mammographic abnormality. If prior sonograms are available, comparison is needed to assess for interval change. Images should be as a standard practice obtained in two perpendicular planes with and without the use of calipers. The size of the lesion should be recorded and location of the lesions in relation to clock face and distance from the nipple has to be documented. The footprint of the transducer is usually 3.5–5 cm and can be used to assess distance from the nipple. The orientation of the lesion in the radial and antiradial planes is notated on the images.

Breast Ultrasound as a Supplemental Modality to Diagnostic Mammography

The two most common indications for the use of breast ultrasound are for characterization of a mammographic mass and further assessment of an area of focal asymmetry that is identified on a mammogram. Sonographic assessment of these findings allows appropriate final categorization of abnormalities (Table 7.1).

Screen-Detected Breast Mass

Breast masses when multiple and bilateral are considered benign with a BI-RADS™ assessment of Category 2 and recommendation for annual screening mammography [16]. Such findings are encountered uncommonly and in one large series represented 1.7 % of screening mammograms [16]. Bilateral similar-appearing masses are often simple or complicated cysts and do not merit a recall. There were only two node-negative cancers among 1440 women in a series reported by Leung and Sickles which is less than the expected interval cancer rate. Recently Berg and others reported that multiple bilateral circumscribed masses are more common at whole-breast US and were seen in 135 of 2,172 women [6.2 %]. There were no malignancies identified in any of these cases at 2 years of follow-up [17]. Annual follow-up by ultrasound may be adequate in these cases if there is no mammographic correlate for a total of 2 years. The malignancy rate among solitary circumscribed masses (complicated cysts; clustered microcysts; circumscribed oval, round, gently lobulated masses) detected at US and with at least 2 years of follow-up has been shown to be low at 0.4 % [17].

The primary role of ultrasound for a finding of a screen-detected mass is to distinguish a simple cyst from a solid lesion. However, a significant proportion of mammographic masses represent a spectrum that ranges between these two findings. This range includes complicated cysts, clustered microcysts, and complex cystic masses.

Simple Cysts

A sharply demarcated anechoic lesion with posterior acoustic enhancement is characteristic of a benign cyst. A thin septa (<0.5 mm) may be seen within a simple cyst. When strict criteria for determination of a cyst are adhered to, the accuracy of ultrasound in making this distinction is 96–100 % [18]. Cysts constitute 25–37 % of all palpable or mammographically detected lesions [3, 19–21]. Simple cysts are epithelial lined and fluid filled that are round or oval shaped and represent dilated terminal ductal–lobular units secondary to obstructed ducts. Cysts are often sharply demarcated on mammography unless obscured by surrounding tissue. The epithelium can be bland or apocrine type; the latter is a tall cuboidal secretory epithelium that can give a fuzzy appearance to the inner wall of the cyst on high-resolution sonography [21]. Cysts are less common in postmenopausal women but may be seen in those women who are on hormone replacement therapy, and in this group they have been reported in 6–29 % [21]. Meticulous attention to gain setting is important to ensure that certain solid masses are not incorrectly diagnosed as cysts which can happen when the gain setting is set at too low. Such a misdiagnosis can happen with circumscribed cancers that have a markedly hypoechogenic internal echotexture. Malignant lesions that can have such an appearance include necrotic invasive ductal cancer, medullary cancer, mucinous cancer, and lymphomatous or metastatic lymph nodes. Metastatic nodes are distinguished by their typical location in the axilla or upper outer quadrant of the breast and some flow on Doppler ultrasound. Margin characterization is also helpful, with malignancies showing at least some focal irregularity; documentation of images without calipers is important so as not to obscure such distinguishing focal irregularities [4, 21].

Complicated Cysts, Clustered Microcysts, and Complex Cystic Masses

These are a common finding on ultrasound and include a spectrum ranging from a cyst with internal septations, clustered cysts, and those with internal echoes and/or intracystic masses [4, 21–25].

Complicated cysts are those with internal debris from cell turnover, bleeding, or infection. Only 2 of 868 lesions [0.23 %] that were thought to represent complicated cysts were proven malignant in multiple series [21]. Complicated cysts when seen with other similar lesions and/or simple cysts are appropriately categorized as benign findings; when solitary, they may be subjected to a short interval follow-up. The distinction is particularly challenging when a lesion is smaller than 4 mm: 21 % were characterized as solid masses in one series [21].

Finding of a fluid debris level or mobile internal echoes allows a confidant determination of a complicated cyst. In the ACRIN6666 trial, 6.1–7.4 % of complicated cysts demonstrated these features [10]. In a complicated cyst without these two features and in which the internal echoes are homogenous, distinction from a solid mass becomes more challenging. It has been reported that about 12 % of such lesions may be solid, and in multiple studies, about 3.1 % of such solid masses have been shown to be malignant [21]. Daly and others found only one cancer in a series of 243 [0.4 %] complicated cysts undergoing aspiration [22]. Presence of internal vascularity is an indication for biopsy since such a finding precludes a cyst. Elastography may also be helpful in distinguishing a benign complicated cyst from a solid mass.

Cystic dilatation of the acini of the terminal ductal-lobular unit leads to formation of clustered microcysts. These are most common in the perimenopausal women and reported in 2.4–5.8 % of women [21]. In the ACRIN6666 trial, there was one 4 mm node-negative invasive lobular cancer among 123 such lesions (0.8 %) [10]. Tissue harmonic imaging by reducing artifactual internal echoes may be helpful in characterizing a lesion as a cyst [26]. Spatial compounding is another tool that can help in this regard. By decreasing speckle and noise, there is better definition of internal structures. An improvement of spatial resolution leads to better recognition of small cysts; posterior acoustic enhancement becomes less apparent when spatial compounding is turned on [27].

These are cysts with walls and/or septations greater than 0.5 mm, intracystic masses or sold masses with cystic areas; such abnormalities are considered suspicious with a recommendation for biopsy. A malignancy rate as high as 36 % has been reported among complex cystic masses [21], although in the ACRIN6666 study no malignancies were found in 20 such lesions. The differential diagnosis of complex cystic mass appears in Box 7.1.

Box 7.1. Differential Diagnosis of Complex Cystic Masses

1. Fat necrosis
2. Papilloma
3. Intracystic carcinoma
4. Abscess
5. Evolving hematoma
6. Galactocele
7. Complex fibroadenoma
8. Phyllodes tumor of the breast

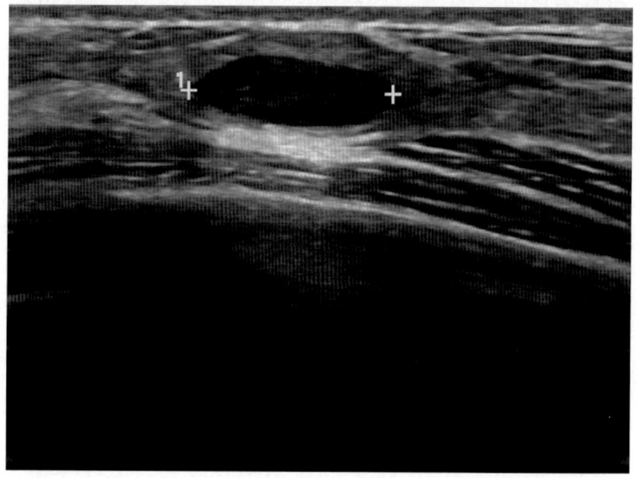

Fig. 7.2 An ovoid mass with a thin echogenic capsule consistent with a benign solid mass. Histological diagnosis: fibroadenoma

Solid Mass

A solid mass is characterized based on ultrasound features that allow a mass to be categorized in one of three groups: benign, probably malignant, or indeterminate. For a mass to be considered benign, one of three findings have to be present: intense uniform hyperechogenicity, ellipsoid shape with a thin echogenic capsule, and two to three gentle lobulations with a thin echogenic capsule (Figs. 7.2 and 7.3). The negative predictive value of intense uniform hyperechogenicity has been reported to be 100 %, a thin echogenic pseudo capsule was 99.2 %, ellipsoid shape was 99.1 %, and four or fewer gentle lobulations was 98.8 % [20].

There are nine malignant features that have been described by Stavros and others; these include the following (positive predictive value for each of the malignant feature is within parenthesis): spiculation [91.8 %], a solid mass that is taller

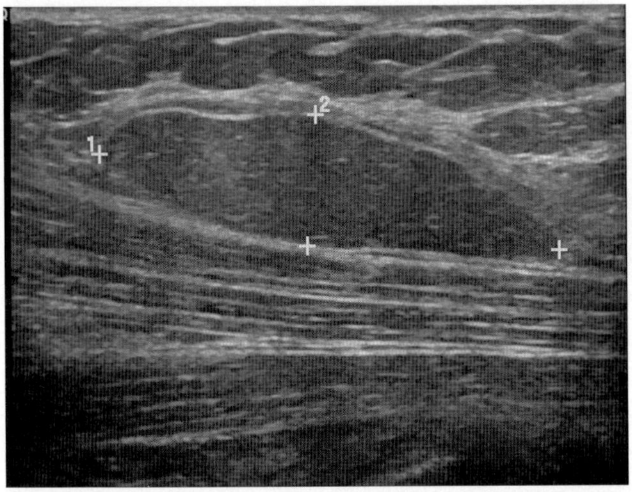

Fig. 7.3 An ovoid mass with a thin echogenic capsule and uniform isoechogenicity consistent with a benign solid mass. Histological diagnosis: lipoma

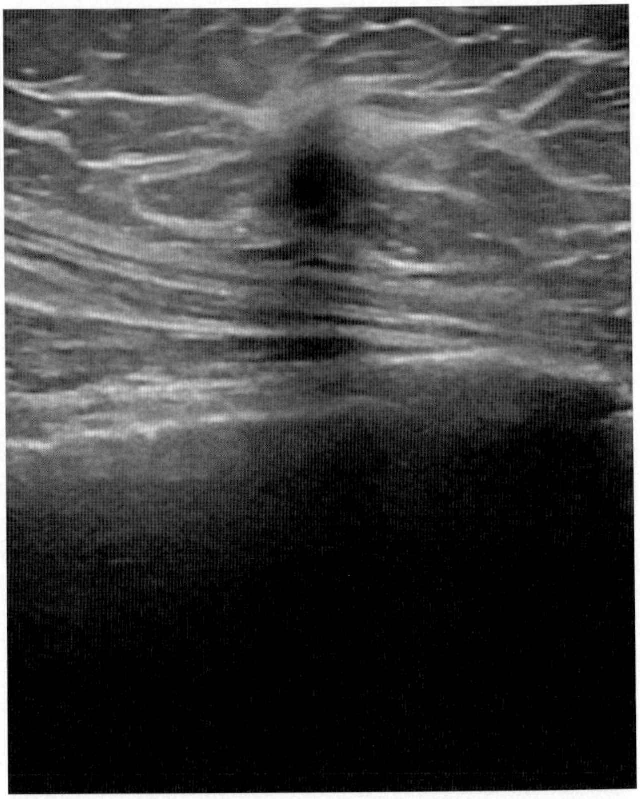

Fig. 7.4 A hypoechogenic mass that is taller than wider. Histological diagnosis: invasive ductal cancer

than wide [81.2 %], a mass with angular margins [67.5 %], one that demonstrates posterior acoustic shadowing [64.9 %], a mass that demonstrates a branching pattern [64 %], hypoechogenicity [60.1 %], calcifications [59.6 %], duct extension [50.8 %], and microlobulations [48.2 %]. A solid mass is initially interrogated for presence of a malignant features, and when absent, the previously described benign features are sought. If benign characteristics are seen, a solid mass is classified as being benign. Solid masses which do not demonstrate malignant or specific benign features are then classified as indeterminate with a recommendation for tissue diagnosis [20] (Figs. 7.4, 7.5, 7.6, and 7.7).

Description of Benign Features [21]

Intense and uniform *hyperechogenicity* refers to markedly hyperechoic tissue compared to the echogenicity of fat. Hyperechogenicity should be uniform and usually corresponds to fibrous tissue; this criterion cannot be applied to masses that have areas of decreased echogenicity within other than fat lobules or ducts or terminal lobular ductal units that are larger than 4 mm.

An *ellipsoid shape* or a *mass that is taller than wider* refers to a sagittal and transverse diameter that is greater than the anteroposterior dimensions. A *thin echogenic capsule* indicates a slow-growing lesion; in order to demonstrate this finding in its entire extent, the transducer will have to be angled and studied in real time in multiple planes. *Gentle lobulations* are gently curving, smooth, and few in number, three or less, as opposed to microlobulations that are a feature of a malignant mass. Since some purely intraductal cancers may have a thin echogenic capsule and a few malignant

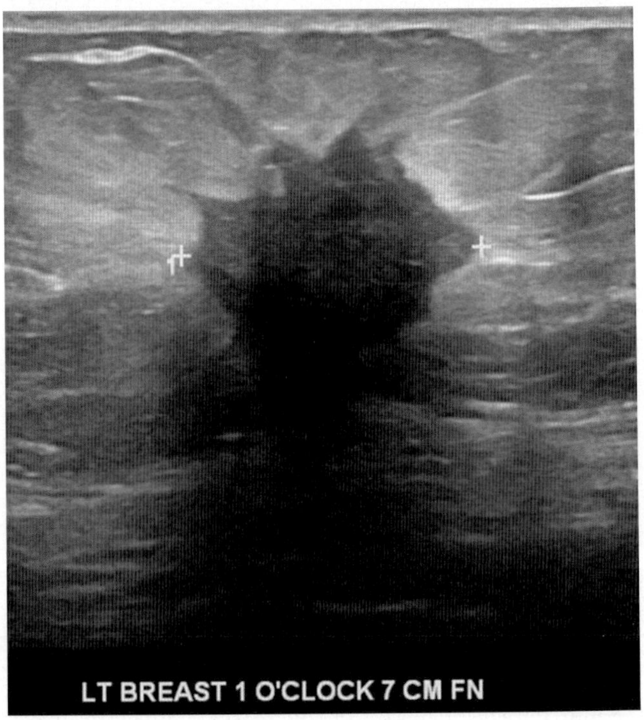

Fig. 7.5 A hypoechogenic mass with angular margins. Histological diagnosis: invasive ductal cancer

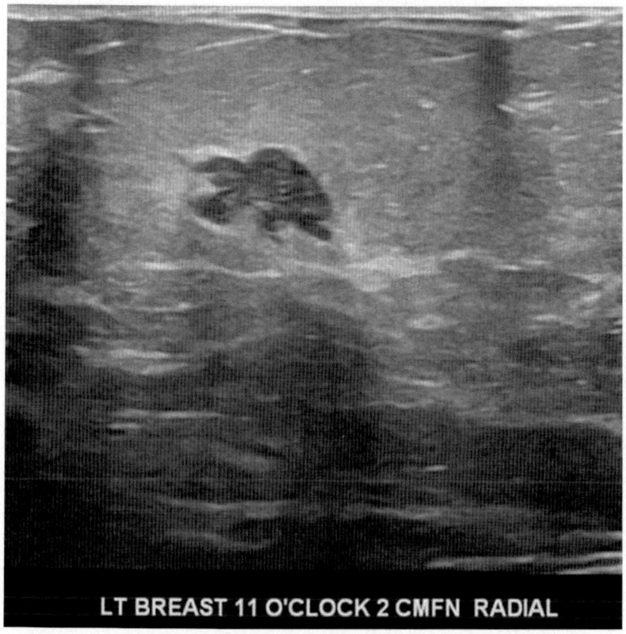

Fig. 7.6 A hypoechogenic mass with a branching pattern. Histological diagnosis: invasive ductal cancer

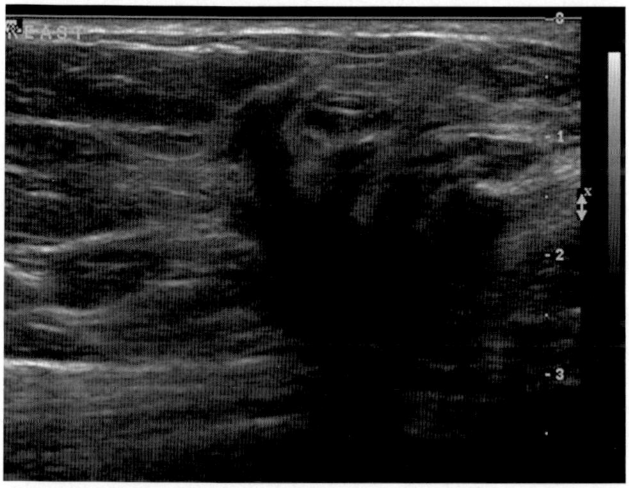

Fig. 7.7 A hypoechogenic mass with a duct extension. Histological diagnosis: ductal carcinoma in situ

ellipsoid masses with gentle lobulations do not have a thin echogenic capsule, using these criteria in combination improves the accuracy of characterizing breast masses [20].

Description of Malignant Features [20]

Spiculation is seen as alternating hyperechoic and hypoechoic lines that radiate from the surface of a mass. The appearance of these spicules is modified depending on whether hyperechoic tissue surrounds the mass. A mass that is *taller than wider* is when any part of a mass is greater in its anteroposterior dimension than in its sagittal or transverse dimension indicating that the tumor is aggressive and transgressing the normal tissue planes of the breast. *Angular margins* refer to the junction between the hypoechoic central portion of the solid mass and the surrounding tissue; this interface may be acute, obtuse, or 90°. *Branching pattern* in a solid mass is akin to duct extension and refers to presence of multiple broad-based projections extending from the surface of the mass. *Marked hypoechogenicity is* a finding described in comparison to the surrounding tissue. *Duct extension* is said to be present when there is radial extension of the tumor either within or along a duct coursing in the direction of the areola. *Posterior acoustic shadowing* is considered present even when mild or present behind a small portion of the mass. *Calcifications* refer to punctate calcifications seen in a mass; these are more suggestive of a malignant process: calcifications are more apparent when a mass is intensely hypoechogenic. *Microlobulations* refer to the presence of 1–2 mm lobulations on the surface of a solid mass.

Using the previously described criteria, Stavros and others, in a series of 750 solid masses, characterized 625 masses as benign (83 %) and 125 as malignant. Mammography did poorly compared with sonography in characterizing a malignant mass. Mammography did not identify 24/125 malignant masses that were correctly characterized by sonography; an additional five malignant masses were classified as probably benign based on mammographic features [20]. The high negative predictive value of sonography in excluding malignancy in a solid mass was proven in this study where only two [0.5 %] of the 426 solid masses that were characterized as benign were malignant, one of which was a metastasis from lung cancer [20]. The malignancy rate among masses classified as malignant was 73 % and the cancer rate in the group considered as indeterminate was 12.3 % [20]. Screen-detected mammographic mass can sometimes be sonographically occult [28]. The accuracy of ultrasound in being able to distinguish benign from malignant masses has been shown in several other studies with similar results [3, 19, 29–33]. The value of sonography in diagnosing malignant palpable masses was reported in a multi-institutional study of palpable masses undergoing sonography; all 293 of 616 palpable masses were correctly characterized as probably malignant by sonography [31]. In a retrospective series of 162 masses undergoing biopsy, three most reliable discriminatory features of a benign mass were round or oval shape (67/71, 94 % benign), circumscribed margins (95/104, 91 % benign), and a width to anteroposterior dimension >1.4 (82/92, 89 %) [19]. Morphological features most suggestive of a malignant mass were an irregular shape (19/31, 61 %), width to anteroposterior ratio of <1.4 (28/70, 40 %), microlobulations (4/6, 67 %), and spiculation (2/3, 67 %). Like others, these investigators found that the internal echotexture of a mass and presence of posterior acoustic enhancement does not help in the distinction between a benign or malignant mass. Uniform hyperechogenicity, although a very useful feature in characterizing a mass as benign, is not very helpful since it is a finding uncommonly encountered in a mass [30, 32]. Some of the descriptors of a mass such as a thin echogenic capsule is a finding that may be subject to considerable interobserver variability [19, 30]. If the three of the most useful sonographic features of a benign solid mass were strictly applied, the positive biopsy ratio would potentially increase from 23 to 39 % [19]. Using benign mass criteria of an oval or lobulated shape; circumscribed margins; internal echogenicity of isoechoic, mildly hypoechoic, or hyperechoic; and a mass that was wider than tall and a non-shadowing mass or one with increased posterior echoes, 144 of 844 solid masses were categorized as benign; there was only one malignant mass in this group, indicating that biopsy avoidance is a feasible alternative when clearly benign sonographic features are demonstrated in a solid mass [19, 30].

Focal Asymmetry

The American College of Radiology has provided separate definitions in the Breast Imaging Reporting and Data System (BI-RADS) lexicon for focal asymmetric density and asymmetric breast tissue. A focal asymmetric density is described as "... a density that cannot be accurately described using the other shapes. It is visible as asymmetry of tissue density with a similar shape on two views, but completely lacking borders and the conspicuity of a true mass. It could represent an island of normal breast, but lack of specific benign characteristics may warrant further evaluation. Additional imaging may reveal a true mass or significant architectural distortion" [34].

"Asymmetric breast tissue is judged relative to the corresponding area in the other breast and includes a greater volume of breast tissue, greater density of breast tissue or more 'prominent ducts.' There is no focal mass formation, no central density, no distorted architecture, and no associated calcifications." A focal asymmetric density should be further evaluated to distinguish it from benign asymmetric tissue and to exclude an underlying mass [34]. Focal asymmetry of the breast can be a mammographic sign of breast cancer [34–39]. Sonography is indicated only after a thorough mammographic workup of focal asymmetry; once the finding is determined to be real based on such a workup, sonography is appropriate to exclude an underlying mass [36]. In the absence of a palpable finding, or a suspicious associated mammographic finding such as microcalcifications or distortion, a negative sonogram can be reassuring in a patient where focal asymmetry is seen on a baseline mammogram or when prior mammograms are not available. A final assessment category of BI-RADS 3 with a recommendation for a short interval follow-up is appropriate since the likelihood of cancer in such cases is less than 1 % [36]. On the other hand, if the finding is new or enlarging, tissue diagnosis is indicated despite lack of an associated physical finding and associated suspicious mammographic features despite absence of a sonographic finding. In those women where the focal asymmetry has been stable for 1 year, a BI-RADS 3 assessment with annual follow-up for 1–2 years is appropriate [36]. The negative predictive value of sonography in excluding cancer was 89.4 % in one series of 36 patients who underwent biopsy [35]. Ultrasound demonstrated a finding in 26 of 36 cases: all 5 solid masses with probable malignant features were invasive ductal cancers. Developing asymmetry has a 13–27 % likelihood of malignancy, and this depends on whether this finding was identified on a screening or a diagnostic mammogram [39].

Breast Ultrasound in the Symptomatic Patient

Palpable Abnormalities of the Breast

The accuracy of clinical evaluation of a palpable abnormality of the breast is limited; signs of breast cancer are not distinctive. It is not possible to reliably distinguish cysts from solid masses on physical examination [34, 35]. A majority of palpable abnormalities of the breast are caused by benign abnormalities especially in women under the age of 40 years. Malignancy has been reported in 4–5 % of patients with breast symptoms and even among palpable lesions undergoing biopsy [40–43]. The role of mammography in patients with palpable breast lumps is to show a benign cause for the palpable abnormality, which, although uncommon, avoids further intervention (calcified involuting fibroadenoma, lipoma, oil cyst, galactocele, and hamartoma), to support earlier intervention for a mass with malignant features, to screen the remainder of the ipsilateral and contralateral breast for additional lesions, and to assess the extent of malignancy when cancer is diagnosed [44].

Mammography has limitations in assessing women with palpable abnormalities; a false-negative rate of mammography for breast cancer in patients with palpable abnormalities of the breast can be high and reported false-negative rates range from 16.5 to 40 % [19, 45]. It is standard practice to assess a palpable abnormality with mammogram and ultrasound with some few exceptions noted previously. Addition of sonography in the imaging evaluation leads to a high degree of accuracy in detecting underlying abnormalities. Multiple studies have shown that the false-negative rate for a combined mammographic and sonographic evaluation varies from 0 to 2.6 % [40–44].

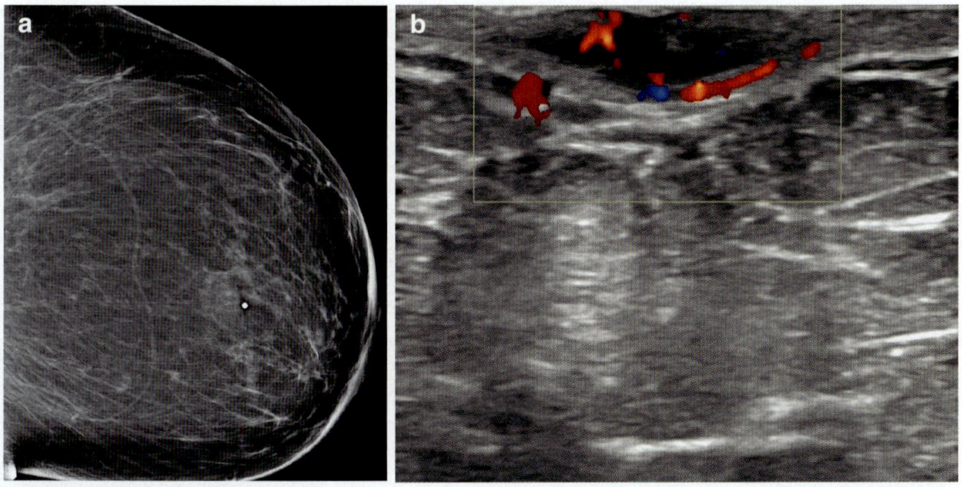

Fig. 7.8 (**a**) Mediolateral view of the left breast demonstrates a focal asymmetry corresponding to the palpable lump. (**b**) A palpable lump that is sonographically determined to be in the dermis and hence benign. A complex cystic abnormality consistent with an infected epidermal cyst. Color Doppler interrogation shows increased peripheral vascularity suggestive of inflammation

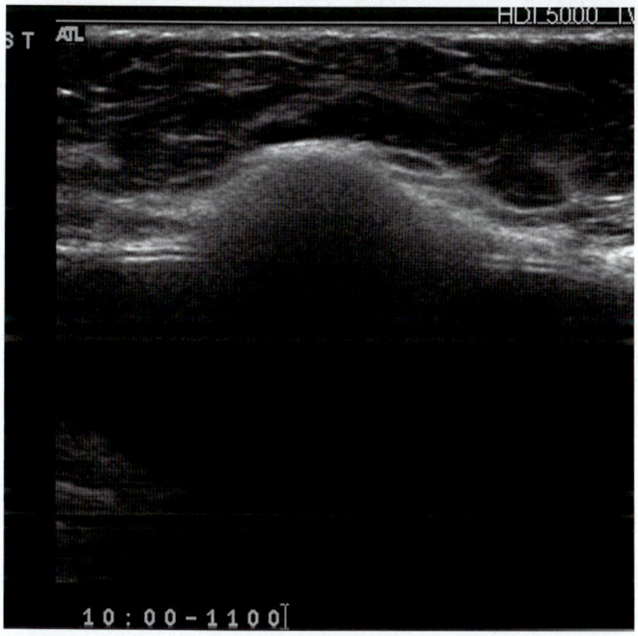

Fig. 7.9 A palpable lump in a patient with a silicone implant reveals it to be caused by localized extravasation of silicone producing a "snow storm" appearance, classic of extracapsular implant rupture

Sonography in addition may obviate the need for intervention by showing benign causes of palpable abnormalities such as cysts, benign intramammary lymph nodes, extravasated silicone, and superficial thrombophlebitis of Mondor's disease of the breast [6, 45–49] (Figs. 7.8a, b and 7.9). Sonography is also able to characterize palpable lesions obscured by dense tissue on mammograms. Moss et al. reported that sonography increased cancer detection by 14 % in symptomatic patients who were evaluated with both mammography and sonography [50]. In a retrospective analysis of 293 palpable malignant lesions, sonography detected all cancers; 18 (6.1 %) of these 293 cancers were mammographically occult [31]. In a consecutive series of 123 cases with palpable breast thickening, sensitivity of sonography for detection of invasive cancer was 100 % [51].

Is Follow-Up of Palpable Solid Masses an Option?

An assessment of a probably benign finding with a recommendation for a short interval follow-up has not been validated for masses in the breast when they are palpable [52–54]. Sickles criteria for such categorization specifically excluded lesions that were palpable. One of the criticisms of the publication of findings on ultrasound characterization of solid masses by Stavros was that the study cases included both palpable and nonpalpable masses [20]. Over the past few years, there has been increasing support for the fact that palpability of solid breast masses need not be criteria for tissue diagnosis [55–60]. Some breast imagers categorize solid palpable breast masses with otherwise benign sonographic features as BI-RADS 4A [2–10 % chance of malignancy] with a recommendation for tissue diagnosis [61] mainly due to the palpability factor. One such series of 41 cases had no cases of cancer [55]. In another series of 312 such masses undergoing biopsy, 310 were benign [99.4 %] lending scientific support for follow-up and biopsy avoidance [56]. Others have also reported that a follow-up protocol for palpable solid breast masses has shown similar results. In a series of 157 palpable breast masses, 112 were followed with interval increase in size in six at follow-up all were proven benign at biopsy. Forty-five masses underwent biopsy without follow-up with no malignancy identified [57]. In yet another larger series of patients in whom noncalcified solid breast masses were followed, there was a malignancy rate of 0.2 % [1 of 448 masses] which was biopsied based on interval enlargement at follow-up [58]. When following solid masses particularly

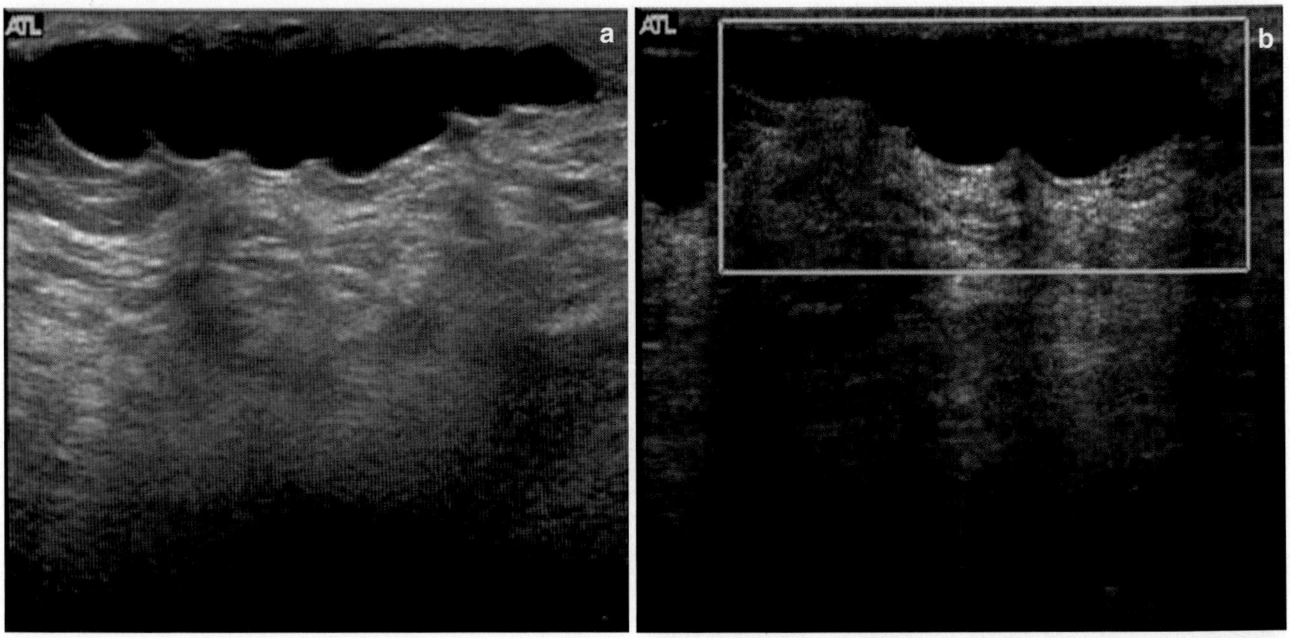

Fig. 7.10 (**a**, **b**) A palpable cord-like tender lump on ultrasound demonstrates a beaded tubular anechoic structure in a non-subareolar location consistent with a thrombosed superficial vein in a patient with Mondor's disease of the breast. Color Doppler image demonstrates no flow and confirms the finding of a thrombosed vessel

those that are palpable, careful inspection of morphologic features is, however, important. Of these features particularly the margins need to be assessed for irregularities; it is not uncommon for masses that may appear mammographically benign to have ill-defined margins on ultrasound for certain special types of cancers such as mucinous cancer (Fig. 7.10a, b). Also, certain cancers that are hyperechoic and initially put on a surveillance protocol on follow-up may be determined not to exhibit strictly benign features, particularly in the case of hyperechoic masses that on close inspection demonstrate internal inhomogeneity (Fig. 7.11a–c).

Breast Pain

There is little justification in imaging a woman with diffuse pain, bilateral pain, or one who is complaining of cyclical pain. Imaging is recommended only when pain is associated with a physical finding [62]. Pain when associated with cancer is likely unrelated to cancer and an incidental finding. Imaging is often justified for patient reassurance, but has been shown to lead to additional evaluation; diagnostic examination in those women without an abnormal clinical finding did not find any cancers [63]. In this series, breast pain accounted for 32 % of referrals for breast symptoms, 12 % of whom had an abnormal physical finding and 25 % of whom were referred for breast imaging. In the absence of a physical finding or an imaging-detected mass, no cases of cancer were reported at the site of pain; breast cancers when reported to be associated are often identified at imaging in an area remote from the pain and/or in the contralateral breast [63–65]. The negative predictive value of ultrasound and mammogram in patients with focal breast pain has been reported to be 100 % [65]. In an observational study, there was no significant incidence of breast cancer in a group of women who presented with breast pain when compared to a control group of asymptomatic women screened [64]. Focal breast pain when associated with a palpable finding should prompt imaging; ultrasound may reveal a cyst under tension which may be relieved if aspirated. In routine practice, imaging reveals no abnormal findings or nonspecific findings of fibrocystic changes such as small cysts.

Nipple Discharge

Nipple discharge is worrisome particularly when unilateral, blood stained, or spontaneous. When bilateral, serous, or expressed, it is more likely physiologic. Nipple discharge is investigated with mammography, sonography, ductography, MRI, or ductoscopy [66–69]. In a series of 357 women with pathologic nipple discharge, the sensitivity of sonography was 72 %, mammography 62.9 %, that of galactography was 81.4 %, and that of ductoscopy was 86.6 % [67]. In one series of 416 cases of nipple discharge, 31 % were considered physiologic [66]. Of the 69 % which had bloody and spontaneous discharge, biopsy or surgery identified an underlying etiology in

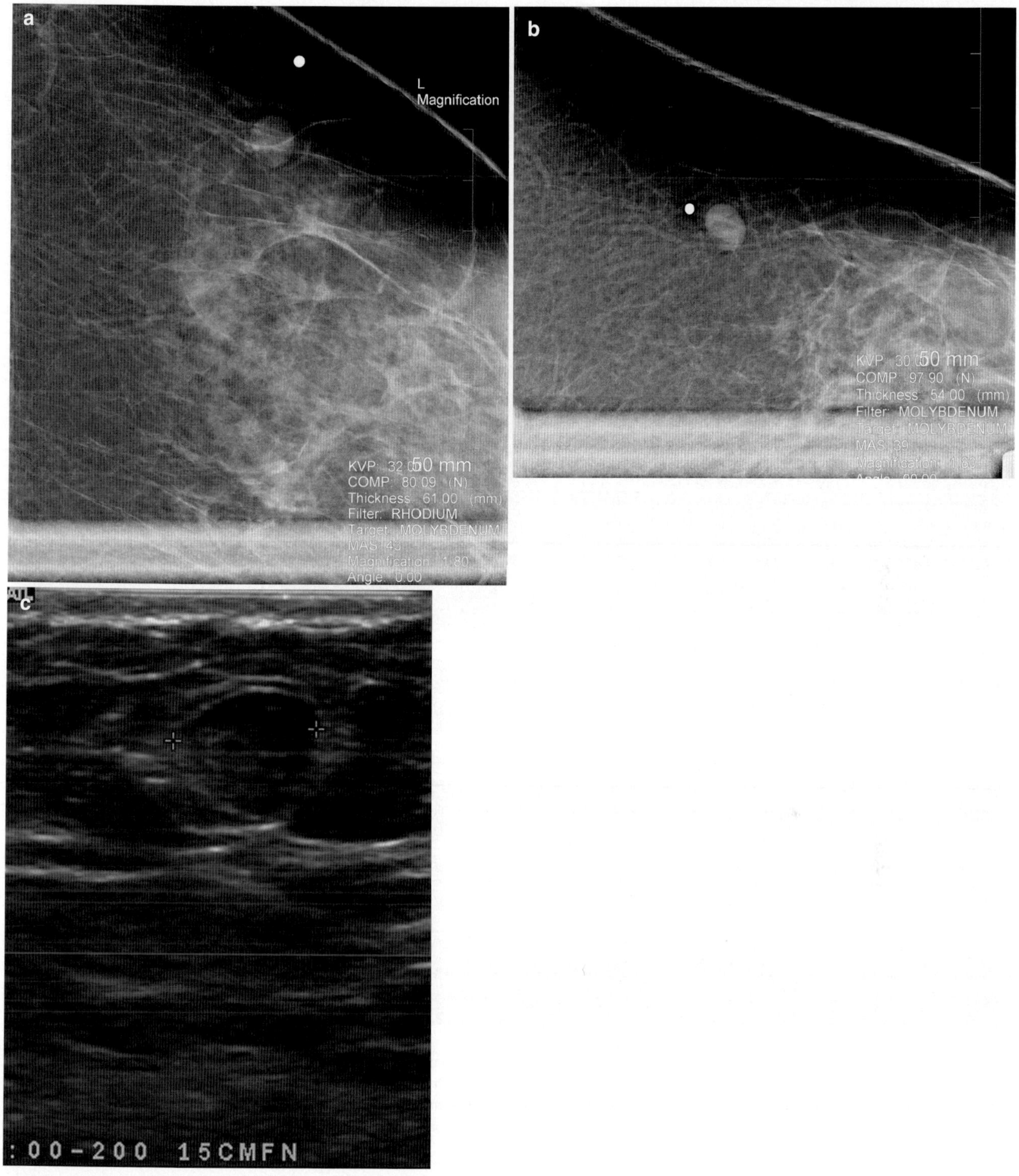

Fig. 7.11 (**a–c**) A 39-year-old with a palpable lump. Histological diagnosis was mucinous carcinoma. (**a**) Magnification mediolateral view demonstrates a benign-appearing round circumscribed isodense mass. (**b**) Magnification craniocaudal view demonstrates a round benign-appearing circumscribed isodense mass. (**c**) Ultrasound demonstrates a heterogeneous solid mass with ill-defined borders

90 % of which 37 % were malignant or high-risk lesions. Sole predictor of malignant or high-risk lesion was the presence of a palpable mass. Preoperative assessment identified 80 % of malignant or high-risk lesions; the remainder of the lesions were identified by duct excision alone [66]. Spontaneous nipple discharge (SND) is defined as a nonphysiologic unilateral nipple discharge from a single duct unit. It is usually benign, caused primarily by

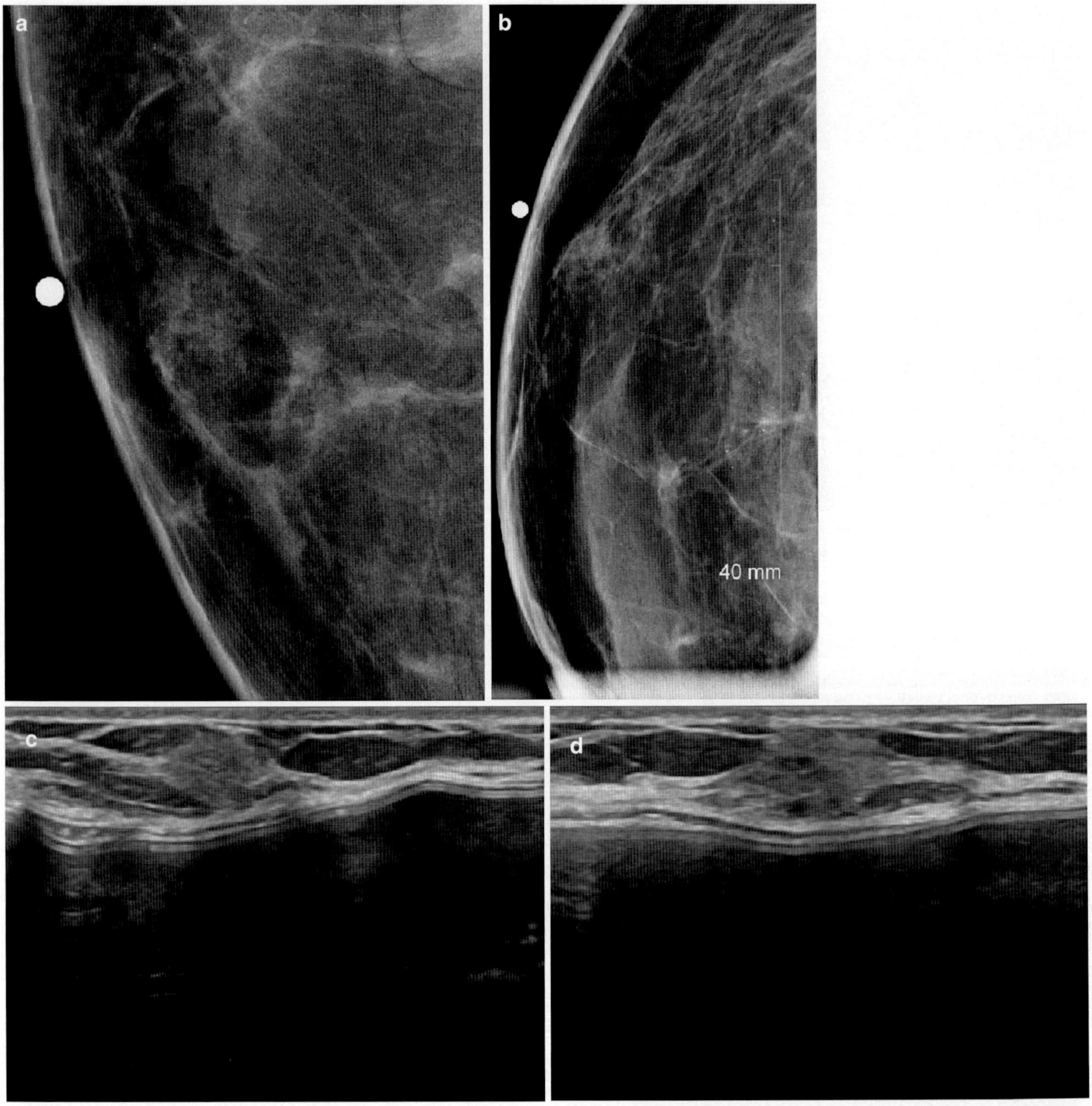

Fig. 7.12 (**a**–**d**) A 35-year-old woman with a right breast palpable lump. Histologically proven to be an invasive ductal cancer. (**a**) Magnification view in the mediolateral oblique projection demonstrates a small focal asymmetry. (**b**) Magnification view in the craniocaudal projection demonstrates a small focal asymmetry. (**c**) Ultrasound demonstrates a hyperechoic mass that was initially assigned a probably benign category. (**d**) Close inspection of the ultrasound image demonstrates that the hyperechogenicity is heterogeneous

intraductal disorders among which papillary lesions (PL) are frequent [70–72]. Intraductal papillary lesions account for 1–2 % of all breast neoplasms and have a wide morphologic spectrum, varying from a single papilloma to a ductal carcinoma in situ (DCIS) and invasive cancer of the breast (Figs. 7.12a–d, 7.13, and 7.14). It is generally accepted that intraductal papillary lesions have to be surgically excised with the duct. There is a 4–11 % risk of cancer development in a solitary papilloma; this risk can be as high as 33 % in atypical papillomas [73, 74].

Nipple discharge therefore can be the result from benign conditions, such as intraductal papilloma, duct ectasia, plasma cell mastitis, or galactorrhea, or caused by malignant conditions such as ductal, lobular, or papillary carcinoma. Techniques used in nipple discharge evaluation include mammography, ultrasound, cytology (which could be assisted

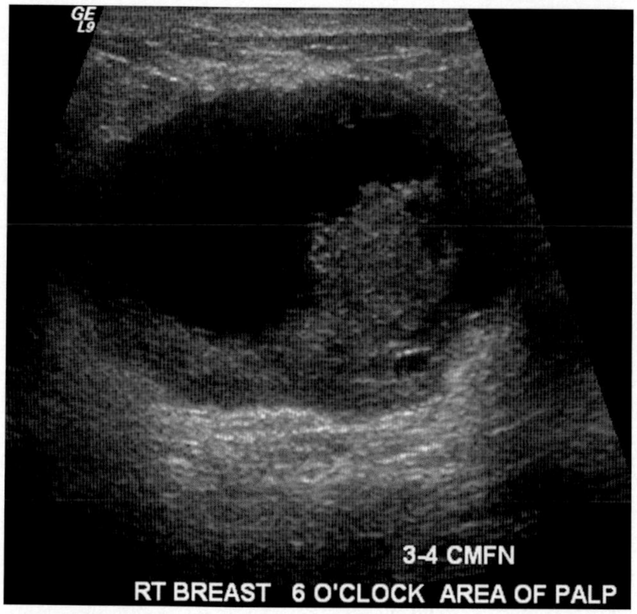

Fig. 7.13 A 44-year-old woman with a bloody nipple discharge and a palpable lump. Ultrasound demonstrates a complex cystic subareolar mass with an irregular mural nodule histologically confirmed to be a benign papilloma

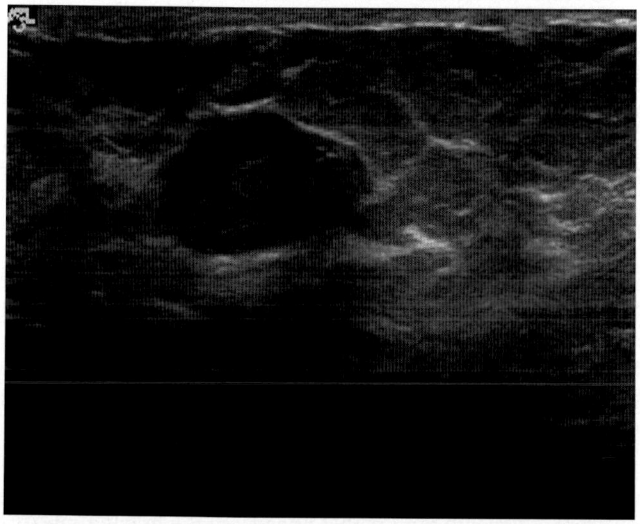

Fig. 7.14 A 72-year-old woman with a bloody nipple discharge. Ultrasound shows a complex cystic subareolar mass with multiple intracystic masses histologically proven at excisional biopsy to be an intracystic papillary cancer

by a mammary pump), duct endoscopy, ductography, immunochemical methods, and at least surgical excision of the pathological ducts for diagnosis and treatment in the same procedure [69]. About 7–22 % of nipple discharge that is clinically suspicious and investigated may have an underlying malignancy [66, 75, 76].

Breast Ultrasound in DCIS

Ductal carcinoma in situ (DCIS) refers to cancerous breast epithelial cells within the ducts and lobules of the terminal ductal–lobular unit [TDLU]. There is an abnormal increase in the growth of the epithelial cells, which accumulate within and greatly expand the ducts and lobules. DCIS is a nonlethal type of cancer by itself but is, however, the immediate precursor of invasive breast cancers, which are potentially lethal [77]. Prior to the widespread introduction of screening mammography, DCIS accounted for only 0.8–5 % of breast cancers, but now it accounts for up to 30 % of cancers in the screened population and 5 % of cancers in the symptomatic women [78–80]. Mammography identifies DCIS with a high sensitivity ranging from 84 to 90 %. The most common mammographic sign is calcifications, and these are seen in 67–88 % of cases of DCIS; the remainder appear as masses, focal asymmetry, or density [81, 82]. Several studies have been published on the sonographic evaluation of DCIS in both asymptomatic and symptomatic women [81–86]. Improvements in image resolution resulting from the use of high-frequency linear array transducers allow for better detection of microcalcifications on ultrasound [87, 88]. The reported range of sensitivity of US for detections of microcalcifications varies from 35 to 74 % [81, 87, 88]. One series showed ultrasound to have as high as 93 % sensitivity in detection of DCIS in a series of 75 biopsy proven cases; 39 of these were DCIS with microinvasion and 36 pure DCIS [84]. Ultrasound is particularly helpful in detecting masses associated with microcalcifications that may not be readily visible or obscured on a mammogram. However, finding of a mass in areas of microcalcifications increases the likelihood of invasive disease. In one prospective study of 46 cases, US sensitivity for detection of microcalcifications associated with invasive and in situ malignancy was 100 % [87]. Ultrasound is less reliable in identifying microcalcifications associated with benign fibrocystic changes.

Unlike mammographic detected DCIS, those that are detected on ultrasound most commonly are masses with or without calcifications, 76 % in a series of 38 cases; only a small percentage appear as pure calcifications unassociated with a mass [15 %]. US identified DCIS has also been shown to be more commonly associated with microinvasion and comedocarcinoma [82]. Overall the most frequently encountered sonographic finding in a case of DCIS is a noncircumscribed oval mass with parallel orientation and normal acoustic transmission [82]. A microlobulated mass with normal acoustic transmission, mild hypoechogenicity, and intraductal extension is also a common ultrasound finding (Fig. 7.15). While noncalcified DCIS appear as masses on ultrasound, those with calcifications tend to appear as masses that are associated with calcifications [81]. In one series, 62 % of DCIS with calcifications appeared as masses on

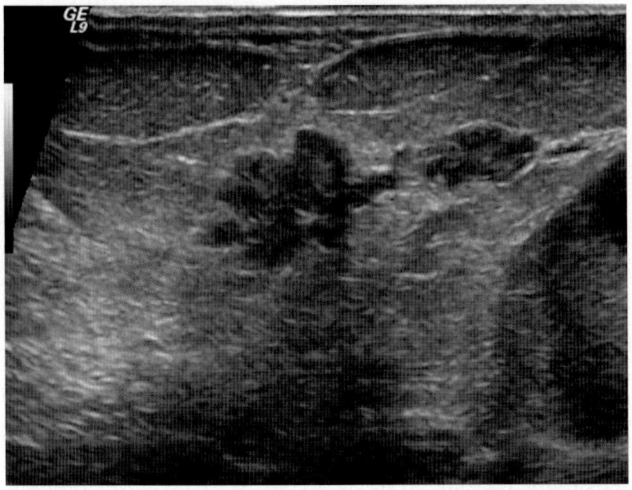

Fig. 7.15 A 53-year-old woman with a tubular and branching solid mass histologically proven to be DCIS

ultrasound, 25 % appeared as calcifications alone, and 13 % were false negative [81]. In the same series, 49 % of noncalcified DCIS was false negative on the mammogram but identified in all cases on ultrasound [81]. Seventy-two percent of false-negative mammograms in noncalcified DCIS had a dense breast parenchyma [81].

Second-look ultrasound with focused evaluation of area of microcalcifications prior to stereotactic biopsy demonstrated calcifications in 35 % of cases; when an associated mass is present, if ultrasound is then chosen to sample, close follow-up even when histology is negative is indicated to avoid delay in breast cancer diagnosis [88]. Interestingly in screen-detected microcalcifications with a low suspicion of cancer that has been assigned BI-RADS 4A, ultrasound may have some role; one study found that 75 % of such cases where US was negative had benign findings [89]. When an invasive cancer is associated with DCIS, spiculated margins, marked hypoechogenicity, thick echogenic rim, and posterior acoustic shadowing are associated. The primary role of ultrasound in screen-detected microcalcifications that are suspicious for malignancy is to determine if US can be used as a modality for tissue diagnosis by core needle biopsy or prior to surgical excision. Additional role for ultrasound is to identify noncalcified DCIS and evaluate the extent of disease in a patient with dense breast [84].

Microcalcifications are less frequent mammographic sign of DCIS in the symptomatic women compared to those in the asymptomatic group [85, 86]. In one series of 60 cases of DCIS in symptomatic women, sensitivity of ultrasound was 90 % and that of mammography was 80 %. Sonographic features of DCIS included a mass [72 %] or ductal changes [23 %] or architectural distortion [7 %] with some lesions demonstrating more than one feature. The most frequent feature of DCIS was a focal mass, low-level intraductal echoes, ductal extension or dilatation, and architectural distortion. In a series of 231 cases of symptomatic and asymptomatic DCIS that had preoperatively undergone mammography and sonography, the false-negative rate with sonography was 10 % for asymptomatic screen-detected DCIS and only 1 % in symptomatic cases. Of the false-negative cases, a majority [10/11] manifested as microcalcifications on mammogram. In the symptomatic group of women, 92 % of DCIS appeared as a mass. Masses were commonly irregular in shape [64 %] and had indistinct margins [51 %] [86]. Extensive DCIS in subareolar location may present with unilateral bloody nipple discharge. Ultrasound may reveal tubular retroareolar masses representing ducts filled with cancer cells. Galactogram will show multiple filling defects (Fig. 7.16a–f).

Ultrasound of the Axilla

The most common palpable masses in the axilla are those due to axillary lymph nodes with metastasis from breast cancer [90]. A detailed description of assessment of the axillary lymph nodes appears in the chapter on staging of breast cancer (Chap. 15). The most frequent cause of lymphadenopathy is nonspecific benign lymphadenopathy followed by metastatic adenopathy [91] and chronic lymphocytic leukemia or well-differentiated lymphocytic lymphoma. Less common etiologies include collagen vascular disease, metastasis from a nonbreast primary, metastasis from an unknown primary, HIV-associated lymphadenopathy, sarcoidosis, or reactive lymphadenopathy related to an infection in the breast [90]. Nonlymph node masses in the axilla include masses that arise in accessory breast tissue such as fibroadenomas, hamartoma, fat necrosis or breast cancers, and soft tissue tumors such as lipomas, hemangiomas, epidermoid cysts, schwannomas, and malignant fibrous histiocytomas [91]. Accessory breast tissue occurs in 0.6 to 6 % of the population, with highest prevalence observed in the Japanese population and lowest in the white population. Breast cancer in the axillary tail of Spence is rare and has been reported to be about 1 % in a series of 839 breast cancer cases [92]. Rarely neurogenic tumors that arise from the brachial plexus can present as an axillary mass and need to be distinguished from an abnormal axillary node to avoid excision that can lead to permanent nerve damage [93, 94]. A central band-shaped increased echogenicity described as the coffee bean sign is characteristic of neurogenic tumors; these appear as enhancing and low T2 signal areas on MRI [93].

Isolated finding of unilaterally enlarged lymph nodes is an uncommon finding. There are no clear guidelines for reporting of abnormal axillary lymph nodes. The BI-RADS atlas includes this under associated findings and states "enlarged non-fatty replaced axillary lymph nodes may be commented on"; however, mammographic assessment of

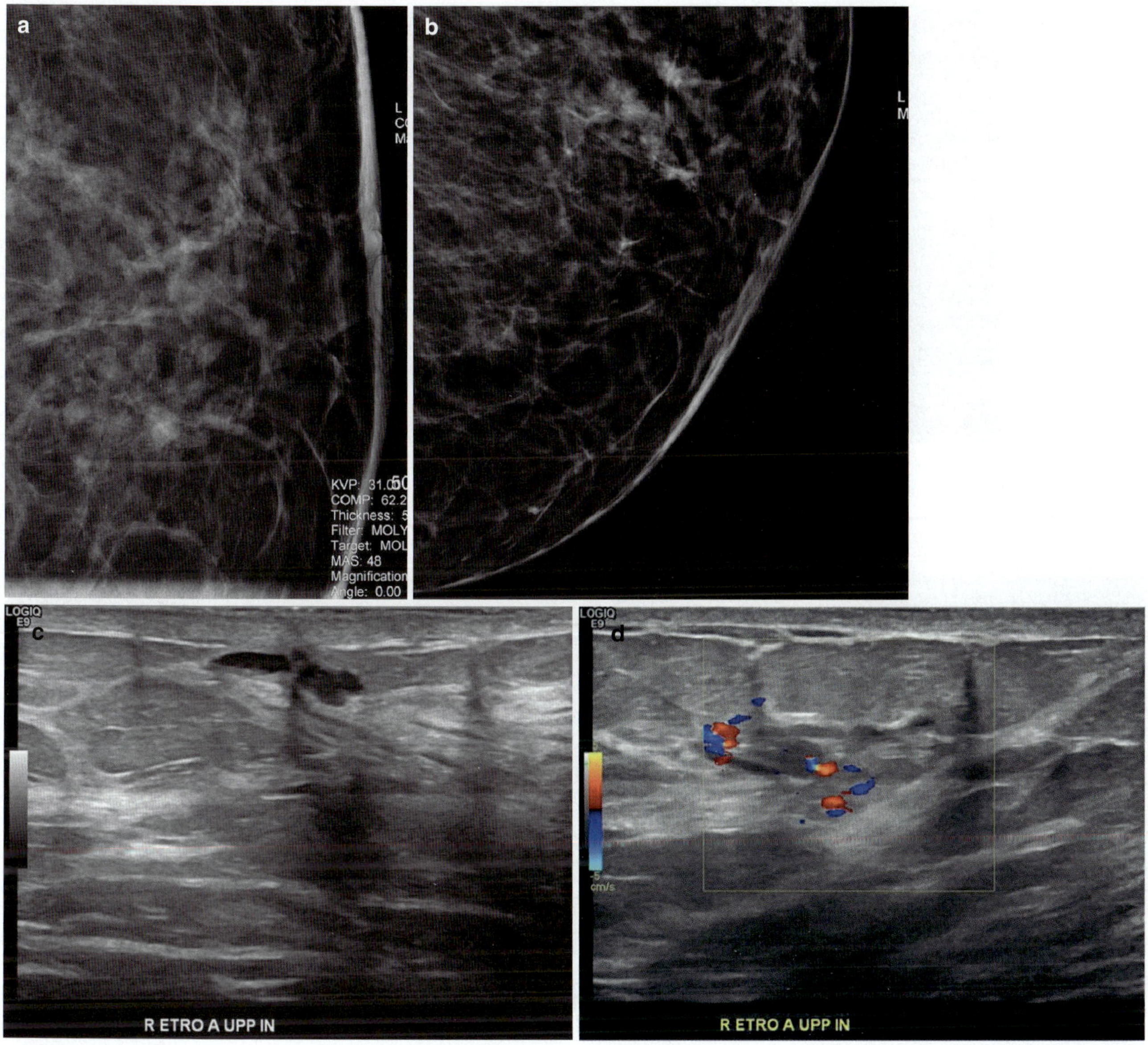

Fig. 7.16 (**a**–**f**) 36-year-old with history of bloody nipple discharge. (**a**) Magnification mediolateral oblique view reveals no abnormality. (**b**) Magnification craniocaudal view reveals no abnormality. (**c**) Ultrasound demonstrates tubular retroareolar masses suggestive of intraductal pathology. (**d**) Ultrasound demonstrates tubular retroareolar masses suggestive of intraductal pathology. (**e**) Ultrasound demonstrates tubular partly cystic retroareolar mass suggestive of intraductal pathology. (**f**) Galactogram reveals intraductal filling defects. Excisional biopsy was performed. Histology showed DCIS

such lymph nodes is unreliable [34]. Abnormal appearance of the lymph nodes include a size greater than 20 mm, absence of a fatty hilum, increased density, and a round shape. When any two of these criteria are fulfilled or when one is present and significant interval increase in size as shown by a greater than 100 % increase, sonographic assessment is useful [95]. Sonographic criteria for abnormal lymph nodes include absence of fatty hilum, abnormal cortex, size greater than 2 cm, and round shape. Malignancy rate in unilateral isolated abnormal lymph nodes has been reported to be between 45 and 58 % [95–97]. When the fatty hilum of an intramammary lymph node is replaced, distinction from a small cancer is impossible. In such cases, tissue diagnosis is the only option. Presence of a vascular pedicle in the region of the hilum prebiopsy may give an indication of a lymph node mass (Fig. 7.17a, b). Assigning a benign category for small low-density nodules when seen in the expected locations of lymph nodes can also lead to a misdiagnosis. Careful inspection of the margins with spot compression views is mandatory for all masses, and sonography helps to characterize the margin characteristics as well (Fig. 7.18a–d).

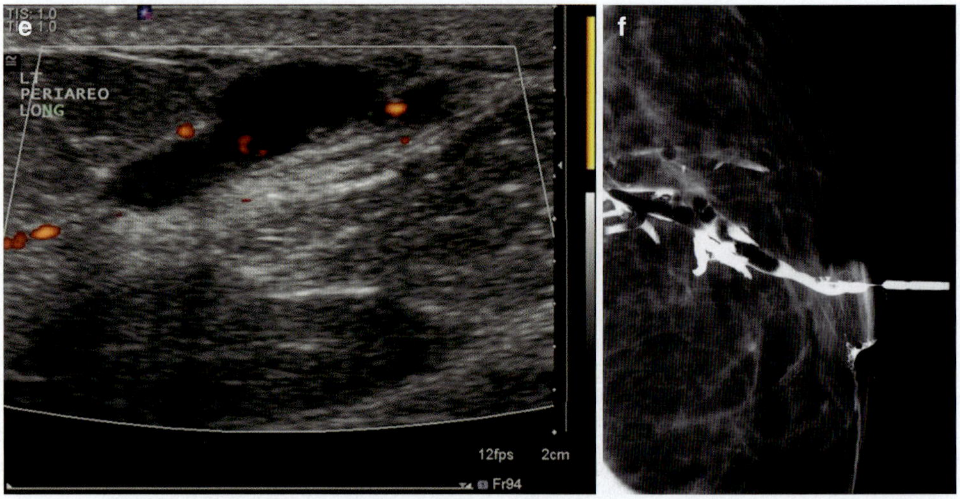

Fig. 7.16 (continued)

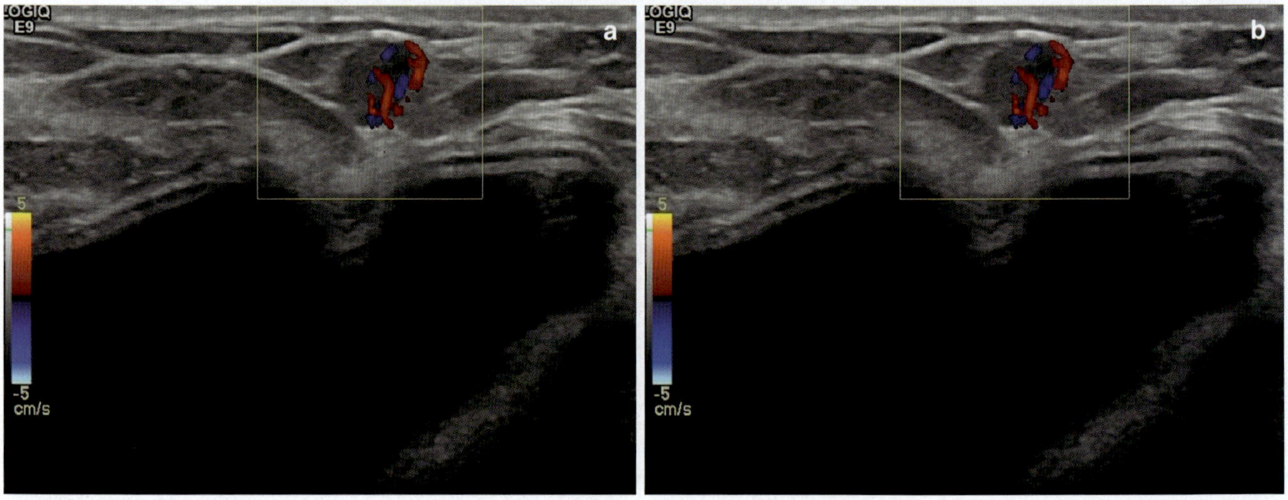

Fig. 7.17 (**a**, **b**) A palpable mass in the upper outer quadrant of the left breast. Histological diagnosis: reactive lymph node with foreign body granulomatous infection. (**a**) A round solid mass in the upper outer quadrant of the left breast. No fatty hilum is visible. (**b**) Color Doppler image demonstrates the hilar vascular pedicle characteristic of lymph nodes

Doppler Sonography of Breast Masses

Neovascularization is a feature of malignant tumors, and hence color and power Doppler imaging has been proposed as a complementary tool in the evaluation of a solid breast mass [98–102].

Color Doppler imaging reflects the mean intravascular frequency shift caused by the Doppler effects of flowing red blood cells, whereas the power Doppler represents the intensities of the Doppler signals within a time period. On ultrasound images, hypervascularity (92.9 %) and presence of irregular vessels (73.2 %) are features of malignant tumors. Other associated features in a malignant mass are the presence of rich vascularization (vessel mass ratio >10 % in 54.2 % of cases) and more than one vascular pole [99]. Typical color Doppler signs of malignancy are intratumoral vessels that are central (86 % in malignancy vs 51 % in benignity), penetrating (65 % vs 34 %), branching (56 % vs 22 %), and disordered (42 % vs 8 %). Power Doppler imaging can be used to depict a significant intratumoral increase in blood flow ($P \leq .0001$) compared with the flow in normal breast tissue [103]; an increased vascularity on power Doppler images in the area of a possible isoechoic nodule in fat increases confidence that the finding indicates an abnormality [102]. However, such a finding is not useful until the presence of a focal isoechoic

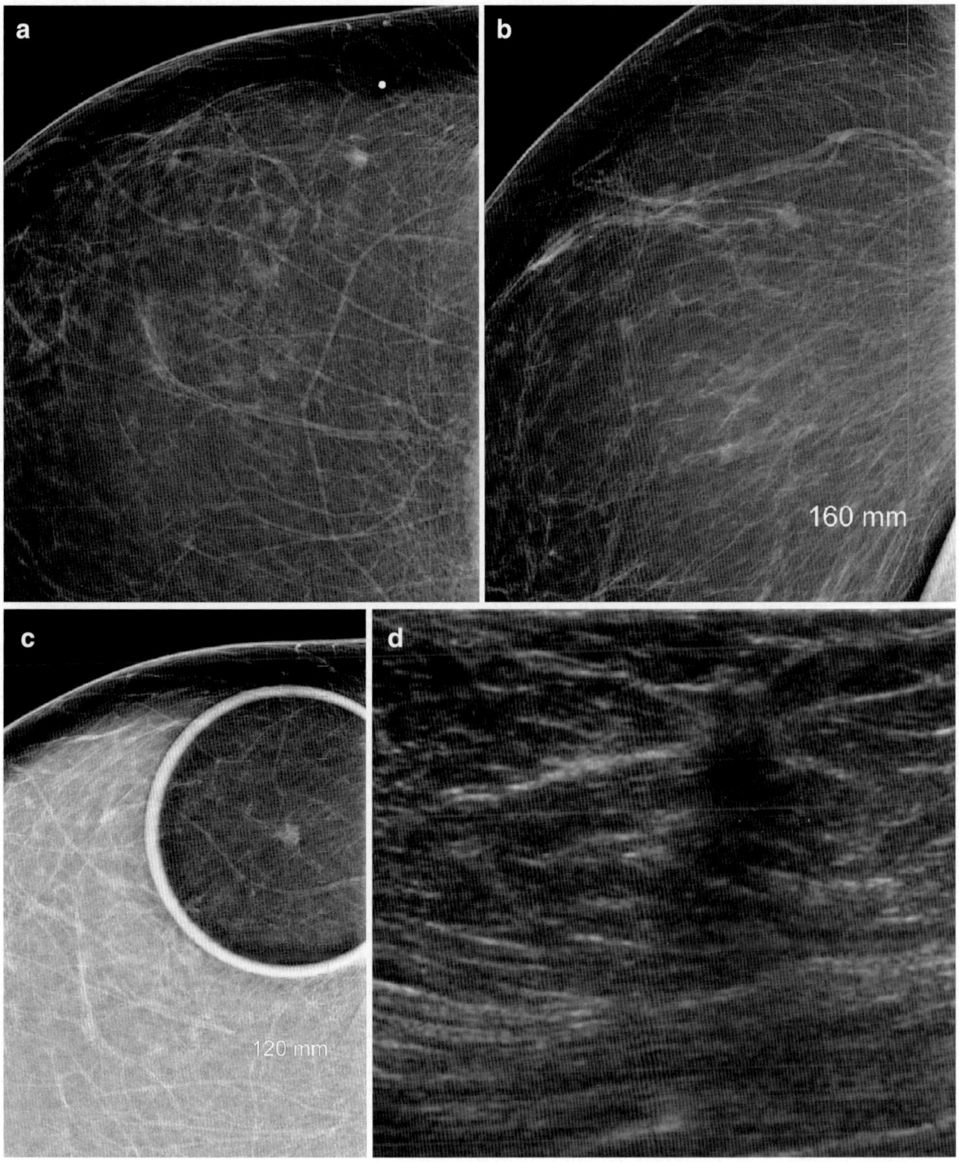

Fig. 7.18 (a–d) A 52-year-old with a palpable mass. Histological diagnosis: invasive ductal cancer. (a) Craniocaudal mammogram demonstrates a benign-appearing small low-density mass with obscured margins in the upper outer quadrant of the breast. (b) Mediolateral view demonstrates a low-density mass with partially obscured margins. (c) Spot compression mammogram demonstrates irregular margins. (d) Ultrasound demonstrates a small irregular mass with malignant features

mass is suspected. False-negative findings at B-mode US screening of the breast are not improved by using Doppler imaging [99]. Isoechoic lesions surrounded by fat can result in false-negative interpretations and a delayed diagnosis of breast cancer. Color and power Doppler imaging in combination with spatial compound imaging, tissue harmonic imaging, and elastography power Doppler fremitus imaging and contrast agent enhancement have been proposed as supplemental techniques to aid in identification of such isoechoic masses [102]. In a series of 25 malignant masses, 21 had either penetrating vessels [17] or peripheral vessels [4] on power Doppler sonography [104]. By using penetrating vessels to indicate malignancy, sensitivity for power Doppler US was 68 %, specificity was 95 %, positive predictive value was 85 %, and negative predictive value was 88 % [103].

Elastography

Sonoelastography is a method that attempts to distinguish benign from malignant masses [104–112]. Tissue compression results in tissue deformation; the extent of this deformation is measured. Elastography has the potential of reducing the unacceptably high false positive that is currently a huge problem in routine use of ultrasound as a screening modality. There are two methods of elastography: one is compression or strain elastography that produces an image that is based on the displacement of the tissue in a mass resulting from external source or patient source. This allows for a qualitative assessment of the lesion. In shear wave elastography, a special "push pulse" is applied which results in shear wave propagation that can be measured as a velocity. Since speed of sound through tissues is dependent on the stiffness of the tissue, a quantitative value of the stiffness can be calculated [104]. Benign lesions measure smaller than cancers on compression elastography than on the corresponding B-mode image. A ratio of elasticity/B-mode size greater than 1.2 has been proposed and tested as diagnostic criteria for malignancy. A multicenter trial of 635 biopsy proven cases reported a sensitivity of 99 % and specificity of 87 % [105].

Shear wave elastography although more objective has both false positives and false negatives. False positives are, however, seen more often in benign masses. Factors affecting false findings are related to lesion size, breast thickness, and lesion depth. Larger benign lesions tended to have a higher false-positive rate, and small malignant lesions also had similar higher false-negative rate. In large breast and deeper lesions accuracy tended to be lower, correspondingly better for more superficial masses [111]. A color scale has been proposed which incorporates a five-point grading scale that combines the ratio change in the size of the lesion and the degree of stiffness of the lesion. A lesion that is hard and greater than the lesion is given a score of 5; 1 that is hard and same size gets a score of 4 and a lesion that is soft gets a score of 1. Lesions with a score of 4 or higher are recommended to undergo biopsy [104, 105]. Combined use of ultrasound elastography and color Doppler sonography has been proposed to improve specificity and reduce false positives [112]. In a series of 367 lesions, when both elastography and Doppler scores were negative, specificity increased for all readers from an average of 25.3–34 % [112].

The rationale and value of techniques such as elastography to reduce false positives and unnecessary biopsies have been questioned. Dempsey points out in an editorial opinion "We cannot, therefore, afford to continue to function in a mindset where we try at all cost to avoid doing a simple, rapid, and accurate needle biopsy by which a definite histologic diagnosis can be made. We must not attempt to substitute one or more time-consuming, physician-inefficient, costly, and often inaccurate imaging studies that, based on data currently available, accomplish nothing more than producing a needless procrastination in a timeline that should be efficiently targeted to quickly establishing a firm diagnosis from which proper patient management can be promptly initiated" [113]. Breast ultrasound is a useful modality for the assessment of the breast in both symptomatic and asymptomatic women. Its role in the diagnosis and differential diagnosis of breast cancer will continue to evolve and grow.

Appendices

Appendix 7A. American College of Radiology ACR Appropriateness Criteria® – Clinical Condition: Palpable Breast Masses

American College of Radiology
ACR Appropriateness Criteria®

Clinical Condition: **Palpable Breast Masses**

Variant 1: **Woman 40 years of age or older, initial evaluation. (See Appendices 1A-1B at http://www.acr.org/~/media/ACR/Documents/AppCriteria/Diagnostic/PalpableBreastMasses.pdf for additional steps in the workup of these patients.)**

Radiologic Procedure	Rating	Comments	RRL*
Mammography diagnostic	9		☢☢
US breast	4	If she had recent mammogram (ie, past 6 months), US may be appropriate.	O
MRI breast without and with contrast	2		O
MRI breast without contrast	1		O
FDG-PEM	1		☢☢☢☢
Tc-99m sestamibi BSGI	1		☢☢☢☢
Image-guided fine needle aspiration breast	1		Varies
Image-guided core biopsy breast	1		Varies
Rating Scale: 1,2,3 Usually not appropriate; 4,5,6 May be appropriate; 7,8,9 Usually appropriate			*Relative Radiation Level

Clinical Condition: **Palpable Breast Masses**

Variant 2: **Woman 40 years of age or older, mammography findings suspicious for malignancy. Next examination to perform. (See Appendix 1A at http://www.acr.org/~/media/ACR/Documents/AppCriteria/Diagnostic/PalpableBreastMasses.pdf for additional steps in the workup of these patients.)**

Radiologic Procedure	Rating	Comments	RRL*
US breast	9		O
MRI breast without and with contrast	2		O
Image-guided core biopsy breast	2		Varies
Mammography short interval follow-up	1		☢ ☢
MRI breast without contrast	1		O
FDG-PEM	1		☢ ☢ ☢ ☢
Tc-99m sestamibi BSGI	1		☢ ☢ ☢ ☢
Image-guided fine needle aspiration breast	1		Varies
Rating Scale: 1,2,3 Usually not appropriate; 4,5,6 May be appropriate; 7,8,9 Usually appropriate			*Relative Radiation Level

Clinical Condition: **Palpable Breast Masses**

Variant 3: **Woman 40 years of age or older, mammography findings probably benign. Next examination to perform. (See Appendix 1A at http://www.acr.org/~/media/ACR/Documents/AppCriteria/Diagnostic/PalpableBreastMasses.pdf for additional steps in the workup of these patients.)**

Radiologic Procedure	Rating	Comments	RRL*
Mammography short interval follow-up	8		☢ ☢
US breast	8	US is frequently performed to confirm correlation of imaging and clinical findings, as well as lesion characterization.	O
MRI breast without and with contrast	2		O
Image-guided core biopsy breast	2		Varies
MRI breast without contrast	1		O
FDG-PEM	1		☢ ☢ ☢ ☢
Tc-99m sestamibi BSGI	1		☢ ☢ ☢ ☢
Image-guided fine needle aspiration breast	1		Varies
Rating Scale: 1,2,3 Usually not appropriate; 4,5,6 May be appropriate; 7,8,9 Usually appropriate			*Relative Radiation Level

Clinical Condition: Palpable Breast Masses

Variant 4: **Woman 40 years of age or older, mammography findings benign (like lipoma) at site of palpable mass. Next examination to perform.**

Radiologic Procedure	Rating	Comments	RRL*
Mammography short interval follow-up	2		☢☢
US breast	2	US may be done if correlation between the clinical examination and mammography is not clear.	O
Image-guided fine needle aspiration breast	2		Varies
MRI breast without and with contrast	1		O
MRI breast without contrast	1		O
FDG-PEM	1		☢☢☢☢
Tc-99m sestamibi BSGI	1		☢☢☢☢
Image-guided core biopsy breast	1		Varies
Rating Scale: 1,2,3 Usually not appropriate; 4,5,6 May be appropriate; 7,8,9 Usually appropriate			*Relative Radiation Level

Clinical Condition: **Palpable Breast Masses**

Variant 5: **Woman 40 years of age or older, mammography findings negative. Next examination to perform. (See Appendix 1B at http://www.acr.org/~/media/ACR/Documents/AppCriteria/Diagnostic/PalpableBreastMasses.pdf for additional steps in the workup of these patients.)**

Radiologic Procedure	Rating	Comments	RRL* Palpable Breast Mass
US breast	9		O
Mammography short interval follow-up	1		☢☢
MRI breast without and with contrast	1		O
MRI breast without contrast	1		O
FDG-PEM	1		☢☢☢☢
Tc-99m sestamibi BSGI	1		☢☢☢☢
Image-guided fine needle aspiration breast	1		Varies
Image-guided core biopsy breast	1		Varies
Rating Scale: 1,2,3 Usually not appropriate; 4,5,6 May be appropriate; 7,8,9 Usually appropriate			*Relative Radiation Level

Clinical Condition: **Palpable Breast Masses**

Variant 6: **Woman younger than 30 years of age, initial evaluation. (See Appendices 2A-2B a t http://www.acr.org/~/media/ACR/Documents/AppCriteria/Diagnostic/PalpableBreastMasses.pdf for additional steps in the workup of these patients.)**

Radiologic Procedure	Rating	Comments	RRL*
US breast	9		O
Mammography diagnostic	3		☢☢
MRI breast without and with contrast	1		O
MRI breast without contrast	1		O
FDG-PEM	1		☢☢☢☢
Tc-99m sestamibi BSGI	1		☢☢☢☢
Image-guided fine needle aspiration breast	1		Varies
Image-guided core biopsy breast	1		Varies
Rating Scale: 1,2,3 Usually not appropriate; 4,5,6 May be appropriate; 7,8,9 Usually appropriate			*Relative Radiation Level

Clinical Condition: **Palpable Breast Masses**

Variant 7: **Woman younger than 30 years of age, US findings suspicious for malignancy. Next examination to perform. (See Appendix 2A a t http://www.acr.org/~/media/ACR/Documents/AppCriteria/Diagnostic/PalpableBreastMasses.pdf for additional steps in the workup of these patients.)**

Radiologic Procedure	Rating	Comments	RRL*
Image-guided core biopsy breast	9	Either mammography or biopsy is appropriate. It depends on the history and findings.	Varies Palpable Breast Mass
Mammography diagnostic	8	Either mammography or biopsy is appropriate. It depends on the history and findings.	☢☢
US breast short interval follow-up	1		O
MRI breast without and with contrast	1		O
MRI breast without contrast	1		O
FDG-PEM	1		☢☢☢☢
Tc-99m sestamibi BSGI	1		☢☢☢☢
Image-guided fine needle aspiration breast	1		Varies
Rating Scale: 1,2,3 Usually not appropriate; 4,5,6 May be appropriate; 7,8,9 Usually appropriate			*Relative Radiation Level

Clinical Condition: **Palpable Breast Masses**

Variant 8: **Woman younger than 30 years of age, US findings probably benign. Next examination to perform. (See Appendix 2B at**

http://www.acr.org/~/media/ACR/Documents/AppCriteria/Diagnostic/PalpableBreastMasses.pdf

for additional steps in the workup of these patients.)

Radiologic Procedure	Rating	Comments	RRL*
US breast short interval follow-up	9		O
Mammography diagnostic	3		☢☢
Image-guided core biopsy breast	3		Varies
MRI breast without and with contrast	2		O
Image-guided fine needle aspiration breast	2		Varies
MRI breast without contrast	1		O
FDG-PEM	1		☢☢☢☢
Tc-99m sestamibi BSGI	1		☢☢☢☢
Rating Scale: 1,2,3 Usually not appropriate; 4,5,6 May be appropriate; 7,8,9 Usually appropriate			*Relative Radiation Level

Clinical Condition: **Palpable Breast Masses**

Variant 9: **Woman younger than 30 years of age, US findings benign (like simple cyst). Next examination to perform.**

Radiologic Procedure	Rating	Comments	RRL*
Mammography diagnostic	2		☢☢
US breast short interval follow-up	2		O
Image-guided fine needle aspiration breast	2		Varies Palpable Breast Mass
MRI breast without and with contrast	1		O
MRI breast without contrast	1		O
FDG-PEM	1		☢☢☢☢
Tc-99m sestamibi BSGI	1		☢☢☢☢
Image-guided core biopsy breast	1		Varies
Rating Scale: 1,2,3 Usually not appropriate; 4,5,6 May be appropriate; 7,8,9 Usually appropriate			*Relative Radiation Level

Clinical Condition: Palpable Breast Masses

Variant 10: **Woman younger than 30 years of age, US findings negative. Next examination to perform.**

Radiologic Procedure	Rating	Comments	RRL*
Mammography diagnostic	3		☢☢
MRI breast without and with contrast	2		O
US breast short interval follow-up	1		O
MRI breast without contrast	1		O
FDG-PEM	1		☢☢☢☢
Tc-99m sestamibi BSGI	1		☢☢☢☢
Image-guided fine needle aspiration breast	1		Varies
Image-guided core biopsy breast	1		Varies
Rating Scale: 1,2,3 Usually not appropriate; 4,5,6 May be appropriate; 7,8,9 Usually appropriate			*Relative Radiation Level

Clinical Condition: **Palpable Breast Masses**

Variant 11: **Woman age 30-39 years of age, initial evaluation. (See Appendix 3 at**

http://www.acr.org/~/media/ACR/Documents/AppCriteria/Diagnostic/PalpableBreastMasses.pdf

for additional steps in the workup of these patients.)

Radiologic Procedure	Rating	Comments	RRL*
US breast	8	If imaged initially with US, see variants 7-10 for additional imaging.	O
Mammography diagnostic	8	If imaged initially with mammography, see variants 2-5.	☢☢
MRI breast without and with contrast	2	Palpable Breast Mass	O
MRI breast without contrast	1		O
FDG-PEM	1		☢☢☢☢
Tc-99m sestamibi BSGI	1		☢☢☢☢
Image-guided fine needle aspiration breast	1		Varies
Image-guided core biopsy breast	1		Varies
Rating Scale: 1,2,3 Usually not appropriate; 4,5,6 May be appropriate; 7,8,9 Usually appropriate			*Relative Radiation Level

Appendix 7B. American College of Radiology ACR Appropriateness Criteria® – Clinical Condition: Nonpalpable Mammographic Findings (Excluding Calcifications)

American College of Radiology
ACR Appropriateness Criteria®

Clinical Condition: **Nonpalpable Mammographic Findings (Excluding Calcifications)**

Variant 1: **Architectural distortion seen on screening mammogram. No history of prior surgery or trauma. Next examination to perform. (See Appendix 1 at http://www.acr.org/~/media/ACR/Documents/AppCriteria/Diagnostic/NonpalpableMammographicFindings.pdf for additional steps in the workup of these patients.)**

Radiologic Procedure	Rating	Comments	RRL*
Mammography diagnostic	9		☢☢
Mammography short-interval follow-up	1		☢☢
US breast	1		O
MRI breast without and with contrast	1		O
MRI breast without contrast	1		O
Image-guided core biopsy breast	1		Varies
Rating Scale: 1,2,3 Usually not appropriate; 4,5,6 May be appropriate; 7,8,9 Usually appropriate			*Relative Radiation Level

Clinical Condition: **Nonpalpable Mammographic Findings (Excluding Calcifications)**

Variant 2: **Architectural distortion seen on screening mammogram. Prior surgery or trauma at area of distortion. No prior examinations available. Next examination to perform. (See Appendix 1 at http://www.acr.org/~/media/ACR/Documents/AppCriteria/Diagnostic/NonpalpableMammographicFindings.pdf for additional steps in the workup of these patients.)**

Radiologic Procedure	Rating	Comments	RRL*
Mammography diagnostic	6	Use of a scar marker on the original screening study may preclude the need for diagnostic evaluation.	☢☢
Return to screening mammography	4	If the area can be confidently determined to be related to prior surgery (ie, by scar marker) or the sequelae of trauma (eg, presence of fat necrosis), consider return to screening mammography.	☢☢
Mammography short-interval follow-up	1		☢☢
US breast	1		O
MRI breast without and with contrast	1		O
MRI breast without contrast	1		O
Image-guided core biopsy breast	1		Varies
Rating Scale: 1,2,3 Usually not appropriate; 4,5,6 May be appropriate; 7,8,9 Usually appropriate			*Relative Radiation Level

Clinical Condition: **Nonpalpable Mammographic Findings (Excluding Calcifications)**

Variant 3: **Mass seen on screening mammogram (assuming mass has not previously been worked up). Indistinct, microlobulated, or spiculated margins. Next examination to perform. (See Appendix 2 at http://www.acr.org/~/media/ACR/Documents/AppCriteria/Diagnostic/NonpalpableMammographicFindings.pdf for additional steps in the workup of these patients.)**

Radiologic Procedure	Rating	Comments	RRL*
Mammography diagnostic	9		☢☢
Mammography short-interval follow-up	1		☢☢
US breast	1		O
MRI breast without and with contrast	1		O
MRI breast without contrast	1		O
Image-guided core biopsy breast	1		Varies
Rating Scale: 1,2,3 Usually not appropriate; 4,5,6 May be appropriate; 7,8,9 Usually appropriate			*Relative Radiation Level

Clinical Condition: **Nonpalpable Mammographic Findings (Excluding Calcifications)**

Variant 4: **Mass seen on screening mammogram (assuming mass has not previously been worked up). Circumscribed margins with no associated suspicious features. New or enlarging compared to prior examinations or no priors available. Next examination to perform. (See Appendix 2 at http://www.acr.org/~/media/ACR/Documents/AppCriteria/Diagnostic/NonpalpableMammographicFindings.pdf for additional steps in the workup of these patients.)**

Radiologic Procedure	Rating	Comments	RRL*
US breast	9		O
Mammography diagnostic	5	In selected cases, spot/magnification views may help elucidate margins, exclude intramammary node as etiology.	☢☢
Mammography short-interval follow-up	1		☢☢
MRI breast without and with contrast	1		O
MRI breast without contrast	1		O
Image-guided core biopsy breast	1		Varies
Rating Scale: 1,2,3 Usually not appropriate; 4,5,6 May be appropriate; 7,8,9 Usually appropriate			*Relative Radiation Level

Clinical Condition: **Nonpalpable Mammographic Findings (Excluding Calcifications)**

Variant 5: **Multiple bilateral masses seen on screening mammogram. No suspicious features in any mass. Baseline examination or no priors available. Next examination to perform. (See Appendix 3 at http://www.acr.org/~/media/ACR/Documents/AppCriteria/Diagnostic/NonpalpableMammographicFindings.pdf for additional steps in the workup of these patients.)**

Radiologic Procedure	Rating	Comments	RRL*
Return to screening mammography	8		☢☢
Mammography short-interval follow-up	3	In selected cases, may be appropriate.	☢☢
US breast	1		O
MRI breast without and with contrast	1		O
MRI breast without contrast	1		O
Image-guided core biopsy breast	1		Varies
Rating Scale: 1,2,3 Usually not appropriate; 4,5,6 May be appropriate; 7,8,9 Usually appropriate			*Relative Radiation Level

Clinical Condition: **Nonpalpable Mammographic Findings (Excluding Calcifications)**

Variant 6: **Multiple bilateral masses seen on screening mammogram. One or more masses suspicious, or a dominant mass is present. Next examination to perform. (See Appendix 3 at http://www.acr.org/~/media/ACR/Documents/AppCriteria/Diagnostic/NonpalpableMammographicFindings.pdf for additional steps in the workup of these patients.)**

Radiologic Procedure	Rating	Comments	RRL*
Mammography diagnostic	9		☢☢
US breast	5	May proceed directly to US if mass in question is seen in two projections.	O
Mammography short-interval follow-up	1		☢☢
MRI breast without and with contrast	1		O
MRI breast without contrast	1		O
Image-guided core biopsy breast	1		Varies
Rating Scale: 1,2,3 Usually not appropriate; 4,5,6 May be appropriate; 7,8,9 Usually appropriate			*Relative Radiation Level

Clinical Condition: **Nonpalpable Mammographic Findings (Excluding Calcifications)**

Variant 7: **Focal asymmetry or asymmetry (single-view finding) seen on screening mammogram. No priors available. Next examination to perform. (See Appendix 4 at http://www.acr.org/~/media/ACR/Documents/AppCriteria/Diagnostic/NonpalpableMammographicFindings.pdf for additional steps in the workup of these patients.)**

Radiologic Procedure	Rating	Comments	RRL*
Mammography diagnostic	8		☢☢
Mammography short-interval follow-up	1		☢☢
Return to screening mammography	1		☢☢
US breast	1		O
MRI breast without and with contrast	1		O
MRI breast without contrast	1		O
Image-guided core biopsy breast	1		Varies
Rating Scale: 1,2,3 Usually not appropriate; 4,5,6 May be appropriate; 7,8,9 Usually appropriate			*Relative Radiation Level

Clinical Condition: **Nonpalpable Mammographic Findings (Excluding Calcifications)**

Variant 8: **Focal asymmetry or asymmetry (single-view finding) seen on screening mammogram. New or enlarging from prior examinations. Next examination to perform. (See Appendix 4 at http://www.acr.org/~/media/ACR/Documents/AppCriteria/Diagnostic/NonpalpableMammographicFindings.pdf for additional steps in the workup of these patients.)**

Radiologic Procedure	Rating	Comments	RRL*
Mammography diagnostic	9		☢☢
Mammography short-interval follow-up	1		☢☢
Return to screening mammography	1		☢☢
US breast	1		O
MRI breast without and with contrast	1		O
MRI breast without contrast	1		O
Image-guided core biopsy breast	1		Varies
Rating Scale: 1,2,3 Usually not appropriate; 4,5,6 May be appropriate; 7,8,9 Usually appropriate			*Relative Radiation Level

References

1. American Institute of Ultrasound in Medicine. AIUM practice guideline for the performance of a breast ultrasound examination. J Ultrasound Med. 2009;28:105–9.
2. Mendelson EB, et al. ACR practice guideline for the performance of a breast ultrasound examination. 1–5. http://www.acr.org/~/media/52D58307E93E45898B09D4C4D407DD76.pdf.
3. Hilton SV, Leopold GR, Olson LK, Willson SA. Real-time breast sonography: application in 300 consecutive patients. AJR Am J Roentgenol. 1986;147:479–86.
4. Hong AS, Rosen EL, Soo MS, Baker JA, et al. BI-RADS for sonography: positive and negative predictive values of sonographic features. AJR Am J Roentgenol. 2005;184:1260–5.
5. Mendelson EB, Baum JK, Berg WA, Merritt CB, Rubin E. Breast imaging reporting and data system BIRADS: ultrasound. In: D'Orsi CJ, Mendelson EB, Ikeda DM, et al., editors. Breast imaging reporting and data system. 1st ed. Reston: American College of Radiology; 2003.
6. Soo MS, Rosen EL, Baker JA, Vo TT, Boyd BA. Negative predictive value of sonography with mammography in patients with palpable breast lesions. AJR Am J Roentgenol. 2001;177:1167–70.
7. Berg WA, Gutierrez L, NessAiver MS, et al. Diagnostic accuracy of mammography, clinical examination, US, and MR imaging in preoperative accuracy of mammography, clinical examination, US, and MR imaging in preoperative assessment of breast cancer. Radiology. 2004;233:830–49.
8. Mendelson EB. Problem-solving ultrasound. Radiol Clin North Am. 2004;42:909–18.
9. Parker SH, Jobe WE, Dennis MA, et al. US-guided automated large-core breast biopsy. Radiology. 1993;187:507–11.
10. Berg WA, Blume JD, Cormack JB, et al. Combined screening with ultrasound and mammography vs mammography alone in women at elevated risk of breast cancer. JAMA. 2008;299:2151–63.
11. Gordon PB. Ultrasound for breast cancer screening and staging. Radiol Clin North Am. 2002;40:431–41.
12. Alvarez S, Anorbe E, Alcorta P, Lopez F, Alonso I, Cortes J. Role of sonography in the diagnosis of axillary lymph node metastases in breast cancer: a systematic review. AJR Am J Roentgenol. 2006;186:1342–8.
13. Esen G, Gurses B, Yilmaz MH, et al. Gray scale and power Doppler US in the preoperative evaluation of axillary metastases in breast cancer patients with no palpable lymph nodes. Eur Radiol. 2005;15:1215–23.
14. D'Orsi C, Mendelson E, Bassett L, et al. American College Of Radiology, ACR appropriateness criteria 2000: work-up of nonpalpable breast masses. Radiology. 2000;215(S):965–72.
15. Evans 3rd WP, Mendelson E, Bassett L, et al. Appropriate imaging work-up of palpable breast masses. American College of Radiology. ACR appropriateness criteria. Radiology. 2000;215(Suppl):961–4.
16. Leung JW, Sickles E. Multiple bilateral masses detected on screening mammography: assessment of need for recall imaging. AJR Am J Roentgenol. 2000;175(1):23–9.
17. Berg WA, Zhang Z, Cormack JB, Mendelson EB. Multiple Bilateral Circumscribed Masses at Screening Breast US: Consider Annual Follow-up. Radiology. 2013;268(3):673–83.
18. Sickles EA. Detection and diagnosis of breast cancer with mammography. Perspect Radiol. 1988;1:36–65.
19. Shetty MK, Shah YP, Sharman RS. Prospective evaluation of the value of combined mammographic and sonographic assessment in patients with palpable abnormalities of the breast. J Ultrasound Med. 2003;22(3):263–8.
20. Stavros AT, Thickman D, Rapp CL, Dennis MA, Parker SH, Sisney GA. Solid breast nodules: use of sonography to distinguish between benign and malignant lesions. Radiology. 1995;196:123–34.
21. Berg WA, Sechtin AG, Marques H, Zhang Z. Cystic breast masses and the ACRIN 6666 experience. Radiol Clin North Am. 2010;48(5):931–87.
22. Rinaldi P, Ierardi C, Costantini M, Magno S, Giuliani M, Belli P, Bonomo L. Cystic breast lesions: sonographic findings and clinical management. J Ultrasound Med. 2010;29(11):1617–26.
23. Daly CP, Bailey JE, Klein KA, Helvie MA. Complicated breast cysts on sonography: is aspiration necessary to exclude malignancy? Acad Radiol. 2008;15(5):610–7.
24. Huff JG. The sonographic findings and differing clinical implications of simple, complicated, and complex breast cysts. J Natl Compr Canc Netw. 2009;7(10):1101–4.
25. Hines N, Slanetz PJ, Eisneberg R. Cystic masses of the breast. AJR Am J Roentgenol. 2010;194:W122–33.
26. Sklair-Levy M, Muradali D, Kulkarni S. Linear transducer harmonic imaging: improved characterization of breast cysts compared to conventional sonography. AJR Am J Roentgenol. 2001;176:6–7.
27. Merritt C, Piccoli C, Forsberg F, Wilkes A, Cavanaugh B, Lee S. Real-time spatial compound imaging of the breast: clinical evaluation of masses. Radiology. 2000;217:491–2.
28. Shetty MK, Watson Jr AB. Sonographically occult screen detected breast masses: a retrospective analysis of cases undergoing biopsy. Clin Imaging. 2008;32(1):28–31.
29. Shetty MK, Watson AW. Mondor's disease of the breast: sonographic and mammographic findings. AJR Am J Roentgenol. 2001;177(4):893–6.
30. Adrada B, Yun W, Yang W. Hyperechoic lesions of the breast: radiologic-histopathologic correlation. AJR Am J Roentgenol. 2013;200:W518–30.
31. Georgian-Smith D, Taylor KJW, Madjar H, et al. Sonography of palpable breast cancer. J Clin Ultrasound. 2000;28:211–6.
32. Mainiero MB, Goldkamp A, Lazarus E. Characterization of breast masses with sonography can biopsy of some solid masses be deferred? J Ultrasound Med. 2005;24(2):161–7.
33. Rahbar G, Sie AC, Hansen GC, et al. Benign versus malignant solid breast masses: US differentiation. Radiology. 1999;213:889–94.
34. D'Orsi CJ, Mendelson EB, Ikeda DM, et al. Breast imaging reporting and data system: ACR BI-RADS – breast imaging atlas. Reston: American College of Radiology; 2003.
35. Shetty MK, Watson AB. Sonographic evaluation of focal asymmetric density of the breast. Ultrasound Q. 2002;18(2):115–21.
36. Sickles EA. The spectrum of breast asymmetries: imaging features, work-up, management. Radiol Clin North Am. 2007;45(5):765–71.
37. Youk JH, Kim EK, Ko KH, Kim MJ. Asymmetric mammographic findings based on the fourth edition of BI-RADS: types, evaluation, and management. Radiographics. 2009;29(1):e33.
38. Samardar P, de Paredes ES, Grimes MM, Wilson JD. Focal asymmetric densities seen at mammography: US and pathologic correlation. Radiographics. 2002;22(1):19–33.
39. Leung JWT, Sickles EA. Developing asymmetry identified on mammography: correlation with imaging outcome and pathologic findings. AJR Am J Roentgenol. 2007;188(3):667–75.
40. Donegan WL. Evaluation of a palpable breast mass. N Engl J Med. 1992;327:937–42.
41. Rosner D, Blair D. What ultrasonography can tell in breast masses that mammography and physical examination cannot. J Surg Oncol. 1985;28:308–13.
42. Barton MB, Elmore JG, Fletcher SW. Breast symptoms among women enrolled in a health maintenance organization: frequency, evaluation, and outcome. Ann Intern Med. 1999;130:651–7.
43. Perdue P, Page D, Nellestein M, Salem C, Galbo C, Ghosh B. Early detection of breast carcinoma: a comparison of palpable and nonpalpable lesions. Surgery. 1992;111:656–9.

44. Kopans DB. Palpable abnormalities and breast imaging. In: Breast imaging. 2nd ed. Philadelphia: Lippincott Williams & Wilkins; 1998. p. 747–59.
45. Coveney EC, Geraghty JG, O'Laoide R, Hourihane JB, O'Higgins NJ. Reasons underlying negative mammography in patients with palpable breast cancer. Clin Radiol. 1994;49:123–5.
46. Dennis MA, Parker SH, Klaus AJ, Stavros AT, Kaske TI, Clark SB. Breast biopsy avoidance: the value of normal mammograms and normal sonograms in the setting of a palpable lump. Radiology. 2001;219:186–91.
47. Weinstein SP, Conant EF, Orel SG, Zuckerman JA, Czeriecki B, Lawton TJ. Retrospective review of palpable breast lesion: negative mammography and sonography. J Womens Imaging. 2000;2:15–8.
48. Moy L, Slantez PJ, Moore R, et al. Specificity of mammography and US in the evaluation of a palpable abnormality. Radiology. 2002;225:176–81.
49. Shetty MK, Shah YP. Prospective evaluation of the value of negative sonographic and mammographic findings in patients with palpable abnormalities of the breast. J Ultrasound Med. 2002;21(11):1211–6; quiz 1217–9.
50. Moss HA, Britton PD, Flower CDR, Freeman AH, Lomas DJ, Warren RML. How reliable is modern breast imaging in differentiating benign from malignant breast lesions in the symptomatic population? Clin Radiol. 1999;54:676–82.
51. Kaiser JS, Helvie MA, Blacklaw RL, Roubidoux MA. Palpable breast thickening: role of mammography and US in cancer detection. Radiology. 2002;223:839–44.
52. Sickles EA. Periodic mammographic follow-up of probably benign lesions: results in 3,184 consecutive cases. Radiology. 1991;179(2):463–8.
53. Vizcaíno I, Gadea L, Andreo L, Salas D, Ruiz-Perales F, Cuevas D, Herranz C, Bueno F. Short-term follow-up results in 795 nonpalpable probably benign lesions detected at screening mammography. Radiology. 2001;219(2):475–83.
54. Dawson JS. Wilson AR Short-term recall for "probably benign" mammographic lesions detected in a three yearly screening programme. Clin Radiol. 1994;49(6):391–5.
55. Kaplan SS, Collado-Mesa F, Ekens J, Thurber M. Palpable solid breast masses with probably benign sonographic features: can biopsy be avoided? Breast J. 2013;19(2):212–4.
56. Park YM, Kim EK, Lee JH, Ryu JH, Han SS, Choi SJ, Lee SJ, Yoon HK. Palpable breast masses with probably benign morphology at sonography: can biopsy be deferred? Acta Radiol. 2008;49(10):1104–11.
57. Graf O, Helbich TH, Fuchsjaeger MH, Hopf G, Morgun M, Graf C, Mallek R, Sickles EA. Follow-up of palpable circumscribed noncalcified solid breast masses at mammography and US: can biopsy be averted? Radiology. 2004;233(3):850–6.
58. Graf O, Helbich TH, Hopf G, Graf C, Sickles EA. Probably benign breast masses at US: is follow-up an acceptable alternative to biopsy? Radiology. 2007;244(1):87–93.
59. Giess CS, Smeglin LZ, Meyer JE, Ritner JA, Birdwell RL. Risk of malignancy in palpable solid breast masses considered probably benign or low suspicion: implications for management. J Ultrasound Med. 2012;31(12):1943–9.
60. Harvey JA, Nicholson BT, LoRusso AP, Cohen MA, Bovbireg VE. Short-term follow-up of palpable breast lesions with benign imaging features: evaluation of 375 lesions in 320 Women. AJR Am J Roentgenol. 2009;193:1723–30.
61. Bent CK, Bassett LW, D'Orsi CJ, Sayre JW. The positive predictive value of BI-RADS microcalcification descriptors and final assessment categories. AJR Am J Roentgenol. 2010;194:1378–83.
62. Morrow M. The evaluation of common breast problems. Am Fam Physician. 2000;61(8):2371–8.
63. Howard MB, Battaglia T, Prout M, Freund K. The effect of imaging on the clinical management of breast pain. J Gen Intern Med. 2012;27(7):817–24.
64. Duijm LEM, Guit GL, Hendriks JHCL, Zaat JOM, Mali WPTM. Value of breast imaging in women with painful breasts: observational follow up study. BMJ. 1998;317:1492–5.
65. Tumyan L, Hoyt AC, Bassett LW. Negative predictive value of sonography and mammography in patients with focal breast pain. Breast J. 2005;11(5):333–7.
66. Morrogh M, Park A, Elkin EB, King TA. Lessons learned from 416 cases of nipple discharge of the breast. Am J Surg. 2010;200(1):73–80.
67. Kamali S, Bender O, Kamali GH, Aydin MT, Karatepe O, Yuney E. Breast diagnostic and therapeutic value of ductoscopy in nipple discharge and intraductal proliferations compared with standard methods. Cancer. 2014;21(2):154–61.
68. Okazaki A, Hirata K, Okazaki M, Svane G, Azavedo E. Nipple discharge disorders: current diagnostic management and the role of fiber-ductoscopy. Eur Radiol. 1999;9(4):583–90.
69. Zervoudis S, Iatrakis G, Economides P, Polyzos D, Navrozoglou I. Nipple discharge screening. Womens Health (Lond Engl). 2010;6(1):135–51.
70. Yamamoto D, Shoji T, Kawanishi H, Nakagawa H, Haijima H, Gondo H, et al. A utility of ductography and fiberoptic ductoscopy for patients with nipple discharge. Breast Cancer Res Treat. 2001;70:103–8.
71. Ueng S, Mezzetti T, Tavassoli FA. Papillary neoplasms of the breast. Arch Pathol Lab Med. 2009;133:893–907.
72. Grunwald S, Heyer H, Paepke S, Schwesinger G, Schimming A, Hahn M, et al. Diagnostic value of ductoscopy in the diagnosis of nipple discharge and intraductal proliferations in comparison to standard methods. Onkologie. 2007;30:243–8.
73. Gioffre FMA, Manganero T, Pollicino A, Paola S, Biagio M. Surgical approach to nipple discharge: a ten-year experience. J Surg Oncol. 1999;71:235–8.
74. Maxwell AJ. Ultrasound-guided vacuum-assisted excision of breast papillomas: review of 6-years experience. Clin Radiol. 2009;64:801–6.
75. Louie LD, Crowe JP, Dawson AE, et al. Identification of breast cancer in patients with pathologic nipple discharge: does ductoscopy predict malignancy? Am J Surg. 2006;192:530–3.
76. Van Zee KJ, Ortega Perez G, Minnard E, Cohen MA. Preoperative galactography increases the diagnostic yield of major duct excision for nipple discharge. Cancer. 1998;82:1874–80.
77. Allred DC. Ductal carcinoma in situ: terminology, classification, and natural history. J Natl Cancer Inst Monogr. 2010; 2010(41):134–8.
78. Schnitt SJ, Silen W, Sadowsky NL, et al. Ductal carcinoma in situ (intraductal carcinoma) of the breast. N Engl J Med. 1988; 318:898–903.
79. Tabar L, Vitak B, Chen HH, et al. The Swedish Two-County Trial twenty years later. Updated mortality results and new insights from long-term follow-up. Radiol Clin North Am. 2000;38:625–51.
80. Stomper PC, Connolly JL, Meyer JE, et al. Clinically occult ductal carcinoma in situ detected with mammography: analysis of 100 cases with radiologic pathologic correlation. Radiology. 1989;172:235–41.
81. Mun HS, Shin HJ, Kim HH, Cha JH, Kim H. Screening-detected calcified and non-calcified ductal carcinoma in situ: Differences in the imaging and histopathological features. Clin Radiol. 2013;68(1):e27–35.
82. Gwak YJ, Kim HJ, Kwak JY, Lee SK, et al. Ultrasonographic detection and characterization of asymptomatic ductal carcinoma in situ with histopathologic correlation. Acta Radiol. 2011;52(4): 364–71.

83. Nagashima T, Hashimoto H, Oshida K, et al. Ultrasound demonstration of mammographically detected microcalcifications in patients with ductal carcinoma in situ of the breast. Breast Cancer. 2005;12(3):216–20.
84. Moon WK, Myung JS, Lee YJ, Park IA, Noh DY, Im JG. US of ductal carcinoma in situ. Radiographics. 2002;22(2):269–80.
85. Yang WT, Tse GMK. Sonographic, mammographic, and histopathologic correlation of symptomatic ductal carcinoma in situ. AJR Am J Roentgenol. 2004;182:101–10.
86. Shin HJ, Kim HH, Kim SM, Kwon GY, Gong G, Cho OK. Screening-detected and symptomatic ductal carcinoma in situ: differences in the sonographic and pathologic features. AJR Am J Roentgenol. 2008;190(2):516–25.
87. Gufler H, Buitrago-Téllez CH, Madjar H. Ultrasound demonstration of mammographically detected microcalcifications. Acta Radiol. 2000;41(3):217–21.
88. Cheung YC, Wan YL, Chen SC. Sonographic evaluation of mammographically detected microcalcifications without a mass prior to stereotactic core needle biopsy. J Clin Ultrasound. 2002;30(6):323–31.
89. Kang SS, Ko EY, Han B, et al. Breast US in patients who had microcalcifications with low concern of malignancy on screening mammography. Eur J Radiol. 2008;67(2):285–91.
90. Kim EY, Ko EY, Han BK, Shin JH. Sonography of axillary masses: what should be considered other than the lymph nodes? J Ultrasound Med. 2009;28(7):923–39.
91. Walsh R, Kornguth PJ, Soo MS, Bentley R, DeLong DM. Axillary lymph nodes: mammographic, pathologic, and clinical correlation. AJR Am J Roentgenol. 1997;168(1):33–8.
92. Ampil F, Caldito G, Henderson B, Li B, Kim RH, Burton G, Chu Q. Carcinoma of the axillary tail of Spence: a case series. Anticancer Res. 2012;32(9):4057–9.
93. Song SE, Seo BK, Choi JW, Son GS, Cho KR, Kim BH. The sonographic "coffee bean" sign helps distinguish an axillary neurofibroma from a lymphadenopathy. J Clin Ultrasound. 2014; 42(1):33–7.
94. Sohn YM, Kim SY, Kim EK. Sonographic appearance of a schwannoma mimicking an axillary lymphadenopathy. J Clin Ultrasound. 2011;39(8):477–9.
95. Shetty MK, Carpenter WS. Sonographic evaluation of isolated abnormal axillary lymph nodes identified on mammograms. J Ultrasound Med. 2004;23(1):63–71.
96. Given-Wilson RM, Murray ME. The clinical importance of axillary lymphadenopathy detected on screening mammography. Clin Radiol. 1997;52:458–61.
97. Bergvist L, Frodis E, Hedborg-Mellander C, Hansen J. Management of accidentally found pathological lymph nodes on routine screening mammography. Eur J Surg Oncol. 1996;22:250–3.
98. Srivastava A, Hughes LE, Woodcock JP, Laidler P. Vascularity in cutaneous melanoma detected by Doppler sonography and histology: correlation with tumour behavior. Br J Cancer. 1989;59(1):89–91.
99. Schroeder RJ, Bostanjoglo M, Rademaker J, Maeurer J, Felix R. Role of power Doppler techniques and ultrasound contrast enhancement in the differential diagnosis of focal breast lesions. Eur Radiol. 2003;13(1):68–79.
100. Giuseppetti GM, Baldassarre S, Marconi E. Color Doppler sonography. Eur J Radiol. 1998;27 Suppl 2:S254–8.
101. Kook SH, Park HW, Lee YR, Lee YU, Pae WK, Park YL. Evaluation of solid breast lesions with power Doppler sonography. J Clin Ultrasound. 1999;27(5):231–7.
102. Milz P, Lienemann A, Kessler M, Reiser M. Evaluation of breast lesions by power Doppler sonography. Eur Radiol. 2001; 11(4):547–54.
103. Raza S, Baum JK. Solid breast lesions: evaluation with power Doppler US. Radiology. 1997;203(1):164–8.
104. Barr RG. Sonographic breast elastography: a primer. J Ultrasound Med. 2012;31(5):773–83.
105. Barr RG, Destounis S, Lackey II LB, Svensson WE, Balleyguier C, Smith C. Evaluation of breast lesions using ultrasound elasticity imaging: a multicenter trial. J Ultrasound Med. 2012;31: 281–7.
106. Kim MJ, Kim JY, Yoon JH, Youk JH, Moon HJ, Son EJ, Kwak JY, Kim EK. How to find an isoechoic lesion with breast US. Radiographics. 2011;31(3):663–76.
107. Zhao QL, Ruan LT, Zhang H, Yin YM, Duan SX. Diagnosis of solid breast lesions by elastography 5-point score and strain ratio method. Eur J Radiol. 2012;81(11):3245–9.
108. Thitaikumar A, Ophir J. Effect of lesion boundary conditions on axial strain elastograms: a parametric study. Ultrasound Med Biol. 2007;33(9):1463–7.
109. Itoh A, Ueno E, Tohno E, et al. Breast disease: clinical application of US elastography for diagnosis. Radiology. 2006;239(2): 341–50.
110. Yoon JH, Jung HK, Lee JT, Ko KH. Shear wave elastography in the diagnosis of solid breast masses: what leads to false-negative or false-positive results? Eur Radiol. 2013;23(9):2432–40.
111. Youk JH, Gweon HM, Son EJ, Han KH, Kim JA. Diagnostic value of commercially available shear-wave elastography for breast cancers: integration into BI-RADS classification with subcategories of category 4. Eur Radiol. 2013;23(10): 2695–704.
112. Cho N, Jang M, Lyou CY, Park JS, Choi HY, Moon WK. Distinguishing benign from malignant masses at breast US: combined US elastography and color doppler US – influence on radiologist accuracy. Radiology. 2012;262(1):80–90.
113. Dempsey PJ. New ultrasound-based imaging technologies are claimed to avoid unnecessary breast biopsies, but what is an "unnecessary" image-guided needle biopsy of the breast? J Clin Ultrasound. 2010;38(3):111–2.

The Basics of Breast MRI

8

Mahesh K. Shetty

Introduction

Magnetic resonance imaging of the breast has been well established as a supplemental imaging modality with proven benefit in breast cancer screening and diagnosis. Dynamic contrast-enhanced MRI of the breast has been shown to be the most sensitive imaging modality in the detection of breast carcinoma. A review of the currently accepted as well as some additional less commonly used indications that have not been rigorously validated is presented. The protocols, techniques of examination, and the artifacts encountered in a breast MRI examination are discussed. The role of MRI in the assessment of breast implants is briefly described. The BI-RADS terminology for breast MRI is presented. Breast MRI in the staging and diagnosis of breast cancer is discussed in Chap. 9.

Clinical Applications of Breast MRI

The role of MRI in the diagnosis of breast cancer has been well established. MRI depicts cancers that are occult on screening mammography, breast ultrasound, and clinical breast examination [1]. This advantage has to be balanced with a less than perfect specificity resulting in high false positives that may be higher in certain patient populations. Cost of exam, lack of widespread availability and expertise in interpretation, significantly longer examination time, need to use intravenous contrast with its attendant complications, and a cumbersome biopsy procedure for lesions that are seen on MRI are additional drawbacks to be borne in mind. Judicious utilization of this modality is therefore required [1]. And for these reasons despite the high sensitivity of MRI in detection of breast cancer it is not recommended for routine screening in women with an average risk for breast cancer. Use of breast MRI should be dictated by scientifically proven accuracy for any particular indication. Box 8.1 lists the currently utilized common indications for the use of breast MRI.

Breast MRI as a Supplemental Screening Modality in Women with an Elevated Risk for Breast Cancer

The value of breast MRI in screening for breast cancer in women at an elevated risk has been shown in several observational studies [1–15]. Currently the American Cancer Society recommends annual screening with MRI for women with a 20–25 % lifetime risk of developing breast cancer [2]

Box 8.1 Appropriate Indications for the Use of Breast MRI

1. As a supplemental modality to screen for breast cancer in women at an elevated risk for breast cancer
2. Known breast cancer patient
   (a) Staging of breast cancer to determine extent of disease to aid in treatment planning
   (b) Monitoring patients undergoing neoadjuvant chemotherapy
3. As a supplemental modality to diagnostic mammography and/or ultrasound in:
   (a) Diagnosis of occult breast cancer in patients metastatic axillary adenocarcinoma with an unknown primary
   (b) Problem-solving assessment in:
      (i) Lesion characterization
      (ii) Sonographically occult one-view-only mammographic finding
4. To assess integrity of breast implants

M.K. Shetty, MD, FRCR, FACR, FAIUM
Department of Radiology, Baylor College of Medicine, Houston, TX, USA

Woman's Center for Breast Care and MRI, Woman's Hospital of Texas, Fannin 7600, Houston, TX 77054, USA
e-mail: mshettymd@womans-clinic.com

M.K. Shetty (ed.), *Breast Cancer Screening and Diagnosis: A Synopsis*,
DOI 10.1007/978-1-4939-1267-4_8, © Springer Science+Business Media New York 2015

Box 8.2 American Cancer Society Guidelines for Breast Screening with MRI as an Adjunct to Mammography

Recommend annual MRI screening (based on evidence*)
- *BRCA* mutation
- First-degree relative of *BRCA* carrier, but untested
- Lifetime risk ~20–25 % or greater, as defined by BRCAPRO or other models that are largely dependent on family history

Recommend annual MRI screening (based on expert consensus opinion)
- Radiation to chest between age 10 and 30 years
- Li-Fraumeni syndrome and first-degree relatives
- Cowden and Bannayan-Riley-Ruvalcaba syndromes and first-degree relatives

Insufficient evidence to recommend for or against MRI screening
- Lifetime risk 15–20 %, as defined by BRCAPRO or other models that are largely dependent on family history
- Lobular carcinoma in situ (LCIS) or atypical lobular hyperplasia (ALH)
- Atypical ductal hyperplasia (ADH)
- Heterogeneously or extremely dense breast on mammography
- Women with a personal history of breast cancer, including ductal carcinoma in situ (DCIS)

Recommend against MRI screening (based on expert consensus opinion)
- Women at less than 15 % lifetime risk

Used with permission from Saslow et al. [2]
*Evidence from nonrandomized screening trials and observational studies

[Box 8.2]. There is insufficient evidence showing benefit in screening women with a 15–20 % lifetime risk, and MRI is not recommended for those with a less than 15 % lifetime risk of developing breast cancer [2]. Women with a genetic BRCA1 and BRCA2 mutations account for about 3 % of all breast cancers. These women and their untested relatives may have a 50–60 % lifetime risk of breast cancer. There is insufficient evidence for routine screening with MRI in women with a personal history of breast cancer, in those diagnosed with atypical ductal or lobular hyperplasia or DCIS, or in those with extremely dense breast. About 5–10 % of breast cancers are truly hereditary [3].

Table 8.1 compares the sensitivity of mammography to breast MRI in screening for breast cancer in high-risk women. MRI is clearly the winner; mammography performs poorly mainly due to reduced sensitivity resulting from dense breast tissue that is more prevalent in these young women who are being screened. One of the initial large observational studies examining the benefits of screening for breast cancer in women at high risk was the Dutch Magnetic Resonance Imaging Screening study undertaken in 2004. Since most women at high risk refused consent for randomization, the study population was compared with a control group of non-screened women from an external source [4]. The multicenter study included 1,909 women of whom 358 were gene carriers, 1,052 had a lifetime risk of 30–50 % [high-risk group], and 499 women had a lifetime risk between 15 and 30 % [moderate-risk group]. There were 19 malignancies in mutation carriers, in the high-risk group there were 15 cancers, and in the moderate-risk group there were 11 cancers. The sensitivity of MRI in this study was 79.5 % and that of mammography was 33.3 %, clearly showing the superiority of breast MRI over screening mammography [4]. The Magnetic Resonance Imaging Breast Screening [MARIBS] trial was a prospective study of 649 high-risk women; in this study, mammography was shown to have a sensitivity of only 40 % compared to 77 % with breast MRI. Combined sensitivity for the two modalities was high at 94 %, justifying the use of both modalities to screen for breast cancer. The High Breast Cancer Risk Italian trial [HIBCRIT] included 278 women, all of whom were BRCA1 and BRCA2 carriers; the sensitivity of MRI was 94 % compared to 59 % with mammography. A recent large trial including 609 women demonstrated a sensitivity of 17 % for whole breast ultrasound, 33 % for film-screen mammography, 39 % for digital mammography, and 71 % for MRI. These studies have also shown the value of MRI in detecting cancer at a more favorable tumor stage. The Dutch trial showed that MRI-screened patients had a significantly higher percentage of small cancers, 10 mm or less in 43 % of women compared with 12.5 % in age- and risk-matched women, and had positive lymph nodes in 21.4 % of women compared to 56.4 % in the non-MRI-screened women. There is, therefore, indirect evidence of a beneficial effect on prognosis; however, in the absence of randomized clinical trials, it is not possible to reach conclusions regarding

Table 8.1 Comparison of sensitivity of screening MRI and mammography for detection of breast cancer in women with an elevated risk

Study	MRI sensitivity	Mammography sensitivity
Kreige et al. [4] $N=1,909$	71.1 %	40
Warner et al. [7]	77.3	36.4
Leach et al. [6] $N=649$	77	40
Saridenelli et al. [8] $N=278$	93.8	58.8
Weinstein et al. [9] $N=609$	71	39
Lehman et al. [12] $N=171$	100	33.3
Morris et al. [11] $N=365$	100	
Podo et al. [10] $N=105$	100	12.5 %

mortality rate reduction or even improved disease-free survival [1].

The role of MRI as a supplement to mammography and whole breast ultrasound has been reported by Berg and others. The supplemental yield of additional cancers was 14.7 per 1,000 women screened using breast MRI. Among women screened with MRI, 2.6 % were diagnosed with breast cancer [15]. The sensitivity and value of MRI has been therefore clearly proven in these studies. The number of screens needed to detect one cancer was 127 for mammography, 234 for supplemental breast ultrasound, and 68 for MRI after a negative mammogram and ultrasound. The sensitivity and PPV3 [positive predictive value] for combined mammography and ultrasound were 44 and 18 %; for combined MRI, mammography, and ultrasound, they were 100 and 19 % [15]. Among the 612 women who had MRI in addition to mammography and ultrasound, the rate of biopsy increased from 6.2 to 13.2 % because of the addition of MRI. The PPV3 for MRI was 19 % [15]. The increased cancer detection rate varied between 1.2 and 6.7 % and was accompanied by a positive predictive value ranging from 23.7 to 60 %. MRI will lead to increased biopsies; the reported range is from 4.6 to 16.1 % [1].

Role of Breast MRI in a Patient with Known Breast Cancer

Indications for use of breast MRI in a patient diagnosed with breast cancer for staging and to assess response to chemotherapy are discussed in detail in Chap. 9.

Breast MRI to Assess Integrity of Implants

There are many different types of breast implants that complicate imaging assessment. About 14 types have been described [16]. Approximately 80 % of the implants are placed for cosmetic reasons and about 20 % are placed as a part of reconstructive surgery. A large majority of breast implants are single-lumen silicone gel implants, about 80 % in a series of nearly 10,000 implants. Saline-filled, dextran-filled, and PVP-filled implants have similar appearances on MR imaging. An understanding of the various types of implants and their component features improves accuracy in assessment of these implants [16]. There are three common types of implants: the single-lumen silicone gel, which consists of an outer silicone capsule containing viscous silicone gel, the single-lumen inflatable saline implant with greater chances of deflation when ruptured, and the double-lumen implants. The latter are of two types, one in which the inner lumen is filled with silicone and the other in which there is a saline-filled inner lumen and silicone-filled outer lumen [17].

Table 8.2 MR signs of breast implant rupture

Definite sign of implant rupture	Possible rupture	Not indicative of a rupture
Linguine sign	Teardrop sign	Irregular margin
Subcapsular line	Noose sign, keyhole sign	Lobulated contour
Train sign	Droplets in silicone	Simple radial folds
Salad oil sign		Complex radial folds
Extracapsular silicone		

Gel leaking or leeching refers to microscopic leakage of silicone through semipermeable membrane leading to capsule formation and contracture [17]. To minimize the chances of this happening decreasing the gel concentration and placement of silicone barriers on the inner surface of the envelope has been tried. Implants may be placed subglandular or subpectoral. The incidence of capsular contraction is higher with the subglandular implants and is likely due to direct contact of the implant with breast tissue. MR imaging is performed to identify implant rupture and has been shown to be the most reliable modality to diagnose implant-related complications [16–23]. The diagnosis of an implant rupture is important because the release of silicone gel and fluid into tissues can lead to local complications [18]. The incidence of implant rupture is 1–2 %; the rate of silent rupture is considerably higher [16]. Rupture may be suspected due to symptoms such as tenderness, palpable nodules, asymmetry, or infection. Implant rupture may be asymptomatic and be discovered during clinical examination, particularly when the rupture is intracapsular, where free silicone remains inside the fibrous capsule that develops around the implant. In an extracapsular rupture, free silicone is seen in the breast tissue outside the implant. Mammography is of limited use in the assessment of implant rupture and is able to diagnose extracapsular rupture only in which case free silicone is seen in the breast parenchyma [17]. Ultrasound is more useful in the assessment of breast implants but is less accurate than is MRI. Diffuse low-level echoes when seen is suggestive of an implant rupture [19]. A contour abnormality is an unreliable sign of implant rupture [19]. Common implant-related complications include hematoma in the early postoperative period, infection, capsule contracture, rupture, and formation of silicone granulomas [19]. More recent studies have reaffirmed the accuracy of MR imaging in assessment of implants [22, 23]. An accuracy of 90–92 %, sensitivity of 89–96 %, specificity of 77–97 %, positive predictive value of 90–99 %, and a negative predictive value of 79–90 % have been reported [22, 23]. The linguine sign and the salad oil signs were statistically the most significant signs [23]. Presence of silicone granulomas, free silicone, and silicone in axillary lymph nodes are suggested as signs that require immediate explantation (Table 8.2) [23]:

- *Linguine Sign/Subcapsular Line*: These two signs are the most reliable signs of an implant rupture and appear as

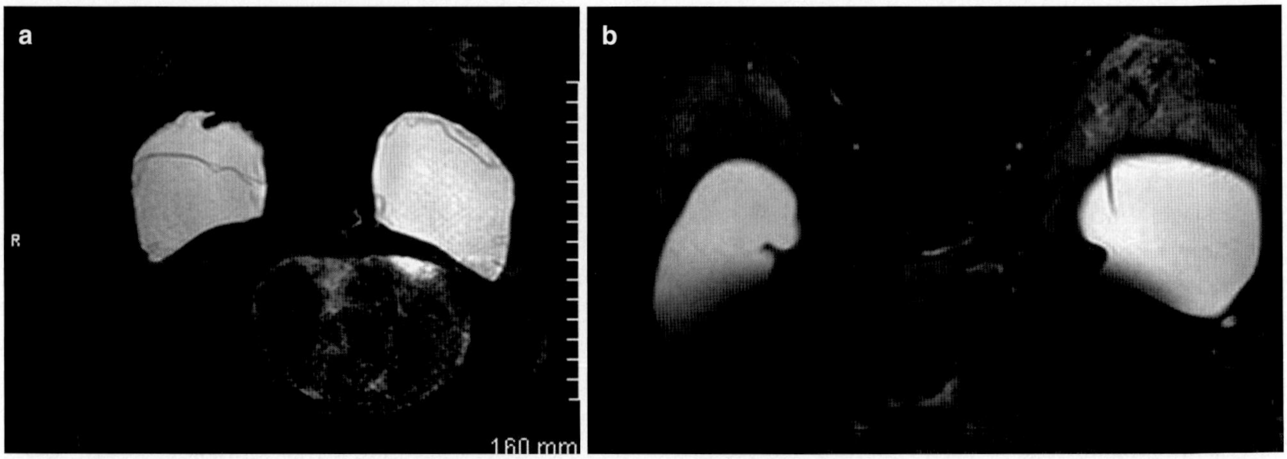

Fig. 8.1 (**a**) A silicone-excited sequence shows bilateral implant rupture with typical "linguine sign" within the implants representing collapsed implant shell. (**b**) A silicone-excited sequence shows normal infolding of the implant shell simulating a "linguine sign"

hypointense lines that are wavy and appear folded within the silicone gel and lie parallel to the fibrous capsule; these represent the ruptured silicone shell floating within the fibrous capsule (Fig. 8.1a, b). Subcapsular line is a prelude to the linguine sign when the detachment from the fibrous capsule is not complete [22].

- *Teardrop Sign, Noose Sign, or Keyhole Sign*: These signs are a result of invagination of the silicone membrane containing a drop of silicone; hence, the membranes are not opposed or touching each other as in folds. This finding depending on the shape may appear as a teardrop, noose, or a keyhole. When such an appearance is seen in more than one image, it is suggestive of an implant rupture.
- *Droplet Sign or the Salad Oil Sign*: Dot-like hypointensity within silicone represents the presence of water or serum droplets within the silicone gel. By itself this sign cannot be considered diagnostic of an implant rupture and may even represent a normal finding if saline steroids or antibiotics are directly injected into the silicone chamber in the perioperative period [23]. When larger this sign is called as the salad oil sign, a finding that is diagnostic of an implant rupture [23].
- *Train Rail Sign*: Two hypointense parallel lines are seen in close proximity forming a double-contoured subcapsular line within the silicone gel indicating that both membranes in a double-lumen implant have ruptured [22].
- *Simple and Complex Radial Folds*: Radial folds represent normal infolding of the implant shell and may simulate the linguine sign of implant rupture; these are normal findings that represent uninterrupted hypointense lines, and these extend almost perpendicularly into the lumen and end blindly (Fig. 8.1b). Complex folds are longer and have a multidirectional course. Use of orthogonal planes and reduced slice thickness or volumetric acquisitions help. Patient motion artifacts can also sometimes cause curvilinear hypointense lines within the implant simulating the linguine sign [22, 23].
- *Contour Change/Irregular Margin*: Contour changes and irregular margin when by itself is not a sign of implant rupture and may indicate herniation of the fibrous capsule. Rupture without collapse has been attributed to some cases of implant rupture that was missed on MR imaging [20]. The ruptured surface elastomer in these cases adhered to the fibrous capsule without producing the linguine sign. The homogenous high signal was maintained within the ruptured implant.
- *Extracapsular Silicone*: This is a sign of extracapsular rupture of an implant. There is free silicone in the soft tissue or a silicone granuloma which may appear as dense rounded or irregular mass.

Breast MRI as a Problem-Solving Tool

MR imaging is not recommended for routine use as a problem-solving tool to supplement diagnostic mammography. There have been studies that have examined the value of MRI as a supplemental modality for equivocal findings on mammography [24–27]. MRI is not recommended for lesion characterization or biopsy avoidance. However, in routine practice occasional use of breast MRI is made to further assess suspected abnormal findings. Judicious use of MRI is important due to the cost and potential for false positives. The ACR Practice Guideline for the Performance of Contrast-Enhanced MRI of the breast includes "additional evaluation of clinical or imaging findings" as one of the indications for performing breast MRI. The guideline specifically states that "breast MRI may be indicated when other imaging examinations, such as ultrasound and mammography, and physical examination are inconclusive for the presence of breast cancer, and biopsy could not be performed." The guideline goes on to caution, however, that "MRI should not supplant careful problem-solving mammographic views or ultrasound in the diagnostic setting" and "should not be used in lieu of biopsy of a mammographically, clinically, and sonographically suspicious finding" [28].

In one series problem solving was an indication for 3.9 % of MRI exams of the breast performed over a 6-year period; there were 115 exams performed for inconclusive findings that represented 0.14 % of the total number of mammograms performed [24]. The most common indication was focal asymmetry [85 %] followed by architectural distortion [10 %] and scar at site of benign breast biopsy [4 %]. A majority of cases were classified as BI-RADS 0 prior to MRI [68 %]; in 19 % an assignment of BI-RADS 4 was made and MRI was performed as a biopsy avoidance tool. Ultrasound was performed in 65 of these 115 cases with no malignancies found. MRI of the breast identified six malignancies and had a sensitivity of 100 %; two of these six cancers were seen on one mammographic view. The positive predictive value of MRI was 14 % [24]. The role of MRI in downgrading BI-RADS 3 lesions has been reported but is not a cost-effective approach for this indication. The negative predictive value of MRI in reported studies for noncalcified BI-RADS 3 lesions was 100 %. For probably benign calcifications, the negative predictive value was 76–97 % for BI-RADS 3 microcalcifications [25]. For this reason there is no justification for use of MRI downgrading BI-RADS microcalcifications. A report on use of MRI as an adjunct to mammography found that MRI had the most benefit in lesions that were characterized as BI-RADS 0 or 3. A significant higher sensitivity was achieved with the use of MRI with nearly similar specificity [26]. Cost-effectiveness remains an issue despite the beneficial findings shown in these few studies and was not addressed. MRI should generally not be used for lesion characterization or for biopsy avoidance since percutaneous biopsy under imaging guidance is relatively safe, less expensive, and readily available [1]. Moreover, for this indication to be valid, MRI has to have a greater than 98 % negative predictive value which has not been the case. A large series of 821 patients with a suspicious mammographic or clinical finding found an NPV of only 85 % with cancer missed in 48 of 329 negative MR examinations [27]. Based on lack of robust data and issue of cost-effectiveness, it seems prudent to use MRI occasionally as a problem-solving tool in cases such as lesions seen on one view and sonographically occult [13].

Breast MRI to Diagnose an Occult Breast Cancer

Uncommonly, adenocarcinoma is identified in axillary lymph nodes with no mammographic evidence of a primary in the breast. Such a presentation is seen in less than 1 % of breast cancer cases [1]. Such metastasis is usually from the ipsilateral breast. Identifying a tumor may result in less radical surgical procedures and/or radiation depending on tumor size, characteristics, and extent [1]. MRI successfully identifies occult primary cancer in 61 % of cases [1]. The European Society of Breast Imaging recommends use of MRI in case of localized metastatic disease such as axillary adenopathy when clinical and conventional imaging fail to identify a breast primary [5]. When metastasis is extensive and prognosis is poor and will not be affected by site of primary tumor, there is no role for the use of breast MRI [5].

MRI BI-RADS Lexicon

Dynamic contrast-enhanced MR mammography is now an accepted modality for screening, diagnosing, and staging of breast cancer. With increasing utilization of breast MRI, there was a need to standardize terminology, reporting, and final assessments to fall in line with what had already been established and used for mammography and breast ultrasound. The American College of Radiology incorporated the BI-RADS™ MRI lexicon into its Breast Imaging and Data System Atlas in 2003 [29]. An updated version is nearly complete and due to be released later this year with significant changes made to the original lexicon [30].

The descriptors are for types of enhancement, location of the lesion, the kinetic time-intensity information, and associated findings [31, 32]. There are two main categories of descriptors of enhancing lesions, namely, the morphology and the enhancement kinetics. There are three morphologic types of enhancing lesions that will be discussed next.

Focus or Foci

Focus or foci are enhancing lesions that are small and typically less than 5 mm; these are often related to hormonal changes and are benign (Fig. 8.2a, b). The finding of a focus or foci is often stable on follow-up examination. Foci may be challenging to assess for enhancement kinetics due to volume averaging effect. The differential diagnosis of such foci includes focal fibrocystic change, small fibroadenoma, papilloma, benign lymph node, or rarely DCIS or a small invasive ductal cancer [32]. In a retrospective study of 666 MR-only detected lesions that underwent histological confirmation, the incidence of cancer among foci was less than 3 %; for this reason biopsy is rarely needed for foci particularly when there are more than one such finding [33].

Masses

A mass is larger than 5 mm and is three dimensional and visible on precontrast images. This may indicate an invasive breast cancer or a benign entity such as a fibroadenoma. The shape, margins, and internal enhancement characteristics are described next.

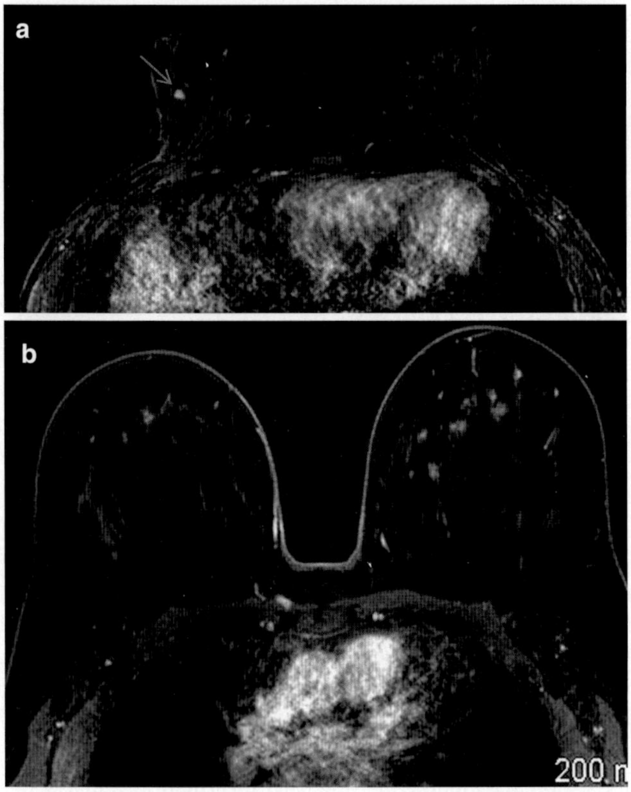

Fig. 8.2 (**a**) Axial postcontrast fat-suppressed T1-weighted subtraction image shows a 4 mm enhancing focus in the right breast. (**b**) Axial postcontrast fat-suppressed T1-weighted subtraction image shows multiple bilateral enhancing foci

Shape of a Mass

This may be described as round, oval, or lobulated when the border is undulating. The shape is considered irregular when it has an uneven shape and cannot be categorized as round, oval, or lobulated. A round mass is circular or ball shaped, an oval mass is elliptical, a lobulated mass can have a scalloped contour.

Margins of a Mass

This feature can be described as being smooth, irregular, or spiculated. The latter is suspicious for cancer or a radial scar. Smooth margin is well defined with sharp demarcation from surrounding tissue (Fig. 8.3a–c). An irregular margin is uneven, ill-defined, or indistinct and can have jagged edges. A spiculated margin has spicules radiating from the surface. An irregular mass or one with an irregular or spiculated margin is commonly associated with invasive breast cancer.

Internal Enhancement Characteristics

There are six patterns of internal enhancement that are encountered: homogenous, heterogeneous, rim, dark internal septations, enhancing internal septations, and central enhancement. They are described as follows:

- A homogenous enhancement pattern is associated with uniform enhancement within the mass.
- A heterogeneous enhancement refers to an inhomogeneous internal enhancement pattern resulting in variable signal intensity.
- Rim enhancement refers to a peripheral rind of enhancement. Dark internal septations are nonenhancing linear areas within a mass.
- Enhancing lines within a mass indicate the presence of internal enhancing septations.
- A central enhancement is when there is more pronounced enhancement at the center of a mass.

Smooth margins, poorly enhanced lobulated masses, and presence of nonenhancing internal septations are predictors of benignity in a mass (Fig. 8.3a–c). The degree of enhancement in a fibroadenoma is variable depending on the fibrotic component and hormonal stimulation of the breast. Myxoid fibroadenomas enhance strongly but tend to washout slow unlike invasive cancers. Phyllodes tumors can show heterogeneous enhancement and may have nonenhancing internal septations (Fig. 8.3c). Although a fibroadenoma can typically demonstrate homogeneous enhancement, this can also be associated with invasive breast cancer.

A lobulated mass without septations or with enhancing septations and moderate to intense enhancement and with washout kinetics is highly suggestive of malignancy and may be characteristically seen in medullary and colloid cancers and also in some invasive ductal and lobular cancers. Rim enhancement has a high predictive value for malignancy, although not a frequent finding (Fig. 8.4a–c). This finding is commonly associated with invasive ductal cancer of a higher grade [32]. Spiculated margins are often seen in invasive ductal cancers and in radial scars; enhancement kinetics may help in the differential diagnosis (Fig. 8.5). Spiculated margins less commonly may be associated with tubular cancers, DCIS, and invasive lobular cancer.

Non-Mass-Like Enhancement [NMLE]

Non-mass-like enhancement refers to areas of enhancement that do not correspond to a defined 3-dimensional mass. Features in such areas of enhancement that are described include the distribution, the internal characteristics or patterns of enhancement, and the presence of symmetry or asymmetry in appearance when bilateral. These areas of enhancement are distinct from the surrounding breast tissue. In general NMLE may be associated with DCIS, invasive lobular cancer, adenosis, fibrocystic change, or inflammation. It is not associated with estrogen receptor-positive cancers [32].

Distribution of NMLE

- Focal enhancement is a single small area of NMLE confined to less than 25 % of a quadrant of the breast (Fig. 8.6a–d).

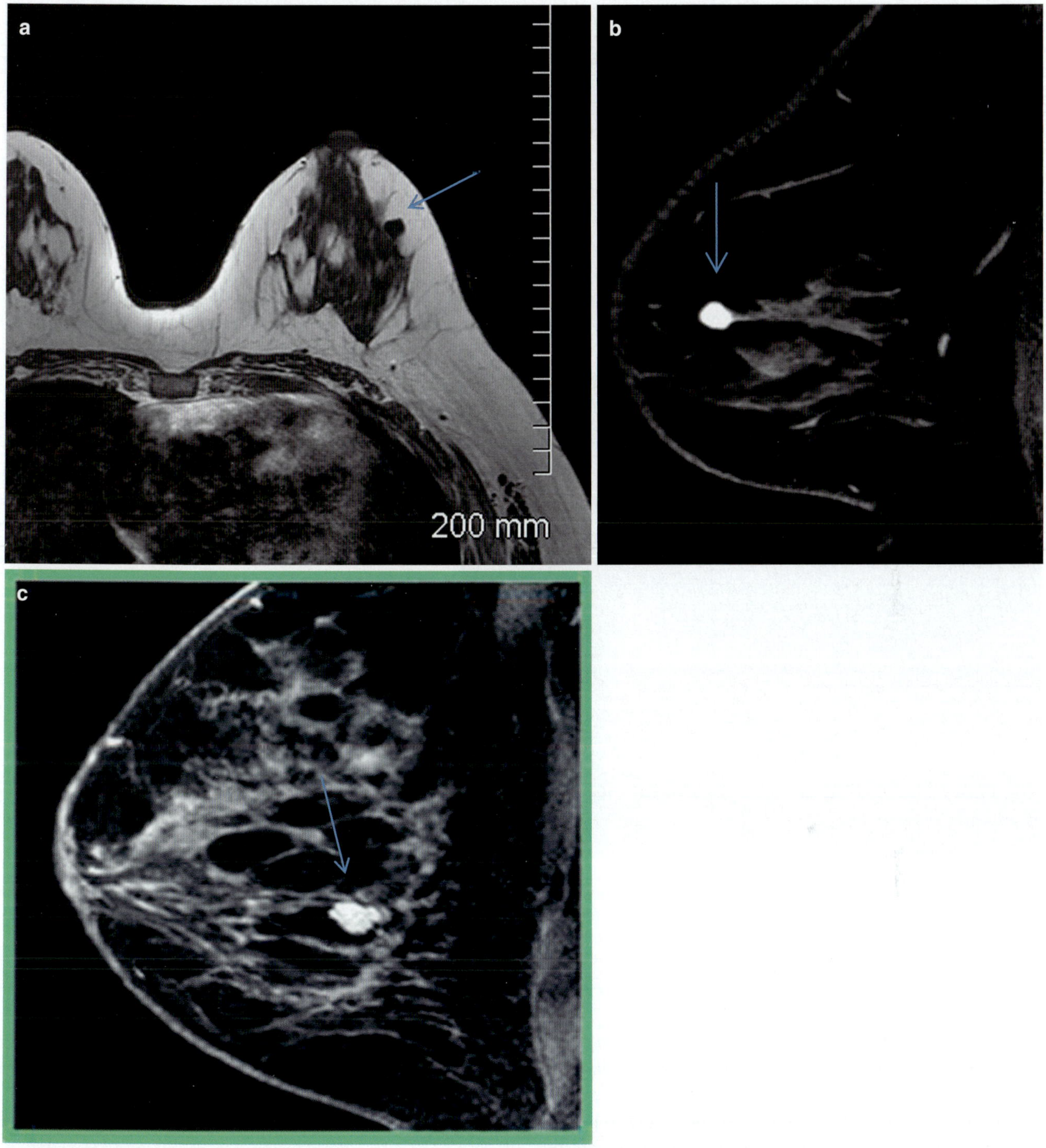

Fig. 8.3 (**a**) Axial T1-weighted image shows an isointense mass with smooth borders in the outer central left breast. (**b**) Sagittal postcontrast fat-suppressed T1-weighted image shows homogenous enhancement and smooth margins suggestive of a benign mass. Histological diagnosis: fibroadenoma. (**c**) Sagittal postcontrast fat-suppressed T1-weighted image shows enhancing mass with dark internal septations and smooth margins suggestive of a benign mass. Histological diagnosis: fibroadenoma

- Linear enhancement is seen along a line but not conforming to a ductal distribution, it may appear sheet like in an orthogonal plane.
- Ductal enhancement occurs along a single duct or in a branching pattern and usually toward the nipple. This pattern of non-mass-like enhancement is highly predictive of malignancy. It is frequently associated with DCIS. It is sometimes associated with benign histology such as atypical ductal hyperplasia and lobular carcinoma in situ (Fig. 8.7).

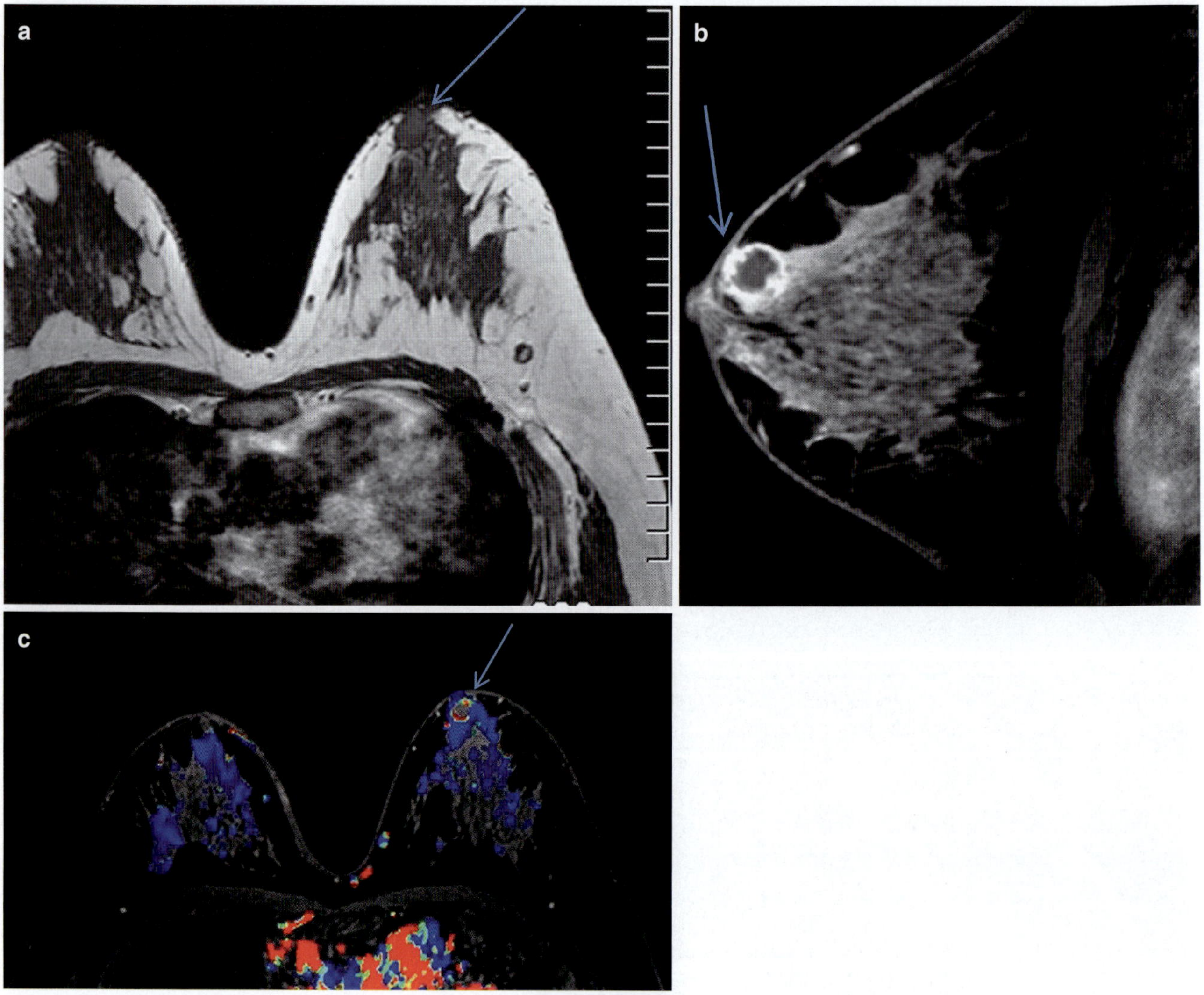

Fig. 8.4 (**a**) Axial T1-weighted image shows an isointense mass with lobulated borders in the subareolar left breast. (**b**) Axial postcontrast fat-suppressed T1-weighted image shows an enhancing lesion with irregular thick rim enhancement suspicious for malignancy. (**c**) Axial postcontrast subtraction image with color overlay demonstrates washout kinetics in the thick irregular rim of the subareolar mass. Histological diagnosis: invasive ductal cancer

- Segmental enhancement refers to enhancement that conforms to a segment drained by a single duct system and may be triangular or cone shaped and pointing toward the nipple. This type of enhancement is highly predictive of malignancy and with linear type represents the most commonly encountered enhancement pattern in DCIS [32].
- Regional enhancement occupies a larger area of enhancement, not confined to a segment and less distinct from surrounding tissue, and may be patchy or geographic. Such enhancements are frequently associated with benign fibrocystic changes.
- Multiple regional enhancements are multiple areas of enhancement in a pattern described previously.
- Diffuse enhancement refers to evenly distributed enhancement throughout the fibroglandular tissue.

Multiple regional and diffuse patterns are nearly always related to benign or hormone-related changes particularly when bilateral. Occasionally when unilateral these patterns may be seen in invasive ductal and lobular cancers.

Internal Characteristics of NMLE

- Homogeneous is confluent and uniform enhancement.
- Heterogeneous is nonuniform NMLE that is separated by areas of nonenhancing normal breast parenchyma.
- Stippled/punctate are multiple dot-like scattered 1–2 mm enhancing foci and not conforming to a duct, and these are strongly associated with a benign process or normal breast tissue.
- Clumped enhancement appears as aggregate of enhancing masses or foci that may appear confluent; such a pattern is strongly associated with DCIS (Fig. 8.7).

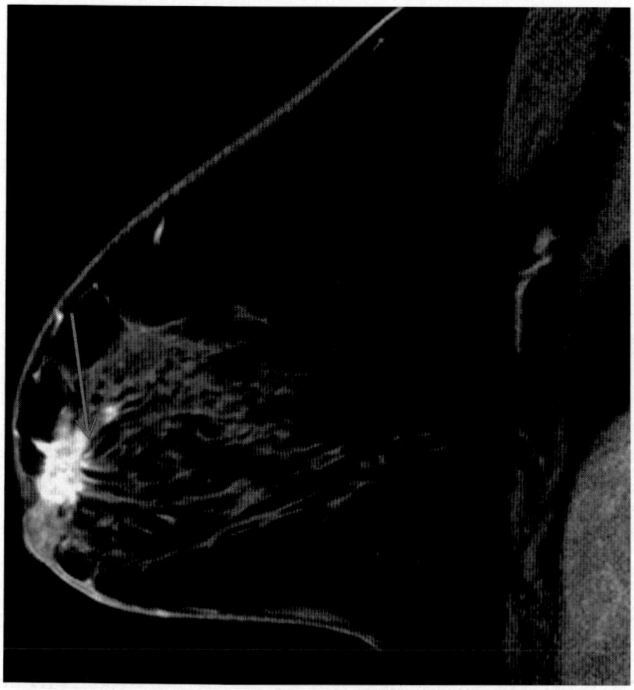

Fig. 8.5 Sagittal postcontrast fat-suppressed T1-weighted image shows an enhancing lesion with spiculated borders suspicious for malignancy in the retroareolar right breast. Histological diagnosis: invasive ductal cancer

- Dendritic/reticular pattern of enhancement appears as strands of enhancement and may represent involuting glandular tissue that leaves behind enhancing tissue between fat.
- Symmetry: When an enhancement pattern has a mirror image in the other breast, it is referred to as a symmetric pattern, and when enhancement is less pronounced in one breast, it is referred to as being asymmetric in distribution. Symmetric enhancement is strongly associated with benign findings.

Associated Findings

These include skin and areolar changes, lymph nodes, chest wall involvement in posterior carcinomas, ductal hyperintensity on precontrast images, cysts, hematoma, and signal void artifact arising from a clip. Enhancement of the nipple areolar complex is seen in the affected breast in Paget's disease of the nipple. Enhancement within the pectoral muscle when contiguous with a posterior carcinoma is suggestive of muscle invasion. Abnormal lymph nodes cannot be discriminated based on enhancement kinetics since they exhibit intense enhancement with washout kinetics similar to cancer. Correlation with T1-weighted images helps in making an accurate diagnosis of a benign lymph node. A short axis dimension of greater than 10 mm, absence of fatty hilum, rounded shape, and cortical abnormalities are predictors of abnormal lymph nodes. Dynamic contrast-enhanced MRI has been found to be useful in evaluating lymph node involvement in patients with known breast cancer [33, 34]. Using specific MRI lymph node findings such as presence of irregular margins, cortical nodularity or thickening, replaced fatty hilum, perinodal edema, rim enhancement, and lymph node asymmetry and with multivariate analysis, it has been reported that axillary lymph node metastasis can be diagnosed with a high diagnostic accuracy [34].

Kinetic Enhancement Curve

The kinetic curve assessment is described from the most suspicious curve pattern selected from the fastest enhancing part of a lesion. The kinetic curve is assessed in two phases, the initial phase and the delayed phase. The initial phase is during the first two minutes after initiation of contrast injection. This phase is described as being slow, medium, or fast. The second or the delayed phase is after the first two minutes or after the kinetic curve begins to change. The delayed phase has three possible patterns: rapid washout, plateau, or persistent. A rapid initial phase is also a feature suspicious for malignancy. Rapid enhancement in the initial phase and washout or plateau delayed phase is commonly associated with invasive cancer, and persistence in the delayed phase is observed in benign lesions. Invasive lobular cancer may demonstrate low magnitude and persistent enhancement kinetics due to weak angiogenesis; therefore, in NMLE, kinetics have to be interpreted with caution never excluding malignancy based purely on kinetics. It is important to bear in mind that morphology always trumps kinetics. DCIS may also demonstrate slow initial phase and variable delayed phase enhancement patterns [31, 32]. Three types of enhancement patterns have been described. Type I refers to progressive enhancement, and this pattern is commonly associated with a benign lesion [83 %] and uncommonly with malignancy [9 %]. Type II curve is a plateau pattern where after initial enhancement there is flattening of the curve. Type III is a washout curve demonstrating an initial increase and a progressive washout. This pattern is characteristic of malignancy with 76 % of such patterns being reportedly associated with cancer; however, sensitivity is low and reported to be about 20 %. The reported range of association of the three types of enhancement with malignancy is as follows: Type I curve has a 5–9 % malignancy rate (Fig. 8.6d); the type II curve has an association of 6–64 % with malignancy; and the type III curve where there is a rapid washout has a 33–85 % association with malignancy. For optimal accuracy morphology has to be combined with enhancement kinetics [35].

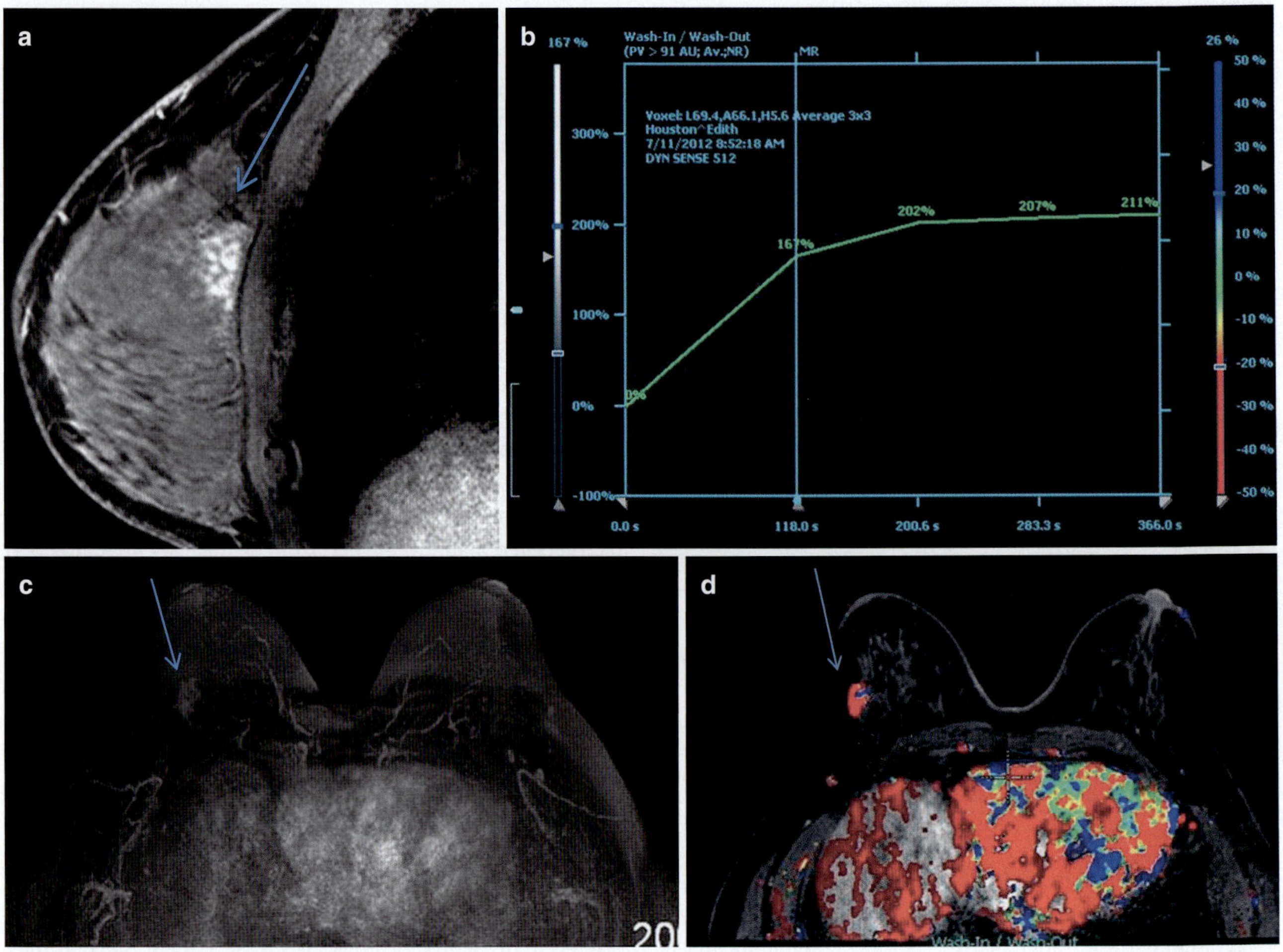

Fig. 8.6 (**a**–**d**) Non-mass-like enhancement [NMLE]. (**a**) Sagittal postcontrast T1-weighted image shows a segmental area of non-mass-like enhancement in the posterior upper right breast. (**b**) Kinetic curve demonstrates slow uptake and progressive enhancement characteristic of a benign abnormality. (**c**) 3D MIP image demonstrates a NMLE in the posterior outer right breast. (**d**) Color overlay demonstrates washout kinetics. Histological diagnosis: invasive ductal cancer

Updated MRI BI-RADS Lexicon

There are several important descriptors in dynamic contrast-enhanced [DCE] breast MR imaging that do not appear in the BI-RADS^{TM} lexicon [36]. "Blooming sign" refers to well-demarcated margins exhibited by malignant lesions that on subsequent delayed scans appear less distinct [36]. Hook sign refers to a hooklike dendrite leading from the center of a malignant lesion and extending to the pectoral muscle on T2-weighted images. Edema appearing as bright T2 signal around a lesion and prominent vessels in relation to a lesion are signs associated with malignancy.

The soon to be released version of the American College of Radiology MRI BI-RADS recommends the use of precontrast T2-weighted sequence. Combined reporting of findings on mammograms, ultrasound, and breast MRI is recommended. A section on breast implants has been added describing findings in normal and ruptured implants. A description of background breast parenchymal enhancement is added since this can affect sensitivity of breast MRI in cancer detection. This can be none, minimal, mild, moderate, or marked. Central and septal enhancements and enhancing septations have been deleted. Clustered ring enhancement has been added. The term non-mass-like enhancement will be replaced with non-mass enhancement. The term irregular margin is to be replaced by uneven margin in masses with an irregular shape. There are no changes in the kinetic terminology in the upcoming BI-RADS^{TM} atlas [36].

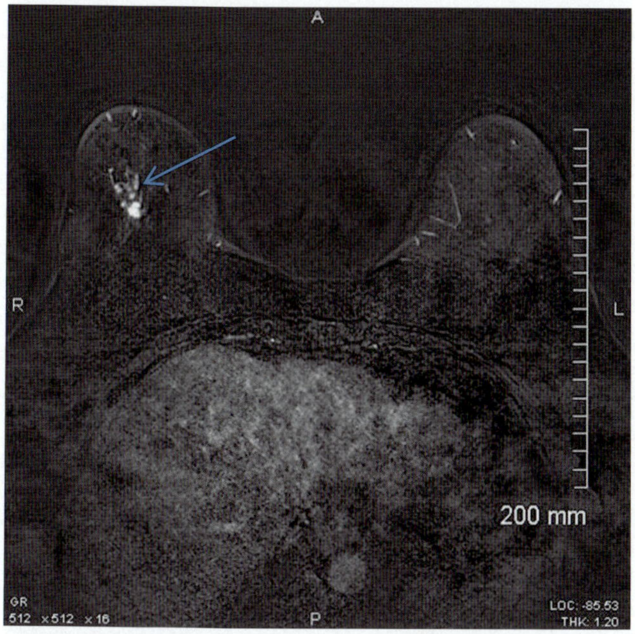

Fig. 8.7 Axial postcontrast subtraction image demonstrates linear clumped enhancement in the posterior central right breast. Histological diagnosis: DCIS

Lesions with Bright T2 Signal

Bright T2 signal lesions may occur in solid tumors that have extensive necrosis, a cystic or microcystic component, an adipose or sebaceous component, mucinous stroma, loose myxoid stroma, stromal edema, and hemorrhagic changes [37]. Mucinous carcinoma may have a lobulated or circumscribed border and bright T2 signal and hence may simulate a benign lesion; however, rim or heterogeneous enhancement may point correctly to a malignant diagnosis. Necrotic invasive ductal carcinoma can also display bright signal on T2-weighted images. Metaplastic carcinoma is rare but also commonly demonstrates bright signal on T2-weighted imaging sequence.

Positive Predictive Value of BI-RADS MRI Assessment

Criteria for Benignity

The absence of a visible lesion on contrast-enhanced MRI corresponding to a palpable or a mammographic lesion is predictive of a benign abnormality. A mass with a smooth margin or internal nonenhancing septa is highly predictive of benignity [NPV=98 %]. A lobulated mass with minimal enhancement has a nearly 100 % likelihood of benignity. Mild regional non-mass-like enhancement has a 92 % NPV for a benign abnormality. T2 hyperintensity within enhancing portions of a tumor is suggestive of a benign abnormality in a lobulated or a mass with smooth margins. Fibroadenomas particularly in younger women tend to be T2 hyperintense. Most cancers tend to appear hypo- or isointense compared to surrounding breast tissue on T2-weighted images [35].

Predictors of Malignancy

In a large prospective multicenter trial of screening breast MR imaging, mass lesions with an irregular shape had a positive predictive value of 30.6 %, spiculated margins had a PPV of 33.3 %, and marked internal enhancement had a PPV of 23 %. Ductal enhancement type of NMLE had a PPV of 50 % [38]. The likelihood of cancer was high with initial rapid enhancement and for both plateau and washout kinetic curve. The PPV for cancer with BI-RADS 4 and 5 was 28 % [38]. A study of enhancement curves in 125 lesions, 42 malignant and 83 benign; there were no significant differences in initial peak enhancement between benign and malignant lesions. Washout was the most suspicious with 45.7 % being malignant compared to 20 % with plateau and 13.3 % with entirely persistent enhancement [39]. It is clear from these data that kinetic curves are useful adjunctive tools but cannot be relied on solely to confirm or exclude malignancy. In a study of 666 nonpalpable mammographically occult MR-detected lesions undergoing MR-guided localization, mean lesion size was 1 cm [40]. Malignancy was present in 22 % of lesions. Frequency of malignancy increased with lesion size, with only one out of 37 lesions under 5 mm being malignant (3 %).

BI-RADS™ 3 Probably Benign Findings Category Lesions on MRI

There are no established criteria in the BI-RADS atlas to categorize lesions on DCE breast MRI as probably benign. In a large series of 106 patients with a BI-RADS 3 assessment, the most common underlying lesion was NMLE [40.7 %], followed by foci [32.4 %] and masses [25.5 %]. In this study there was no malignancy detected at 2 years of follow-up in 78 % of women, and the remainder of the patients had a tissue diagnosis due to either patient preference or interval change. There was one case of DCIS in this group leading to a malignancy rate of 0.9 % in the BI-RADS 3 category [41]. In a series that evaluated MRI BI-RADS 3 lesions, such an assessment was given in 20 % of 809 exams, and in them there was only one cancer with a malignancy rate of 1 in 160 [0.6 %] [42]. In another series, 260 [10.1 %] of 2,569 consecutive examinations had an assignment of BI-RADS 3; cancer yield was 0.85 % with both cases being DCIS.

There were no cancers in 69 foci with persistent enhancement [43]. In a series of 44 patients comprising of 6.3 % of consecutive breast examination, one malignancy was identified which was a malignant phyllodes tumor [44]. The overall malignancy rate in several studies of MR BI-RADS 3 lesions varies from 0.7 to 10 % [43]. The criteria for BI-RADS 3 categorization on a breast MRI examination have not been established or validated. These studies were retrospective studies and none provide an explanation for including lesions with suspicious morphology or kinetics in the study group. The low malignancy yield has to be considered with caution because of lack of uniformity in selection criteria to categorize lesions as BI-RADS 3. Based on data available it seems prudent to categorize foci with persistent kinetics as BI-RADS 2. Regional NMLE when unilateral seems to be a type of lesion that can be categorized as BI-RADS 3. There is need for more robust data from well-designed prospective studies for establishing criteria to categorize lesions on DCE breast MRI with adequate follow-up as has been done for mammographic BI-RADS 3 lesions.

Breast MRI: Methodology and Protocol

Breast MRI protocol has to be optimized to capitalize on the high sensitivity of mammography to detect breast cancer. There are certain basic prerequisites to optimize the quality of the morphology and kinetics of abnormalities seen on breast MR examination [45]:

- Bilateral dedicated breast coil has to be used and patient scanned in the prone position. Bilateral imaging is now the accepted standard of care. This allows for accurate identification of bilateral symmetric physiologic changes and also detection of occult contralateral cancers.
- MR imaging system with a high field strength and with a magnetic field that is homogeneous across the whole field of view covering both breasts to allow for uniform fat suppression.
- Mild compression of the breast is helpful to decrease motion that prevents misregistration artifacts and decreases the image acquisition times in axial and sagittal plane.
- Dedicated multichannel breast coils provide high signal to noise ratios and uniform image resolution. Vendors currently offer 7, 12, and 16 channel dedicated breast coils. Multichannel coil imaging also allows a reduction in image acquisition times.
- Protocol typically includes the following sequences:
  1. A T1-weighted sequence to assess masses and lymph nodes, a T2-weighted sequence to identify cysts, and a 3-D imaging using spoiled gradient-echo T1-weighted imaging with fat suppression prior to and following intravenous contrast administration. Frequency-selective fat suppression is needed for homogeneous fat suppression.
  2. The imaging thickness should be less than 3 mm and pixel size less than 1 mm in each plane.
  3. Intravenous administration of gadolinium chelate at a dose of 0.1–0.2 mmol/kg is injected at 1–2 cc/s.
  4. Four to five postcontrast acquisition are obtained following one prior to contrast. Imaging continues to about 7 min after injection, each acquisition lasting 1–2 min.
  5. Peak contrast enhancement in a malignant lesion typically occurs between 90 and 180 s after injection of the contrast agent requiring an optimal temporal resolution of less than 2 min to assess the kinetic curve of enhancement. Since data from postcontrast images are subtracted from the precontrast image, it is critical to keep imaging parameters identical on both these sets of images. To evaluate the shape of the enhancement curve scanning is continued for 6–7 min with multiple acquisitions.
  6. Time enhancement curves assess the pattern of enhancement of lesions by displaying signal intensity over time. The signal intensity is color coded. The region of interest [ROI] is placed on the part of the lesion showing maximum enhancement on the non-subtracted image. The threshold level is typically set around 60 % increase in signal intensity from precontrast images. It is critical to document and take into account the most suspicious of the kinetic curve [45].

Potential Pitfalls and Artifacts in MR Imaging [46, 47]

False Positive

- *False Enhancement*: This occurs due to movement of the breast between pre- and postcontrast images leading to an area of pseudoenhancement that appears at the edge of fat parenchyma interface. Movement most often is related to contraction of the pectoral muscle which may be apparent on inspection of the appearance of the muscle on the images. When movement occurs in the same plane as the slice, the artifact is more readily apparent since an area of bright signal corresponding to pseudoenhancement appears next to an area of dark signal. However, problem arises when the displacement occurs in a plane that is not the same as that of the MRI image acquisition. Pre- and postcontrast source images need to be carefully reviewed to identify motion artifacts causing pseudoenhancement.
- *Normally Enhancing Structures*: These include blood vessels, lymph nodes and the nipple, and hormone-related enhancement of breast parenchyma [48–50]. Blood vessels

Table 8.3 Differential diagnosis of abnormalities in the breast

	Benign	Probably benign	Suspicious
Mass	Cyst	Smooth borders, uniform enhancement, T2 hyperintensity, benign kinetics in a non-BRCA patient	Irregular margins, heterogeneous or rim enhancement
	Lymph node		Washout kinetic curve
	Fat necrosis		
Non-mass-like enhancement	Bilateral symmetric, benign kinetics	Diffuse unilateral or regional patchy or stippled	Regional clumped, ductal, heterogeneous
			Segmental
Focus	Multiple or bilateral, single without washout	Single, washout, in non-BRCA patient	Single, washout in a BRCA patient

are easily recognized due to their course and bright signal on T2 images. Lymph nodes are predominantly seen in the upper outer quadrant of the breast. They can demonstrate intense rapid enhancement with washout kinetics. T1-weighted images demonstrate the fatty hilum and allow for a confident diagnosis of a lymph node. The rich vascularity of the nipple areolar complex may produce enhancement in the nipple that can be confusing particularly when the nipple is displaced or flattened against the coil. Precontrast images, comparison with the opposite nipple and 3-D reformatting is helpful in making an accurate assessment [47]. Normal breast parenchyma may also show mild enhancement; however, especially in the second half of the cycle or during menstruation, multiple bilateral foci of enhancement may be seen predominantly in the outer breasts, and these may also be seen in post menopausal women on hormonal therapy. Cessation of hormonal therapy 4–6 weeks prior to MRI and scanning menstruating women during the first part of the menstrual cycle are advised whenever feasible.

False Negative

- *Nonenhancing Cancer*: Detection of cancer in breast MRI is based on the presence of neovascularity and tumor angiogenesis that causes cancers to enhance and be identified. The degree of angiogenesis is variable and is lower in DCIS and invasive cancers that are smaller than 5 mm [51, 52]. About 2/3 of nonenhancing cancers are DCIS [51]. Occasionally, cancers larger than 5 mm do not enhance, and this has been reported in inflammatory breast cancer [53]. A lesion that is considered suspicious based on mammographic or sonographic characteristics should not be downgraded based on lack of enhancement.
- *Missed Enhancement*: Careful analysis of the images is important to ensure that contrast has been injected by identifying normally enhancing structures such as the heart and blood vessels. Motion can lead to misregistration artifacts, and areas of true enhancement may be missed by being subtracted out. A strong background parenchymal enhancement can also be a cause of missing a small enhancing cancer. In one series 83 % of false-negative cases were attributed to a strong surrounding enhancement pattern [51].
- *Misinterpretation Enhancement*: This occurs due to morphological characteristics or kinetic curve pattern that may have benign features or in cases where a lesion was considered benign due to being stable.

To minimize the likelihood of missing breast cancer on an MRI examination, it is important to assess both morphology and the kinetic curve pattern, and, keeping in mind that the kinetic curve pattern may have significant overlap between benign and malignant lesions, it is important not to solely rely on the enhancement curve pattern to exclude cancer. Table 8.3 summarizes the common imaging features of benign, probably benign, and malignant lesions on a breast MRI.

MRI of the breast when appropriate is a useful breast imaging tool. Although controversies continue on its use in staging the extent of disease in a known breast cancer patient, it is useful in screening women at an elevated risk for breast cancer, for assessment of implants, and occasional use for problem-solving tool as a supplement to mammography and sonography.

References

1. DeMartini W, Lehman C. A review of current evidence-based clinical applications for breast magnetic resonance imaging. Top Magn Reson Imaging. 2008;19(3):143–50.
2. Saslow D, et al. American Cancer Society guidelines for breast screening with MRI as an adjunct to mammography. CA Cancer J Clin. 2007;57(2):75–89.
3. Boetes C. Update on screening breast MRI in high-risk women. Obstet Gynecol Clin North Am. 2011;38(1):149–58.
4. Kriege M, Brekelmans CT, Boetes C, et al. Efficacy of MRI and mammography for breast-cancer screening in women with a familial or genetic predisposition. N Engl J Med. 2004;351(5):427–37.
5. Sardanelli F, et al. Magnetic resonance imaging of the breast: recommendations from the EUSOMA working group. Eur J Cancer. 2010;46(8):1296–316.

6. Leach MO, Boggis CR, Dixon AK, et al. Screening with magnetic resonance imaging and mammography of a UK population at high familial risk of breast cancer: a prospective multicentre cohort study (MARIBS). Lancet. 2005;365(9473):1769–78.
7. Warner E, Plewes DB, Hill KA, et al. Surveillance of BRCA1 and BRCA2 mutation carriers with magnetic resonance imaging, ultrasound, mammography, and clinical breast examination. JAMA. 2004;292(11):1317–25.
8. Sardanelli F, Podo F, D'Agnolo G, et al. Multicenter comparative multimodality surveillance of women at genetic-familial high risk for breast cancer (HIBCRIT study): interim results. Radiology. 2007;242(3):698–715.
9. Weinstein SP, Localio AR, Conant EF, et al. Multimodality screening of high-risk women: a prospective cohort study. J Clin Oncol. 2009;27(36):6124–8.
10. Podo F, Sardanelli F, Canese R, et al. The Italian multi-centre project on evaluation of MRI and other imaging modalities in early detection of breast cancer in subjects at high genetic risk. J Exp Clin Cancer Res. 2002;21:115–24.
11. Morris EA, Liberman L, Ballon DJ, et al. MRI of occult breast carcinoma in a high-risk population. AJR Am J Roentgenol. 2003;181:619–26.
12. Lehman CD, Isaacs C, Schnall MD, et al. Cancer yield of mammography, MRI, and ultrasound in high risk women: prospective multi-institution breast cancer screening study. Radiology. 2007;244:381–8.
13. Sutcliffe 3rd JB, Otto PM. Controversies in breast MRI. Curr Probl Diagn Radiol. 2013;42(4):149–63.
14. Warner E, et al. Systematic review: using magnetic resonance imaging to screen women at high risk for breast cancer. Ann Intern Med. 2008;148(9):671–9.
15. Berg WA. Detection of breast cancer with addition of annual screening ultrasound or a single screening MRI to mammography in women with elevated breast cancer risk. JAMA. 2012;307(13):1394–404.
16. Middleton MS, McNamara Jr MP. Breasts implant classification with MR imaging correlation. Radiographics. 2000;20(3):1–72.
17. DeAngelis GA, de Lange EE, Miller LR, Morgan RF. MR imaging of breast implants. Radiographics. 1994;14(4):783–94.
18. Bondurant S, Ernster V, Herdman R, editors. Safety of silicone breast implants. Report produced by the Committee on the Safety of Silicone Breast Implants, Institute of Medicine, National Academy of Sciences; 1999.
19. Steinbach BG, Hardt NS, Abbitt PL, Lanier L, Caffee HH. Breast implants, common complications and concurrent breast disease. Radiographics. 1993;13(1):95–118.
20. Berg WA, et al. Diagnosing breast implant rupture with MR imaging, US, and mammography. Radiographics. 1993;13(6):1323–36.
21. Piccoli CW, Greer JG, Mitchell DG. Breast MR imaging for cancer detection and implant evaluation: potential pitfalls. Radiographics. 1996;16(1):63–75.
22. Hölmich LR, Vejborg I, Conrad C, Sletting S, McLaughlin JK. The diagnosis of breast implant rupture: MRI findings compared with findings at explantation. Eur J Radiol. 2005;53(2):213–25.
23. Vestito A, Mangieri FF, Ancona A, Minervini C, Perchinunno V, Rinaldi S. Study of breast implant rupture: MRI versus surgical findings. Radiol Med. 2012;117(6):1004–18.
24. Moy L, et al. Is breast MRI helpful in the evaluation of inconclusive mammographic findings? AJR Am J Roentgenol. 2009;193(4):986–93.
25. Dorrius MD, Pijnappel RM, Jansen-van der Weide MC, Oudkerk M. Breast magnetic resonance imaging as a problem-solving modality in mammographic BI-RADS 3 lesions. Cancer Imaging. 2010;10(Spec no A):S54–8.
26. Benndorf M, Baltzer PA, Vag T, Gajda M, Runnebaum IB, Kaiser WA. Breast MRI as an adjunct to mammography: does it really suffer from low specificity? A retrospective analysis stratified by mammographic BI-RADS classes. Acta Radiol. 2010;51(7):715–21.
27. Bluemke DA, Gatsonis CA, Chen MH, et al. Magnetic resonance imaging of the breast prior to biopsy. JAMA. 2004;292:2735–42.
28. ACR practice guideline for the performance of contrast-enhanced magnetic resonance imaging (MRI) of the breast. American College of Radiology. Revised 2008 (Resolution 25). Section II, 1, a. Available from: http://www.acr.org/SecondaryMainMenuCategories/quality_safety/guidelines/breast/mri_breast.aspx.
29. Ikeda DM, Hylton NM, Kuhl CK, et al. BI-RADS: magnetic resonance imaging. In: D'Orsi CJ, Mendelson EB, Ikeda DM, editors. Breast imaging reporting and data system: ACR BI-RADS – breast imaging atlas. 1st ed. Reston: American College of Radiology; 2003.
30. Ikeda DM. Updated breast MRI Lexicon. Eur J Radiol. 2012;81 Suppl 1:S63.
31. Erguvan-Dogan B, Whitman GJ, Kushwaha AC, Phelps MJ, Dempsey PJ. BI-RADS-MRI: a primer. AJR Am J Roentgenol. 2006;187(2):W152–60.
32. Agrawal G, Su MY, Nalcioglu O, Feig SA, Chen JH. Significance of breast lesion descriptors in the ACR BI-RADS MRI lexicon. Cancer. 2009;115(7):1363–80.
33. Baltzer PA, Dietzel M, Burmeister HP, et al. Application of MR mammography beyond local staging: Is there a potential to accurately assess axillary lymph nodes? Evaluation of an extended protocol in an initial prospective study. AJR Am J Roentgenol. 2011;196:W641–7.
34. Rahbar H, Partridge SC, Javid SH, Lehman CD. Imaging axillary lymph nodes in patients with newly diagnosed breast cancer. Curr Probl Diagn Radiol. 2012;41(5):149–58.
35. Macura KJ, Ouwerkerk R, Jacobs MA, Bluemke DA. Patterns of enhancement on breast MR images: interpretation and imaging pitfalls. Radiographics. 2006;26(6):1719–34.
36. Kelcz F. It is not all in the CAD or BI-RADS. Eur J Radiol. 2012;81 Suppl 1:S76–7.
37. Santamaría G, et al. Radiologic and pathologic findings in breast tumors with high signal intensity on T2-weighted MR images. Radiographics. 2010;30(2):533–48.
38. Mahoney MC, Gatsonis C, Hanna L, DeMartini WB, Lehman C. Positive predictive value of BI-RADS MR imaging. Radiology. 2012;264(1):51–8.
39. Wang LC, DeMartini WB, Partridge SC, Peacock S, Lehman CD. MRI-detected suspicious breast lesions: predictive values of kinetic features measured by computer-aided evaluation. AJR Am J Roentgenol. 2009;193(3):826–31.
40. Liberman L, Mason G, Morris EA, Dershaw DD. Does size matter? Positive predictive value of MRI-detected breast lesions as a function of lesion size. AJR Am J Roentgenol. 2006;186:426–30.
41. Weinstein SP, et al. Frequency of malignancy seen in probably benign lesions at contrast-enhanced breast MR imaging: findings from ACRIN 6667. Radiology. 2010;255(3):731–7.
42. Eby PR, et al. Cancer yield of probably benign breast MR examinations. J Magn Reson Imaging. 2007;26(4):950–5.
43. Eby PR, DeMartini WB, Gutierrez RL, Saini MH, Peacock S, Lehman CD. Characteristics of probably benign breast MRI lesions. AJR Am J Roentgenol. 2009;193(3):861–7.
44. Hauth E, Umutlu L, Kümmel S, Kimmig R, Forsting M. Follow-up of probably benign lesions (BI-RADS 3 category) in breast MR imaging. Breast J. 2010;16(3):297–304.
45. Rausch DR, Hendrick RE. How to optimize clinical breast MR imaging practices and techniques on Your 1.5-T system. Radiographics. 2006;26(5):1469–84.
46. Millet I, Pages E, Hoa D, Merigeaud S, Curros Doyon F, Prat X, Taourel P. Pearls and pitfalls in breast MRI. Br J Radiol. 2012;85(1011):197–207.

47. Harvey JA. Breast MR, imaging artifacts: how to recognize and fix them. Radiographics. 2007;27 Suppl 1:S131–45.
48. Ojeda-Fournier H, Choe KA, Mahoney MC. Recognizing and interpreting artifacts and pitfalls in MR imaging of the breast. Radiographics. 2007;27:S147–64.
49. Friedman EP, Hall-Craggs MA, Mumtaz H, Schneidau A. Breast MR and the appearance of the normal and abnormal nipple. Clin Radiol. 1997;52:854–61.
50. Spillane AJ, Donnellan M, Matthews AR. Clinical significance of intramammary lymph nodes. Breast. 1999;8:143–6.
51. Obdeijn IM, Loo CE, Rijnsburger AJ, Wasser MN, Bergers E, Kok T, et al. Assessment of false-negative cases of breast MR imaging in women with a familial or genetic predisposition. Breast Cancer Res Treat. 2010;119:399–407.
52. Teifke A, Hlawatsch A, Beier T, Werner Vomweg T, Schadmand S, Schmidt M, et al. Undetected malignancies of the breast: dynamic contrast-enhanced MR imaging at 1.0 T. Radiology. 2002;224:881–8.
53. Kurz KD, Roy S, Modder U, Skaane P, Saleh A. Typical atypical findings on dynamic MRI of the breast. Eur J Radiol. 2010;76:195–210.

Breast MRI for Diagnosis and Staging of Breast Cancer

9

Riham H. El Khouli, Michael A. Jacobs,
and Katarzyna J. Macura

Introduction

Breast MRI has an established role in the surveillance, workup, and follow-up of breast cancer. In recent years there has been widespread adoption of this technology, especially with the increasing number of studies and significant multicenter trials showing the higher accuracy of MRI compared to mammography and ultrasound in detecting and characterizing breast cancer. The rapid acceptance of breast MRI is due to the superior sensitivity of MRI for detection of ductal carcinoma in situ (DCIS) and also invasive carcinoma compared to mammography and ultrasound. Current efforts are directed toward developing and applying advanced techniques to improve the specificity of MRI and consequently prevent unnecessary biopsy, as well as to tailor treatment regimens with better assessment of treatment response.

R.H. El Khouli, MD, PhD
Department of Radiology and Radiological Sciences,
The Johns Hopkins University School of Medicine,
Baltimore, MD 21287, USA
e-mail: relkhou2@jhmi.edu

M.A. Jacobs, PhD
The Russell H. Morgan Department of Radiology and Radiological Sciences, Sidney Kimmel Comprehensive Cancer Center,
The Johns Hopkins University School of Medicine,
Traylor Blg, Rm 309, 712 Rutland Avenue, Baltimore,
MD 21205, USA
e-mail: mikej@mri.jhu.edu

K.J. Macura, MD, PhD (✉)
The Russell H. Morgan Department of Radiology and Radiological Sciences, The Johns Hopkins University,
601 N. Caroline Street, Baltimore, MD 21287, USA
e-mail: kmacura@jhmi.edu

Clinical Indications for Breast MRI

In the practice guidelines released by the American College of Radiology (ACR) in 2008 and 2013 [1], the indications for breast MRI are listed under three main categories: screening, extent of disease, and additional evaluation of clinical or imaging findings (Box 9.1). Indications are summarized next.

Screening

1. *Women with high lifetime risk for breast cancer (>20% lifetime risk by Gail model)*, such as in cases of family history of breast cancer and genetic predisposition due to mutations of tumor suppression genes BRCA 1 and 2.

Box 9.1 Clinical Indications of Breast MRI

Screening
- Women with high lifetime risk of breast cancer
- Women newly diagnosed with breast cancer to screen the contralateral breast
- Women post breast augmentation

Extent of disease
- Multifocality and multicentricity
- Extension to chest wall and skin
- Residual breast cancer
- Treatment response evaluation

Additional evaluation
- Inconclusive and equivocal breast exam
- Recurrence
- Metastatic disease and lymphadenopathy with suspected breast primary but negative physical exam and mammography
- MRI-guided intervention for lesions seen only with MRI

M.K. Shetty (ed.), *Breast Cancer Screening and Diagnosis: A Synopsis*,
DOI 10.1007/978-1-4939-1267-4_9, © Springer Science+Business Media New York 2015

2. *Women with newly diagnosed breast cancer to screen the contralateral breast* to detect 3–5 % of cases where there is an occult contralateral breast cancer.
3. *Women post breast augmentation* with silicone or saline breast implants and those with injections of free silicone, paraffin, or polyacrylamide gel that would be difficult to screen with mammography and are preferably screened with contrast-enhanced MRI. The assessment of integrity of the implant, on the other hand, is done with non-contrast MRI.

Extent of Disease

1. *Multifocality*, the presence of two or more tumor foci within the same quadrant of the breast, and *multicentricity*, the presence of two or more tumor foci in different quadrants of the same breast, are common in both invasive breast cancer and DCIS. The accurate assessment of the extent of breast cancer can change the management significantly; hence, the improved accuracy of MRI over mammography in evaluating the extent of breast cancer makes it a preferable modality for this purpose.
2. *Extension of breast cancer to the chest wall and skin* is an important factor in breast cancer staging. MRI offers better visualization and assessment of breast cancer invasion and its relation to the deep fascia.
3. *Residual breast cancer*: MRI is used to evaluate the residual disease in cases of lumpectomy with positive margins in pathology.
4. *Treatment response evaluation*: MRI can be used to evaluate the response to treatment during and after the course of chemotherapy and to evaluate the residual tumor before the surgical intervention. A baseline exam, before the start of treatment, is critical to achieve that goal. Also, the placement of a tissue marker within the tumor before the start of treatment is essential to be able to identify its location in cases of complete response.

Additional Evaluation of Clinical or Imaging Findings

1. *Inconclusive and equivocal breast exam with mammography and ultrasound*
2. *Breast cancer recurrence*, to include patients with breast reconstruction surgery (tissue transfer flaps)
3. *Metastatic disease or axillary lymphadenopathy* when the breast primary is suspected with negative physical exam and mammography
4. *MRI-guided intervention, biopsy, and wire localization* for breast lesions visualized only with MRI and undetectable with other modalities

Breast Cancer Diagnosis

The clinical breast MRI examination is based on the assessment of the breast lesion morphology and breast tissue perfusion evaluated with the dynamic contrast-enhanced (DCE) MRI. In addition, breast glandular tissue composition, nipple, skin, chest wall, and axillae are also evaluated.

Breast Composition (Density)

A subjective assessment of the fibroglandular tissue density of the breast is usually the initial step in the evaluation of the breast MRI. The importance of breast density assessment arises from the correlation between higher breast density and risk of breast cancer [2–4]. According to the ACR BI-RADS, breast composition is categorized into four groups (Fig. 9.1) [5]:

1. *Almost entirely fatty* with glandular tissue density <25 %
2. *Scattered fibroglandular* with glandular tissue density of 25–50 %
3. *Heterogeneous fibroglandular densities* with glandular tissue density of 51–75 %
4. *Mostly fibroglandular (extremely dense)* with glandular tissue density >75 %

Breast Lesion Morphological Assessment

In the clinical breast MRI exam, a high spatial resolution (0.5 mm) and high temporal resolution (15 s) contrast-enhanced imaging are included to optimize morphological evaluation of the breast tissue and enable assessment of breast tissue perfusion. When setting up a breast MRI protocol, the high spatial resolution sequences are used to scan patients pre- and post-contrast injection, which allows subtraction of the images for improved visualization of the resultant morphology of enhancing lesions. Acquiring high spatial resolution breast MRI is needed for the accurate clinical interpretation of size, shape, borders, and internal architecture of the lesion. The American College of Radiology (ACR) Breast Imaging and Reporting Data System-MRI (BI-RADS-MRI) classifies MRI breast lesions into three categories (Box 9.2):

1. *Focus*: A tiny spot of enhancement <5 mm in diameter is identified as a focus as it is so small that it would be difficult to classify it under other categories and it is also difficult to further assess its borders and internal characteristics. Foci are typically associated with benign fibrocystic changes.
2. *Mass*: It is a three-dimensional space-occupying lesion that should have a distinct border with a describable shape

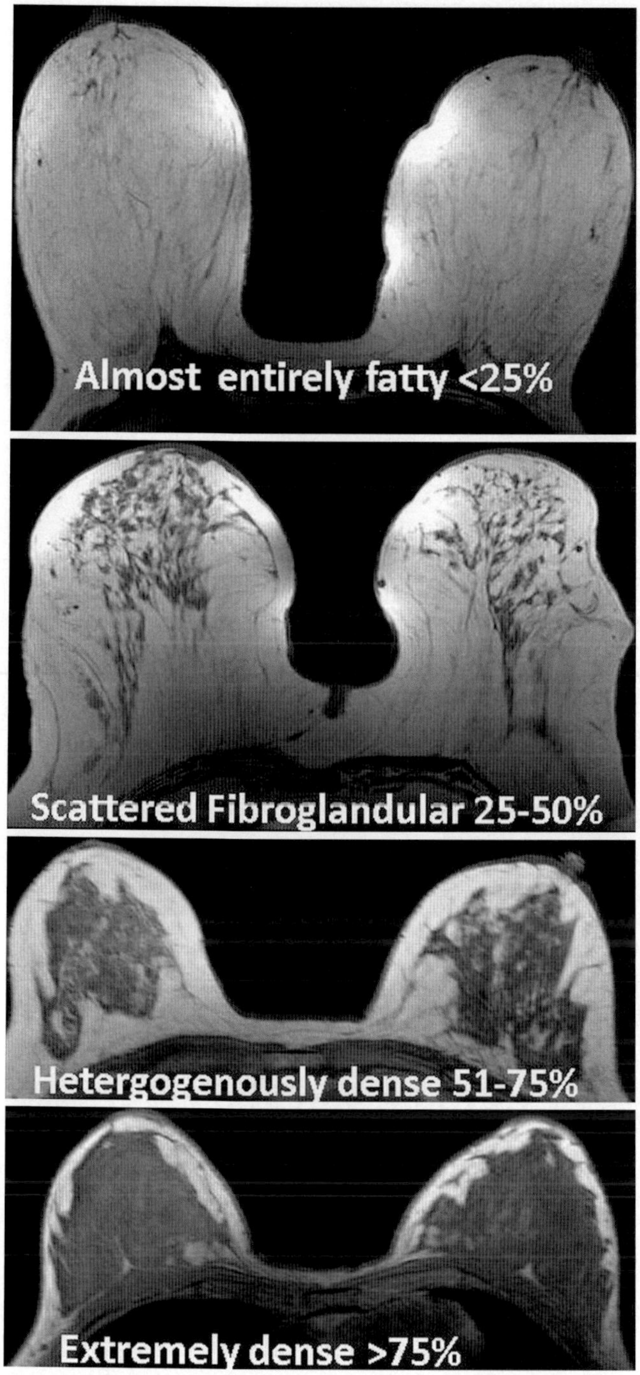

Fig. 9.1 Breast composition (breast density) categorization according to the ACR BI-RADS classification

and usually can be identified on non-enhanced T1 and T2 sequences (Box 9.2 and Fig. 9.2).

3. *Non-mass-like enhancement* (*NMLE*): It is an enhancement seen after contrast injection that does not have distinct border and cannot be separated from the surrounding glandular tissue. It is usually not detected on pre-contrast images even when correlated with post-contrast images, and it follows the distribution of glandular tissue (Fig. 9.2). This entity is unique to MRI and it is usually not detected with mammography or ultrasound.

Box 9.2 Breast Lesion Morphological Assessment

Breast lesion

Focus: a tiny enhancing spot <5 mm

Mass: 3D space-occupying lesion that has distinct borders and shape

- *Shape*: round, oval, lobulated, or irregular
- *Margins*: smooth, lobulated, irregular, or spiculated
- *Internal enhancement pattern*: homogeneous, heterogeneous, or rim
- *Benign features*: non-enhancing T2 dark septations and fatty hilum

Non-mass-like enhancement (*NMLE*): an area of enhancement seen only after contrast injection and following the glandular distribution

- *Pattern of distribution*: focal, linear, ductal, segmental, regional, multiple regions, or diffuse
- *Internal enhancement pattern*: homogeneous, heterogeneous, stippled, clumped, or reticular
- *Symmetry*

There are some differences in the reporting system when assessing morphology of masses versus NMLE; therefore, we will discuss their features separately.

Mass

Masses should be assessed for size, shape, margins, and internal enhancement pattern (Box 9.2):

1. *Size*: It is recommended to report the three dimensions of the mass: anteroposterior (AP), supero-inferior (SI), and right to left (RL).
2. *Location*: There are two systems used to define the lesion location within the breast; the first is the quadrant system, where the breast is divided into five regions: four quadrants (upper outer, upper inner, lower outer, and lower inner) + the nipple and retroareolar region. The second system is the clockwise system where the lesion location is defined as the clock hand position (Fig. 9.3).
3. *Shape*: Shape of the mass can be round, oval, lobulated, or irregular.
4. *Margins*: Margins of the mass may be smooth, lobulated, irregular, or spiculated. The strongest predictor of cancer is spiculated margin with a very high positive predictive value (PPV) 91–94 % [6–8] (Fig. 9.4).
5. *Internal enhancement pattern*: Internal enhancement pattern can be homogeneous, heterogeneous, or rim enhancement (Fig. 9.5). Rim enhancement is the strongest predictor of cancer, with PPV of 70–88 % [7, 9]. It is also important to mention that the total lack of enhancement has a very high negative predictive value that approaches 100 % in some reports [9] (Fig. 9.5).

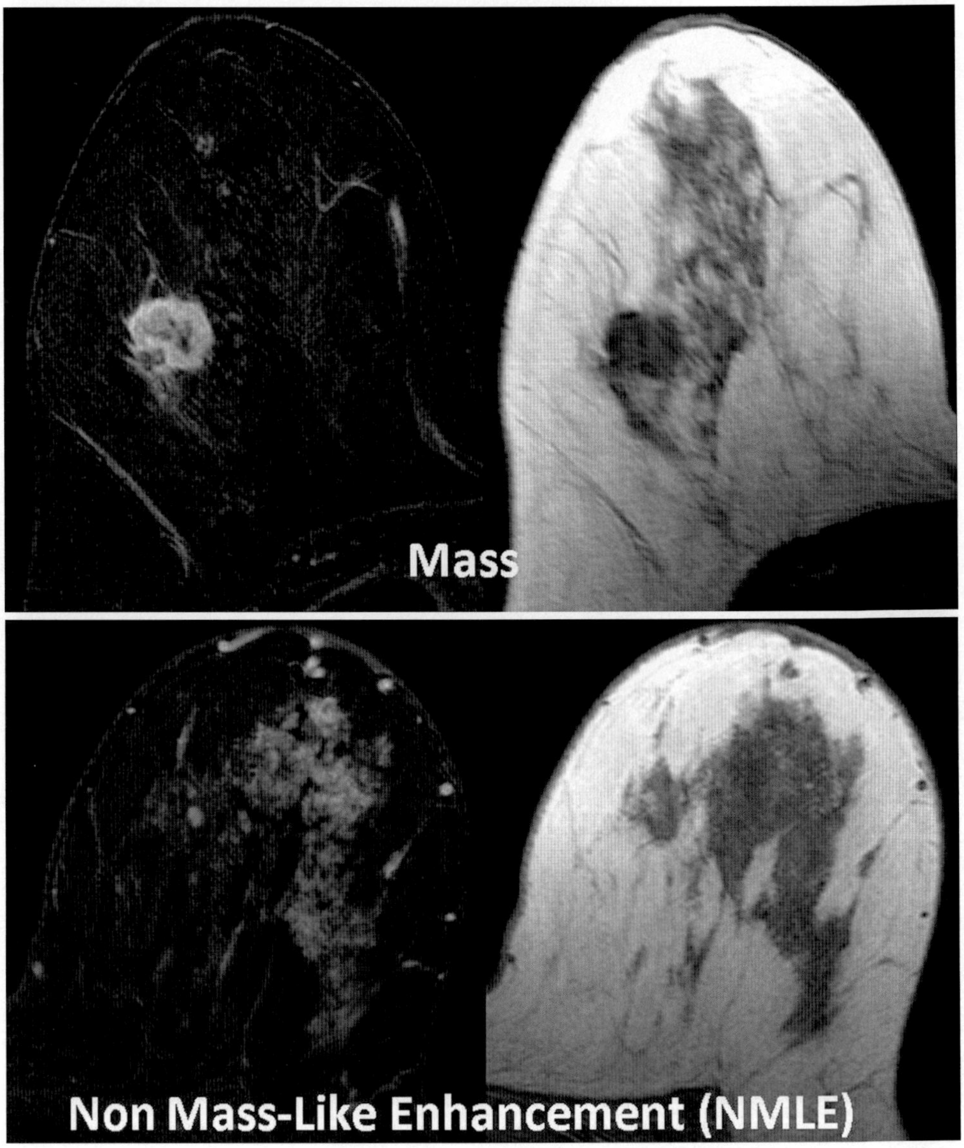

Fig. 9.2 Difference between mass- and non-mass-like enhancement (*NMLE*). A mass is a space-occupying lesion that has distinct borders and a describable shape. The NMLE is an enhancement that follows the distribution of the glandular tissue with no distinct border or describable shape. Notice that on the non-contrast and non-fat-suppressed T1-weighted image (*right side of figure*), the mass is recognizable with convex border while the NMLE is not

6. *Specific benign features of breast masses*:
   (i) *Non-enhancing T2 dark septations*: Non-enhancing septations with low T2 signal are highly suggestive of fibroadenoma [7]. Other features when combined might be associated with fibroadenoma as well such as smooth or lobulated borders with increased T2 signal and a progressive pattern of enhancement. See Fig. 9.6.
   (ii) *Fatty hilum*: A fatty hilum is characteristic of a benign lymph node. Lymph nodes usually have high T2 signal and a smooth margin.

Non-Mass-Like Enhancement (NMLE)

For the NMLE breast lesions, the three-dimensional size and location of the NMLE lesion should be reported, in a similar fashion to masses. Additional lesion modifiers are used to describe patterns of distribution and enhancement (Box 9.2):

1. *Pattern of distribution* (Fig. 9.7): The pattern of NMLE distribution can be described as focal, linear, ductal, segmental, regional, multiple regions, or diffuse. *A focal area of enhancement* usually encompasses <25 % of a single quadrant. *Linear enhancement*, as the name implies, corresponds to a line of enhancement. *Ductal enhancement* can be in a linear or branching pattern and usually radiates toward the nipple and is believed to conform to a duct. *Segmental enhancement* is a triangular or cone-shaped enhancement with its apex at or directed toward the nipple. *Regional enhancement* involves a larger area of enhancement than focal or segmental and has an irregular geographic outline. Multiple regions and diffuse enhancement are even larger and involve the whole or most of the breast. The difference between these two types is that in *multiple regions of enhancement*, areas of

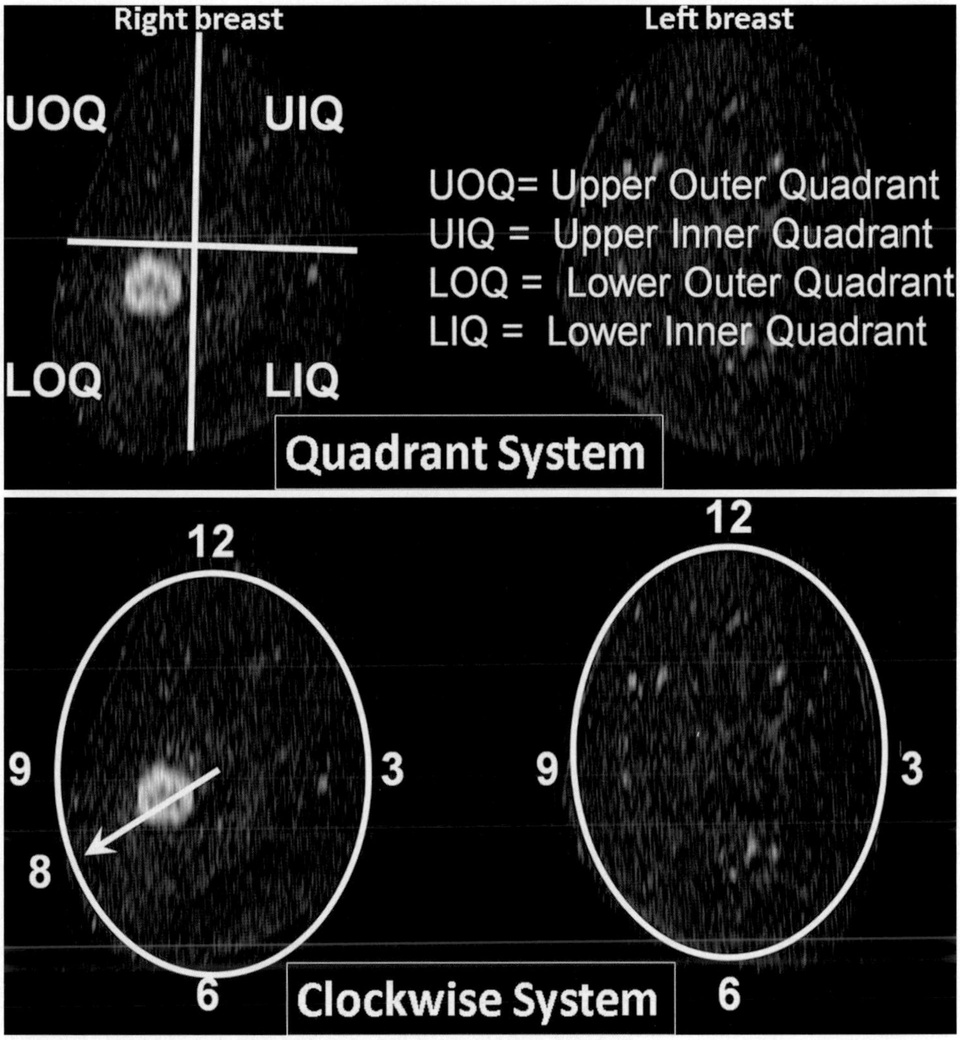

Fig. 9.3 Illustration of the two systems used to define the breast lesion location on coronal reconstructed MR images. The top row is the quadrant system, which divides the breast into four quadrants and the retroareolar region (not shown). The bottom row is the clockwise system, which imagines the breast in coronal orientation as a clock and describes the lesion location as the clock hand position. Notice that the right breast mass is located in the lower outer quadrant or at the 8 o'clock position

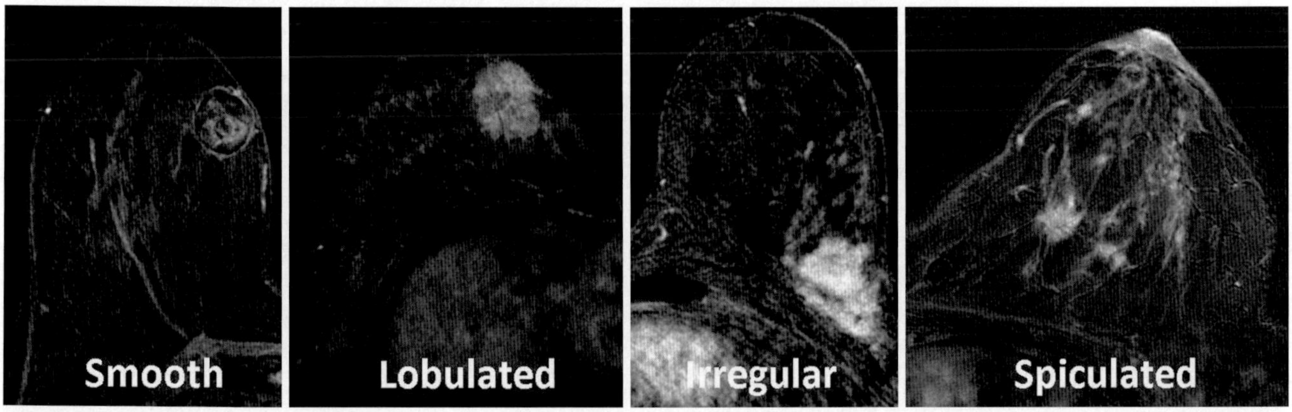

Fig. 9.4 Demonstration of different margins of masses

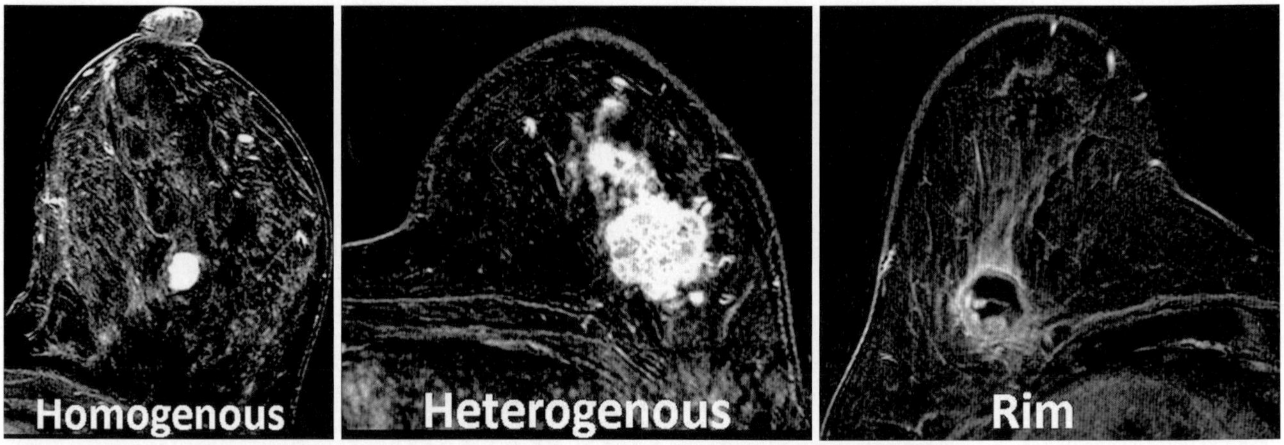

Fig. 9.5 Demonstration of different internal enhancement patterns of masses

Fig. 9.6 A T2 or STIR bright mass demonstrates dark and non-enhancing septations (*arrows*), a benign sign that is highly correlated with a fibroadenoma. *STIR* (short T1 inversion recovery) and *SUB* (post-contrast subtraction) images

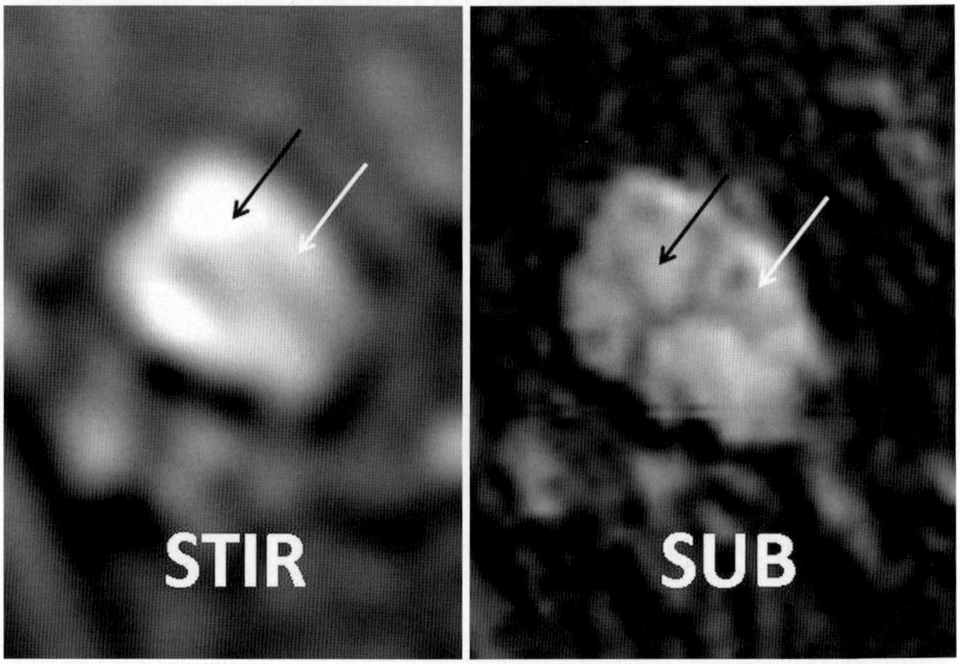

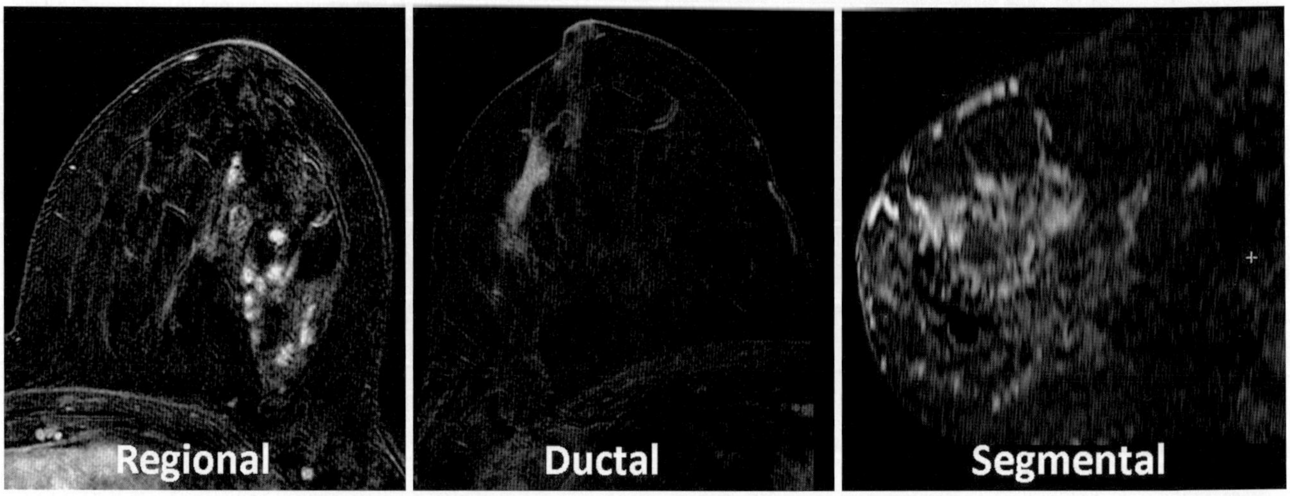

Fig. 9.7 Examples of patterns of distribution of NMLE lesions

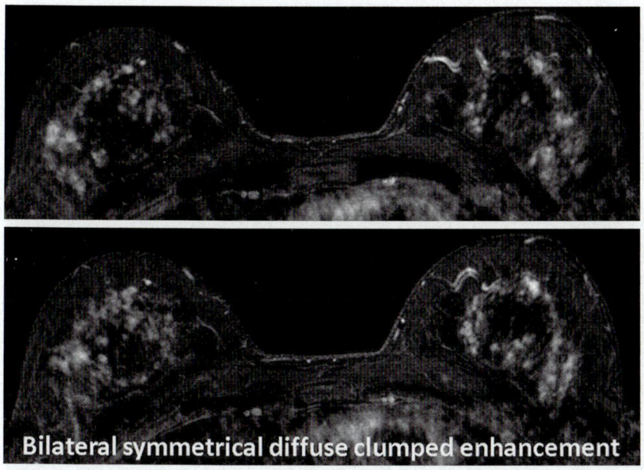

Fig. 9.8 Bilateral T1-weighted fat-saturated images after contrast administration show bilateral symmetrical diffuse confluent enhancement. Although the pattern of NMLE is clumped, which is a suspicious pattern, the symmetricity and diffuse distribution of the enhancement lower the level of suspicion. Pathology revealed dense fibrous benign breast tissue

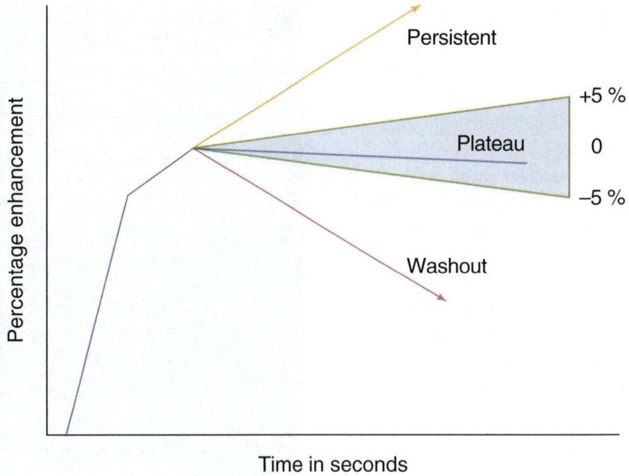

Fig. 9.9 Demonstration of the difference between stippled (scattered punctate, similar appearing enhancing foci) and clumped (cobblestone-like, confluent) enhancement patterns

normal glandular or fat tissues separate the multiple regions, while in *diffuse enhancement* it is widely distributed throughout the breast following the glandular tissue distribution (Fig. 9.8).

Ductal and segmental enhancements are strong predictors of DCIS with a wide range of positive predictive value (PPV) between 24 and 67 % [8, 10]. It is also important to mention that although there is wide variation in the reported PPV of these two patterns, they are unique to MRI and contribute to the added value of MRI with the high sensitivity in detecting DCIS.

2. *Internal enhancement pattern* (Fig. 9.9): The internal enhancement pattern of NMLE can be homogeneous, heterogeneous, stippled, clumped, or reticular. *Stippled enhancement* corresponds to innumerable small (1–2 mm) punctate dots scattered and widely separated within the enhancing area. This is usually an indicator of benign, fibrocystic changes. *Clumped enhancement* corresponds to clusters or foci that tend to coalesce. Clumped enhancement is concerning for DCIS, especially if following the segmental distribution. *Reticular enhancement* corresponds to a dendritic pattern with loss of normal curving pattern of glandular tissue. It is usually found in women experiencing some degree of glandular tissue involution with replacement by fat resulting in scattered glandular tissue within fat.
3. *Symmetry*: The symmetry of enhancement is an important indicator of normal glandular tissue distribution and might indicate scanning in the wrong time of the menstrual cycle (Fig. 9.8), i.e., in the secretory phase in the second half of menstrual cycle. Lack of symmetry of the enhancement may raise the suspicion of NMLE.

Dynamic Contrast-Enhanced (DCE) MRI Interpretation

Dynamic contrast-enhanced MRI is an essential component of the clinical breast MRI [11–15] exam. The purpose of the DCE-MRI is to observe the uptake and washout of intravenously injected contrast material of the tissue as an indicator of the perfusion and vascular pattern of the tissue of interest. There are several specific DCE parameters that can be extracted from the DCE imaging series. The main parameter that is universally used in the clinical practice is the time signal intensity curve (commonly called the kinetic curve) [15].

Time Signal Intensity Curve (Kinetic Curve Type)

The kinetic curve type is constructed by plotting the change in signal intensity (SI) resulting from contrast injection (on the *Y*-axis) over time (on the *X*-axis) (Fig. 9.10). Most breast centers use the percentage enhancement rather than the crude SI. The percentage enhancement method has many distinct advantages over the SI method by normalizing the SI in the post-contrast image to the baseline SI (pre-contrast), this eliminates the confounding effect of many factors that may influence the SI in both the patient and scanner. Moreover, using the percentage enhancement can measure the initial uptake within the lesion.

The percentage enhancement is calculated according to the following universal equation [13, 16]:

$$\frac{\text{SI post} - \text{SI pre}}{\text{SI pre}} * 100$$

where SI pre is the signal intensity in the pre-contrast image, while SI post is the signal intensity in the post-contrast image.

The shape of the kinetic curve is the most widely used parameter to differentiate benign from malignant enhancement patterns and is categorized into three different types (Fig. 9.10):

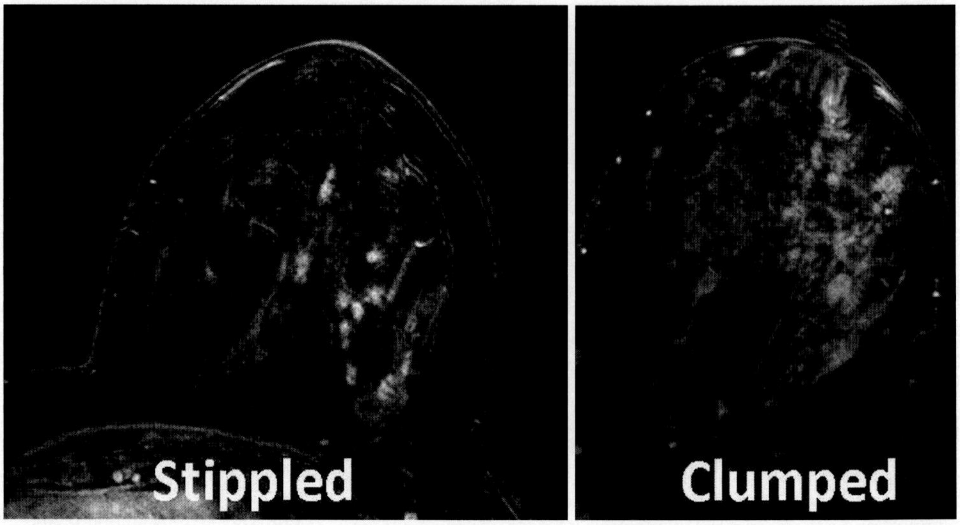

Fig. 9.10 The time to % enhancement graph demonstrates three types of kinetic curve shape. It also illustrates the semiquantitative method for kinetic curve-type categorization based on the change from the peak enhancement to the delayed phase, 5 % on both sides (positive and negative) defined as a plateau, and considering an increase or a decrease of more than 5 % defined as persistently enhancing or washout, respectively

- *Type 1 (persistently enhancing)*: Where there is gradual slow and continuous enhancement along the DCE series time. This type is further categorized into type 1A and type 1B according to the enhancement pattern in the first 2 min. In type 1A the enhancement is slowly progressing, while in type 1B there is an early marked enhancement, sometimes exceeding 80 % percentage enhancement, followed by a slower continuous enhancement (Fig. 9.10). Both types 1A and 1B are considered a good predictor of a benign enhancement pattern with a 94 % negative predictive value (NPV) [15] unless morphological features indicate otherwise.
- *Type 2 (plateau)*: Where there is an intense early enhancement (in the first 2 min) ≥80 % percentage enhancement followed by persistence of enhancement along the rest of the DCE series. This type of curve carries intermediate probability as this enhancement pattern has been demonstrated in both benign and malignant lesions. When morphological features are suggestive of malignant process, this kinetic curve shape is considered supportive of malignancy; however, when morphological features are indeterminate, further workup should be considered.
- *Type 3 (washout)*: Where there is an intense early enhancement ≥80 % followed by a decrease in the percentage enhancement (washout). This type reflects the expected vascular pattern of malignant tumors and is considered a strong indicator of malignancy with 87 % PPV [15].

Although kinetic curve shape is the most important parameter of DCE-MRI interpretation, it is commonly assessed qualitatively (subjectively). The qualitative assessment of kinetic curve shape is frequently reported to widely vary among readers and even among different readings of the same radiologist and is expected to depend on the experience of the radiologists [11, 14, 15, 17].

Semiquantitative Method (Fig. 9.10)

The assessment of the kinetic curve shape can be performed with a more quantitative (objective) approach which makes it independent of observer's subjectivity, as was proposed in the literature [18]. Two parameters were calculated from the kinetic curves: the average washout slope and the absolute washout percentage enhancement difference. The enhancement difference is an easier and more practical method and it is calculated as the difference between the peak percentage enhancement and the mean value of the last three time points (in the high temporal resolution DCE series). The percentage enhancement cutoff point is 5 %, so if the percentage enhancement difference is between −5 and +5 %, the kinetic curve shape is categorized as plateau (type 2), while if it is > +5 %, the curve type is 1 for persistently enhancing. An example of the semiquantitative categorization is shown in Fig. 9.10.

The Wash-In Rate and Early Peak Percentage Enhancement

Wash-in rate is the rate of change of the tissue SI over time in seconds within the first 2 min after contrast injection, while the peak percentage enhancement is the highest enhancement within the first 2 min. Wash-in rate is categorized into *slow* (initial enhancement <60 %), *intermediate* (initial enhancement 60–80 %), or *fast* (initial enhancement >80 %) [15]. Lesions that show early intense enhancement are highly suspicious for malignancy. The *percentage enhancement >80 % in the first 2 min* is suspicions for malignancy.

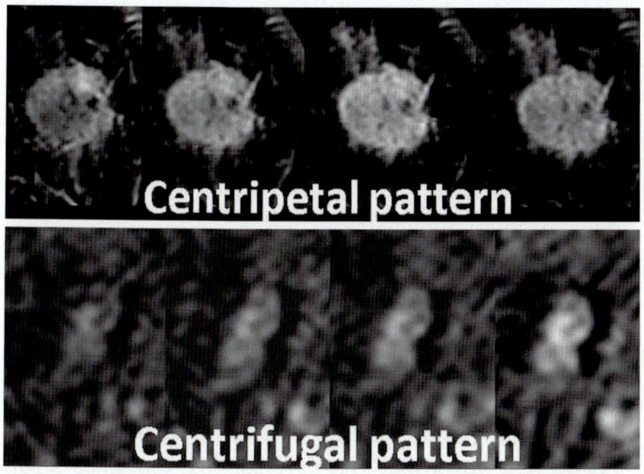

Fig. 9.11 Demonstration of the two enhancement patterns: centripetal (from the periphery to the center) and centrifugal (from the center to the periphery). The *top row* is an invasive ductal carcinoma and the *bottom row* is a fibroadenoma

Washout Rate

Washout rate is a quantitative assessment of the delayed phases of the DCE series (washout portion). Washout curves (type 3) showing negative washout rates are considered high predictor for malignancy, while persistently enhancing (positive washout rates) curves type 1 are considered a good predictor of benign behavior.

Enhancement Pattern

The enhancement pattern describes the direction of filling (enhancement) of the enhancing lesion through different phases of the DCE-MRI series [16, 19]. The pattern of enhancement can be described as centripetal or centrifugal:

- *In centripetal pattern*, the lesion starts enhancing from the periphery and progresses to the central portion and may suggest malignant pattern of enhancement (Fig. 9.11).
- *In centrifugal pattern*, the lesion starts enhancing from the center and progresses to the periphery and may suggest a benign pattern (Fig. 9.11).

Unilateral Increased Vascularity

To assess the breast vascularity, a maximum intensity projection (MIP) image can be generated [20, 21], and vascularity of both breasts can be compared. Breast vascularity scoring is then determined [21] depending on number of vessels per breast that are ≥3 cm in length and ≥2 mm in maximum transverse diameter (Table 9.1). When the difference in number of vessels between the two breasts was ≥2, it was considered positive for unilateral increased vascularity of the breast, and the breast with a higher number of vessels was considered suspicious for harboring a malignant lesion (Fig. 9.12).

Table 9.1 Vascularity map scoring

Vascularity map scoring	
Score 0	Absent or very low vascularity (no vessels[a])
Score 1	Low vascularity (only one vessel[a])
Score 2	Moderate vascularity (2–4 vessels[a])
Score 3	High vascularity (>5 vessels[a])

[a]Vessels ≥3 cm long and ≥2 mm diameter

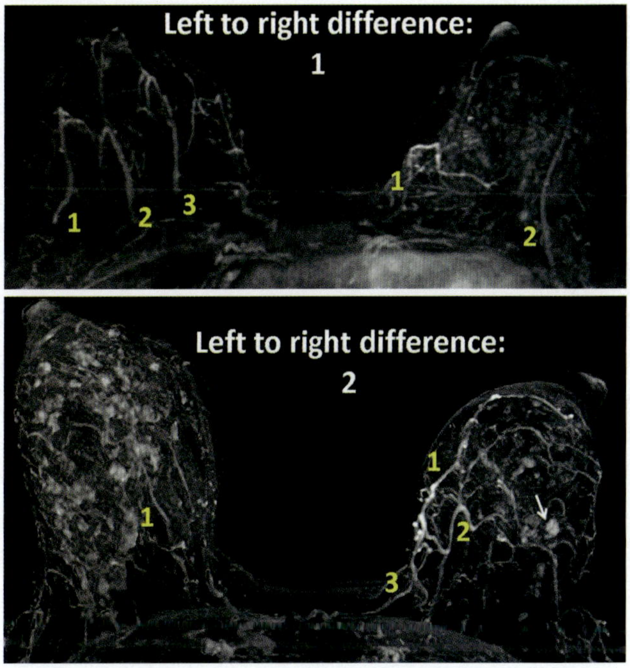

Fig. 9.12 Illustration of the unilateral increased vascularity sign. Vessels that meet two criteria (length 3 cm or longer and thickness 2 mm or thicker) are counted on each side (*yellow numbers*). Then the difference between the side of interest (with a suspicious lesion) and the contralateral side is calculated. A difference of two or more increases the suspicion of malignancy. The *top image* shows a difference of one, and the lesion in the left side was found to be benign. The *bottom image* shows that the left breast has two more vessels meeting the criteria which denote a positive left-side unilateral increased vascularity and the lesion (*arrow*) was proven to be infiltrating ductal carcinoma

ACR BI-RADS-MRI Impression

The overall assessment of the breast MRI exam should be reported according to the following BI-RADS classification:

- *BI-RADS 0*: *Need additional imaging evaluation*. That may include repeating the MRI scan if not technically satisfactory or getting a second-look ultrasound.
- *BI-RADS 1*: *Negative*. This indicates normal exam with a recommendation to return to routine screening.
- *BI-RADS 2*: *Benign findings*. This indicates that lesions with benign features but no lesions with malignant features were noted with a recommendation to return to routine screening.

- *BI-RADS 3*: *Probably benign with low probability of malignancy*. Short interval follow-up would be recommended.
- *BI-RADS 4*: *Suspicious findings*. Lesion has moderate probability of malignancy but no confirmatory method was performed. Biopsy should be considered.
- *BI-RADS 5*: *Highly suggestive of malignancy and appropriate action should be taken.*
- *BI-RADS 6*: *Known biopsy proved malignancy and appropriate action should be taken.*

Future Directions

Pharmacokinetic Modeling

Pharmacokinetic modeling is based on the analysis of the enhancement kinetics to characterize tissue perfusion. Pharmacokinetic modeling offers many advantages over the typical qualitative assessment of the DCE-MRI studies; it provides quantitative parameters that reflect physiological and anatomical information about the lesion. These parameters are expected to be more independent of the scanner hardware and software. They allow characterization of breast lesions and enable the assessment of treatment response in a setting of neoadjuvant therapy of breast cancer [22, 23].

Scanning Recommendation

1. *The baseline T1 mapping sequence*: Pharmacokinetic modeling relies on accurate calculation of contrast material concentration within the tissue of interest in each dynamic phase. The simplest way to measure the change in contrast material concentration along time is to assume that the change in T1 is directly proportional to the contrast material concentration with the tissue of interest. Because of the fact that the relationship between the contrast concentration and SI is not linear, a baseline T1 map is generated for an accurate measurement of contrast concentration [24–27].
2. *The dynamic series*: It is recommended to include a large blood vessel within the field of view of the DCE series to allow measurement of the vascular input function (VIF), contrast material concentration in the plasma over time. The VIF is used to calculate the contrast material concentration gradient (between the blood and lesion), which enables accurate pharmacokinetic modeling analysis [28, 29].

Pharmacokinetic Parameters

The three main quantitative parameters that are extracted from the DCE-MRI data using the pharmacokinetic analysis are as follows:

1. K^{trans} (*transfer constant*): the rate of contrast agent transfer from plasma compartment to extravascular extracellular spaces (wash-in rate).
2. K_{ep} (*rate constant*): the rate of escape of contrast agent from the extracellular spaces to the plasma compartment (washout rate). K_{ep} is the ratio of the transfer constant to the extravascular extracellular space fractional volume (v_e).
3. V_e (*extravascular extracellular space volume*): volume of the interstitial tumor space.
4. *Peak enhancement*: maximum tissue enhancement.
5. *Initial area under the curve* (*IAUC*): Another method for quantitative assessment of DCE-MRI is the measurement of IAUC of the contrast agent concentration across the early acquisition phase (within the initial 2 min after contrast injection). It was reported to be reproducible and correlated well with tissue permeability, especially when normalized to the surrounding normal tissue [30].

Visual Display (Fig. 9.13)

1. *Color maps*: Pharmacokinetic model while attempting to simulate the physiology of the MRI contrast agent distribution within the breast tissue calculates multiple parameters that describe contrast delivery, accumulation, and washout. To simplify the clinical interpretation of this complicated multiparametric analysis, color maps reflecting pharmacokinetic information were introduced into clinical settings. Color maps are constructed by representing the combined values of K^{trans} (permeability) and V_e (extracellular volume fraction (EVF)) on a voxel level, using cutoff values. Color red indicates high permeability and low extracellular volume fraction typically seen in cancer, while color blue indicates low permeability and high extracellular volume fraction typically seen in benign tissues. Color green reflects intermediate values for permeability and extracellular volume fraction. Color maps enable radiologists to accurately place the ROI on the most suspicious part of the lesion instead of the usual method of placing ROI randomly (Fig. 9.13).
2. *Joint histogram* (Fig. 9.13): A 2D table that shows the combined value of K^{trans} (on the *Y*-axis) and V_e (on the *X*-axis). Cutoff lines based on research cases separate three areas: red, green, and blue.
3. *Histograms*: Another way to display pharmacokinetic information is by constructing histograms of the calculated parameters (K^{trans}, K_{ep}, and V_e) to document frequency distribution of voxels (Fig. 9.13).
4. *Percentage distribution charts*: The percentage distribution of each color and color hue (depth) within a single lesion is displayed on percentage charts. It has been suggested that when red color pixel percentage distribution is more than 16 %, the rate of malignancy is higher. On the other hand, blue color percentage distribution of more than 20 % increases the probability of benign tissue (Fig. 9.13) [12, 31–37].

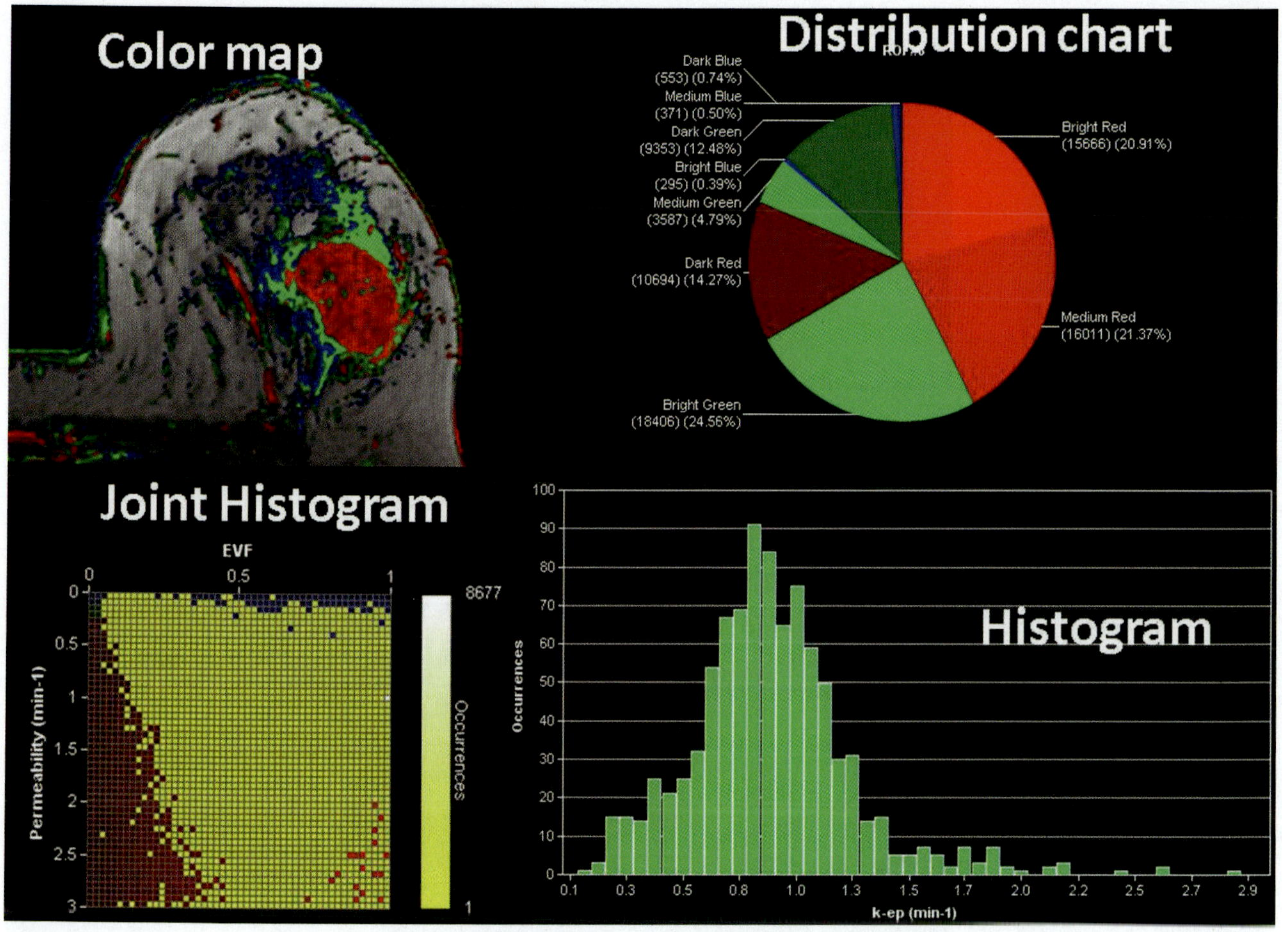

Fig. 9.13 Computer-assisted diagnosis (CAD) demonstrates different visual display options of the quantitative data from the pharmacokinetic analysis of DCE-MRI series, a color map, pixel color distribution chart, joint histogram of permeability and extracellular volume fraction EVF, and a *k*-ep histogram

Diffusion-Weighted Imaging (DWI)

Principle

DWI has the potential to provide physiological information about the functional environment and movement of water in normal versus pathological tissue. DWI is sensitive to changes in the microdiffusion of water within the intracellular spaces and extracellular spaces [38]. Differences in the apparent diffusion coefficient (ADC) values of benign and malignant breast lesions have been reported [39–44]. Malignant breast lesions are expected to have lower ADC values than benign lesions, indicating restricted diffusion of water with increased cellular density in malignant lesions [41–45].

Technical Consideration

The b-Value: DWI imaging uses b-values to discern the changes in the motion of water by varying the two different gradient pulses around the 180° pulse. This application of the gradient allows for the dephasing of the spins. The *b-values* are determined by the following equation ($b=\gamma^2G^2\delta^2(\Delta-\delta/3)$), (s/mm^2)), γ = gyromagnetic ratio, G = gradient strength, δ = diffusion gradient duration, and Δ = time between diffusion gradient pulses.

ADC Map Generation: ADC maps are created on a pixel-by-pixel basis for quantitative analysis according to the equation

$$\mathrm{ADC}=\sum_{i=1}^{n}\frac{\ln\left(\dfrac{S_i}{S_0}\right)}{b_i} \tag{9.1}$$

where b_i = the diffusion gradient values, S_0 = 1st image ($b=0$), and S_i = ith image. The *b*-value specifies the sensitivity of diffusion. Correctly assigning the *b*-value for a breast DWI is critical because it directly affects the ability to detect water molecular diffusion. As the *b*-value increases, the amount of diffusion weighting increases, and sensitivity to diffusion

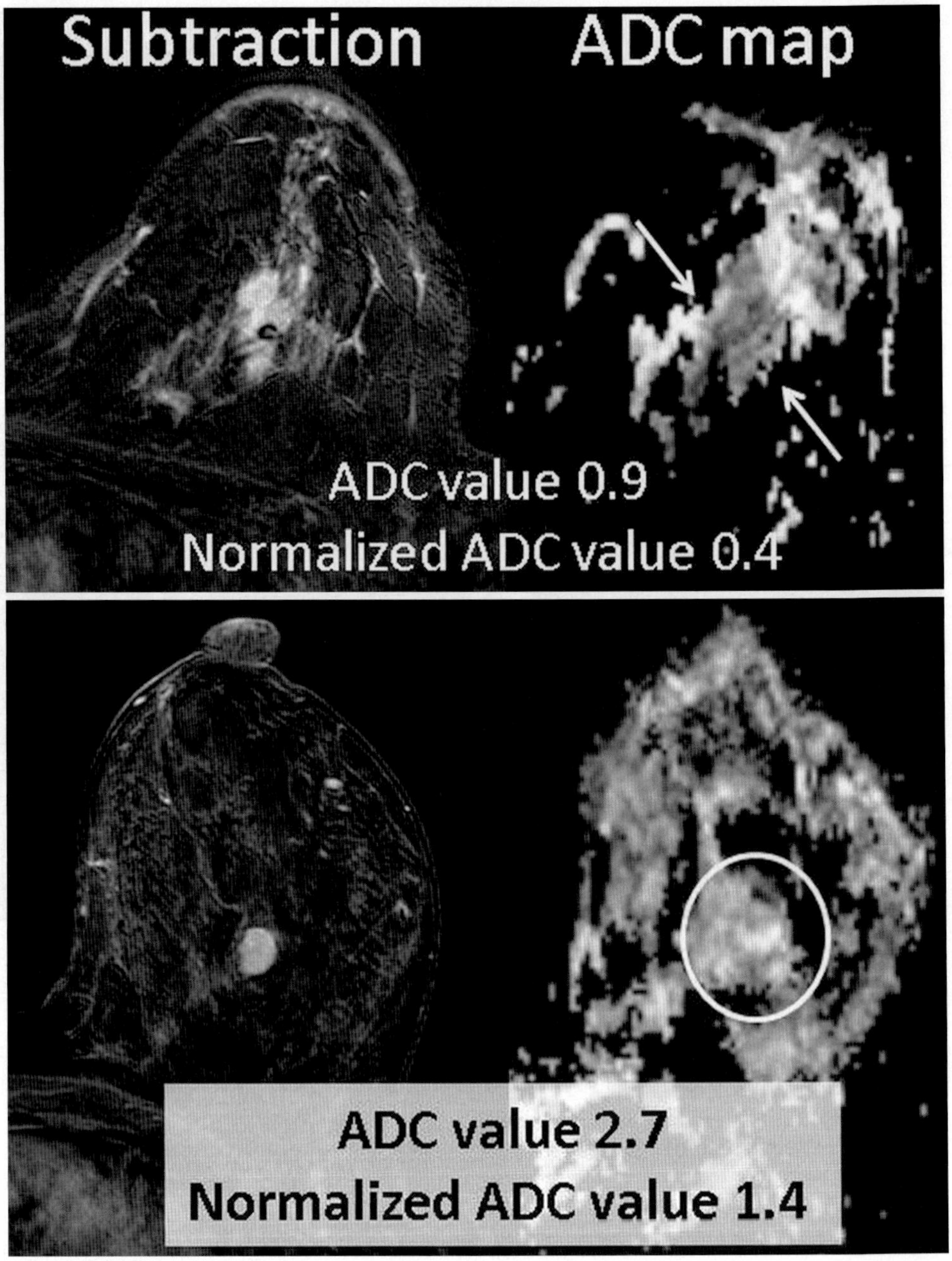

Fig. 9.14 Comparison of T1-weighted fat-suppressed postcontrast images (*left*) and ADC maps (*right*) from a malignant (*top*) and a benign (*bottom*) lesion. Figure shows the utilization of DWI in characterizing breast lesions. Localization of breast lesion is done using the high spatial resolution images (subtraction images on the *left side*). The *top row* images show a lobulated heterogeneously enhancing mass with an ADC value of 0.9 (suspicious using the two suggested cutoff values of 1.3 and 1.6) and a normalized ADC value of 0.4 (suspicious using the suggested cutoff value of 0.7). The lesion was proven to be in situ and infiltrating ductal carcinoma. The *bottom row* images show a well-defined mass with smooth margin with homogeneous internal enhancement. The ADC value is 2.7 (benign according to the cutoff values of 1.3 and 1.6) and a normalized ADC value of 1.4 (benign using the cutoff value of 0.7). The lesion was proven to be fibroadenoma

increases. At high *b*-value, DWI represents the molecular diffusion of water almost exclusively. As the *b*-value increases, it prolongs the gradient RF pulse, thus increasing TE value, and the quality of the DWI is degraded and the signal-to-noise ratio decreases accordingly. The smaller the *b*-value, the higher is the quality and SNR of the DWI images.

The range of *b*-values (s/mm^2) reported in the literature varies for breast DWI and is 0–1,000. The two *b*-values method is a more common method due to the shorter scanning time compared to the multiple (three or more) *b*-values method, yet some studies suggest that at least three *b*-values are needed for an accurate ADC value calculation. This is because the use of only two *b*-values gives a straight line slope and may underestimate the ADC map. Examples of the recommended *b*-values method are a low *b*-value (0–50) and at least two higher *b*-values >500–750 [46] and 50–850 [47].

Clinical Application of Apparent Diffusion Coefficient

Potential ADC Cutoff Values to Differentiate Benign from Malignant Breast Lesions: Few ADC values cutoffs to differentiate benign from malignant breast lesions have been suggested such as 1.3 and 1.6×10^{-3} mm^2/s [42, 45, 48]; ADC values above 1.3×10^{-3} mm^2/s are considered likely benign, whereas breast lesions with ADC values below 1.3×10^{-3} mm^2/s are considered likely malignant. See Fig. 9.14. However, there may be considerable overlap between the benign and malignant breast lesion ADC values.

Normalized ADC Value: A method to decrease potential overlap of ADC values is to use a reference tissue to normalize to the lesion ADC values. For example, normalizing breast lesion to the normal ipsilateral glandular tissue (GT) ADC value was demonstrated to decrease the overlap in absolute ADC values and increase the accuracy of interpretation of the DWI exam. The normalized ADC value is calculated by the equation $\text{Normalized AD value} = \dfrac{\text{Lesion ADC value}}{\text{GT ADC value}}$ [45]. This normalization approach is expected to overcome many factors affecting the ADC map values due to normal physiological body changes (hormonal variation across menstrual cycle [49]) as well as scanning parameters. The suggested normalized ADC map value cutoff to differentiate malignant from benign lesions was 0.7 [45] (Fig. 9.14).

Breast Cancer Treatment Response Assessment

To date, there is no cure for breast cancer. The key to effective treatment to reduce mortality is early detection, diagnosis, and treatment monitoring. Unfortunately, many patients still succumb to cancer, despite the improvement in quality of targeted oncologic therapeutics. For example, in breast cancer, treating 100 % of patients with drugs to achieve a 10–15 % response rate exposes many cancer patients to the expense and the toxicity of these aggressive therapies without any benefit. However, a fundamental challenge for determining early treatment response in breast cancer is characterizing the underlying tumor microenvironment during the initial treatment cycles and developing a tissue signature of these characteristics for accurate treatment response prediction. Fortunately, remarkable progress has occurred in the diagnosis and detection using advanced radiological imaging of breast cancer, and these methods can lead to more efficient monitoring of treatment response. Moreover, breast lesions are very heterogeneous and composed of phenotypically and functionally distinct cell populations. This heterogeneity within breast tumor does result in different radiological image characteristics and functional MRI parameters that have biological significance and are needed to better discern these tumor characteristics. For example, malignant lesions commonly show a rapid uptake followed by washout due to increased vascularity and permeability, and DCE-MRI can image this behavior. In addition, DWI with the ADC can provide functional and metabolic information about the changes in the diffusion of endogenous water molecules within the intra- and intercellular environments that can be assessed at the baseline and during treatment. The ADC map as a quantitative biophysical parameter derived from DWI and a measure of cellularity of the lesion can be used to monitor changes within the tumor cellular makeup.

Tumor Size

Change in tumor size is the single basic well-established radiological criterion for treatment response assessment.

Table 9.2 Treatment response categories according to WHO and RECIST

		WHO	RECIST
Complete response CR	Disappearance of all lesions confirmed at 4 weeks	–	–
Partial response PR	Partial decrease in tumor size confirmed at 4 weeks	50 % decrease	30 % decrease
Progressive disease PD	Increase in tumor size without a previous CR or PR *New lesion	25 % increase	20 % increase
Stable disease SD	If criteria do not meet neither PR nor PD	–	–

Two main classifications are widely used: the World Health Organization (WHO) and Response Evaluation Criteria In Solid Tumors (RECIST). Both classifications assess the treatment response based on percent change of measurable tumor size; the main differences are demonstrated in Table 9.2 [50, 51]. Both WHO and RECIST classified response to treatment into four categories: complete response (CR), partial response (PR), stable disease (SD), and progressive disease (PD) (Table 9.2 and Fig. 9.15). The most important difference between the WHO and RECIST classification is the method of tumor size measurement; the WHO classification is based on the bidimensional approach measuring the longest diameter (D_1) and the longest perpendicular diameter (D_2) and multiplying the two numbers ($D_1 \times D_2$), while the RECIST classification is based on a unidimensional approach (the longest diameter D_1) [52, 53].

Tumor Volumetric Assessment

Three-dimensional cross-sectional methods for assessing tumor volumes all over the body such as on CT and MRI have been established, and more efforts have been directed toward assessing the value of volumetric assessment in breast imaging rather than uni- or bidimensional approaches that were limited to the 2D imaging modalities such as mammography. Three-dimensional volume change of a mass on MRI seems to be a promising approach to predict recurrence-free survival in patients undergoing neoadjuvant chemotherapy [54]. Three-dimensional tumor volume can be calculated as:

$$\text{Tumor volume} = (\pi / 6) \times d_1 \times d_2 \times d_3$$

DCE-MRI Analysis (Pharmacokinetic Parameters)

DCE-MRI as a functional imaging tool plays a role in treatment response assessment. The advantage of DCE-MRI over conventional size assessment is in its ability to predict treatment response early in the treatment course, usually after the first cycle of therapy, where the conventional size assessment is usually performed mid-treatment (usually after third to fourth cycle). Differences in PK-DEC parameters of vascular density, perfusion (K^{trans}), and vascular permeability (K_{ep}) are

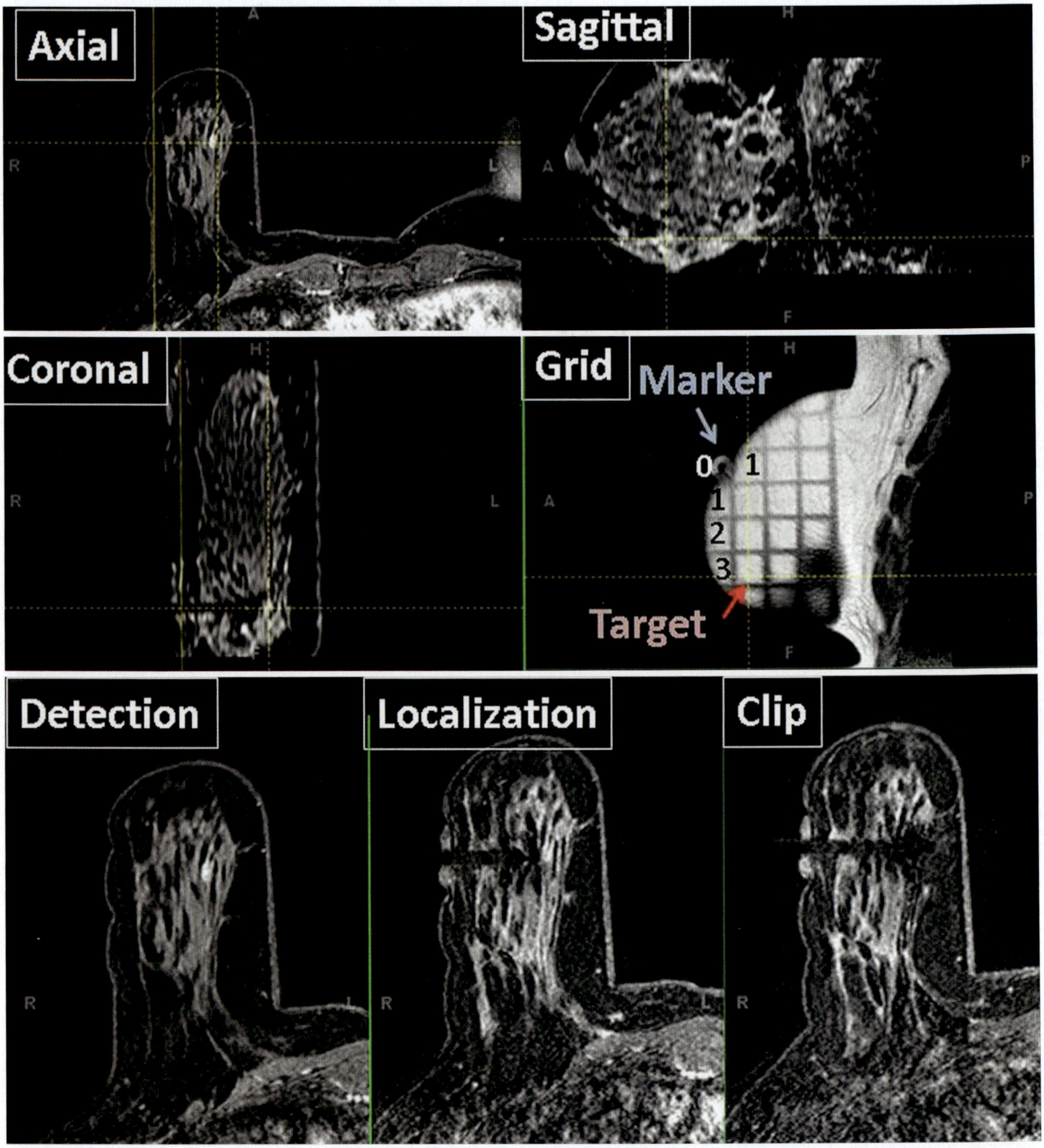

Fig. 9.15 Illustration of the basic steps of MRI-guided biopsy procedure. The *top two rows* of images show the multiplanar reconstruction window, where the mass is visualized in three planes (axial, coronal, and sagittal). The forth image is the sagittal T1 non-fat-suppressed image that is used to visualize the grid compressing the breast. Having the coordinates crossed on the lesion on three planes guides the operator to where the lesion location corresponds to on the grid. Placing the marker away from the lesion enables the operator to use it as a reference to where the lesion is located relative to the marker. Using the grid image, the operator plans the path for the needle access to the target (need to move 1 square toward the chest wall and 3 squares toward the foot). The *bottom row* images show the sequential imaging needed for lesion visualization (*left*), for confirmation of correct positioning of the needle tip relative to the lesion prior to biopsy (*middle*), and for a postbiopsy clip placement confirmation (*right*)

suggested to differentiate responders (pathological complete responders) from nonresponders (progressive disease) (Table 9.3 and Fig. 9.15). Several reports have begun to combine the architectural and dynamic features with PK-DCE-MRI with promising results that provide important functional information [54–61].

Table 9.3 DCE-MRI pharmacokinetic parameters change in response to treatment

	Pretreatment	Post-treatment
K^{trans}	Higher values correlated with higher response probability	Significant reduction from baseline seen in RESPONDERS
K_{ep}	NA	Significant reduction from baseline seen in RESPONDERS
V_e	Higher values correlated with higher response probability	Significant increase in V_e correlated value seen in NONRESPONDERS

Data from Padhani et al. [58]; Wasser et al. [60]; Pickles et al. [61]

Diffusion-Weighted Imaging with ADC Mapping

Diffusion-weighted imaging (DWI) with ADC mapping can bring additional valuable information to determine treatment response [62–64] (Fig. 9.16). ADC value has been shown to be useful in assessing both the early (after one cycle) [65, 66] and the late (after three cycles) [67] treatment response compared to tumor volume [66] and dynamic contrast-enhanced MRI parameters [68]. Typically, an increase in the ADC map value after the first cycle of treatment confers a potential pathological response. For example, reports have indicated that ADC map values with increases of 50 % were sufficient

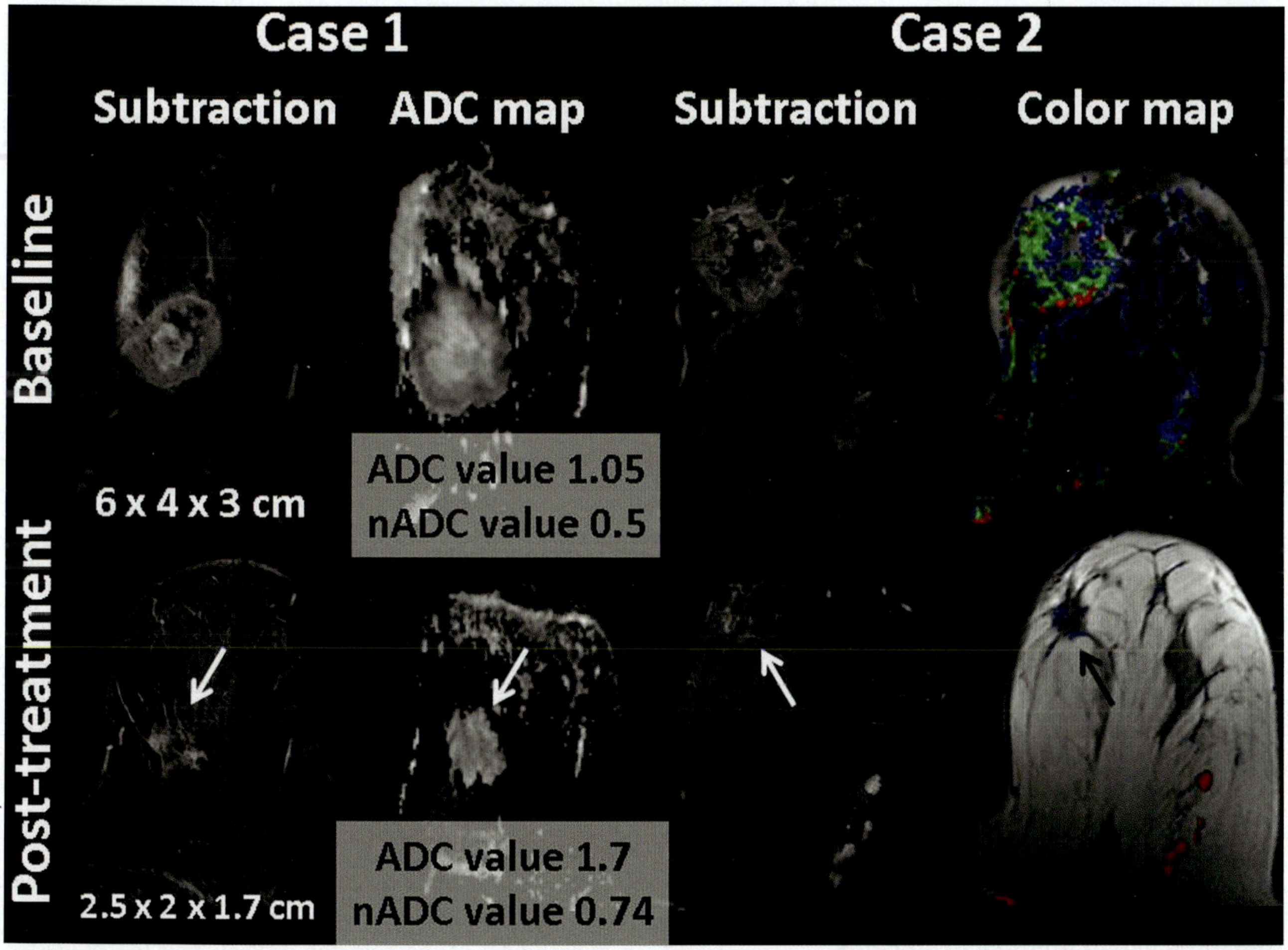

Fig. 9.16 Two examples of patients with breast cancer undergoing chemotherapy. *Case 1*: A 56-year-old female diagnosed with infiltrating ductal carcinoma with a baseline exam showing a large (6×4×3 cm) mass with rim enhancement and an ADC value of 1.05 and normalized ADC value of 0.54 (both suspicious). The post-treatment MRI exam showed significant reduction of mass size (58.3 % reduction of the unidimensional measurement and 79 % reduction of the bidimensional measurement) denoting partial response by both WHO and RECIST classifications, respectively. Both ADC and normalized ADC value showed significant increase in the post-treatment scans compared to baseline scan denoting favorable response. Patient underwent lumpectomy and pathology revealed partial response with scattered foci of carcinoma. *Case 2*: A 52-year-old female diagnosed with stage IIIA infiltrating ductal carcinoma with a baseline MRI exam revealing a large (5.6×5.2×4.1 cm) mass with rim enhancement and suspicious pharmacokinetic parameters (*top right* images (subtraction and color map)). The post-treatment exam shows complete regression of the mass (*arrow*) with significant reduction in enhancement (*bottom images*). Patient underwent lumpectomy after the breast MRI exam, and the pathology report revealed complete regression of the tumor with no neoplastic cells detected

Table 9.4 Examples and practical tips of breast MRI artifacts

Artifact	How to detect it?	How to correct it?
Improper positioning	Areas of high signal intensity where breast tissue is adjacent to coil elements	Breast should be centered within the coil
Motion	Misregistration errors in subtraction images	1. Explaining the importance of staying still to the patient 2. Ensuring a comfortable patient position 3. Sedation for claustrophobic patients
Susceptibility artifact (metallic artifact)	Local signal intensity void and distortion	1. Removing any metallic objects if possible. 2. Using titanium (MR-compatible) clips instead of the regular ferromagnetic once
Wraparound artifact	Tissues outside the FOV become superimposed on structures within the FOV	Increase FOV
Zebra artifact	Black and white bands within the image	1. Increase FOV 2. Apply phase over-sampling
Chemical shift artifact	Bright or dark band perpendicular to frequency-encoding direction at the fat and water interface	Increase bandwidth per pixel of the imaging sequence

for differentiating responders from nonresponders with high sensitivity (>90 %; 95 % CI 0.82–0.97) and moderate specificity (82 %: 95 % CI 0.70–0.9 [66, 69]).

Technical Requirements for Breast MRI

Breast MRI Scan Timing

Due to the effect of hormonal changes across the menstrual cycle on the MRI quality and different parameters such as glandular tissue enhancement and DWI, the optimal imaging time had to be determined. It is now widely accepted that the optimum time for breast MRI imaging is the second week of the menstrual cycle (between 7 and 14 days from the start of menstrual cycle), which corresponds to the proliferative phase.

Field Strength

Although 1.5 T magnetic field strength is still the most widely used in the clinical practice, more interest has been directed toward 3 T magnets to benefit from the higher magnetic field, in terms of the higher signal-to-noise ratio (SNR) and higher spatial resolution achievable in a shorter scanning time (higher temporal resolution) [70–72]. However, with the higher magnetic field come challenges such as the magnification of susceptibility and chemical shift artifacts.

Unilateral Versus Bilateral Acquisition

It is now widely accepted that bilateral image acquisition for breast MRI is more beneficial for comparison purposes, as symmetry is an important benign feature, and for detection of contralateral occult breast cancer; 4 % of women with recently diagnosed breast cancer were found to have a contralateral invasive breast cancer detected on MRI and otherwise undetectable by other breast imaging modalities [73]. The axial plane of scanning is preferable to achieve simultaneous bilateral breast visualization. It also enables acquisition with an extended field of view to include the axillary tail and axilla for lymph node assessment.

Fat Suppression Versus Subtraction

Subtraction images are the easiest way to screen the breast quickly for any enhancing lesions. The lack of enhancement has been reported to carry a very high negative predictive value, which means that a lesion that does not enhance is most probably not a cancer. However, it is important to review the original high spatial resolution post-contrast images to complete the evaluation. Some breast cancer subtypes, such as colloid cancer, tend not to enhance or enhance very weakly. Therefore, these lesions would most probably be missed if the original post-contrast images were not reviewed along with the corresponding subtraction series. Another reason to pay special attention to the high-resolution images is that morphological parameters carry the highest predictive value in cancer detection and characterization and are considered the foundation of MRI interpretation with the advanced techniques improving the specificity.

Breast MRI Artifacts

It is important to be aware of the common artifacts that might affect the accuracy of breast MRI interpretation. Table 9.4 explains some of the common artifacts and the suggested methods to correct them [74].

Temporal Resolution Versus Spatial Resolution

When developing breast MRI protocol, one of the important considerations is addressing the trade-offs between the high spatial resolution needed for morphological evaluation and high temporal resolution needed for quantitative

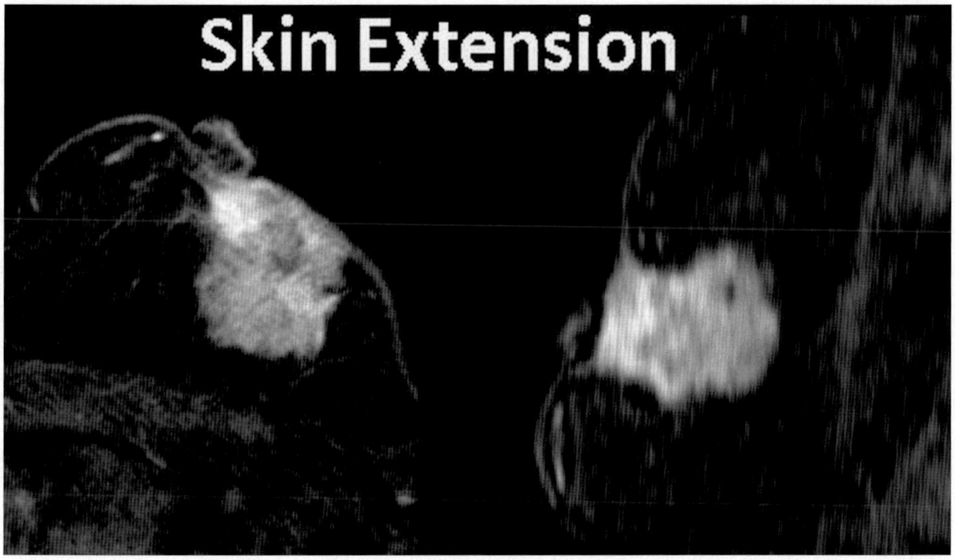

Fig. 9.17 Two views from subtraction of T1-weighted fat-suppressed postcontrast images in axial and sagittal planes demonstrate the value of MRI in the staging of breast cancer. The lesion seen on the images is a 3 cm mass extending to the skin and nipple. According to the size only, it would be assigned to a T3 category. Yet, because of the skin involvement, it should be assigned to a T4 category

assessment of perfusion with DCE-MRI. Two main approaches are widely used. The first is the trade-off approach, in which the important role of morphological characteristics of breast lesion is emphasized [6, 9, 75] with focus on the high spatial resolution image acquisition. In this approach, a modest temporal resolution is accepted for a better spatial resolution [6, 7, 17]. The second approach is the hybrid protocol approach, where two sets of pre-/postcontrast images are acquired: one with the high spatial and one with the high temporal resolution. In this approach, there is a gap in the DCE series created to acquire postcontrast high spatial resolution images. One of the important factors that increased the need to this approach is the introduction of the pharmacokinetic modeling techniques [76–78]. Pharmacokinetic analysis accuracy has been always linked to the need for a high temporal resolution acquisition (<20 s/acquisition) [27, 76–79].

Gadolinium Contrast Agent

There are many contrast agents available with different relaxivities. MRI contrast shortens the T1 time of the tissue which results in higher signals on T1 weighted. The type of contrast and magnetic field may affect the contrast enhancement of tissues, especially when pharmacokinetic analysis is performed. *Nephrogenic systemic fibrosis* (*NSF*) or nephrogenic fibrosing dermatopathy is a newly discovered (in 1997) rare but serious syndrome that has been associated with the administration of gadolinium-based contrast agents in patients with impaired kidney functions that involve skin, joints, and other organs. It was also connected to administering higher doses of contrast (multiple standard doses). To prevent the occurrence of this syndrome, the ACR Committee on MR Safety [80] recommended that glomerular filtration rate (GFR) has to be measured within 1 month of the examination and should be >60 for certain patient groups before the administration of gadolinium contrast to them (age of 60 years and above, diabetes, hypertension, systemic lupus erythematosus, history of renal disease, liver disease, multiple myeloma).

Staging

Breast MRI can offer valuable information that can significantly affect the overall staging decision as it provides [81, 82] accurate size assessment which is important in the determination of the T component of the tumor nodes metastasis (TNM) classification system. MRI has a very high sensitivity in assessing the extent of tumor to the chest wall and skin. Tumors of any size that extend to the chest wall or skin are assigned the highest T category (T4) in the TNM classification system (Fig. 9.17). Lymph node (LN) assessment is a basic part of the TNM classification. MRI can provide information on the axillary as well as internal mammary lymph node features and raise suspicion toward LN metastasis. The sentinel node and histopathologic examination remain the gold standard that is clinically accepted for final staging.

MR-Guided Biopsy

The need for MRI-guided biopsy procedure originated from the MRI's ability to detect two breast lesion categories that are not detectable by other modalities, such as small breast lesions (even 1 mm) and non-mass-like enhancement (NMLE).

The accuracy of MRI-guided core biopsy is high, ranging from 95 to 100 % with cancer yield ranging from 5 to 61 % depending on the patient population.

MRI-Guided Breast Biopsy Technique (Fig. 9.15)

Different devices and software are available for breast MRI-guided biopsy and clip placement [83, 84]. There are, however, a few basic steps that are applied routinely regardless of the technical differences. These are as follows:

1. Patients are usually positioned in prone position for a lateral approach with mild breast compression with a grid plate.
2. While positioning the patient, sterile skin preparation of the breast with the index lesions is performed.
3. An MR marker is placed on one of the grid holes expected to be far from the lesion location to be then used as a reference during the biopsy planning.
4. Initial localizing scans, sagittal T1 non-fat-suppressed scan, and axial pre- and post-contrast 3DT1-weighted GRE acquisitions are obtained for target lesion localization.
5. Multiplanar planning of the biopsy on a 3D workstation is used with mapping of the target to the external compression grid.
6. An introducer is advanced to the target lesion with confirmation of correct position of the introducer tip on repeated axial 3DT1 scan.
7. After acquiring the tissue specimens with vacuum biopsy devices, a clip is placed at the biopsy site.
8. Finally, a post-biopsy scan is acquired to confirm the location of the clip for future reference.

Summary

Breast MRI has gained a wide acceptance in the clinical breast imaging community because of its extremely high sensitivity, improved specificity, and the unique functional information that it provides without exposing women to the harmful ionizing radiation. The side effects of the gadolinium-based contrast agent can be avoided with a proper clinical screening. Breast MRI is the only MRI exam clinically used for screening purposes since the issuing of the National Cancer Association guideline in 2007 that recommended using MRI as an adjunct to mammography for breast cancer annual screening in high-risk women. Beside breast lesion detection and characterization, breast MRI offers an excellent tool for pretreatment assessment as well as treatment response evaluation of breast cancer. MRI offers not only the standard temporal assessment of size change but also a method for temporal assessment of change in functional parameters during and after the completion of treatment. Breast MRI is a fast developing tool with large opportunities for introduction of new imaging sequences, post-processing tools, and novel contrast agents for improved breast tissue characterization.

References

1. Glunde K, Jacobs MA, Pathak AP, Artemov D, Bhujwalla ZM. Molecular and functional imaging of breast cancer. NMR Biomed. 2009;22(1):92–103.
2. Kerlikowske K, Cook AJ, Buist DS, Cummings SR, Vachon C, Vacek P, et al. Breast cancer risk by breast density, menopause, and postmenopausal hormone therapy use. J Clin Oncol. 2010;28(24):3830–7.
3. McCormack VA, dos Santos Silva I. Breast density and parenchymal patterns as markers of breast cancer risk: a meta-analysis. Cancer Epidemiol Biomarkers Prev. 2006;15(6):1159–69.
4. Yaghjyan L, Colditz GA, Collins LC, Schnitt SJ, Rosner B, Vachon C, et al. Mammographic breast density and subsequent risk of breast cancer in postmenopausal women according to tumor characteristics. J Natl Cancer Inst. 2011;103(15):1179–89.
5. American College of Radiology. Breast imaging and reporting data system. 5th ed. Reston: American College of Radiology; 2004.
6. Nunes LW, Schnall MD, Orel SG. Update of breast MR imaging architectural interpretation model. Radiology. 2001;219(2):484–94.
7. Schnall MD, Rosten S, Englander S, Orel SG, Nunes LW. A combined architectural and kinetic interpretation model for breast MR images. Acad Radiol. 2001;8(7):591–7.
8. Liberman L, Morris EA, Lee MJ, Kaplan JB, LaTrenta LR, Menell JH, et al. Breast lesions detected on MR imaging: features and positive predictive value. AJR Am J Roentgenol. 2002;179(1):171–8.
9. Nunes LW, Schnall MD, Siegelman ES, Langlotz CP, Orel SG, Sullivan D, et al. Diagnostic performance characteristics of architectural features revealed by high spatial-resolution MR imaging of the breast. AJR Am J Roentgenol. 1997;169(2):409–15.
10. Morakkabati-Spitz N, Leutner C, Schild H, Traeber F, Kuhl C. Diagnostic usefulness of segmental and linear enhancement in dynamic breast MRI. Eur Radiol. 2005;15(9):2010–7.
11. Bluemke DA, Gatsonis CA, Chen MH, DeAngelis GA, DeBruhl N, Harms S, et al. Magnetic resonance imaging of the breast prior to biopsy. JAMA. 2004;292(22):2735–42.
12. El Khouli RH, Macura KJ, Kamel IR, Jacobs MA, Bluemke DA. 3-T dynamic contrast-enhanced MRI of the breast: pharmacokinetic parameters versus conventional kinetic curve analysis. AJR Am J Roentgenol. 2011;197(6):1498–505.
13. Kaiser WA, Zeitler E. MR imaging of the breast: fast imaging sequences with and without Gd-DTPA. Preliminary observations. Radiology. 1989;170(3 Pt 1):681–6.
14. Kinkel K, Helbich TH, Esserman LJ, Barclay J, Schwerin EH, Sickles EA, et al. Dynamic high-spatial-resolution MR imaging of suspicious breast lesions: diagnostic criteria and interobserver variability. AJR Am J Roentgenol. 2000;175(1):35–43.
15. Kuhl CK, Mielcareck P, Klaschik S, Leutner C, Wardelmann E, Gieseke J, et al. Dynamic breast MR imaging: are signal intensity time course data useful for differential diagnosis of enhancing lesions? Radiology. 1999;211(1):101–10.
16. Kaiser WA, Deimling M. [A new multislice measurement sequence for the complete dynamic MR examination of the larger organs: application to the breast]. Eine neue Multischicht-Messsequenz fur die komplette dynamische MR-Untersuchung an grosseren Organen: Anwendung an der Brust. Rofo. 1990;152(5):577–82.
17. Kuhl CK, Schild HH, Morakkabati N. Dynamic bilateral contrast-enhanced MR imaging of the breast: trade-off between spatial and temporal resolution. Radiology. 2005;236(3):789–800.
18. El Khouli RH, Macura KJ, Jacobs MA, Khalil TH, Kamel IR, Dwyer A, et al. Dynamic contrast-enhanced MRI of the breast: quantitative method for kinetic curve type assessment. AJR Am J Roentgenol. 2009;193(4):W295–300.
19. Boetes C, Barentsz JO, Mus RD, van der Sluis RF, van Erning LJ, Hendriks JH, et al. MR characterization of suspicious breast lesions

with a gadolinium-enhanced TurboFLASH subtraction technique. Radiology. 1994;193(3):777–81.
20. Mahfouz AE, Sherif H, Saad A, Taupitz M, Filimonow S, Kivelitz D, et al. Gadolinium-enhanced MR angiography of the breast: is breast cancer associated with ipsilateral higher vascularity? Eur Radiol. 2001;11(6):965–9.
21. Sardanelli F, Iozzelli A, Fausto A, Carriero A, Kirchin MA. Gadobenate dimeglumine-enhanced MR imaging breast vascular maps: association between invasive cancer and ipsilateral increased vascularity. Radiology. 2005;235(3):791–7.
22. Jackson A, O'Connor JP, Parker GJ, Jayson GC. Imaging tumor vascular heterogeneity and angiogenesis using dynamic contrast-enhanced magnetic resonance imaging. Clin Cancer Res. 2007; 13(12):3449–59.
23. O'Connor JP, Jackson A, Parker GJ, Jayson GC. DCE-MRI biomarkers in the clinical evaluation of antiangiogenic and vascular disrupting agents. Br J Cancer. 2007;96(2):189–95.
24. Brix G, Semmler W, Port R, Schad LR, Layer G, Lorenz WJ. Pharmacokinetic parameters in CNS Gd-DTPA enhanced MR imaging. J Comput Assist Tomogr. 1991;15(4):621–8.
25. Taylor JS, Tofts PS, Port R, Evelhoch JL, Knopp M, Reddick WE, et al. MR imaging of tumor microcirculation: promise for the new millennium. J Magn Reson Imaging. 1999;10(6):903–7.
26. Evelhoch JL. Key factors in the acquisition of contrast kinetic data for oncology. J Magn Reson Imaging. 1999;10(3):254–9.
27. Tofts PS, Brix G, Buckley DL, Evelhoch JL, Henderson E, Knopp MV, et al. Estimating kinetic parameters from dynamic contrast-enhanced T(1)-weighted MRI of a diffusable tracer: standardized quantities and symbols. J Magn Reson Imaging. 1999;10(3): 223–32.
28. Parker GJ, Roberts C, Macdonald A, Buonaccorsi GA, Cheung S, Buckley DL, et al. Experimentally-derived functional form for a population-averaged high-temporal-resolution arterial input function for dynamic contrast-enhanced MRI. Magn Reson Med. 2006;56(5):993–1000.
29. Buonaccorsi GA, Roberts C, Cheung S, Watson Y, O'Connor JP, Davies K, et al. Comparison of the performance of tracer kinetic model-driven registration for dynamic contrast enhanced MRI using different models of contrast enhancement. Acad Radiol. 2006;13(9):1112–23.
30. Roberts C, Issa B, Stone A, Jackson A, Waterton JC, Parker GJ. Comparative study into the robustness of compartmental modeling and model-free analysis in DCE-MRI studies. J Magn Reson Imaging. 2006;23(4):554–63.
31. Huang W, Li X, Morris EA, Tudorica LA, Seshan VE, Rooney WD, et al. The magnetic resonance shutter speed discriminates vascular properties of malignant and benign breast tumors in vivo. Proc Natl Acad Sci U S A. 2008;105(46):17943–8.
32. Haris M, Husain N, Singh A, Awasthi R, Singh Rathore RK, Husain M, et al. Dynamic contrast-enhanced (DCE) derived transfer coefficient (ktrans) is a surrogate marker of matrix metalloproteinase 9 (MMP-9) expression in brain tuberculomas. J Magn Reson Imaging. 2008;28(3):588–97.
33. Yankeelov TE, Luci JJ, Lepage M, Li R, Debusk L, Lin PC, et al. Quantitative pharmacokinetic analysis of DCE-MRI data without an arterial input function: a reference region model. Magn Reson Imaging. 2005;23(4):519–29.
34. Yankeelov TE, Rooney WD, Huang W, Dyke JP, Li X, Tudorica A, et al. Evidence for shutter-speed variation in CR bolus-tracking studies of human pathology. NMR Biomed. 2005;18(3):173–85.
35. Jackson A, Jayson GC, Li KL, Zhu XP, Checkley DR, Tessier JJ, et al. Reproducibility of quantitative dynamic contrast-enhanced MRI in newly presenting glioma. Br J Radiol. 2003;76(903):153–62.
36. Bhujwalla ZM, Artemov D, Glockner J. Tumor angiogenesis, vascularization, and contrast-enhanced magnetic resonance imaging. Top Magn Reson Imaging. 1999;10(2):92–103.
37. Mussurakis S, Buckley DL, Horsman A. Dynamic MRI of invasive breast cancer: assessment of three region-of-interest analysis methods. J Comput Assist Tomogr. 1997;21(3):431–8.
38. Le Bihan D, Breton E, Lallemand D, Grenier P, Cabanis E, Laval-Jeantet M. MR imaging of intravoxel incoherent motions: application to diffusion and perfusion in neurologic disorders. Radiology. 1986;161(2):401–7.
39. Englander SA, Ulug AM, Brem R, Glickson JD, van Zijl PC. Diffusion imaging of human breast. NMR Biomed. 1997; 10(7):348–52.
40. Guo Y, Cai YQ, Cai ZL, Gao YG, An NY, Ma L, et al. Differentiation of clinically benign and malignant breast lesions using diffusion-weighted imaging. J Magn Reson Imaging. 2002;16(2):172–8.
41. Sinha S, Lucas-Quesada FA, Sinha U, DeBruhl N, Bassett LW. In vivo diffusion-weighted MRI of the breast: potential for lesion characterization. J Magn Reson Imaging. 2002;15(6):693–704.
42. Woodhams R, Matsunaga K, Iwabuchi K, Kan S, Hata H, Kuranami M, et al. Diffusion-weighted imaging of malignant breast tumors: the usefulness of apparent diffusion coefficient (ADC) value and ADC map for the detection of malignant breast tumors and evaluation of cancer extension. J Comput Assist Tomogr. 2005; 29(5):644–9.
43. Woodhams R, Matsunaga K, Kan S, Hata H, Ozaki M, Iwabuchi K, et al. ADC mapping of benign and malignant breast tumors. Magn Reson Med Sci. 2005;4(1):35–42.
44. Park MJ, Cha ES, Kang BJ, Ihn YK, Baik JH. The role of diffusion-weighted imaging and the apparent diffusion coefficient (ADC) values for breast tumors. Korean J Radiol. 2007;8(5):390–6.
45. Ei Khouli RH, Jacobs MA, Mezban SD, Huang P, Kamel IR, Macura KJ, et al. Diffusion-weighted imaging improves the diagnostic accuracy of conventional 3.0-T breast MR imaging. Radiology. 2010;256(1):64–73.
46. Pereira FP, Martins G, Figueiredo E, Domingues MN, Domingues RC, da Fonseca LM, et al. Assessment of breast lesions with diffusion-weighted MRI: comparing the use of different b values. AJR Am J Roentgenol. 2009;193(4):1030–5.
47. Bogner W, Gruber S, Pinker K, Grabner G, Stadlbauer A, Weber M, et al. Diffusion-weighted MR for differentiation of breast lesions at 3.0 T: how does selection of diffusion protocols affect diagnosis? Radiology. 2009;253(2):341–51.
48. Marini C, Iacconi C, Giannelli M, Cilotti A, Moretti M, Bartolozzi C. Quantitative diffusion-weighted MR imaging in the differential diagnosis of breast lesion. Eur Radiol. 2007;17(10):2646–55.
49. Partridge SC, McKinnon GC, Henry RG, Hylton NM. Menstrual cycle variation of apparent diffusion coefficients measured in the normal breast using MRI. J Magn Reson Imaging. 2001;14(4):433–8.
50. James K, Eisenhauer E, Christian M, Terenziani M, Vena D, Muldal A, et al. Measuring response in solid tumors: unidimensional versus bidimensional measurement. J Natl Cancer Inst. 1999;91(6):523–8.
51. Therasse P. Measuring the clinical response. What does it mean? Eur J Cancer. 2002;38(14):1817–23.
52. Tran LN, Brown MS, Goldin JG, Yan X, Pais RC, McNitt-Gray MF, et al. Comparison of treatment response classifications between unidimensional, bidimensional, and volumetric measurements of metastatic lung lesions on chest computed tomography. Acad Radiol. 2004;11(12):1355–60.
53. Park JO, Lee SI, Song SY, Kim K, Kim WS, Jung CW, et al. Measuring response in solid tumors: comparison of RECIST and WHO response criteria. Jpn J Clin Oncol. 2003;33(10):533–7.
54. Partridge SC, Gibbs JE, Lu Y, Esserman LJ, Tripathy D, Wolverton DS, et al. MRI measurements of breast tumor volume predict response to neoadjuvant chemotherapy and recurrence-free survival. AJR Am J Roentgenol. 2005;184(6):1774–81.
55. Jacobs MA, Stearns V, Wolff AC, Macura K, Argani P, Khouri N, et al. Multiparametric magnetic resonance imaging, spectroscopy and multinuclear ((2)(3)Na) imaging monitoring of preoperative

chemotherapy for locally advanced breast cancer. Acad Radiol. 2010;17(12):1477–85.
56. Marinovich ML, Sardanelli F, Ciatto S, Mamounas E, Brennan M, Macaskill P, et al. Early prediction of pathologic response to neoadjuvant therapy in breast cancer: systematic review of the accuracy of MRI. Breast. 2012;21(5):669–77.
57. Wiener JI, Schilling KJ, Adami C, Obuchowski NA. Assessment of suspected breast cancer by MRI: a prospective clinical trial using a combined kinetic and morphologic analysis. AJR Am J Roentgenol. 2005;184(3):878–86.
58. Padhani AR, Hayes C, Assersohn L, Powles T, Makris A, Suckling J, et al. Prediction of clinicopathologic response of breast cancer to primary chemotherapy at contrast-enhanced MR imaging: initial clinical results. Radiology. 2006;239(2):361–74.
59. Jacobs MA, Ouwerkerk R, Wolff AC, Gabrielson E, Warzecha H, Jeter S, et al. Monitoring of neoadjuvant chemotherapy using multiparametric, (2)(3)Na sodium MR, and multimodality (PET/CT/MRI) imaging in locally advanced breast cancer. Breast Cancer Res Treat. 2011;128(1):119–26.
60. Wasser K, Klein SK, Fink C, Junkermann H, Sinn HP, Zuna I, et al. Evaluation of neoadjuvant chemotherapeutic response of breast cancer using dynamic MRI with high temporal resolution. Eur Radiol. 2003;13(1):80–7.
61. Pickles MD, Lowry M, Manton DJ, Gibbs P, Turnbull LW. Role of dynamic contrast enhanced MRI in monitoring early response of locally advanced breast cancer to neoadjuvant chemotherapy. Breast Cancer Res Treat. 2005;91(1):1–10.
62. Malayeri AA, El Khouli RH, Zaheer A, Jacobs MA, Corona-Villalobos CP, Kamel IR, et al. Principles and applications of diffusion-weighted imaging in cancer detection, staging, and treatment follow-up. Radiographics. 2011;31(6):1773–91.
63. Chenevert TL, Stegman LD, Taylor JM, Robertson PL, Greenberg HS, Rehemtulla A, et al. Diffusion magnetic resonance imaging: an early surrogate marker of therapeutic efficacy in brain tumors. J Natl Cancer Inst. 2000;92(24):2029–36.
64. Chenevert TL, Meyer CR, Moffat BA, Rehemtulla A, Mukherji SK, Gebarski SS, et al. Diffusion MRI: a new strategy for assessment of cancer therapeutic efficacy. Mol Imaging. 2002;1(4): 336–43.
65. Partridge SC, DeMartini WB, Kurland BF, Eby PR, White SW, Lehman CD. Quantitative diffusion-weighted imaging as an adjunct to conventional breast MRI for improved positive predictive value. AJR Am J Roentgenol. 2009;193(6):1716–22.
66. Sharma U, Danishad KK, Seenu V, Jagannathan NR. Longitudinal study of the assessment by MRI and diffusion-weighted imaging of tumor response in patients with locally advanced breast cancer undergoing neoadjuvant chemotherapy. NMR Biomed. 2009;22(1): 104–13.
67. Park SH, Moon WK, Cho N, Song IC, Chang JM, Park IA, et al. Diffusion-weighted MR imaging: pretreatment prediction of response to neoadjuvant chemotherapy in patients with breast cancer. Radiology. 2010;257(1):56–63.
68. Woodhams R, Kakita S, Hata H, Iwabuchi K, Kuranami M, Gautam S, et al. Identification of residual breast carcinoma following neoadjuvant chemotherapy: diffusion-weighted imaging – comparison with contrast-enhanced MR imaging and pathologic findings. Radiology. 2010;254(2):357–66.
69. Wu LM, Hu JN, Gu HY, Hua J, Chen J, Xu JR. Can diffusion-weighted MR imaging and contrast-enhanced MR imaging precisely evaluate and predict pathological response to neoadjuvant chemotherapy in patients with breast cancer? Breast Cancer Res Treat. 2012;135(1):17–28.
70. Kuhl CK, Jost P, Morakkabati N, Zivanovic O, Schild HH, Gieseke J. Contrast-enhanced MR imaging of the breast at 3.0 and 1.5 T in the same patients: initial experience. Radiology. 2006;239(3): 666–76.
71. Rakow-Penner R, Daniel B, Yu H, Sawyer-Glover A, Glover GH. Relaxation times of breast tissue at 1.5 T and 3 T measured using IDEAL. J Magn Reson Imaging. 2006;23(1):87–91.
72. Rausch DR, Hendrick RE. How to optimize clinical breast MR imaging practices and techniques on Your 1.5-T system. Radiographics. 2006;26(5):1469–84.
73. Lehman CD, Blume JD, Thickman D, Bluemke DA, Pisano E, Kuhl C, et al. Added cancer yield of MRI in screening the contralateral breast of women recently diagnosed with breast cancer: results from the International Breast Magnetic Resonance Consortium (IBMC) trial. J Surg Oncol. 2005;92(1):9–15; discussion 15 6.
74. Harvey JA, Hendrick RE, Coll JM, Nicholson BT, Burkholder BT, Cohen MA. Breast MR imaging artifacts: how to recognize and fix them. Radiographics. 2007;27 Suppl 1:S131–45.
75. Nunes LW, Schnall MD, Orel SG, Hochman MG, Langlotz CP, Reynolds CA, et al. Breast MR imaging: interpretation model. Radiology. 1997;202(3):833–41.
76. Tofts PS. Modeling tracer kinetics in dynamic Gd-DTPA MR imaging. J Magn Reson Imaging. 1997;7(1):91–101.
77. Tofts PS, Berkowitz B, Schnall MD. Quantitative analysis of dynamic Gd-DTPA enhancement in breast tumors using a permeability model. Magn Reson Med. 1995;33(4):564–8.
78. Collins DJ, Padhani AR. Dynamic magnetic resonance imaging of tumor perfusion. Approaches and biomedical challenges. IEEE Eng Med Biol Mag. 2004;23(5):65–83.
79. Dale BM, Jesberger JA, Lewin JS, Hillenbrand CM, Duerk JL. Determining and optimizing the precision of quantitative measurements of perfusion from dynamic contrast enhanced MRI. J Magn Reson Imaging. 2003;18(5):575–84.
80. Kanal E, Barkovich AJ, Bell C, Borgstede JP, Bradley Jr WG, Froelich JW, et al. ACR guidance document for safe MR practices: 2007. AJR Am J Roentgenol. 2007;188(6):1447–74.
81. Braun M, Polcher M, Schrading S, Zivanovic O, Kowalski T, Flucke U, et al. Influence of preoperative MRI on the surgical management of patients with operable breast cancer. Breast Cancer Res Treat. 2008;111(1):179–87.
82. Mameri CS, Kemp C, Goldman SM, Sobral LA, Ajzen S. Impact of breast MRI on surgical treatment, axillary approach, and systemic therapy for breast cancer. Breast J. 2008;14(3):236–44.
83. Meeuwis C, Veltman J, van Hall HN, Mus RD, Boetes C, Barentsz JO, et al. MR-guided breast biopsy at 3 T: diagnostic yield of large core needle biopsy compared with vacuum-assisted biopsy. Eur Radiol. 2012;22(2):341–9.
84. El Khouli RH, Macura KJ, Barker PB, Elkady LM, Jacobs MA, Vogel-Claussen J, et al. MRI-guided vacuum-assisted breast biopsy: a phantom and patient evaluation of targeting accuracy. J Magn Reson Imaging. 2009;30(2):424–9.

Optimizing Mammographic Screening and Diagnosis of Breast Cancer

10

Mahesh K. Shetty

Introduction

A robust quality assurance mechanism needs to be in place and rigorously enforced to ensure consistently high-quality screening mammography. Such a quality assurance program has three principal components, namely, the mammographic equipment, image quality issues, and interpretative accuracy. There are regulatory processes in place at both the national and state levels mandated by law that are aimed at achieving this objective [1–3], and these are presented in these direct citations that follow:

> The Mammography Quality Standards Act (MQSA) was passed by the United States Congress on October 27, 1992, to establish national quality standards for mammography. The MQSA requires that to provide mammography services legally after October 1, 1994, all facilities, except facilities of the Department of Veterans Affairs, must be accredited by an approved accreditation body and certified by the Secretary of Health and Human Services (the Secretary). The authority to approve accreditation bodies and to certify facilities was delegated by the Secretary to the FDA (Food and drug administration). [1]
> The FDA is responsible for developing final standards, approving accrediting bodies, certifying all mammography facilities in the U.S., evaluating the effectiveness of the program, and implementing sanctions for noncompliant facilities. FDA is allowed to adopt existing standards from the American College of Radiology [ACR], HCFA [Health care financing Administration] and state regulations. The final Rules have additional changes in the Quality Assurance (QA) Sections (900.12 d and e) and direct facilities as to how to conduct document and evaluate the results of Quality assurance [QA] tests, taking responsibility for establishing and maintaining a QA program. [1]
> The FDA [Food and Drug Administration] uses mandatory language, such as shall, must, and require, when referring to statutory or regulatory requirements. The FDA uses non-mandatory language, such as should, may, can, and recommend when referring to guidance. It is the responsibility of the facility to read, understand, and follow the final regulations. Under its own authority, a State may impose more stringent requirements beyond those specified under MQSA and its implementing regulations. A facility needs to check with the State or local authorities regarding their requirements. [1]
> MQSA aims to ensure safety, reliability, clarity and accuracy of the mammography services performed in each and every facility in the USA. The rules also specify the roles of interpreting physicians, medical physicists and quality control technologists. Data indicates that such regulation has improved mammography in the U.S. By January 1997, the Government Accounting Office reported that 1,500 facilities had undergone two rounds of MQSA inspections. During the first year of MQSA, 26 percent had significant violations, while only 10 percent did on the second round. [2]
> The MQSA regulations are written by the FDA and are the national standards for quality of Mammography services. Adherence to these stated standards is the law and not optional. For lawful operation each facility and the Mammography unit has to be certified. [1]
> To obtain this certificate the facility has to fulfill the quality standards that is outlined in the section 900.12 of the final rule, in addition each facility has to be accredited by an approved entity which is designated by FDA. Currently the American College of Radiology and the States of Texas, Arkansas, Iowa and California have been authorized by MQSA to be the accreditation bodies, the State bodies are allowed to accredit facilities in their respective states. The accreditation body is responsible for reviewing the equipment, procedures, personnel and the Medical Physicist. Personnel including the radiologist and the technologists are reviewed to ensure compliance in qualifications and training as required by MQSA regulations. The physicist survey of the equipment includes dosimetry, quality control tests on the equipment, evaluation of the phantom images as well as clinical images of patients. Based on a facility fulfilling all of the requirements outlined in the MQSA, the accreditation process is complete. The accreditation body notifies the MQSA and the latter body issues a certificate. This certificate is valid for three years. However, annual inspection is conducted by the MQSA to ensure continued compliance. [1]

Certification for Interpreting Physicians and Radiologic Technologists

The following is an outline of the requirements as stated in the MQSA manual describing the requirements of the various components to obtain MQSA certification to operate a

M.K. Shetty, MD, FRCR, FACR, FAIUM
Department of Radiology, Baylor College of Medicine, Houston, TX, USA

Woman's Center for Breast Care and MRI, Woman's Hospital of Texas, Fannin 7600, Houston, TX 77054, USA
e-mail: mshettymd@gmail.com

M.K. Shetty (ed.), *Breast Cancer Screening and Diagnosis: A Synopsis*,
DOI 10.1007/978-1-4939-1267-4_10, © Springer Science+Business Media New York 2015

mammography unit and provide screening and diagnostic mammography to patients [1]:

Interpreting Physicians

Interpreting physicians initially qualifying on or after the April 28, 1999 effective date of the final regulations must meet all of the following requirements. Physicians who qualified under FDA's interim regulations (prior to April 28, 1999) are considered to have met the initial requirements listed in items 2 through 4. They may continue to interpret mammograms if they continue to meet the licensure requirement in item 1, the new modality training requirement for item 5 (if applicable), and the continuing experience and continuing education requirements for items 6 and 7.

1. **Licensure**: Be licensed to practice medicine in a State.

AND

2. a. **Board Certification**: Be certified in radiology or diagnostic radiology by any of the following bodies:
   - The American Board of Radiology (ABR)
   - The American Osteopathic Board of Radiology (AOBR)
   - The Royal College of Physicians and Surgeons of Canada (RCPSC)

   OR

   b. **Initial Training**: Have had at least 3 months of documented formal training in the interpretation of mammograms and in topics related to mammography (to include instruction in radiation physics, including radiation physics specific to mammography, radiation effects, and radiation physics.

AND

3. **Initial Category I Education**: Have a minimum of 60 hours of documented category I medical education in mammography (including instruction in the interpretation of mammograms and education in basic breast anatomy, pathology, physiology, technical aspects of mammography, and quality assurance and quality control in mammography). At least 15 of the required 60 hours must have been acquired within the 3 years immediately before the physician's initial qualification date. These 60 hours may be included in the 3 months of training specified in 2.b. Hours received in residency training are considered equivalent to category I.

AND

4. **Initial Experience**: Have interpreted or multi-read, under direct supervision of a qualified interpreting physician, at least 240 mammographic examinations within the 6-month period immediately before the date that the physician qualifies as an interpreting physician (or in any 6-month period during the last 2 years of a diagnostic radiology residency for physicians who become appropriately board certified at the first allowable time, as defined by the board).

AND

5. **New Mammographic Modality**: Before an interpreting physician may begin independently interpreting mammograms produced by any mammographic modality in which the interpreting physician was not previously trained (e.g., xeromammography, digital mammography, screen-film mammography), the physician must have at least 8 hours of training in that mammographic modality.

AND

6. **Continuing Experience**: Have interpreted or multi-read at least 960 mammographic examinations during the 24 months immediately preceding the date of the facility's annual MQSA inspection, or the last day of the calendar quarter preceding the inspection, or any date in between the two.

   The beginning date for meeting the continuing experience requirement is the later of October 1, 1994, or the individual's actual starting date (the date on which an individual met all applicable requirements to begin independently providing mammography services). Failure to meet the continuing experience requirement will not be considered a noncompliance until at least 24 months after the individual's starting date.

AND

7. **Continuing Education**: Have taught or completed at least 15 category I continuing medical education (CME) credits in mammography during the 36 months immediately preceding the date of the facility's annual MQSA inspection, or the last day of the calendar quarter preceding the inspection, or any date in between the two. CME credits earned through teaching a course can be counted only once toward meeting the 15 credits required in any 36-month period. Such training shall include at least 6 credits of category I CME in each mammographic modality used by the interpreting physician. *The beginning date for meeting the continuing education requirement is the later of October 1, 1994, or the individual's actual starting date (the date on which an individual met all applicable requirement to begin independently providing mammography services). Failure to meet the continuing education requirement will not be considered a noncompliance until at least 36 months after the individual's starting date.*

   FDA permits multi-reading/interpreting of mammograms and summing of readings/interpretations from different facilities in calculating the total mammographic examinations for items 4 and 6. Multi-reading is defined as two or more physicians, at least one of whom is a fully qualified interpreting physician, interpreting the same mammogram. Multi-reading includes reading comparison mammograms not previously read by the physician. So that facilities are aware of potential problems, FDA recommends that facilities update education and experience records at least quarterly." [1]

Radiologic Technologist

Radiologic technologists initially qualifying on or after the April 28, 1999 effective date of the final regulations must meet all of the following requirements. Radiologic technologists, who qualified under FDA's interim regulations (before April 28, 1999), are considered to have met the initial training requirements listed in item 2. They may continue to perform mammograms if they continue to meet the licensure or certification requirements of item 1, any applicable new modality training requirement from item 3, and the continuing experience and education requirements of items 4 and 5.

1. a. **Licensure**: Have a general/full license to perform radiographic procedures issued by a State.

   OR

   b. **Board Certification**: Be certified by either of the following bodies:
   - The American Registry of Radiologic Technologists (ARRT)
   - The American Registry of Clinical Radiography Technologists (ARCRT)

AND

2. **Initial Training in Mammography**: Have at least 40 contact hours of mammography training, including breast

anatomy, physiology, positioning, compression, quality assurance/quality control techniques, imaging of patients with breast implants, and the performance of 25 supervised examinations. The actual time spent performing supervised examinations may be included in the 40 hour total. As guidance, however, no more than 12.5 hours of the required 40 should come from the performance of examinations.

AND

3. **New Mammographic Modality**: Before a radiologic technologist may independently perform mammographic examinations using any mammographic modality in which the radiologic technologist was not previously trained (e.g., xeromammography, digital mammography, screen-film mammography), the radiologic technologist must have at least 8 hours of training in the modality.

AND

4. **Continuing Experience**: Have performed a minimum of 200 mammography examinations during the 24 months immediately preceding the date of the facility's annual MQSA inspection, or the last day of the calendar quarter preceding the inspection, or any date in between the two.

AND

5. **Continuing Education**: Have taught or completed at least 15 continuing education units in mammography during the 36 months immediately preceding the date of the facility's annual MQSA inspection, or the last day of the calendar quarter preceding the inspection, or any date in between the two. At least 6 of these CEUs must be in each of the mammographic modalities used by the technologist. CEUs earned through teaching a course can be counted only once towards meeting the units required in any 36-month period.

The beginning date for meeting the continuing education requirements is the later of October 1, 1994, or the individual's actual starting date (date on which the individual initially qualifies to work independently), whichever is later. Failure to meet the continuing education requirements will not be considered a noncompliance until at least 36 months after the technologist's starting date. [1]

Regulations for Medical Records

The following is an outline of the requirements as stated in the MQSA manual describing the requirements of the various components to obtain MQSA certification as regards patient permanent records [1]:

Patient Permanent Records

Medical records must contain certain required types of information. To ensure that both the mammographic images and reports are being retained as required, and to verify they contain the information outlined in this section, the inspector will randomly select records for review. In general, the inspector will request reports from those examinations performed since the last MQSA inspection, or since the facility's certification, whichever is the most recent. However, inspectors may examine records from other time frames. The inspector will not attempt to assess the correctness of these reports, but will determine that the records are being generated, properly maintained and identify the interpreting physician who originally interpreted the mammograms. For those mammography medical reports created on or after April 28, 1999, the inspector will also verify that one of the following assessment categories appears in each: "Negative," "Benign," "Probably Benign," "Suspicious," "Highly suggestive of malignancy," or "Incomplete: Need additional imaging evaluation."

These are based on the assessment categories as outlined in the American College of Radiology BI-RADS™ atlas [4].

The facility is also required to communicate the results, within 30 days of the examination, to the referring health care provider and to the patient (lay summary). In the case of self-referred patients, if a health care provider (or a responsible designee) is not named or is unavailable, then the report must be provided to the patient. Communications to the patient, if there is no health care provider, must include (1) the complete report of findings referenced previously and (2) the summary written in lay terms that is required for all patients.

When the assessment is "Suspicious" or "Highly suggestive of malignancy," the facility is required to communicate the results, as soon as possible, to the referring health care provider and to the patient (lay summary) and depending on health care provider availability, may need to send the complete report to the patient). Facility personnel should be prepared to explain the facility's procedure for communicating results to referring physicians and to patients and their mechanism for providing quick response for cases requiring such action.

FDA's concern is not the details of the communication system but rather:

- that one has been established by the facility,
- that it is in place, and
- that it meets the requirements of the regulations.

The inspector will verify that the communication system meets these criteria and that lay summaries are available. If patient records are stored in an electronic format, the inspector will ask the facility to assist in the selection and retrieval of the records to be inspected. The inspector will also examine the audit system for the inclusion of the previously-mentioned items, ascertain how biopsy results are obtained, and request to see examples of biopsy results that the facility has obtained. If biopsies were recommended but no results were obtained, the facility must provide documentation of attempts to get this information. [1]

Follow-Up for Additional Imaging or Biopsy

Most facilities perform significantly better than required under MQSA in following up after a recommendation for additional imaging or for a biopsy after a diagnostic work-up. A study that looked at the timeliness of follow-up care following a recommendation for additional imaging in 214,897 women at 118 facilities and 35,622 recommendations for breast biopsy or surgical consultation found that the median time to subsequent follow-up care after additional imaging recommendation was 14 days and 16 days after a recommendation for breast biopsy or surgical consultation. Timely follow-up was associated with larger volume of the recommended procedures. Most patients returned within 3 weeks for follow-up care [5].

The time to follow up after an abnormal screening or diagnostic mammogram may also be influenced by woman-level characteristics. In a large series of 20,060 screening and

3,184 diagnostic studies after an abnormal screening mammogram, later follow-up was observed among older women and Asians and in those who had a college degree. For diagnostic mammograms, presence of symptoms or being obese was associated with earlier follow-up [6].

Recommendations Outside the USA

Similar to the MQSA, the Europe against cancer has developed a European guideline for quality control and quality assurance in breast cancer screening and diagnosis. The purpose of such a rigorous quality assurance program in breast cancer screening was to diminish the potential harm that can result from mammography such as unnecessary anxiety and morbidity, inappropriate economic cost, and the use of ionizing radiation [7]. The guidelines emphasize that a breast cancer screening program should aim to avoid unnecessary work-up of clearly benign abnormalities so as to reduce unnecessary anxiety and maintain a cost-effective program. Somewhat similar to the mandated requirements in the USA, the European guidelines for quality assurance recommend the need for quality assurance on all mammography units, implementation of a robust accreditation of all screening programs, and the need for all staff to hold professional qualifications to perform and interpret mammograms and to undertake specialist training and participate in CME and updates and participate in external quality assessment schemes. Each screening unit is required to have a lead professional to oversee overall quality assurance and performance of the screening mammography program. Strict adherence to such national and regional guidelines is critical for a successful screening program, and many countries where screening programs are in place or are being implemented adopt similar measures to ensure quality [7].

Mammography Audit

The goal of screening mammography is to detect clinically occult breast cancer. A mammography audit aims to measure the success of such a program. An audit of a mammography practice essentially looks at the appropriateness and interpretive accuracy of a facility and the individual physicians [4, 8, 9]. The MQSA-mandated mammography audit is quite basic; the American College of Radiology on the other hand outlines both a basic and a comprehensive audit process in its BI-RADS™ atlas. The expanded mammography audit as outlined in the American College of Radiology Breast Imaging and Data Systems is a comprehensive method of analyzing the quality of performance of a breast cancer screening and diagnostic program and of the individual physicians [4]. See Boxes 10.1 and 10.2.

Box 10.1. Basic Clinical Mammography Audit

Raw data

- Time period being audited and the total number of examinations during that time
- Number of screening and number of diagnostic examinations and separate audit for each of these two groups
- Number of BI-RADS Category 0 assessment
- Number of BI-RADS Category 4 and 5 assessment [MQSA mandated]
- Biopsy results for fine needle, core biopsy, and open surgical biopsy
- Cancer staging: size of the tumor, histological type, nodal status, and grading
- All cases of known false-negative mammograms have to be analyzed and mammograms prior to the diagnosis of cancer should be reviewed [MQSA mandated]

Derived data

- True positives
- False positives
- Positive predictive value [PPV1, PPV2, PPV3]
- Cancer detection rate for screening examinations
- Percentage of minimal cancers [DCIS or invasive cancers 1 cm or less]
- Node-negative cancers
- Abnormal interpretation rates

Data from D'Orsi et al. [4]

Box 10.2. Complete Mammography Audit

Additional data to be collected for a complete mammography audit

- Risk factors
- Patients' age
- Breast cancer history: personal and family
- Hormone replacement therapy
- Previous biopsy proven atypia or lobular carcinoma in situ
- Baseline, routine follow-up or short interval follow-up examination
- Mammographic assessment
- BI-RADS Category 1, negative, and BI-RADS Category 2 benign findings
- Short interval follow-up: BI-RADS Category 3
- Cancer data
- Mammographic findings: mass, calcifications, indirect signs of cancer, no mammographic signs of cancer
- Palpable or not

Derived data to be calculated from the more complete mammographic audit

- True negatives, false negatives
- Sensitivity
- Specificity

Cancer detection rate
Prevalent vs. incident cancer detection rates for screening
Cancer detection rate for diagnostic examinations
Rates for various age groups
Percentages of nonpalpable cancers calculated separately for screening and diagnostic examinations
Percentage of minimal cancers separately for screening and diagnostic examinations
Percentage of node-negative cancers separately for screening and diagnostic examinations
Abnormal interpretation rate for diagnostic examinations

Mammography Audit Definitions [4]

It is important to understand the definitions of the types of a breast imaging studies and the parameters that are used in a mammography audit. These are outlined next as they appear in the BI-RADS™ atlas [4]:

- A *screening examination* is defined as an examination performed on asymptomatic woman to detect early, clinically unsuspected cancer. The screening group also includes special sub-groups namely women with augmented breast who need additional views optimized to assess breast and women with a personal history of breast cancer.
- A *diagnostic mammographic* examination is performed when there are clinical signs and symptoms that suggest breast cancer, and on a woman with an abnormal screening examination
- A *tissue diagnosis* is a pathologic diagnosis rendered after any type of biopsy, percutaneous or open surgical with or without image guidance and or localization.
- A *positive screening examination* includes one for which a recall is initiated or a tissue diagnosis is recommended. It is to be noted that the MQSA final rules includes only those that have been recommended for tissue diagnosis as being a positive screening examination.
- A *positive diagnostic examination* is one that requires a tissue diagnosis
- A *negative screening examination* is one that is negative or benign findings (BI-RADS Category 1 or 2)
- A *negative diagnostic examination* includes, a negative, benign or probably benign assessment (BI-RADS Category 1, 2, 3)
- *Cancer diagnosis* refers to Ductal carcinoma in situ or any type of primary invasive breast carcinoma, metastatic carcinoma is not included.
- *True positive* (*TP*) is when there is a tissue diagnosis of cancer within one year of a positive examination. (BI-RADS Category 0, 4, or 5 for screening study and BI-RADS Category 4 or 5 for diagnostic study).
- *True negative* (*TN*) is when there is no tissue diagnosis of cancer within one year of a negative examination (BI-RADS Category 1 or 2 for screening; BI-RADS Category 1, 2 or 3 for diagnostic).
- *False negative* (*FN*) is when there is a tissue diagnosis of cancer within one year of a negative examination (BI-RADS Category 1 or 2 for screening; BI-RADS Category 1,2 or 3 for diagnostic).
- *False positive* (*FP*) has three definitions:

  FP 1: No known tissue diagnosis of cancer within one year of a positive screening examination
  (BI-RADS Category 0, 4, or 5)
  FP 2: No known tissue diagnosis of cancer within one year after recommendation for biopsy or surgical consultation resulting from a positive examination (BI-RADS Category 4, or 5)
  FP3: A benign tissue diagnosis of cancer within one year after recommendation for biopsy or surgical consultation resulting from a positive examination (BI-RADS Category 4, or 5)
- *Positive Predictive Value* (*PPV*)

  PPV 1: The percentage of all positive screening examinations with a tissue diagnosis of cancer within one year (BI-RADS Category 0, 4, or 5). It is very unusual yet possible to assign a category 4 or 5 on an initial screening assessment.
  PPV 2: The percentage of all positive screening or diagnostic examinations that were recommended for biopsy or surgical consultations and with a tissue diagnosis of cancer within one year (BI-RADS Category 4, or 5).
  PPV 3: The percentage of all known biopsies done as a result of a positive screening or diagnostic examinations [BI-RADS 4 and 5] that resulted in a tissue diagnosis of cancer within one year.
- Sensitivity is the probability of detecting cancer when a cancer exists or the number of cancers diagnosed after being identified at mammography in a population within one year of the imaging examination divided by all cancers present in the population in the same time period. Sensitivity = TP/TP + FN
- Specificity: The probability of interpreting a mammogram as negative when cancer does not exist or the number of true negative mammograms in a population divided by all actual negative cases in the population. Specificity = TN/TN + FP
- *Cancer detection rate*: The number of cancers correctly detected at Screening Mammography per 1,000 patients and if calculated for diagnostic mammography should be reported separate from Screening Mammography.
- *Abnormal Interpretation Rate*: This is the rate of examinations that are positive, for screening examinations this will include BI-RADS Category 0, 4 and 5 assessments and BI-RADS 4 or 5 for diagnostic mammography. For the most part abnormal interpretation rate is the same as recall rate; the only rare exception is when a BI-RADS 4 or 5 assessments is given on a screening mammogram. Even in cases of obvious suspicious findings, additional imaging is generally needed to determine extent of disease and to plan type of image guidance for biopsy.

MQSA-Mandated Mammography Audit

MQSA requires that each facility designate a lead interpreting physician who is responsible for reviewing medical audit outcomes yearly. Results have to be analyzed and individual radiologists and the facility have to be notified. The audit data have to be maintained for at least 24 months and longer if required to do so by state regulatory bodies. A system should be in place to collect and review outcome data on all mammograms performed. Follow-up on all positive mammograms is required. A system needs to be in place to attempt obtaining pathology results on all mammograms with a recommendation for biopsy with correlation of biopsy results with the mammographic findings. Outcome data analysis is required for individual physicians as well as for the facility. Computerized tracking and analyzing system is acceptable and desirable but not required. FDA requires only determining that the biopsy is benign or malignant. Any case with a benign or negative assessment with a breast cancer diagnosis within a year, considered as false negative, should be analyzed.

The MQSA basic audit is likely to be expanded in the near future. The United States Congress has commissioned the Institute of Medicine [IOM] to produce a report to enhance quality of breast imaging practice [10]. The IOM report has conclude that the current requirements are inadequate for measuring or improving the quality of mammographic interpretation [10].

Box 10.3. Summary of Recommendations to Improve Breast Imaging Quality

1. Revise and standardize the required medical audit component of MQSA
2. Facilitate a voluntary advanced medical audit with feedback
3. Designate specialized Breast Imaging Centers of Excellence and undertake demonstration projects and evaluations within them
4. Further study the effects of CME, reader volume, double reading, and CAD
5. Revise MQSA regulations, inspections, and enforcement
6. Modify regulations to clarify their intent and address current technology
7. Streamline inspections and strengthen enforcement for patient protection
8. Ensure an adequate workforce for breast cancer screening and diagnosis
9. Collect and analyze data on the mammography workforce and service capacity
10. Devise strategies to recruit and retain highly skilled breast imaging professionals
11. Make more effective use of breast imaging specialists
12. Improve breast imaging quality beyond mammography by mandating accreditation for nonmammographic breast imaging methods that are routinely used for breast cancer detection and diagnosis, such as ultrasound and magnetic resonance imaging (MRI)

Data from Institute of Medicine [10]

IOM Recommendations to Improve Interpretative Performance [10]

The institute of medicine in its manual on improving breast imaging quality standards has recommended carrying out studies to determine what additional approaches would improve the quality of mammography interpretation since the currently available data not sufficient to justify regulatory changes. Among the suggested studies to be undertaken are those that would demonstrate the efficacy of continuing medical education specifically dedicated to improving interpretive skills and effects of reader volume on interpretive performance, measuring the impact of double reading and computer-aided detection on interpretive performance over time and at different levels of experience and in different practice setting. The funding for such studies is recommended to be granted by the National Cancer Institute.

An outline of the recommendations appears in Box 10.3. The summary of these recommendations follows:

Include PPV2, cancer detection rate, and abnormal interpretation rate in the required basic medical audit.

- In addition to tracking BI-RADS 4 and 5 assessments, all women for whom additional imaging has been recommended should also be tracked. [BI-RADS 0; incomplete assessment, needs additional imaging].
- All performance measures should be measured separately for screening and diagnostic mammography.
- Each interpreting physician should be allowed to combine audit data from all facilities that he or she is interpreting.
- Encourage facilities to participate in a voluntary enhanced mammography audit that would collect data on patient characteristics and tumor staging information from pathology reports. This should be tied into a central data and statistical coordinating center that would collect data from interpreting physicians and provide feedback for quality assurance and improvement. Implementation of such an audit needs to be incentivized by tying in pay for performance by Centers for Medicare & Medicaid Services [CMS] and payors by providing higher reimbursement rates for those meeting performance criteria that are set by a group of experts and patient advocates and periodically updates. Exempting such facilities from FDA inspection of medical audit data is an additional incentive.

Given the fact that the current MQSA-required audit is bare bones, it is desirable for each breast imaging facility to perform at a minimum the BI-RADS basic audit. Unlike the USA, in countries where organized screening is in place, a more stringent audit is mandated by government regulatory bodies. Additionally audit results should be examined for the facility as a whole as well as for individual radiologists interpreting mammograms. There are several commercially available software programs that continually accumulate data and produce metrics at defined intervals. The lead interpreting

Table 10.1 Mammography interpretative performance benchmarks for screening mammography

Measure	Minimal acceptable criteria
Sensitivity	<75 %
Specificity	<88 % or greater than 95 %
Recall rate	<5 % or greater than 12 %
PPV2	<20 % or greater than 40 %
Cancer detection rate	<2.5 % per 1,000 screens

Data from Carney et al. [12]

radiologist should monitor metrics of his or her colleagues and initiate remedial measures if performance metrics falls significantly out of the expected benchmarks (Table 10.1).

Audits are meaningful when performed separately for diagnostic and screening mammographic examinations due to expected variation in outcomes [11, 12]. In an analysis of 51,805 mammographies where screening and diagnostic examinations were audited separately, expected outcomes for various mixes were calculated based on a known mix of 79 and 21 % in the study group. For a screening diagnostic mix of 90 and 10 %, compared to a 50–50 % mix, the expected rate of abnormal findings was 6–11 %, rate of positive biopsy findings was 38 % vs. 42 %, cancer detection rate was 10 per 10,000 to 30 per 10,000, invasive cancer size was 14.4 vs. 16.0 mm, nodal metastasis was 8–11 %, and rate of stage 0 and stage 1 cancers was 87 % vs. 82 %. Among diagnostic mammographic examinations, a higher percentage for all these numbers is expected for those with palpable findings [11]. Extrapolation from known outcomes is suggested when audit data for screening and diagnostic examinations are combined. As was shown in this study, the mix of screening and diagnostic, as well as the type of indication for a diagnostic examination, will influence the outcomes [11].

Mammographic Interpretation, Interpretive Accuracy, and Benchmarks

Benchmarks that are used to determine interpretive performance may be derived from expert panels or derived from published large samples of data from clinical practice. The introduction and implementation of MQSA has had the intended effect of improving the technical quality of mammographic examinations; however, there has not been a corresponding improvement in the interpretative quality of mammograms as judged by sensitivity and specificity [10].

Minimally acceptable criteria for interpretive performance for screening and diagnostic mammography have been published [11–16]. One of these studies examined minimally acceptable performance standards for interpreting screening mammograms: a sensitivity of less than 75 %, a specificity that was less than 88 % or greater than 95 %, a recall rate that was less than 5 % or greater than 12 %, PPV2 of less than 20 % or greater than 40 %, and cancer detection rate of 2.5 per 1,000 interpretations as indicating low performance (Table 10.1). If underperforming physicians moved into the acceptable range by additional training, detection of an additional 14 cancers per 100,000 women screened and a reduction in the number of false-positive examinations by 880 per 100,000 women screened would be expected [12]. Radiologists interpreting moderate (1,001–2,000) and those with high volume (>2,000) had a higher sensitivity [12].

Reducing Recall and False Positives

The recall rate remains one of the most important benchmark of interpretive performance in screening mammography. A high recall rate leads an increased false-positive rate which is one of the most frequently cited as a cause of unnecessary patient anxiety and a shortcoming of mammography. Recall rate is used as an indicator of quality of imaging performance in the National Accreditation Program for Breast Centers as well as in the National Quality Benchmarks for Breast Centers. False-positive mammogram not only causes increased anxiety; it also leads to excess costs and morbidity from subsequent biopsies, many of which result in a benign diagnosis. The rate of recall for screening mammography in the USA is twice the recall rate in the UK (e.g., 12.5–14.4 % vs. 7.6 %), with no difference in cancer detection rate [17]. One of the contributory factors for this difference maybe the practice of defensive medicine; failure to diagnose breast cancer is the leading cause of malpractice litigation in the USA [18]. Additional factor that is in play is the higher interpretive volume of screening mammography among breast imagers in the UK [17, 19].

In a study that looked at three groups of radiologists interpreting mammograms, the sensitivity in the group considered as high-volume readers which included those who read >301 mammograms each month was significantly higher than in those who read <100 or those who read between 100 and 300 mammograms. The specificity was also better among high-volume readers although was not statistically significant [19, 20]. In the USA the minimum number of mammograms required to be read per MQSA regulations is 480/year compared to 5,000/year required in the UK [17]. Others have also shown that increasing minimum interpretive volume requirements in the USA while adding a minimal requirement for diagnostic interpretation could reduce the number of false-positive work-ups without hindering cancer detection [20].

Several studies have been published describing ways of optimizing recall rate in screening mammography. Large studies of performance metrics for radiologists in community practice have shown that cancer outcomes for the majority of radiologists exceed the set benchmarks except for recall rate which has been shown to be outside of the recommended range in greater than half of the radiologists studied [21]. Baseline mammography or when no comparison is available also contributes to a higher rate of recall. The false-positive rate is significantly higher, 16.3 % in one large series on the initial screening round than at subsequent mammography, and the same applies to false-positive biopsy rate which was shown to be 2.5 % at first and 1.0 % at subsequent examinations. Having prior films available was shown to halve the odds of a false-positive examination. Over a 10-year period of annual screening, more than 50 % of women received a false-positive recall and 7–9 % a false-positive biopsy recommendation. These investigators also found a lower rate in those undergoing biennial mammography albeit with a small absolute increase in the probability of being diagnosed with late stage of cancer [22]. Availability of comparison mammograms not only is beneficial in reducing recall rate but has been shown to permit cancer detection at an early stage for screening mammograms. An analysis of 48,281 consecutive mammography examinations for which previous mammography (9,825 diagnostic, 38,456 screening) had been performed between 1997 and 2001 reported that for screening mammography, comparison with previous examinations significantly decreases false positives and permits detection of cancers at an earlier stage. For diagnostic mammography, comparison with previous examinations increases true-positive findings. In the diagnostic setting, comparison with previous examinations increases the biopsy yield from 38 to 51 % and the overall cancer detection rate from 11/1,000 to 39/1,000. A significant decrease in the frequency of axillary node metastasis and the cancer stage for screening mammography was observed [23].

Educational Intervention to Improve Recall

Several investigators have looked into the value of improving recall rate by educational intervention [24–26]. In a study where, among a group of 31 radiologists, 22 received 1 h Web-based training and 9 radiologists in the control group received none, there was no positive benefit seen in the group that received the training. A multi-institutional study that used a tailored Web-based intervention to assess radiologist's ability to set goals to improve recall rates had better results. Peer comparison data that profiled breast cancer risk in the radiologist's patient populations was provided to the radiologists. Such an intervention was successful in helping radiologists develop goals that ultimately reduce unnecessary recall. There have been other studies evaluating effectiveness of a more rigorous and comprehensive intervention [27, 28]. The UK national health program evaluated a 2-week multidisciplinary course with a specialist training at high-volume screening sites which was combined with breast disease–related meetings and personal and group audit reports inclusive of cancer detection rate, recall rate, and PPV2. An impressive reduction in the recall rate from 7 to 4 % was observed with an increase in the small invasive cancer detection rate from 1.6 per 1,000 women screened to 2.5 per 1,000 women screened [27]. In the USA, a study group of 21 radiologists were provided personal and group audits and attended a self-assessment, case review sessions and were required to interpret 8,000 mammogram annually. An improvement in sensitivity from 70 to 80 % was noted with a mean cancer detection rate of 7.5/1,000 and a mean recall rate of 7 % [28].

Interpretative Benchmarks for Diagnostic Mammograms

Monitoring clinical outcome is well accepted as a measure of quality of interpretation and is a requirement in a basic form by the MQSA. However, performance benchmarks need to be separate for screening and diagnostic studies since the expected outcomes are significantly different for these two categories of breast imaging studies [12, 13, 15]. A large series of 332,926 diagnostic mammography examinations derived from six mammography registries that submitted data to the Breast Cancer Surveillance Consortium (BCSC) looked at the mean performance parameter values and reported an abnormal interpretation rate of 8 %, PPV2 of 31.5 %, PPV3 of 39.5 %, and cancer detection rate of 25.3 % per 1,000 examinations; invasive cancer size was 20.2 mm, the percentage of minimal cancers was 42 %, percentage of node-negative cancers was 73.6 %, and percentage of early-stage [stage 0 and I] cancers was 62.4 % [15]. A recently published article outlined minimally acceptable interpretive performance criteria for diagnostic mammography [13]. Simulations and normative data from the BCSC were used to help a panel of breast imaging expert radiologists to identify the impact of cutoff points and estimate the expected clinical impact from setting of performance thresholds. Thresholds were determined for work-up of screen-recalled abnormalities separately from those being worked up for a breast lump. In the former group minimum acceptable threshold was set as a sensitivity less than 80 %, specificity less than 80 % or greater than 95 %, abnormal interpretation rate of less than 8 % or greater than 25 %, PPV2 of less than 15 % or greater than 40 %, PPV3 of less than 20 % or greater than 45 %, and a cancer diagnosis rate of less than 20 per 1,000 interpretations. Following work-up of breast lump, the thresholds were sensitivity less than 85 %, specificity less than 83 % or greater than 95 %, abnormal interpretation rate of less than 10 % or greater than 25 %, a PPV2 less than 25 % or greater than 50 %, PPV3 less than 30 % or greater than 55 %, and a cancer diagnosis rate of less than 40 per 1,000 interpretations. These cutoff points for performance benchmarks were expected to lead to 16–34 % of interpreting physicians and 11–24 % of facilities being recommended for additional training in diagnostic mammography following abnormal screening examinations and 21–42 % of radiologists and 14–54 % of facilities for additional training in diagnostic mammography performed to evaluate a breast lump. Those radiologists who fell outside the acceptable threshold would benefit from remedial training and consequently be expected to diagnose an additional 186 cancers per 100,000 screening examinations and reduce the number of false-positive examinations by 1,067 per 100,000 women and, following work-up of a breast lump, would be expected to diagnose an additional 335 cancers per 100,000 women with a reduction of false-positive examinations by 634 per 100,000 women [13]. Published goals are important guidelines but making radiologists aware of these goals is a challenge; a study found that many radiologists' understanding of the desirable goals for interpretative accuracy in fact falls outside of the published benchmarks. Those who were in academic practice and receive breast imaging CME and receive annual feedback were more likely to report desirable PPV2 goals. Cancer detection rates were also higher among those who have had >10 years of experience reading mammograms and in those who read >1,000 mammograms per year [16].

The Breast Cancer Surveillance Consortium [BCSC] [29]

The National cancer Institute [NCI], USA, outlines a "discovery-development-delivery" approach to cancer research [29]. "Discovery is the process of generating new information about fundamental cancer processes from the genetic to the population level. Development is the process of creating and evaluating tools and interventions that are valuable in detecting, diagnosing, predicting, treating, and preventing cancer. Delivery involves promoting and facilitating the application of evidence-based cancer interventions" [29]. The Breast Cancer Surveillance Consortium [BCSC] was established by the NCI in 1994. The benefits of screening mammography have been well established in large randomized clinical trials; however, there was a need to study the effectiveness of screening mammography more thoroughly in routine clinical practice. It was also recognized that useful information could only be obtained by linking screening patterns and performance parameters as outlined by national bodies and professional societies such as the American College of Radiology, with cancer outcomes. At the present time seven data collection and research centers and the statistical coordinating center comprise the BCSC. A key program of NCI's Division of Cancer Control and Population Sciences focuses on the delivery component, and its research wing aims to promote adoption of proven intervention methods in clinical and public health practice. The BCSC links surveillance data on breast screening practices with data from population-based cancer registries. Most recent data, which include data on screening mammography performed from 2002 to 2006 and analyzed in 2009, show a cancer detection rate of 4.6 per 1,000 women among 1,960,500 mammograms performed. Sensitivity and specificity for 2,264,089 screening mammography examinations from 2002 to 2006—based on BCSC data as of 2009—are 84.1 % and 90.4 %, respectively. The recall rate was 10 %. PPV 2 was 23.6 % [cases where biopsy was recommended], and PPV 3 was 28.9 % [cases where biopsy was performed within 1 year] [29]. An analysis of the results of 47,798 screening and 13,286 diagnostic mammograms found that radiologists that are specialized in breast imaging detected more cancers and more early-stage cancers, recommended more biopsies, and had lower recall rates than did the general radiologists. Cancer detection rate of specialists was 6 % compared to 3.4 % for generalists. A database of such large samples of screened population allows the consortium to study and publish several key features of community-based breast cancer screening programs such as characteristics of women that affect the performance of screening mammography; characteristics of radiologist, radiology facility, or mammographic technologists affecting performance of screening mammography; and characteristics of mammography equipment that affects the performance of screening mammography. The low-contrast detectability was studied using a full-field digital mammography system in terms of and compared with results obtained from an optimized screen-film system. Results showed that using a softer x-ray beam for thin breasts and a harder x-ray beam for thick breasts improved digital mammography's ability to detect low-contrast lesions when the average glandular dose was kept constant. Under this constraint, optimum low-contrast lesion detection with digital mammography was superior to that of conventional screen-film mammography for all but the thinnest breasts [30].

Mammographic Interpretative Accuracy: Film vs. Digital Mammography [30, 31]

About 2/3 of all mammography equipment in the USA is digital, predominantly full-field digital systems. In one study, a total of 49,528 asymptomatic women presenting for screening mammography at 33 sites in the USA and Canada underwent both digital and film mammography [30]. The overall diagnostic accuracy of full-field digital mammography [FFDM] and screen-film mammography [SFM] as a means of screening for breast cancer was found to be similar, but digital mammography was found to be more accurate in women under the age of 50 years, women with radiographically dense breasts, and premenopausal or perimenopausal women [28]. Another study that compared the miss rate of breast cancer found no difference in those who underwent screen-film mammography from those who underwent full-field digital mammography. The missed cancers in the SFM group of 52,444 women had microcalcifications on the prior mammograms in 34 %, compared to 18 % in the FFDM group of 35,127 women; focal asymmetry at the site of cancer was seen more frequently at the site of missed cancers in women who underwent FFDM, 27 % compared to 10 % in those who underwent SFM [30, 31].

Attaining Excellence in Comprehensive Breast Cancer Care

The importance of a multidisciplinary approach in managing the breast cancer patient is well recognized. There are both discipline-specific programs and breast center–specific programs. Professional organizations have taken on the task of ensuring excellence in breast cancer care in multidisciplinary breast centers. There are several major voluntary accreditation programs in the USA, some discipline specific and some conducted by national professional bodies. Notable of these are the American College of Radiology program for accreditation of Breast Imaging Centers of Excellence, the National Quality Measures for Breast Centers Program, and the National Accreditation Program for Breast Centers.

Breast Imaging Center of Excellence [American College of Radiology]

The American College of Radiology recognizes breast imaging centers that achieve excellence by seeking and earning accreditation in the ACR's entire voluntary breast imaging accreditation programs and modules in addition to the mandatory Mammography Accreditation Program by providing them a certificate that identifies them as a Breast Imaging Center of Excellence [32].

In order to receive the ACR's Breast Imaging Center of Excellence designation, a center must be fully accredited in [32]:

- Mammography by the ACR (or an FDA-approved state accrediting body)
- Stereotactic breast biopsy by the ACR
- Breast ultrasound by the ACR (including the Ultrasound-Guided Breast Biopsy module)

National Quality Measures for Breast Centers™ (NQMBC™)

The National Quality Measures for Breast Centers™ Program (NQMBC™) is a free interactive Internet model for breast centers to track and measure quality performance in more than 30 separate quality indicators. The NQMBC™ Program identifies quality care measures and provides immediate access to information that allows participating breast centers to compare performance with other centers across the USA. The NQMBC™ Program is a result of the National Consortium of Breast Centers' (NCBC) commitment to increase the quality of breast health care provided by professionals to their patients [http://www.nqmbc.org/] [33, 34]. There are three levels of designation: participant [data should be supplied for 40 % of the measures], quality breast center [data should be supplied for 75 % of the measures], and breast center of excellence [data should be supplied for 90 % of the measures]:

- The breast center must have supplied data for 40–90 % of the measures for which their quality breast center type should be able to measure performance.
- This quality data being considered for evaluation must span two consecutive data collection periods. (A data period is a 6-month range during which time data is collected according to the parameters of the indicator.)
- These two consecutive data collection periods being audited for certification must be within the last 3 years.
- After the initial certification at this level, the two consecutive data periods being audited for certification must be after the two consecutive data collection periods and within the last 2 year's data. A data period may be audited only once for certification.

Box 10.4 summarizes the performance measures required for a screening and diagnostic breast center to achieve NQMBC™ quality certification.

National Accreditation Program for Breast Centers [NAPBC] [34–37]

Breast care quality can be assessed by three measures, an outcome of care, structure of care, or process of care. Outcome care that needs long-term data on survival, morbidity, and mortality is not useful to assess breast care due to its complexity. Structural measurements include an interdisciplinary breast conference, having a sentinel node protocol, and having a standardized synoptic pathology reporting system. These elements lead to a higher quality of care. Of greater importance is a process measurement that evaluated the type of care that is actually provided [34]. NAPBC was developed by a multidisciplinary team which combined its expertise in breast health care to create a validation process for breast programs. This program focuses on the process of care that includes self-monitoring of process measures, peer compari-

Box 10.4. Summary of Performance Measures for Screening and Diagnostic Breast Center to Achieve NQMBC™ (National Quality Measures for Breast Centers) Quality Certification

Screening breast center
- Mammography call back rate

Diagnostic breast center
- Imaging timeliness of care: time between screening and diagnostic mammogram
- Mammography call back rate
- Surgical timeliness of care: time between diagnostic and open surgical biopsy
- Imaging timeliness of care: time between diagnostic mammogram and core needle biopsy
- Core needle biopsy rate
- Pathology timeliness of care: time between initial breast biopsy excluding open surgical biopsy and pathology results

Used with permission of the National Consortium of Breast Centers, Inc. From http://www.nqmbc.org/QualityPerformanceYouShouldMeasure.htm

Box 10 5. Summary of Breast Imaging Specific Components of NAPBC (National Accreditation Program for Breast Centers)

1. Community outreach program to educate on benefits of screening mammography
2. Screening mammography and diagnostic mammography are performed at Mammography Quality Standards Act (MQSA)-certified facilities and interpreted by MQSA-certified physicians
3. Palpation-guided or image-guided needle biopsy is the initial diagnostic approach rather than open biopsy. Diagnostic ultrasound and/or ultrasound-guided needle biopsy are performed at an American College of Radiology (ACR)-accredited facility or by an American Society of Breast Surgeons (ASBS)-certified physician

son, and local intervention that is aimed at improvement in the process of care. The NAPBC is a consortium of national, professional organizations focused on breast health, dedicated to the improvement of the quality of care and outcomes of patients with diseases of the breast through evidence-based standards, and patient and professional education [35]. From a breast imagers' perspective, there are components of the requirements to be accredited that are listed in Box 10.5. An analysis of the NAPBC 2-year data suggests that a wide variety of BC models adequately provide a high level of care and services for patients across the nation [37].

Summary

Benefits of a breast cancer screening and diagnostic program can only be realized by maintaining a rigorous quality assurance program that encompasses image quality, personnel qualifications, and interpretive accuracy. MQSA ensures quality of mammographic screening for breast cancer in the USA. Continuing monitoring of performance of image quality and radiologists' interpretive performance is needed to maintain the highest possible quality. Accreditation programs offered by professional societies offer a voluntary opportunity for breast centers to achieve excellence in breast care and be recognized for being one.

References

1. Mammography Quality Standards Act of 1992. Mammography facilities requirement for accrediting bodies, and quality standards and certifying requirements: interim rules (21 CFR 900). 1993; 58:57558–72.
2. Butler PF. MQSA (Mammography Quality Standards Act) update–focusing on quality assurance. Radiol Manage. 1998;20(4):40–50.
3. Bassett LW, Hendrick RE, Bassford TL, et al. Quality determinants of mammography. Clinical practice guideline no. 13. AHCPR publication no. 95–0632. Rockville: Agency for Health Care Policy and Research, Public Health Service, U.S. Department of Health and Human Services; 1994.
4. D'Orsi CJ, Bassett LW, Feig SA, et al. Breast imaging reporting and data system. 3rd ed. Reston: American College of Radiology; 1998.
5. Rosenberg RD, Haneuse SJ, Geller BM, Buist DS, Miglioretti DL, Brenner RJ, Smith-Bindman R, Taplin SH, Breast Cancer Surveillance Consortium. Timeliness of follow-up after abnormal screening mammogram: variability of facilities. Radiology. 2011;261(2):404–13.
6. Wernli KJ, Aiello Bowles EJ, Haneuse S, Elmore JG, Buist DS. Timing of follow-up after abnormal screening and diagnostic mammograms. Am J Manag Care. 2011;17(2):162–7.
7. Perry N, Broeders M, Wolf CD, Tornberg S, Holland R, Karsa LV. European guidelines for quality assurance in breast cancer screening and diagnosis. Fourth edition-summary document. Ann Oncol. 2008;19:614–22.
8. Sickles EA. Auditing your breast imaging practice: an evidence-based approach. Semin Roentgenol. 2007;42(4):211–7.
9. Monsees BS. The Mammography Quality Standards Act. An overview of the regulations and guidance. Radiol Clin North Am. 2000;38(4):759–72.
10. Institute of Medicine. Improving breast imaging quality standards. Washington, DC: National Academies Press; 2005. p. 1–16.
11. Sohlich RE, Sickles EA, Burnside ES, et al. Interpreting data from audits when screening and diagnostic mammography outcomes are combined. AJR Am J Roentgenol. 2002;178:681–6.
12. Carney PA, Sickles EA, Monsees BA, Bassett LA, et al. Identifying minimally acceptable interpretive performance criteria for screening mammography. Radiology. 2010;255(2):354–61.
13. Carney PA, Parikh J, Sickles EA, Feig SA, Monsees B, Bassett LW, Smith RA, Rosenberg R, Ichikawa L, Wallace J, Tran K, Miglioretti DL. Diagnostic mammography: identifying minimally acceptable interpretive performance criteria. Radiology. 2013;267(2): 359–67.

14. Rosenberg RD, Yankaskas BC, Abraham LA, Sickles EA, et al. Performance benchmarks for screening mammography. Radiology. 2006;241(1):55–66.
15. Sickles EA, Miglioretti DL, Ballard-Barbash R, et al. Performance benchmarks for diagnostic mammography. Radiology. 2005;235:775–90.
16. Jackson SL, Cook AJ, Miglioretti DL, et al. Are radiologists goals for mammography accuracy consistent with published recommendations? Acad Radiol. 2012;19(3):289–95.
17. Smith-Bindman R, Chu PW, Miglioretti DL, et al. Comparison of screening mammography in the United States and the United Kingdom. JAMA. 2003;290:2129–37.
18. Elmore JG, Taplin SH, Barlow WE, et al. Does litigation influence medical practice? The influence of community radiologists' medical malpractice perceptions and experience on screening mammography. Radiology. 2005;236:37–46.
19. Esserman L, Cowley H, Eberle C, Kirkpatrick A, Chang S, Berbaum K, et al. Improving the accuracy of mammography: volume and outcome relationships. J Natl Cancer Inst. 2002;94(5):369–75.
20. Elmore Carney PA. Does practice make perfect when interpreting mammography? J Natl Cancer Inst. 2002;94(5):321–3.
21. Buist DS, Anderson ML, Haneuse SJ, et al. Influence of annual interpretive volume on screening mammography performance in the United States. Radiology. 2011;259(1):72–84.
22. Hubbard RA, Kerlikowske K, Flowers CI, et al. Cumulative probability of false-positive recall or biopsy recommendation after 10 years of screening mammography. Ann Intern Med. 2011;155(8):481–92.
23. Burnside ES, Sickles EA, Sohlich RE, Dee KE. Differential value of comparison with previous examination in diagnostic versus screening mammography. AJR Am J Roentgenol. 2002;179(5):1173–7.
24. Carney PA, Abraham L, Cook A, Feig SA, Sickles EA, Miglioretti DL, Geller BM, Yankaskas BC, Elmore JG. Impact of an educational intervention designed to reduce unnecessary recall during screening mammography. Acad Radiol. 2012;19(9):1114–20.
25. Carney PA, Bowles EJ, Sickles EA, Geller BM, Feig SA, Jackson S, Brown D, Cook A, Yankaskas BC, Miglioretti DL, Elmore JG. Using a tailored web-based intervention to set goals to reduce unnecessary recall. Acad Radiol. 2011;18(4):495–503.
26. Carney PA, Geller BM, Sickles EA, Miglioretti DL, Aiello Bowles EJ, Abraham L, Feig SA, Brown D, Cook AJ, Yankaskas BC, Elmore JG. Feasibility and satisfaction with a tailored web-based audit intervention for recalibrating radiologists' thresholds for conducting additional work-up. Acad Radiol. 2011;18(3):369–76.
27. Perry NM. Breast cancer screening–the European experience. Int J Fertil Womens Med. 2004;49(5):228–30.
28. Adcock KA. Initiative to improve mammogram interpretation. Perm J. 2004;8(2):12–8.
29. National Cancer Institute. Breast Cancer Surveillance Consortium: evaluating screening performance in practice. NIH publication no. 04–5490. Bethesda: National Cancer Institute, National Institutes of Health, U.S. Department of Health and Human Services; 2004. Available at: http://breastscreening.cancer.gov/espp.pdf.
30. Pisano ED, Gatsonis C, Hendrick E, et al. Diagnostic performance of digital versus film mammography for breast-cancer screening. N Engl J Med. 2005;353(17):1773–83.
31. Hoff SR, Abrahamsen A-L, Samset JH, Vigeland E, Klepp O, Hofvind S. Breast cancer: missed interval and screening-detected cancer at full-field digital mammography and screen-film mammography—results from a retrospective review. Radiology. 2012;264:378–86.
32. American College of Radiology: Breast Imaging Center of Excellence. http://www.acr.org/quality-safety/accreditation/bicoe.
33. Kaufman C, Shockney L, Rabinowitz B, et al. National Quality Measures for Breast Centers (NQMBC): a robust quality tool. Ann Surg Oncol. 2010;17:3377–85.
34. Kaufman C. Validating quality breast care: three new validation programs for 2007. Am J Surg. 2007;194:515–7.
35. American College of Surgeons: National Accreditation Program for Breast Centers. http://napbc-breast.org/.
36. Winchester DP. The National Accreditation Program for Breast Centers: quality improvement through standard setting. Surg Oncol Clin N Am. 2011;20(3):581–6.
37. Moran MS, Kaufman C, Burgin C, Swain S, Granville T, Winchester DP. What currently defines a breast center? Initial data from the national accreditation program for breast centers. J Oncol Pract. 2013;9(2):e62–70.

Imaging of the Symptomatic Breast in the Young, Pregnant, or Lactating Woman

11

Mahesh K. Shetty

Palpable Breast Masses in the Pediatric and Adolescent Population

The spectrum of abnormalities in the pediatric and adolescents is different from those encountered in older women. Masses may be related to normal or abnormal development of the breast. Breast cancer is exceedingly rare in this age group. Infection, trauma, and cyst formation account for most of the masses prior to puberty and fibroadenoma after [1]. Some of the commonly encountered abnormalities, non-neoplastic and neoplastic, are described next.

Non-neoplastic

Mammary Duct Ectasia

Mammary duct ectasia may occur in infants and be associated with a bloody nipple discharge; associated infection is rare but has been reported [1–3]. Ultrasound demonstrates subareolar ecstatic ducts with debris if infected. Persistent symptoms are rare and if present may require surgical excision [2, 3].

Galactocele

Galactoceles, typically seen in lactating women, may occasionally appear in infants or older boys. Sonographically, these appear as complex cysts, with fat component appearing hyperechoic and water component hypoechoic. Aspiration if performed reveals a milky fluid [1].

M.K. Shetty, MD, FRCR, FACR, FAIUM
Department of Radiology, Baylor College of Medicine, Houston, TX, USA

Woman's Center for Breast Care and MRI, Woman's Hospital of Texas, Houston, TX 77054, USA
e-mail: mshettymd@gmail.com

Retroareolar Cysts

A mass at the edge of the areola in adolescents may result from obstruction of the glands of Montgomery. These lumps can be painful. Ultrasound may not be needed for a diagnosis but if performed reveals cysts less than 2 cm; these cysts are often bilateral.

Abscess and Mastitis

Mastitis may occur in adolescents and may be caused by duct obstruction, an immune-compromised state, or nipple injury. Presentation may be with a painful lump with or without fever. The most common pathogen is *Staphylococcus aureus*. Sonographic appearance is that of a typical abscess characterized by a complex cystic mass with peripheral increased vascularity [1, 2].

Hematomas

Hematomas commonly result from sports or iatrogenic trauma and result in lumps that are sonographically complex and whose appearance will depend on the stage of hemorrhage; in the acute phase, these lesions are hyperechoic and progressively become cystic as the hematoma evolves. Mammograms are seldom performed and, when done, demonstrate a hyperattenuating mass in the acute phase with ill-defined margins; in the chronic phase, reactive changes around the hematoma may cause spiculation [1].

Neoplastic

Benign Breast Masses

Fibroadenoma, Juvenile Fibroadenoma

Fibroadenoma is a benign fibroepithelial neoplasm and the most common cause of a solid mass in girls younger than 20 years, accounting for well over 50 % of all such masses, 10/17 in one series and 91 % in another [4]. Fibroadenoma represents 91 % of all solid breast masses in girls younger than 19 years [5]. Presentation usually is a slowly enlarging mass that is mobile and nontender on clinical examination.

M.K. Shetty (ed.), *Breast Cancer Screening and Diagnosis: A Synopsis*,
DOI 10.1007/978-1-4939-1267-4_11, © Springer Science+Business Media New York 2015

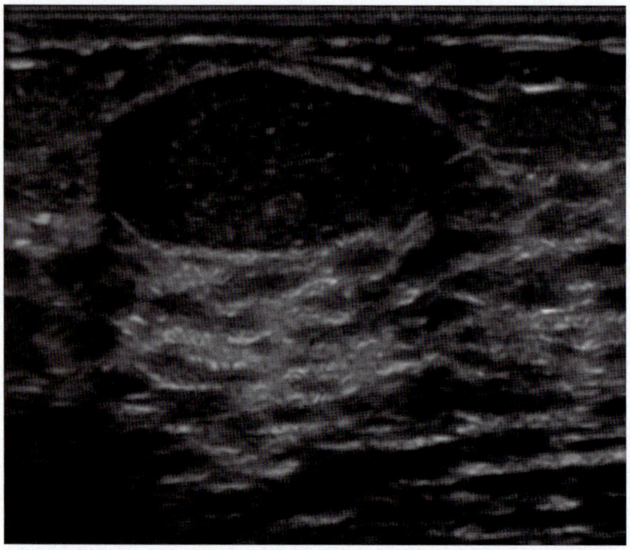

Fig. 11.1 A 16-year-old with a palpable mass histologically proven to be a fibroadenoma at core-needle biopsy. Ultrasound shows an ovoid circumscribed mass with homogenous internal echotexture

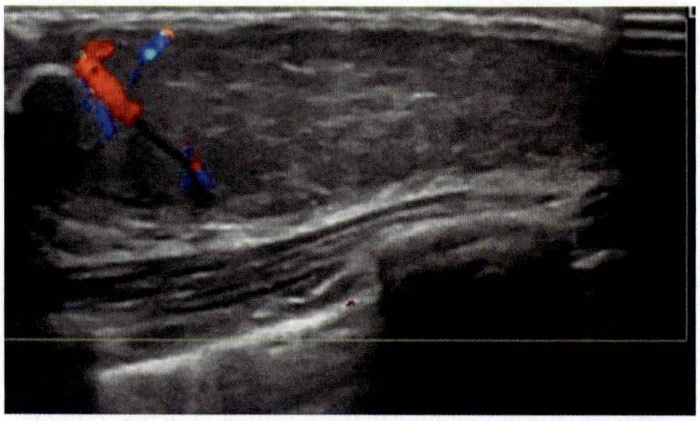

Fig. 11.2 A 15-year-old with a large palpable mass histologically proven to be a juvenile fibroadenoma. Ultrasound shows a large circumscribed ovoid mass with a peripheral cleft and vascularity

A fibroadenoma can undergo faster growth in pregnancy. These benign tumors appear sonographically as circumscribed oval-shaped masses with uniform echogenicity measuring 2–5 cm (Fig. 11.1). About 7–10 % of these belong to a special type referred to as a juvenile or cellular fibroadenoma that tends to grow rapidly and attain a size of 5–10 cm when it is also referred to as a giant fibroadenoma [1, 6]. When seen, slender cystic spaces and clefts are characteristic of juvenile fibroadenoma. Juvenile fibroadenomas can have a macrolobulated appearance (Fig. 11.2). They are more commonly seen in African American girls and may be multiple and bilateral. Fibroadenomas are generally avascular although there may be occasional central vascularity. Histologically, juvenile fibroadenoma is characterized by cellular proliferation of stroma consisting of spindle cells in a myxoid stroma [1]. At imaging distinction between juvenile fibroadenoma and phyllodes tumor is difficult; peripheral cysts are more suggestive of the latter. Rapidly enlarging breast masses are generally excised due to difficulty in differentiating the two entities. Histological distinction between cellular fibroadenomas and benign phyllodes tumor can be challenging. For masses that are smaller and not rapidly growing, sonographic and clinical surveillance is all that is needed. About 10 % of the fibroadenomas in young girls can spontaneously regress [7]. Unnecessary intervention should be avoided so as not to damage the developing breast that can lead to aplasia or hypoplasia [8].

Pseudoangiomatous Stromal Hyperplasia (PASH)

Pseudoangiomatous stromal hyperplasia (PASH) is an entity that is generally seen in older women. It is histologically characterized by hormonally stimulated proliferations of myofibroblasts; rarely they may be seen in late adolescence and uncommonly grow rapidly. Clinically and on imaging, these lesions can have features similar to fibroadenomas. The mean size of these tumors is 4.2 cm with a range between 1 and 11 cm [9]. The name is derived from the characteristic histological feature of anastomosing slit-like channels lined by flat myofibroblastic cells that resemble endothelial cells and is surrounded by dense stroma [1]. When red blood cells are seen within these slit-like spaces on a core biopsy, it can be confused with an angiosarcoma [10]. On sonography, these masses appear as an oval circumscribed mass with margins that may be less well defined than a typical fibroadenoma; there may be a posterior acoustic enhancement associated with this mass. Conservative management after a diagnosis of PASH is recommended with excision reserved for symptomatic or enlarging masses.

Juvenile Papillomatosis

Juvenile papillomatosis is a localized benign proliferative disorder that is uncommonly seen in teens with a mean age of diagnosis at 19 years [11]. Histologically, there are multiple cysts and dilated ducts in a dense stroma, an appearance that has been characterized as "Swiss cheese disease." Mammography may show an area of focal asymmetry or microcalcifications [12]. At sonography, an ill-defined mass with multiple cystic areas of varying sizes is seen at the periphery of the lesion [12]. Juvenile papillomatosis is a marker for familial breast cancer. About 5–15 % of patients have concurrent breast cancer and 33–58 % of cases have a positive family history of breast cancer [13, 14].

Intraductal Papilloma

Intraductal papillomas are rare in children and when seen appear as solitary circumscribed masses in a dilated duct and may be outlined by secretions within a duct. These tend to occur in the larger subareolar ducts. In 25 % of cases, papillomas may be bilateral [2]. Nipple discharge may be a presenting symptom. Histologically, these papillomas resemble juvenile papillomatosis.

Granular Cell Tumor

Granular cell tumor is a rare benign tumor; about 5–6 % of these occur in the breast and most commonly in premenopausal African American women [15]. These account for 1 % of breast tumors in children and originate from perineural cells. Granular cell tumors appear as 1–2 cm superficially located firm masses and may be associated with skin fixation or retraction. At mammography, they may appear as a spiculated mass or as a circumscribed mass. On ultrasound, the spiculated mass may demonstrate posterior acoustic shadowing and appear malignant. These are treated with wide excision when a histological diagnosis is achieved with percutaneous biopsy.

Malignant Tumors

Phyllodes Tumor

Phyllodes tumor is the most common primary breast malignancy in the adolescents. It is a stromal tumor arising from the lobular connective tissue [7]. A higher incidence has been reported in those with an Asian heritage. These tumors present as rapidly enlarging breast lumps. The benign types of phyllodes are more common in this age group. Phyllodes tumors occur predominantly in older women; however, about 5 % of these tumors are seen in girls younger than 20 years. Clinically, pathologically, and at imaging, these tumors may resemble a juvenile type of fibroadenoma [1]. Most tumors are larger than 6 cm with an average range of 8–10 cm [2]. A size less than 4 cm has a favorable prognosis as does presence of pushing rather than infiltrative borders, lack of necrosis, and lesser than three mitosis per high power field [1].

At sonography, these masses are circumscribed but tend to have a heterogeneous internal echotexture with clefts and cystic spaces compared to the more homogenous areas within a fibroadenoma (Fig. 11.3a, b). Mammography demonstrates a hyperdense circumscribed mass without calcifications; malignant types may exhibit pleomorphic microcalcifications. Recurrence is a feature noticed in both benign and malignant types; the former recurs about 10–25 % of the time and the recurrence rate in malignant phyllodes is greater than 40 % even following a wide excision [4]. About 5–24 % of phyllodes in those less than 20 years of age are malignant. Metastasis is uncommon but when present is hematogenous and to the lungs. Malignant types are histologically associated with sarcomatous elements, infiltrative margins, necrosis, cellular atypia, and increased stromal cellularity.

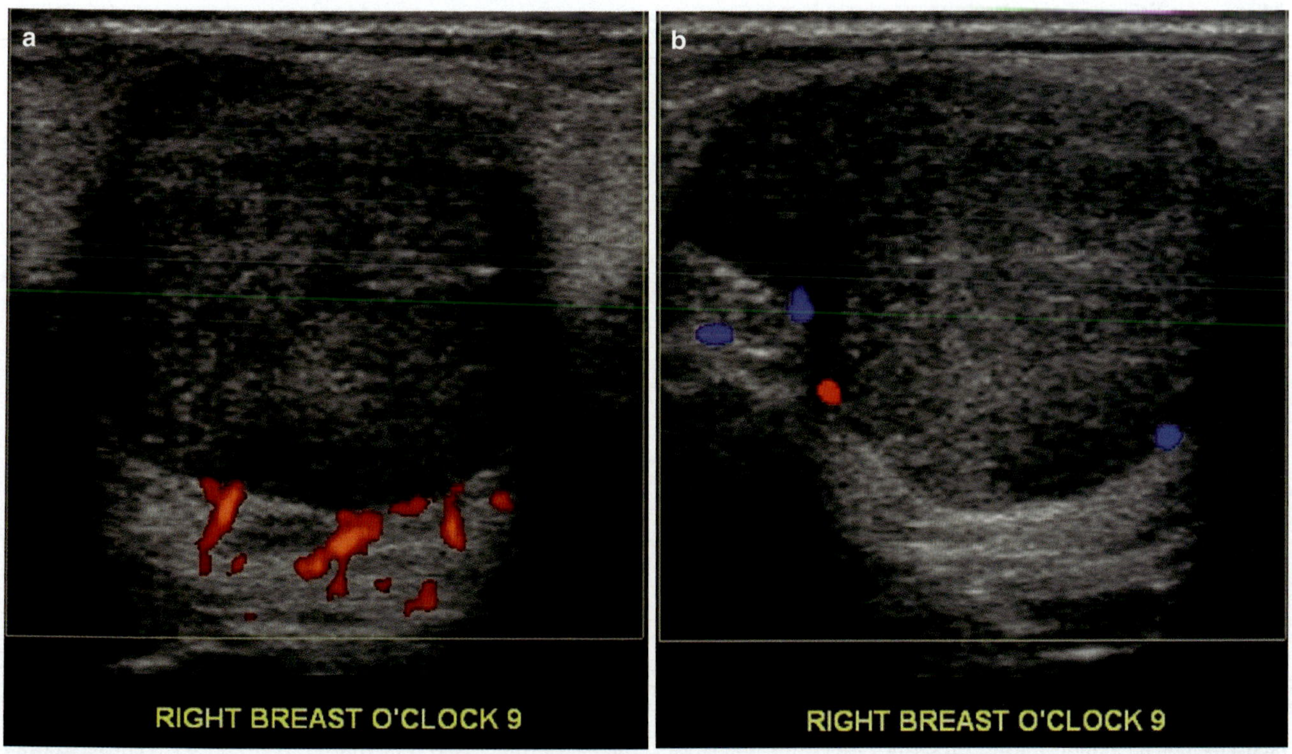

Fig. 11.3 (**a**, **b**) An 18-year-old with a rapidly enlarging palpable mass histologically proven to be a benign phyllodes tumor at excisional biopsy. Ultrasound demonstrates a round solid mass with ill-defined margins

Carcinoma

Breast carcinoma in girls under the age of 20 years is exceedingly rare, and based on the National Cancer Institute's Surveillance Epidemiology and End Results data from 2006 to 2010, 0.0 % was diagnosed [16]. Less than 1 % of breast lesions in children is caused by breast cancer [17]. The most common type is the secretory carcinoma that presents as a circumscribed mass less than 3 cm and with a pseudo capsule [1, 11]. Prognosis is favorable. Breast cancer in these girls may be related to inherited BRCA1 and BRCA2 mutations [11]. Sonographic appearance is that of a malignant mass with irregular margins, taller than wide and with posterior acoustic shadowing.

Metastasis

The most prevalent malignant tumors in the breast in children and adolescents are metastasis. The most common tumors metastasizing to the breast are rhabdomyosarcoma, neuroblastoma, and hematolymphoid malignancies [1, 18]. Breast metastasis has been reported in 6 % of patients with rhabdomyosarcoma [18]. Metastasis are frequently bilateral and multiple although a solitary mass may also be seen. Clinically, masses may exhibit rapid growth and be painful. Sonographic appearance is variable and may exhibit a spectrum of appearance leading to an indeterminate morphology prompting a tissue diagnosis.

Pregnancy and Lactation: Benign Abnormalities of the Breast

The physiologic changes occurring in pregnancy are induced by high circulating levels of estrogen and progesterone, and these lead to increase in breast size, its firmness, and increased nodularity. These changes continue for 3 months after cessation of lactation. Physical examination is difficult as a result of these changes in the breast and it is advised that a baseline clinical breast exam is performed during the first visit to the obstetrician [19]. Mammographic increase in density of the breast also limits its value during pregnancy and lactation. Pumping of the breast prior to a mammogram is also helpful. Ultrasound demonstrates diffuse increase in the echogenicity of normal breast tissue during pregnancy and lactation. During lactation, one sees distended ducts as hypoechoic tubular structures. Increased vascularity is also an expected feature [20].

The most common symptoms prompting imaging in pregnancy and lactation are a palpable lump, mastitis, and a bloody nipple discharge. Ultrasound is the initial imaging modality of choice and often the only modality that is utilized. Mammography is generally not performed in pregnancy although the radiation risk to the developing fetus is insignificant [21]. MRI of the breast is not an option during pregnancy since the safety of intravenous gadolinium has not been established in pregnancy. During lactation, MRI may be used if needed with instructions to stop breastfeeding for 24 h after [21].

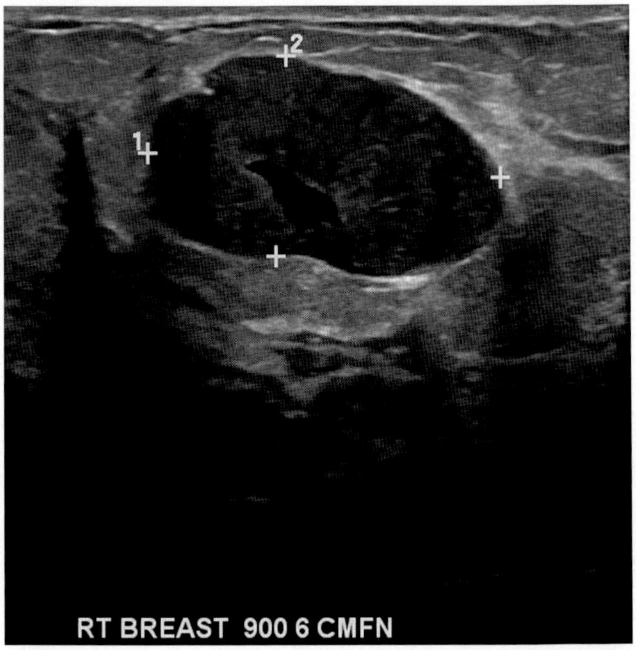

Fig. 11.4 A 28-year-old pregnant woman with a palpable lump. Ultrasound demonstrated a circumscribed ovoid solid mass with a central tubular cystic structure consistent with gravidic fibroadenoma

Spontaneous Nipple Discharge in Pregnancy

Nipple discharge in pregnancy is uncommon; cytological examination of spontaneous nipple discharge is performed. If no pathology is seen and physical and ultrasound examination is normal, clinical follow-up is advised. If pathologic results are seen on cytology, galactography may be indicated to exclude an intraductal lesion such as a papilloma. Nipple discharge is an uncommon manifestation of pregnancy-associated breast cancer [21].

Fibroadenoma

Fibroadenomas being hormone-sensitive tumors may manifest varied appearances in pregnancy and lactation due to superimposition of hormone-induced and or lactational changes. Previously unsuspected fibroadenomas may be discovered in pregnancy due to enlargement and becoming palpable or symptomatic. Palpable fibroadenomas generally require tissue diagnosis that is best achieved with percutaneous core biopsy. Nonpalpable solid masses without suspicious morphology may be followed. The appearance of a fibroadenoma on ultrasound in pregnancy and lactation is varied and the following descriptions have been used [21]. Gravid fibroadenomas may demonstrate large cysts, dilated ducts, or increased vascularity (Fig. 11.4). Fibroadenoma with infarction may present as a painful tender mass. Intravascular thrombi have been identified on occasion in these fibroadenomas; this occurs usually in the third trimester.

A more lobulated contour, heterogeneous architecture and posterior acoustic shadowing may be seen in such tumors as a result of infarction. Fibroadenoma with lactational changes and secretory hyperplasia demonstrates dilated ducts within, hyperechogenicity, and cystic changes. Aspiration may sometimes reveal milk as in a galactocele; distinction from a lactating adenoma may be difficult as well although this is not a management issue. Lactational adenoma histologically lacks the myoepithelial proliferation that is characteristic of fibroadenoma.

Galactocele

Galactoceles are the most common benign breast lesions in lactating women but are more frequently seen after cessation of lactation due to stagnation and retention of milk in the breast [21]. These are cysts that are lined with flat or cuboidal epithelium containing fluid that resembles milk that contains a variable amount of protein, fat, and lactose. The underlying etiopathogenesis is ductal dilatation, surrounding fibrous wall, and varying degrees of inflammation. Aspiration is diagnostic and therapeutic. The imaging appearance is variable depending on the contents:

- Pseudolipoma is when the entire content is fat in which case mammographically a lucent circumscribed mass is encountered that sonographically appears uniformly hyperechoic or hypoechoic (Figs. 11.5a–c and 11.6a–c). Cystic mass with fat fluid level is when there is a mixture of fat that rises on top of water contents leading to a fat fluid level seen on mediolateral mammograms and on ultrasound. This sign is characteristic of a galactocele but may occasionally be seen in fat necrosis (Fig. 11.7a–f).
- Pseudohamartoma is an appearance more often seen in chronic galactocele where a mixed fat and soft tissue density mass is seen resembling a hamartoma. Galactoceles can get infected and painful; aspiration in such cases may reveal purulent material with positive culture.

Galactocele can have a complex cystic mass with thick internal septations. Aspiration causes the lesion to partially collapse and reveals milk-like aspirate (Figs. 11.7a–f and 11.8a, b).

Lactating Adenoma

Lactating adenomas are benign tumors of the breast typically seen in the third trimester and during lactation [20]. These masses resemble fibroadenoma clinically and on imaging appear as circumscribed mobile oval-shaped masses. When infracted, they appear as firm tender masses [22]. Histologically unlike a fibroadenoma, these have very little stromal elements and consist predominantly of epithelial elements. These elements consist of mature tubules containing actively secreting cells filling up the acini with secretions [22]. Lactating adenomas uniquely tend to regress after cessation of breastfeeding [23]. At sonography, posterior acoustic enhancement and increased lesion compressibility is characteristic likely due to large amount of secretions in the acini (Figs. 11.9a, b, 11.10a–c, and 11.11a–c) [22]. Infarction leads to appearance of irregular margins and posterior acoustic shadowing.

Juvenile Papillomatosis

There is an increased frequency of benign proliferative disease during pregnancy and lactation [21]. Juvenile papillomatosis is generally seen in young women. An association with pregnancy has been proposed based on finding 5 cases of this entity in a series of 18 pregnant patients [21]. On ultrasound, juvenile papillomatosis appears as an ill-defined mass that is composed of multiple cysts surrounded by fibrous septa and well demarcated histologically from surrounding tissue. The cystic and ductal hyperplasia is associated with papillary hyperplasia lining the cystic spaces [24]. Definitive treatment is by surgical excision with negative margins required to avoid local recurrence [21]. In young women, juvenile papillomatosis is a risk factor for breast cancer with a reported association with breast cancer in 15 % of cases and a reported incidence of breast cancers in up to 50 % of female relatives [21, 24].

Granular Cell Tumor

This is a rare benign tumor seen in young women. About 5–6 % are seen in the breast and more commonly seen in African American women. They arise from perineural cells. Clinically, these present as superficial firm masses and there may be associated skin changes [1]. Histologically, they tend to form an infiltrative growth and simulate an infiltrative carcinoma, clinically and on imaging. At sonography, these appear as 1–2 cm irregular masses with posterior acoustic shadowing and tend to exhibit characteristics of a malignant mass (Fig. 11.12a, b). At mammography, these may appear as spiculated masses and simulate invasive ductal cancers; these can also appear as well-circumscribed masses. Despite the malignant appearance on imaging, these tumors are benign and preoperative diagnosis is important to treat appropriately with wide excision [1].

Granulomatous Mastitis

Granulomatous mastitis is a rare chronic inflammatory condition of the breast of unknown etiology. It affects women of childbearing age who most commonly present with an inflamed breast mass with or without pain. This condition

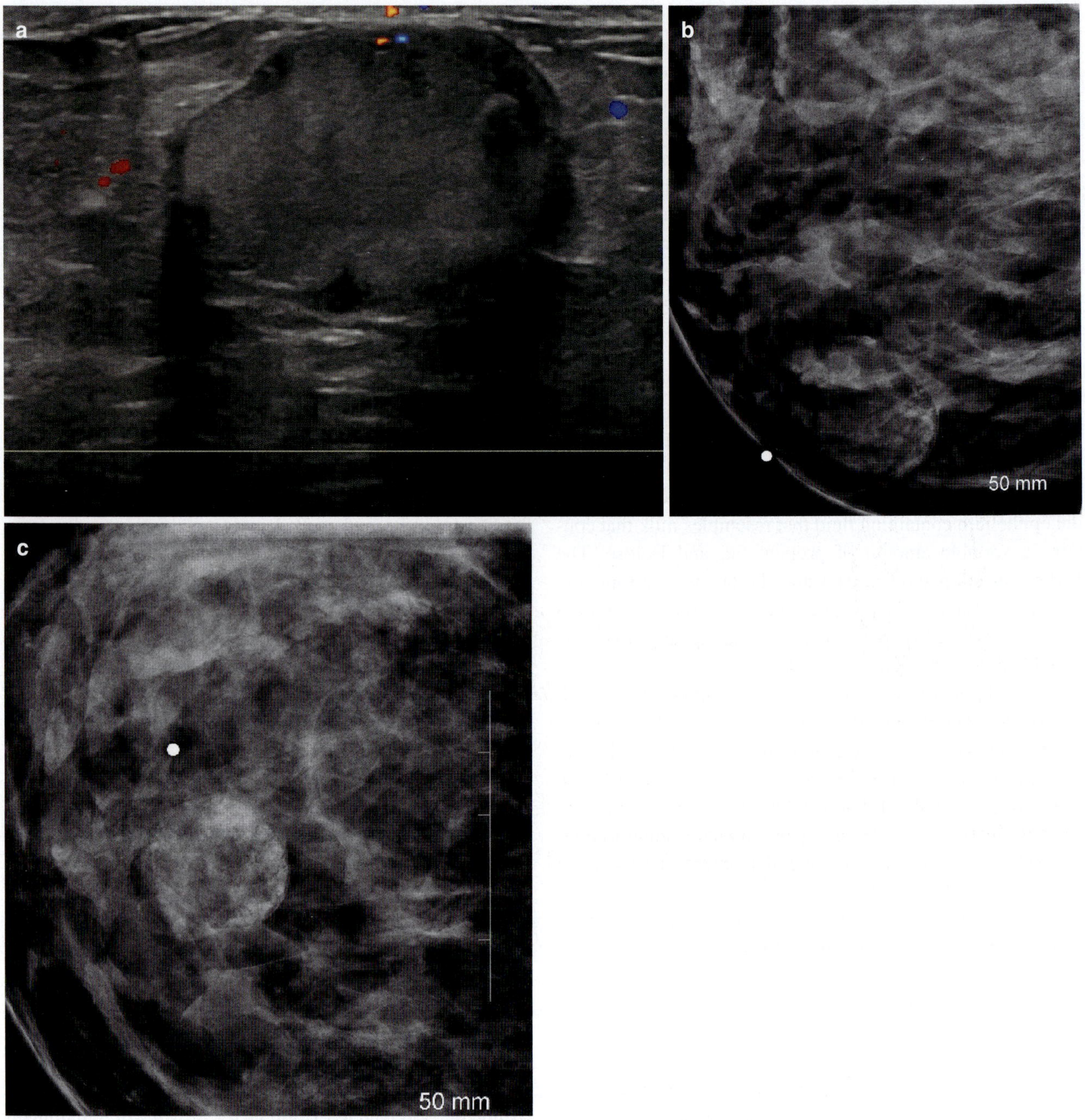

Fig. 11.5 (**a–c**) A 31-year-old lactating woman with a palpable lump histologically proven to be a galactocele. (**a**) Ultrasound demonstrated a hyperechoic circumscribed solid mass. (**b**) Spot compression view in the mediolateral projection shows a mixed fat and soft tissue mass. (**c**) Spot compression view in the craniocaudal projection shows a mixed fat and soft tissue mass

is benign but needs to be differentiated from inflammatory breast cancer and other chronic inflammatory conditions of the breast. There has been reported association with tuberculosis and HIV infection [25]. In one of the largest reported series of 41 cases seen over a period of 10 years, affliction was predominantly unilateral (95 %); a mass was found in 78 % on clinical examination and in 52 % on mammography and ultrasound. Tenderness (41 %) and erythema were less common (29 %); the subareolar region is typically spared. At ultrasound, multiple clustered tubular hypoechoic structures or poorly defined large hypoechoic masses may be seen and often mistaken for malignancy. Mammography may not demonstrate an abnormal finding especially in a dense breast or may show a mass or a focal asymmetry [21]. Reactive lymphadenopathy has been seen in 15 % of cases. Histologically at core biopsy, abundance of epithelioid

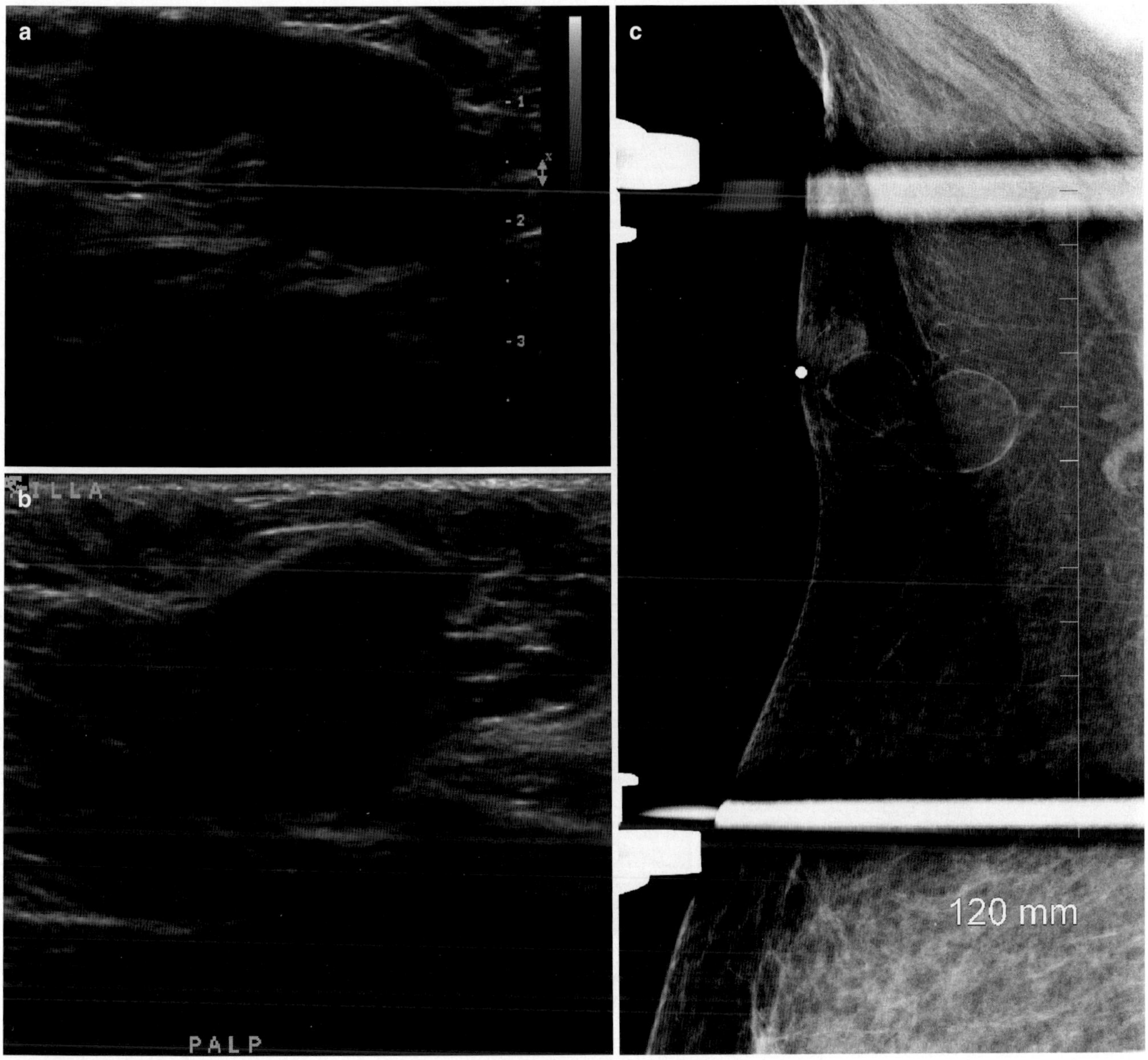

Fig. 11.6 (**a–c**) A 31-year-old with a palpable lump in the right axilla adjacent to an accessory nipple consistent with a galactocele. (**a**) Ultrasound demonstrates a circumscribed solid hypoechoic mass with a shape simulating an enlarged abnormal axillary lymph node. (**b**) Ultrasound demonstrates a circumscribed solid hypoechoic mass with a shape simulating an enlarged abnormal axillary lymph node. (**c**) Spot compression mammographic view shows the ultrasound solid-appearing mass to be radiolucent mass consistent with a benign finding. The round density contiguous with this lesion corresponded to the accessory nipple

histiocytes among a predominantly neutrophilic background is characteristic. Noncaseating granuloma formation within the breast parenchyma centered on breast lobules is typically seen. Prognosis is good; steroid therapy and excisional biopsy have been shown to be effective [21].

Fat Necrosis and Inflammation

Minor trauma to the breast may result in fat necrosis and inflammation. Presentation is with a painful lump. Ultrasound may show a solid hyperechoic mass; mammogram may reveal a partly radiolucent mass or an iso- or high-density mass interspersed with fat (Fig. 11.13a–c).

Mastitis and Breast Abscess

Infection of the breast predominantly affects young women and occurs most commonly during lactational period. *Staphylococcus aureus* is the most common causative organism followed by streptococcus. Staphylococcus infection

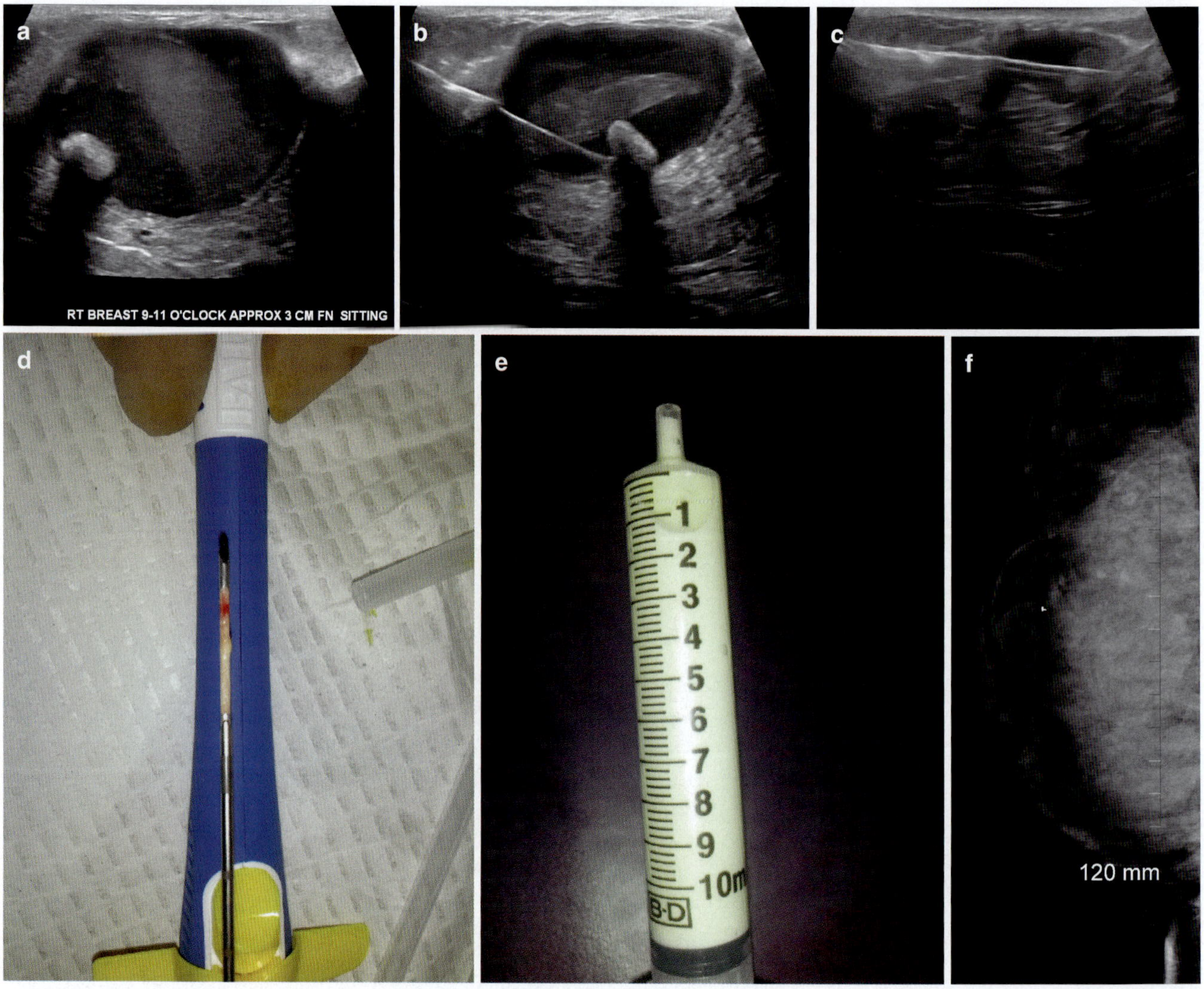

Fig. 11.7 (a–f) A 28-year-old lactating woman with a painful palpable lump histologically proven to be a galactocele. (**a**) Ultrasound demonstrated a complex cystic mass with echogenic contents and a mural nodule showing posterior acoustic shadowing. (**b**) US-guided aspiration with needle in the cystic mass and within the mural nodule. (**c**) Post core-needle biopsy, the cavity is partially collapsed. (**d**) Core specimen from the mural nodule and cyst wall. (**e**) Milky aspirate from the galactocele in a syringe. (**f**) Post-biopsy mediolateral oblique view demonstrates a fat density mass with the post-biopsy clip and a fat fluid level

tends to be invasive and localized with a greater propensity for abscess formation, whereas streptococcus infection presents as diffuse mastitis with abscess formation seen only in late phases [26]. There are several types of clinical presentation, and these are discussed next.

Puerperal Mastitis

Mastitis is said to occur in 1–24 % of breastfeeding women [27]. Breast abscess is reported to complicate puerperal mastitis in 5–11 % of cases [28]. The organism gains entry through cracked nipples during lactation originating from the nasopharynx or mouth of the infant and proliferates in the stagnant lactiferous ducts. Breastfeeding is encouraged during mastitis to drain such engorged ducts. Breastfeeding cessation is only advised following surgical drainage or if the mother is on an antibiotic that is contraindicated for the newborn [26].

Central Nonpuerperal Abscess

In women who are not lactating, the most common type of abscess is the central nonpuerperal type. These occur predominantly in young women who are smokers. Cessation of smoking should be strongly advised, and in those over 35 years of age, mammography is indicated to exclude malignancy. Cigarette smoke induced changes in the epithelium of the retroareolar ducts leading to formation of keratin plugs, periductal mastitis, distension and obstruction of the ducts,

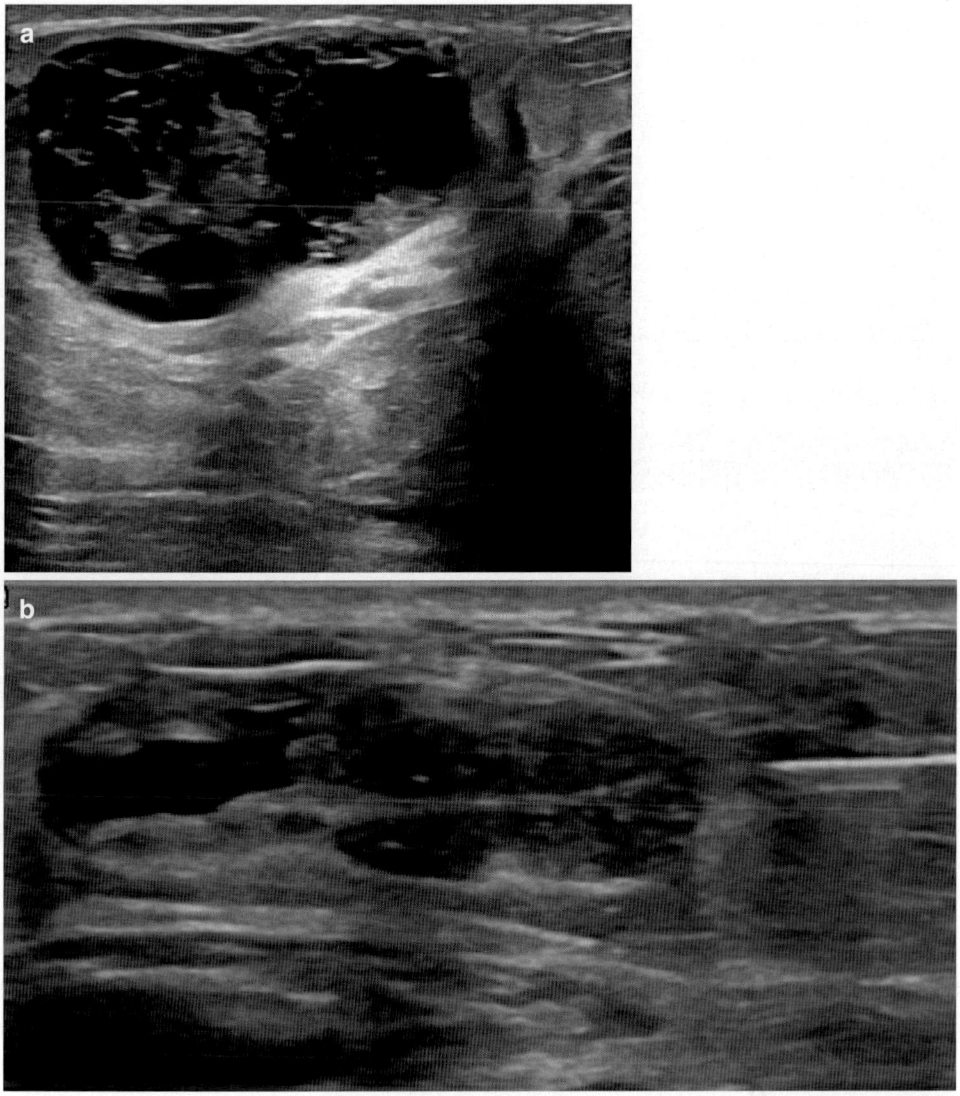

Fig. 11.8 (**a**, **b**) A 32-year-old woman with a palpable tender lump during lactation revealed a complex galactocele at biopsy. (**a**) Ultrasound demonstrates a complex cystic mass with thick internal septations. (**b**) Post ultrasound-guided core biopsy, the lesion is partially collapsed

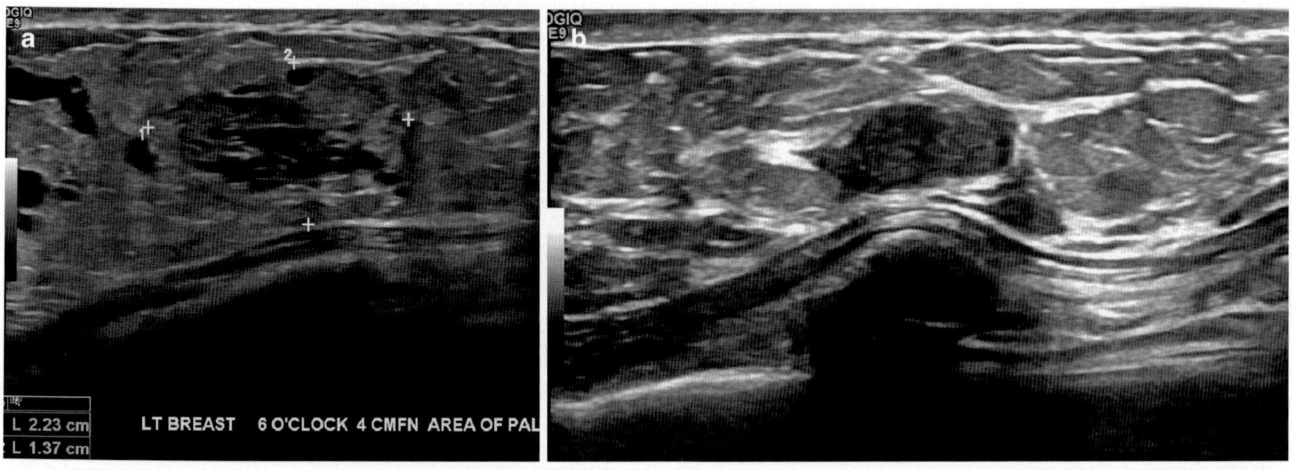

Fig. 11.9 (**a**, **b**) A 34-year-old woman with a palpable lump during lactation revealed a lactating adenoma. (**a**) Ultrasound demonstrates a solid mass with multiple tubular cystic structures within representing dilated ducts. (**b**) Follow-up ultrasound at 12 months reveals the mass being smaller and without the lactational changes of dilated ducts

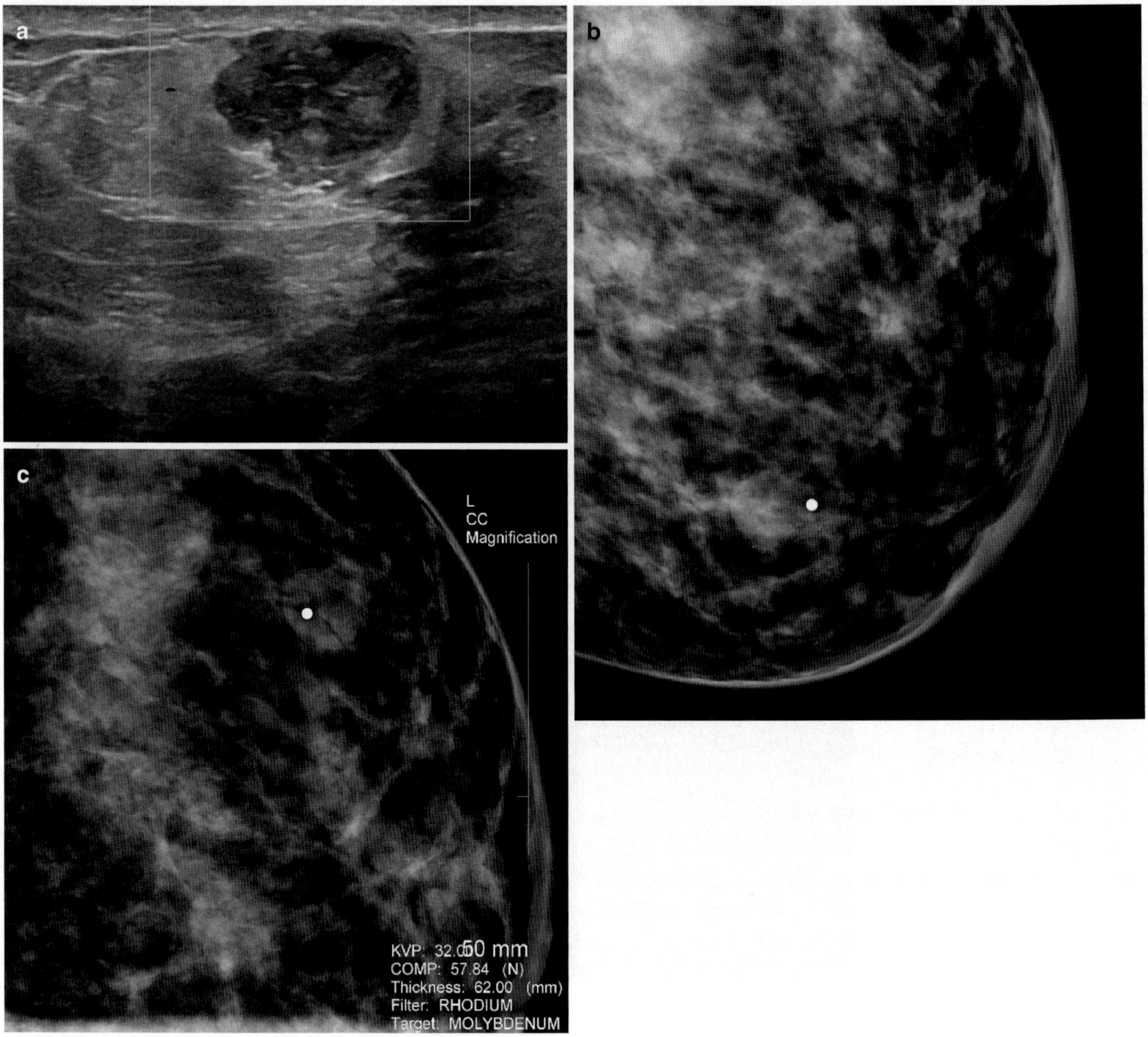

Fig. 11.10 (**a**–**c**) A 34-year-old with a palpable lump histologically proven to be an infracted lactating adenoma. (**a**) Ultrasound demonstrated a solid indeterminate mass. (**b**) Mediolateral oblique mammogram shows a round dense mass with obscured borders. (**c**) Craniocaudal mammogram shows a round dense mass with obscured borders

and stagnation, and infection ensues [26]. Treatment is by means of percutaneous drainage. Bilaterality is common and reported in 25 % of cases and recurrence also occurs in 25–40 % of cases.

Peripheral Nonpuerperal Abscess

These are less common and seen in older women. These may be seen in women with chronic underlying conditions such as diabetes mellitus or rheumatoid arthritis. Steroid therapy or recent breast interventions are also potential underlying factors [26]. In most women with nonpuerperal peripheral mastitis, there is no underlying condition. Treatment is by drainage and antibiotics and recurrence is rare.

Imaging in Mastitis and Breast Abscess

Pain, redness, heat, and palpable lumps are frequently seen in those with mastitis and abscess; fever is uncommon. In a series of breast abscesses with lumps, 80 % were painful and 71 % were associated with redness of the overlying skin with only 12 % associated with fever [29]. Abscess is seen in 40–65 % of cases on ultrasound and at more than one site in 21 % of cases [27].

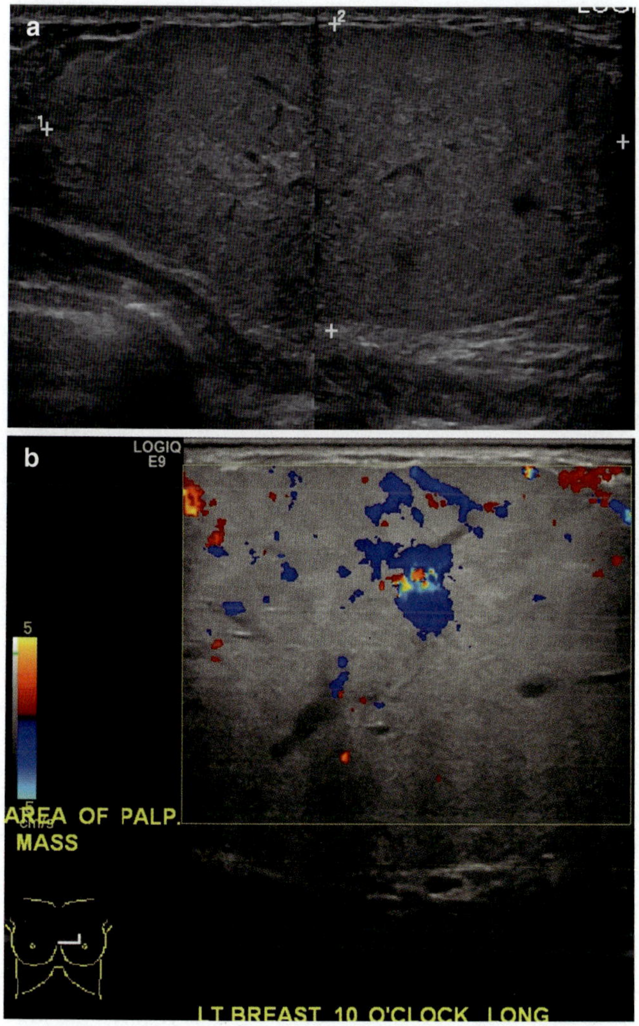

Fig. 11.11 (**a**, **b**) A 36-year-old with a palpable lump in the left breast with histologically proven infracted lactating adenoma. Ultrasound demonstrates a superficially located solid mass with heterogeneous echotexture and circumscribed lobulated borders. Appearance was consistent with an indeterminate mass with a recommendation for ultrasound-guided core biopsy

At ultrasound which is the initial and often the only imaging modality that is used for diagnosis and management, mastitis appears as ill-defined areas of increased echogenicity in the fat lobules and as areas of decreased echogenicity in the glandular parenchyma. Skin thickening is frequently observed. Reactive lymphadenopathy is seen as lymph nodes that are enlarged with diffuse thickening of the cortex and preservation of the fatty hilum and increased vascularity. Abscess is seen as an irregular fluid collection with multiloculation, posterior acoustic enhancement, and sometimes with a hyperechoic rim showing increased vascularity (Fig. 11.14a, b). Mammography is performed in older women, in those not responding to treatment, or for those who are not lactating mainly to exclude malignancy. Mammography is deferred until the acute phase has subsided to avoid the added discomfort of compression. Skin thickening, focal asymmetry or a mass are signs that may be present but are nonspecific and do not help in the distinction from malignancy. Presence of suspicious microcalcifications, however, is worrisome and should prompt biopsy. In a series of 975 cases of suspected mastitis, there were 6 cases of inflammatory breast cancer (IBC) [26]. In two of these cases, there were suspicious microcalcifications seen at mammography. Mastitis that is seen in a nonpuerperal setting or one that is not responding to treatment should raise the suspicion of IBC particularly in older women. Pain in IBC is generally less severe than in mastitis; skin thickening is also more localized than in IBC. Suspicious microcalcifications are seen in up to 47 % of cases of IBC and hence when seen is the most specific sign of an underlying malignancy [26]. The finding of a mass on mammography and more frequently on an ultrasound is also more indicative of an underlying malignancy. There can still be some overlap in the imaging findings between mastitis and abscess and IBC posing diagnostic challenges [30].

Pregnancy-Associated Breast Cancer

Breast cancer that is diagnosed during pregnancy or within 1 year after childbirth is included in the definition of pregnancy-associated breast cancer (PABC) [31]. PABC has been traditionally associated with poor prognosis and an advanced stage at presentation mainly due to delay in diagnosis [32, 33]. In an analysis of 104 PABC among 652 women under the age of 35 years with breast cancer, there was found to be no statistically significant difference in locoregional recurrence, distant metastasis, or in overall survival among women with PABC compared to those in nonpregnant women. It was, however, noted in this retrospective study that pregnancy caused a delay in diagnosis, evaluation, and treatment [34]. The authors found that any treatment intervention during pregnancy resulted in improved survival when compared to those whose treatment was delayed due to pregnancy. Primary care physicians and obstetricians should aggressively pursue workup of breast symptoms in pregnancy for a prompt diagnosis of breast cancer and appropriate initiation of multidisciplinary treatment. The spectrum of the imaging appearance of PABC has been well described in literature [31, 35–37]. PABC is rare and has been reported in 0.3 per 1000 pregnancies [38]. About 2/3 of these cancers are diagnosed in the postpartum period [35].

Imaging Evaluation in PABC

Under the influence of hormones estrogen, progesterone, and prolactin, there is proliferation of ducts and lobules, increased secretion, and enlargement of the lobular acini with

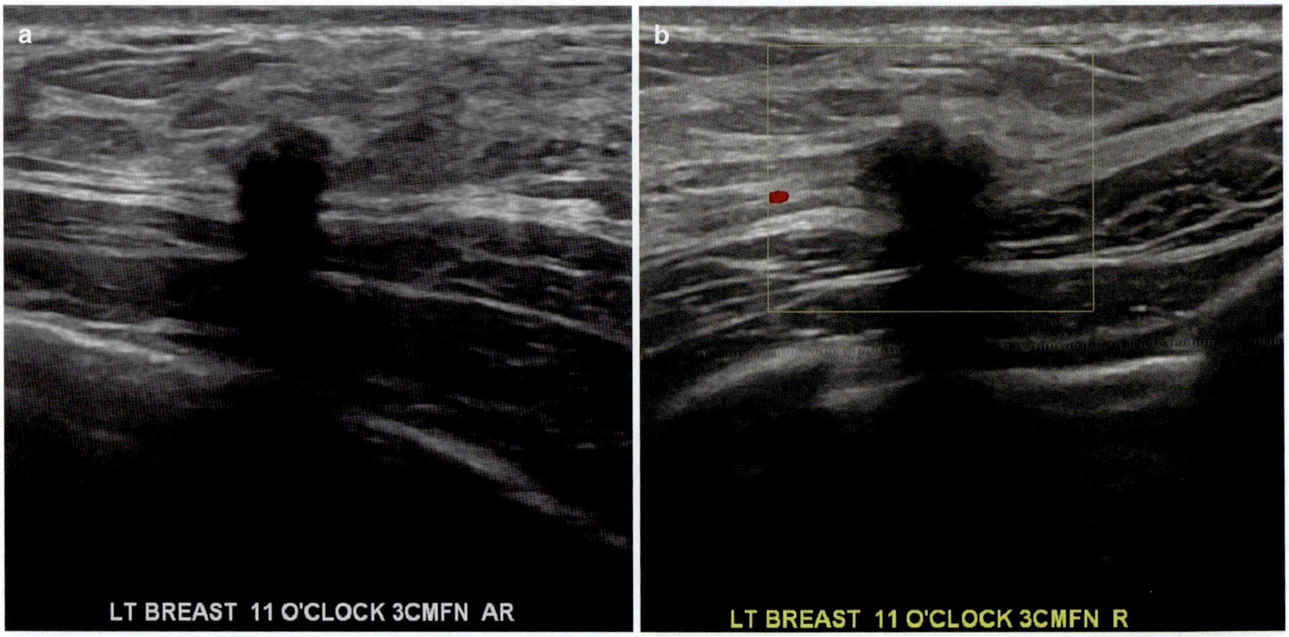

Fig. 11.12 (**a**, **b**) A 29-year-old woman postpartum with a hard palpable lump histologically proven to be a granular cell tumor. Ultrasound demonstrates a small irregular hypoechogenic mass with posterior acoustic shadowing that was prebiopsy categorized as highly suggestive of malignancy

colostrums. These changes in the breast parenchyma lead to a marked increase in the breast density and make it nodular with decreased fat tissue [36]. Clinical evaluation is limited for these reasons. This also causes significantly decreased sensitivity of mammography. A persistent localized palpable finding needs to be further evaluated by imaging. Sonography is the imaging modality of choice. Abnormal mammographic findings when seen in PABC include masses, asymmetric density, suspicious calcifications, skin and trabecular thickening, and axillary adenopathy. Widespread calcifications have been reported in 26 % of cases of PABC [37]. Sonography is the initial imaging modality for the evaluation of breast symptoms in pregnancy with a reported sensitivity of 100 % for the diagnosis of breast cancer [36]. The negative predictive value of sonography is 100 % [36]. Sonography is useful in distinguishing benign changes from a solid tumor and can predict malignancy accurately using morphologic criteria described by Stavros (Fig. 11.15a, b) [39]. However, there are certain features that are more commonly associated with benign masses that may be more commonly associated with PABC. Parallel orientation is one such feature that was found in 58 % of cancers in one series [36]. Due to rapid growth and increased vascularity, cystic changes may also be encountered in PABC; hence, complex cystic masses in pregnancy need a tissue diagnosis so as not to mistake PABC for a galactocele or an abscess. Similarly, posterior acoustic enhancement is a more commonly encountered feature of a mass in PABC compared to those in a nonpregnant patient [36]. Mammography reveals positive findings in 74–87 % despite sensitivity being reduced due to increased breast density [36, 37]. A negative sonographic study should prompt biopsy when the mass is clinically suspicious. Mammography is generally performed when initial evaluation is suspicious for malignancy. Invasive ductal cancers constitute a large percentage of PABC accounting for 58–91 % of cases [36, 37]. Ultrasound of the axilla is useful in identifying metastatic nodes in patients with PABC. Some authors have found ultrasound of the axilla more useful [40] than others [37]. Inflammatory breast cancer is not more prevalent in pregnancy; about 2–18 % of breast cancers in pregnancy are inflammatory breast cancer [36, 41]. However, since mastitis is more prevalent during lactation, having a high index of suspicion for IBC is important particularly in cases not responding to treatment (Fig. 11.16a, b).

Breast Cancer in the Young Woman

There has been a steady improvement in the outcomes of treatment for breast cancer with 5-year disease-free survival being 75–85 %. Most of the improvement in the outcome is attributed to early detection due to the widespread use of screening mammography. More than half of all patients that are screened with mammography have stage 0 or stage I disease [42, 43]. Conversely, 71 % of breast cancer deaths were reported to be in women who had not undergone screening

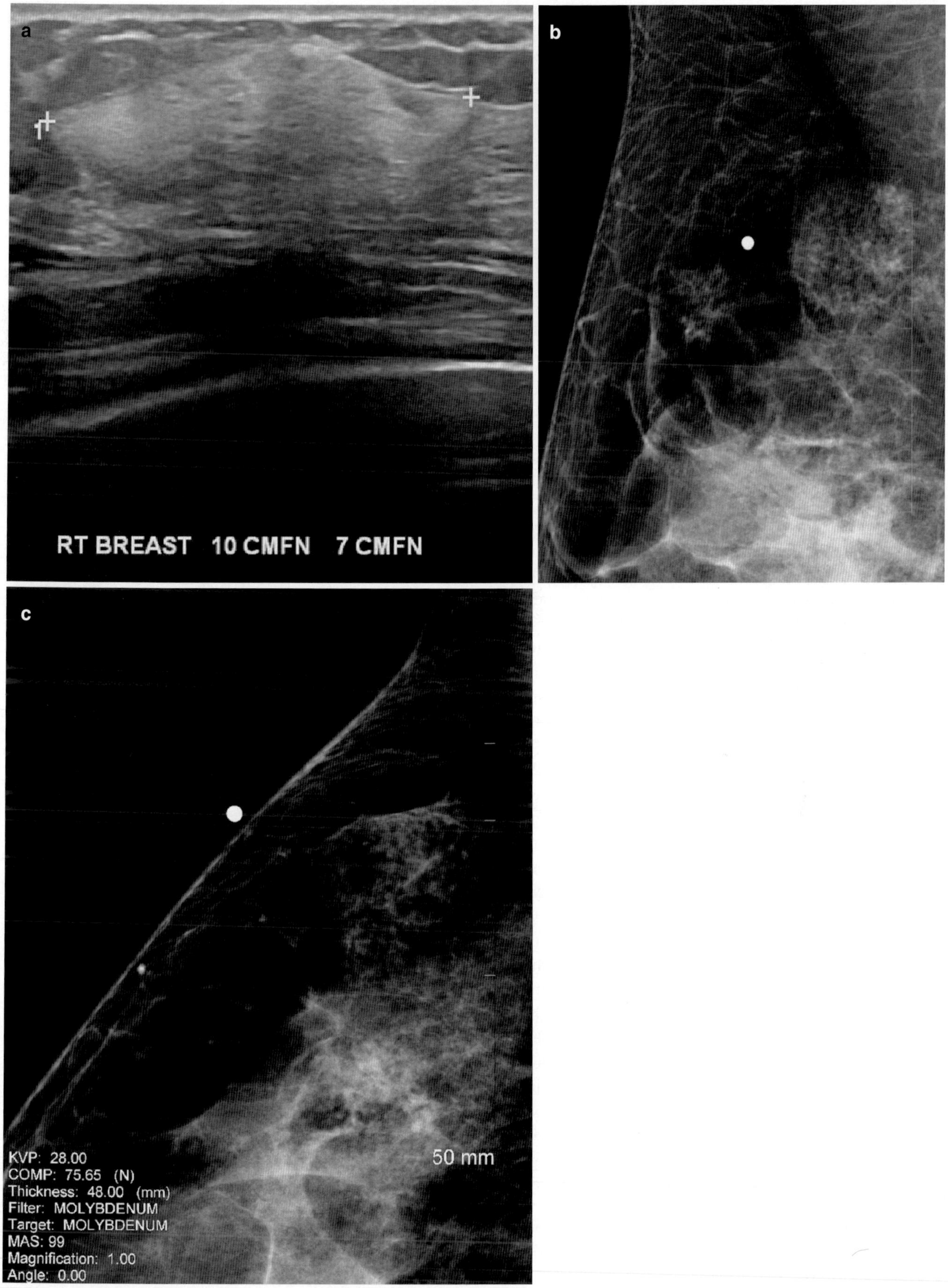

Fig. 11.13 (**a**–**c**) A 27-year-old woman during lactation with a painful palpable lump in the right breast histologically proven to be fat necrosis with inflammatory changes. (**a**) Ultrasound demonstrates an ovoid hyperechoic mass. (**b**) Spot magnification view in the mediolateral oblique view demonstrates a mixed density mass. (**c**) Spot magnification view in the craniocaudal view demonstrates a mixed density mass

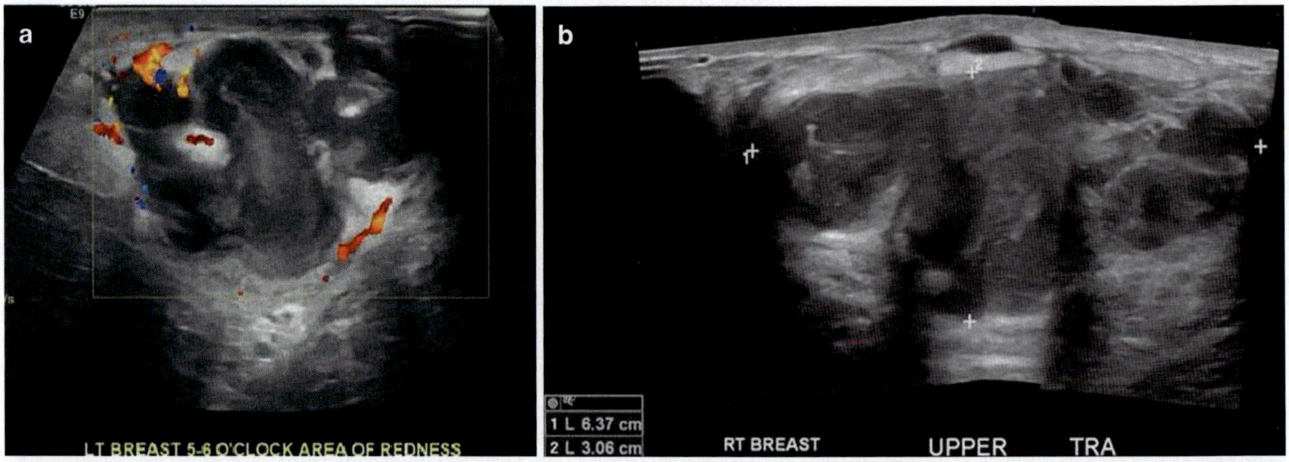

Fig. 11.14 (**a**, **b**) A 35-year-old woman during lactation with a painful lump associated with mastitis. (**a**, **b**) Ultrasound demonstrates a complex fluid collection consistent with an abscess

mammography compared to 29 % in women who had undergone regular screening mammography [44]. The benefit of screening does not apply to women under the age of 40 years in whom screening for breast cancer is not recommended for those at average risk for breast cancer. A low prevalence of breast cancer combined with reduced sensitivity of mammography makes this modality not a cost-effective intervention in young women. There has been no improvement in breast cancer survival over the years in women under the age of 40 years.

Breast cancer occurs less frequently in women under the age of 40 years. The prevalence of cancer in this group of women who are not routinely screened when at average risk is low. Interestingly, the risk of developing cancer in women under 40 years of age is similar throughout the world including the developing nations that have seen a dramatic increased incidence of breast cancer in recent years [45]. The worldwide average for developing breast cancer before 40 years of age is 0.3 % and is similar in Japan, Canada, Bangladesh, and Nigeria [45, 46]. The cumulative risk of breast cancer to age 39 in the USA is 0.45 and in Canada 0.38 [45]. The low prevalence of disease means that screening is not a feasible or cost-effective tool to detect cancers at an early stage. Risk factors in young women include a lean body habitus and recent use of contraceptives [46]. In the USA, based on estimates of the American Cancer Society, there will be 230,000 women who will receive a diagnosis of invasive breast cancer, only 5 % of which will be in women under 40 years of age [47]. Breast cancer in young women tends to be aggressive, of higher grade with a greater proportion of triple-negative tumors. Additionally, young age is an independent negative predictor of cancer-specific survival. Local recurrence and contralateral disease are higher. Increasing breast cancer awareness may lead to diagnosing cancers when smaller than 2.0 cm with consequent improved mortality. A study compared the risk factors, clinical presentation, pathologic findings, tumor characteristics, extent of disease, treatment, and outcomes for 101 women under the age of 36 treated for breast cancer with 631 patients 36 years or older. Patients under the age of 36 years diagnosed with breast cancer presented more often with a palpable mass; cancers were more aggressive and advanced (Figs. 11.17a–e and 11.18a–d). Despite aggressive treatment with chemotherapy and mastectomy, local and distant metastases were higher; local and distant failure rates were also higher. A majority of patients younger than 36 years were diagnosed with stage II or stage III disease, whereas majority of cancers in women greater than 36 years of age were diagnosed with stage 0 or stage I disease [48].

Due to the fact that mammographic screening is not routinely offered or recommended in women under the age of 40 years, breast cancer awareness is of importance to detect cancer at an earlier stage. The size of the cancer being the predictor of long-term survival, increasing awareness may potentially lead to young women seeking earlier attention for breast symptoms.

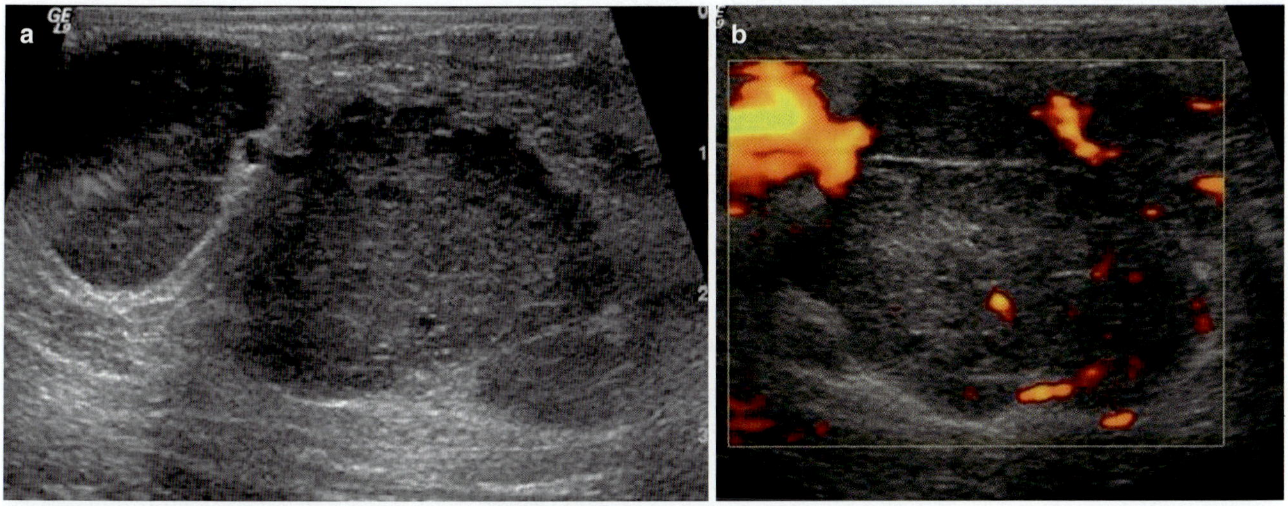

Fig. 11.15 (**a**, **b**) A 28-year-old woman with a palpable lump in her right breast initially misinterpreted as a cyst (images not shown). Mass continued to enlarge. Subsequent biopsy revealed an infiltrating carcinoma. (**a**) Ultrasound shows a large solid mass with lobulations and ill-defined borders. (**b**) Doppler imaging demonstrates peripheral and internal vascularity

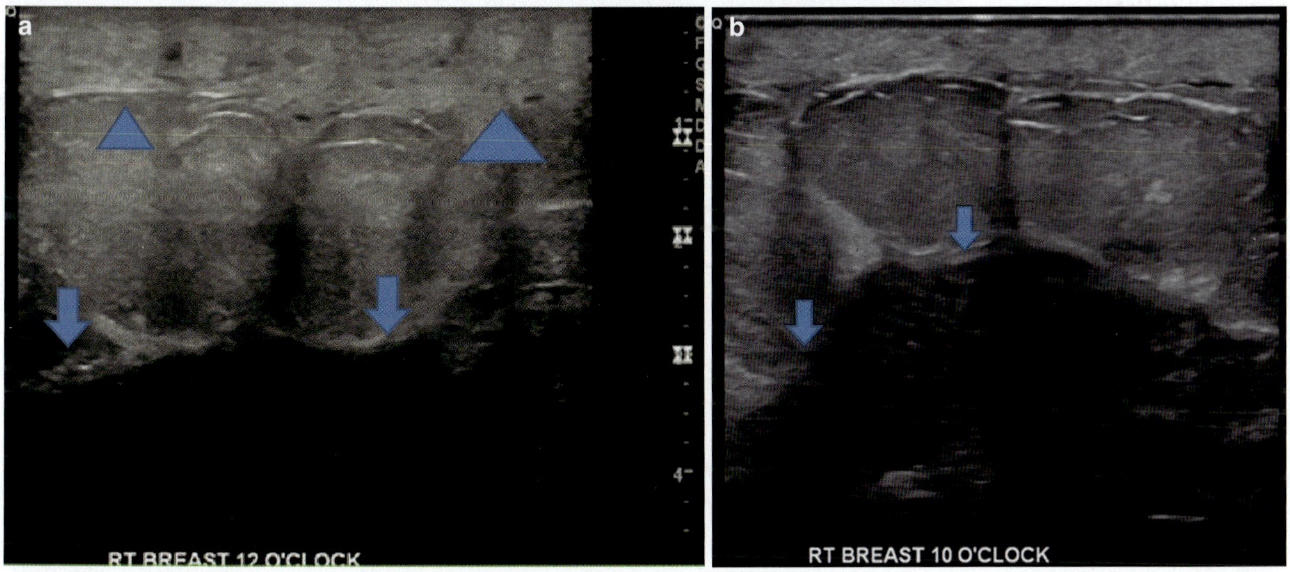

Fig. 11.16 (**a**, **b**) A 29-year-old woman with a progressively enlarging mass and skin changes during pregnancy histologically proven inflammatory breast cancer. (**a**, **b**) Ultrasound of the affected breast performed following childbirth demonstrates a very large irregular hypoechoic mass (*arrows*). There is marked thickening of the skin (*arrowheads*)

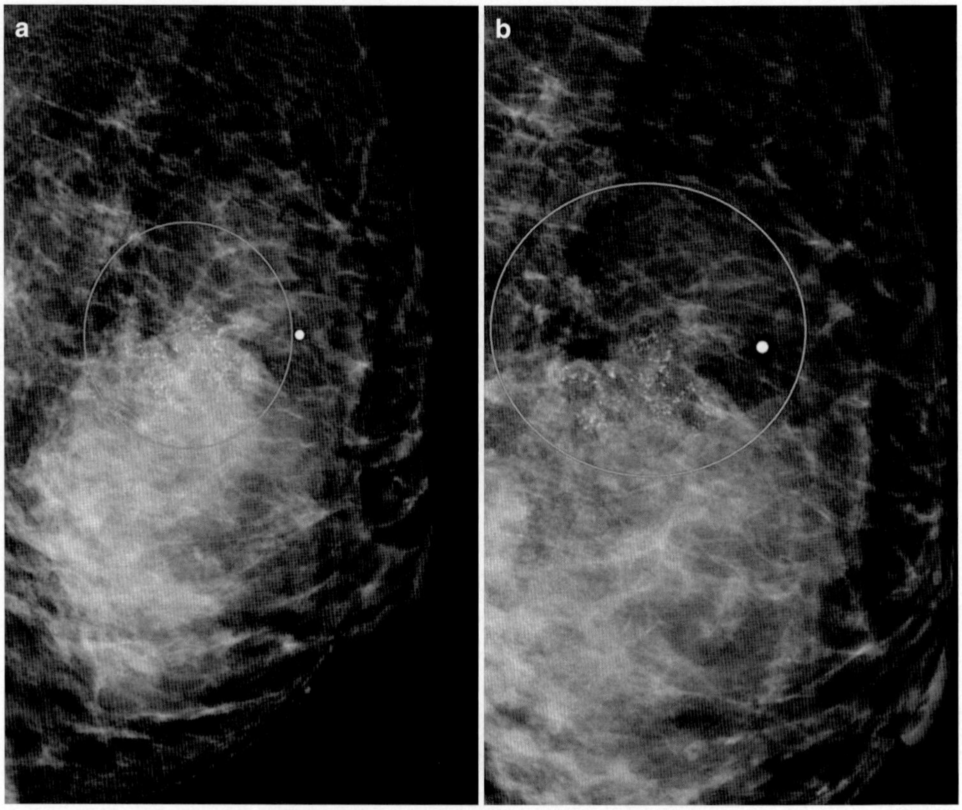

Fig. 11.17 (**a–e**) A 31-year-old woman with a palpable lump in the left breast histologically proven to be DCIS with invasive component. (**a**) Left mediolateral oblique view demonstrates extensive pleomorphic calcifications in the area of palpable abnormality. (**b**) Left craniocaudal projection view demonstrates extensive pleomorphic calcifications in the area of palpable abnormality. (**c**) Magnification view in the mediolateral projection demonstrates pleomorphic calcifications in a segmental distribution highly suggestive of malignancy. (**d**) Magnification view in the craniocaudal projection demonstrates pleomorphic calcifications in a segmental distribution highly suggestive of malignancy. (**e**) Ultrasound demonstrates a solid mass with intraductal calcifications

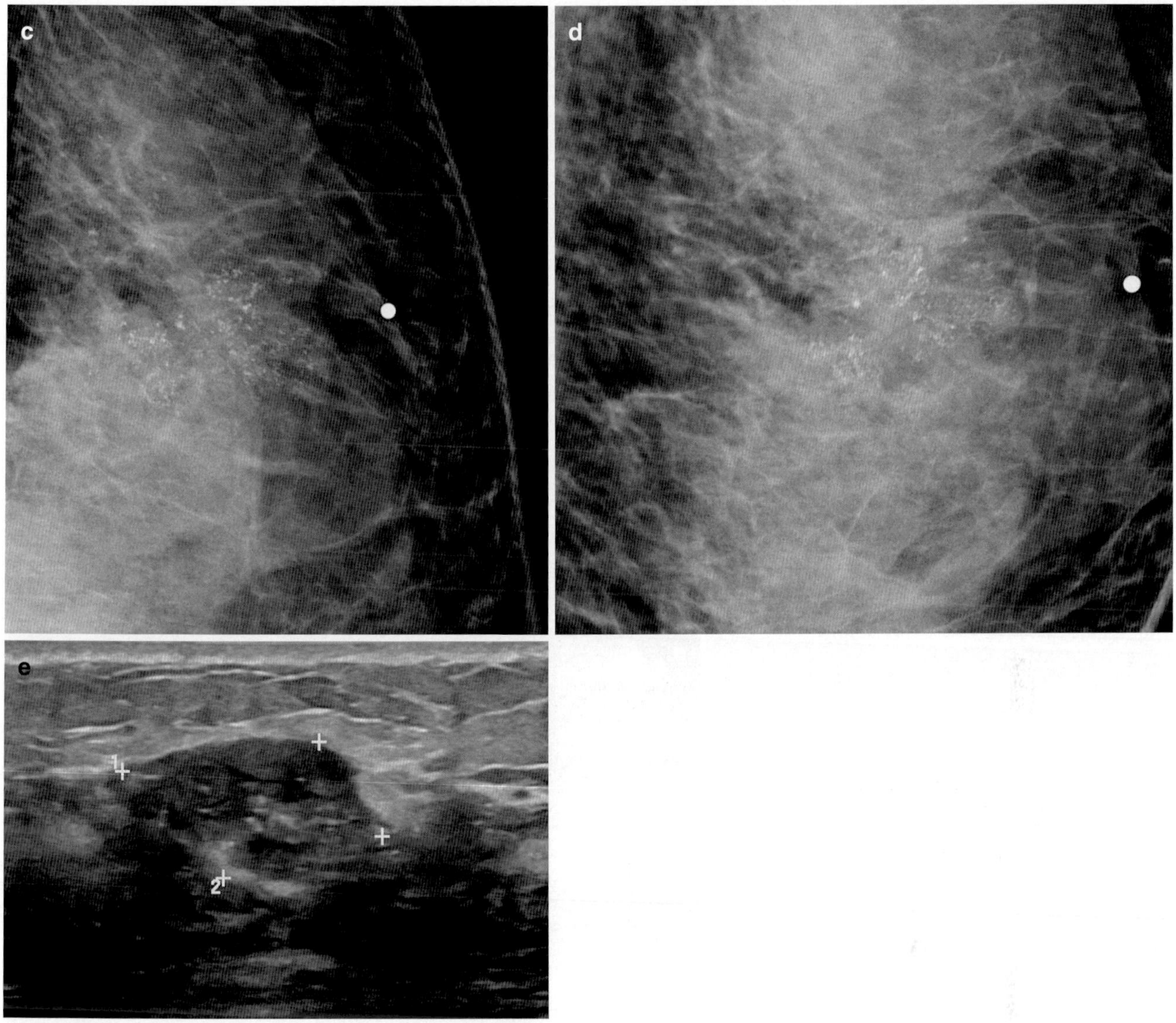

Fig. 11.17 (continued)

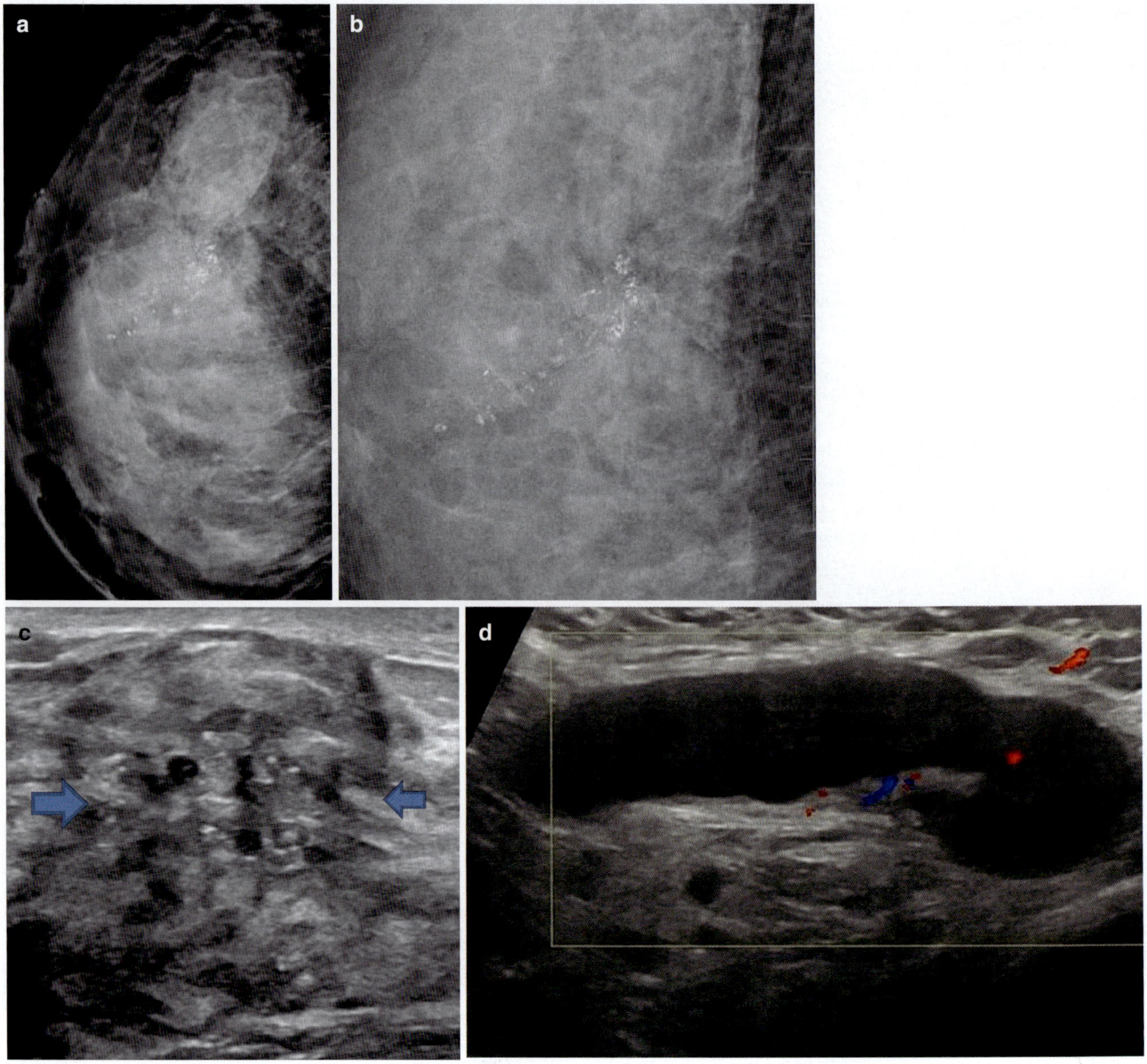

Fig. 11.18 (**a**–**d**) A 24-year-old woman with a family history of cancer and a palpable lump in the right breast histologically proven to be invasive ductal cancer. (**a**) Right mediolateral oblique view demonstrates pleomorphic microcalcifications highly suggestive of cancer. (**b**) Magnification view shows linearly distributed pleomorphic calcifications in greater detail. (**c**) Ultrasound demonstrates a poorly defined hypoechoic area with intraductal microcalcifications (*arrows*). (**d**) Ultrasound of the right axilla demonstrates a markedly enlarged lymph node with replacement of the fatty hilum proven at fine-needle aspiration biopsy to be a metastatic lymphadenopathy

References

1. Chung EM, Cube R, Hall GJ, González C, Stocker JT, Glassman LM. From the archives of the AFIP: breast masses in children and adolescents: radiologic-pathologic correlation. Radiographics. 2009;29(3):907–31.
2. Greydanus DE, Matytsina L, Gains M. Breast disorders in children and adolescents. Prim Care. 2006;33:455–502.
3. Welch ST, Babcock DS, Ballard ET. Sonography of pediatric male breast masses: gynecomastia and beyond. Pediatr Radiol. 2004;34:952–7.
4. Vade A, Lafita VS, Ward KA, Lim-Dunham JE, Bova D. Role of breast sonography in imaging of adolescents with palpable solid breast masses. AJR Am J Roentgenol. 2008;191(3):659–63.
5. Sanchez R, Ladino-Torres MF, Bernat JA, Joe A, DiPietro MA. Breast fibroadenomas in the pediatric population: common and uncommon sonographic findings. Pediatr Radiol. 2010;40: 1681–9.
6. Sklair-Levy M, Sella T, Alweiss T, Craciun I, Libson E, Mally B. Incidence and management of complex fibroadenomas. AJR Am J Roentgenol. 2008;190:214–8.
7. West KW, Rescoria FJ, Scherer III LR, Grosfeld JL. Diagnosis and treatment of symptomatic breast masses in the pediatric population. J Pediatr Surg. 1995;30:182–6; discussion, 186–7.
8. García CJ, Espinoza A, Dinamarca V, et al. Breast US in children and adolescents. Radiographics. 2000;20:1605–12.
9. Ferreira M, Albarracin CT, Resetkova E. Pseudoangiomatous stromal hyperplasia tumor: a clinical, radiologic and pathologic study of 26 cases. Mod Pathol. 2008;21:201–7.
10. Kaneda HJ, Mack J, Kasales CJ, Schetter S. Pediatric and adolescent breast masses: a review of pathophysiology, imaging, diagnosis, and treatment. AJR Am J Roentgenol. 2013;200(2):W204–12.
11. Coffin CM. The breast. In: Stocker JT, Dehner LP, editors. Pediatric pathology. 2nd ed. Philadelphia: Lippincott Williams & Wilkins; 2002. p. 993 1015.
12. Sabate JM, Clotet M, Torrubia S, et al. Radiologic evaluation of breast disorders related to pregnancy and lactation. Radiographics. 2007;27(Spec Issue):S101–24.
13. Bazzocchi F, Santini D, Martinelli G, et al. Juvenile papillomatosis (epitheliosis) of the breast: a clinical and pathologic study of 13 cases. Am J Clin Pathol. 1986;86:745–8.
14. Rosen PP, Kimmel M. Juvenile papillomatosis of the breast: a follow-up study of 41 patients having biopsies before 1979. Am J Clin Pathol. 1990;93:599–603.
15. Adeniran A, Al-Ahmadie H, Mahoney MC, Robinson-Smith TM. Granular cell tumor of the breast: a series of 17 cases and review of the literature. Breast J. 2004;10:528–31.
16. Howlader N, Noone AM, Krapcho M, Garshell J, Neyman N, Altekruse SF, Kosary CL, Yu M, Ruhl J, Tatalovich Z, Cho H, Mariotto A, Lewis DR, Chen HS, Feuer EJ, Cronin KA, editors. SEER cancer statistics review, 1975–2010. Bethesda: National Cancer Institute. http://seer.cancer.gov/csr/1975_2010/, based on November 2012 SEER data submission, posted to the SEER web site, 2013.
17. Gains M. Breast disorders in children and adolescents. Prim Care. 2006;33:455–502.
18. Howarth CB, Caces JN, Pratt CB. Breast metastases in children with rhabdomyosarcoma. Cancer. 1980;46:2520–4.
19. Gemignani ML, Petrek JA. Pregnancy-associated breast cancer: diagnosis and treatment. Breast J. 2000;6:68–73.
20. Vashi R, Hooley R, Butler R, Geisel J, Philpotts L. Breast imaging of the pregnant and lactating patient: physiologic changes and common benign entities. AJR Am J Roentgenol. 2013;200(2):329–36.
21. Sabate JM, Clotet M, Torrubia S, Gomez A, Guerrero R, de las Heras P, Lerma E. Radiologic evaluation of breast disorders related to pregnancy and lactation. Radiographics. 2007;27 Suppl 1: S101–24.
22. Stavros AT. Breast ultrasound. Philadelphia: Lippincott Williams & Wilkins; 2004.
23. Sumkin JH, Perrone AM, Harris KM, Nath ME, Amortegui AJ, Weinstein BJ. Lactating adenoma: US features and literature review. Radiology. 1998;206:271–4.
24. Rosen PP. Breast tumors in children. In: Rosen PP, editor. Rosen's breast pathology. 2nd ed. Philadelphia: Lippincott-Raven; 2001. p. 729–48.
25. Mohammed S, Statz A, Lacross JS, Lassinger BK, Contreras A, Gutierrez C, Bonefas E, Liscum KR, Silberfein EJ. Granulomatous mastitis: a 10 year experience from a large inner city county hospital. J Surg Res. 2013;184(1):299–303.
26. Trop I, Dugas A, David J, El Khoury M, Boileau JF, Larouche N, Lalonde L. Breast abscesses: evidence-based algorithms for diagnosis, management, and follow-up. Radiographics. 2011;31(6): 1683–99.
27. Ulitzsch D, Nyman MK, Carlson RA. Breast abscess in lactating women: US-guided treatment. Radiology. 2004;232(3):904–9.
28. Thomsen AC, Espersen T, Maigaard S. Course and treatment of milk stasis, noninfectious inflammation of the breast, and infectious mastitis in nursing women. Am J Obstet Gynecol. 1984;149(5): 492–5.
29. Leborgne F, Leborgne F. Treatment of breast abscesses with sonographically guided aspiration, irrigation, and instillation of antibiotics. AJR Am J Roentgenol. 2003;181(4):1089–91.
30. Renz DM, Baltzer PAT, Böttcher J, et al. Magnetic resonance imaging of inflammatory breast carcinoma and acute mastitis: a comparative study. Eur Radiol. 2008;18(11):2370–80.
31. Vashi R, Hooley R, Butler R, Geisel J, Philpotts L. Breast imaging of the pregnant and lactating patient: imaging modalities and pregnancy-associated breast cancer. AJR Am J Roentgenol. 2013;200(2):321–8.
32. Treves N, Holleb AI. A report of 549 cases of breast cancer in women 35 years of age or younger. Surg Gynecol Obstet. 1958;107: 271–83.
33. Woo JC, Yu T, Hurd TC. Breast cancer in pregnancy: a literature review. Arch Surg. 2003;138:91–8.
34. Beadle BM, et al. The impact of pregnancy on breast cancer outcomes in women<or=35 years. Cancer. 2009;115(6):1174–84.
35. Ayyappan AP, Kulkarni S, Crystal P. Pregnancy-associated breast cancer: spectrum of imaging appearances. Br J Radiol. 2010;83(990):529–34.
36. Ahn BY, Kim HH, Moon WK, Pisano ED, Kim HS, Cha ES, Kim JS, Oh KK, Park SH. Pregnancy- and lactation-associated breast cancer : mammographic and sonographic findings. J Ultrasound Med. 2003;22(5):491–7.
37. Taylor D, Lazberger J, Ives A, Wylie E, Saunders C. Reducing delay in the diagnosis of pregnancy-associated breast cancer: how imaging can help us. J Med Imaging Radiat Oncol. 2011;55(1): 33–42.
38. Keleher AJ, Theriault RL, Gwyn KM, Hunt KK, Stelling CB, Singletary SE, et al. Multidisciplinary management of breast cancer concurrent with pregnancy. J Am Coll Surg. 2002;194:54–64.
39. Stavros AT, Thickman D, Rapp CL, Dennis MA, Parker SH, Sisney GA. Solid breast nodules: use of sonography to distinguish between benign and malignant lesions. Radiology. 1995;196:123–34.
40. Yang WT, Dryden MJ, Gwyn K, Whitman GJ, Theriault R. Imaging of breast cancer diagnosed and treated with chemotherapy during pregnancy. Radiology. 2006;239:52–60.
41. Petrek JA. Breast cancer during pregnancy. Cancer. 1994;74:518–27.
42. Osteen RT, Cady B, Chmiel JS, et al. 1991 national survey of carcinoma of the breast by the Commission on Cancer. J Am Coll Surg. 1994;178:213–9.

43. Tartter PI. Prognosis. In: Hermann G, Schwartz IS, Tartter PI, editors. Nonpalpable breast cancer: diagnosis and management. New York: Igaku-Shoin Medical Publishers; 1992. p. 112–9.
44. Webb ML, Cady B, Michaelson JS, Bush DM, Calvillo KZ, Kopans DB, Smith BL. A failure analysis of invasive breast cancer. Cancer. 2013. doi:10.1002/cncr.28199.
45. Ferlay J et al. GLOBOCAN 2008 v1.2, cancer incidence and mortality worldwide: IARC cancer base no. 10. Lyon: International Agency for Research on Cancer [online]; 2010. http://globocan.iarc.fr.
46. Narod SA. Breast cancer in young women. Nat Rev Clin Oncol. 2012;9(8):460–70.
47. Peres J. Advanced breast cancer in young women. J Natl Cancer Inst. 2013;105(17):1257–8.
48. Gajdos C, Tartter PI, Bleiweiss IJ, Bodian C, Brower ST. Stage 0 to stage III breast cancer in young women. J Am Coll Surg. 2000; 190(5):523–9.

Breast Intervention

12

Nan M. Garrett, Candace E. Roberts, Karen E. Gerlach, and Mahesh K. Shetty

Introduction

Breast intervention has evolved over the last two decades from being confined to image guidance for surgical excision biopsy of nonpalpable abnormalities to minimally invasive per cutaneous biopsy procedures performed under mammographic, ultrasound, and MRI guidance. The rate of open surgical biopsy has seen a dramatic drop during this time period and is now used for specific indications only.

This chapter provides an overview of breast interventional procedures in four sections:

- Ultrasound-guided breast biopsy
- MRI-guided biopsy
- Presurgical needle wire localization
- Stereotactic breast biopsy

N.M. Garrett, MD • K.E. Gerlach, MD, MS
Department of Radiology, Woman's Hospital of Texas, Houston, TX 77054, USA
e-mail: nan.garrett@hcahealthcare.com; karengerlachmd@hotmail.com

C.E. Roberts, MD
Department of Radiology, Woman's Hospital of Texas, Houston, TX 77054, USA

Department of Radiology, Baylor College of Medicine, Houston, TX 77054, USA
e-mail: candace.roberts@hcahealthcare.com

M.K. Shetty, MD, FRCR, FACR, FAIUM (✉)
Department of Radiology, Baylor College of Medicine, Houston, TX 77054, USA

Woman's Center for Breast Care and MRI, Woman's Hospital of Texas, Houston, TX 77054, USA
e-mail: mshettymd@gmail.com

Ultrasound-Guided Breast Interventional Procedure

Ultrasound-guided breast interventional procedures may be performed for either diagnostic or therapeutic purposes. Diagnostic indications include sampling of suspicious lesions, and therapeutic indications include cyst aspiration and abscess drainage. Ultrasound-guided core needle biopsy is the current method of choice for performing breast biopsies of most sonographically visualized lesions.

Image-guided percutaneous biopsy is safe, accurate, and minimally invasive. It causes minimal breast deformation and scarring, has few complications, and is faster and less expensive than surgical biopsy. Women diagnosed with breast cancer by core needle biopsy require significant fewer surgical procedures than those diagnosed by open surgical biopsy [1–9]. Image-guided percutaneous biopsy has become increasingly common as the number of nonpalpable breast lesions found on screening exams has increased. The majority (70–80 %) of breast lesions referred for biopsies are benign [4].

As per the American College of Radiology Practice guidelines, the indications for US-guided intervention in the breast include:

1. Simple and complicated cysts
2. Complex and solid masses
3. Repeat biopsy
4. Presurgical localization
5. Biopsy of axillary/axillary tail lymph nodes in known or suspected malignancy

US-Guided Core Needle Biopsy

Ultrasound in particular offers many advantages over other guidance techniques. These include nonionizing radiation, low cost, visualization of the needle in real time, accessibility, patient comfort, and speed. Percutaneous biopsy devices and techniques have evolved over time. What began with

M.K. Shetty (ed.), *Breast Cancer Screening and Diagnosis: A Synopsis*,
DOI 10.1007/978-1-4939-1267-4_12, © Springer Science+Business Media New York 2015

simple fine-needle aspirations progressed to large core needles, then to automated spring-loaded (ASL) core needles, and on to vacuum-assisted (VA) core needle biopsy. Ultrasound-guided core needle biopsy (CNB) is used to evaluate ultrasound-detected suspicious and highly suspicious (BI-RADS 4 and 5) lesions to establish a diagnosis and to optimize surgical planning or neoadjuvant therapy when indicated. For probably benign lesions (BI-RADS 3), ultrasound-guided CNB allows patients to avoid more costly, invasive surgical biopsy.

A rapid, accurate evaluation of suspicious and highly suspicious lesions is extremely important. Studies have shown that the period surrounding the diagnosis of breast cancer is one of the most stressful times for women [10]. Reducing the period of uncertainty between the discovery of a breast tumor and histological diagnosis significantly decreases a woman's anxiety. Since the majority of woman will have a benign diagnosis, breast teams strive to provide an answer as soon as possible. And for patients with a malignant diagnosis, the uncertainty period may be decreased to allow for focus on therapy and treatment options. Ultrasound-guided CNB has a sensitivity of 92–97.5 %, a specificity of 99–100 %, and an accuracy of 96–99 %. False-negative rates overall are 0.4 %, with a range from 0 to 9 %. The false-negative rate correlates well with the false-negative rate of surgical biopsy of nonpalpable lesions, 2 % (range 0–8 %) [2, 6, 9, 11–14].

There are very few contraindications for ultrasound-guided CNB. Inability to visualize the lesion sonographically is the only absolute contraindication. Patients must be able to cooperate. Patients with severe psychiatric disorders or combative patients may not be able to safely undergo biopsy. Rarely, very superficial lesions or certain lesions in patients with implants or other implanted devices may make ultrasound-guided intervention challenging. Although anticoagulation is not an absolute contraindication to biopsy, temporarily holding or altering anticoagulation when clinically feasible is preferred. Consultation with the referring physician is advised to assess the risks/benefits of holding or altering anticoagulation.

Principles and Techniques of US CNB

Equipment Needed

A high-resolution ultrasound unit with a 12.5-MHz linear array transducer should be used to perform optimal ultrasound-guided CNB. (ACR guidelines call for a minimum of a 10-MHz transducer [15].) Multiple commercially available automated spring-loaded (ASL) core needle devices (aka biopsy guns) are available (Fig. 12.1). These devices obtain tissue by firing a stylet at high speed into the target lesion, rapidly followed by a cutting cannula (Fig. 12.2). Although many variations are available, a 14 G with a throw of 2.2 cm is the "gold standard" [16] and the most commonly used [2]. Cores obtained with a 14 gauge are

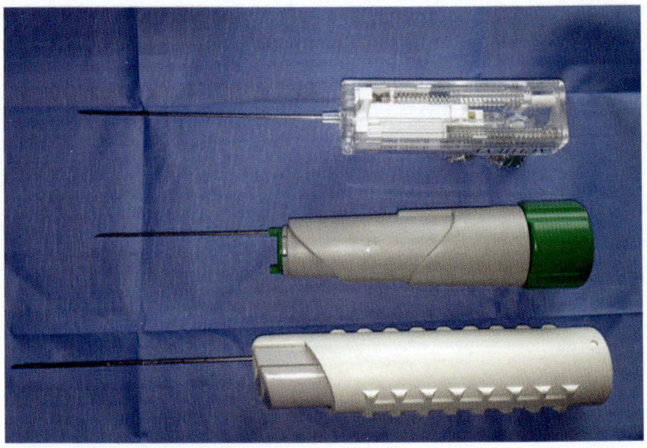

Fig. 12.1 Multiple automated spring-loaded biopsy guns are commercially available. Gauges range from 12 to 18

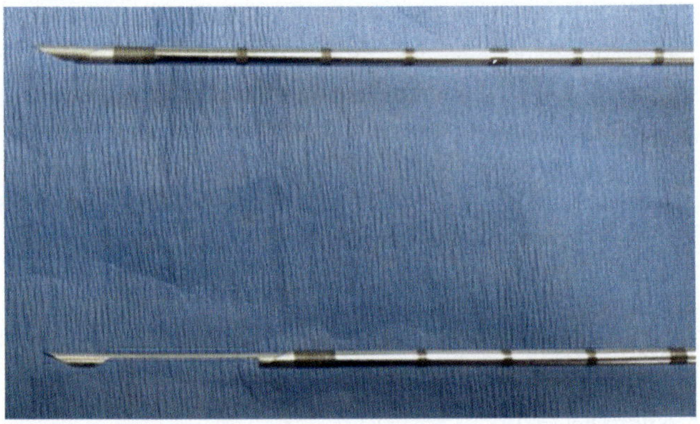

Fig. 12.2 Automated spring-loaded core needle tip in the unfired (*top*) and fired (*bottom*) position

sustainably larger than those obtained with a 16 gauge (Fig. 12.3). Several handheld vacuum-assisted (VA) core needle devices are also available. Like spring-loaded devices, many sizes are available, with 10–12 G commonly used. After the needle is positioned, the vacuum pulls the tissue into the biopsy aperture. An internal rotating cutter then shears off a tissue specimen. The specimen is then transported to the specimen port for collection. Currently at our institution we employ either a 14-gauge Max-Core® device (Bard, Tempe, AZ) or a 12-gauge ATEC® device (Hologic, Indianapolis, IN).

Patient Preparation

Explanation, Stress Reduction, and Consent

Undergoing a breast biopsy can be a very stressful event for a patient. Typically the psychological stress is far more bothersome than the physical discomfort experienced during the procedure. Although we routinely offer premedication with anxiolytics for our stereotactic patients, premedication of our US patients is more variable. Music is routinely used in our procedure rooms or patients may bring in their own music/ listening devices. Studies have shown both music and anxiolytics decrease procedure-related anxiety in breast biopsy patients [17]. 5–10 mg of valium or 0.25–0.5 mg of alprazolam are often used for outpatient procedures. Medications are given in the department approximately 30 min prior to the procedure and after informed consent has been obtained. We require all patients to have someone available to drive them home.

In our department patients usually undergo a prebiopsy consultation, ideally performed the same day as the diagnostic imaging that resulted in a biopsy recommendation. The aim is to discuss the biopsy, answer any questions, go over consents, address stress reduction techniques, etc. Patients are instructed to avoid aspirin and NSAIDs (such as ibuprofen) prior to biopsy. Patients referred from outside facilities may be consulted over the phone. When the patient arrives in the biopsy suite, the procedure is discussed in detail with the patient, if this has not been done ahead of time. Informed consent must be obtained from the patient. Risks, benefits, and alternatives should be discussed as well as a thorough discussion of what the patient should expect during the biopsy. Immediately prior to the procedure, a universal "time-out" is performed.

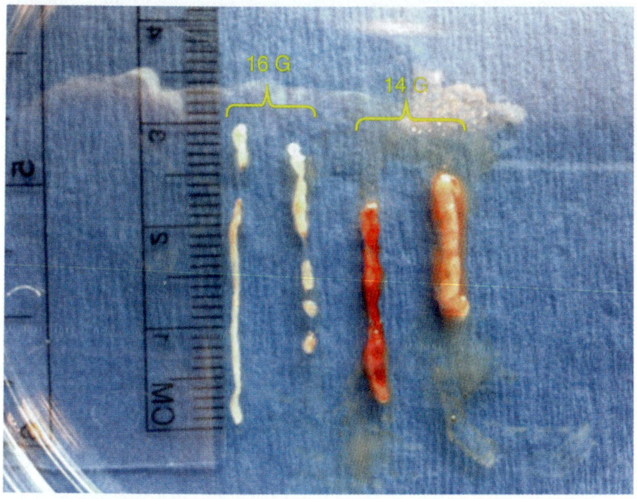

Fig. 12.3 Size of a 14-gauge samples versus 16-gauge samples obtained with an automated spring-loaded core device

US Approach and Positioning

The patient is placed supine on the table, with the ipsilateral arm elevated above the head. The physician then scans to confirm lesion location and determine the best approach to use. If needed the patient may be repositioned to an oblique angle for better access to a lateral lesion. Needles will pass more easily through fatty and glandular tissue than dense echogenic fibrous tissue. As such, finding an approach path with fatty tissue rather than dense tissue is preferred when possible (Fig. 12.4a, b). Use of Doppler may be helpful to avoid vessels. The subareolar region should be avoided if possible as this tends to be a very tender and sometime challenging area to anesthetize. If the mass is located in the subareolar region, a "nipple block" may be performed with topical lidocaine (such as EMLA®, AstraZeneca) with an occlusive dressing, followed by intradermal injection of lidocaine circumferentially around the nipple-areolar complex [18].

As a general rule, the shortest distance from the skin to the lesion should be used, keeping in mind the basic principles of ultrasound guidance. Although a vertical approach may be the shortest distance, a more lateral or oblique approach is required for ultrasound visualization. The intensity of the echoes produced by the needle increases as the angle of incidence

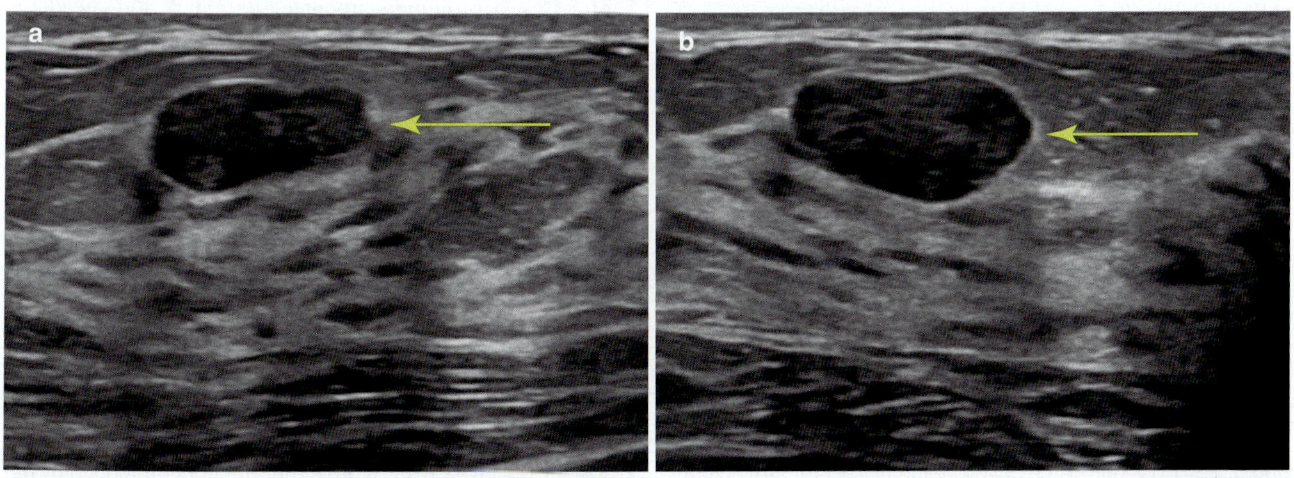

Fig. 12.4 (**a**, **b**) Planning your approach: the breast should be scanned from various angles to choose the optimal path of the needle (*arrow*). Transversing dense breast tissue with the needle (**a**) is more difficult than transversing fatty tissue (**b**)

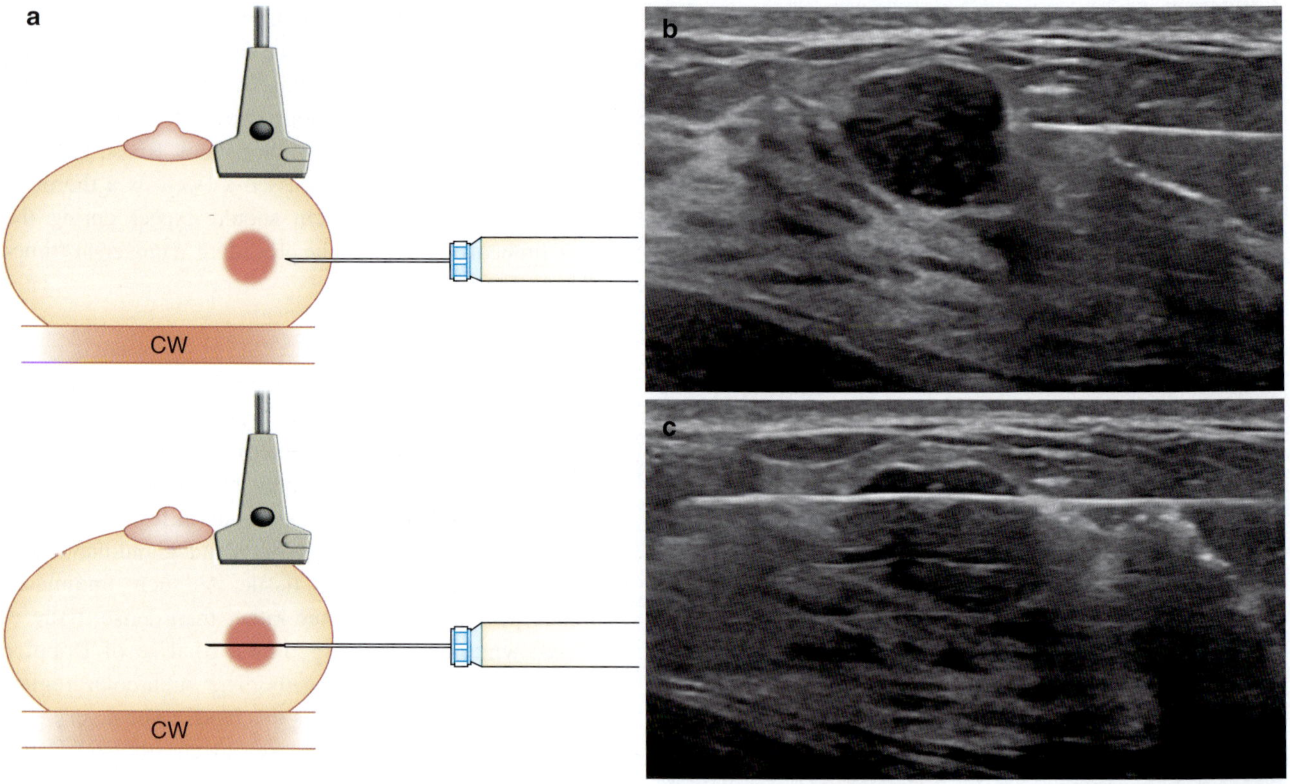

Fig. 12.5 (**a**) Transducer should be parallel to the needle to allow for maximum visualization of the needle and needle tip. Chest wall (*CW*). (**b**) Prefire location. (**c**) Postfire location

decreases, with the most useful specular reflections taking place when the ultrasound beam strikes the reflector at 90° to the surface of the needle. The needle must be parallel to the long axis of the transducer to produce the maximal number of reflected echoes for visualization. The needle should also be as parallel to the chest wall as possible (Fig. 12.5a–c).

Images should be obtained documenting lesion location, approach, and any pertinent findings (adjacent chest wall, skin, implant, etc.).

Biopsy Procedure: ASL

Skin Prep, Anesthesia, and Incision

After choosing the best approach, the biopsy tray is assembled as per physician preference. The tray and supplies should be positioned to ensure maximum accessibility and ease of use (Fig. 12.6). When setting up the tray, one should always be cognizant of accidental needle sticks or contamination. Examining your equipment prior to use to ensure no defects is always good practice. Many radiologists perform a test firing of the biopsy device to confirm proper function. This also provides an opportunity to warn the patient of the sound to avoid a startle reaction during the actual procedure. It should be noted, however, that some device manuals specifically precaution "never test the product by firing into the air" [19]. The breast is prepped and draped in the normal sterile fashion. Betadine solution is used to cleanse the skin and a sterile drape is placed. The transducer is routinely cleansed or a sterile probe cover can be used. One percent lidocaine (with or without epinephrine 1:100,000) is used for local anesthesia. Use of lidocaine with epinephrine can decrease bleeding and subsequent bruising. We prefer to buffer our lidocaine to decrease the pain associated with dermal injection. Ten milliliters of 1 % lidocaine (with or without epinephrine) is diluted with 1 mL of 8.4 % sodium bicarbonate [20, 21]. A 30-G needle is used for the initial superficial injection which also significantly reduces discomfort, with most patients reporting minimal to no pain with injection. This is followed by deeper injection with a 25-G 1 ½ needle. Ultrasound guidance should be used while giving anesthesia as this gives the radiologist a feel for the angle and approach that will be needed for the actual biopsy, a sort of trial run. Additionally any distortion (fluid pockets or hemorrhage) caused by the lidocaine can be seen real time so as not to confuse the subsequent biopsy. The lidocaine syringe should be well flushed before use to avoid introduction of air into the target field, which could obscure lesion visualization. The lidocaine placement can also be used to "move" the lesion as necessary, such as elevating a deep lesion off the chest wall by injecting the lidocaine deep to the lesion and "pushing" it more superiorly. Alternatively it can be used to make a shallow lesion "deeper."

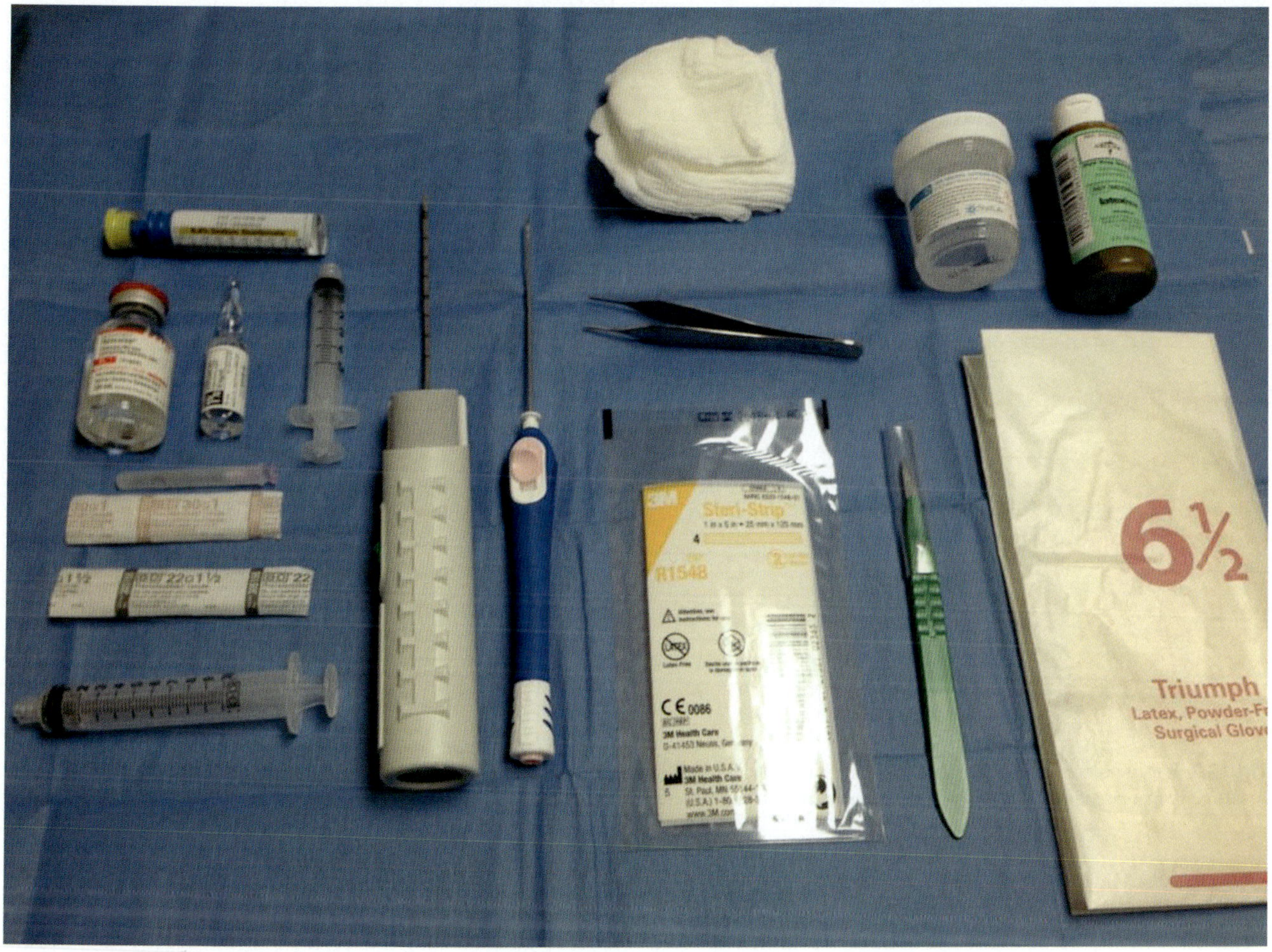

Fig. 12.6 Supplies for ultrasound-guided core needle biopsy

Insertion, Correct Positioning, and Firing of the Needle

A small skin nick is made with a #11 blade scalpel. Although targeting systems are available, the freehand method is preferred by most radiologists and is used at our institution. The physician holds the transducer in one hand (usually the non-dominant hand) and the biopsy device in the other. Alternately, a well-trained technologist can hold the transducer allowing the physician to have both hands free for the biopsy. The skin entry point should be shallow, located 1–2 cm from the edge of the transducer to ensure a needle path that is parallel with the transducer (Figs. 12.7, 12.8a–e, 12.9a, b, and 12.10a, b). As such, the angle of incidence is zero, creating maximal specular reflection and allowing visualization of the entire needle and tip. Steep angles and short axis imaging can lead to inaccurate needle tip location and poor sampling.

The needle is inserted and advanced under the long axis of the transducer. The transducer hand should now be fixed and still. Your eyes should be in the habit of mostly looking at the breast, not the screen. With a "mental image" of where the mass is, the needle is moved to the transducer. Once in position, a prefire image is obtained for documentation. The needle should be positioned in or at the edge of the mass. Prefire positioning depends on several variables. First you must be aware of the penetration depth or "throw" of the needle. Most throws are ~2.2 cm, meaning the needle tip will be advanced 2.2 cm from the original prefire tip location. The length of the sample notch is ~1.9 cm. There is also a small ~6–7-mm dead space at the needle tip. It is important to be aware of the throw, dead space length, and notch size of whatever needle you are using (Fig. 12.11a, b). If sampling a large lesion, the prefire position may be just in front of the mass to sample both the edge (perilesional) and the center portion of the lesion (Fig. 12.12). Alternatively the tip can be placed within the lesion, especially if the mass moves and the needle "bounces off" the mass. In smaller lesions, the needle tip must be further away from the mass to ensure the mass lies within the sample notch postfire. Prior

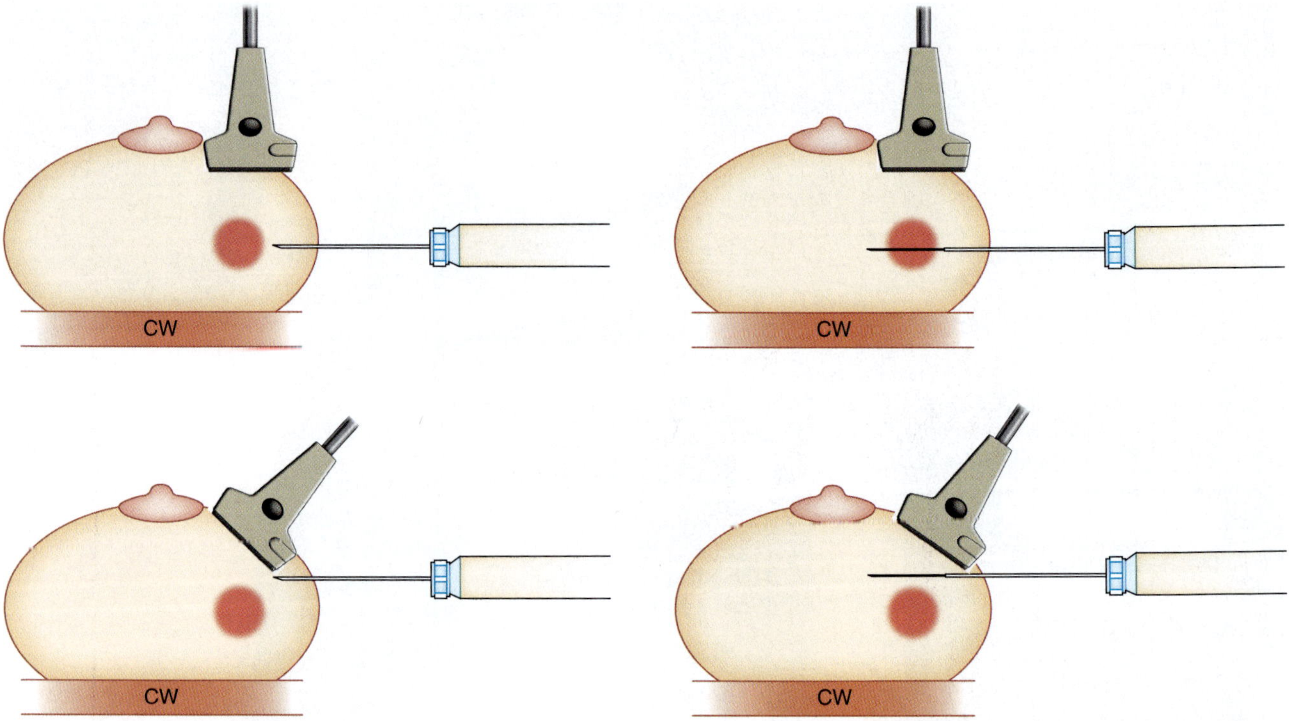

Fig. 12.7 It is important to keep the transducer parallel (*top*) to the needle to ensure proper targeting of the lesion. If the plane of the transducer is not parallel (*bottom*) to the needle, then although it may appear that the needle is in/in front of the lesion, errors in targeting will occur chest wall (*CW*)

to firing the needle, one must estimate the postfire needle position to insure no unwanted structures are in the expected path.

Obtaining a rim of normal perilesional tissue can aid the pathologist in making the correct diagnosis. Multiple areas of the lesion should be sampled to decrease sampling error and improve diagnosis (Fig. 12.13a, b). Another key point to remember is to use the spring to your advantage. Some lesions tend to be "pushed away" from the needle as it is advanced. The rapid forcefully fired spring mechanism can help combat this in many cases (Fig. 12.14a, b). Another useful trick in very dense tissue is using a 16 G instead of a 14 G. The smaller diameter will often pierce the tissue better and achieve nice specimens, especially of "hard" lesions.

A coaxial introducer may be used in conjunction with the biopsy gun. The introducer is placed similar to the needle placement described previously. Introducers are typically extremely sharp and do not usually require a skin incision. The trochar is then removed and the biopsy needle is placed through the introducer and into proper position to obtain a sample. This allows multiple samples to be obtained with only a single skin puncture. It decreases trauma to the surrounding tissue and can be very useful in dense, difficult to penetrate tissue.

In cases where automatic deployment is not safe, a device with a manual mode is advantageous. The Achieve® biopsy device (Cardinal Health, Dublin, OH) is available in several gauges, and the stylet can be deployed independently from the cutting cannula. An introducer must first be placed. The device, with the stylet prefired, is placed thru the cannula and the sample notch can be positioned as desired within the mass. The cutting cannula is then deployed directly over the stylet, with no additional needle tip forward advancement. This can be very useful in cases with masses very near implants or other sensitive structures.

Inspection of Specimen and Number of Cores

After obtaining a sample the needle is removed. Manual pressure should be applied over the incision by the technologist while the needle is out to aid in hemostasis and decrease bleeding. Care should be taken to maintain sterile technique. Tweezers or the tip of a needle can be used to remove the specimen from the sample notch and place it into formalin. Care should be taken not to crush or damage the specimen. A small amount of normal saline from a sterile syringe can also be used to "wash" the specimen out of the notch. The needle should not be placed directly into the formalin, as this would introduce a caustic substance into the patient. Some centers prefer to swish the needle tip in a small test tube of normal saline to remove the specimen. This can subsequently be transferred to a formalin container.

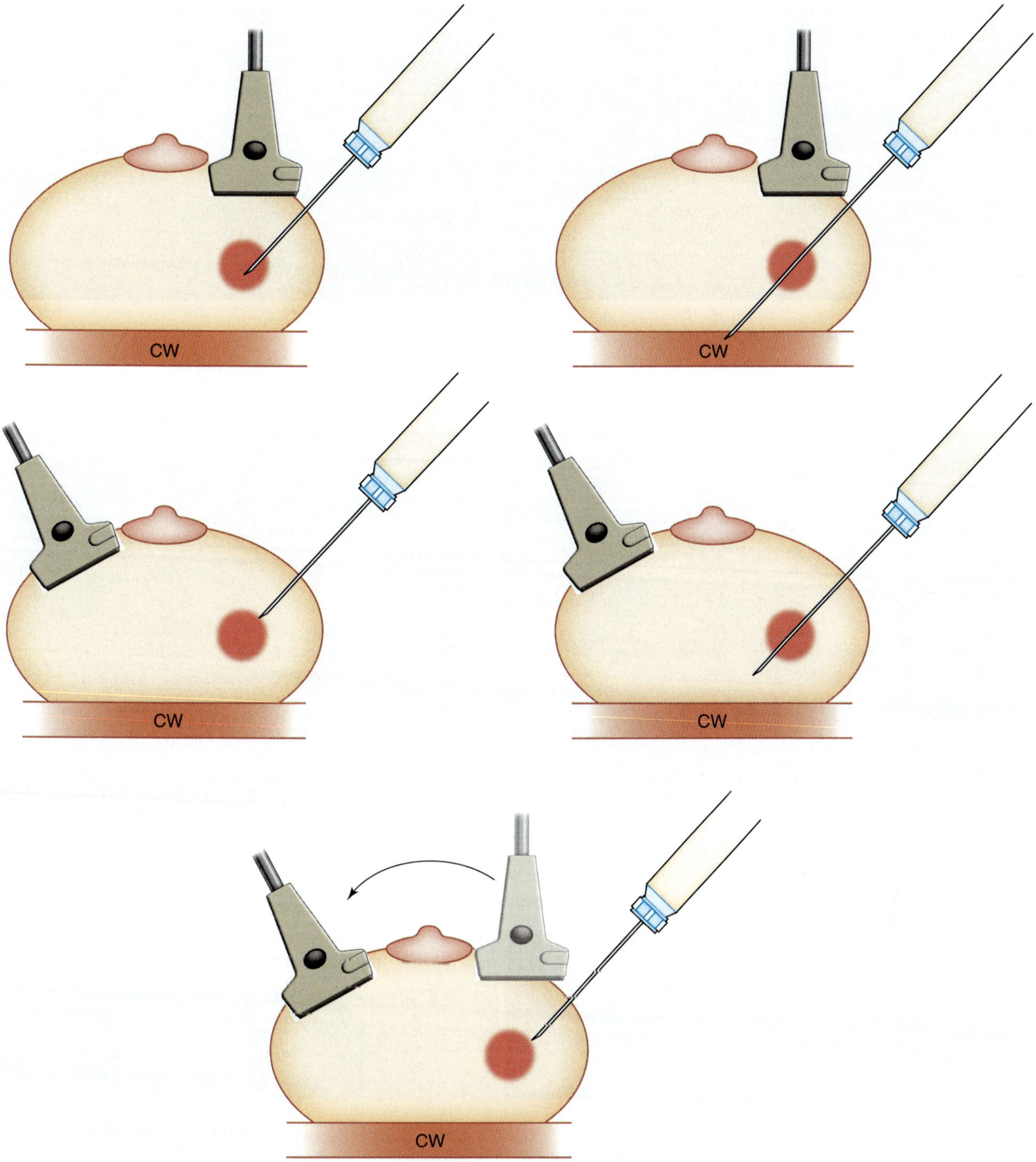

Fig. 12.8 (**a–e**) If a steep-angled approach is necessary, caution must be used to avoid piercing the chest wall (*CW*). Prefire (**a**) and postfire (**b**) show incorrect probe angle for a steep approach. The angle of the probe must be changed (**c**). Prefire (**d**) and postfire (**e**) correct angle and accurate biopsy

The macroscopic evaluation of the specimen can yield important information regarding quality. Intact, firm, white or dark red-brown cores that sink are favorable signs. Fragmented, yellow, floating oily cores are less likely to yield a conclusive diagnosis.

As per the ACR Guidelines, 3–6 core samples are generally recommended [15]. Several authors have advised not be "dogmatic" about the number of cores, with the exact number based on case-by-case assessment. Decisions regarding the optimal number of specimens should take into account

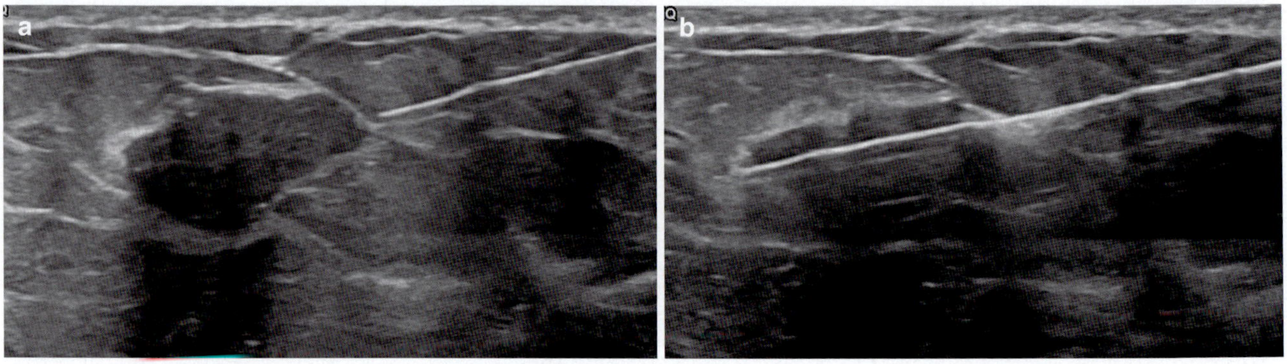

Fig. 12.9 (**a**, **b**) Pre- (**a**) and postfire (**b**) images demonstrating proper targeting

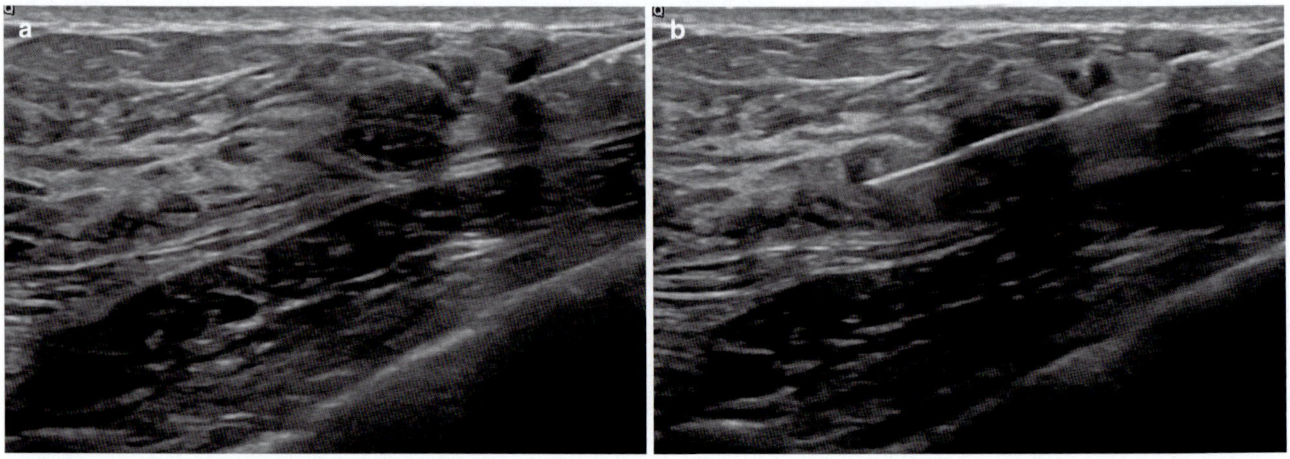

Fig. 12.10 (**a**, **b**) Pre- (**a**) and postfire (**b**) images demonstrating proper targeting

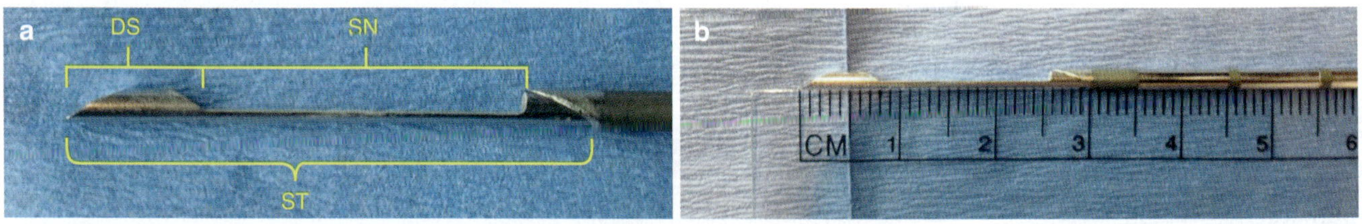

Fig. 12.11 (**a**, **b**) Close-up of the cutting notch. The stylet (ST) advances into the lesion and a sample falls into the notch (SN). A sheath is then closed over the notch, coring a sample of tissue in the notch. The dead space of the needle (DS) is also depicted

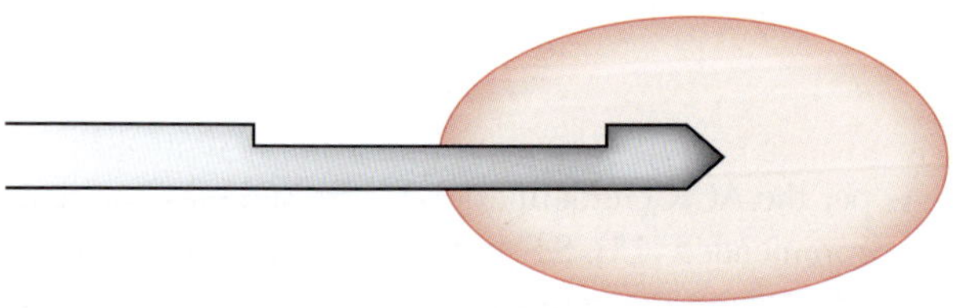

Fig. 12.12 Biopsy needle shown with the cutting notch encompassing both the lesion and the perilesional tissue

the radiologist overall confidence in the specimens. Factors to consider include how well the lesion was seen before and during the procedure, needle location pre- and postfire, and visual evaluation of the specimen [16, 22].

Biopsy Procedure: VAC

Vacuum-assisted core needle biopsy may also be performed. Ultrasound-guidance principles are the same as automated

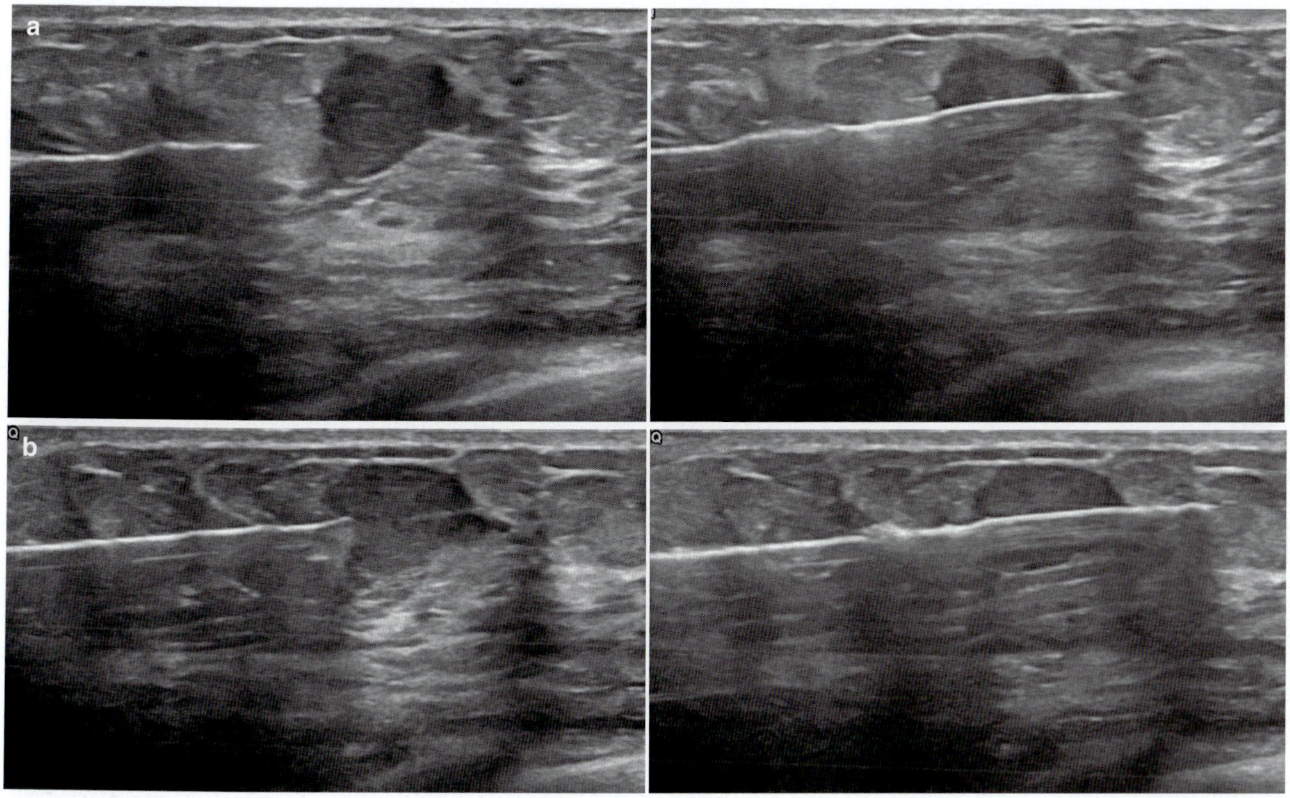

Fig. 12.13 (**a**, **b**) It is helpful to sample the edge of the lesion, including some the normal margin to aid the pathologist in diagnosis. (**a**) This can be accomplished by positioning the needle slightly away from the mass to ensure the notch captures some normal breast tissue before entering the mass. (**b**) If positioned close to the mass, the entire sample will likely arise within the mass

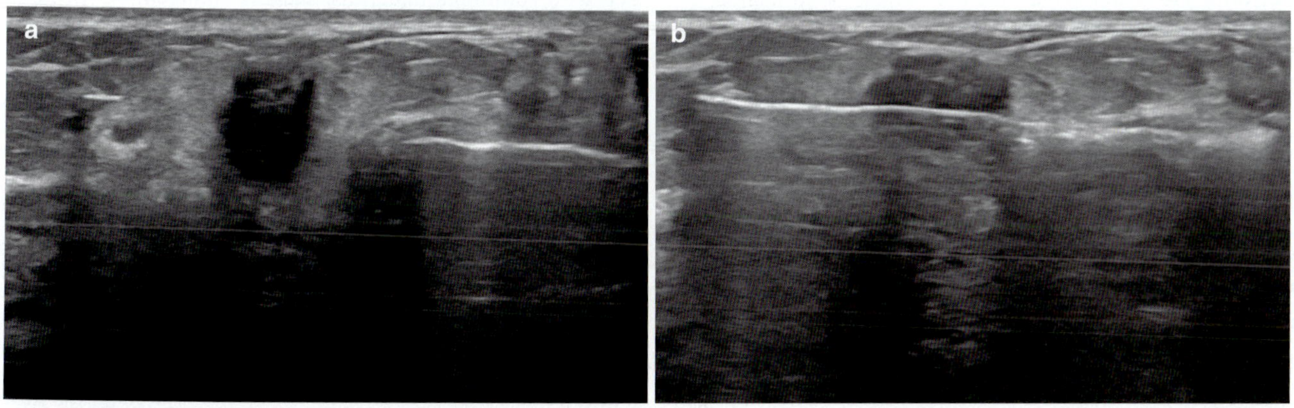

Fig. 12.14 (**a**) As seen on the image, the tissue can "bunch up" in front of the needle, as the lesion tries to move away from the advancing needle tip. (**b**) The spring action of the needle helps to eliminate this problem

spring-loaded devices. A range of needle sizes are available (7–14 gauge). The needle is usually positioned at the inferior margin of the lesion in the case of small lesions (Fig. 12.15). For larger lesions or non-mass-like areas, the needle may be centrally located within the mass. When the needle is in correct position, the vacuum is activated; the specimen is then pulled into the shaft and cut. The sample moves back down the needle to the container and the biopsy aperture is ready to obtain another specimen. Multiple samples can be obtained

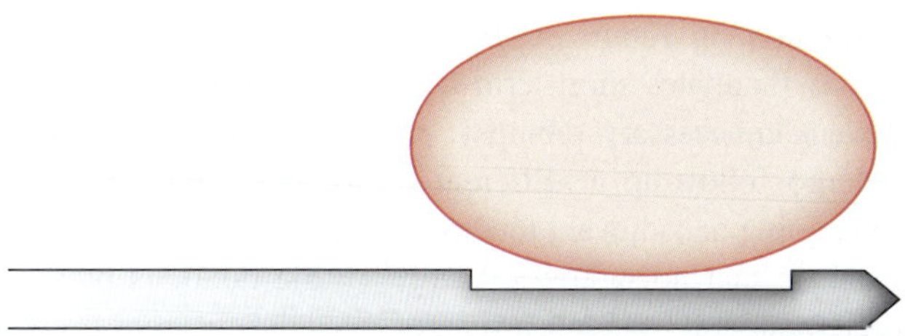

Fig. 12.15 The vacuum-assisted biopsy needle is usually placed along the undersurface of the lesion to be sampled

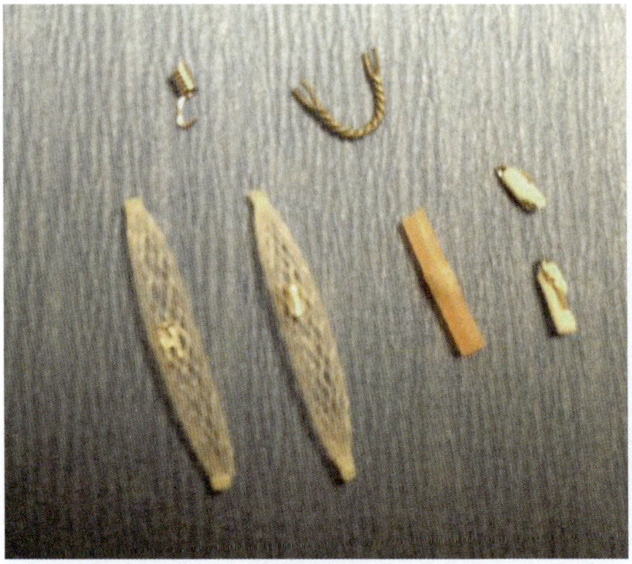

Fig. 12.16 Gross image of a sample of available breast markers

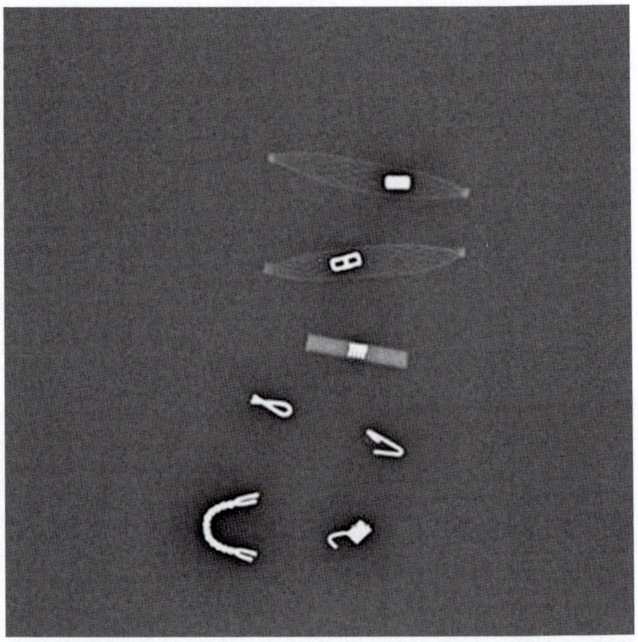

Fig. 12.17 Mammographic image of a sample of available breast markers

without moving the needle as the vacuum action continually sucks the lesion into the aperture. The shaft of the needle can also be rotated (directional control) to obtain specimens from various clock faces. Vacuum-assisted devices allow rapid acquisition of large volume specimens with a single insertion. An average of six cores is usually taken [6], although like spring-loaded cores numbers will vary. After the biopsy has been completed, lavage and aspiration of the biopsy cavity are performed to decrease bleeding and hematoma formation.

Marker Placement

Biopsy marker placement is essential for optimal patient management. Marker placement benefits [23]:

- Marking multiple lesions
- Insuring correlation across different imaging modalities
- Follow-up of benign lesions
- Monitoring neoadjuvant therapy
- Preoperative surgical localization and postoperative specimen evaluation

Multiple lesions often reveal varying pathological analysis and require different treatments/intervention. The vast array of marker shapes (Figs. 12.16 and 12.17) allow for easy identification of multiple lesions. Occasionally correlation across varying modalities may be in doubt prior to biopsy; marker placement can help verify. Marker placement aids in correlation on future exams as well. Marking of benign lesions facilitates short-term follow-up as well as helps to prevent unnecessary rebiopsy, particularly in patients who undergo follow-up at different institutions. Some patients undergoing neoadjuvant therapy may have such an excellent response that no radiographically visible tumor is present after treatment, making a marker essential to preoperative localization of the original tumor bed.

There are multiple commercially available markers on the market today. Some are designed to be deployed through the biopsy device (often the case in vacuum-assisted devices) others by freehand. Most markers are very small, 2–3 mm, and made of titanium or stainless steel. They may be imbedded with additional materials, such as collagen, PLA (polylactic acid), PGA (polyglycolic acid), interwoven polymer, or hydrogel to increase US visualization and decrease clip migration.

Choosing which marker to use is highly institution dependant. Different-shaped markers should be used when biopsying multiple areas with clear documentation in the report regarding which marker was placed into which lesion. Consideration may also be given to how one desires the marker to be visualized on subsequent exams. All commercial markers are seen well mammographically. However, some are better seen than others on US and MRI. US visualization can be increased with various embedding material such as woven polymer or hydrogel. MRI appearance depends on type (stainless steel creates a larger artifact than titanium), shape, and imaging parameters. Some marker material/shape combination will produce almost no MRI artifact with routine sequences, while others produce a fairly large MRI artifact. One that produces a clearly detectable but small artifact is usually best.

Marker placement utilizes the same basic ultrasound-guidance principles as described for CNB. In freehand placement, the tissue marker needle tip is advanced into the lesion/biopsy bed. A pre-deployment image is obtained. Under direct ultrasound visualization the marker is deployed.

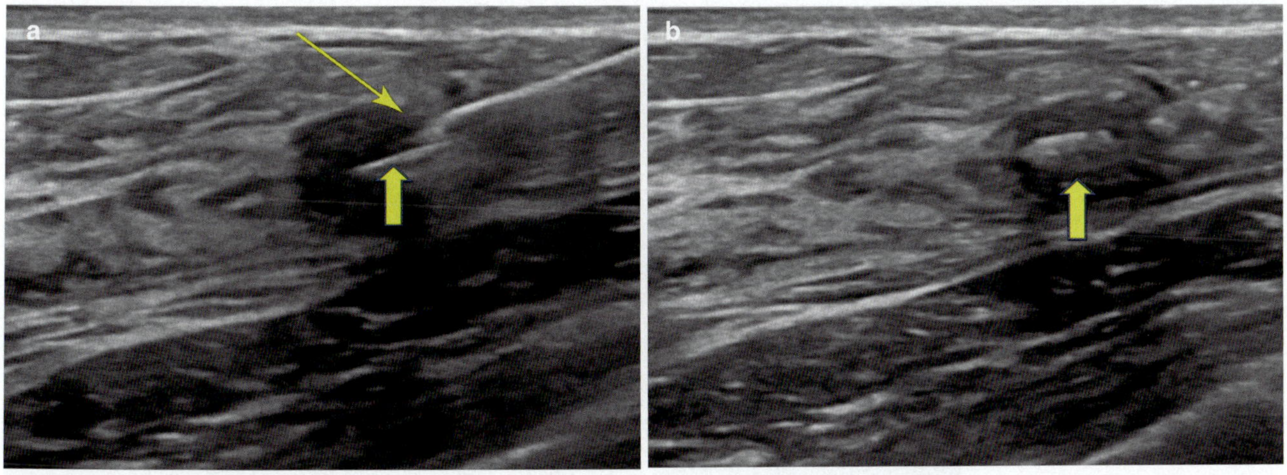

Fig. 12.18 (**a**, **b**) Clip deployment. (**a**) The breast tissue marker needle tip is inserted into the mass under direct ultrasound visualization. Clip (*thick arrow*) is deployed from the tip (*thin arrow*) or distal side port. (**b**) Clip (*thick arrow*) is well visualized within the mass following deployment

It should be seen extruding from the tip of the device (Fig. 12.18a). The needle is then removed and a post marker placement image is obtained (Fig. 12.18b). Care should be taken when removing the needle to ensure that it does not "drag" the marker back out, down the biopsy tract. It is good practice to inspect the deployment device after removal.

For vacuum-assisted devices, after the specimens have been obtained, the inner needle is usually removed and a compatible marker clip device is placed through the outer introducer sheath and deployed. Markers may also be placed freehand. As the marker is not anchored to the wall of the biopsy cavity, it can move within the breast tissue and result in clip migration. The marker should be within 1 cm of the lesion following placement. Causes of clip migration include the "accordion effect." This refers to clip migration along the *z* axis. It can occur during decompression of the breast with stereotactic or MRI biopsy. Hematoma formation and distortion caused by excess bleeding may also cause migration. Fatty breasts may have more migration than dense breasts. Larger-gauge needles and larger biopsy cavities have also been implicated in increased risk of clip migration.

A PubMed literature review demonstrated no definite documented cases of breast marker allergic reaction. Two case reports show a possible exacerbation of preexisting atopic dermatitis with titanium breast clips. There are rare reports of titanium allergy with pacemaker contact sensitivity and some orthopedic implants [23, 24]. Markers may be removed under stereotactic guidance if needed [25].

Hemostasis, Post-biopsy Mammograms, and Post-Biopsy Care

Following marker placement, direct manual pressure is applied to the biopsy site for approximately 10 min to achieve hemostasis. The skin is then cleaned and a Steri-Strip™ (3 M) bandage is applied. The patient undergoes immediate postbiopsy mammogram. Craniocaudal and 90° lateral views are routinely obtained (Fig. 12.19a, b). Additional views may occasionally be required to visualize the marker. Marker placement and mammographic correlation are confirmed. A small ice pack is placed over the biopsy site. The patient is instructed on routine postbiopsy care and provided with written information. This includes keeping the wound clean and dry. Strenuous activity should be avoided for 24 h, and PRN ice packs (first 24 h) and heating pads (after 24 h) may be used. The patient is instructed to keep the wound dry for 24 h and avoid swimming pools and hot tubes for 1 week following the biopsy to allow for complete wound closure. OTC medications (acetaminophen) are advised for postbiopsy discomfort, which should be minimal. Aspirin and NSAIDs should be avoided for 48 h.

Follow-Up

Imaging/pathology concordance is critical to assure appropriate patient care. The pathology report should be reviewed by the radiologist for concordance. (Please see Chap. 13 for discussion.) The patient and/or referring physician should be notified of the pathology and recommended follow-up. Concordant malignant findings should be referred to appropriate surgical/oncological consultation, as should discordance.

No BI-RADS recommendations exist regarding imaging surveillance for benign concordant core needle biopsy. Since CNB involves sampling, not removing lesions, imaging is required to demonstrate stability. However, there is no consensus regarding the timing of follow-up, with recommendations ranging from 6 months to 1 year. Salkowski et al. [26] found that rebiopsy recommendation rates and PPVs did not

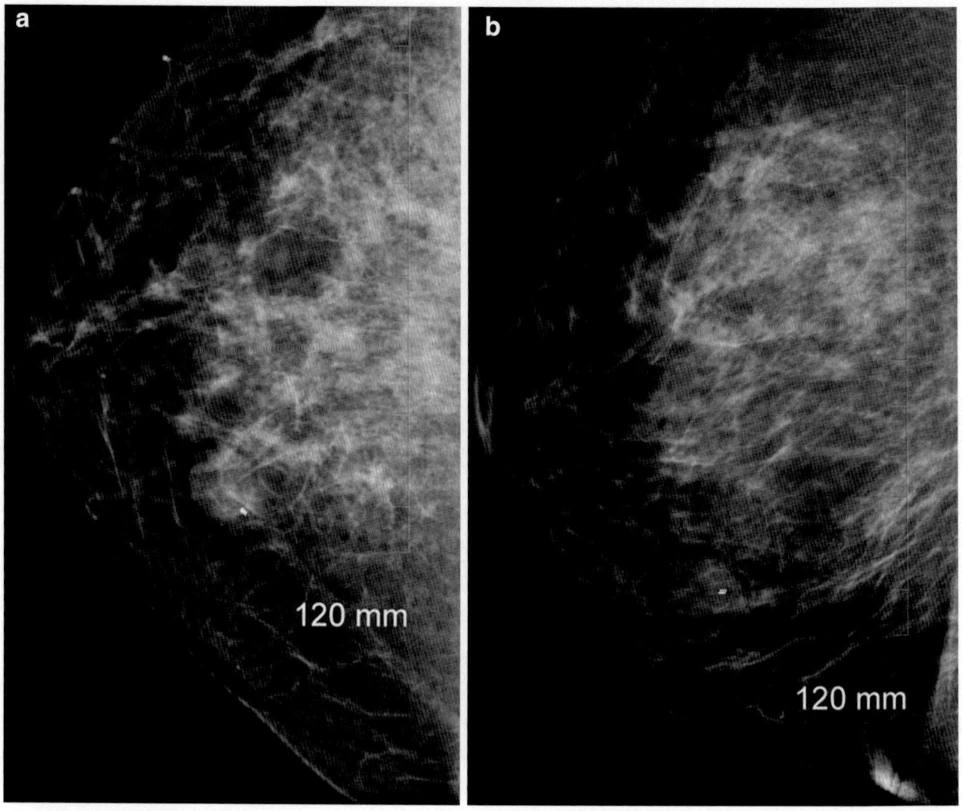

Fig. 12.19 (**a**, **b**) Post-biopsy mammogram (**a**, CC; **b**, LM) showing marker within the breast mass

differ in the 6- and 12-month groups. They suggest yearly follow-up may be more appropriate, lower costs, decrease patient anxiety, and lower radiation dose. Practice at our institution varies between 6 months and 1 year. Several factors are taken into account, including but not limited to specific pathology, image findings, and patient/physician preference.

Biopsy Report

As per ACR guidelines, the radiologist report should include the following [15]:

1. Procedure performed
2. Left and/or right breast
3. Description and location of the lesion with standard lexicon
4. Type and amount of local anesthesia
5. Gauge of needle and type of device
6. Complications and treatment, if any
7. Specimen radiographs or ultrasounds, if any
8. Marker placement, if performed
9. Postprocedure mammogram/ultrasound documenting marker placement and location of marker relative to sampled lesion
10. Recommendations based on tissue sampling results, imaging information, and concordance
11. Record of communication with the patient and/or referring physician

Complications of US CNB

The risk of complications in ultrasound-guided core needle biopsy is minimal. The reported risk of complications for automated spring-loaded CNB has been reported as less than 1 % [4, 27]. Complications with vacuum-assisted biopsy are reported as higher, ranging from 0 to 10 %, with a mean of 2.5 % [11, 27, 28]. The risk of severe complications (requiring surgical intervention) is lower with CNB (automated spring loaded or vacuum assisted) than with open surgical procedures, <1 % versus 2–10 % [1]. The most common complications include pain, bleeding, hematoma formation, and infection. Rare complications include pneumothorax, implant rupture/damage to implanted devices, and milk fistula/galactocele formation.

Pain

A study by Szynglarewicz [29] found a median pain rate of 4 (on an 11-point visual analogue scale of pain; 0 = none 10 = extreme) in women undergoing US-guided core biopsy. Specifically they compared pain experienced by patients undergoing US-guided biopsy with either a 14-gauge automated core needle or an 11-gauge vacuum-assisted CNB. Despite the larger gauge, the study found that less pain was experienced in the VA biopsy group. The authors believe this is due to contiguous collection of tissue without removing the needle. They reference similar findings in other studies.

They also point out that while some studies indicate more pain with an 11-G VA needle biopsy than with a 14-G ASL needle biopsy, these studies were comparing 11 stereotactic procedures with 14-G US-guided procedures. The findings may be related to inherent differences in stereotactic guidance versus US guidance (longer procedure time, prone positioning, compression, etc.).

Hematoma/Bleeding

Most studies indicate hematoma formation and bleeding are more common in VA biopsies than in ASL biopsies [1, 5, 27, 30]. The fairly straightforward argument holds that a larger biopsy cavity creates more bleeding. A few studies demonstrate that hematoma/bleeding is less common (or equal) in VA biopsies compared to ASL biopsies [29, 31]. These authors argue that although more tissue is removed, the single insertion with subsequent decreased tissue trauma and the ability to evacuate the biopsy cavity with vacuum actually decreases hematoma formation.

Implant Injury

Although implant rupture is a risk, it is very low given the real-time imaging capability. In addition, manual devices such as the previously mentioned, Achieve®, and VA devices that do not require a "throw" can be helpful in challenging cases. Both stereotactic and US-guided biopsies are safe and accurate in augmented breasts [32].

Tumor Cell Displacement

Seeding of biopsy needle track with viable malignant cells was an initial concern with all diagnostic breast needle procedures. Tissue seeding has been reported in 37 % ultrasound-guided ASL biopsy and in 23 % of the cases following VA biopsy [16]. In a prospective study from the Netherlands [33], seeding was not felt to be clinically significant, as radiotherapy is performed and conclusions were that tumor cells do not survive displacement.

Table 12.1 Needle gauge comparison chart

Needle gauge	Nominal outer diameter (mm)
8	4.2
9	3.8
10	3.4
11	3.1
12	2.8
13	2.4
14	2.1
15	1.9
16	1.7
17	1.5
18	1.3

Adapted from http://Wikipedia.org/wiki/needle_gauge_comparison_chart. http://creativecommon.org/licenses/by-sa/3.0/

Table 12.2 Volume of tissue obtained with various CNB devices

Gauge	Core needle biopsy (CNB) device type	Volume of tissue obtained (mg)
16	ASL	5.3
14	ASL	12.7–17
14	VA	34–40
11	VA	94–100
7	VA	250

Data from Lai et al. [14], Liberman [4], and O'Flynn et al. [6]
ASL automated spring loaded, *VA* vacuum assisted

Size and Type Argument: VA Biopsy Versus ALS CNB

The volume of tissue removed with vacuum-assisted core (VAC) devices is significantly greater than the volume obtained with automated spring-loaded core devices (ASLC). (See Tables 12.1 and 12.2.) Although this has proved invaluable in stereotactic biopsy of calcifications, overall utility in ultrasound lesions is not as clear.

When choosing between the use of a 14-gauge automated spring-loaded core needle biopsy and a vacuum-assisted core needle biopsy (usually 9–11 gauge), many things should be considered [34, 35]. While the accuracy of biopsy is increased with VAC [1], there is also a significant increase in cost and complications (although increased complication rate seems to be under debate) [4, 11, 27, 28]. Increased accuracy may not justify the routine use of VAC. VAC may not be as accessible as ASLC. In the diagnosis of high-risk lesions (such as ADH, radial scar, papillomas), ASLCN is more likely to underestimate the presence of DCIS than VAC. Invasive carcinoma is more likely to be underestimated in DCIS specimens with ASLCN than VAC. However, as standard of care is to send these lesions to surgical excision, no carcinomas are missed. Verifying concordance also ensures carcinomas are not missed. In larger lesions where the overall outcome is very unlikely to be different; the increased cost, resources, and patient discomfort of VAC would argue against its routine use.

However, others argue that with increased large volume samples, select high-risk lesions may not require surgical excision when appropriately reviewed in a multidisciplinary setting. If so, this may justify the increased use of vacuum-assisted biopsy. There is also a fairly strong argument for using VAC in small (less than 1.5–1 cm) lesions [29]. As there is inherently increased risk for sampling error in smaller lesions, the use of VAC may beneficial. As detailed in the complications section of this chapter, there are a few studies that demonstrate decreased pain and complications with VAC compared to ASLC [29, 36]. Overall, VAC shows significant improved accuracy with calcifications, non-mass-like areas, and small masses (not larger masses) and cost more than ASLC. Results of pain and complication rates between the

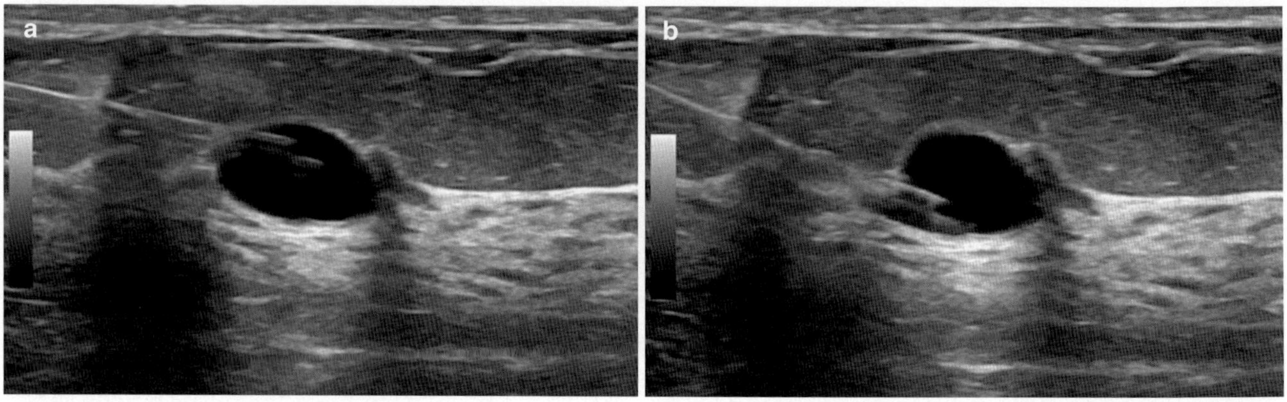

Fig. 12.20 (**a**, **b**) "Rocking" the needle tip. The needle tip can be moved up (**a**) and down (**b**) within the cyst. If this were a solid mass, rocking the needle up or down would move the entire mass up and down and the needle would remain in the same location within the mass

two procedures show varying results. More studies should be performed in addressing the optimum choice in various clinical scenarios.

Cyst Aspiration

Although aspiration of a simple cyst is not necessary for diagnostic purposes, tender or painful cysts may be aspirated for symptomatic relief. For a suspected but not definitive simple cyst by ultrasound criteria, cyst aspiration may be performed to confirm the cystic nature of the lesion. If such lesions prove solid, then the procedure can easily be converted to a core needle biopsy. Complex cysts with mural nodules or irregular septations should not be aspirated as cytology from such is often falsely negative even in the presence of intracystic carcinoma. In dealing with such lesions, vacuum-assisted CNB or surgical excision is advised. Cyst aspiration may also be performed to help improve clinical exam or help clarify imaging findings.

Preparation, local anesthesia, and guidance principles are the same for cyst aspiration as they are for the previously described ultrasound-guided core needle biopsy. Under direct ultrasound guidance an 18-G needle with an attached syringe is advanced into the cyst. You should usually be able to "feel" the needle enter the cyst, which is confirmed with images and documented. Being able to "freely rock" the needle tip within the lesion is very good indicator of a cystic or fluid component (Fig. 12.20a, b). The contents are then aspirated and inspected (Fig. 12.21a, b). Complete or near-complete resolution of the cyst should be confirmed with real-time imaging. *Tip: It is often possible to aspirate a simple small cyst with the lidocaine needle/syringe, sparing the patient an additional stick.* Occasionally when an aspirate is unable to be obtained, despite strong suspicion of a cystic nature, an attempt can be made with a 16-G needle. If this fails, we will usually proceed to core needle biopsy.

Fine-Needle Aspiration (FNA) of Lymph Nodes

Ultrasound is increasingly being used in the evaluation of lymph nodes in the breast. Documenting lymph node metastasis is an important step in breast cancer management. Sentinel node biopsy is often performed to asses for metastatic disease of the axilla. Ultrasound and FNA can help select patients avoid the time, cost, and stress of sentinel lymph node biopsy. Fine-needle aspiration cytology involves collecting cells from a suspicious lymph node with a small hypodermic needle. FNA is fast, inexpensive, and minimally invasive. It can easily be performed when the patient undergoes CNB of their primary breast lesion. A screening ultrasound is performed of the axilla and the most suspicious lymph node is chosen for biopsy.

For evaluation of metastatic or suspected metastatic disease of the axilla, most studies describe the use of FNA. There have been reports of core needle biopsy as well, although much fewer in number. Ultrasound combined with CNB or FNA has specificity reported to be as high as 100 %. FNA sensitivities range from 21 to 95 %, and CNB have reported similar results, 40–91 % [37]. Preparation, local anesthesia, and guidance principles are the same for fine-needle aspiration as they are for the previously described ultrasound-guided core needle biopsy. Using ultrasound guidance, a small hypodermic needle (usually 21–25 gauge) can be used to obtain aspiration cytology. Larger 18-gauge needles are also sometimes used. The needle tip is advanced into the lymph node under ultrasound guidance. Once confirmed and documented in place, negative pressure is applied to the needle with an attached syringe as the tip is moved around in the mass to collect cells (Fig. 12.22a–d). No aspiration should be applied when removing the needle. This may add nonlesional material and increases track seeding [38]. Others prefer to use the capillary action of the needle, where cells are detached by the cutting edge of the needle and are conducted into the lumen by capillary force rather

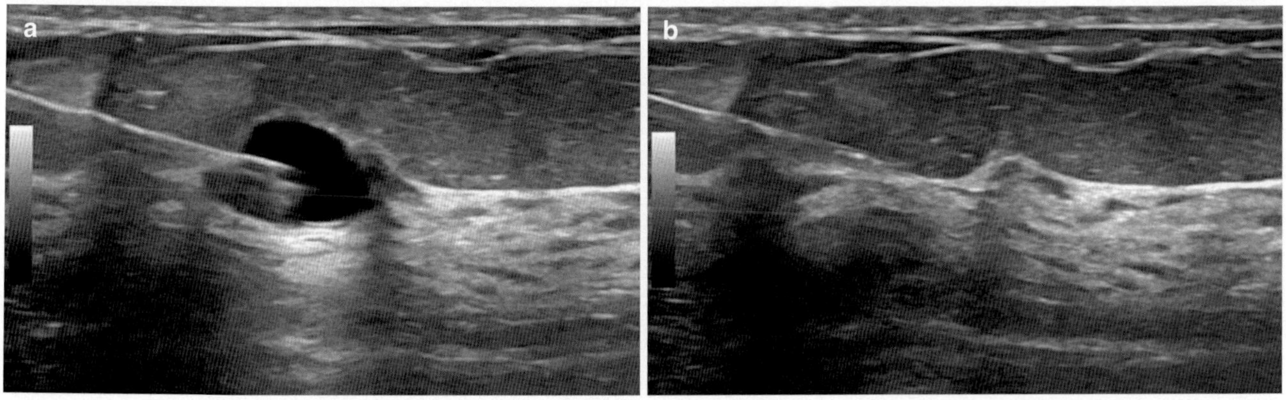

Fig. 12.21 (**a**, **b**) Cyst aspiration. (**a**) The needle tip is inserted into the cyst. (**b**) The cyst is then completely aspirated

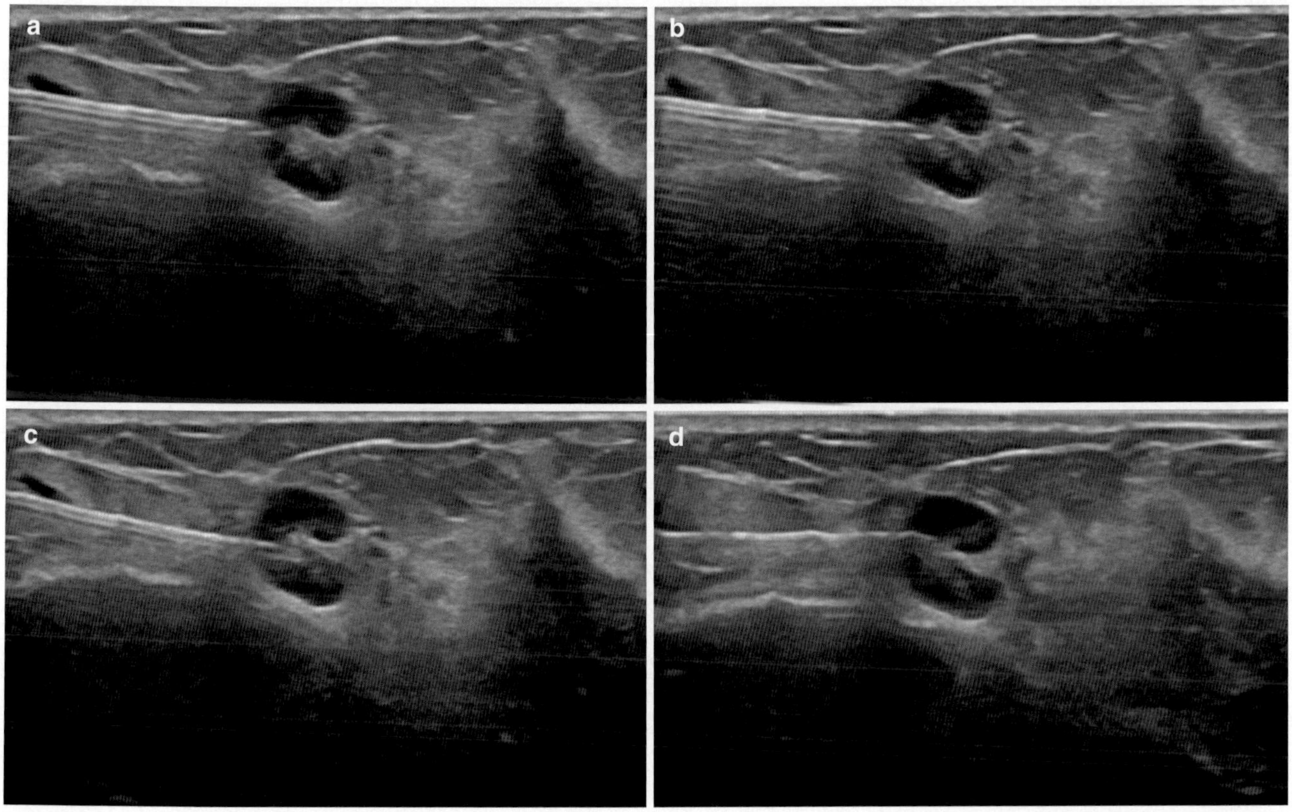

Fig. 12.22 (**a**–**d**) The needle is advanced into the lymph node and gently moved to and fro within the node to obtain cells from various locations

than aspiration. Typically between two and five needle passes are performed per suspicious lymph node. However, studies have shown that after four passes, the gain is minimal [39]. Having a cytologist immediately available to inspect the specimens for adequacy is very helpful in obtaining optimum FNAs.

Abscess Drainage

Abscess drainage is most often performed surgically as percutaneous drainage does not offer the amount of complete drainage possible with a surgical incision. However, there are times when percutaneous abscess drainage may be helpful; when surgery is not feasible or samples are needed for culture. A large bore 16- or 18-gauge hypodermic needle attached to a syringe is used to aspirate pus or fluid form the abscess.

MRI-Guided Breast Biopsy

A lesion may be seen on MRI and not visualized by mammography, ultrasound, or clinical examination. In this case, MRI-guided biopsy may be the only option for tissue diagnosis. A second-look ultrasound and possible diagnostic mammogram are recommended to check if lesions are amendable to biopsy using other methods, particularly when the lesion is greater than 1 cm. Ultrasound-guided biopsy is generally more comfortable from the patient standpoint, more rapid, and more cost effective. However, per Morris, an ultrasound correlate was found in only 23 % of cases [40].

Percutaneous biopsy is advantageous over surgical excisional biopsy with decreased morbidity, faster recovery, improved cosmetic result, and decreased scarring on subsequent mammograms. Percutaneous biopsy has decreased the number of benign findings from surgical excision. If cancer is diagnosed by percutaneous biopsy, better surgical planning with fewer surgeries result. Additionally, monitoring a patient's response to neoadjuvant treatment is also possible. The accuracy of percutaneous biopsy approaches that of surgical biopsy [41, 42].

Indications

Indications for percutaneous MRI-guided biopsy per the American College of Radiology include MRI lesions with no correlate on mammogram or ultrasound. This includes suspicious lesions or lesions highly suggestive of malignancy (BI-RADS® Category 4 or 5 in the Breast Imaging Reporting and Data System). Probably benign lesions (BI-RADS® Category 3) may be biopsied if there are valid clinical indications or if short-term interval imaging follow-up would be difficult. A repeat MRI-guided biopsy may also be performed in nondiagnostic or discordant cases [42].

Contraindications

Contraindications include lesion nonvisualization following contrast injection. Allergies to gadolinium are rare but also are a contraindication. The continued use of aspirin, anticoagulants, or other agents affecting bleeding times or bleeding diatheses is also discouraged. Basic MRI safety precautions and gadolinium risk assessments should be followed. Also, patient size should also be considered. Patients should also be able to tolerate prolonged, still positioning [42].

Prebiopsy Considerations

Ideally, breast MRI biopsy should be performed in the same location as the initial MRI imaging. The use of identical protocols decreases the need for repeat MRI imaging which might occur when comparing images from different centers. If different centers must be used, the protocols and technical factors should be replicated to avoid duplicated examinations. Additionally, the physicians MRI interpretive ability is improved when the pathology correlate is known. Before an MRI-guided biopsy is performed, the lesion should be correlated with prior imaging such as mammography or ultrasound to insure this is not a stable, benign mass. If prior imaging is not available, diagnostic mammography and focused breast ultrasound may further characterize the finding. If the lesion is amendable to ultrasound-guided biopsy, this will be more rapid, comfortable, and less costly. Of note, masses are usually easier to demonstrate versus non-mass-like enhancement. Of note, second-look ultrasound may fail to visualize a correlate up to 77 % of cases [40, 43]. When comparing different modalities, the lesion distance from the nipple may vary due to differing positions in mammography, ultrasound, and MRI. It might be more helpful to describe the findings as anterior, middle, or posterior in position. Landmarks may also prove useful when correlating different modalities [44].

Consent

Informed consent should be documented and include risks, benefits, limitations, and alternatives. Complications can occur in less than 5 % of cases. These include bleeding which might require compression, suture placement, surgical drainage, large hematoma, infection, and damage to surrounding tissue and organs and vasovagal reactions [40].

The Joint Commission's Universal Protocol for Preventing Wrong Site, Wrong Procedure, Wrong Person Surgery is also required. The biopsy site should be marked and confirmed and a time-out performed [42].

Equipment Needed

A 1.5 T MRI machine is typically utilized with a breast coil and several commercial options are available. A guidance method is used which includes a grid and pillar and post. Some clinicians utilize CAD or a worksheet system.

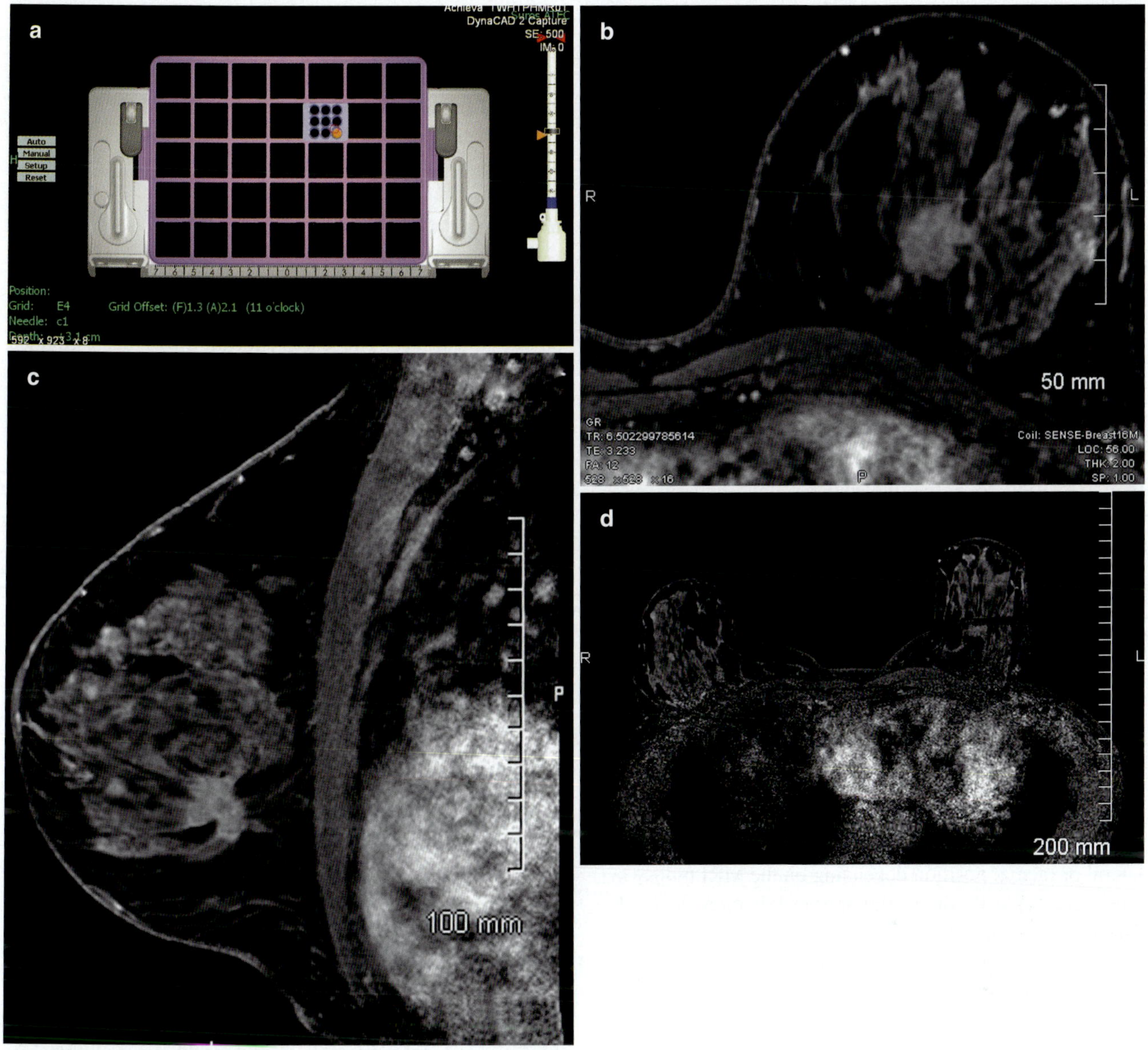

Fig. 12.23 (**a–d**) MR-guided biopsy of a lesion in the left breast. Histological diagnosis: invasive ductal cancer. (**a**) Pre-biopsy localization of the lesion using a CAD system that displays a lateral grid on the monitor identifying the location of the lesion to be biopsied and its depth. (**b**) T1-weighted axial image following gadolinium injection shows a spiculated mass in the left breast. (**c**) T1-weighted axial image following gadolinium injection shows a spiculated mass in the left breast. (**d**) Subtraction image demonstrates the biopsy needle in satisfactory position within the mass to be biopsied

A coaxial system comprised of an introducer sheath, trochar, obturator, and biopsy needle helps minimizes needle deflection and decreases repeated trauma to the breast parenchyma. A vacuum-assisted core biopsy device is used to obtain the sample. The MRI compatible biopsy kit contains a white introducer with 5-mm markings to adjust the depth. The trochar is placed through the introducer which will be inserted in to the breast. The obturator replaces the trochar during imaging to confirm placement with a black dot at the intended biopsy location. The vacuum-assisted biopsy needle has a sampling notch, and the samples are collected in a specimen collecting cup. Tubing connects the hand piece to the control module which remains outside the MRI room. A biopsy clip must also be available and is placed through the introducer after the biopsy is complete (Fig. 12.23a–d).

Pretreatment

Generally, we do not pretreat the patient unless the patient is unable to tolerate the procedure. With proper explanation prior to the procedure, we find most patients tolerate it well.

If pretreatment is required, oral benzodiazepines may be used. This includes diazepam (Valium®, Roche), 5 mg oral, 1–2 doses, or lorazepam (Ativan™, Baxter), 0.5 mg oral, 1–2 doses prior to the procedure [40].

Medication

Prior to scheduling the procedure, the patient should be asked about anticoagulants.

The risks and benefits of stopping Coumadin should be discussed with the patient and her referring clinician. Coumadin® (Bristol-Myers Squibb) may be discontinued approximately 4 days prior to biopsy and INR (international normalization ratio) checked prior to biopsy. Coumadin therapy can resume after the biopsy. If patient is high risk, patient may transition to a low-molecular-weight heparin which may be discontinued prior to biopsy [40]. Anticoagulant management should be performed under the direction of the patient's referring clinician. Other anticoagulants include aspirin which should be discontinued 1 week prior to the examination. NSAIDS should be discontinued 48 h prior to the examination.

Patient Positioning

Patient is placed in the prone position with the breast in an open breast coil. The biopsy is usually performed from the lateral or medial position depending on the MRI biopsy system used. Typically the lateral approach is more accessible. The breast is placed between a grid device. Compression should be adequate for visualization. Over compression should be avoided which can effect contrast enhancement.

Lesion Localization

The MRI should be high resolution and replicate the initial MRI examination as closely as possible. The grid contains a fiduciary marker. The marker should be visualized on the localization images. The lesion should be also included in the field of view. Initial localizer sequences are performed in the sagittal and axial positions. If positioning is satisfactory, Pre- and postcontrast T1-weighted fat-saturated images are performed using axial and sagittal images. Fat saturation images may assist finding the lesion in the event the patient moves between examinations causing misregistration in the subtraction images. The standard gadolinium contrast bolus is 0.1 mmol/L/kg of body weight. It is administered as a rapid bolus with a subsequent 10 cc saline flush. Images are obtained rapidly before the contrast washes out of the lesion. The scan time should not exceed 4 min. The presence and location of the lesion is confirmed in two planes. If the lesion is not seen, please refer to the troubleshooting section. Adjacent landmarks may also be utilized to confirm the region of interest is visualized. The *X*, *Y*, and *Z* coordinates are then calculated.

MR Guidance Methods

MR-guided biopsy was first attempted in the freehand manner. Cutaneous markers such a vitamin E capsule was placed on the skin surface. The lesion's location was then estimated [45]. Current methods involve guidance through a grid. A square insert is placed in the grid and the software will calculate the square fenestration the needle should pass through [46].

Procedure

The biopsy area is prepared in the normal fashion using betadine solution, provided the patient is not allergic. If patient is sensitive to betadine, chlorhexidine solution is substituted.

The superficial and deep area is anesthetized using approximately 10 mL sterile 1 % lidocaine (Xylocaine). Some practitioners prefer 10 mL 1 % lidocaine 10 mg/mL with epinephrine 1:100,000. The skin entry site is nicked with a scalpel. While cutting trochars are available which do not require a skin nick, we have had better results using an initial nick .The introducer and trochar are passed as a unit to the calculated depth through the needle guide using a twisting motion. The trochar is replaced with the obturator. The breasts are subsequently scanned to confirm that the introducer/obturator placement corresponds to the lesion. This can be visualized as a black dot. Axial and sagittal T1-weighted fat-saturated images without contrast are performed. If adjustments are needed, additional T1-weighted fat-saturated sequences without contrast may be performed at this time to confirm placement.

If placement is satisfactory, the obturator is removed and a 9- or 11-gauge vacuum-assisted biopsy needle is carefully placed through the introducer. When the biopsy needle is placed at the hub of the introducer, the biopsy needle tip will protrude through the introducer tip at the site of the lesion. Vacuum-assisted biopsy is more accurate than fine-needle aspiration and offers more tissue sample compared to core biopsy. The samples are obtained in a 360° (12 sample) or 180° (6 sample) configuration, depending on the biopsy needle position relative to the lesion. The biopsy needle is rotated one clock face step each time a beep is heard while stepping on the foot pedal. Approximately 100–150 mg of tissue is obtained depending on the biopsy needle used [47].

The biopsy samples are removed and placed in a prelabeled vial containing formalin solution, per pathology specifications. The biopsy site is then flushed with saline. The biopsy needle is replaced with the obturator and a noncontrast fat-saturated T1 image is performed.

A clip is placed to assist with future localization techniques or monitoring, depending on the pathology results. The clip device is placed through the introducer to its hub and deployed. The clip introducer is rotated, removed, and inspected to ensure deployment [40].

An additional postbiopsy sequence is performed. There can be difficulty in distinguishing the clip and postbiopsy air. For this reason, craniocaudal and lateral mammogram projections help confirm the clip position in the event wire localization is needed in the future. In the event of clip migration, mammographic landmarks may assist future wire localization.

Post-biopsy Care

Direct compression is applied for 10 min along the biopsy tract. Antibiotic ointment, Steri-Strips, and overlying gauze bandages are applied. The patient is offered an icepack and compression netting. Post-procedural care instructions are provided which include keeping the wound dry for 48 h and no heavy lifting. Signs and symptoms of infection are explained to the patient. It is also helpful for the patient to be aware that some bruising is expected. The radiologist's contact information is provided should concerns develop.

A postbiopsy visit may be scheduled to inspect the incision site and relay biopsy results to the patient. If this is not possible, the results must be conveyed to the patient and documented and patient referred for follow-up as appropriate. Follow-up recommendations may assist the referring clinicians, particularly if they are not breast surgeon specialists.

Follow-Up Pathology Concordance

If the results are benign and concordant with the imaging findings, the patient may return to screening mammography. If there is any concern of biopsy accuracy, follow-up MRI is recommended in 6 months. If the lesion is considered high risk or discordant, breast surgeon consultation is recommended to discuss excisional biopsy. Medical audits should also document false-negative and false-positive results [42].

Troubleshooting

Lesion Is Not Visualized at Time of Biopsy

If a lesion is not visualized at time of percutaneous MRI biopsy, the MRI images should be evaluated for evidence of contrast opacification of the heart and internal mammary arteries. Other sources of nonvisualization include breast overcompression which hinders contrast enhancement. Additionally, if the images were obtained too soon, a delayed image may show contrast enhancement. If the lesion is still not visualized, this might be due to hormonal effects and should be correlated with the menstrual cycle. Landmarks may also be helpful in evaluating the region of concern. Some clinicians may administer additional contrast but we typically reschedule the biopsy on another day. If the lesion is still not able to be visualized, MRI follow-up in 6 months is recommended to confirm that the lesion is not visualized.

Lesion Appears Not to Have Been Sampled

The MRI images performed after the biopsy may indicate that the area of concern was not sampled. In this case, the introducer unit may be repositioned. If the lesion is superficial, the introducer and trochar are advanced to the appropriate position. If the introducer is too deep, the introducer and obturator unit are pulled back to the appropriate depth. The new position is confirmed on MRI and additional tissue is obtained and placed in a separate formalin vial [40].

Posterior Lesion

Some lesions may be located far posteriorly. In these cases, patient positioning with a technologist experienced in stereotactic biopsy may be invaluable. Decreased cushioning might be considered if the patient is amendable to this. The needle may be placed either in the posterior grid or posterior to the grid [40]. In the event of a nondiagnostic biopsy, the biopsy clip may be useful to help guide an excisional biopsy. The lesion position relative to the clip should be documented and conveyed to the breast surgeon. The patient should be made aware of the possibility of a nondiagnostic biopsy in these cases.

Medial Lesion

If a medial approach is not permitted by the MRI biopsy system, the sample is obtained from the lateral approach. Alternatively, the breast may be positioned in the contralateral opening in a thin patient. The medial breast will now abut the lateral aspect of the contralateral coil. This may also assist accessing a posterior lesion in the medal breast [48]. A slight oblique position may also be helpful. The MRI technologist should be informed of the patient's positioning in this case so appropriate image annotations may be performed.

Dense Tissue

It is important to be aware that a snowplow effect may occur when the dense tissue and possibly skin are pushed by the needle rather than cutting through the breast parenchyma. Stereotactic biopsy can overcome this using a firing system to advance the needle into place. MRI-guided systems do not have this feature and appropriate pressure needs to be used to advance the introducer and trochar [48].

Thin Breasts

Similar to stereotactic-guided biopsy, thin breasts may pose a challenge. Care must be taken to ensure that the full thickness of the needle biopsy chamber is well within the parenchyma and clear of the skin. Recommendations are similar to stereotactic biopsy. Minimal compression and a generous wheal of anesthetic may be helpful. A grid on the opposite side might allow for enough skin and subcutaneous displacement to enable the procedure to be performed [40].

Multiple Lesions in the Same Breast

If there are multiple lesions in the same breast, the needles are placed consecutively after a single IV contrast bolus [48]. If patient will not tolerate multiple biopsies, the more suspicious lesion might be biopsied first and hopefully help guide management of the other lesions.

Bilateral Breast Lesions

Bilateral breast lesions may be biopsied in the same session. The breasts may be distinguished by using one fiducial marker on the right grid and two fiducial markers on the left grid [48].

Patient Motion

Clear instructions to the patient are critical prior to the procedures start. Oftentimes, the patient is unaware that even slight shoulder movement may affect the biopsy procedure. It is sometimes helpful to mark the skin at the grid border to confirm the patient has not moved mid-procedure. In the event of motion after the skin nick, the obturator may be left in place and another attempt to confirm the biopsy site may be performed using adjacent landmarks. If the lesion is close to the obturator (within 5 mm), the biopsy needle may be oriented to sample in the direction of the lesion [48]. If there is question of an inadequate sample, the biopsy clip may assist mammographic-guided needle localization if surgical excision is indicated. Alternatively, if the skin is intact and there are no reliable landmarks, the patient may be rescheduled on another day when contrast can be administered. If patient has difficulty tolerating the procedure, premedication might be considered to decrease motion.

Implants

It is our practice to diligently confirm whether the lesion is amendable to ultrasound-guided biopsy under direct visualization or whether mammographic-guided wire localization and excision are more safely performed. There are reports of stereotactic-guided biopsies in the literature [49].

Presurgical Localization of Breast Lesions

Presurgical localization of breast lesions was initially performed to obtain histological diagnosis of mammographic screen-detected nonpalpable abnormalities of the breast. Over the last two decades, there has been a dramatic drop in the number of these procedures due to widespread use of minimally invasive percutaneous biopsy procedures performed under ultrasound or stereotactic mammographic guidance. Apart from the morbidity factor, the cost benefit of performing imaging-guided percutaneous procedures has been shown by multiple studies [50–53]. Preoperative diagnosis of cancer decreases or eliminates positive operative margins and need to re-excise tissue. Stereotactic percutaneous biopsy has been recommended as the procedure of choice for mammographically detected abnormalities [50].

Presurgical localization is now performed for selected indications, such as in those patients with a biopsy-proven cancer, in those who have imaging pathological discordance at core needle biopsy, in those with high-risk lesions diagnosed at percutaneous biopsy, or in those where core needle biopsy is not an option or fails to provide a definitive histological diagnosis. It has been reported that with selective use of excisional biopsy for indications noted previously, missed diagnosis of breast cancer is rare [50]. Compared with surgical excisional biopsy, preoperative diagnosis by core needle biopsy allows for wider margins of excision, fewer positive margins, and fewer surgical procedures to achieve adequate treatment than diagnosis by surgical excisional biopsy alone would permit [50]. A study testing the cost-effectiveness of stereotactic biopsy versus needle-localized open surgical biopsy reported that there was no difference in cost benefit in cases where there are lesions highly suggestive of breast cancer (BI-RADS 5) or those cases suspicious for ductal carcinoma in situ [53]. However, in cases of intermediate risk lesions classified as BI-RADS 4, these investigators noted significant cost savings when stereotactic percutaneous biopsy was performed instead of needle-localized breast biopsy [53].

Mammographic-Guided Needle Wire Localization

Mammographic guidance is used for lesions that are seen well only on mammography. In this method there are three variables to be considered, the type of needle wire, the length of the needle, and the type of approach. A modified hook wire system with a reinforced 2-cm segment 1.2 cm from its hook is commonly used for all procedures regardless of whether localization was performed under mammographic or sonographic guidance. A 5-, 7-, or 9-cm needle length is used depending on the depth of the abnormality being localized in the breast. All procedures are performed using the parallel-to-the-chest-wall approach; a freehand approach has been described [54].

Two kinds compression paddles can be used; the alphanumeric grid is the one that is most commonly used. The alternate Swiss cheese paddle is a smaller paddle with multiple holes and is useful in women with small breasts, for lesions in the subareolar region, those high up in the axilla or close to the chest wall, where the small size of the paddle allows for easier access and optimal immobilization.

Informed consent is obtained routinely following explanation of the procedure and a description of the potential complications including informing the patient of the possibility of failure to adequately excise the abnormality localized. Local anesthesia is not administered at our institution for mammographic-guided localization procedures but is used in most instances for an ultrasound-guided localization. The decision to use local anesthesia for sonographic-guided localization procedure is dependent on both physician and patient preference.

For the parallel-to-the-chest-wall approach, the breast is positioned such that the lesion to be localized is closest to the skin surface through which the needle wire combination is to be introduced. For a lesion at the 12 o'clock position in the upper breast, for instance, the approach is superior with the breast placed in the craniocaudal position, and a lesion at the 3 o'clock position of the right breast is best approached medially with the breast in compression in the mediolateral position. The length of the needle selected depended on the depth of the lesion, keeping in mind that the final wire placement should be such that the tip of the wire extends beyond the lesion and is ideally with 0.5 cm from the abnormality. Once the approach and length of the needle is decided, the breast is placed under compression. The lesion coordinates are obtained from this initial mammogram based on its location within the alphanumeric grid (Fig. 12.24a). Using the collimator cross hairs, the point of entry is determined and the needle wire is advanced to the predetermined depth, satisfactory placement of the needle wire is determined by obtaining two views in the orthogonal plane, and needle position is adjusted based on these two views as needed (Fig. 12.24b, c). Once this is satisfactory, the wire is advanced so that the hook wire anchors to the tissue and the needle is gently withdrawn. A final two-view mammogram is obtained to confirm that the wire tip is located within 5 mm of the lesion (Fig. 12.24d–f). The patient is then transported to the operating suite with the films showing the position of the localizing wire so that the surgeon can see review prior to performing the excisional biopsy. Similar procedure is followed for masses that are localized under mammographic guidance (Fig. 12.25a–f).

Ultrasound-Guided Localization

When an abnormality is seen well on ultrasound and concordance with mammographic finding has been proven for those abnormalities that are seen on mammograms, sonographic localization is the preferred modality for localization. These lesions are usually solid masses. The same needle wire utilized for mammographic localization is used when localizing abnormalities under ultrasound guidance. The needle wire is introduced through a point on the skin determined to be the shortest to the lesion. Under real-time guidance, the needle wire is advanced 1 cm beyond the lesion, and once position is determined to be satisfactory, the wire is advanced over the wire and the needle is withdrawn gently taking care not to withdraw the wire with the needle. An image with wire in satisfactory position is obtained and sent with the patient for the surgeon. In both types of presurgical localization procedures, the wire is taped firmly in position, and the patient is advised not to move the arm in question to avoid movement of the wire during transportation to the operating room. All surgical excisional procedures were performed under general anesthesia.

Presurgical localization is performed generally for nonpalpable abnormalities considered suspicious for breast cancer based on mammographic and or sonographic workup of screen-detected breast abnormalities. Mammographic abnormalities localized for excisional biopsy may include microcalcifications, solid or complex cystic masses, areas of architectural distortions, or focal asymmetry. In some instances a surgeon may request imaging guidance prior to surgical excision of palpable abnormalities to ensure optimal correlation between clinical and mammographic or sonographic findings [54]. The hook wire technique using the parallel-to-the-chest-wall approach that we use at our institution for needle localization is the most commonly used method and is described in the materials and methods section of this article. An alternate approach using the hook wire is the freehand technique or an anterior approach. In this method the radiologist extrapolates the location of the abnormality from the mammograms to a decompressed breast and advances the needle blindly towards the chest wall. Two-view mammograms are obtained and repeated as needed after repositioning until the wire is seen to be within 1 cm of the lesion being localized. This technique requires more time and tends to have a higher complication rate [54]. Other techniques have been described that have also been used to localize breast abnormalities under mammographic guidance. When an abnormality is located within 1 cm of the skin surface, placing a BB on the skin overlying the abnormality may be adequate to perform localization. The position of the BB is then be confirmed by a two-view mammogram. Skin localization is, however, not recommended for lesions at a depth greater than 1 cm and may lead to excision of unacceptably

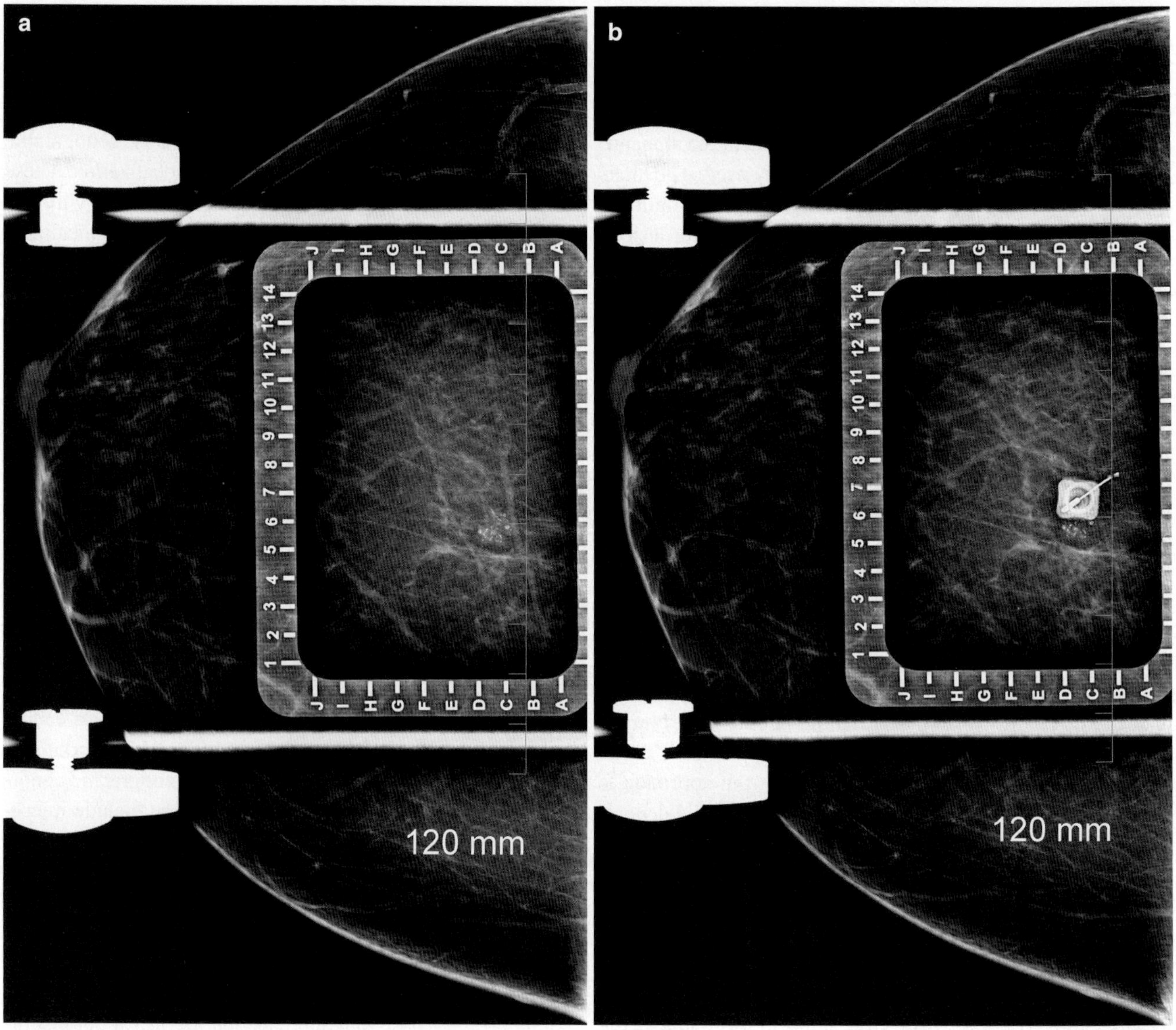

Fig. 12.24 (**a**–**f**) Mammographic presurgical localization for clustered microcalcifications that were histologically proven to be DCIS. (**a**) Craniocaudal view with breast under compression with an alphanumeric grid showing microcalcifications at 6D coordinate. (**b**) Craniocaudal view with breast under compression with an alphanumeric grid and needle wire in satisfactory position. (**c**) Mediolateral view confirming satisfactory placement of the needle wire. (**d**) Mediolateral view following showing satisfactory deployment of the wire. (**e**) Craniocaudal view showing satisfactory position of the wire. (**f**) Specimen radiograph showing the wire adjacent to the localized microcalcifications

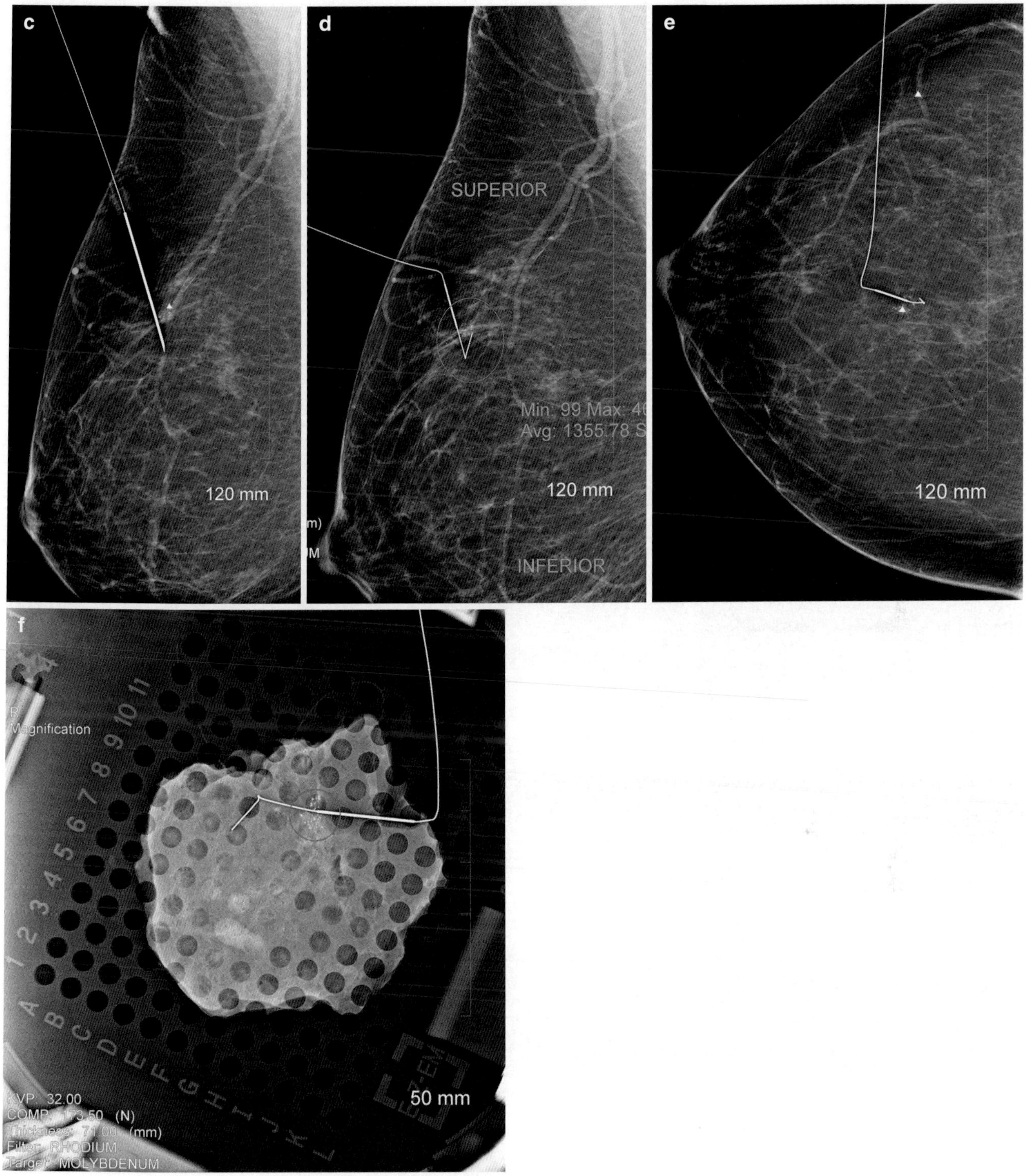

Fig. 12.24 (continued)

large volume of tissue. The dye method of localization involves injection of 0.2 mL of dye through a needle positioned under mammographic guidance near the abnormality localized. As the needle is withdrawn, a dye outlined track is left behind which the surgeon uses as a guide to find the abnormality. Methylene blue dye or alcian blue dye can be used; care should be taken to inject not more than 0.2 mL to avoid dye diffusion. The advantage of this method is that there is no need to leave a wire in the breast and hence avoids the problem of potential wire displacement or migration

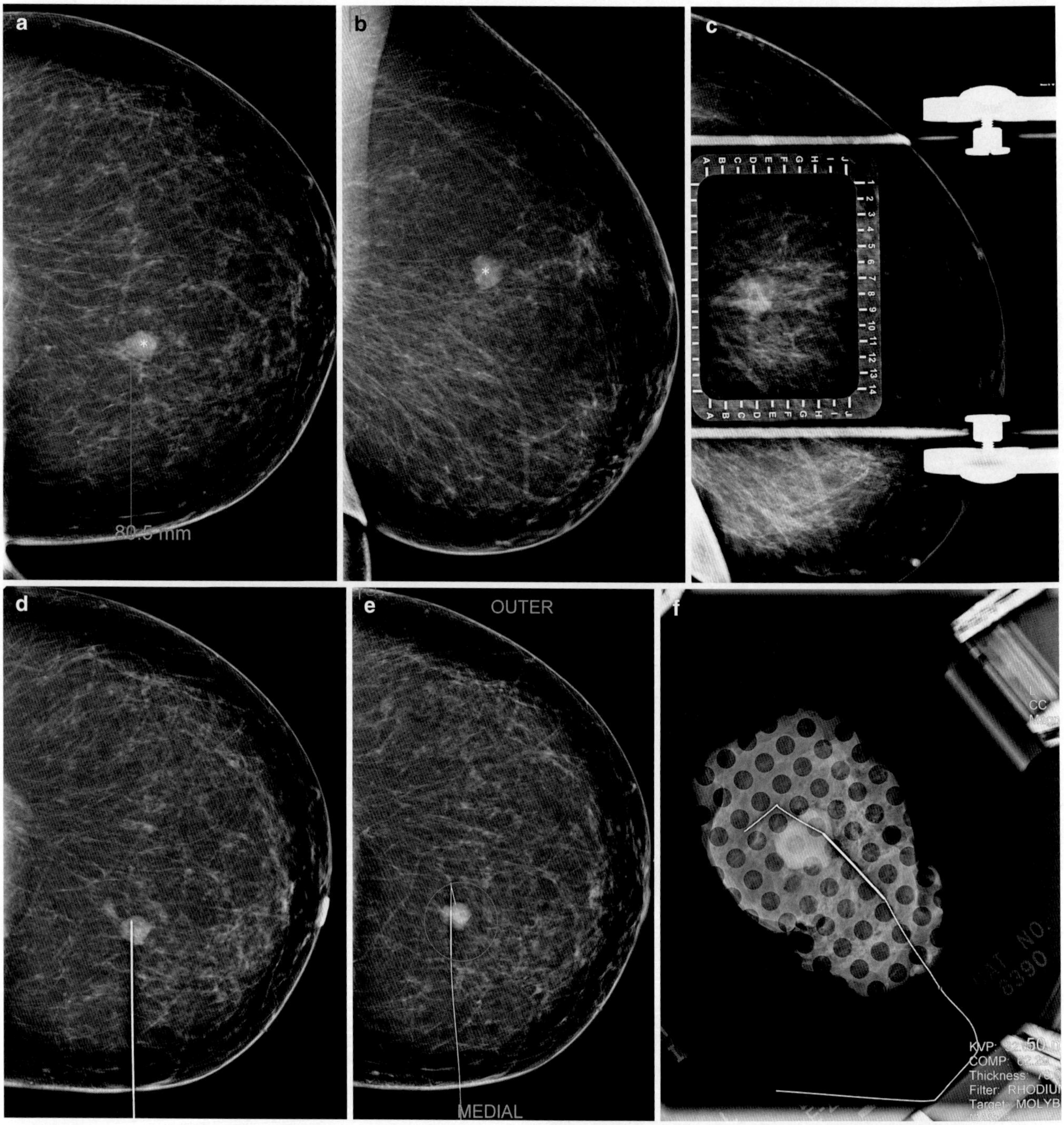

Fig. 12.25 (**a**–**f**) Mammographic presurgical localization for a mass that was histologically proven to be a fibroadenoma. (**a**). Craniocaudal view showing the mass. (**b**) Mediolateral view showing the mass. (**c**) Mediolateral view with breast under compression in a fenestrated paddle with an alphanumeric grid. (**d**) Craniocaudal view with satisfactory placement of the needle wire. (**e**) Craniocaudal view showing satisfactory position of the wire. (**f**) Specimen radiograph showing the wire adjacent to the localized mass

during transfer to the operating suite [54]. The practice of using local anesthetic prior to introduction of the needle wire is variable. At our institution we do not use local anesthetic during mammographic localizations and often do for sonographic-guided procedures. The value of local anesthetic has been questioned. In a study of 89 patients undergoing mammographic localized excisional biopsy, 46 patients received local anesthetic and 43 did not. Patients who did not receive the local anesthetic reported a lower mean pain score than those who did [55].

Complications of the presurgical imaging-guided localization procedures may involve failure to excise the localized abnormality or procedure-related complications. A failure to excise the localized mammographic abnormality has been reported in 2.5–6.7 % of cases. Jackman and Marzoni looked at a series of 280 lesions undergoing presurgical localization [56]. Failure to localize occurred in 7 (2.5 %), 21 lesions that were not initially excised were done so on repeat excision of more than one tissue specimen in 14 of 21 cases where specimen radiography did not demonstrate the abnormality [56]. These authors concluded that failure was more likely with two lesions, small breast, for microcalcifications, small specimen, and small lesions [56]. In another study Abrahamson and others reported a success rate of 93.3 % (254 of 272 lesions) and concluded that placement of the localization wire within 5 mm was a significant predictor of successful removal of the localized lesion and that failure rate was higher when wire was greater than 5 mm from the lesion, in small breasts and in small specimen [57]. Potential reasons for failure to excise include placement of the wire greater than 1 cm from the lesion, placing the wire short of the lesion or advancing the wire significantly beyond the lesion, wire movement during patient transfer to the operating suite, and bleeding leading to hematoma formation.

Procedure-related complications are relatively rare. Of the known complications, the most common ones are vasovagal reactions and bleeding, both of which are self-limited and easy to manage and almost never lead to cancellation or failure of the procedure. Migration of the wire, fragmentation of the wire, and pneumothorax are very rare complications [58, 59]. There has been a report of a hook wire causing delayed cardiac injury by penetrating the pericardium and myocardium and lodging in the aorta with patient presenting with chest pain. Following an echocardiogram and CT scan, the wire was surgically removed [58]. We did not encounter any procedure-related complications during the 1-year study period,

Specimen radiography following imaging-guided localization is performed for several reasons. Primarily it verifies that the entire lesion has been removed. It provides a guide for the pathologist to the location of the lesion in the specimen. It verifies that the wire has been removed from the breast. Other advantages include detecting additional abnormalities that may not have been suspected and is a good learning tool to correlate lesion morphology with histology [54]. At our institution we routinely perform specimen radiography on almost all cases undergoing mammographic localizations, and less commonly so when ultrasound is used to localize masses, the decision is surgeon driven. The benefit of specimen radiography has been questioned, in one study only 3 of 165 patients (1.8 %) benefited from performance of specimen radiography [60]. A technique of immersion ultrasonography of excised specimens has been reported for lesions localized under ultrasound guidance and those that are not mammographically visible [61]. The diagnostic accuracy of the procedure is excellent and reported to be 100 % when the localized lesion is seen on the specimen radiograph and available for histopathology evaluation. A study looking at the diagnostic accuracy of needle-localized open breast biopsy reported 96 % accuracy at 5-year follow-up. A review of the cases of missed breast cancer revealed that six of the seven that were missed were in fact failure to excise the localized abnormalities and in one instance the cancer was noted to have developed after the surgical excision [62].

Imaging-guided presurgical localization of non-palpable mammographic screen-detected abnormalities of the breast is a simple, safe, and accurate way of diagnosing early-stage breast cancers. Over the last two decades, a rapid decrease in the number of these procedures has been noted due to advent of minimally invasive percutaneous biopsy procedures performed under mammographic or sonographic guidance. Nevertheless it still remains a useful method and is now indicated in selected cases where a cancer diagnosis has been made based on a needle biopsy, when there is imaging pathological discordance following needle biopsy or in those patients where imaging-guided biopsy is not an option due to patient related factors.

Stereotactic Breast Biopsy

Since its description in the 1970s, image-guided breast biopsy has become increasingly utilized for the diagnosis of breast lesions. Stereotactic biopsy can be performed on suspicious calcifications as well as masses and areas of parenchymal distortion not visualized by ultrasound. Most women undergoing breast biopsies do not have cancer; therefore methods for diagnosis should be minimally invasive. Stereotactic biopsy has been shown to be safe, accurate, and cost effective [63]. Successful biopsy is dependent on proper patient selection and understanding of the equipment and procedure by those performing the biopsies.

Advantages of Stereotactic Biopsy

Stereotactic biopsy is a less invasive procedure which can be performed quickly at less cost than open biopsy. It causes minimal or no scarring and recovery is quicker. Few significant complications occur. Accuracy is comparable to open biopsy [63]. With the introduction of large-gauge vacuum-assisted biopsy devices, more accurate diagnoses can be made with fewer false-negative results. For benign lesions there is no need for excisional biopsy and malignant lesions can undergo a single surgery.

Indications

Lesions amenable to stereotactic biopsy are ACR BI-RADS Category 4 and 5 calcifications, masses, and areas of architectural distortion. ACR BI-RADS Category 3 lesions should undergo short-term follow-up unless the patient is considered to be at high risk for breast cancer, cannot comply with follow-up recommendations, or has undue anxiety.

Contraindications

Patients must be able to lie still during the procedure. Any medical, physical, or mental condition that would interfere is a contraindication. Prone table also have a weight limit, while upright units do not. Anticoagulant therapy is a relative contraindication especially if the medication cannot be temporarily withheld. Consultation with referring physicians should be made on a case-by-case basis.

Patient Selection

The lesion must be able to be properly targeted to perform the procedure. Beware of patients referred for stereotactic biopsy who have not been thoroughly evaluated. Lesions visible by ultrasound should undergo ultrasound-guided biopsy. As already noted prone tables have a weight restriction and adherence to its limits will prevent unsuccessful procedures.

For biopsies on a prone table, the patient must be able to lie without moving for the length of the procedure. A history of congestive heart failure, severe gastroesophageal reflux, arthritis, shoulder or spine injury, or psychiatric illness may preclude the patient's cooperation.

Prior to the procedure a history should be obtained and if necessary a "trial run" to position the patient on the table to determine if the patient can cooperate. Patient educational material such as brochures or videos can be helpful in reducing anxiety.

Qualifications for Performing the Procedure

The American College of Radiologists have set forth the qualifications for performing stereotactic biopsies for physicians, medical physicists, radiologist assistants, and radiologic technologists [64].

Stereotaxis

The ability to determine the position in space of a fixed point can be calculated by the apparent shift of that point on stereotactic image pairs. The stereotactic table compresses the breast between a compression plate and the image detector. The stereotactic image pairs are taken by convention at $+15°$ and $-15°$ around the x axis of a Cartesian coordinate system. The z axis or depth is then calculated by the computer. The principle of stereotaxis and errors and problems that can be encountered have been described in depth.

The Equipment

Most stereotactic biopsies are now performed on dedicated prone table or upright systems that can be used with mammographic units. These upright "add-on" units now have the capability for the patient to lie in the lateral decubitus position reducing the likelihood of vasovagal reactions.

Each of the available systems has proscribed procedures for localizing breast lesions. Before performance of a stereotactic biopsy, one must become familiar with the specific equipment and its requirements to ensure a successful biopsy. Core needle biopsy devices may be spring loaded or vacuum assisted and come in sizes ranging from 16 to 8 gauge.

Patient Preparation

Educational material such as brochures or videos may help relieve anxiety for the patient. At our institution we ask the patient to come in for a consultation at which time the patient is shown the stereotactic room and table. We also make sure the patient understands that a biopsy tissue marker will be placed at the time of the procedure. Any questions the patent has can be answered. We also take the opportunity to assess the patient by asking pertinent medical history, reviewing medications, and obtaining vital signs as indicated. Patients are instructed to take medications (except for anticoagulants) the day of the procedure. If the patient desires anxiolytics (diazepam 5–10 mg), arrangements are made for the patient to pick the medication up at her pharmacy and bring it the day of the procedure. We instruct the patients to make arrangements to have someone be available to take them home.

Informed consent should be obtained prior to the procedure. Antianxiety medications can be taken by the patient after informed consent has been obtained. Ensuring the patient has voided, is in comfortable clothing, and is comfortable on the table will help the patient remain still during the procedure. Patients do not have to be NPO and are encouraged having a light meal a few hours prior to the procedure.

The Procedure

The patient is positioned on the table with the breast containing the area of interest positioned through the opening. The technologist positions the area of interest in the open field of view. It is important to place the area of interest in the center of the field especially in the x axis to ensure the target remains visible on the stereotactic pairs. A scout image is obtained. The stereotactic pairs are obtained and the lesion is targeted. It is important at this step to ensure the area targeted in the two images is the same. If different points are targeted, there is a greater likelihood of a failed procedure. The computer calculates the depth and the coordinated are transferred to the table. One staff member reads the coordinates from the computer and a second staff member verbally confirms the coordinates. As the physician performing the biopsy, it is well worth your time to "double-check" these coordinates.

At this point prior to anesthesia instillation, it is important to determine that there will be adequate tissue between the tip of the needle and the back of the breast after the needle is fully deployed. This is noted as the stroke margin and is the compressed breast thickness minus the calculated z depth – 6 (a safety margin). The stroke margin must be positive or the needle will exit the breast and enter the back breast support. Newer equipment has an audible signal if the needle is placed in the prefire position that will result in a negative stroke margin.

The breast is prepped with a skin antiseptic; the most common is an iodine-based solution. A skin weal is made with buffered lidocaine. Deeper anesthesia is given centrally then in four sites around the center of the area of interest (i.e., 12, 3, 6, and 9 o'clock) in equal amounts so as not to move the underlying target. Repeat stereotactic images can be obtained to ensure the target has not been displaced by the anesthetic. A small skin incision is then made at the expected entrance of the biopsy needle. The needle is then manually advanced into the breast. Quite often there is tenting of the breast, and it is important to have the needle through the breast and for the skin to return to its normal configuration. The needle is then positioned in the prefire position. Repeat stereotactic pairs are obtained. It is at this time the final assessment can be made before placing the biopsy needle at the target. The needle is placed, and "postfire" position of the target is determined by repeat images before samples are obtained.

The number of samples obtained is determined by the needle gauge, size of the lesion, and patient tolerance. Vacuum-assisted devices can be rotated to obtain samples from multiple directions. The samples are then placed in a container suitable for specimen imaging to confirm presence of calcifications. Specimen x-ray obtained for masses or areas of distortion can be made on a case-by-case preference. At our institution the specimens containing the calcifications are sent separately from those without calcifications.

Marker Placement

A tissue marker is deployed and confirmation with one image is made prior to removal of the biopsy needle. Marker placement is vital for further patient management. If a lesion is benign, the markers can be used for follow-up of the area and to mark the area as biopsied if the patient is seen at another institution in the future. If the lesions are one such as atypical ductal hyperplasia that should be further evaluated or is malignant, the marker can be used for preoperative localization or as follow-up to neoadjuvant therapy. Different markers are available and should be compatible with the biopsy system. These markers are small (2–3 mm) and made of titanium or stainless steel. Since some patients have multiple lesions or may have had previous biopsies with marker placement, it is important to ensure the marker is unique to each procedure. Marker migration can occur, and it is important to denote with measurements and location the length and direction of any movement.

Post-biopsy

After the biopsy marker is deployed and confirmed by typically a single image, the introducer is removed and manual compression is held for 20 min to ensure hemostasis. A visual inspection of the breast is made and further compression is performed if indicated. The breast is then cleaned and a Steri-Strip™ is applied and the area is bandaged. A two-view mammogram (cranial caudal and 90° lateral) with minimal compression is obtained for confirmation of the tissue marker position and to assess the postbiopsy appearance of the targeted area.

Post-biopsy Instructions/Care

A cold pack is given to the patient for the trip home. Patients are asked not to soak in a bath, swim in either a pool or ocean or submerge the biopsied breast in a hot tub/spa for 5–7 days. Other postbiopsy instructions include how to recognize early signs of infections, and the patients are given contact numbers as well as written instructions. For pain, over-the-counter pain relievers are recommended such as acetaminophen. Use of aspirin and nonsteroidal antiinflammatory drugs are discouraged because of the potential for bleeding. The patient is asked to avoid strenuous activity for 24 h and then resume activities as tolerated.

Complications

Report of the Procedure

Per ACR guidelines permanent retrievable images documenting the procedure should be obtained with the normal identification. The report of the procedure per the guidelines includes very specific items and which should be included. A template within a reporting system is very helpful to ensure all items are reported. At our institution, a workflow sheet is kept by one of the staff during the procedure and includes time medication such as diazepam is taken, time patient is placed on table, approach used, amount of anesthesia used, number and clock face of core sample obtained, time specimens are placed in formalin, type of biopsy tissue marker placed, time of deployment of the marker, and length of time the breast is compressed for hemostasis. The staff also records any immediate complications and the time and to whom the patient is discharged [63].

Postprocedure Follow-Up

Any complication (significant hematoma, infections, etc.) should be documented. The radiologist is also required to report on the concordance of the pathology with the imaging finding. These reports should be in compliance with the ACR Practice guidelines for reporting and communication of diagnostic imaging findings [65]. Further management of the patient should be based on concordance of findings and pathology results. The findings are then communicated to the referring physician and patient.

Concordance/Discordance of Pathology

It is incumbent upon the radiologist to determine whether the pathology is concordant or discordant with the mammographic/biopsied area.

A benign concordant biopsy is followed up short term (6–12 months) to ensure sampling error has not occurred. At our institution 6 months is the typical time frame.

For a discordant result the patient may undergo a second biopsy or surgical excision.

Concordant malignant results should be referred for further surgical/oncological management.

Elsewhere in this book are discussions on imaging pathological correlation (Chap. 13).

Reasons for Failed Biopsy

Proper maintenance of the equipment as well as daily calibration is important to ensure successful biopsies.

Failure to bring the target area into the field of view can happen if it is near the chest wall or in the extreme outer breast.

During the targeting on the stereotactic pairs, it is possible to target different calcifications on each image causing the needle not be ideally placed. If there are many calcifications scattered in the breast beside the target group, one may select a calcification outside of the target group.

References

1. Bruening W, Fontanarosa J, Tipton K, Teadwell JR, Launders J, Schoelles K. Systemic review: comparative effectiveness of core-needle and open surgical biopsy to diagnose breast lesions. Ann Intern Med. 2010;152(4):238–46.
2. Apesteguia L, Pina LJ. Ultrasound-guided core needle biopsy of breast lesions. Insights Imaging. 2011;2(4):493–500.
3. Hoagland L, Hitt R. Technique for ultrasound-guided, percutaneous core-needle breast biopsy. Appl Radiol. 2013;42:14–9.
4. Liberman L. Percutaneous image-guided core breast biopsy. Radiol Clin North Am. 2002;40(3):483–500.
5. Nakano S, Sakamoto H, Ohtsuka M, Mibu A, Sakata H. Evaluation and indications of ultrasound-guided vacuum-assisted core needle biopsy. Breast Cancer. 2007;14(3):292–6.
6. O'Flynn EA, Wilson AR, Michell MJ. Image-guided breast biopsy: state of the art. Clin Radiol. 2010;65(4):259–70.
7. Parker S, Jobe W, Dennis M, Stavros A, Johnson K, Yakes W, truell J, Price J, Kortz A, Clark D. US-guided automated large core breast biopsy. Radiology. 1993;187:507–11.
8. Parker S, Lovin J, Jobe W, Luethke J, Hopper K, Yakes W, Burke B. Stereotactic breast biopsy with a biopsy gun. Radiology. 1990;176:74–747.
9. Prutki M, Stern-Padovan R, Jakic-Razumovic J, Potocki K, Badovinac—Crnjevic T, Golubic AT. Ultrasound guided breast biopsy—a retrospective study and literature review. Lijec Vjesn. 2012;134(9–10):270–5.
10. Mueller-Holzner E, Frede T, Daniaux M, Ban M, Taucher S, Schneitter A, Zeimet A, Marth C. Ultrasound-guided core needle biopsy of the breast: does frozen section give an accurate diagnosis? Breast Cancer Res Treat. 2007;106:399–406.
11. Cassano E, Urban L, Pizzamiglio M, Abbate F, Maisonneuve P, Renne G, Viale G, Bellomi M. Ultrasound-guided vacuum-assisted core breast biopsy: experience with 406 cases. Breast Cancer Res Treat. 2007;102:103–10.
12. Ciatto S, Houssami N, Ambrogetti D, Bianchi S, Bonardi R, Brancato B, Catarzi S, Risso GG. Accuracy and underestimation of malignancy of breast core needle biopsy: the florence experience of over 4000 consecutive biopsies. Breast Cancer Res Treat. 2007;101:291–7.
13. Fajardo LL, Pisano ED, Caudry DJ, Gatsonis CA, Berg WA, Connolly J, Schnitt S, Page DL, McNeil BJ, Radiologist Investigators of the Radiologic Diagnostic Oncology Group V. Stereotactic and sonographic large-core biopsy of nonpalpable breast lesions: results of the Radiologic Diagnostic Oncology Group V study. Acad Radiol. 2004;11(3):293–308.
14. Lai HW, Wu HK, Kuo SJ, Chen ST, Tseng HS, Tseng LM, Chen DR. Differences in accuracy and underestimation rates for 14- vs 16-gauge core needle biopsies in ultrasound-detectable breast lesions. Asian J Surg. 2013;36(2):83–8.
15. ACR Practice guideline for the performance of ultrasound-guided percutaneous breast interventional procedures. American College of Radiology. 2009. Available at http://www.acr.org/quality-safety/standards-guidelines. Accessed 14 Jul 2013.
16. Schueller G, Schueller-Weidekamm C, Helbich TH. Accuracy of ultrasound-guided, large-core needle breast biopsy. Eur Radiol. 2008;18(9):1761–73.
17. Bugbee M, Wellisch D, Arnott I, Maxwell J, Kirsch D, Sayre D, Bassett L. Breast core-needle biopsy: clinical trial of relaxation technique versus medication versus no intervention for anxiety reduction. Radiology. 2005;234(1):73–8.
18. Flowers C. Breast biopsy: anesthesia, bleeding prevention, representative sampling, and rad/path concordance. Appl Radiol. 2012;41:9–14.
19. Bard®Max-Core® Disposable core biopsy instrument instructions for use. Tempe: Bard.
20. Matsumoto A, Reifsnyder A, Hartwell G, Angle J, Selby JB, Tegtmeyer C. Reducing the discomfort of lidocaine administration through pH buffering. J Vasc Interv Radiol. 1994;5(1):171–5.
21. Pascuet E, Donnelly R, Garceau D, Vaillancourt R. Buffered lidocaine hydrochloride solution with and without epinephrine: stability in polypropylene syringes. Can J Hosp Pharm. 2009;62(5):375–80.
22. Kirshenbaum K, Keppke A, Hou K, Dickerson M, Gajjar M, Kirshenbaum G. Reassessing specimen number and diagnostic

yield of ultrasound guided breast core biopsy. Breast J. 2012; 18(5):464–9.
23. Thomassin-Naggara I, Lalonde L, David J, Darai E, Uzan S, Trop I. A plea for the biopsy marker: how, why, and why not clipping after breast biopsy. Breast Cancer Res Treat. 2012;132:881–93.
24. Tamai K, Mitsumari M, Fujishiro S, Kokubo M, Ooya N, Nagata Y, Sasai K, Hiraoka M, Inamoto T. A case report of allergic reaction to surgical metal clips inserted for postoperative boost irradiation in a patient undergoing breast conserving therapy. Breast Cancer. 2001;8(1):90–2.
25. Brenner RJ. Percutaneous removal of postbiopsy marking clip in the breast using stereotactic technique. Am J Roentgenol. 2001;176(2):417–9.
26. Salkowski LR, Fowler AM, Burnside ES, Sisney GA. Utility of 6-month follow-up imaging after a concordant benign breast biopsy result. Radiology. 2011;258(2):380–7.
27. Uematsu T. How to choose needles and probes for ultrasonographically guided percutaneous breast biopsy: a systemic approach. Breast Cancer. 2012;19(3):238–41.
28. Abbate F, Cassano E, Menna S, Viale G. Ultrasound-guided vacuum-assisted breast biopsy: use at the European Institute of Oncology in 2010. J Ultrasound. 2011;14(4):177–81.
29. Szynglarewicz B, Matkowski R, Kasprzak P, Forgacz J, Zolnierek A, Halon A, Kornafel J. Pain experienced by patients during minimal-invasive ultrasound-guided breast biopsy: vacuum-assisted vs core-needle procedure. Eu J Surg Oncol. 2011;37(5):398–403.
30. Vandromme MJ, Umphrey H, Krontiras H. Image-guided methods for biopsy of suspicious breast lesions. J Surg Oncol. 2011;103(4): 299–305.
31. Povoski SP, Jimenez RE, Wang WP. Ultrasound-guided diagnostic breast biopsy methodology: retrospective comparison of the 8-gauge vacuum-assisted biopsy approach versus spring-loaded 14-gauge core biopsy approach. World J Surg Oncol. 2011;9:87.
32. Uematsu T. Screening and diagnosis of breast cancer in augmented women. Breast Cancer. 2008;15:159–64.
33. Hoorntje L, Schipper M, Kaya A, Verkooijen H, Klinkenbijl J, Borel RI. Tumor cell displacement after 14G breast biopsy. Eur J Surg Oncol. 2004;30:520–5.
34. Suh YJ, Kim MJ, Kim EJ, Moon HJ, Kwak JY, Koo HR, Yoon JH. Comparison of the underestimation rate in cases with ductal carcinoma in situ at ultrasound-guided core biopsy:14-gauge automated core-needle biopsy vs 8- or 11-gauge vacuum-assisted biopsy. Br J Radiol. 2012;85(1016):e349–56.
35. Zhang C, Lewis DR, Nasute P, Hayes M, Warren LJ, Gordon PB. The negative predictive value of ultrasound-guided 14-gauge core needle biopsy of breast masses: a validation study of 339 cases. Cancer Imaging. 2012;12:488–96.
36. Szynglarewicz B, Kasprzak P, Kornafel J, Forgacz J, Pudelko M, Majewski A, Matkowski R. Duration time of vacuum-assisted biopsy for nonpalpable breast masses: comparison between stereotactic and ultrasound-guided procedure. Tumori. 2011;97(4): 517–21.
37. Ojeda-Fournier H, Nguyen JQ. Ultrasound evaluation of regional breast lymph nodes. Semin Roentgenol. 2011;46(1):51–9.
38. Pagani C, Coscia DR, Dellabianca C, Bonardi M, Alessi S, Calliada F. Ultrasound guided fine-needle aspiration cytology of breast lesions. J Ultrasound. 2011;14(4):182–7.
39. Vargas H, Agbunag R, Khalkhali I. State of the art of minimally invasive breast biopsy: principles and practice. Breast Cancer. 2000;7(4):370–9.
40. Morris E, Liberman L. Breast MRI. New York: Springer; 2005.
41. Bassett L, Winchester D, Caplan R, et al. Stereotactic core-needle biopsy of the breast: a report of the Joint Task Force of the American College of Radiology, American College of Surgeons, and College of American Pathologists. CA Cancer J Clin. 1997;47:171–90.
42. Morris E. ACR practice guideline for the performance of magnetic resonance imaging-guided breast interventional procedures. Am Coll Radiol [serial online]. 2011.
43. LaTrenta L, Menell J, Morris E, et al. Breast lesions detected with MR imaging utility and histopathologic importance of identification with US. Radiology. 2003;227:856–61.
44. Philpotts L. MR intervention: indications, techniques, and histologic. In: Moy L, Mercado C, editors. Magnetic resonance imaging clinics of North America. Philadelphia: W.B. Saunders Company; 2010. p. 323–32.
45. Fisher U, Practical MR. Mammography. New York: Thieme; 2004.
46. Cardenosa G. Breast imaging companion. Philadelphia: Lippincott Williams & Wilkins; 2008.
47. Wilson R, Kavia S. Comparison of large-core vacuum-assisted breast biopsy and excision systems. In: Brun del Re R, editor. Minimally invasive breast biopsies. New York: Springer; 2009.
48. Ojeda-Fournier H. MRI-guided breast biopsy. In: Presented at the 10th clinical breast imaging 2013 symposium, Tampa, 2013.
49. Jackman R, Lamm R. Stereotactic histologic biopsy in breasts with implants. Radiology. 2002;222:157–64.
50. Yim JH, Barton PM, Weber B, Radford D, et al. Mammographically detected breast cancer. Benefits of stereotactic core vs wire localization biopsy. Ann Surg June. 1996;223(6):688–700.
51. White RR, Halperin TJ, Olson AJ, et al. Impact of core-needle biopsy on the surgical management of mammographic abnormalities. Ann Surg. 2001;233(6):769–77.
52. Whitten TM, Wallace TW. Image guided core biopsy has advantages over needle localization biopsy for the diagnosis of nonpalpable breast cancer. Am Surg. 1997;63:1072.
53. Fahy BN, Bold RJ, Schneider PD, Khatri V, Goodnight JE. Cost-benefit analysis of biopsy methods for suspicious mammographic lesions. Arch Surg. 2001;136:990–4.
54. Cardenosa G. Breast imaging companion. Philadelphia: Lippincott Williams & Wilkins; 2001. p. 414–33.
55. Reynolds HE, Jackson VP, Musick BS. Preoperative needle localization in the breast: utility of local anesthesia. Radiology. 1993;187:503–5.
56. Jackman RJ, Marzoni FJ. Needle localized breast biopsy. Why do we fail? Radiology. 1997;204(3):677–84.
57. Abrahamson PE, Dunlap LA, Amamoo MA, Schell MJ, Braeuning MP, Pisano ED. Factors predicting successful needle-localized breast biopsy. Acad Radiol. 2003;10:601–6.
58. Martinez SR, Gelfand M, Hourani HS, Sorrento JJ, Mohan EP. Cardiac injury during needle localized surgical breast biopsy. J Surg Oncol. 2003;82(4):261–5.
59. Helvie MA, Ikeda DM, Adler DD. Localization and needle aspiration of breast lesions: complications in 370 cases. AJR Am J Roentgenol. 1991;157:711–4.
60. Bimston DN, Bebb GG, Wagman LD. Is specimen mammography beneficial? Arch Surg. 2000;135:1083–8.
61. Lee KY, Seo BK, Ann Y, et al. Immersion ultrasonography of excised non palpable breast lesion specimens after ultrasound-guided needle localization. Korean J Radiol. 2008;9:312–9.
62. Verkooijen HM, Peeters PHM, Pijnappel RM, Koot VCM, Schipper MEI, Borel Rinkes IHM. Diagnostic accuracy of needle-localized open breast biopsy for impalpable breast disease. Brit J Surg. 2000;87:344–7.
63. Carr JJ, Hemler PF, Halford PW, Freimanis RI, Choplin RH, Chen MY. Stereotactic localization of breast lesions: how it works and methods to improve accuracy. Radiographics. 2001;21(2):463–73.
64. Available at http://www.acr.org/~/media/ACR/Documents/PGTS/guidelines/Stereotactically_Guided_Breast.pdf.
65. Kushner DC, Lucey LL. Diagnostic radiology reporting and communication: the ACR guideline. J Am Coll Radiol. 2005; 2(1):15–21.

Bibliography

Bassett LW, Mahoney MC, Apple SK. Interventional breast imaging: current procedures and assessing for concordance with pathology. Radiol Clin North Am. 2007;45(5):881–94.

Bitencourt AG, Cohen MP, Graziano L, Souza JA, Marques EF, Brites MR, Chojniak R. Pseudoaneurysm after ultrasound-guided vacuum-assisted core breast biopsy. Breast J. 2012;18(2):177–8.

Bulte J, Polman L, Schlooz-Vries M, Werner A, Besselink R, Sessink K, Mus R, Lardenoije S, Imhof-Tas M, Bulten J, van Eagen-van Grunsven ACH, Schaafsma E, Strobbe LJA, Bult P, De Wit JHW. One-day core needle biopsy in a breast clinic: 4 years experience. Breast Cancer Res Treat. 2013;137:609–16.

Dempsey P. New ultrasound-based imaging technologies are claimed to avoid unnecessary breast biopsies, but what is an "unnecessary" image-guided needle biopsy of the breast? J Clin Ultrasound. 2010;38(3):111–2.

Kibil W, Hodorowicz-Zaniewska D, Kulig J. Mammotome biopsy under ultrasound control in the diagnostics and treatment of nodular breast lesions- own experience. Pol Przegl Chir. 2012;84(5):242–6.

Koo JS, Han K, Kim MJ, Moon HJ, Kim EK, Park BW. Can additional immunohistochemistry staining replace the surgical excision for the diagnosis of papillary breast lesions classified as benign on 14-gage core needle biopsy? Breast Cancer Res Treat. 2013;137(3):797–806.

Kurita T, Tsuchiya S, Wtarai Y, Yamamoto Y, Harada O, Yanagihara K, Iida S, Yamashita K, Haga S, Uchida E. Roles of fine-needle aspiration and core needle biopsy in the diagnosis of breast cancer. Breast Cancer. 2012;19:23–9.

Lein BC, Alex WR, Zebley DM, Pezzi CM. Results of needle localized breast biopsy in women under age 50. Am J Surg. 1996;171:356–9.

Markopoulos C, Phil M, Kakisis J, et al. Management of nonpalpable, mammographically detectable breast lesions. World J Surg. 1999;23:434–89.

Murray MP, Luedtke C, Liberman L, Nehhozina T, Akram M, Brogi E. Classic lobular carcinoma in situ and atypical lobular hyperplasia at percutaneous breast core biopsy: outcomes of prospective excision. Cancer. 2013;119(5):1073–9.

Nasrinossadat A, Ladan F, Fereshte E, Asieh O, Reza C, Akramossadat S, Golshan M. Marking non-palpable breast masses with injected methylene blue dye, an easy, safe and low cost method for developing countries and resource limited areas. Asian Pac J Cancer Prev. 2011;12(5):1189–92.

Smetherman DH. Screening, imaging, and image-guided biopsy techniques for breast cancer. Surg Clin North Am. 2013;93(2):309–27.

Son EJ, Oh KK, Kim EK. Pregnancy-associated breast disease: radiologic features and diagnostic dilemmas. Yonsei Med J. 2006;47(1):34–42.

Stavros AT. Breast ultrasound. Philadelphia: Lippincott Williams & Wilkins; 2004.

Taskin F, Unsal A, Ozbas S, Erkus M, Karaman C. Fibrotic lesions of the breast: radiological findings and core-needle biopsy results. Eur J Radiol. 2011;80(3):e231–6.

Tran DQ, Wilkerson DK, Namm J, Zeis MA, Cottone FJ. Needle-localized breast biopsy for mammographic abnormalities: a community hospital experience. Am Surg. 1999;65:281–7.

Wiratkapun C, Treesit T, Wibulpolprasert B, Lertsithichai P. Diagnostic accuracy of ultrasound-guided core needle biopsy for breast lesion. Singapore Med J. 2012;53(1):40–5.

Yao F, Li J, Wan Y, Zhong Y, Wei W, Tu Y, Tong H, Sun S. Sonographically guided vacuum-assisted breast biopsy for complete excision of presumed benign breast lesions. J Ultrasound Med. 2012;31(12):1951–7.

Youk JH, Kim EK, Kim MJ, Lee JY, Oh KK. Missed breast cancers at US-guided core needle biopsy: how to reduce them. Radiographics. 2007;27:79–94.

Imaging Pathological Correlation in Breast Imaging

13

Mahesh K. Shetty

Introduction

Screening mammography aims to find early-stage breast cancer and its efficacy in reducing mortality from breast cancer has been proven [1, 2]. The recall rate from a screening mammogram should ideally range between 7 and 12 %. About one in four diagnostic recalls leads to an assignment of a BI-RADS™ 4 or 5 categories with a recommendation for biopsy leading to a cancer diagnosis in 25–35 % of cases that undergo biopsy [3–5]. Screen-recalled cases with an assessment of BI-RADS™ 3 with recommendation for a short-interval follow-up have a less than 2 % likelihood of cancer [6]. A thorough understanding of commonly encountered pathology affecting the breast and the spectrum of imaging findings associated with these lesions is critical for a breast imager. It is important to be familiar with the pathology of breast diseases so as to correlate the mammographic and sonographic appearance and make management decisions following minimally invasive biopsy. Such an understanding is needed, for example, when excisional biopsy of certain histological diagnosis is indicated either due to known risk of underestimating disease or risk of a lesion being premalignant. In certain cases minimally invasive biopsy may not be the best option and excisional biopsy may be a better option such as when imaging appearance is suggestive of a radial scar or a papilloma.

M.K. Shetty, MD, FRCR, FACR, FAIUM
Department of Radiology,
Baylor College of Medicine, Houston, TX, USA

Woman's Center for Breast Care and MRI,
Woman's Hospital of Texas,
Houston, TX 77054, USA
e-mail: mshettymd@gmail.com

Pathological Correlation in the Probably Benign Assessment Category

Up to 11 % of screening mammograms may be assigned a probably benign BI-RADS™ 3 assessment category with a commonly reported range of 1.2–9.8 % [7]. In a study that included 2,927 of 58,408 eligible women who had recommendations for short-interval follow-up, the incidence of breast cancer was 1.0 % at 2 years compared to incidence of 0.6 % for women with BI-RADS™ 2, benign assessment, and 0.5 % for women with a BI-RADS™ 1, negative assessment [7]. Despite a probably benign assessment, tissue diagnosis may still be obtained in a small percentage of women. An evaluation of cases with a BI-RADS™ 3 assessment that underwent tissue diagnosis found only three cancers in a study group of 288 cases [1 %] [8]. In some European countries such as the United Kingdom and Sweden, a probably benign assessment category is not used; there is instead either a recommendation for routine follow-up or a tissue diagnosis [8]. Most cancers in the probably benign assessment category are diagnosed within the first 12 months. The proportion of stage II or more advanced cancers are reportedly higher in the probably benign recommendation that is based solely on a screening mammogram when compared to those that are assigned such an assessment category after a diagnostic workup [9, 10]. The small numbers of cancers that do develop in patients who are on a short-interval follow-up tend to be detected by interval enlargement and before they are clinically palpable. These therefore generally tend to be early-stage cancers [11, 12]. It is to be noted that unlike in mammography where scientific validation has been established for outcomes based on BI-RADS™ lexicon, such is not yet the case for the BI-RADS™ ultrasound lexicon [10, 12, 13].

M.K. Shetty (ed.), *Breast Cancer Screening and Diagnosis: A Synopsis*,
DOI 10.1007/978-1-4939-1267-4_13, © Springer Science+Business Media New York 2015

Imaging Pathological Correlation in the BI-RADS™ 4 Assessment Category

A BI-RADS™ 4 assessment category is based on a suspicious finding seen on a mammogram and or an ultrasound and tissue diagnosis is obtained in most instances. The final histological diagnosis can either be benign or malignant. The commonly encountered types of benign and malignant histological diagnosis are discussed next. There are in addition some unusual and uncommon tumors of the breast that may be revealed on histological sampling of image-detected abnormalities in the breast:

A. Benign histology: fibrocystic changes, sclerosing adenosis, fibroepithelial tumors
B. Malignant histology: invasive ductal cancer; invasive lobular cancer; tubular, mucinous, medullary cancer; papillary cancers, Paget's disease of the breast
C. Unusual tumors of the breast

BI-RADS™ 4 with Benign Histology

Two of the most common benign histological diagnosis in lesions that are categorized as BI-RADS™ 4 and undergoing biopsy are fibrocystic change and fibroepithelial lesions.

Focal Fibrocystic Change and Sclerosing Adenosis

Fibrocystic change of the breast is the most common benign condition of the breast and has been reported in up to 58 % of premenopausal women [14]. Histologically fibrocystic change includes macrocysts, microcysts, adenosis, apocrine change, fibrosis, or ductal hyperplasia [15]. Imaging findings in fibrocystic change and related histological changes have been reported [16–19]. In a series of 58 cases with fibrocystic change as the histological diagnosis, 46 % appeared as solid masses, half of which were indeterminate [16].

Sclerosing adenosis is defined as a benign lobulocentric lesion of disordered acinar, myoepithelial, and connective tissue elements, which can mimic infiltrating carcinoma both grossly and microscopically [17, 20]. Histologically compressed and attenuated tubules and sclerotic stroma are the hallmark. Overinterpretation leading to false positives on cytological evaluation of palpable nodular adenosis has been known to occur [21]. A mass is seen in 11–53 % of cases of sclerosing adenosis and these masses may be circumscribed or have ill-defined margins. The term nodular adenosis is used when confluent areas of sclerosing adenosis form a mass and these may be palpable [16, 19]. Calcification is also a common mammographic sign of sclerosing adenosis and has been reported in 47–56 % of cases [17, 18]. Calcifications may be either clustered or diffusely scattered in distribution; these are commonly amorphous, pleomorphic, or less commonly punctate [17, 18]. Sclerosing adenosis less commonly may appear as an area of focal asymmetry or architectural distortion.

Fibroepithelial Tumors

Fibrous tumors of the breast are benign abnormalities that are composed of stromal elements and variable amounts of glandular epithelium. These include fibroadenoma, sclerosing lobular hyperplasia, and benign mesenchymal tumors. Benign mesenchymal tumors exhibit dense stromal elements and include stromal fibrosis, pseudoangiomatous hyperplasia, fibromatosis, phyllodes tumor, and fibrous mastopathy. With the exception of phyllodes tumor and fibromatosis, the remainder of fibroepithelial lesions need not undergo excisional biopsy following histological confirmation by means of percutaneous biopsy [22].

Fibroadenoma

The most common type among fibroepithelial tumors of the breast is the fibroadenoma. These are frequently palpable; although more common in the childbearing age, up to 44 % may be seen in postmenopausal women [22, 23]. Fibroadenomas arises from the terminal ductal lobular units. There has been some debate as to the increased risk for breast cancer in those diagnosed with fibroadenoma. There has been a report of increased risk in women with complex fibroadenomas, proliferative disease, or a family history of breast cancer in a study that included fibroadenomas that were surgically excised [24]. Another study that included fibroadenomas that were either excised or followed-up questioned the increased risk. A meta-analysis of studies examining the cancer risk with fibroadenomas has also questioned the increased risk [25]. The relative risk of developing breast cancer in patients who have had surgical excision of a fibroadenoma does increase in the presence of atypical hyperplasia or a family history of breast cancer (in a first-degree relative). Increased risk of breast cancer persists for over 20 years after the diagnosis. However, no study to date has reliably studied the increased risk of breast cancer in excised, nonexcised, or asymptomatic fibroadenomas [26]. Carcinoma within a fibroadenoma is exceedingly rare but has been reported. A total of 120 such cases have been reported. Malignant foci were confined to the fibroadenoma in more than half of the cases. Most of the "cancer" diagnosis reported was LCIS or DCIS [27, 28].

Fibroadenomas may be multiple in up to 15 % of cases. The most common imaging appearance is a circumscribed oval mass, on mammography and sonography. On ultrasound the mass is wider than taller and may be associated with posterior acoustic shadowing, is iso- or hypoechoic, and often demonstrates homogenous internal echoes (Fig. 13.1a, b). Calcifications when seen appear as small peripheral dots that later on lead to the appearance of classical popcorn type of

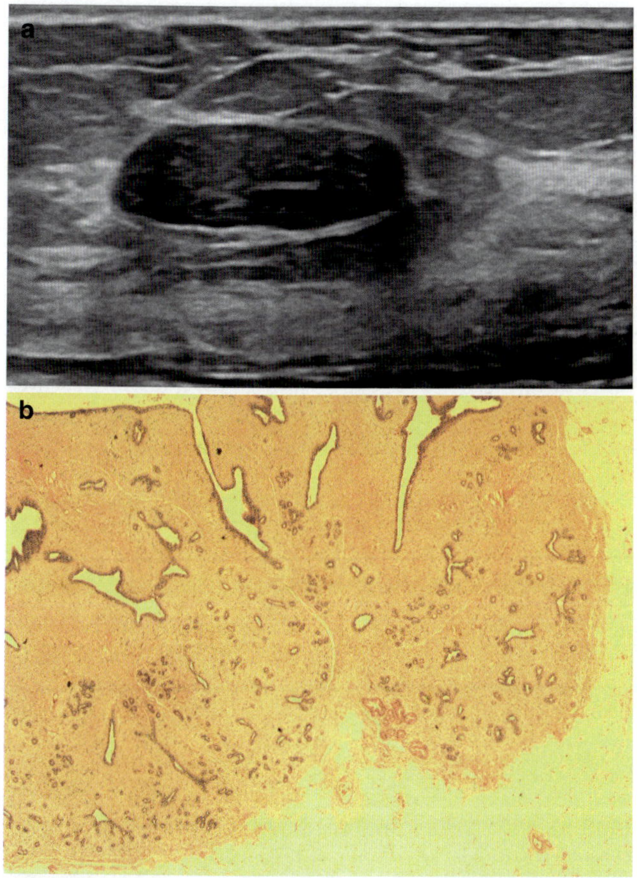

Fig. 13.1 A 35-year-old with a palpable lump histologically proven to be a fibroadenoma. (**a**) Ultrasound demonstrates an ovoid solid mass with circumscribed borders. (**b**) Histology demonstrates pericanalicular type of fibroadenoma

coarse calcifications. When a mass with such characteristic popcorn calcifications are seen an assessment of a benign fibroadenoma with no need for tissue diagnosis is appropriate. Occasionally on a mammogram small punctate, pleomorphic calcifications may be seen and particularly when associated with a mass should prompt a biopsy. Large fibroadenomas may be seen in the juvenile population or in young women and when larger than 5 cm the term giant fibroadenoma is used. In this type of a fibroadenoma, there is increased cellularity in the stroma with epithelial element proliferation. Histologically fibroadenomas are of two types, the intracanalicular type where dense stroma compresses the ducts into appearing like slit spaces and the pericanalicular type where there is no compression of the ducts.

Phyllodes Tumor

These are fibroepithelial tumors that present as large tumors and are commonly seen in young women. The average diameter of phyllodes tumor has been reported to be 5 cm, and the median patient age of presentation is 40 years; these masses are frequently palpable [29, 30]. Phyllodes tumors are composed of a hypercellular connective tissue stroma and epithelial elements. Histologically it is possible to distinguish between the benign type and the malignant type, the latter metastasizes in about 25 % of cases. Phyllodes tumor of the breast are locally aggressive tumors. Irrespective of the histological type, these tumors tend to recur after local excision. It is not possible to predict histologically the type that can locally recur. Following local excision nearly half of borderline phyllodes and two-thirds of malignant phyllodes tumors recurred; even following wide local excision 29–36 % of borderline and malignant phyllodes tumors recur [31]. Even the benign type recurs after local excision (21 %) and wide local excision (8 %). It is clear from these data that since patients with benign phyllodes tumor treated with breast-conserving surgery rarely die from their tumor (0.3 %), wide local excision is the preferred procedure for benign phyllodes tumor and mastectomy is the preferred treatment for malignant phyllodes tumor; a recurrence rate of 12 % has been reported even after mastectomy [31]. Phyllodes tumors of the breast are, however, rare tumors of the accounting for less than 1 % of all breast neoplasms [32, 33]. Majority of these tumors are benign particularly in the younger women; about 31 % of phyllodes tumors are borderline or malignant [32, 34]. On mammography, phyllodes tumor appears as a large circumscribed lobulated hyperdense mass, with calcifications rarely associated. On ultrasound these masses are circumscribed and heterogeneously hypoechoic and may have cleft-like or cystic spaces, being indistinguishable from a fibroadenoma [32] (Fig. 13.2a–f). Sonographic differentiation between benign and malignant types is unreliable. A diagnosis of phyllodes on a core needle biopsy is an indication for excisional biopsy. One study found that complex cystic echogenicity, presence of cleft, and a higher final BI-RADS™ assessment were more common in malignant phyllodes tumor [32].

The treatment of nonmetastatic phyllodes tumors of the breast is complete surgical resection with wide resection margins. Lumpectomy or partial mastectomy is the preferred surgical therapy. Local failure rate is high and 22–25 % of malignant phyllodes tumors metastasize, most frequently to the lungs. Factors that are predictive of an increased risk of recurrence include positive surgical margins, increased stromal cellularity, stromal overgrowth, stromal atypia, and increased mitotic activity [35].

Focal Fibrosis

This entity is also referred to as stromal fibrosis. Histologically focal fibrosis is composed of dense collagenous stroma with sparse glandular and vascular elements [22]. Focal fibrosis has been reported in 2–15 % of breast lesions undergoing tissue diagnosis [36–40]. On a mammogram focal fibrosis appears as a mass or a focal asymmetry; calcifications are rare (Fig. 13.3a, b). Masses are the most common mammographic appearance and have been reported to be seen in

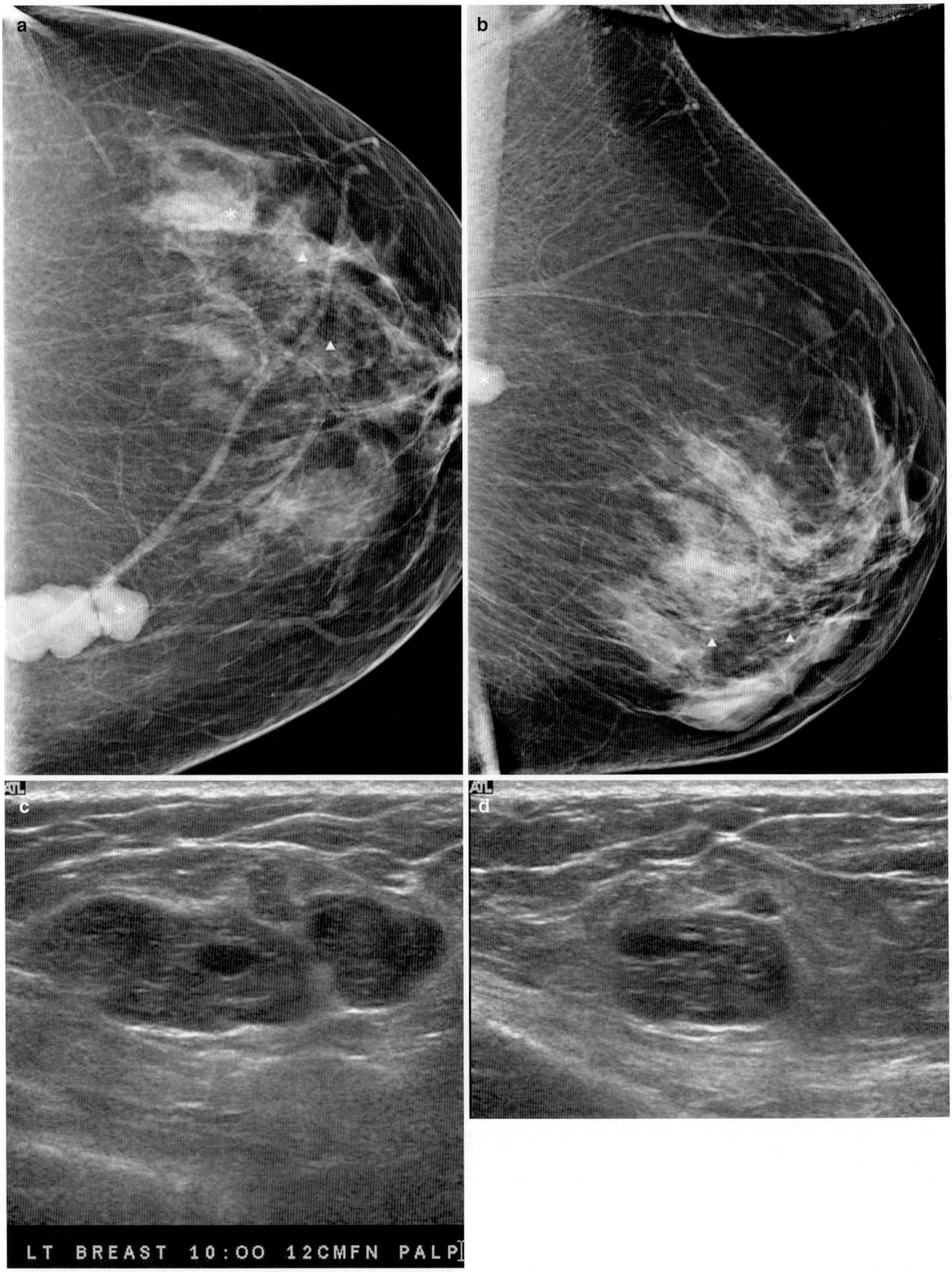

Fig. 13.2 A 55-year-old woman being worked by for excisional biopsy of suspicious calcifications with an incidental mass subsequently proven to be malignant Phyllodes tumor. (**a**) Craniocaudal view demonstrates a high-density lobulated mass in the inner breast whose posterior margin could not be included on the mammogram. (**b**) Mediolateral oblique view demonstrates only a part of the mass. (**c**, **d**) Ultrasound demonstrates a solid mass with cystic changes and ill-defined borders. (**e**, **f**) Histological slides

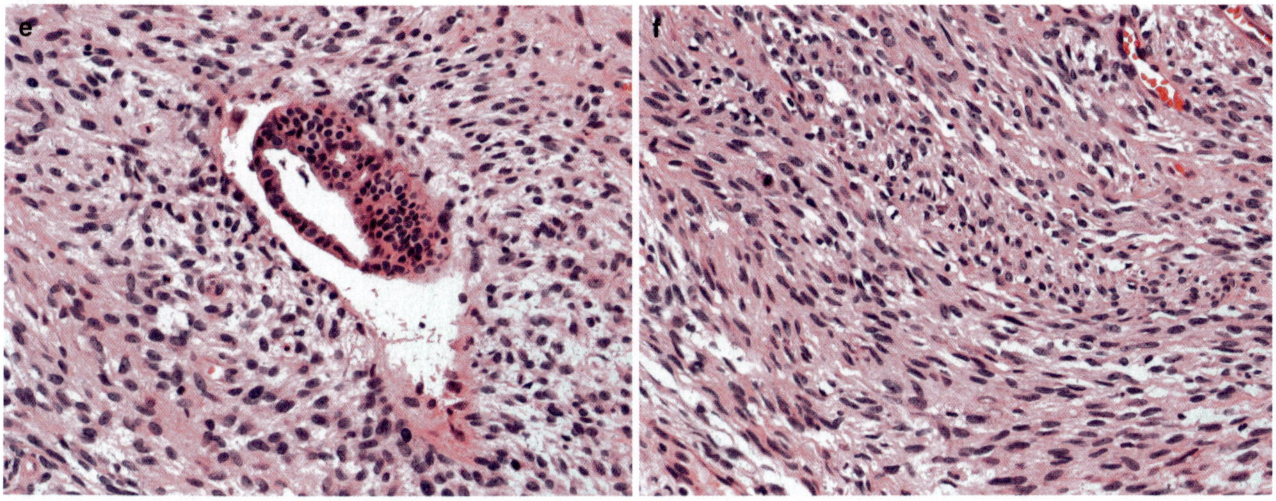

Fig. 13.2 (continued)

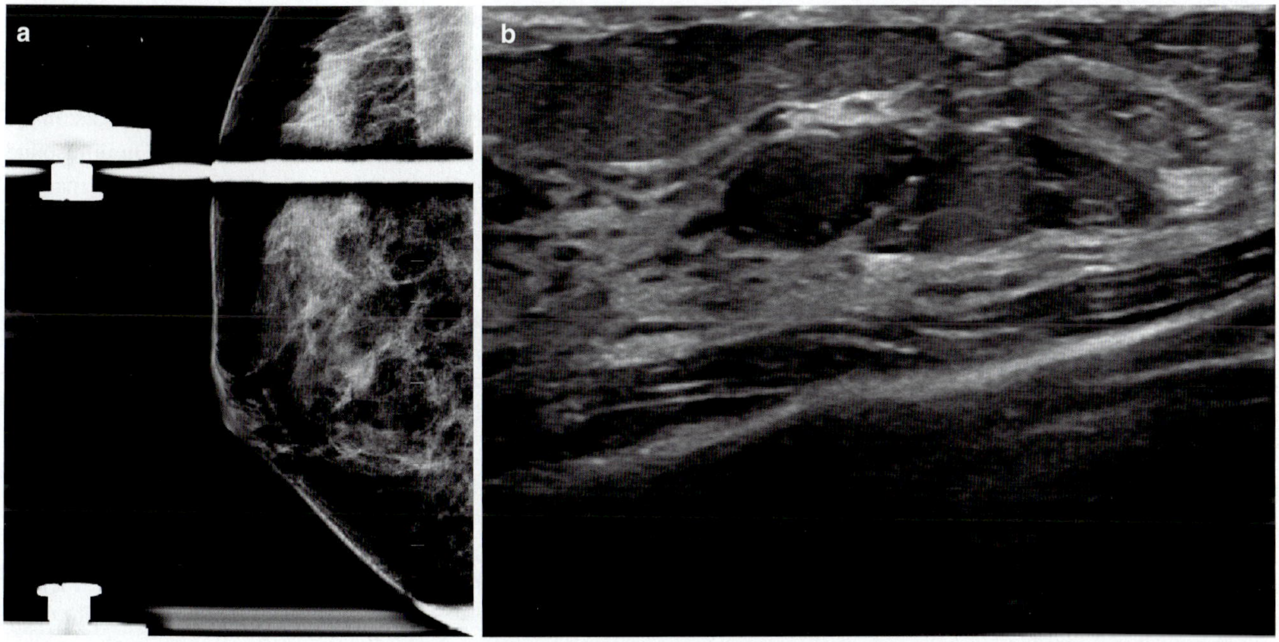

Fig. 13.3 A 47-year-old woman with an abnormality in the right breast histologically proven to be focal fibrosis. (**a**) Mediolateral oblique view with spot compression demonstrates a focal asymmetry. (**b**) Ultrasound demonstrates an ovoid solid mass with indeterminate sonographic features

46–75 % of cases [36, 38–40]. Focal asymmetry has been reported in 10–39 % of cases [36, 39, 40]. Architectural as a sign of focal fibrosis is less common and is seen in 5–12 % of cases [36, 39]. The diagnosis of focal fibrosis on core needle biopsy can be considered concordant for a mass exhibiting well-circumscribed or partially obscured margins. Imaging findings discordant with focal fibrosis, such as marginal spiculation, require excisional biopsy [36].

In 10 % of cases these lesions are mammographically occult and are identified on ultrasound [36]. At ultrasound focal fibrosis frequently demonstrates a mass with indeterminate features prompting a biopsy [16, 36–40]. Sonographically, 72 % ($n=36$) of cases of focal fibrosis presented as masses with three echotexture patterns: hypoechoic, isoechoic, and centrally echogenic with a peripheral hypoechoic rim. The sonographic margins were well circumscribed ($n=21$), lobulated ($n=10$), or ill defined ($n=5$). Histological review revealed three morphological patterns of collagen deposition: perilobular, septal, and haphazard fibrosis. Correlation with the imaging findings shows that the septal and perilobular fibrosis pattern is most often associated with a hypoechoic or a centrally echogenic mass, whereas the haphazard form of fibrosis is associated with architectural distortion [36]. Calcifications, although considered rare, have been reported in 9 % of cases in one series [40].

PASH: Pseudoangiomatous Hyperplasia

Pseudoangiomatous hyperplasia may be seen in up to 25 % of breast biopsy specimens with a probable hormonal cause in premenopausal women [41]. Histological features are similar to a fibroadenoma with predominant finding of sheets of benign ductal cells interspersed with anastomosing slit-like spaces that are lined by spindle cells unlike vascular channels that are lined by endothelial cells and contain red blood cells [42]. PASH is believed to be hormonally induced and accompanied by benign epithelial proliferation in ducts and lobules [43]. The imaging features in PASH have been reported in several studies [43–46]. Two series of 149 and 73 cases reported that on mammography a noncalcified mass or focal asymmetry described as localized increased stroma was the most common finding [43, 44]. There is no risk of malignancy and a diagnosis of PASH at core needle biopsy should be followed by a routine follow-up. Risk of recurrence is low and about 2 % has been reported [43]. At mammography PASH appears as a circumscribed mass or focal asymmetry (Fig. 13.4a–d). Substantial numbers can be mammographically occult. Architectural distortion and calcifications are rare. Majority of lesions are asymptomatic; however, 29 % of lesions were palpable in one series [44]. On ultrasound it appears as a circumscribed mass without malignant features, and increased through transmission has been reported in 69–81 % of cases [43]. Presence of a suspicious finding such as associated calcifications or spiculated borders should be considered discordant and excisional biopsy is advised since a small percentage of PASH can be associated with invasive cancer.

Sclerosing Lobular Hyperplasia or Fibroadenomatoid Mastopathy

This is a benign proliferative lesion seen most often in young black females with a mean age presentation of 32 years [22]. A common appearance is that of a circumscribed noncalcified mass resembling a noncalcified fibroadenoma. Histologically it is characterized by enlargement of lobules, increased number of intralobular ductules, and sclerosis of the intralobular septa [47].

Imaging Pathological Correlation in the BI-RADS™ 5 Assessment Category

BI-RADS™ 5 Assessment with Benign Histology

Mammary Fibromatosis (Desmoid Tumor)

Fibromatosis or desmoid tumor of the breast is rare comprising 0.2 % of breast tumors. It is a benign, nonmetastasizing low-grade spindle cell stromal tumor, which usually presents as a spiculated locally invasive tumor that is often palpable. Average age of presentation is 37 years. There is often a history of trauma or surgery. Recurrence rate is about 25 %. Wide excisional biopsy is recommended. Histologically there is profuse collagen and spindle cells. Absence of mitotic figures distinguishes from fibrosarcoma. Mammographically a desmoid tumor appears as a dense irregular noncalcified spiculated mass. On ultrasound an irregular hypoechoic mass with spiculated borders is typical [22, 48, 49] (Fig. 13.5a–d).

Diabetic Mastopathy

Diabetic mastopathy is characterized by stromal proliferation and is found in women with juvenile-onset insulin-dependent diabetes. Breast lesions are seen in about one half of all female patients with type 1 diabetes [22]. Palpable hard nontender fibrous masses that are frequently multiple and bilateral are encountered. Histologically these are collagenous stroma with increased number of spindle cells and scattered epithelial cells and associated lymphocytic infiltrate in the perivascular spaces [50]. There is no associated risk of breast cancer. Eighty-five percent of lesions were palpable in one series [51]. Diabetic mastopathy appears on the mammogram as a mass or focal asymmetry. On ultrasound these masses are hypoechoic and may have irregular margins corresponding to histological findings of poorly circumscribed and irregular margins. Vascular calcifications are present in a substantial number of cases in the excisional specimen suggesting that vascular damage and wound healing process may contribute to the pathogenesis of this entity [51]. Diabetic mastopathy is often seen in premenopausal women with diabetic complications such as retinopathy. MRI is helpful in diagnosing the benign nature of these masses [51]. Histologically there is lymphocytic lobulitis and ductitis with glandular atrophy as well as lymphocytic and mononuclear perivascular inflammation and dense fibrosis with or without epithelioid-like fibroblasts [51]. Fibrous mastopathy may also occur in nondiabetic patients, in those with autoimmune disease, or in healthy subjects. Recurrence may be seen in up to a quarter of cases [52]. Up to 39 % had an ultrasound appearance of malignancy in one series [52]. Fibrous mastopathy may simulate breast carcinoma on clinical examination, mammography, and ultrasound [53].

Radial Scars

Radial scar of the breast is a benign lesion that mimics a cancer on mammography, sonography, and histologically. There are two types of radial scars that one needs to be aware of: incidental microscopic radial scars that are encountered in breast biopsy specimens and the macroscopic ones identified at imaging. The latter when less than 1 cm are referred to as radial scars and when greater than 1 cm is called complex sclerosing lesions. These larger lesions carry a risk of coexisting carcinoma and can be histologically difficult to distinguish from tubular carcinoma. The incidental microscopic

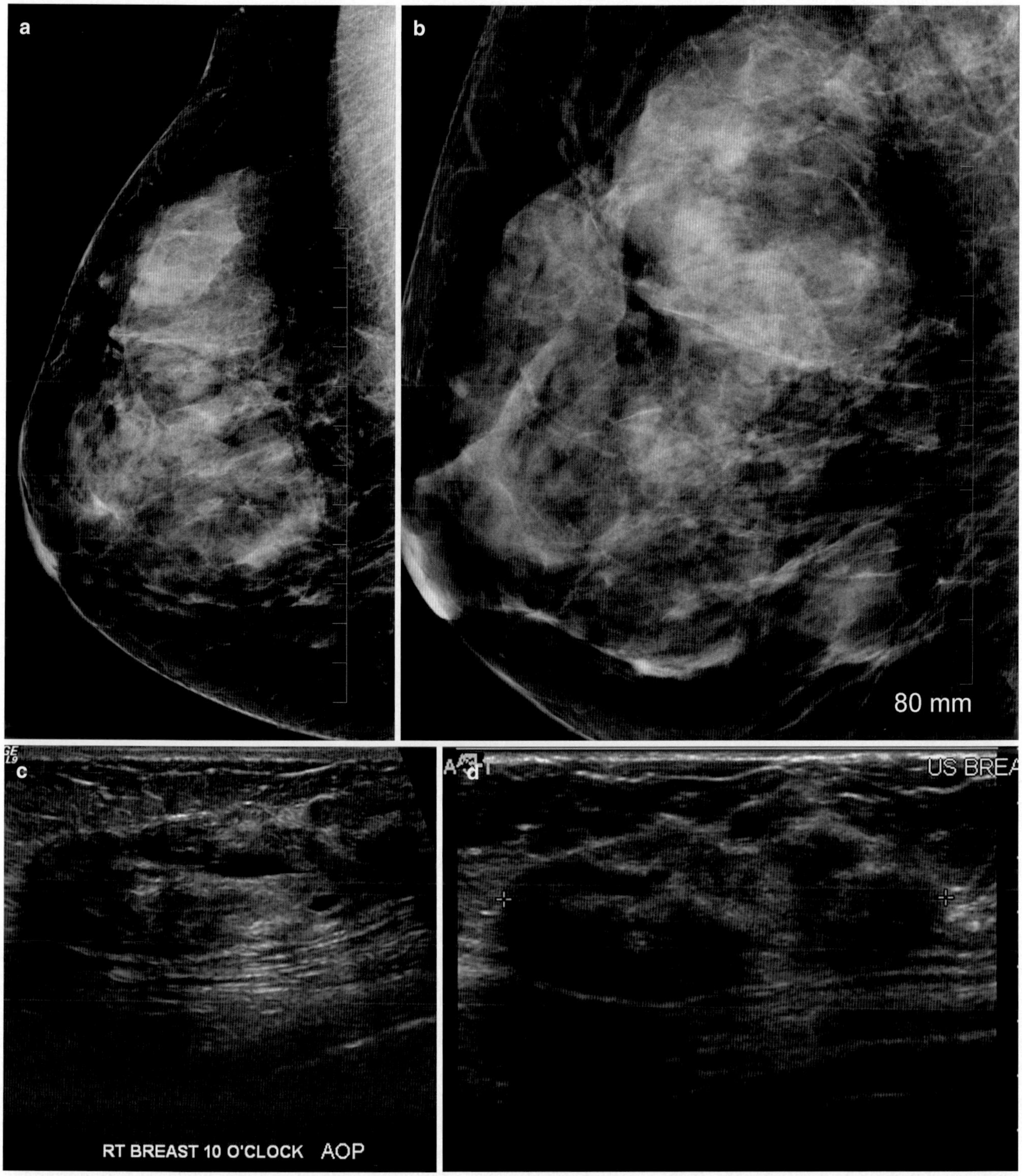

Fig. 13.4 A 53-year-old woman with a palpable mass in the right breast histologically proven to be PASH. (**a**) Mediolateral oblique view with spot compression shows a large focal asymmetry in the upper posterior part of the right breast. (**b**) Craniocaudal view demonstrates the focal asymmetry in the outer breast. (**c**, **d**) Ultrasound demonstrates an ovoid mass with heterogeneous echotexture and ill-defined margins

radial scars do not carry an increased risk for associated breast cancer [54]. Radial scars are histologically characterized by the presence of a central fibroelastic core containing entrapped glandular elements and radiating ductal elements that gives the lesion a characteristic stellate appearance. Radial scars due to presence of entrapped glands in the central portion can mimic tubular carcinoma; however, they can be differentiated by special stains that identify myoepithelial

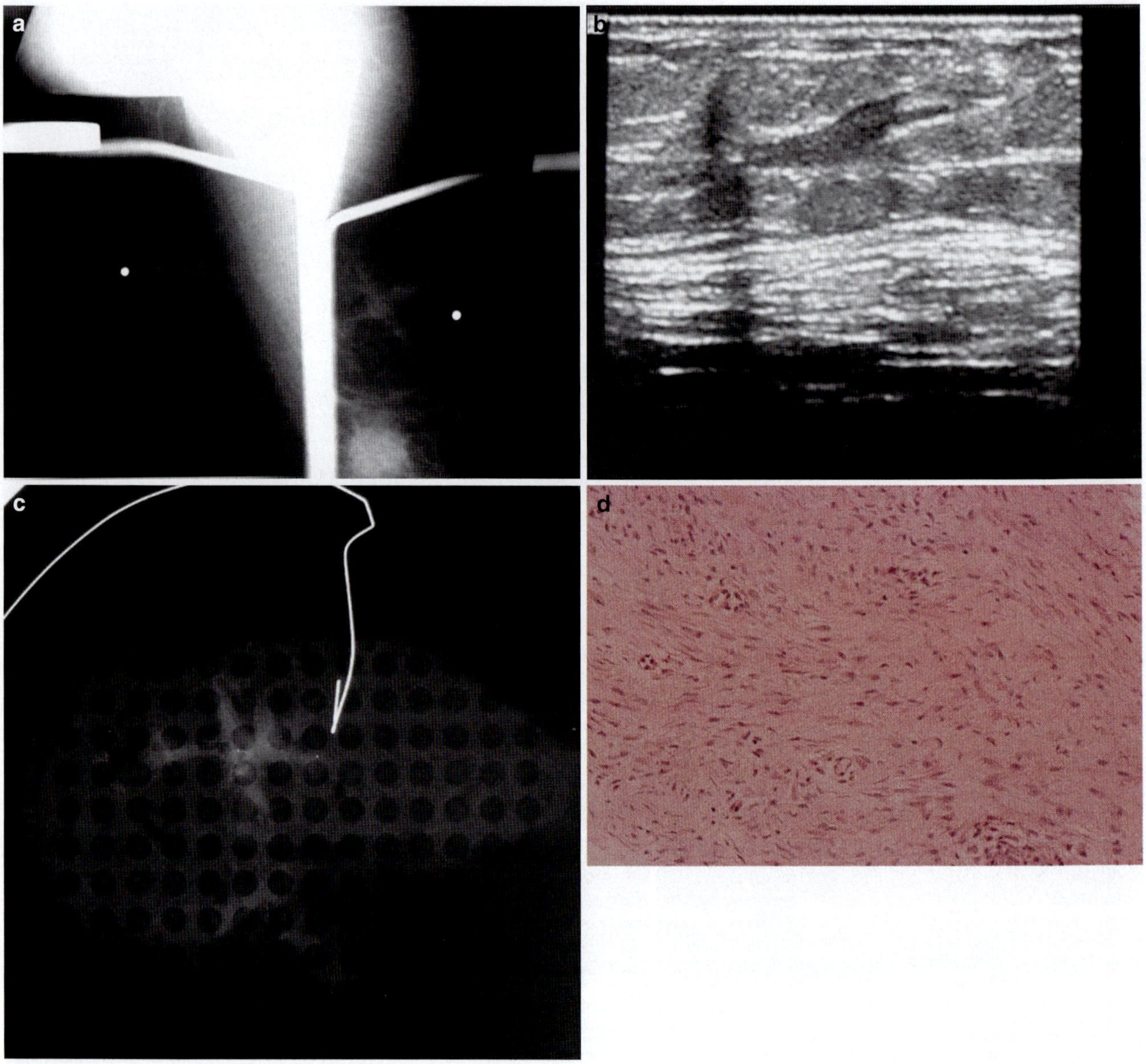

Fig. 13.5 A 46-year old with a palpable lump in left breast. Excisional biopsy revealed mammary fibromatosis (desmoid tumor). (**a**) Spot compression magnification views show an irregular mass. (**b**) Ultrasound demonstrates a hypoechoic solid mass with a branching pattern. (**c**) Specimen radiograph demonstrates the dense irregular mass. (**d**) Hematoxylin and eosinophil staining showing interlacing bundles of spindle cells characteristic of a desmoid tumor

cells in radial scars [55]. An association of radial scar with breast cancer has been reported in 32–46 % of cases, being higher in symptomatic cases [54, 56]. In the screen-detected group, association with breast cancer has been reported in 8 % of cases. There have been no differences in the rate of associated cancers between radial scars and complex sclerosing lesions [56].

Radial scars of the breast are benign lesions that are usually detected incidentally on screening mammography and are difficult to distinguish from breast cancer on mammography. The typical mammographic appearance of radial scars of the breast has been described as showing an absence of a central opacity often substituted by a radiolucent area, presence of multiple, elongated, thin spicules radiating from the center of the lesion, varying appearance in different projections, and absence of a palpable abnormality (Fig. 13.6a, b). Although reported in up to 28 % of benign breast biopsy specimens, they are much less frequently identified on mammograms. A detection rate of three per 1,000 mammograms was reported in one series [57–60]. Because mammographic appearance is suspicious and because of the known risk of coexisting breast cancer, excisional biopsy is indicated even

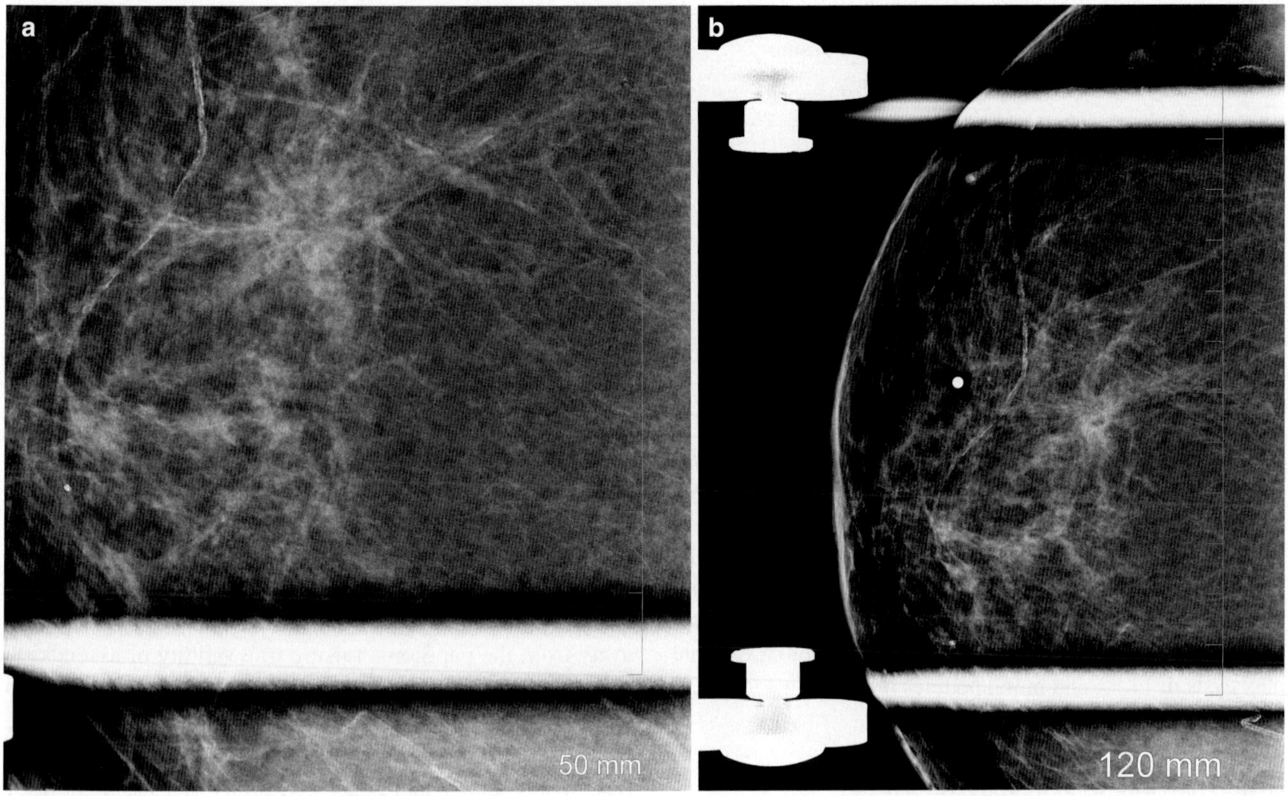

Fig. 13.6 A 57-year-old woman with a histologically proven radial scar in her right breast. (**a**) Spot compression mediolateral oblique view demonstrates an area of distortion and spicules radiating from an area of decreased density. (**b**) Spot compression craniocaudal view demonstrates an area of distortion and spicules radiating from an area of decreased density

when the mammographic appearance is suggestive of a radial scar [54–56].

Sonography is generally considered to have no role in the imaging of lesions mammographically suggestive of a radial scar. However, there have been reports of its value particularly when seen only one view and for guidance of biopsy [57]. On ultrasound a radial scar can have an appearance that is highly suggestive of malignancy or appear as round solid masses or area of shadowing without a focal mass [57]. The incidence of incidental microscopic radial scars in benign breast biopsy specimens has been reported to be 7.1 % [99/1,396] and had a median size of 4 mm [61].

Fat Necrosis

Fat necrosis in the breast is a benign condition that results most commonly as a consequence of iatrogenic trauma to the breast tissue as a result of percutaneous biopsy or breast surgical procedures and uncommonly secondary to anticoagulant therapy or collagen vascular diseases [62]. It may be palpable or incidentally identified on screening mammogram. Fat necrosis can mimic cancer on imaging studies. Histologically it is characterized by destruction of fat cells with hemorrhage and development of vacuoles filled with necrotic lipid material that leads to an inflammatory cell infiltrate with histiocytes that phagocytose necrotic debris within these vacuoles [62–64]. During the next phase of repair fibroblasts proliferate at the periphery of the lesion thereby surrounding areas of fat and necrotic debris. During this phase characteristic calcifications appear. At mammography the spectrum of appearance ranges from the commonly encountered oil cyst that appears as a radiolucent mass that can be confidently categorized as a benign finding to a mass with spiculated borders which in the absence of an area of radiolucency may appear as a suspicious mammographic finding. Presence of coarse dystrophic calcifications are common and can be characterized as benign; however, not uncommonly one may see amorphous or pleomorphic calcifications that may lead to a biopsy recommendation. Ultrasound appearance on the other hand is more often indeterminate and in the absence of correlation with a more frequently associated characterized benign features on mammography may prompt a biopsy.

On ultrasound one may find a sharply demarcated anechoic mass without posterior acoustic enhancement or even posterior acoustic shadowing, an irregular mass with a spiculated border, a complex cystic mass, or an oval or round indeterminate solid mass. The intracystic contents may represent hemorrhage or necrosis and spiculated borders may

Box 13.1. Histology at Core Needle Biopsy Where Excisional Biopsy Is Generally Indicated

Atypical ductal hyperplasia
Papillary lesions
Radial scars
Flat epithelial atypia
Atypical lobular Hyperplasia
Mucocele-like lesions of the breast
Lobular carcinoma in situ

represent the phase of fibrosis. Less than 2 % of breast biopsies result in a diagnosis of fat necrosis at excisional biopsy [64]. About 27 % of fat necrosis appears as a radiolucent oil cyst; about 12 % appear as a round mass; focal asymmetry has been reported in 16 % of cases. Suspicious findings such as pleomorphic calcifications are seen in less than 4 % of cases. Ultrasound shows solid masses in about 14 % of cases, complex cysts in 11 %, and mural nodules in less than 4 % [65].

High-Risk Lesions: Excisional Biopsy Following CNB

These are lesions that carry a risk of associated cancer that may be underestimated on percutaneous core needle biopsy and hence are managed with excisional biopsy [66, 67] (Box 13.1). In this group we have the radial scar, atypical ductal hyperplasia, benign papilloma, lobular neoplasia, flat epithelial atypia, and mucocele-like lesion. Most of the studies that have examined the risk of an upgrade to malignancy have design flaws which make it difficult to draw conclusions on the real risks [66]. These limitations include lack of data on follow-up of all lesions that are not surgically excised or inclusion of cases with imaging pathological discordance [66]. These are retrospective studies that are also limited by the small number of cases studied since these high-risk lesions are small in number and statistical significance is hard to establish [66].

Radial Scars

Due to the risk of missing an associated cancer and the difficulty in distinguishing it from a tubular cancer, all cases of radial scar found on percutaneous biopsy are generally recommended to undergo excisional biopsy. The rate of associated cancer is between 5 and 9 % with a lower rate when larger 11-g needle samples are obtained [68, 69]. This rate is not reduced in radial scars without atypia, and hence irrespective of associated atypia, all radial scars diagnosed at CNB are recommended to undergo surgical excisional biopsy [69]. When atypia is associated with a radial scar, the risk of associated cancer is significantly increased and can be as high as 28 % [55]. This increased risk of cancer, however, does not apply to incidentally identified microscopic foci of radial scars or papillomas that are encountered in otherwise benign histology [70]. In such cases routine imaging follow-up is advised. Becker and others reported no risk of missing an associated cancer using an 11-g vacuum assisted but had a clearly unacceptable number of samples of 32 per lesion [71]. When a 14-g needle was used, the upgrade to cancer was reported in 8 % of lesions [71].

Papilloma

Following a diagnosis of a papilloma on a core needle biopsy, an upgrade to cancer has been reported to vary from 9 to 19% [72–75]. In one series all cases of cancers were identified either as interval enlargement on follow-up or development of symptoms; no cancers were seen in asymptomatic patients or in those with stable findings at follow-up [72]. In some of these studies, cancers were found near a papilloma with a study reporting subsequent of a cancer that was even 3 cm away from the papilloma raising true validity of association with a cancer [75]. One large series of 120 cases showed no cancer at excisional biopsy or on follow-up [73]. Size of the lesion has also been suggested as helpful factor in assessing risk of associated malignancy. Lesions that are 1.4 cm or greater have been shown to have a higher risk of cancer, whereas benign papillomas had a mean size of 0.9 cm (Fig. 13.7a–e). Lesions in the periphery of the breast also had a higher risk of malignancy [76, 77].

Lobular Neoplasia

Atypical lobular neoplasia and lobular carcinoma in situ carry an elevated risk for association with malignancy with LCIS having a stronger association. Atypical lobular hyperplasia is when less than 50 % of the acinar units in a lobule are distended with lobular neoplastic cells. Distension requires at least eight cells within an individual acinar unit. Reported incidence of an upgrade to malignancy in lobular neoplasia varies from as low as 1 % [78] to as high as 23 % [79]. LCIS can present as masses or calcifications [66]. One large series of 278 cases reported an upgrade to malignancy in 25 % of cases of LCIS and 22 % of ALH [78]. The overestimation of the risk of malignancy missed on a core needle biopsy in some of these series happens since cases with imaging pathological discordance or those pleomorphic or nonclassic forms of LCIS are included in the study group. In a study of LCIS upgraded to malignancy, with 9 cases of LCIS, six were in imaging pathological discordance and three included pleomorphic variant of LCIS for which surgical treatment similar to DCIS is routinely recommended [78]. Based on these findings there may not be a real justification in recommending excisional biopsy for classic forms of lobular neoplasia where there is no imaging pathological concordance. Instead imaging and clinical follow-up alone may be appropriate [78].

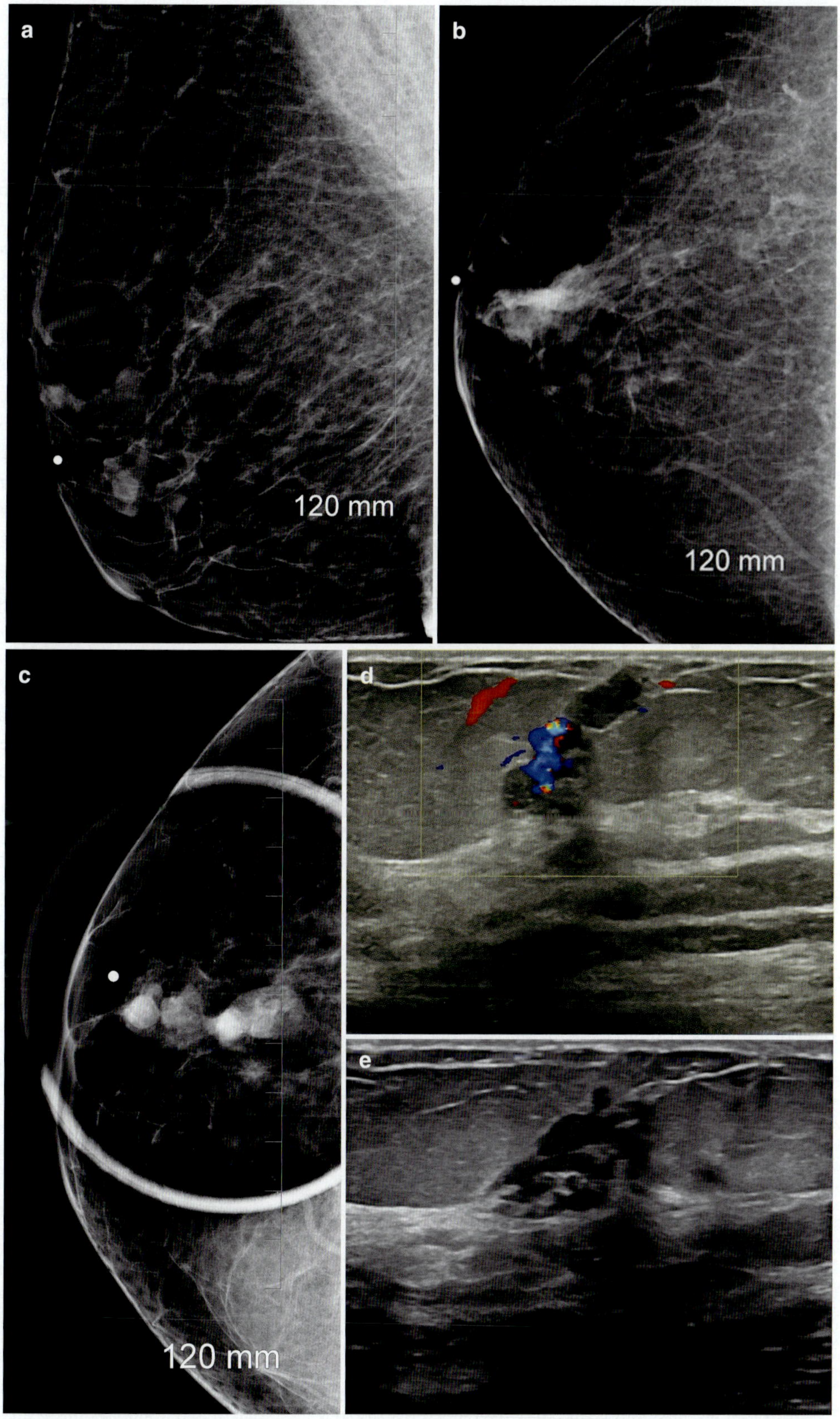

Fig. 13.7 A 67-year-old woman with a history of spontaneous bloody right nipple discharge with histologically proven papilloma associated with DCIS. (**a**) Mediolateral oblique view shows a retroareolar irregular tubular density. (**b**) Craniocaudal view shows a retroareolar irregular tubular density. (**c**) Spot compression craniocaudal view shows a high-density retroareolar irregular tubular density. (**d**) Ultrasound demonstrates an irregular intraductal mass with prominent internal vascularity. (**e**) Ultrasound demonstrates an irregular intraductal mass with a branching pattern

Flat Epithelial Atypia

Flat epithelial atypia or columnar cell change with atypia refers to presence of cystically dilated ducts that are lined by one to several layers of monomorphic but enlarged round to oval cells with low-grade cytologic atypia. Unlike that seen in ADH or DCIS, micropapillary or cribriform growth patterns are not observed in flat epithelial atypia [66]. Reported rate of DCIS and invasive cancer in flat epithelial atypia on excisional biopsy is 6–17 % [80, 81]. Mammographic microcalcifications are the most common underlying finding reported in 69 % of cases in one series followed by ultrasound finding of a hypoechoic mass in 25 % [80]. The mean size of the abnormality was 8 mm. A systematic review of 24 studies determined that the underestimation risk of DCIS in columnar cell change without atypia was 1.5 %, with atypia was 9 %, and with atypical hyperplasia was 20 %. Based on these findings it has been recommended that all cases of CCC with atypia or atypical hyperplasia undergo open surgical biopsy and lesions that demonstrate CCC without atypia can be followed [82].

Imaging Pathological Discordance

Ultrasound- and stereotactic-guided minimally invasive procedure to biopsy abnormalities in the breast has been established alternative to open surgical biopsy [83, 84]. Up to 96 % of cancers are diagnosed at initial US-guided biopsy [83]. Reasons for failed biopsy include sampling error, failure to recognize imaging pathological discordance, and lack of follow-up after benign biopsy results [83]. A large series of 1,352 cases reported a false-negative rate of 1.6 % for lesions undergoing US-guided core biopsy using a 14-g needle [84]. Imaging pathological correlation can have five different outcomes [85]. These are concordant malignancy, discordant benignity, discordant malignancy, discordant benignity, and high-risk lesions:

- In concordant malignancy a lesion that was suspicious on imaging is malignant. Prompt communication to the referring clinician and the breast imager performing the biopsy or the referring clinician should contact the patient and arrange a referral to an oncologist or a breast surgeon.
- In case of discordant malignancy, a lesion with benign imaging features results in a malignant histology; this should lead to management protocol as in the earlier scenario with the added step of careful review of the imaging findings as a second look to seek morphological features that may have suggested malignancy such as areas of ill-defined borders that were initially missed or associated features that are suspicious and may have been overlooked.
- Concordant benignity is when a lesion considered benign is proven benign histologically. Verbal and or written communication with the referring clinician is adequate with a mechanism in place to confirm receipt of the results and proper notification of the patient with recommendation for follow-up.
- Discordant benignity is when lesions are categorized as BI-RADS™ 5 or otherwise considered as suspicious for malignancy but result in nonspecific diagnosis such as benign breast tissue or fibrocystic change. There are few benign lesions that may appear probably malignant but are benign such as the desmoid tumor, fat necrosis, diabetic mastopathy, stromal fibrosis, or radial scar. However, it is safe practice to recommend excisional biopsy on all discordant benignity.

The rate of malignancy in discordant cases has been reported to be between 6.8 and 17.6 % [86–88]. The rate of malignancy in the concordant group has been reported to be low and around 0.4 % [88]. In the discordant group the upgrade was statistically significant for larger masses, in symptomatic cases, and those with a higher BI-RADS™ assessment [86–88]. In the concordant upgrade group, lesion size and symptoms were significant but not the BI-RADS™ assessment [88].

Special Histological Types of Breast Cancer

Heterogeneity of breast cancer is well recognized; about 25 % of invasive breast cancers are of special histological types [89]. Invasive ductal cancer of no special type or not otherwise specified constitutes 60–75 % of all breast cancers and is diagnosed by exclusion which is one that does not fit any special histological type [90]. At least 17 distinct entities are recognized [91]. There are also several interesting phenotypic-genotypic correlations described within this group of special tumor types; a detailed discussion on this is beyond the scope of this chapter but is described by Weigelt et al. [89]. The imaging features of the following special types are discussed here: secretory carcinoma, papillary carcinoma, mucinous carcinoma, medullary carcinoma, and tubular carcinoma. Invasive lobular cancer is discussed in the chapter on mammographic signs of malignancy (Chap. 5).

Secretory Carcinoma

Secretory carcinoma was formerly known as juvenile breast cancer and was renamed since it can occur in a wide range of age group (11–86 years). This very rare form of cancer presents at an early stage and has an indolent course. Only 120 cases have been reported in the literature [92]. The diagnosis of secretory carcinoma is made by the characteristic microscopic appearance of the tumor, with cells containing vacuolated cytoplasm and abundant intra- and extracellular secretory material. Imaging features in small series have been described and is nonspecific; lesions may be palpable or screen detected. Most commonly ultrasound demonstrates circumscribed round or oval mass either as a single nodule or multiple nodules [93].

Tubular Carcinoma

Tubular carcinomas are frequently diagnosed when small, frequently diagnosed in a younger population and have a favorable prognosis with a lower incidence of axillary metastasis. These types of cancers are rare and account for less than 2 % of breast cancers. Tubular carcinoma of the breast is a specific type of Infiltrating carcinoma that is characterized histologically by the presence of 75 % tubular structures that are lined by well-differentiated epithelial cells. The pure type is one where there are more than 90 % tubular elements and a mixed type is where there are 50–90 % tubular elements. Imaging appearances of tubular carcinoma of the breast has been reported [94–99]. Tubular carcinomas frequently appear as irregular masses with spiculated margins on mammography and are commonly visible on ultrasound as hypoechoic masses with ill-defined borders and posterior acoustic shadowing [94] (Fig. 13.8a–g). Majority are palpable [59–85 %] and appear as masses [72 %] [95, 96]. The pure type has a better prognosis and is more likely to be mammographically occult and tends to be oval shaped, whereas the mixed type is more likely to be irregular in shape and have posterior acoustic shadowing on ultrasound [97].

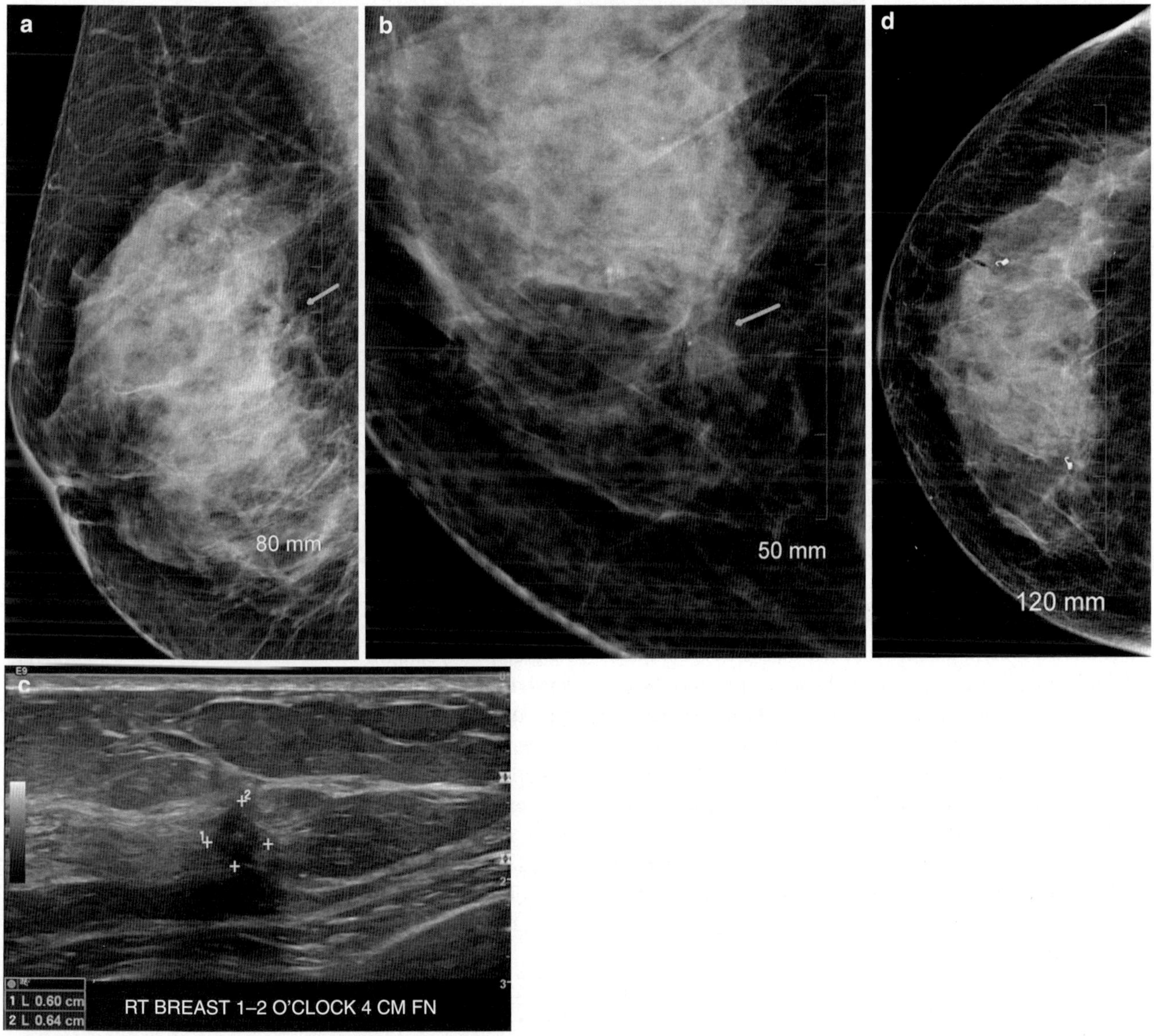

Fig. 13.8 A 46-year-old woman with histologically proven tubular cancer in the right breast. (**a**) Mediolateral oblique view demonstrates a subtle spiculated mass and distortion at the 1–2 o'clock position. (**b**) Craniocaudal view demonstrates a subtle spiculated mass and distortion at the 1–2 o'clock position associated with calcifications. (**c**) Ultrasound demonstrates an irregular small mass. (**d**) Postbiopsy craniocaudal view with a tissue marker in place. The second tissue marker corresponds to a second cancer that was histologically proven to be an invasive lobular cancer. (**e**) Postbiopsy mediolateral view with a tissue marker in place. The second tissue marker corresponds to a second cancer that was histologically proven to be an invasive lobular cancer. (**f**, **g**) Histology demonstrates well-defined glands with round, oval, or angulated contours, open lumina, absence of myoepithelial cell layer, and absence of necrosis or mitoses. *Arrow* indicates the mass described

Fig. 13.8 (continued)

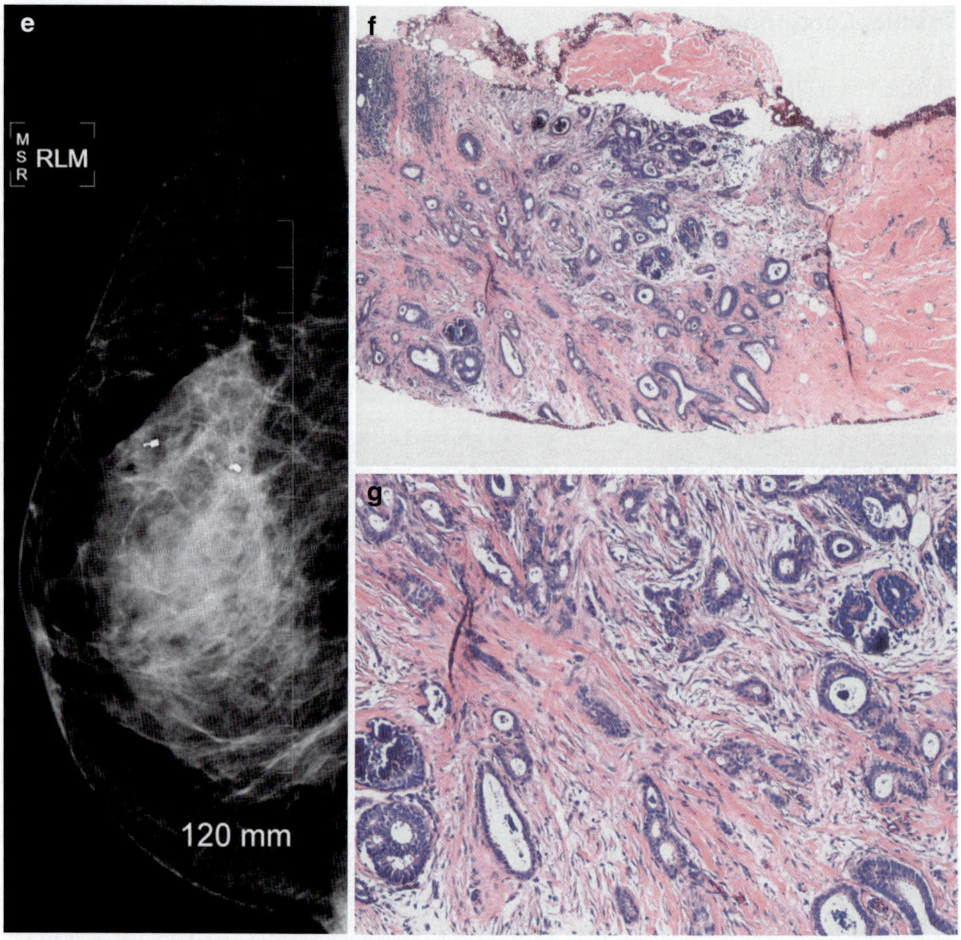

Mucinous Carcinoma

Pure mucinous breast carcinoma is rare, occurs in older women, and is known to have a better short-term prognosis compared with infiltrating ductal cancer. It rarely presents with nodal disease and when it does it is the single significant predictor of poor prognosis. It represents about 1–4 % of breast cancer cases [100]. A large retrospective series of over 11,000 cases showed a 5-year survival rate of 94 %. The favorable outcome is maintained after 20 years; 10-, 15-, and 20-year survival rates were 89, 85, and 81 % compared to 72, 66, and 62 % for IDC [100]. Histologically there are two types, the pure type and the mixed type. Imaging features of mucinous carcinoma of the breast have been reported [101–103]. Not all mucinous carcinomas are mammographically visible; in one series 21 % were not seen on a mammogram [101]. The most common mammographic appearance is that of a circumscribed or microlobulated mass particularly in the pure mucinous type; in the mixed type the margins are ill defined or spiculated [101, 102]. At sonography the pure type of mucinous cancer is isoechoic, with posterior acoustic enhancement in a majority of cases, 63 % in one series [103] (Fig. 13.9a–e). Mixed cystic and solid components and microlobulated borders have also been described [101]. Internal echotexture tends to be homogenous in the pure type of mucinous carcinoma and hypoechogenic in the mixed type [101, 102].

Fig. 13.9 A 39-year-old with two palpable masses in right breast both of which were histologically proven to be mucinous carcinoma. (**a**) Spot compression mediolateral oblique view of the right breast demonstrates an ill-defined focal asymmetry in upper breast corresponding to one of the palpable lumps. (**b**) Spot compression mediolateral oblique view of the right breast demonstrates an ill-defined focal asymmetry adjacent and slightly posterior and corresponding to the second area palpable abnormality. (**c**) Ultrasound demonstrates an ill-defined hyperechoic mass. (**d**) Ultrasound demonstrates the second palpable lump to be a round heterogenous mass with posterior acoustic enhancement. (**e**) Irregular nests and clusters of tumor cells are surrounded by pools of extracellular mucin

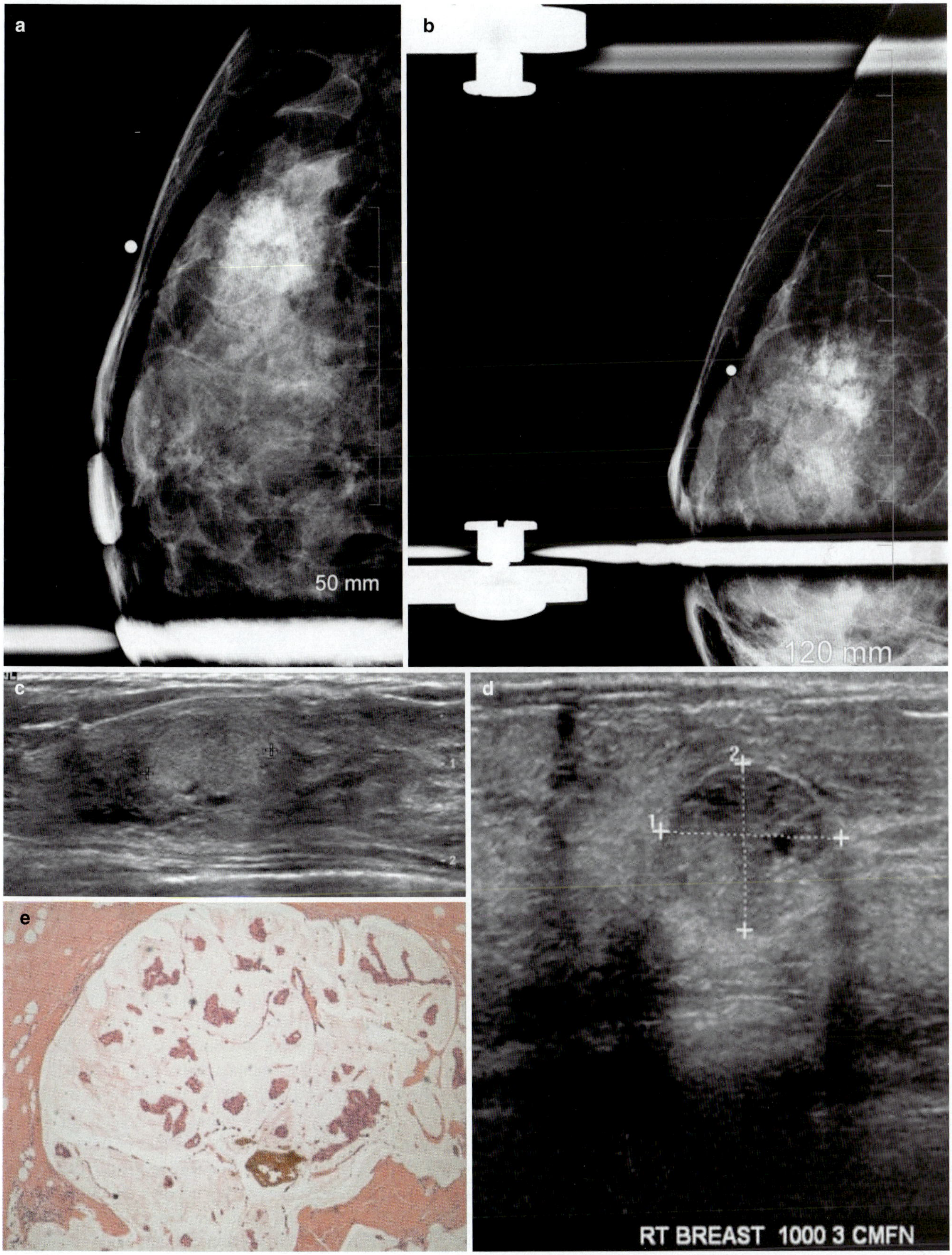
a
b
50 mm
120 mm
c
d
e
RT BREAST 1000 3 CMFN

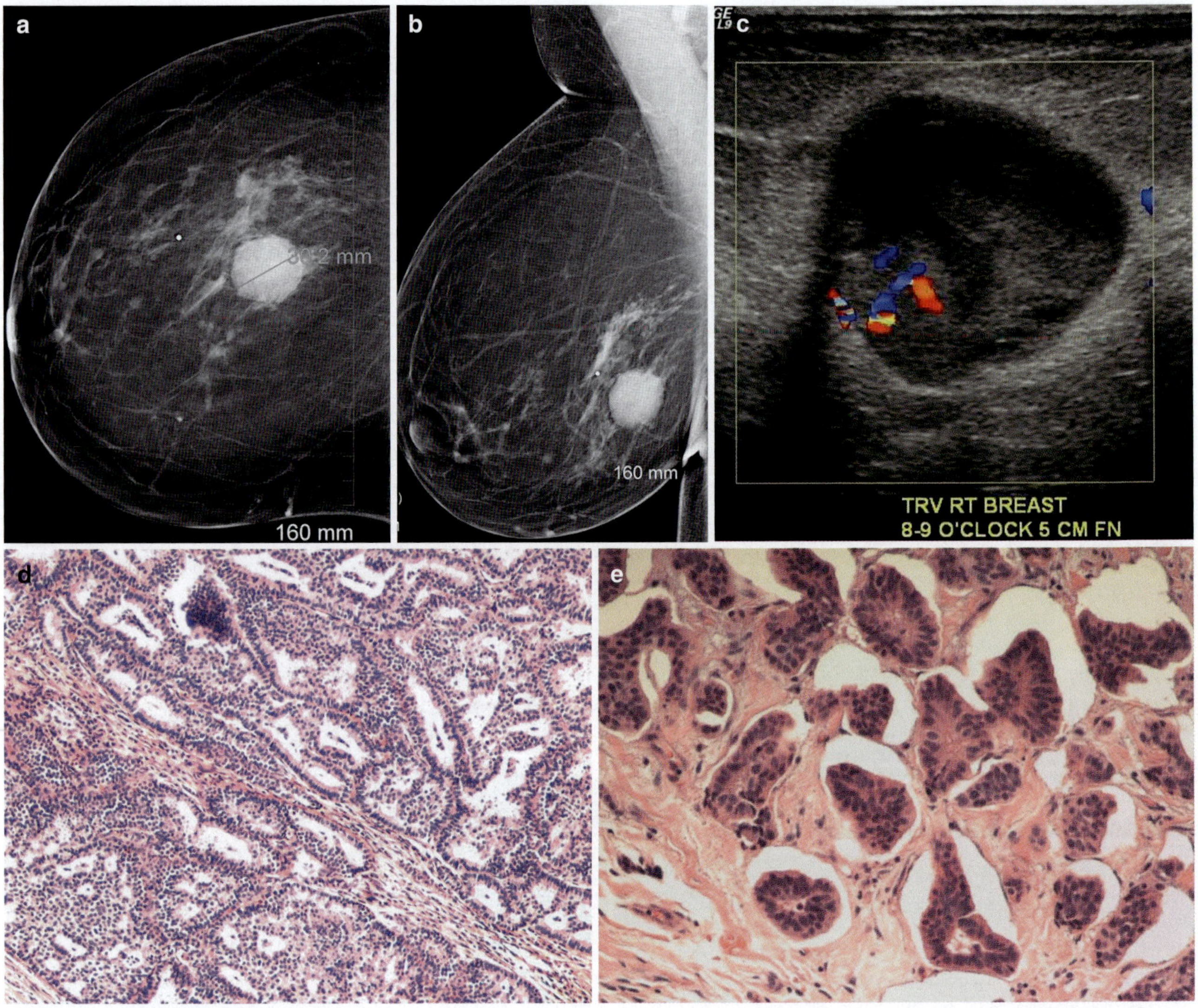

Fig. 13.10 A 50-year-old woman with a painful palpable lump in the right breast. This was histologically proven to be a low-grade invasive papillary cancer. (**a**) Craniocaudal view demonstrates a round dense mass with circumscribed borders. (**b**) Mediolateral view demonstrates a round dense mass with circumscribed borders. (**c**) Ultrasound demonstrates a complex cystic mass with vascular mural nodules. (**d**) Proliferating epithelial cells assume cribriform and micropapillary patterns. (**e**) Epithelial cells display round to oval and hyperchromatic nuclei, some of which exhibit distinct nucleoli

Papillary Cancer

This constitutes about 2–5 % of all breast cancers and is more frequently found in older premenopausal women; bloody nipple discharge is a common presenting clinical feature that has been reported in 22–34 % of cases. There are two types: intraductal papillary cancer or, when a large cystic component is associated, intracystic papillary cancer. Additional classification is based on whether invasive carcinoma is present or not; these invasive components are often at the periphery of these lesions and are at risk of being missed on core biopsies that may target and/or sample the center of a lesion. Invasive papillary carcinoma of the breast accounts for about 0.5–2 % of breast cancer [104–109]. Intracystic papillary cancer is rare, and although literature quotes an incidence of 1–2 % of all breast carcinomas, it is rare occurrence in routine clinical practice and there are mostly single or small case series reports only. These tumors arise within dilated ducts and are called intracystic due to focal dilatation of ducts that simulates a breast cyst with a mural nodule (Fig. 13.10a–e). Tumor may be unifocal or multifocal, it may be in a pure form or be associated with DCIS or invasive cancer. It usually occurs in older women with an average age of onset of 69.5 years [27–99 years]. Clinically it may be asymptomatic or present as an enlarging mass or with a bloody nipple discharge [104, 105]. Histologically there is seen to be proliferation of cells arranged around fibrovascular cores grossly forming circumscribed mass seen on a mammogram as an isodense or hyperdense mass and as a complex cystic mass or a cyst with an intracystic mass. Imaging-identified masses are often subareolar up to 50 % of cases [110]. Presence of indistinct margins may indicate an invasive component. Microcalcifications when seen are pleomorphic and these may indicate not only DCIS but also infarction, fibrosis, or hemorrhage [111]. Papillary cancers on ultrasound may appear as hypoechoic solid masses or a complex cyst with septations or intracystic masses; anechoic areas may represent exuded fluid or hemorrhage. Doppler imaging often shows internal vascularity or feeding vessels [111].

Medullary Carcinoma of the Breast

Medullary carcinomas constitute about 3–5 % of all cancers and are characterized by prominent syncytial growth, circumscribed borders, and a diffuse lymphoid infiltrate and an absence of intraductal component or microglandular features [112]. Survival rate is significantly better than in infiltrating ductal cancer and a 10-year survival rate of 84 % has been reported. In a series of 3,348 cases, advancing age, black race, regional metastasis, distant metastasis, and increasing tumor size and number of lymph node metastasis were associated with decreased survival, and PR-positive patients had a better survival rate [113]. Medullary carcinoma accounts for 11 % of breast carcinomas in women younger than 35 years [114]. The mammographic and sonographic features have been reported [115–117]. Due to increased prevalence in younger women and its imaging appearance, it can be mistaken for a fibroadenoma; medullary cancers tend to be larger than fibroadenoma and have more frequently a round or lobular shape with focally thick walls and anechoic cystic spaces within, a finding unusual in a fibroadenoma in nonpregnant women [115]. It has been suggested that imaging helps to distinguish typical histological types from the more atypical types. Medullary carcinomas that have typical histological features tend to have a smooth outline and demonstrate posterior acoustic enhancement. Medullary cancers with atypical histological features demonstrate irregular borders and posterior acoustic shadowing [116]. Others have not found these sonographic features to be helpful although at mammography most of the typical types of medullary cancers exhibited circumscribed borders [117].

Non-masslike Abnormalities on US

The ultrasound BI-RADS™ lexicon describes lesions on ultrasound under three headings of a mass, calcifications, or special cases [118]. It does not describe small clinically occult nonmasses that appear as hypoechoic areas and do not fit the standard description of a mass [119]. These small nonmasses can be of two types ductal or nonductal. Ductal hypoechoic structure can be single or multiple. A nonductal hypoechoic area is a lesion that differs from the surrounding tissue or same area in the contralateral breast. These nonmasslike abnormalities may represent DCIS or invasive lobular cancers.

Unusual Breast Lesions

Breast Metastasis

Breast metastasis from extra-mammary malignancy is rare. Based on the literature an incidence of 0.4–1.3 % is reported [120]. In adults, the most frequent types of tumors metastasizing in the breast are malignant melanoma and neuroendocrine-like tumors, especially small cell carcinoma and carcinoid. In children, rhabdomyosarcoma is the most common [121]. Mammographically metastasis may be seen as single or multiple masses or as diffuse skin thickening, and on ultrasound metastatic lesions tend to be circumscribed with low-level internal echoes. On clinical examination metastasis appears similar to their actual sizes compared to breast cancer which feels larger than its actual size. Metastasis tends to be more frequently bilateral and multiple and is more common in the subcutaneous plane rather than in the glandular tissue.

Primary Breast Lymphoma

Primary breast lymphoma appears as noncalcified circumscribed mass or as an indistinctly marginated mass [122]. Skin thickening may be an associated feature—cell lymphoma is more common than the T-cell lymphoma [122]. Lymphoma of the breast is rare and presents most commonly as a unilateral breast mass that may be tender. Bilaterality occurs in 10 % of cases and in 15 % metachronous lesions are reported [123]. Solitary mass is more common and reported in 69 76 % of cases compared to multiple masses (Fig. 13.11a–e). Global asymmetry has been described in 16 % of cases. On ultrasound a solid mass is seen in majority of cases; these masses are irregular, hypoechoic, and hypervascular with indistinct margins. Posterior acoustic shadowing is unusual. An infiltrative pattern with architectural distortion is seen in those with extensive involvement of the breast (Fig. 13.12a–e).

Metaplastic Carcinoma

Metaplastic carcinoma is a heterogeneous malignancy containing mixed epithelial and mesenchymal differentiation [124]. Metaplastic changes include squamous cell, spindle cell, and heterologous mesenchymal growth. These present as rapidly growing palpable masses in women older than 50 years; axillary metastasis is infrequent [124].

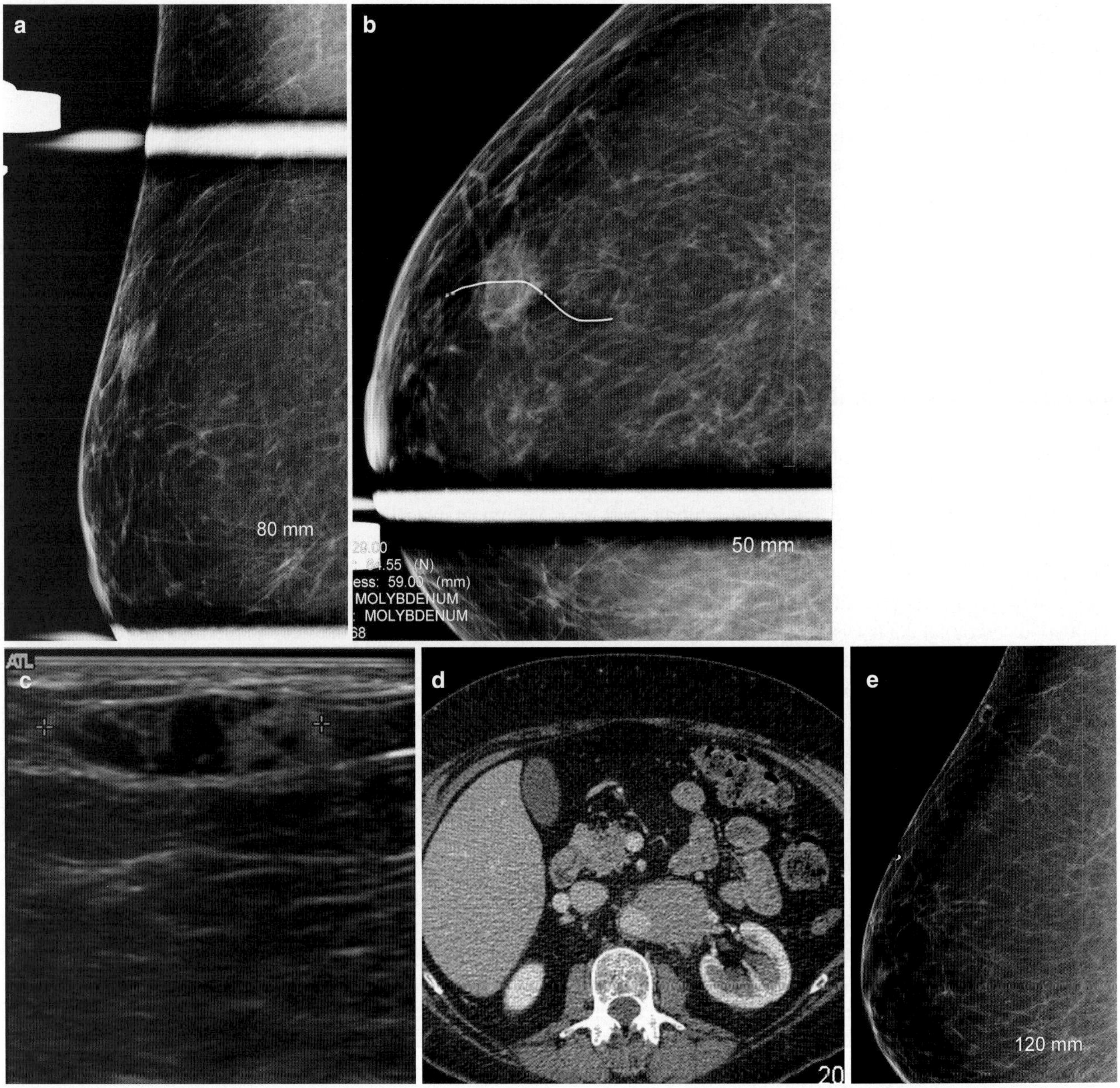

Fig. 13.11 A 38-year-old woman with a palpable lump in the right breast histologically proven to be a breast lymphoma. (**a**) Spot compression mediolateral oblique view demonstrates a focal asymmetry in the anterior upper breast. (**b**) Spot compression craniocaudal view demonstrates a focal asymmetry in the anterior outer breast. (**c**) Ultrasound demonstrates an ill-defined solid mass with cystic changes. (**d**) An axial CT scan through the upper abdomen demonstrates left para-aortic retroperitoneal adenopathy. (**e**) Posttreatment resolution of the breast abnormality. A postbiopsy clip is seen at the site of the mass

Hemangioma of the Breast

Hemangioma of the breast appears as masses smaller than 2 cm, perilobular in location; malignant vascular tumors are more common, of larger size with angiosarcoma being the most common. Histologically dilated blood-filled channels of the capillary or cavernous type are lined by endothelial cells. Mammographically a small circumscribed lobulated mass may be seen. Internal calcifications may result from phleboliths or calcified thrombus. On ultrasound well-defined hypoechoic or hyperechoic masses are seen. Diagnosis of hemangioma on a core needle biopsy need not prompt a recommendation for excisional biopsy [125].

Neurofibromas

Neurofibromas in the breast may uncommonly be seen in Neurofibromatosis type 1 as multiple benign appearing circumscribed masses portions of which may be rimmed with

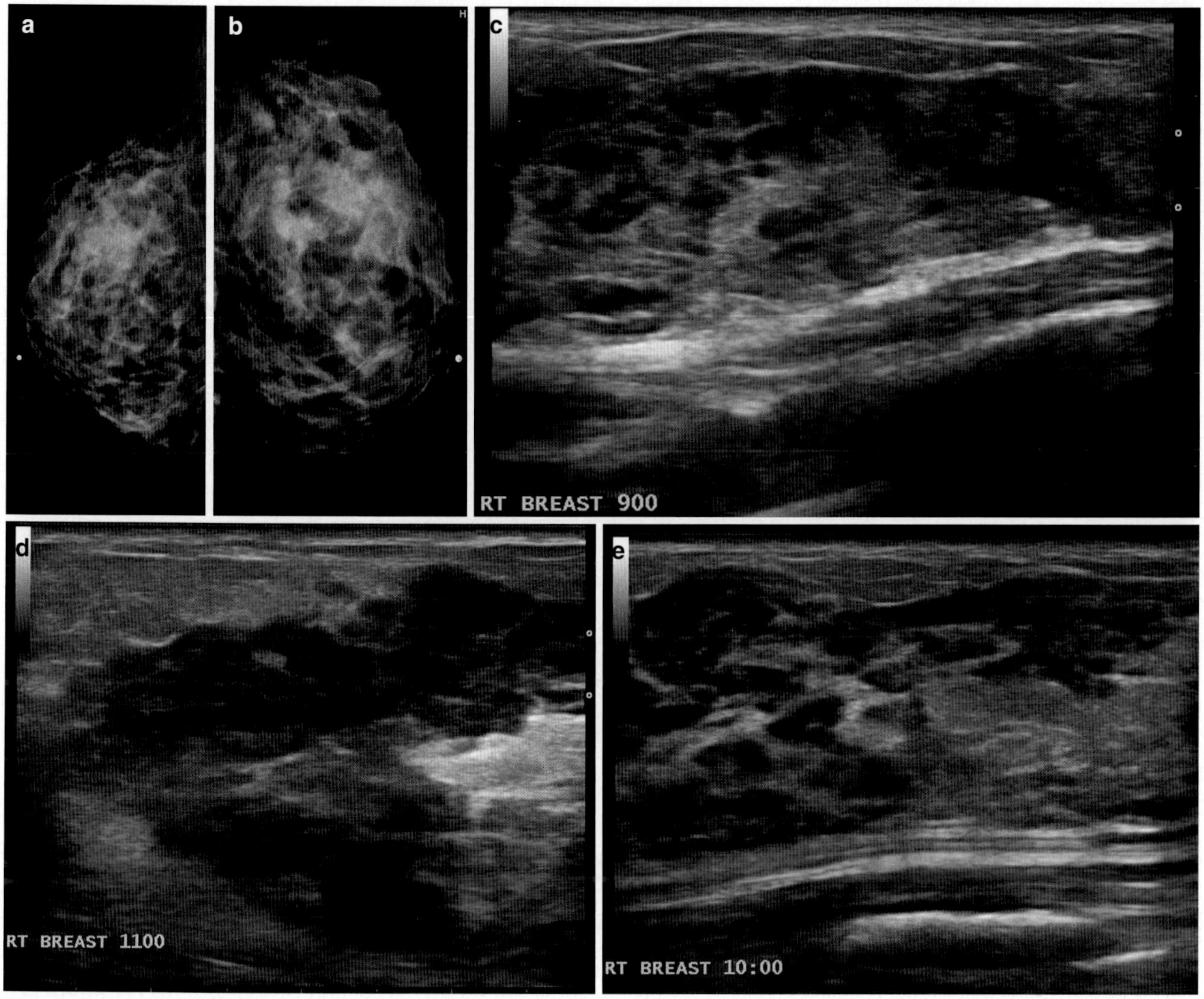

Fig. 13.12 A 43-year-old female with bilateral hard lumps in each breast. Histologically diagnosed to have bilateral breast lymphoma. (**a**) Right breast mediolateral oblique view of a baseline mammogram demonstrates a dense breast parenchymal pattern without a specific mass seen. (**b**) Left breast mediolateral oblique view of a baseline mammogram demonstrates a dense breast parenchymal pattern without a specific mass seen. (**c**–**e**) Right breast ultrasound demonstrates a large ill-defined hypoechoic infiltrative mass

air due to the superficial location. On ultrasound well-defined hypoechoic masses are seen located in the subcutaneous tissue with posterior acoustic enhancement and appear similar to a fibroadenoma [125] (Fig. 13.13a, b).

Mucocele-Like Lesions of the Breasts

Mucocele-like lesions of the breast are uncommon and are characterized by the presence of mucin-filled ducts or cysts with extrusion of the mucin into the surrounding stroma in a core biopsy specimen [126]. Excisional biopsy is indicated especially when there is atypical ductal proliferation. In a small series of ten cases undergoing excisional biopsy, 30 % were malignant [126]. These may present as calcifications on a mammogram or as a mass on ultrasound and may indicate presence of ductal mucinous or invasive mucinous carcinoma.

Angiosarcoma of the Breast

Angiosarcoma of the breast is a rare tumor of the breast that is often seen as a delayed consequence of radiotherapy to the breast in the setting of chronic lymphedema after axillary dissection or as a primary tumor. Presentation is as a palpable mass. Mammographically the tumor is difficult to delineate and appears to be of fat density; on ultrasound a hyperechoic mass is seen; it is likely to be mistaken for a benign lipoma [127, 128] (Fig. 13.14a–f). An enlarging tumor, clinically suspicious should hence be biopsied despite benign appearances on a mammogram and ultrasound. MRI is more accurate in the diagnosis.

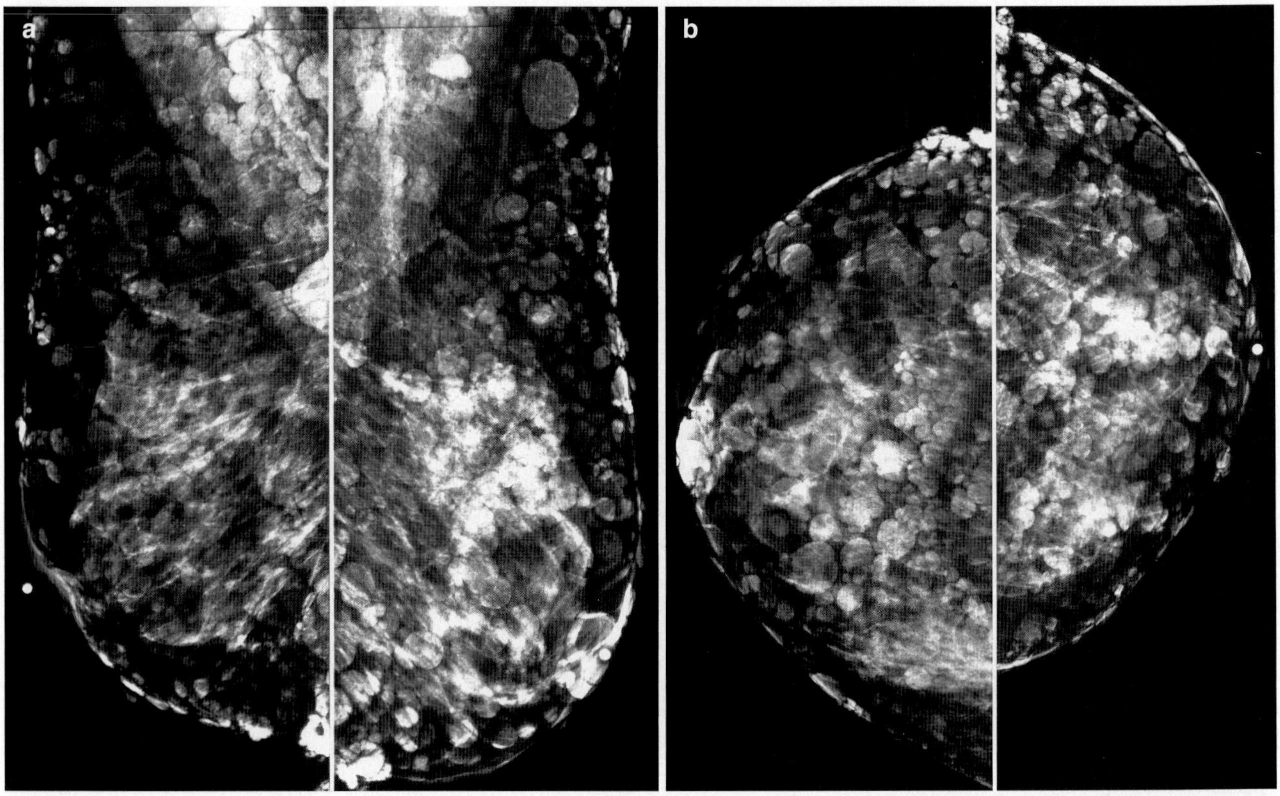

Fig. 13.13 A 47-year-old with history of neurofibromatosis. (**a**) Mediolateral oblique view demonstrates numerous circumscribed subcutaneous masses suggestive of neurofibromas. (**b**) Craniocaudal view demonstrates numerous circumscribed subcutaneous masses suggestive of neurofibromas

Paget's Disease of the Nipple

This is a rare type of cancer that is characterized by the presence of intradermal cancer cells. There is often an underlying DCIS or invasive cancer [129]. Patient presents with eczema and ulceration of the nipple. An underlying cancer has been reported in 79 % of cases prior to surgery. One hundred and seventeen women had noninvasive cancer and 68 women had invasive cancer. Long-term outcome and survival was best in women with noninvasive disease [129] (Fig. 13.15a–e).

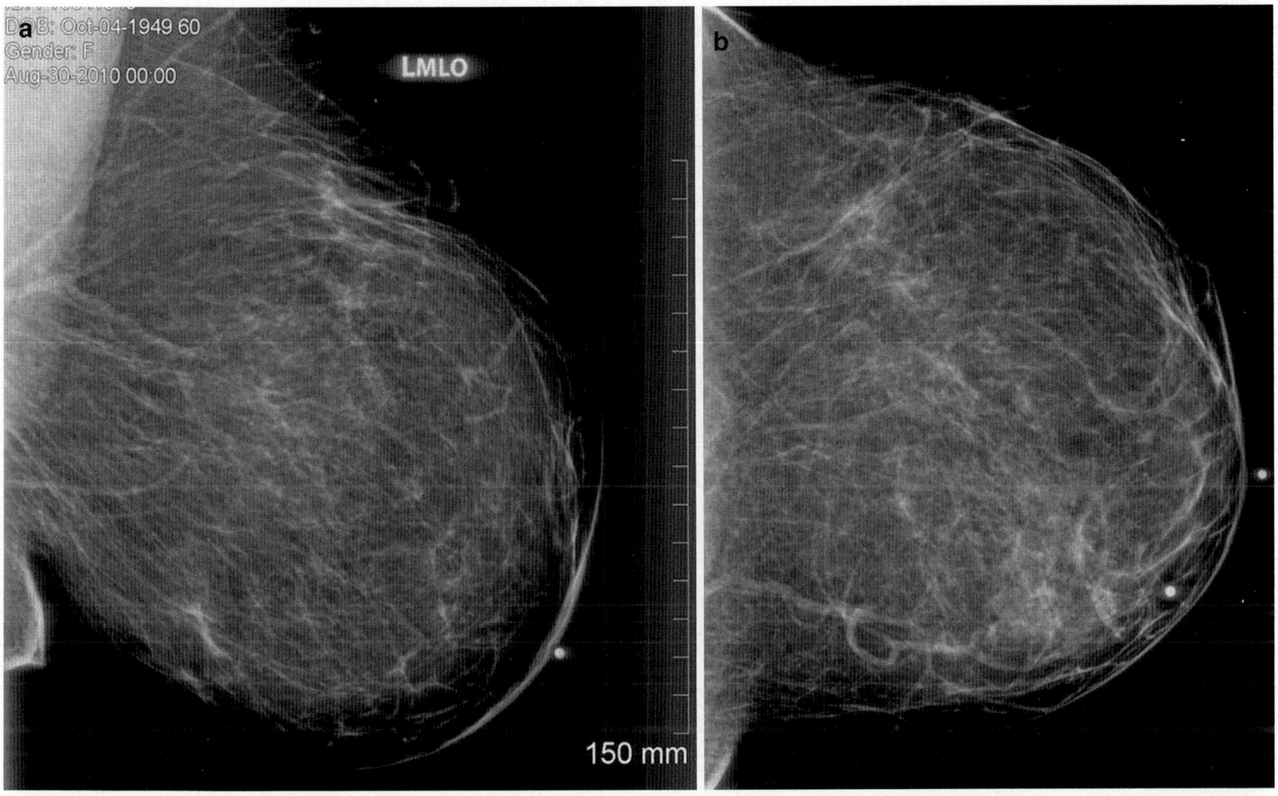

Fig. 13.14 A 60-year-old woman with a large mass in the left breast which at surgical excision proved to be a primary angiosarcoma of the breast Left Mediolateral Oblique view (*LMLO*). (**a**) Mediolateral oblique view of the left breast reveals no discrete mass in a predominantly fat replaced breast. (**b**) Craniocaudal view of the left breast reveals no discrete mass in a predominantly fat replaced breast. (**c**) Ultrasound demonstrates a large hyperechoic mass with ill-defined borders. (**d–f**) Histology slides demonstrates proliferations of atypical vessels that are lined by enlarged hyperchromatic mitotically active nuclei with macronuclei

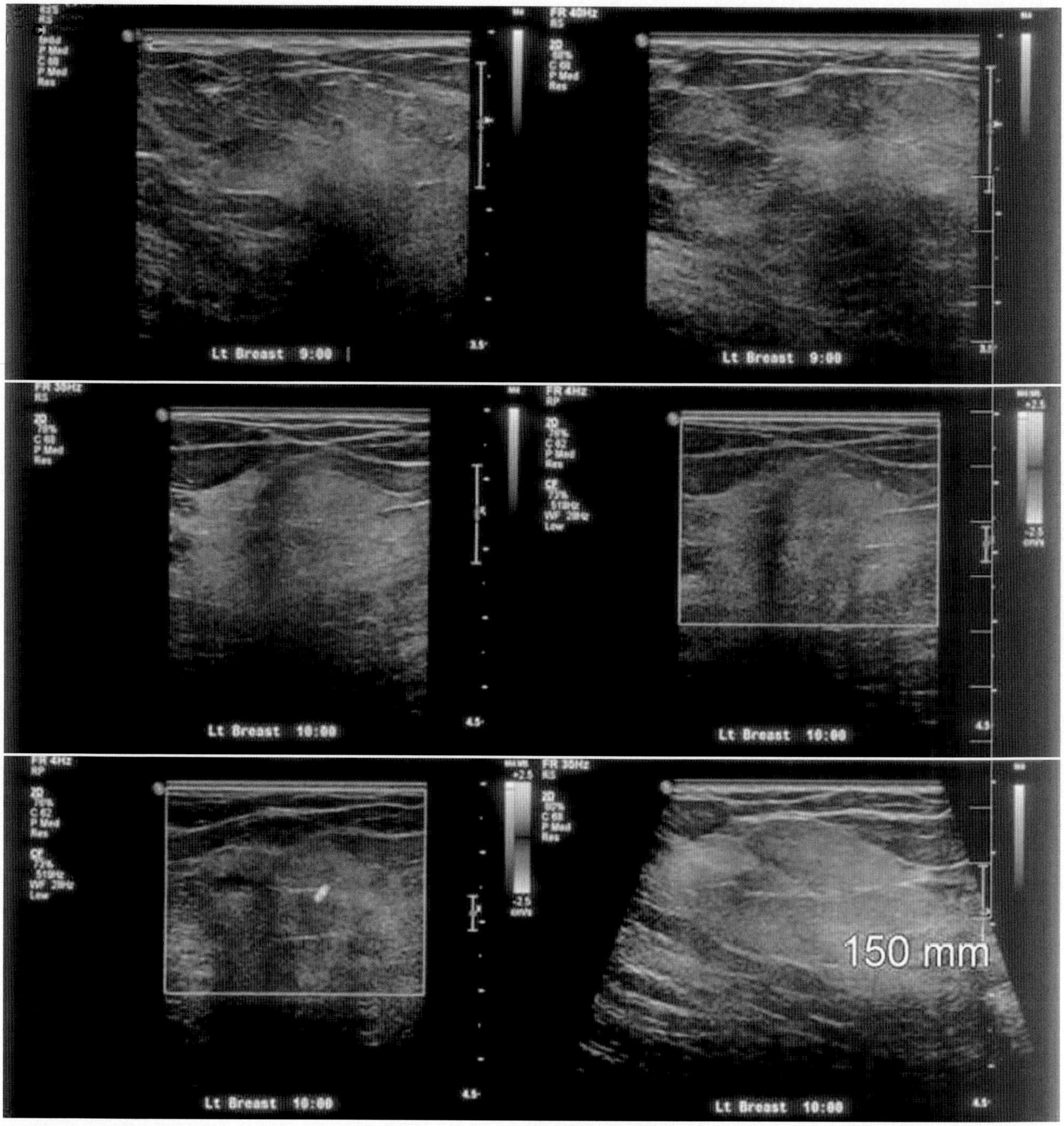

Fig. 13.14 (continued)

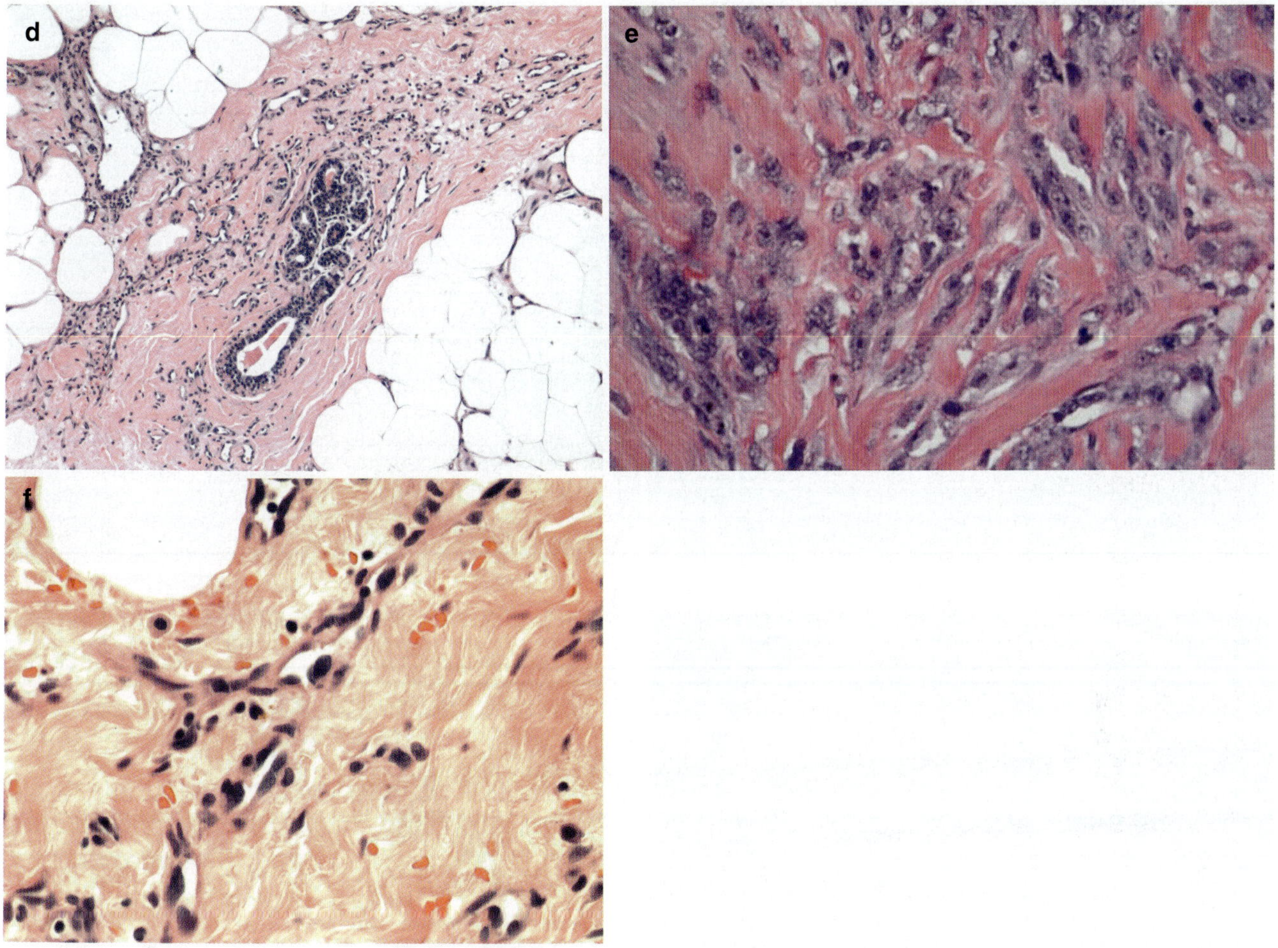

Fig. 13.14 (continued)

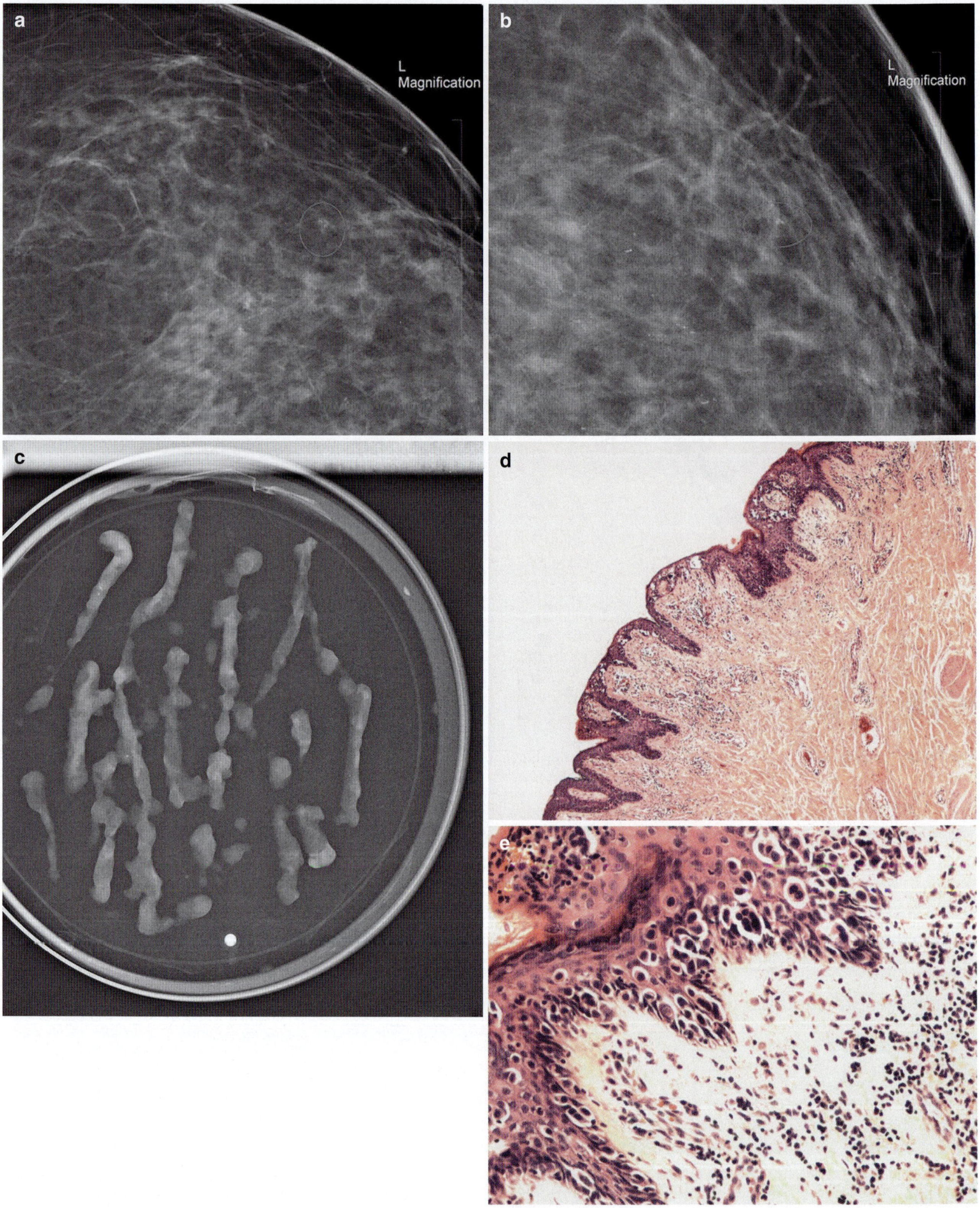

Fig. 13.15 A 44-year-old woman with itching and eczema of the left nipple with a histological diagnosis of DCIS. (**a**) Magnification view in the mediolateral oblique projection demonstrates an area of clustered microcalcifications. (**b**) Magnification view in the craniocaudal projection demonstrates an area of clustered microcalcifications. (**c**) Specimen radiograph of stereotactic biopsy specimen demonstrates microcalcifications. (**d**) Histology specimen demonstrates cancer cells in the dermis (×10). (**e**) Histology specimen demonstrates cancer cells in the dermis (×20)

References

1. Tabár L, Fagerberg CJG, Gad A, et al. Reduction in mortality from breast cancer after mass screening with mammography: randomized trial from the breast cancer screening working group of the Swedish national board of health and welfare. Lancet. 1985; 1:829–32.
2. Tabar L, Fagerberg G, Chen HH, et al. Efficacy of breast cancer screening by age. New results from the Swedish two county trials. Cancer. 1995;75:2507–17.
3. National Cancer Institute. Breast cancer surveillance consortium: evaluating screening performance in practice. NIH Publication No. 04-5490. Bethesda: National Cancer Institute, National Institutes of Health, U.S. Department of Health and Human Services. 2004. Available at: http://breastscreening.cancer.gov/espp.pdf.
4. Carney PA, Parikh J, Sickles EA, Feig SA, Monsees B, Bassett LW, Smith RA, Rosenberg R, Ichikawa L, Wallace J, Tran K, Miglioretti DL. Diagnostic mammography: identifying minimally acceptable interpretive performance criteria. Radiology. 2013;267(2):359–67.
5. Carney PA, Sickles EA, Monsees BA, Bassett LA, et al. Identifying minimally acceptable interpretive performance criteria for screening mammography. Radiology. 2010;255(2):354–61.
6. Sickles EA. Periodic mammographic follow-up of probably benign lesions: results in 3,184 consecutive cases. Radiology. 1991;179(2):463–8.
7. Yasmeen S, et al. Frequency and predictive value of a mammographic recommendation for short-interval follow-up. J Natl Cancer Inst. 2003;95(6):429–36.
8. Gruber R, et al. Histologic work-up of non-palpable breast lesions classified as probably benign at initial mammography and/or ultrasound (BI-RADS category 3). Eur J Radiol. 2013;82(3): 398–403.
9. Kerlikowske K, et al. Breast cancer yield for screening mammographic examinations with recommendation for short-interval follow-up. Radiology. 2005;234(3):684–92.
10. Varas X, Leborgne JH, Leborgne F, Mezzera J, Jaumandreu S. Revisiting the mammographic follow-up of BI-RADS category 3 lesions. AJR Am J Roentgenol. 2002;179:691–5.
11. Vizcaino I, Gadea L, Andreo L, et al. Short-term follow-up results in 795 nonpalpable probably benign lesions detected at screening mammography. Radiology. 2001;219:475–83.
12. Raza S, Goldkamp AL, Chikarmane SA, Birdwell RL. US of breast masses categorized as BI-RADS 3, 4, and 5: pictorial review of factors influencing clinical management. Radiographics. 2010;30(5):1199 213.
13. Raza S, Chikarmane SA, Neilsen SS, Zorn LM, Birdwell RL. BI-RADS 3, 4, and 5 lesions: value of US in management–follow-up and outcome. Radiology. 2008;248(3):773–81.
14. Davis HH, Simons M, Dais JB. Cystic disease of the breast: relationship to carcinoma. Cancer. 1964;17:957–78.
15. Love SM, Gelman RS, Silen W. Fibrocystic "disease" of the breast—a nondisease? N Engl J Med. 1982;307:1010–4.
16. Shetty MK, Shah YP. Sonographic findings in focal fibrocystic changes of the breast. Ultrasound Q. 2002;18(1):35–40.
17. Günhan-Bilgen I, Memiş A, Ustün EE, Ozdemir N, Erhan Y. Sclerosing adenosis: mammographic and ultrasonographic findings with clinical and histopathological correlation. Eur J Radiol. 2002;44(3):232–8.
18. Gill HK, Ioffe OB, Berg WA. When is a diagnosis of sclerosing adenosis acceptable at core biopsy? Radiology. 2003;228(1): 50–7.
19. DiPiro PJ, Gulizia JA, Lester SC, et al. Mammography and sonographic appearances of nodular adenosis. AJR Am J Roentgenol. 2000;175:31–4.
20. Jensen RA, Page DL, Dupont WD, Rogers LW. Invasive breast cancer risk in women with sclerosing adenosis. Cancer. 1989;64:1977–83.
21. Kundu UR, Guo M, Landon G, Wu Y, Sneige N, Gong Y. Fine-needle aspiration cytology of sclerosing adenosis of the breast: a retrospective review of cytologic features in conjunction with corresponding histologic features and radiologic findings. Am J Clin Pathol. 2012;138(1):96–102.
22. Goel NB, Knight TE, Pandey S, Riddick-Young M, de Paredes ES, Trivedi A. Fibrous lesions of the breast: imaging-pathologic correlation. Radiographics. 2005;25(6):1547–59.
23. Foster ME, Garrahan N, Williams S. Fibroadenoma of the breast: a clinical and pathological study. J R Coll Surg Edinb. 1998; 33:16–9.
24. Dupont WD, et al. Long-term risk of breast cancer in women with fibroadenoma. N Engl J Med. 1994;331:10–5.
25. Ciatto S, Bonardi R, Zappa M, Giorgi D. Risk of breast cancer subsequent to histological or clinical diagnosis of fibroadenoma–retrospective longitudinal study of 3938 cases. Ann Oncol. 1997;8(3):297–300.
26. El-Wakeel H, Umpleby HC. Systematic review of fibroadenoma as a risk factor for breast cancer. Breast. 2003;12(5):302–7.
27. Yoshida Y, Takaoka M, Fukumoto M. Carcinoma arising in fibroadenoma: case report and review of the world literature. J Surg Oncol. 1985;29(2):132–40.
28. Psarianos T, Kench JG, Ung OA, Bilous AM. Breast carcinoma in a fibroadenoma: diagnosis by fine needle aspiration cytology. Pathology. 1998;30(4):419–21.
29. Pietruszka M, Barnes L. Cystosarcoma phyllodes. Cancer. 1978;41:1974–83.
30. Haagensen C. Cystosarcoma phyllodes. In: Haagensen C, editor. Diseases of the breast. 3rd ed. Philadelphia: WB Saunders; 1986. p. 284–312.
31. Barth Jr RJ. Histologic features predict local recurrence after breast conserving therapy of phyllodes tumors. Breast Cancer Res Treat. 1999;57(3):291–5.
32. Youn I, Choi SH, Moon HJ, Kim MJ, Kim EK. Phyllodes tumors of the breast: ultrasonographic findings and diagnostic performance of ultrasound-guided core needle biopsy. Ultrasound Med Biol. 2013;39(6):987–92.
33. Liberman L, Bonaccio E, Hamele-Bena D, Abramson AF, Cohen MA, Dershaw DD. Benign and malignant phyllodes tumors: mammographic and sonographic findings. Radiology. 1996;198: 121–4.
34. Guillot E, et al. Management of phyllodes breast tumors. Breast J. 2011;17(2):129–37.
35. Khosravi-Shahi P. Management of non metastatic phyllodes tumors of the breast: review of the literature. Surg Oncol. 2011; 20(4):e143–8.
36. Venta LA, Wiley EL, Gabriel H, Adler YT. Imaging features of focal breast fibrosis: mammographic-pathologic correlation of noncalcified breast lesions. AJR Am J Roentgenol. 1999;173:309–16.
37. Taskin F, Unsal A, Ozbas S, Erkus M, Karaman C. Fibrotic lesions of the breast: radiological findings and core-needle biopsy results. Eur J Radiol. 2011;80(3):e231–6.
38. You JK, Kim EK, Kwak JY, Kim MJ, Oh KK, Park BW, Yang WI. Focal fibrosis of the breast diagnosed by a sonographically guided core biopsy of nonpalpable lesions: imaging findings and clinical relevance. J Ultrasound Med. 2005;24(10):1377–84.
39. Revelon G, Sherman ME, Gatewood OM, Brem RF. Focal fibrosis of the breast: imaging characteristics and histopathologic correlation. Radiology. 2000;216(1):255–9.
40. Rosen EL, Soo MS, Bentley RC. Focal fibrosis: a common breast lesion diagnosed at imaging-guided core biopsy. AJR Am J Roentgenol. 1999;173(6):1657–62.

41. Ibrahim RE, Sciotto CG, Weidner N. Pseudoangiomatous hyperplasia of mammary stroma. Cancer. 1989;63:1154–60.
42. Vuitch MF, Rosen PP, Erlandson RA. Pseudoangiomatous hyperplasia of mammary stroma. Cancer Hum Pathol. 1986;17:185–91.
43. Hargaden GC, Yeh ED, Georgian-Smith D, Moore RH, Rafferty EA, Halpern EF, McKee GT. Analysis of the mammographic and sonographic features of pseudoangiomatous stromal hyperplasia. AJR Am J Roentgenol. 2008;191(2):359–63.
44. Celliers L, Wong DD, Bourke A. Pseudoangiomatous stromal hyperplasia: a study of the mammographic and sonographic features. Clin Radiol. 2010;65(2):145–9.
45. Polger MR, Denison CM, Lester S, Meyer JE. Pseudoangiomatous stromal hyperplasia: mammographic and sonographic appearances. AJR Am J Roentgenol. 1996;166:349–52.
46. Cohen MA, Morris EA, Rosen PP, Dershaw DD, Liberman L, Abramson AF. Pseudoangiomatous stromal hyperplasia: mammographic, sonographic, and clinical patterns. Radiology. 1996; 198:117–20.
47. Poulton TB, de Paredes ES, Baldwin M. Sclerosing lobular hyperplasia of the breast: imaging features in 15 cases. AJR Am J Roentgenol. 1995;165:291–4.
48. Rosen PP, Ernsberger D. Mammary fibromatosis: a benign spindle-cell tumor with significant risk for local recurrence. Cancer. 1989;63:1363–9.
49. Brodt JK, Rhodes DJ, Glazebrook KN, Hruska C, O'Connor M, Boughey JC. Radiologic and pathologic images of mammary fibromatosis. Breast J. 2011;17(2):207–9.
50. Dorokhova O, Fineberg S, Koenigsberg T, Wang Y. Diabetic mastopathy, a clinicopathological correlation of 34 cases. Pathol Int. 2012;62(10):660–4.
51. Thorncroft K, Forsyth L, Desmond S, Audisio RA. The diagnosis and management of diabetic mastopathy. Breast J. 2007;13(6):607–13.
52. Pereira MA, et al. Fibrous mastopathy: clinical, imaging, and histopathologic findings of 31 cases. J Obstet Gynaecol Res. 2010;36(2):326–35.
53. Mackey SP, Sinha S, Pusey J, Chia Y, McPherson GA. Breast carcinoma in diabetic mastopathy. Breast. 2005;14:392–8.
54. King TA, Scharfenberg JC, Smetherman DH, Farkas EA, Bolton JS, Fuhrman GM. A better understanding of the term radial scar. Am J Surg. 2000;180(6):428–32.
55. Brenner RJ, et al. Percutaneous core needle biopsy of radial scars of the breast: when is excision necessary? AJR Am J Roentgenol. 2002;179:1179–84.
56. Patterson JA, Scott M, Anderson N, Kirk SJ. Radial scar, complex sclerosing lesion and risk of breast cancer. Analysis of 175 cases in Northern Ireland. Eur J Surg Oncol. 2004;30(10):1065–8.
57. Shetty MK. Radial scars of the breast: sonographic findings. Ultrasound Q. 2002;18(3):203–7.
58. Tabar L, Dean PB. Teaching atlas of mammography. Stuttgart: Thieme-Verlag; 1985. p. 88–9.
59. Neilsen M, Christensen L, Anderson J. Radial scars in women with breast cancer. Cancer. 1987;59:1019–25.
60. Ciatto S, Morrone D, Catarzi S, et al. Radial scars of the breast: review of 38 consecutive mammographic diagnoses. Radiology. 1993;187:757–60.
61. Jacobs TW, Byrne C, Colditz G, et al. Radial scars in benign breast biopsy specimens and the risk of breast cancer. N Engl J Med. 1999;340:430–6.
62. Chala LF. Fat necrosis of the breast: mammographic, sonographic, computed tomography, and magnetic resonance imaging findings. Curr Probl Diagn Radiol. 2004;33(3):106–26.
63. Rosen PP. Inflammatory and reactive tumors. In: Rosen PP, editor. Rosen's breast pathology. 1st ed. Philadelphia: Lippincott-Raven; 1997. p. 23–56.
64. Hogge JP, Robinson RE, Magnant CM, Zuurbier RA. The mammographic spectrum of fat necrosis of the breast. Radiographics. 1995;15(6):1347–56.
65. Bilgen IG, Ustun EE, Memis A. Fat necrosis of the breast: clinical, mammographic and sonographic features. Eur J Radiol. 2001;39(2):92–9.
66. Georgian-Smith D, Lawton TJ. Variations in physician recommendations for surgery after diagnosis of a high-risk lesion on breast core needle biopsy. AJR Am J Roentgenol. 2012;198(2): 256–63.
67. Degnim AC, King TA. Surgical management of high-risk breast lesions. Surg Clin North Am. 2013;93(2):329–40.
68. Linda A, Zuiani C, Furlan A, Londero V, Girometti R, Machin P, Bazzocchi M. Radial scars without atypia diagnosed at imaging-guided needle biopsy: how often is associated malignancy found at subsequent surgical excision, and do mammography and sonography predict which lesions are malignant? AJR Am J Roentgenol. 2010;194(4):1146–51.
69. Bianchi S, et al. Radial scar without associated atypical epithelial proliferation on image-guided 14-gauge needle core biopsy: analysis of 49 cases from a single-centre and review of the literature. Breast. 2012;21(2):159–64.
70. Lee KA, Zuley ML, Chivukula M, Choksi ND, Ganott MA, Sumkin JH. Risk of malignancy when microscopic radial scars and microscopic papillomas are found at percutaneous biopsy. AJR Am J Roentgenol. 2012;198(2):W141–5.
71. Becker L, Trop I, David J, et al. Management of radial scars found at percutaneous breast biopsy. Can Assoc Radiol J. 2006;57:72–8.
72. Liberman L, Tornos C, Huzjan R, et al. Is surgical excision warranted after benign, concordant diagnosis of papilloma at percutaneous breast biopsy? AJR Am J Roentgenol. 2006;186:1328–34.
73. Bennett LE, Ghate SV, Bentley R, Baker JA. Is surgical excision of core biopsy proven benign papillomas of the breast necessary? Acad Radiol. 2010;17:553–7.
74. Skandarajah AR, Field L, Yuen Larn Mou A, et al. Benign papilloma on core biopsy requires surgical excision. Ann Surg Oncol. 2008;15:2272–7.
75. Bernik SF, Troob S, Ying BL, et al. Papillary lesions of the breast diagnosed by core needle biopsy: 71 cases with surgical follow-up. Am J Surg. 2009;197:473–8.
76. Chang JM, Moon WK, Cho N, et al. Risk of carcinoma after subsequent excision of benign papilloma initially diagnosed with an ultrasound (US)-guided 14-g core needle biopsy: a prospective observational study. Eur Radiol. 2010;20:1093–100.
77. Kil WH, Cho EY, Kim JH, et al. Is surgical excision necessary in benign papillary lesions initially diagnosed at core biopsy? Breast. 2008;17:258–62.
78. Hwang H, Barke LD, Mendelson EB, et al. Atypical lobular hyperplasia and classic lobular carcinoma in situ in core biopsy specimens: routine excision is not necessary. Mod Pathol. 2008;21:1208–16.
79. Brem RF, Lechner MC, Jackman RJ, et al. Lobular neoplasia at percutaneous breast biopsy: variables associated with carcinoma at surgical excision. AJR Am J Roentgenol. 2008;190:637–41.
80. Biggar MA, Kerr KM, Erzetich LM. Bennett IC Columnar cell change with atypia (flat epithelial atypia) on breast core biopsy-outcomes following open excision. Breast J. 2012;18(6):578–81.
81. David N, Labbe-Devilliers C, Moreau D, et al. Lesions de metaplasie cylindriques atypiques (MCA) diagnostiquees par macrobiopsies assistees par aspiration: opportunite d'une exerese chirugicale? J Radiol. 2006;87:1671–7.
82. Verschuur-Maes AH, van Deurzen CH, Monninkhof EM, van Diest PJ. Columnar cell lesions on breast needle biopsies: is surgical excision necessary? A systematic review. Ann Surg. 2012;255(2):259–65.
83. Youk JH, Kim EK, Kim MJ, Lee JY, Oh KK. Missed breast cancers at US-guided core needle biopsy: how to reduce them. Radiographics. 2007;27(1):79–94.
84. Schueller G, et al. US-guided 14-gauge core-needle breast biopsy: results of a validation study in 1352 cases. Radiology. 2008;248(2): 406–13.

85. Parikh J, Tickman R. Image-guided tissue sampling: where radiology meets pathology. Breast J. 2005;11:403–9.
86. Kim MJ, Kim EK, Lee JY, Youk JH, Park BW, Kim SI, Kim H, Oh KK. Breast lesions with imaging-histologic discordance during US-guided 14G automated core biopsy: can the directional vacuum-assisted removal replace the surgical excision? Initial findings. Eur Radiol. 2007;17(9):2376–83.
87. Kim MJ, Kim EK, Park SY, Jung HK, Park BW, Kim H, Oh KK. Imaging-histologic discordance at sonographically guided percutaneous biopsy of breast lesions. Eur J Radiol. 2008;65(1):163–9.
88. Son EJ, Kim EK, Youk JH, Kim MJ, Kwak JY, Choi SH. Imaging histologic discordance after sonographically guided percutaneous breast biopsy: a prospective observational study. Ultrasound Med Biol. 2011;37(11):1771–8.
89. Weigelt B, Geyer FC, Reis-Filho JS. Histological types of breast cancer: how special are they? Mol Oncol. 2010;4(3):192–208.
90. Ellis P, Schnitt SJ, Sastre-Garau X, Bussolati G, Tavassoli FA, Eusebi V, et al. Invasive breast carcinoma. In: Tavassoli FA, Devilee P, editors. WHO classification of tumours. Pathology and genetics of tumours of the breast and Female genital organs. Lyon: Lyon Press; 2001.
91. Reis-Filho JS, Lakhani SR. Breast cancer special types: why bother? J Pathol. 2008;216(4):394–8.
92. Horowitz DP, Sharma CS, Connolly E, Gidea-Addeo D, Deutsch I. Secretory carcinoma of the breast: results from the survival, epidemiology and end results database. Breast. 2012;21(3):350–3.
93. Mun SH, Ko EY, Han BK, Shin JH, Kim SJ, Cho EY. Secretory carcinoma of the breast: sonographic features. J Ultrasound Med. 2008;27(6):947–54.
94. Sheppard DG, Whitman GJ, Huynh PT, Sahin AA, Fornage BD, Stelling CB. Tubular carcinoma of the breast: mammographic and sonographic features. AJR Am J Roentgenol. 2000;174(1):253–7.
95. Günhan-Bilgen I, Oktay A. Tubular carcinoma of the breast: mammographic, sonographic, clinical and pathologic findings. Eur J Radiol. 2007;61(1):158–62.
96. Günhan-Bilgen I, Oktay A. Tubulolobular carcinoma of the breast: clinical, mammographic and sonographic findings. Eur J Radiol. 2006;60(3):418–24.
97. Shin HJ, Kim HH, Kim SM, Kim DB, Lee YR, Kim MJ, Gong G. Pure and mixed tubular carcinoma of the breast: mammographic and sonographic differential features. Korean J Radiol. 2007;8(2):103–10.
98. Daniele S, Imbriaco M, Riccardi A, Selva G, di Nuzzo L, Salvatore M, Sodano A. Mammographic and sonographic features of tubular breast carcinoma. Tumori. 2003;89(4):417–20.
99. Zandrino F, Calabrese M, Faedda C, Musante F. Tubular carcinoma of the breast: pathological, clinical, and ultrasonographic findings. A review of the literature. Radiol Med. 2006;111(6):773–82.
100. Di Saverio S, Gutierrez J, Avisar E. A retrospective review with long term follow up of 11,400 cases of pure mucinous breast carcinoma. Breast Cancer Res Treat. 2008;111(3):541–7.
101. Lam WW, Chu WC, Tse GM, Ma TK. Sonographic appearance of mucinous carcinoma of the breast. AJR Am J Roentgenol. 2004;182(4):1069–74.
102. Memis A, Ozdemir N, Parildar M, Ustun EE, Erhan Y. Mucinous (colloid) breast cancer: mammographic and US features with histologic correlation. Eur J Radiol. 2000;35(1):39–43.
103. Kaoku S. Sonographic and pathologic image analysis of pure mucinous carcinoma of the breast. Ultrasound Med Biol. 2013;39(7):1158–67.
104. Lam WW, Tang AP, Tse G, Chu WC. Radiology-Pathology conference: papillary carcinoma of the breast. Clin Imaging. 2005;29(6):396–400.
105. Rodríguez MC, Secades AL, Angulo JM. Best cases from the AFIP: intracystic papillary carcinoma of the breast. Radiographics. 2010;30(7):2021–7.
106. Rosen PP. Papillary carcinoma. In: Rosen's breast pathology. Philadelphia: Lippincott-Raven; 1997. p. 335–54.
107. Dogan BE, Whitman GJ, Middleton LP, Phelps M. Intracystic papillary carcinoma of the breast. AJR Am J Roentgenol. 2003;181:186.
108. Soo MS, Williford ME, Walsh R, Bentley RC, Kornguth PJ. Papillary carcinoma of the breast: imaging findings. AJR Am J Roentgenol. 1995;164:321–6.
109. Pal SK, et al. Papillary carcinoma of the breast: an overview. Breast Cancer Res Treat. 2010;122(3):637–45.
110. Eiada R, Chong J, Kulkarni S, Goldberg F, Muradali D. Papillary lesions of the breast: MRI, ultrasound, and mammographic appearances. AJR Am J Roentgenol. 2012;198(2):264–71.
111. Brookes MJ, Bourke AG. Radiological appearances of papillary breast lesions. Clin Radiol. 2008;63(11):1265–73.
112. Ridolfi RL, Rosen PP, Port A, Kinne D, Mike V. Medullary carcinoma of the breast: a clinicopathologic study with 10 year follow-up. Cancer. 1977;40(4):1365–85.
113. Martinez SR, Beal SH, Canter RJ, Chen SL, Khatri VP, Bold RJ. Medullary carcinoma of the breast: a population-based perspective. Med Oncol. 2011;28(3):738–44.
114. Rosen PP, Lesser ML, Kinne DW, et al. Breast carcinoma in women 35 years of age or younger. Ann Surg. 1984;199:133.
115. Cho N, Oh KK, Lee S. Medullary Carcinoma of the Breast: Sonographic Features distinguishing it from Fibroadenoma. J Med Ultrasound. 2002;10(4):191–6.
116. Cheung YC, Chen SC, Lee KF, Wan YL, Ng SH. Sonographic and pathologic findings in typical and atypical medullary carcinomas of the breast. J Clin Ultrasound. 2000;28(7):325–31.
117. Yilmaz E, Lebe B, Balci P, Sal S, Canda T. Comparison of mammographic and sonographic findings in typical and atypical medullary carcinomas of the breast. Clin Radiol. 2002;57(7):640–5.
118. Uematsu T. Non-mass-like lesions on breast ultrasonography: a systematic review. Breast Cancer. 2012;19(4):295–301.
119. Mendelson EB, Baum JK, Berg WA, et al. BI-RADS: ultrasound. In: D'Orsi CJ, Mendelson EB, Ikeda DM, et al., editors. Breast imaging reporting and data system: ACR BIRADS– breast imaging atlas. 1st ed. Reston: American College of Radiology; 2003.
120. Maounis N, et al. Metastasis to the breast from an adenocarcinoma of the lung with extensive micropapillary component: a case report and review of the literature. Diagn Pathol. 2010;5:82.
121. Vergier B, Trojani M, de Mascarel I, Coindre JM, Le Treut A. Metastases to the breast: differential diagnosis from primary breast carcinoma. J Surg Oncol. 1991;48(2):112–6.
122. Feder JM, de Paredes ES, Hogge JP, Wilken JJ. Unusual breast lesions: radiologic-pathologic correlation. Radiographics. 1999;19 Spec No:S11–26.
123. Porter GJ, Evans AJ, Lee AH, Hamilton LJ, James JJ. Unusual benign breast lesions. Clin Radiol. 2006;61(7):562–9.
124. Yang WT, Lane DL, Le-Petross HT, Abruzzo LV, Macapinlac HA. Breast lymphoma: imaging findings of 32 tumors in 27 patients. Radiology. 2007;245(3):692–702.
125. Karan B, Pourbagher A, Bolat FA. Unusual malignant breast lesions : imaging-pathological correlations. Diagn Interv Radiol. 2012;18(3):270–6.
126. Carder PJ, Murphy CE, Liston JC. Surgical excision is warranted following a core biopsy diagnosis of mucocoele-like lesion of the breast. Histopathology. 2004;45(2):148–54.
127. Meroni S, Moscovici O, Menna S, Renne G, Sosnovskikh I, Rossi V, Cassano E. Ultrasound challenge: secondary breast angiosarcoma mimicking lipoma. Breast J. 2013;19(4):437–8.
128. Hui A, Henderson M, Speakman D, Skandarajah A. Angiosarcoma of the breast: a difficult surgical challenge. Breast. 2012;21(4):584–9.
129. Dalberg K, Hellborg H, Wärnberg F. Paget's disease of the nipple in a population based cohort. Breast Cancer Res Treat. 2008;111(2):313–9.

Challenges in Breast Imaging

14

Mahesh K. Shetty

Introduction

Breast imaging is fraught with unique challenges in decision making and patient management. The objective of not missing early-stage disease so as to fulfill the prime goal of diagnosing nonpalpable cancers to be balanced with keeping false positives low presents unique practice patterns and challenges. The list of controversies in breast imaging is long; some of the important ones are discussed in this chapter:

- Inappropriate indications for mammography
- Breast intervention
  - Intraductal masses
  - Follow-up after concordant biopsy results
  - Cytology of cyst aspirates
- Dense breast law
- Double reads
- Clinical breast exam during screening
- Imaging the male breast
- Overdiagnosis of breast cancer with screening mammography
- Isolated abnormal axillary nodes

Inappropriate Indications for Mammography

Screening mammography has proven benefits in reducing breast cancer mortality and attention to proper methodology, and appropriate use is critical to optimize these benefits [1]. Some of the controversial indications for use of mammography in asymptomatic women are discussed next.

M.K. Shetty, MD, FRCR, FACR, FAIUM
Clinical Professor of Radiology, Baylor College of Medicine, Houston, TX, USA

Woman's Center for Breast Care and MRI, Woman's Hospital of Texas, Houston, TX 77054, USA
e-mail: mshettymd@gmail.com

Prior to and Following Breast Augmentation

There is no reason for routine use of mammography prior to placement of breast augmentation other than in those who are in the age group where annual screening mammography is recommended by American Cancer Society. It has been suggested that preoperative mammogram will detect abnormalities that could be potentially biopsied during implant placement surgery and to serve as a baseline prior to augmentation. These reasons have not been validated in any published study. Similarly the need for postaugmentation mammogram 6–12 months after surgery has been suggested to serve as a baseline for future follow-up. Although a need for such an examination has also never been validated, there may be some justification since postsurgical changes may be mistaken for signs of malignancy and having a baseline will serve to minimize false positive biopsies [2].

In a series of 1,149 cases of cosmetic surgery of the breast performed from 1973 to 1989, early diagnosis of breast cancer in 34 cases was possible by relying mainly on the use of mammography for the diagnosis. Based on these findings the authors recommended that a policy of mandatory preoperative mammography be implemented so that all patients can be protected from a lethal disease that has a far better prognosis when detected early [3]. This study did not have adequate information on the age group, presence of symptoms, or risk factors in cases of breast cancer that was identified on the mammogram. The findings of this study therefore do not justify routine use of mammography preimplant placement in women under the age of 40 years who are at an average risk.

Imaging Surveillance in the Postmastectomy Patient

There is insufficient evidence for mammographic surveillance in women who have undergone mastectomy or in those who have undergone mastectomy with breast reconstruction or augmentation. The one exception is in women who have

M.K. Shetty (ed.), *Breast Cancer Screening and Diagnosis: A Synopsis*,
DOI 10.1007/978-1-4939-1267-4_14, © Springer Science+Business Media New York 2015

undergone nipple-sparing subcutaneous mastectomy in whom the nipple-areolar complex and the tissue behind are left behind. The annual recurrence rate of cancer in those who have undergone nipple-sparing mastectomy has been reported to be 6.7 % [4]. The yield of nonpalpable cancers in women who have undergone mastectomy is low. Ultrasound and mammography are indicated in the symptomatic patient postmastectomy and reconstruction, with fat necrosis being the most common benign finding in both the symptomatic and the asymptomatic women. In one series of the 227 patients who had undergone mastectomy with breast reconstruction, one cancer was detected among 116 who underwent mammographic surveillance. The recall rate was 4 %. In the symptomatic group of 54 women on the other hand, there were 4 cancers; the most common cause of a palpable finding was fat necrosis [5]. Others have recommended the routine surveillance of the mastectomy side since it is impossible to know how much of glandular tissue has been left behind. A recurrence rate of as high as 7 % has been reported and has been cited as the rationale behind routine surveillance of the postmastectomy breast [6]. Routine surveillance has also been recommended in those patients who undergo postmastectomy reconstruction with transfer of a musculocutaneous flap; recurrence of cancer after 5 years was found by surveillance in a small group of patients [7, 8].

Mammography for Breast Pain

Women seek attention when afflicted with breast pain due to concern of breast cancer. In our practice mammography is frequently ordered in women who present with breast pain; a majority of these women fall in the nonscreened group most commonly in their 30s. As a means of reassurance in those without clinical findings, we perform ultrasound only particularly in those under 30 years old. In one series breast pain accounted for 32 % of new patient referrals, 60 % were in women under the age of 40 years. There was no increased reassurance in excluding malignancy. Although six cancers were detected in the study group of 916 women during a 1-year study period, none were found in patients not associated with clinical breast abnormalities. There is no rationale in imaging the breast for a complaint of pain in the absence of clinical breast abnormalities [9]. In a primary care setting, 45–70 % of breast complaints are attributed to breast pain. When breast pain is the sole complaint, the risk of breast cancer is very low and reported to be 0–3 % [10–12]. Imaging is not justified although commonly used as a means of patient reassurance. Cyclic pain and or diffuse or bilateral breast pain should not prompt imaging in the absence of a clinical abnormality.

Breast Intervention

Intraductal Masses

Intraductal masses are frequently papillomas that are generally recommended to undergo excisional biopsy due to known association with DCIS, an upgrade to malignancy of 4–14 % has been reported [13, 14]. Mammography shows a tubular density with or without branching usually in a subareolar location; calcifications may be associated. Ultrasound may reveal an intraductal mass with or without calcifications and may reveal vascularity on Doppler imaging (Fig. 14.1a–d). A series of 163 intraductal masses reported a malignancy rate of 8 %, 10 of which were DCIS and three invasive cancers. Malignancy was more often associated with symptoms and personal history of cancer. Distinguishing sonographic features in malignant masses included intraductal masses that filled the lumen, extended outside the duct or extended into a branch. Malignant masses were larger than benign intraductal masses [15]. In our practice all papillomas are recommended to undergo excisional biopsy, and on imaging if a papilloma or a papillary lesion is suspected based on the presence of an intraductal mass particularly in a subareolar location, excisional biopsy is recommended at the outset bypassing the step of percutaneous biopsy. It has been suggested that excision be suggested only in those cases where atypia is associated or when the size of the papilloma is greater than 1.5 cm [13].

Follow-up After Concordant Percutaneous Biopsy

Calcifications

For benign concordant pathologic results, a single 6-month follow-up is adequate with magnification views to ensure that calcifications are stable [16]. In case of a specific diagnosis such as a fibroadenoma, a 12-month follow-up may be sufficient. At follow-up if there is no increase in the number of calcifications or a change to a suspicious morphology, no further follow-up is warranted.

Masses

There is no consensus on follow-up after a benign concordant biopsy. Some advocate that no follow-up is needed, while others recommend a 6-, 12-, and 24-month follow-up;, the latter seems excessive. At our institution a single 6-month follow-up is performed for benign concordant histology. If there is a significant increase in the size of the mass or if there are new morphologic features that are suspicious such as marginal irregularity, excisional biopsy is appropriate [16].

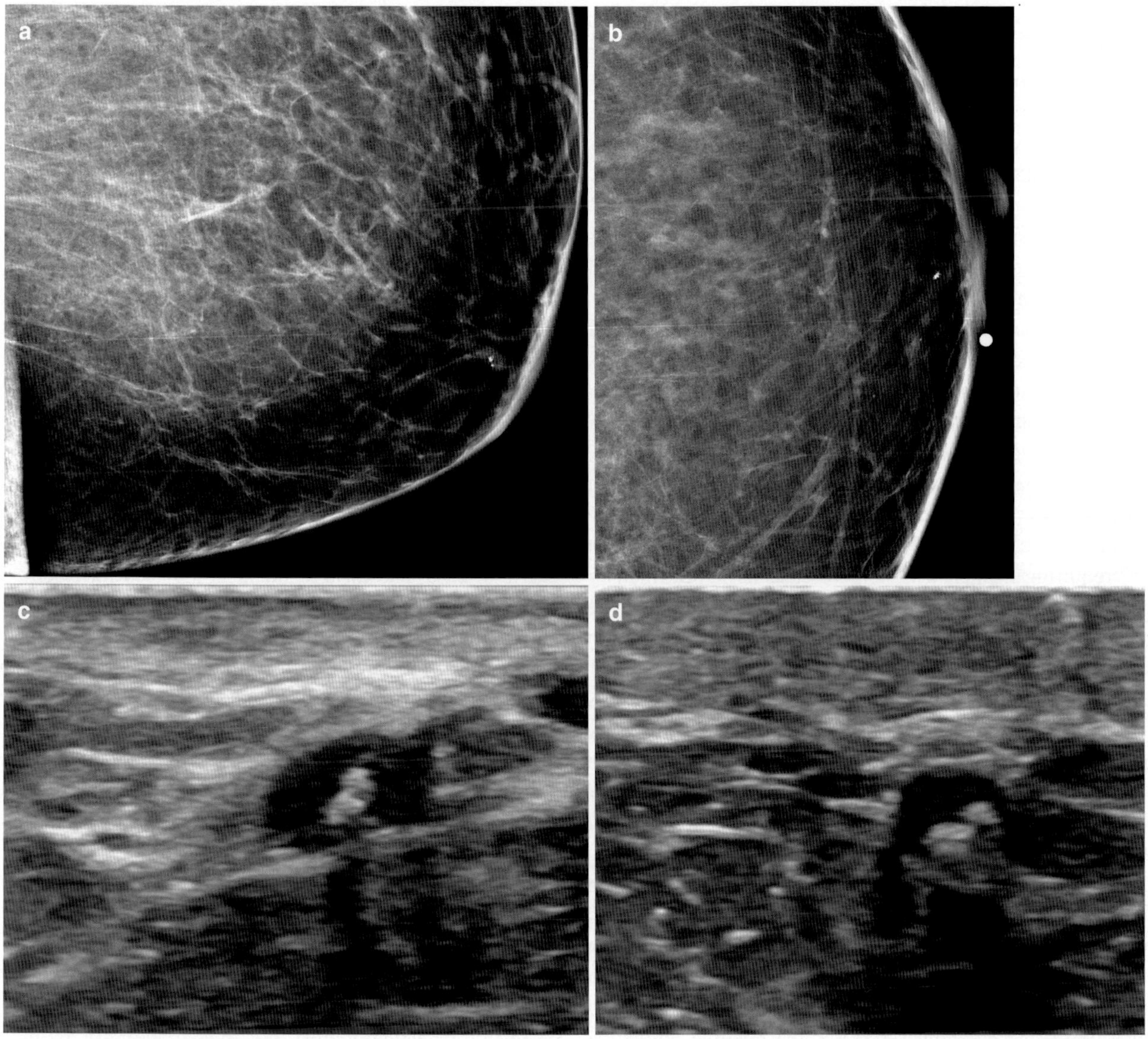

Fig. 14.1 Intraductal papilloma in a 44-year-old female with a spontaneous unilateral serous nipple discharge. (**a**) Mediolateral oblique view of the left breast demonstrates a branching subareolar tubular density with calcifications. (**b**) Craniocaudal view showing a similar finding. (**c**) Ultrasound image of the subareolar region showing a distended duct with an intraductal mass in the radial plane. (**d**) Ultrasound image of the subareolar region showing a distended duct with an intraductal mass in the antiradial plane

Aspiration of Cysts

A simple cyst is a benign finding and requires intervention only for symptomatic relief. Complicated cysts are those which do not fulfill all of the criteria of a simple cyst such as when internal echoes or septations are seen within a cyst or when there is no increased through transmission. These are mostly benign and may not require aspiration. In one series only 1 of 243 lesions (0.4 %) proved malignant; this lesion was 1 of 33 complicated cysts that did not yield fluid [17]. Even when cytology yields atypical cells, the final histology is mostly benign [17]. In a large series of 6,782 cyst aspirations over a 7-year period, the incidence of intracystic papillomas was 5 [0.1 %] [18]. All cases of papilloma showed blood-stained fluid. Overall only 2 % of cyst fluids were blood stained. Cytology of six cases of papilloma was positive in two, negative in two, and falsely positive in two cases [18]. These investigators recommended cytology only when aspirate is blood stained. A cyst that demonstrates thick indistinct walls, thick internal septations, or mixed solid and cystic components requires core biopsy sampling. Clustered microcysts and septate cysts are generally benign [19]. A recently published large series of 5,375 aspirations performed over a 16-year period of noncomplex cysts reported a malignancy rate of 0.3 % [20]. Atypical cytology revealed malignancy in 21 % of cases. All atypical results should undergo further workup. Malignant cytology revealed malignancy in 91 % of cases and hence all patient with malignant histology need to undergo biopsy [20].

Dense Breast Law

Sensitivity of mammography in women with dense breasts has been reported to be as low as 48 % [21]. About 41 % of women may have dense breasts on a mammogram [22]. Increased breast density is an independent risk factor for breast cancer and increased the risk by a factor of 5 [23]. Supplemental ultrasound has been shown to detect additional cancers in women with dense breasts in those with an elevated risk as well in those with an average risk [24–27].

Recently based on these facts and a public campaign undertaken by a breast cancer survivor, several states have passed a law called the "Henda's law" or the "dense breast law" requiring women with dense breasts to be informed by their clinician about their breast density and discussing the option of undergoing supplemental screening depending on their risk factors.

The ACRIN 6,666 trial showed that 4.2 additional cancers were identified by ultrasound in women with an elevated risk for breast cancer [24]. The dense breast law passed in Connecticut requires notification of women with a greater than 50 % density and recommendation for supplemental screening ultrasound; the law also required insurance to pay for supplemental ultrasound screening. A study from Connecticut looking at such women showed that ultrasound lead to an additional yield of 3.25 cancers per 1,000 in women with dense breasts, normal mammograms, and no additional risk factors [25]. Although the NPV [99.9 %] and sensitivity was very high [96.6 %], the positive predictive value was low at 6.7 % [25]. Yet in another study of 5,519 women with dense breasts who underwent sonographic screening, the supplemental yield was only 1.8 per 1,000 and positive predictive value was low at 5.5 %, and mean tumor size was 9.7 mm [26]. Post enactment of the Connecticut law, a study that looked at women with low risk [614/935], intermediate risk [149/935, 15.9 %], and high risk [87/935, 9.3 %] found one cancer in each of the three groups. All of these three cancers were small solid masses in postmenopausal women for a cancer detection rate of 3.2 per 1,000 women screened again with an expected low positive predictive value of only 6.5 % [27].

Double Reads

About half of the countries that use screening mammography have implemented double reading, although direct evidence of its effectiveness in the context of a national screening program is lacking [28]. Analysis of ten cohort studies showed that overall double reading increases the cancer detection rate by 3–11 per 10,000 women screened and most of the cancers thus found are small cancers. The effect on recall rate depended on the methodology. Double reading with unilateral recall increased the number of women recalled from 38 to 149 per 10,000 women screened. In programs where a consensus or arbitration policy was in place, the recall rate decreased between 61 and 269 per 10,000 women screened [28]. In a large majority of cases, double reads do not lead to disagreement; when there is one mutual consultation, this further diminishes the number of recall. In some facilities cases with disagreement are referred to an arbitration panel. The effectiveness of this methodology of referral to an arbitration panel has been studied. In a series from Netherlands involving screening of 65,779 women, there was concordance in the reads of double readers in 98.7 % of women, and there was agreement on the need for referral in 0.8 % of cases and disagreement on the need for referral in 0.5 % of cases which decreased to 0.3 % after mutual consultation. These 183 studies were referred to the arbitration panel which referred 89 of these for further workup that resulted in a cancer diagnosis in 20/89 [22 %]. Among the 94 cases that were not referred, there were 3 cancers [3 %] at the site of the discrepant mammographic findings [29]. Screening mammograms with discrepant findings form a small but significant subset that may lead to a diagnosis of breast cancer.

Double Reads vs Single Reads With CAD

The effectiveness of double reading has been compared to single reader using a CAD [computerized aided detection] by several investigators [30–32]. In a study of 10,267 mammograms, single reading with CAD led to a cancer detection rate that was higher albeit with a higher recall rate of 8.6 % vs 6.5 % achieved with a double read [30]. The cancer detection rate though increased in the CAD group by 15 %. Others have reported similar results. A meta-analysis of ten studies that looked at efficacy of single readers using CAD vs single readers' found that CAD did not significantly increase the cancer detection rate and increased the recall rate. The same report in a meta-analysis of 17 studies that assessed the value of double reads over single reads found that double reads increased both cancer detection rate and the recall rates; however, double read with arbitration increased cancer detection rate with decreased recall [31]. A literature review of six studies that compared single reads with CAD vs double reads showed that three of these studies did not show any differences in sensitivity or specificity: one showed increased sensitivity with same specificity, one showed higher specificity with the same sensitivity, and one had higher sensitivity with lowered specificity [32].

Cost-Effectiveness of Double Reading

The cost-effectiveness resulting from double reading has also been studied [33, 34]. Double reading followed by consensus involving 33,734 consecutive screening mammograms detected an additional 9 cancers per 10,000 women screened. A nonconsensus double reading policy detected an additional 10 cancers per 10,000 women screened. However, nonconsensus double reading resulted in a recall rate was significantly higher than single read; recall rate in consensus double read was significantly lower than with single reads. From a cost-effectiveness perspective consensus double read costs less than single reading (4,853 £ saved per 10,000 women screened) and nonconsensus double reading costs more than single reading (difference of 19,259 £ per 10,000 women screened) [33]. The cost-effectiveness in terms of the cost per cancer detected has also been studied. Data from 255,000 women from Scotland showed that costs per cancer detected by double reading compared to single reading range from $ 1,859 to $ 3,553 [34].

Clinical Breast Exam with Screening Mammography [35–37]

Clinical breast examination [CBE] in conjunction with screening mammography can be implemented concurrently when administered in a breast center by a registered nurse or when a screening mammogram is done following a well woman exam as is more often the case. The former has been studied to determine the added benefit of increasing cancer detection. There were 232,515 women in the group receiving CBE and 57,715 in the group undergoing screening mammogram without a clinical breast exam. Sensitivity in the CBE group was 94.9 % vs 88.6 % for the screened group without CBE. However, the false positive was also higher for those women who had CBE with screening mammography compared to those who did not receive CBE [12.5 % vs 7.4 %] [35]. Another large study with dual screening in 300,303 women, CBE increased the rate of detection of small invasive cancer by 2–6 %. Without the concurrent use of CBE, three cancers would be missed for every 10,000 screens [36]. The cost-effectiveness of offering CBE in a comprehensive breast center was reported in a cohort of 60,000 women who received CBE by a nurse practitioner. Four hundred and seventy four had a positive exam leading to a diagnostic evaluation. Forty-six cancers were identified, 32 of which would have been identified by mammography alone, and only 14 were not seen on a mammogram. The cost of CBE was 122,598 per cancer detected based solely on CBE findings [37].

Imaging of the Male Breast

A male breast is composed of subcutaneous tissue, atrophic ducts, and stromal elements with preponderance of fat [38]. Conditions that affect the male breast are therefore related to ductal and stromal proliferation and include the most commonly encountered gynecomastia, invasive ductal carcinoma, and papillary neoplasm. Most commonly men are referred for a breast lump, breast enlargement, or tenderness. Mammography is the initial imaging and may be the only modality needed. If abnormality cannot be imaged on mammography or if findings are questionable, sonography is indicated. The most common cause of breast symptoms are due to gynecomastia.

Gynecomastia

Gynecomastia is the most common breast problem in a male patient and has been reported to be between 87 and 90 % of cases [39, 40]. There are three patterns of gynecomastia, nodular, dendritic, and diffuse glandular. The nodular pattern represents the early florid phase of ductal and stromal proliferation and is seen in the first year of onset and accounts for 34–36 % of gynecomastia [39, 40]. At mammography it produces a fan-shaped subareolar density that blends into surrounding parenchyma (Fig. 14.2a–d). Ultrasound is not needed when mammographic appearance is characteristic. Ultrasound may show the area of gynecomastia as an irregular mass prompting a recommendation for a biopsy of a benign abnormality and should be avoided for this reason (Fig. 14.2d). The presentation is in the form of a painful mass and the process is reversible if the inciting factor is withdrawn [38]. The dendritic phase is the fibrotic quiescent phase characterized by stromal fibrosis and ductal proliferation. This accounts for 31–35 % of cases of gynecomastia [39, 40]. This represents irreversible phase of gynecomastia. Diffuse glandular type accounts for 31–33 % of cases and is seen in patients receiving estrogen therapy and represents a combination of dendritic and diffuse nodular types. Gynecomastia tends to be bilateral in 55–65 % of cases [39, 40].

Male Breast Cancer

Breast cancer accounts for 1–8 % of symptomatic breast disease in males [39–41]. About 0.7 % of all breast cancers are diagnosed in men [38]. In 2010 based on cancer statistics, 1,970 new cases of male breast cancers were diagnosed [42]. Mass without calcifications is seen in 86 % of breast cancer cases in men and as calcifications in 7 % [39]. Mean size of the mass is 2.4 cm; prognosis is generally poor due to late

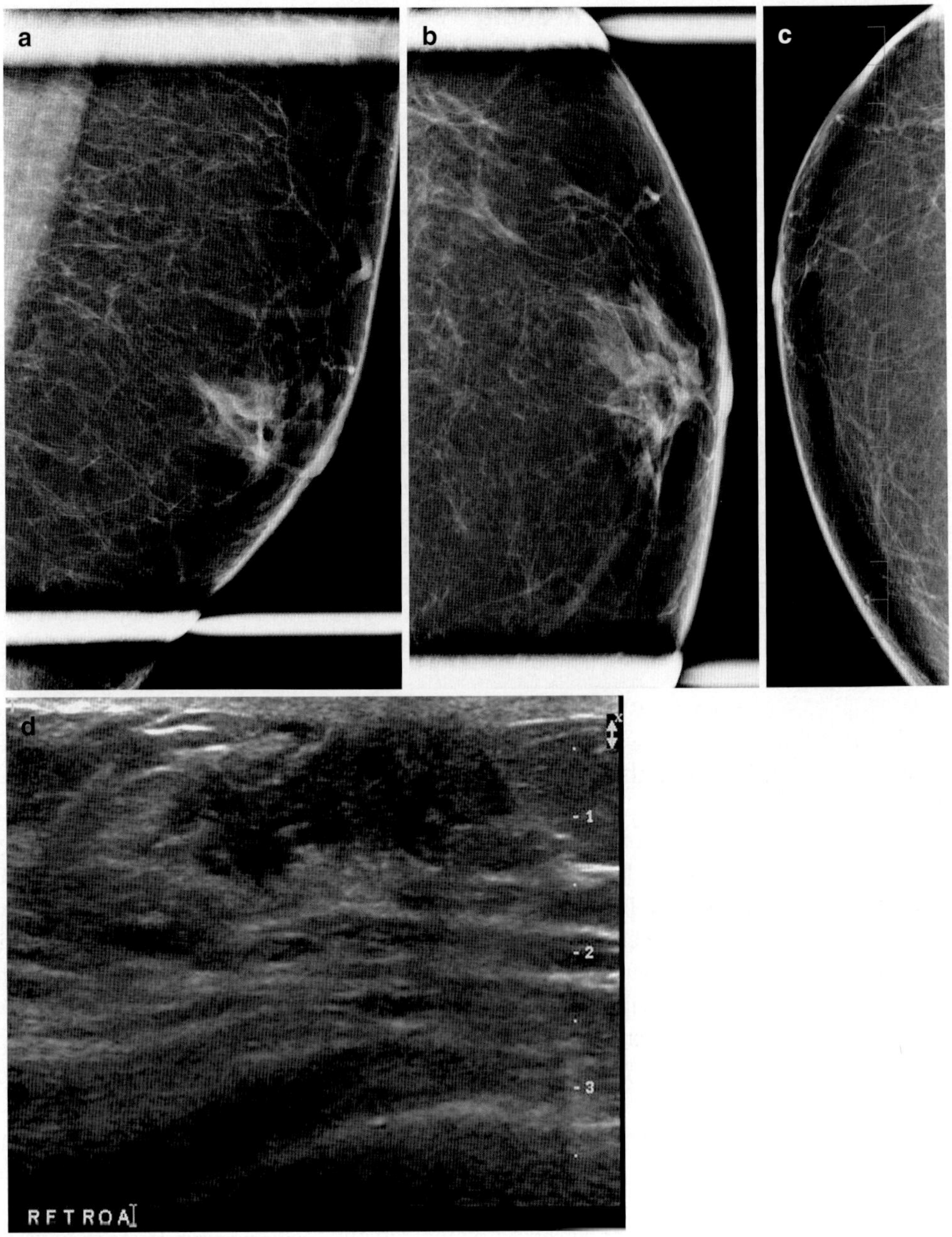

Fig. 14.2 A 65-year-old male with history of liver disease presenting with left breast swelling. (**a**) Mediolateral oblique view of the left breast demonstrates a fan-shaped subareolar density consistent with gynecomastia. (**b**, **c**) Craniocaudal views of the left breast demonstrate a fan-shaped subareolar density consistent with gynecomastia. (**d**) Ultrasound demonstrates an irregular hypoechoic mass-like abnormality representing gynecomastia

stage of presentation. Risk factors for breast cancer in males include Klinefelter syndrome, BRCA1 or BRCA2 mutation, family history of breast cancer in a first-degree male or female relative, hyperestrogenism, exogenous estrogen for feminization purposes, advanced age, and history of chest radiation. Breast cancer typically presents at an age on an average 10 years later than in women, the mean age at diagnosis being 67 years [38]. The disease is often at an advanced stage at diagnosis with axillary node metastasis seen at initial evaluation in 50 % of cases [38]. Secondary signs of breast cancer occur earlier in the male breast because of the smaller size of the breast. These include nipple retraction, skin ulceration and thickening, and axillary adenopathy [41]. Cystic lesions in a male breast have to be worked up as potentially malignant since cystic lesions commonly demonstrate malignant findings. Breast cancer most often presents as a discrete mass with malignant features on a mammogram or ultrasound. The relationship of the mass to the nipple is helpful; an eccentric mass is highly suspicious for cancer [41].

The differential diagnosis of male breast includes gynecomastia, lipoma, epidermal inclusion cyst, pseudoangiomatous hyperplasia, and intraductal papilloma. The most common histological type of breast cancer is the infiltrating ductal cancer accounting for 80 % of all cancers, ductal carcinoma in situ accounts for 5 % of cancers, and rarer types include papillary cancer [38].

Overdiagnosis of Breast Cancer with Screening Mammography

The term *overdiagnosis* of breast cancer by screening mammography in population-based studies refers to the difference between cancer detection and subsequent treatment of abnormal findings and the corresponding effect on mortality. The percentage of overdiagnosis represents the estimated percentage of cases that were detected and treated but that would not have affected mortality if had been left alone. In other words mammography identifies cancers that are nonlethal and do not lead to mortality [43, 44]. Bleyer and Belch used a model for expectation values and estimated that 31 % of cancers that are diagnosed breast cancer represent overdiagnosis [43]. They then concluded that the reduction in mortality can be attributed to improvements in therapy and not to early diagnosis [43]. In an opinion article in response to this theory, Gur and Sumkin correctly point out that once a decision to screen is made, the role of a breast imager should be to detect disease early and towards this end due diligence is needed to detect and correctly diagnose all abnormalities at the earliest stage possible. It is then the responsibility of other specialties to make the best use of the information provided by the radiologist to decide how best to use the information in the appropriate management of the patient. They state that there can only be a "correct, partially correct or an incorrect diagnosis and there can only be optimally managed, suboptimally managed and mismanaged and over treated disease" [44]. They go on to appropriately state "There should not be any doubt that the overall objective of a screening program is to first and foremost detect, correctly diagnose, and appropriately treat early preclinical cancers that, if left alone, would become life threatening cancers" [44]. This seems to be a reasonable and appropriate response to the criticism of overdiagnosis of breast cancer.

Mammographically Occult Breast Cancer with Axillary Metastasis

Axillary metastatic lymphadenopathy with no primary tumor identified in the breast on physical examination or mammography is rare, and only three such cases of mammographically occult breast cancer were reported in one study over a 10-year period [45]. In another reported series, isolated enlarged axillary nodes were present in 72 of 200,716 women screened [46]. Thirteen patients had no reason for recall, and of the 59 patients recalled, only 13 had malignancy, 4 were metastatic breast cancer, and 9 were lymphoma; the remainder of the cases had a benign etiology for the presence of isolated abnormal axillary lymph nodes [46]. Fine needle aspiration biopsy with definitive cytological diagnosis precludes need for excisional biopsy in most cases. It has been suggested that such cases of axillary metastasis from occult breast cancer can be managed with axillary node clearance and chemotherapy with a possible role for radiation treatment to the ipsilateral breast [45]. Metastatic axillary adenocarcinoma with an occult breast cancer is uncommon type of stage II breast cancers. Prognosis is not as grave as is believed for individual patients. In the largest reported series of 48 patients with an axillary mass proven to be metastatic adenocarcinoma consistent with mammary origin, patients were followed for 5 years. All primary cancers were clinically occult and mammographically occult in 28 women [76 %]. In nine patients metastasis was positive for estrogen and progesterone receptors [ER, PR +] and in 10 patients [ER, PR –]. Mastectomy with axillary dissection was carried out in 38 of 48 patients, 21 received adjuvant chemotherapy [47]. Pathologically a primary breast cancer was found in the mastectomy specimen in 36/48 [75 %] of cases; seven of these cancers were histologically noninvasive. Tumor size ranged from 1 mm to 6.5 cm. In 20 of 48 patients, there were 1–3 positive axillary nodes [47].

An isolated abnormal lymph node in the axilla identified on a screening mammogram is optimally imaged with ultrasound [48]. A size greater than 2 cm, absence of fatty hilum, a rounded shape, and focal or diffuse cortical thickening are recognized abnormal sonographic criteria for classifying a lymph node as abnormal with a recommendation for biopsy (Fig. 14.3a, b). In one series 10 of 17 with such abnormal features were histologically proven to be malignant. Six of these ten cases were metastatic adenocarcinoma and three were lymphoma and one was undifferentiated sarcoma [48]. Apart from metastatic breast cancer and lymphoma most commonly non-Hodgkin's type, metastasis from malignant melanoma, lung carcinoma, stomach carcinoma, or ovarian carcinoma should be considered [49]. Breast MRI is useful in further evaluation of a patient with a biopsy-proven metastatic adenocarcinoma in an axillary lymph node with a mammographically and clinically occult ipsilateral breast cancer [50]. In a review of eight retrospective studies, MRI was able to detect cancers in more than two-thirds of patients; in 80 % of these cases, a second-look ultrasound was able to find the MRI-detected abnormality. MRI provided a possibility of a breast-conserving surgery in one-third of these patients [50]. A finding of an isolated abnormal axillary lymph and a normal mammogram is best managed by a whole breast and axillary ultrasound followed by fine needle or a core needle biopsy under ultrasound guidance. If metastatic adenocarcinoma is found, an MRI is indicated to identify an occult cancer.

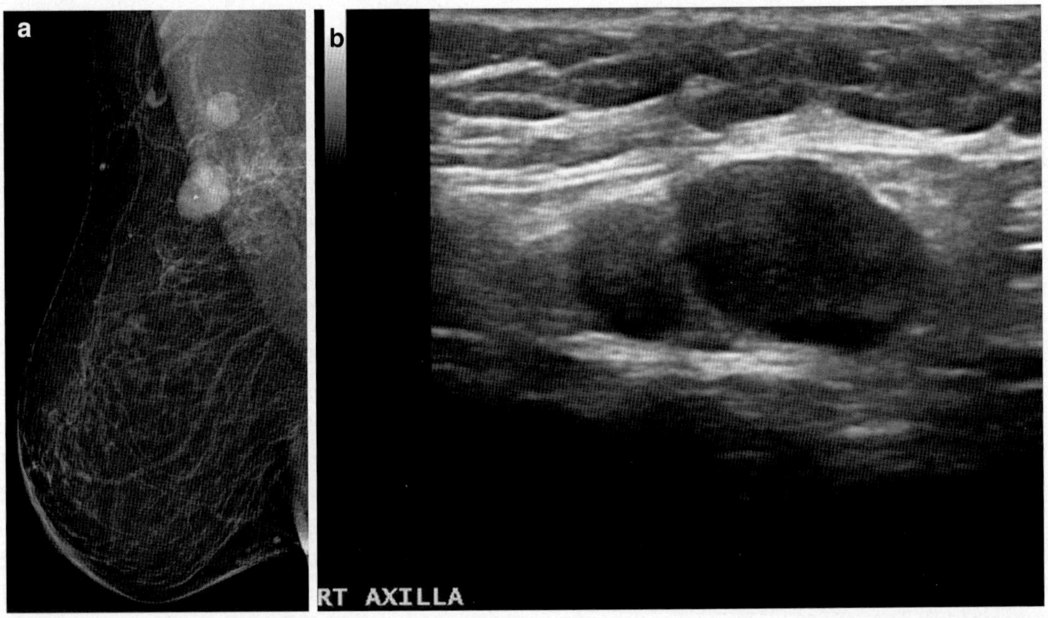

Fig. 14.3 Isolated enlarged right axillary lymph node histologically proven to be benign reactive follicular hyperplasia. (**a**) Right breast mammogram with an enlarged dense fat replaced lymph node with a post-biopsy clip within. There was no mammographic or clinical abnormality in the right breast. (**b**) Ultrasound demonstrates an abnormal enlarged lymph node with absence of fat hilum

Challenges in breast imaging are many, and these challenges often may not have a standardized management protocol; decisions may have to be made based on available resources and expertise as well as the individual patient. Some of the commonly encountered challenges have been discussed previously. Management decisions will continue to evolve as our knowledge in understanding the many facets of breast cancer screening and diagnosis unfolds in the future as technologies and expertise evolves.

References

1. Di Maggio C. State of the art of current modalities for the diagnosis of breast lesions. Eur J Nucl Med Mol Imaging. 2004;31 Suppl 1:S56–69.
2. Shiffman MA. Mammograms in cosmetic breast surgery. Indian J Plast Surg. 2005;38:100–4.
3. Perras C. Fifteen years of mammography in cosmetic surgery of the breast. Aesthetic Plast Surg. 1990;14(2):81–4.
4. Kroll SS, Schusterman MA, Tadjalli HE, Singletary SE, Ames F. Risk of recurrence after treatment of early breast cancer with skin-sparing mastectomy. Ann Surg Oncol. 1997;4(3):193–7.
5. Sim YT, Litherland JC. The use of imaging in patients post breast reconstruction. Clin Radiol. 2012;67(2):128–33.
6. Destounis S, Morgan R, Arieno A, Seifert P, Somerville P, Murphy P. A review of breast imaging following mastectomy with or without reconstruction in an outpatient community center. Breast Cancer. 2011;18(4):259–67.
7. Helvie MA, Wilson TE, Roubidoux MA, Wilkins EG, Chang AE. Mammographic appearance of recurrent breast carcinoma with TRAM flap breast reconstructions. Radiology. 1998;209:711–5.
8. Helvie M, Bailey J, Roubidoux M, Pass H, Chang A, Pierce L, et al. Mammographic screening of TRAM flap breast reconstructions for detection of non-palpable recurrent cancer. Radiology. 2002;224:211–6.
9. Howard MB, Battaglia T, Prout M, Freund K. The effect of imaging on the clinical management of breast pain. J Gen Intern Med. 2012;27(7):817–24.
10. Lumachi F, Ermani M, Brandes AA, et al. Breast complaints and risk of breast cancer. Population-based study of 2,879 self-selected women and long-term follow-up. Biomed Pharmacother. 2002;56(2):88–92.
11. Smith RL, Pruthi S, Fitzpatrick LA. Evaluation and management of breast pain. Mayo Clin Proc. 2004;79(3):353–72.
12. Duijm LEM, Guit GL, Hendriks JHCL, Zaat JOM, Mali WPTM. Value of breast imaging in women with painful breasts: observational follow up study. Br Med J. 1998;317(7171):1492–5.
13. Chang JM, Moon WK, Cho N, Han W, Noh DY, Park IA, Jung EJ. Risk of carcinoma after subsequent excision of benign papilloma initially diagnosed with an ultrasound (US)-guided 14-gauge core needle biopsy: a prospective observational study. Eur Radiol. 2010;20(5):1093–100.
14. Liberman L, Tornos C, Huzjan R, Bartella L, Morris EA, Dershaw DD. Is surgical excision warranted after benign, concordant diagnosis of papilloma at percutaneous breast biopsy? AJR Am J Roentgenol. 2006;186:1328–34.
15. Kim WH, Chang JM, Moon WK, Cho N, Yi A, Koo HR, Kim SJ. Intraductal mass on breast ultrasound: final outcomes and predictors of malignancy. AJR Am J Roentgenol. 2013;200(4):932–7.
16. Shin S, Schneider HB, Cole Jr FJ, Laronga C. Follow-up recommendations for benign breast biopsies. Breast J. 2006;12(5):413–7.
17. Daly CP, Bailey JE, Klein KA, Helvie MA. Complicated breast cysts on sonography: is aspiration necessary to exclude malignancy? Acad Radiol. 2008;15(5):610–7.
18. Ciatto S, Cariaggi P, Bulgaresi P. The value of routine cytologic examination of breast cyst fluids. Acta Cytol. 1987;31(3):301–4.

19. Berg WA, Campassi CI, Ioffe OB. Cystic lesions of the breast: sonographic-pathologic correlation. Radiology. 2003;227(1):183–91.
20. Sanders LM, Lacz NL, Lara J. 16 year experience with aspiration of noncomplex breast cysts: cytology results with focus on positive cases. Breast J. 2012;18(5):443–52.
21. Gottlieb S. Ultrasound plus mammography may detect more early cancers. BMJ. 2002;325:678.
22. Stomper PC, D'Souza DJ, DiNitto PA, Arredondo MA. Analysis of parenchymal density on mammograms in 1353 women 25–79 years old. AJR Am J Roentgenol. 1996;167:1261–5.
23. Boyd NF, Guo H, Martin LJ, et al. Mammographic density and the risk and detection of breast cancer. N Engl J Med. 2007;356: 227–336.
24. Berg WA, Blume JD, Cormack JB, et al. Combined screening with ultrasound and mammography vs mammography alone in women at elevated risk of breast cancer. JAMA. 2008;299:2151–63.
25. Weigert J, Steenbergen S. The Connecticut experiment: the role of ultrasound in the screening of women with dense breasts. Breast J. 2012;18(6):517–22.
26. Parris T, Wakefield D, Frimmer H. Real world performance of screening breast ultrasound following enactment of Connecticut Bill 458. Breast J. 2013;19(1):64–70.
27. Hooley RJ, Greenberg KL, Stackhouse RM, Geisel JL, Butler RS, Philpotts LE. Screening US in patients with mammographically dense breasts: initial experience with Connecticut Public Act 09–41. Radiology. 2012;265(1):59–69.
28. Dinnes J, Moss S, Melia J, Blanks R, Song F, Kleijnen J. Effectiveness and cost-effectiveness of double reading of mammograms in breast cancer screening: findings of a systematic review. Breast. 2001;10(6):455–63.
29. Duijm LE, Groenewoud JH, Hendriks JH, de Koning HJ. Independent double reading of screening mammograms in The Netherlands : effect of arbitration following reader disagreements. Radiology. 2004;231(2):564–70.
30. Gilbert FJ, Astley SM, McGee MA, Gillan MG, Boggis CR, Griffiths PM, Duffy SW. Single reading with computer-aided detection and double reading of screening mammograms in the United Kingdom National Breast Screening Program. Radiology. 2006;241(1):47–53.
31. Taylor P, Potts HW. Computer aids and human second reading as interventions in screening mammography: two systematic reviews to compare effects on cancer detection and recall rate. Eur J Cancer. 2008;44(6):798–807.
32. Bennett RL, Blanks RG, Moss SM. Does the accuracy of single reading with CAD (computer-aided detection) compare with that of double reading?: A review of the literature. Clin Radiol. 2006;61(12):1023–8.
33. Brown J, Bryan S, Warren R. Mammography screening: an incremental cost effectiveness analysis of double versus single reading of mammograms. BMJ. 1996;312(7034):809–12.
34. Cairns J, Van Der Pol M. Cost-effectiveness of non-consensus double reading. Breast. 1998;7(5):243–6.
35. Chiarelli AM, Majpruz V, Brown P, Thériault M, Shumak R, Mai V. The contribution of clinical breast examination to the accuracy of breast screening. J Natl Cancer Inst. 2009;101(18):1236–43.
36. Bancej C, Decker K, Chiarelli A, Harrison M, Turner D, Brisson J. Contribution of clinical breast examination to mammography screening in the early detection of breast cancer. J Med Screen. 2003;10(1):16–21.
37. Feigin KN, Keating DM, Telford PM, Cohen MA. Clinical breast examination in a comprehensive breast cancer screening program: contribution and cost. Radiology. 2006;240(3):650–5.
38. Nguyen C, Kettler MD, Swirsky ME, Miller VI, Scott C, Krause R, Hadro JA. Male breast disease : pictorial review with radiologic-pathologic correlation. Radiographics. 2013;33(3):763–79.
39. Günhan-Bilgen I, Bozkaya H, Ustün E, Memiş A. Male breast disease: clinical, mammographic, and ultrasonographic features. Eur J Radiol. 2002;43(3):246–55.
40. Adibelli ZH, Oztekin O, Gunhan-Bilgen I, Postaci H, Uslu A, Ilhan E. Imaging characteristics of male breast disease. Breast J. 2010;16(5):510–8.
41. Chen L, Chantra PK, Larsen LH, Barton P, Rohitopakarn M, Zhu EQ, Bassett LW. Imaging characteristics of malignant lesions of the male breast. Radiographics. 2006;26(4):993–1006.
42. Jemal A, Siegel R, Xu J, Ward E. Cancer statistics, 2010. CA Cancer J Clin. 2010;60(5):277–300.
43. Bleyer A, Welch HG. Effect of three decades of screening mammography on breast-cancer incidence. N Engl J Med. 2012; 367(21):1998–2005.
44. Gur D, Sumkin JH. Screening for early detection of breast cancer: overdiagnosis versus suboptimal patient management. Radiology. 2013;268(2):327–8.
45. Lanitis S, Behranwala KA, Al-Mufti R, Hadjiminas D. Axillary metastatic disease as presentation of occult or contralateral breast cancer. Breast. 2009;18(4):225–7.
46. Patel T, Given-Wilson RM, Thomas V. The clinical importance of axillary lymphadenopathy detected on screening mammography: revisited. Clin Radiol. 2005;60(1):64–71.
47. Rosen PP, Kimmel M. Occult breast carcinoma presenting with axillary lymph node metastases: a follow-up study of 48 patients. Hum Pathol. 1990;21(5):518–23.
48. Shetty MK, Carpenter WS. Sonographic evaluation of isolated abnormal axillary lymph nodes identified on mammograms. J Ultrasound Med. 2004;23(1):63–71.
49. Görkem SB, O'Connell AM. Abnormal axillary lymph nodes on negative mammograms: causes other than breast cancer. Diagn Interv Radiol. 2012;18(5):473–9.
50. de Bresser J, de Vos B, van der Ent F, Hulsewé K. Breast MRI in clinically and mammographically occult breast cancer presenting with an axillary metastasis: a systematic review. Eur J Surg Oncol. 2010;36(2):114–9.

Staging of Breast Cancer

15

H. Carisa Le-Petross and Abigail S. Caudle

Introduction

Breast cancer remains the second most frequently diagnosed cancer in women (after skin cancer) in part owing to screening programs and advances in both diagnostic and treatment technology. Approximately 232,670 newly diagnosed cases of invasive breast cancer in women and 2,360 in men are expected in the United States during the year 2014 [1]. Even though breast cancer remains the number one cause of new cancer cases in the United States, data from one cancer institution indicate that the overall survival of patients has steadily improved over the past six decades [2]. The 5-year relative survival rate for women with invasive breast cancer has improved from 75 % in the mid-1970s to 90 % today. In the rest of the world, the implementation of screening programs has been suggested to reduce the detection of the breast cancer lesion from a palpable lesion to a non-palpable and radiographic lesion only. This outcome is likely related to several factors including early detection and diagnosis, development of systemic therapies, preoperative chemotherapy, and better local control with surgery and radiation therapy [2]. Therefore, accurate staging is important in predicting prognosis and clinical outcome as well as for treatment planning.

H.C. Le-Petross, MD, FRCPC (✉)
Department of Radiology, University of Texas MD Anderson Cancer Center, 155 Pressler St, Houston, TX 77030, USA
e-mail: hlepetross@mdanderson.org

A.S. Caudle, MD, MS
Department of Surgical Oncology, University of Texas MD Anderson Cancer Center,
1515 Holcombe Blvd, Unit 1484, Houston, TX 77030, USA
e-mail: ascaudle@mdanderson.org

Staging and Guidelines

When a breast cancer is initially diagnosed, the patient undergoes staging evaluation to determine the extent and severity of the cancer, to define the best individual care for that patient, and to estimate the prognosis and risks of recurrence and mortality. Staging also enables physicians to identify those patients who are eligible for clinical trials. Of the three classification systems used in the United States, the tumor, node, metastasis (TNM) system is the most clinically relevant. In the latest (seventh) edition of the American Joint Committee on Cancer Staging Manual, the TNM system acknowledges the increasing use of neoadjuvant therapy. Therefore, the TNM system incorporates both clinical and pathological features with initial or clinical staging (c) performed prior to surgery or neoadjuvant therapy, and pathology staging (p) usually follows the first treatment modality or surgery. After neoadjuvant therapy, the post-therapy pathological staging is recorded as "yp." The clinical tumor stage is based on tumor size (measured in centimeters) as determined by physical examination and imaging modalities, such as mammography, ultrasound (US), or magnetic resonance imaging (MRI). The other two systems are the Extent of Disease system used by the National Cancer Institute Surveillance, Epidemiology, and End Results Program (SEER) and the Summary Stage system used by state cancer registries. In this chapter, we will refer to only the TNM system.

The TNM system (Table 15.1) includes the primary breast tumor size, the spread of cancer to the regional lymph nodes, and the spread of cancer to distant sites [3]. The pathological staging is based on the tumor size of the final pathology specimen. When there are multiple synchronous ipsilateral primary breast carcinomas, the largest tumor is used. For patients treated with neoadjuvant therapy, pathological or post-therapy size is designated with "ypT" and defined as the largest contiguous focus of invasive cancer with a subscript to indicate the presence of multifocal disease. Once the tumor size, node status, and presence of metastatic disease

M.K. Shetty (ed.), *Breast Cancer Screening and Diagnosis: A Synopsis*,
DOI 10.1007/978-1-4939-1267-4_15, © Springer Science+Business Media New York 2015

Table 15.1 AJCC TNM classification of breast cancer

T	*Primary tumor*
Tx	Primary tumor cannot be assessed
To	Primary tumor cannot be detected
Tis	[a]DCIS, LCIS, Paget disease of the nipple with no tumor
T1	Tumor ≤ 2 cm in the greatest dimension
T1mic	Microinvasion ≤0.1 cm in the greatest dimension
T1a	Tumor >0.1 cm but ≤0.5 cm in the greatest dimension
T1b	Tumor >0.5 cm but ≤1 cm in the greatest dimension
T1c	Tumor >1 cm but ≤2 cm in the greatest dimension
T2	Tumor > 2 cm but ≤5 cm in the greatest dimension
T3	Tumor > 5 cm in the greatest dimension
T4	Tumor of any size with direct extension to chest wall or skin
T4a	Extension to the chest wall, but not pectoralis muscle
T4b	Edema (including peau d'orange or ulceration of the skin of the breast or satellite skin nodules confined to the same breast)
T4c	Both T4a and 4b
T4d	Inflammatory carcinoma
N	*Regional lymph nodes*
Nx	Regional lymph nodes cannot be assessed
N0	No regional lymph node metastasis
N1	Micrometastasis
	Metastases in 1–3 axillary lymph nodes ± internal mammary nodes
N2	Metastases in 10 or more axillary lymph nodes
	Infraclavicular lymph nodes (level III)
	Clinically detected internal mammary lymph nodes
	>3 axillary lymph nodes and internal mammary nodes
	Ipsilateral supraclavicular lymph nodes
N3	Metastases in 10 or more axillary lymph nodes
	Metastases to infraclavicular lymph nodes (level III)
M	*Distant metastases*
M0	No distant metastases
cM0 (i+)	Circulating tumor cells or microscopic tumor cells in the bone marrow
	No clinical or radiological distant metastasis
M1	Distant metastases

Used with permission from Edge et al. [3]
[a]DCIS, ductal carcinoma in situ; LCIS, lobular carcinoma in situ

Table 15.2 AJCC stage grouping classification of breast cancer

Stage grouping	
Stage 0	Tis N_0 M_0
Stage I	T_1 N_0 M_0
Stage IIA	T_0 N_1 M_0
	T_1* N_1 M_0
	T_2 N_0 M_0
Stage IIB	T_2 N_1 M_0
	T_3 N_0 M_0
Stage IIIA	T_0 N_2 M_0
	T_1* N_2 M_0
	T_2 N_2 M_0
	T_3 N_1 M_0
	T_3 N_2 M_0
Stage IIIB	T_4 N_0 M_0
	T_4 N_1 M_0
	T_4 N_2 M_0
Stage IIIC	Any T N_3 M_0
Stage IV	Any T Any N M_1

Used with permission from Edge et al. [3]

have been determined, one of the five breast cancer stages is assigned (Table 15.2). Stage 0 is assigned to precancerous lesions or carcinoma in situ with no local or distant metastasis; this stage is associated with a cure rate of nearly 100 %. Stage I is assigned to small cancers confined to the breast; patients with stage I disease have an excellent prognosis. Stage II cancers have regional lymph node metastases, and stage III breast cancers have large tumors or locally advanced disease at the time of initial diagnosis. Stages II and III are associated with a poor prognosis. Stage IV cancers have a distant metastasis and are associated with a poor survival.

The prognostic factors to estimate the chance of recurrent disease and distant metastases include tumor size, histological grade, and lymph node status. Breast cancer cells can spread via the lymphatic system to the regional lymph nodes, involving the low axillary lymph nodes (level I) first followed by the mid- (level II) and high axillary lymph nodes (level III) (Fig. 15.1). Level I lymph nodes are lateral to the lateral border of the pectoralis minor muscle. Level II lymph nodes are between the medial and lateral borders of the pectoralis minor muscle and also include interpectoral lymph nodes (Rotter's nodes). Level III lymph nodes are nodes medial to the medial margin of the pectoralis minor muscle and inferior to the clavicle and are not commonly resected due to an increased risk of lymphedema. The standard approach to staging lymph nodes via axillary nodal dissection often involves removal of the low and mid-axillary lymph nodes. 12–25 % of breast cancer patients have internal mammary drainage with approximately 9–30 % with internal mammary nodal metastases, often those with large and deep medially located breast cancer, who can have a 5-year survival of 95 % after appropriate therapy [4, 5]. The seventh edition of the TNM staging manual considers internal mammary lymph nodes to be axillary nodes for the purposes of staging (cN2b or cN2c). If supraclavicular nodes are involved, then this is designated as N3 disease with poorer prognosis, because patients with infraclavicular and supraclavicular nodal disease tend to have increased tumor burden compared with those with only axillary nodal disease.

The National Comprehensive Cancer Network (NCCN) Guidelines for Breast Cancer are statements and consensus from experts regarding current acceptable approaches to the treatment of breast disease. The use of imaging in the staging evaluation of breast disease is also included. For example, the latest version (3.2013) of the NCCN guidelines includes breast MRI as an optional imaging work-up added for the

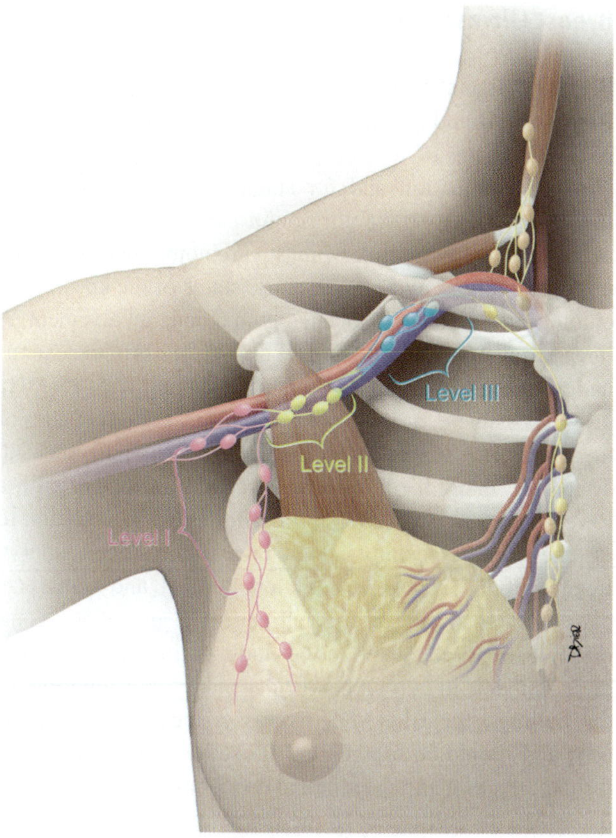

Fig. 15.1 Regional lymph node staging in breast cancer. Level I lymph nodes (*pink color*): nodes lateral to the pectoralis minor muscle (*brown muscle*). Level II lymph nodes (*yellow color*): nodes between the medial and lateral margins and posterior to the pectoralis minor muscle. Rotter's nodes are located between the pectoralis major and minor muscles. Level III lymph nodes (*sky blue color*): nodes medial to the pectoralis minor muscle and inferior to the clavicle (Courtesy of David Bier, Medical Illustrator, The University of Texas MD Anderson Cancer Center)

ductal carcinoma in situ (DCIS) staging evaluation. For invasive breast cancer, the uses of optional breast MRI for mammographically occult tumors, bone scan, or sodium fluoride PET/CT for clinical stage IIIA were added or modified [6].

Local Staging of Breast Cancer by Imaging

Mammography

Diagnostic mammography or problem-solving mammography is performed when a patient presents with a palpable finding or when a suspicious finding is detected with screening mammography. A radiopaque BB or skin marker may be placed directly over the suspicious region before the mammogram is obtained. Many facilities have adopted a filmless practice and have successfully converted from conventional film mammography to digital mammography. For both conventional and digital mammography, a standard examination consists of a mediolateral oblique and a craniocaudal view for each breast. Additional views may be indicated to properly evaluate the abnormality. These additional views include a 90° lateral view to triangulate the abnormality and spot compression views, in craniocaudal and lateral projections, and to evaluate a possible mass, asymmetric density, or superimposition of normal breast parenchyma. Magnification views, commonly performed in craniocaudal and lateral projections, facilitate characterization of microcalcifications. With advances in digital acquisition and processing technology, digital tomosynthesis is being incorporated into mammography systems and may provide a solution to the problem of distinguishing overlapping structures in the breast, increasing the sensitivity and specificity of mammography for cancer detection and diagnosis [7]. Clinical trials are currently under way to establish the efficacy of digital breast tomosynthesis and to define its role in future practice.

In contrast to a screening mammography examination, a diagnostic mammogram can also provide valuable information during the staging work-up of a newly diagnosed breast cancer. If a patient has DCIS with associated microcalcifications, then magnification views are needed to determine the extent of the microcalcifications, the multifocal or multicentric distribution, and the proximity of the calcifications to the nipple. The accuracy of this information is very important because this disease has a favorable prognosis if there is no progression to invasive carcinoma, and the treatment options for DCIS include breast-conserving surgery with radiation therapy or mastectomy. Accurate size measurement of the area of involvement can help clinicians determine the best surgical approach. In general, an axillary lymph node dissection is not necessary, but a sentinel lymph node biopsy would be performed. If noncontiguous groups of suspicious microcalcifications are identified during the staging evaluation, then mammographic-guided breast interventions such as stereotactic-guided core biopsy using vacuum-assisted devices would be suggested. Prior to surgery, mammographic-guided needle localization of multiple sites or bracketing of a large area is commonly performed to assist surgeons in obtaining negative margins at surgery (Fig. 15.2). Immediately after resection of the targeted lesion, the biopsy or surgically resected specimen can be imaged while the patient is still under anesthesia in order to verify the margins. This "specimen radiography" is very helpful, not only to optimize the chance of obtaining final negative margins but also to provide additional information in patients who had a complete response to preoperative chemotherapy, as the only image-detectable finding is often the biopsy clip placed at the time of the initial biopsy or residual calcifications (Fig. 15.3). Radioactive seed localization is being incorporated into several practices, replacing wire localization prior to surgery, due to several advantages. These advantages include precise knowledge of the tumor with the radioactive seed, allowing the surgeon to determine the incisional site. Also, the radiologist's localization approach can be independent of the surgeon's incisional approach, and the seed(s) can be placed days prior to surgery [8].

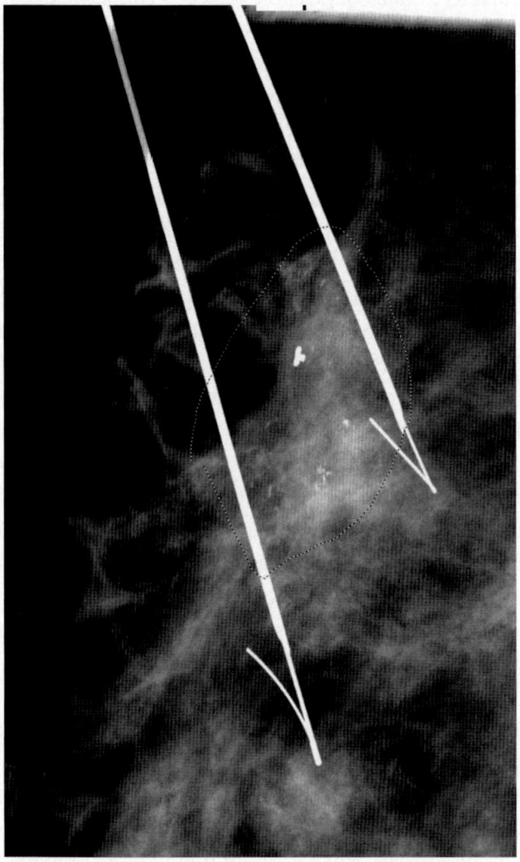

Fig. 15.2 Preoperative needle localization. A 57-year-old female with a diagnosis of ductal carcinoma in situ (DCIS) of the breast. The 3 cm area of pleomorphic calcifications (area demarcated with faint *doted circle*) was bracketed on the day of surgery using two Kopans localization needles. Final pathology confirmed a 3.5 cm area of DCIS successfully resected with final negative surgical margins

Breast Ultrasound

Primary Breast Site

Breast ultrasound is commonly used as a diagnostic tool for characterization of lesions detected via mammography or clinical examination and for staging of newly diagnosed breast cancer. A breast ultrasound examination can determine the size of the index breast carcinoma; determine the unifocal, multifocal, or multicentric status of the known carcinoma; and evaluate associated lymph node involvement. A linear array transducer should be used to perform the examination utilizing the highest center frequency (7.5–18-MHz probe) possible in order to provide high-resolution images of the breast. However, penetration to the chest wall is needed. Therefore, many facilities have a second transducer with a lower frequency (2–5-MHz probe) for better penetration to the chest wall, especially in large breasts with deep lesion(s). Images of the lesion in both longitudinal and transverse planes or radial and orthogonal antiradial planes are commonly used to characterize the findings, in order to obtain measurements in two perpendicular planes. For reporting of the findings, the BI-RADS risk assessment categories are used and should be adhered to [9]. At our facility, the entire ipsilateral breast and the regional nodal basins are scanned to determine the full extent of the index lesion, any associated satellite or synchronous lesions, and associated nodal disease.

Breast tumors are usually hypoechoic solid masses, with irregular margins, posterior acoustic shadowing, and internal vascularity on color Doppler imaging (Fig. 15.4). Unlike invasive ductal carcinoma, invasive lobular carcinoma does not tend to form a dominant or palpable mass but presents as vague architectural distortion or focal asymmetry on mammography [10, 11]. This is likely due to the microscopic single-file growing pattern of the tumor cells and their infiltrative nature, which result in high false-negative rates on mammography. US has been reported to have higher sensi-

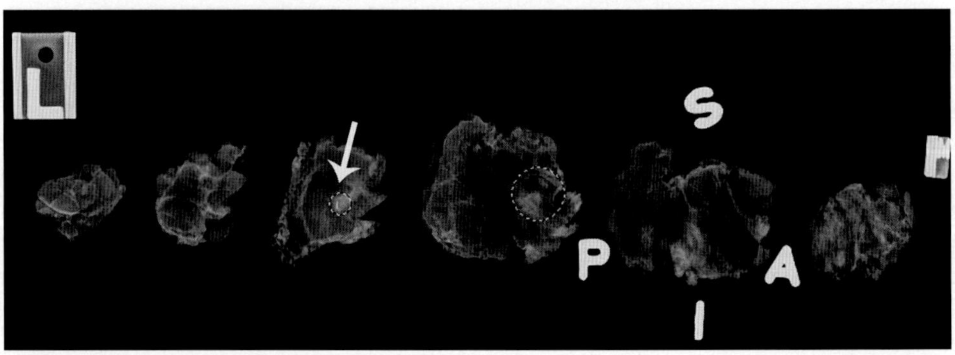

Fig. 15.3 Specimen x-ray. A 56-year-old female with invasive ductal carcinoma of the breast who received segmentectomy after completion of neoadjuvant chemotherapy. The biopsy clip: and the doted circles (*white arrow and the doted circles*) visible on the specimen radiograph confirmed the site of biopsy-proven carcinoma. Final pathology revealed no residual tumor. *S* superior margin, *P* posterior margin, *I* inferior margin, *A* anterior margin

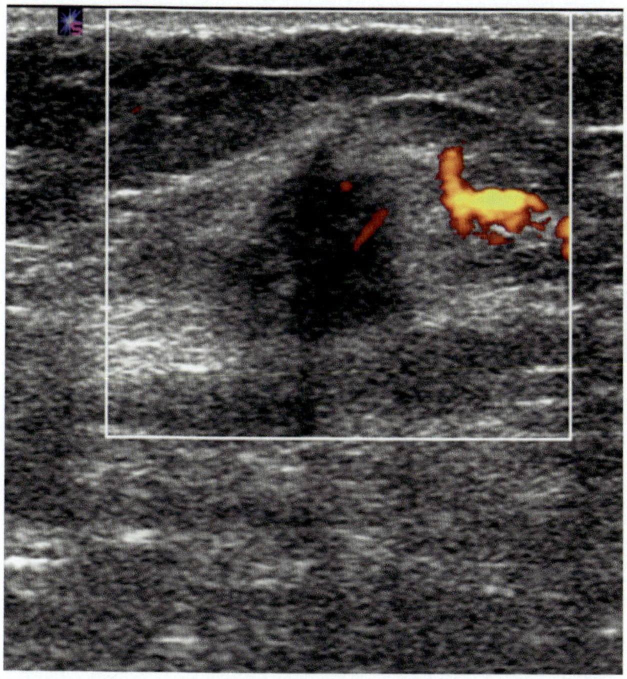

Fig. 15.4 Ultrasound of breast carcinoma. Power Doppler ultrasound of the right breast (*white box*) in a 58-year-old female showing a 1.6 cm hypoechoic solid mass with posterior shadowing and internal vascularity, which was biopsy-proven carcinoma

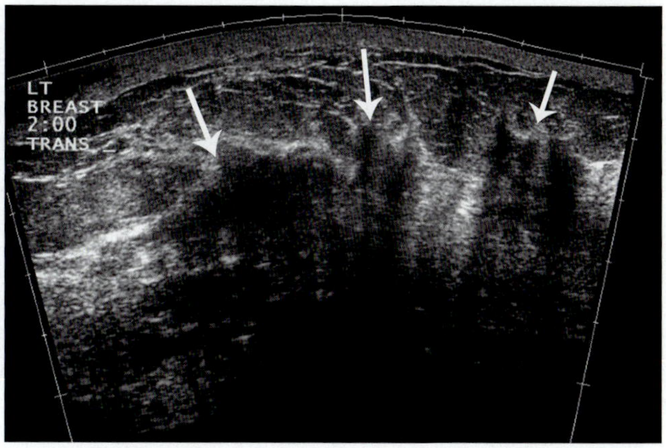

Fig. 15.5 Extended-field-of-view ultrasound. A 43-year-old female with multicentric invasive ductal breast carcinoma. Extended-field-of-view ultrasound imaging of the left breast demonstrates multiple areas (*arrows*) of heterogeneous shadowing tissue and distortion of the normal tissue. Biopsy confirmed invasive ductal carcinoma at 2 sites and final pathology at mastectomy showed a 9×5 cm area of tumor

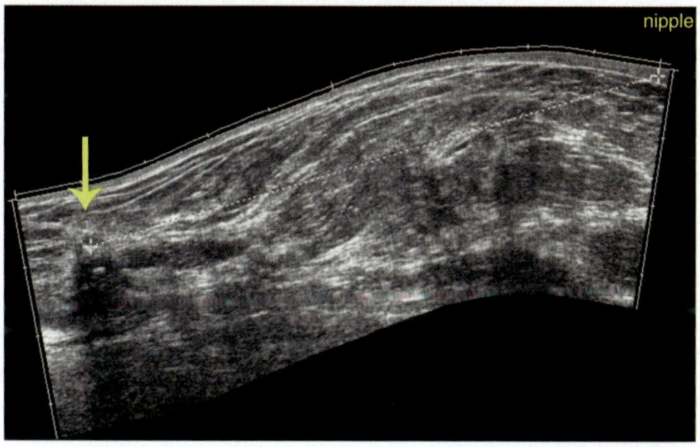

Fig. 15.6 Ultrasound: distance from nipple. Extended-field-of-view ultrasound imaging of the right breast demonstrates how the measurement of the distance from the hypoechoic irregular carcinoma (*yellow arrow*) to the nipple is measured

tivity in the detection of invasive lobular carcinoma, with the most common imaging feature being a hypoechoic mass or masses with posterior acoustic shadowing, in an infiltrative pattern [12–16].

Most invasive carcinomas have a mixture of invasive and noninvasive or intraductal components. The intraductal components or DCIS may present as linear hypoechoic long ductal extensions with an extensive branching pattern from the index mass towards the nipple, or linear extensions between hypoechoic masses. Sometimes the calcifications associated with DCIS can be detected on ultrasound as smaller hyperechoic foci within distended ducts or within a suspicious mass [17]. Some DCIS present as intraductal or intracystic masses [18]. In addition, US can be used as an adjuvant modality to detect any associated invasive carcinoma in patients with newly diagnosed DCIS, and ultrasound-guided biopsy is performed. For multicentric disease in which the lesions are more than 5 cm apart or the multiple tumor foci lie in different quadrants of the breast, extended field of view is commonly used in some facilities (Fig. 15.5). This technology allows the radiologist to present a wider field of view than is available using standard real-time transducers. In addition to imaging multiple lesions on one image, the extended field of view also enables the operator to provide an image documenting the distance of the index mass from the nipple (Fig. 15.6).

Regional Lymph Nodes

Nodal Staging y Imaging

Ultrasound of the nodal basins is being performed at more facilities now than previously, in both academic and private practices. In many places, sonographic evaluation of the ipsilateral axilla is conducted for all newly diagnosed breast cancer cases to assess the size and morphology of any suspicious or abnormal nodes. When a lymph node is infiltrated with tumor, the size of the lymph node is usually increased in addition to the change in the cortical morphology of that node. Abnormal cortical morphology includes eccentric cortical thickening with focal cortical lobulation, or diffuse hypoechoic lymph node with the loss of the central echogenic hilum [19, 20]. The morphology of the lymph node is suggested to be more specific (88.4–98.1 %) than the lymph

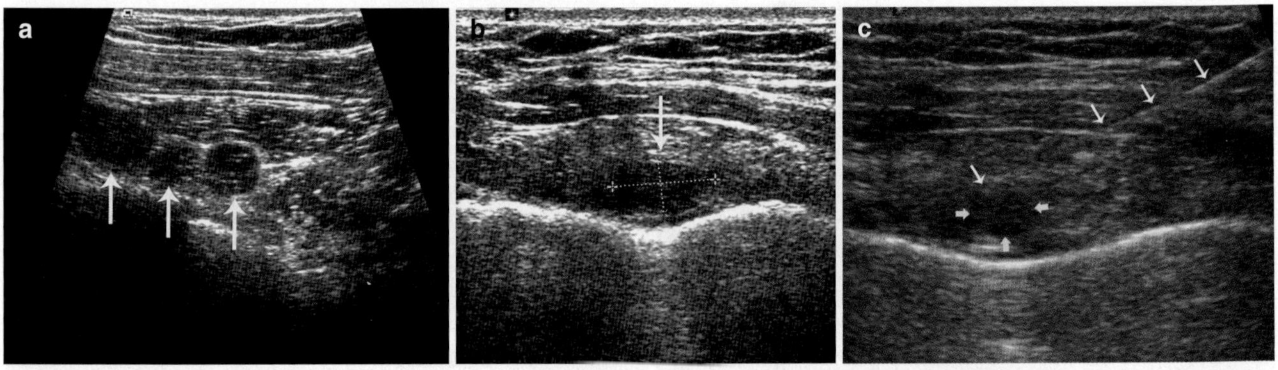

Fig. 15.7 (**a**–**c**) Staging ultrasound of the infraclavicular and internal mammary nodal basins. (**a**) Transverse grayscale ultrasound shows abnormal round hypoechoic infraclavicular lymph nodes (*three arrows*) without central fatty hila. (**b**) Transverse grayscale ultrasound shows an abnormal enlarged hypoechoic lymph node (*single arrow and doted lines*) in the first internal mammary space. (**c**) Fine-needle aspiration biopsy (*white arrows along needle shaft*) confirmed metastatic lymph node (*yellow arrows*)

node size (55.6–97.3 %) [21]. Upon detection of an abnormal lymph node, pathology confirmation of nodal malignancy can be performed prior to surgery by ultrasound-guided core biopsy or fine-needle aspiration biopsy. This information may assist the surgeon in the decision to proceed directly to an axillary lymph node dissection (ALND) as opposed to a sentinel lymph node biopsy (SLND). Radiological marker placement at the time of the ultrasound-guided biopsy can aid in facilitating subsequent confirmation of biopsy-proven metastatic node recovery or in ensuring the complete removal of the breast cancer that has disappeared after the completion of neoadjuvant chemotherapy. At our institution, the infraclavicular and internal mammary nodal basins are also evaluated at the initial staging sonographic examination of all newly diagnosed breast cancer cases (Fig. 15.7a–c).

Nodal Staging by Surgery

Sentinel lymph node dissection (SLND) is based on the concept that the breast has an orderly pattern of lymphatic drainage with specific lymph nodes, or sentinel nodes, that drain the breast first, followed by drainage to the remaining nodal basin. This idea was first reported by Braithwaite over 100 years ago after observing the lymphatic drainage pattern of a gangrenous appendix. The first clinical applications were presented in the 1970s for penile cancer, although the technique did not become widely used because of its difficulty [22]. In the early 1990s, a more facile technique was created for melanoma that allowed for widespread implementation [23]. Previously, women had usually undergone ALND for staging of axillary nodes, with associated morbidities including functional deficits, chronic pain, and development of lymphedema. Unfortunately, many of these patients had no nodal metastases and thus suffered the morbidities without an oncologic benefit. Thus, there was tremendous interest in applying SLND to breast cancer patients, and SLND was quickly validated as an accurate technique for staging nodal basins in breast cancer patients with increased sensitivity and decreased risks [24–26]. There are many variations in the SLND technique, although all involve the basic principle of injecting the breast with a mapping agent or combination of agents (usually radioisotope and blue dye), which is then allowed to drain to the nodal regions and collect in the sentinel node(s). This can be performed preoperatively or intraoperatively. At the time of surgery, any node collecting the mapping agent (as determined by being blue if blue dye is used or being "hot," i.e., having increased radioactivity by handheld Geiger probe if radioisotope is injected) are removed and sent for pathological evaluation.

In clinically node-negative patients who are undergoing surgery as the first component of their breast cancer treatment, SLND is the standard surgical approach to axillary staging. Multiple studies have demonstrated that an SLN can be identified in 93–99 % of patients with a false-negative rate (i.e., number of patients with axillary metastases in which no cancer is seen in the SLN) of 5–11 % [27, 28]. If the SLN is negative for metastases, then no further axillary surgery is required and the remaining lymph nodes can be left in place. While initially all patients with axillary metastases underwent ALND, this paradigm has shifted since the American College of Surgeons Oncology Group (ACOSOG) Z0011 trial, which demonstrated that ALND can be safely omitted in carefully selected patients with early-stage breast cancer who undergo breast-conservation therapy and whole-breast radiation [7, 29]. ALND is still recommended for patients who do not meet the eligibility criteria for this trial, such as those with large tumors or extensive nodal involvement, those who have received neoadjuvant chemotherapy (NCT), or those undergoing mastectomy [30].

Axillary lymph node dissection is now performed only if there is confirmation of axillary metastases, either by ultrasound and needle biopsy or by SLND. ALND allows for a more thorough staging of the axillary nodes because all

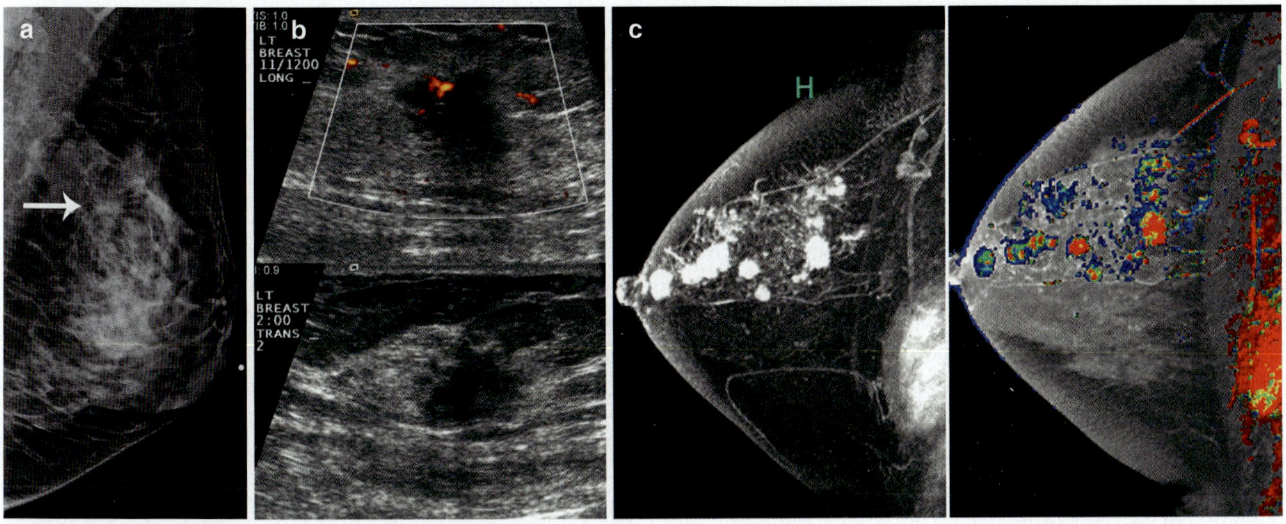

Fig. 15.8 (**a–c**) MRI detects additional lesions. (**a**) Right mediolateral oblique mammogram shows an architectural distortion (*white arrow*) at the 12 o'clock position. (**b**) Grayscale ultrasound reveals two irregular suspicious masses at 12 and 2 o'clock positions. (**c**) Sagittal maximum-intensity projection images show over 6 masses in the superior breast, and final pathology at mastectomy confirms multicentric disease

nodes are removed and the total number of involved nodes can be counted. In addition to being a diagnostic procedure, there is also a therapeutic advantage to ALND in node-positive women [31]. Standard ALND involves the removal of the level I and II axillary lymph nodes. Level III nodes are not routinely removed unless there is evidence of their involvement. Unfortunately, ALND is associated with significant short- and long-term morbidities. Short-term effects include the need for uncomfortable postoperative drains and the potential for seromas. Ligation of intercostobrachial nerves, which often occurs during the resection, can lead to pain and neuropathies that can be permanent. Functional limitations of arm abduction are common in the immediate postoperative period and may persist even with aggressive physical therapy. Perhaps the most significant effect is the possibility of lymphedema, which requires aggressive and time-consuming therapy with physical therapy, diet modifications, and compression garments and which carries an increased risk of cellulitis [32].

Breast MRI

Technique

A breast MRI is performed with the patient lying in a prone position within a 1.5 T or higher magnetic field strength scanner. Only breast-dedicated multiphase array coils should be used to ensure adequate spatial resolution. The examination usually utilizes bilateral imaging techniques for several reasons, including the ability to assess asymmetric enhancement between the breasts as well as evaluation for contralateral carcinoma in patients with newly diagnosed breast cancer. Common sequences of a standard examination include a precontrast T1-weighted pulse sequence to delineate fat from a lesion or lymph node, a precontrast T2-weighted pulse sequence with fat suppression to separate cysts from most solid masses, a time series of contrast-enhanced T1-weighted sequences to enhance detection of breast masses, or a dynamic contrast-enhanced series. This series usually consists of a minimum of three time points over a 6–8-min period after intravenous administration of the contrast medium. The minimal imaging parameter requirements for the dynamic acquisition as recommended by the American College of Radiology include a slice thickness ≤3 mm and in-plane resolution ≤1 mm to facilitate the evaluation of essential morphological details such as lesion margins, spiculations, and internal enhancement [33]. Interpretation is based on the descriptors from the BI-RADS MRI lexicon [34].

Role of MRI in Breast Cancer Staging

During the last decade, breast MRI was routinely used in the preoperative evaluation of newly diagnosed breast cancer cases for assessing the extent of the primary tumor site and for identifying mammographically or sonographically occult multicentric and contralateral cancers [Fig. 15.8a–c]. In the last few years, this practice has been heavily scrutinized, and the role of MRI in staging remains a source of considerable discussion. MRI can be helpful in defining the extent and size of the primary breast carcinoma and in detecting additional foci of malignancy within the ipsilateral breast in up to 16 % of patients, and MRI can detect malignancies that were occult on mammography within the contralateral breast in up to 4 % of patients [35, 36]. A meta-analysis of 19 studies and prospective randomized trials consisting of 2,610 patients reported that the addition of MRI-detected lesions resulted in more extensive surgery than planned, with conversion from breast-conserving surgery to mastectomy or a larger excision in 19 % of patients [35]. No benefit on the reoperation rate was reported [35, 37]. Initially, there was an assumption that treatment of additional foci of tumor visible only on MRI would result in better clinical and survival outcomes. A retrospective study of 756 women with breast cancer comparing women who had preoperative breast MRI and women who did not have breast MRI reported no significant difference in the local recurrence rate ($P=0.51$) after a median follow-up of 4.6 years [38]. Two years later, the COMICE (comparative effectiveness of MRI in breast cancer) multicenter trial from the United Kingdom reported no significant reduction in the reoperation rate in the women who were randomly assigned to receive MRI compared with those who did not receive MRI ($P=0.77$) [37]. While these publications suggested that preoperative MRI is not necessarily indicated for every patient, the ability of MRI to detect additional tumor foci and contralateral cancer not detected via physical examination or mammography should not be discounted. Lehman et al. [39] reported a 3.1 % incidence of contralateral malignancy detected by MRI only and not seen with mammography or clinical examination. The effect of preoperative MRI-based decisions on recurrent disease or overall survival remains unclear and is a subject for future clinical research. Breast MRI is still recommended for selected cases of invasive lobular carcinoma or inflammatory breast cancer, to assess tumor involvement in the skin, nipple, and/or chest wall (Fig. 15.9a, b) [40, 41]. Because of the diffuse infiltrative growth pattern of invasive lobular carcinoma, MRI may allow better visualization of the tumor in a background of extensive fibrosis and help facilitate a more effective biopsy and surgical plan. At our institution, all patients who present with adenocarcinoma in the axilla without a diagnosis of a primary carcinoma but with tumor markers raise the suspicion of an occult breast primary tumor, and MRI is recommended (Fig. 15.10a, b). This has been demonstrated to be beneficial in identifying the primary tumor [42]. When a primary breast lesion can be detected, proper staging can be performed, facilitating targeted therapy or consideration for breast conservation therapy in conjunction with radiotherapy, depending on the stage of the carcinoma.

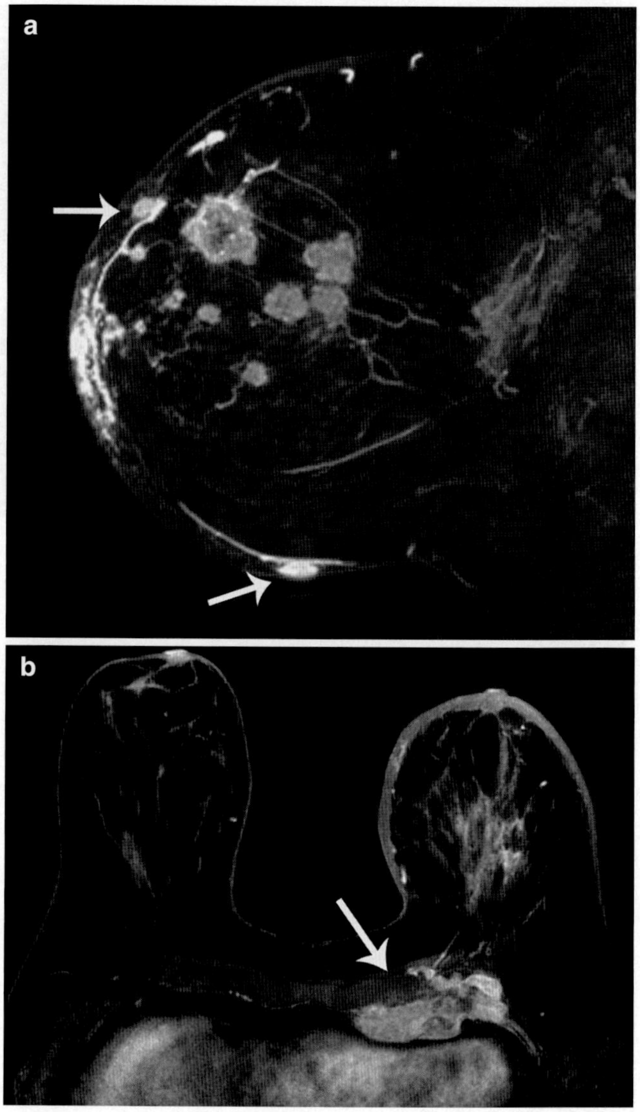

Fig. 15.9 (**a**, **b**) MRI detects skin and chest wall involvement. (**a**) Sagittal maximum-intensity projection MR image of the left breast in a patient with inflammatory breast carcinoma showing multiple enhancing lesions in the skin (*white arrows*). (**b**) Axial contrast-enhanced MR image shows an irregular chest wall mass extending into the anterior mediastinal region (*white arrow*) in a patient with invasive ductal carcinoma

DCIS is a noninvasive malignancy, and the patient is often asymptomatic; however, DCIS is associated with increased risk of developing invasive carcinoma that can involve multiple sites and intervening normal tissue. The prevalence of DCIS diagnoses in the United States has increased with the introduction of screening mammography and currently comprises 25–30 % of all reported breast cancers. However, mammography tends to underestimate both the size and extent of DCIS, especially when the DCIS is not associated with the characteristic pleomorphic microcalcifications [43]. MRI, on the other hand, has a reported sensitivity of 67–100 % for the detection of DCIS, whereas mammography has a sensitivity of 70–80 % [44, 45]. Common MRI features indicative of DCIS include clumped or heterogeneous enhancement in a linear, ductal, or segmental distribution. Despite these highly specific morphological features, current MRI techniques poorly differentiate benign proliferative disease from DCIS; thus, the specificity of MRI in the detection of DCIS remains low due to a high rate of false-negative findings [46]. Ultimately, MRI may be useful in cases in which mammography, ultrasound, and clinical findings are inconclusive and no focal finding is apparent; currently, approximately 95 % of DCIS cases are diagnosed via calcifications identified on mammography.

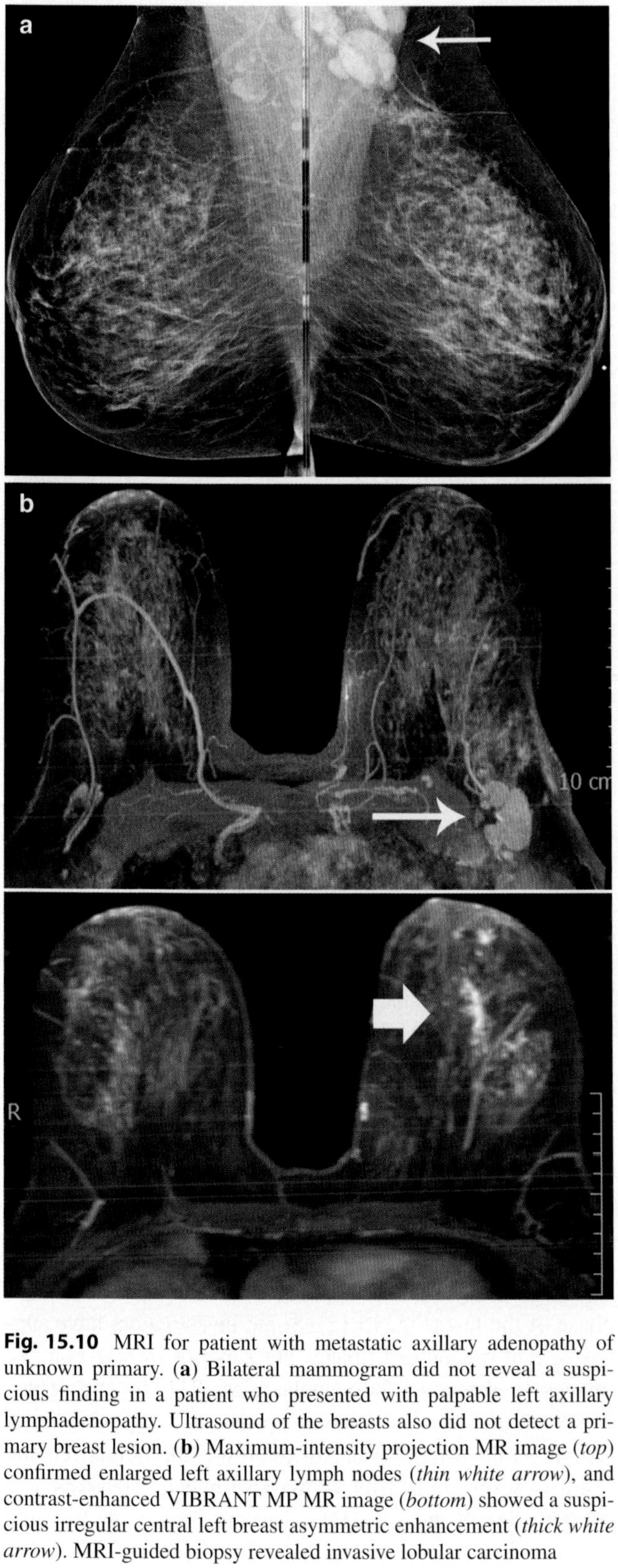

Fig. 15.10 MRI for patient with metastatic axillary adenopathy of unknown primary. (**a**) Bilateral mammogram did not reveal a suspicious finding in a patient who presented with palpable left axillary lymphadenopathy. Ultrasound of the breasts also did not detect a primary breast lesion. (**b**) Maximum-intensity projection MR image (*top*) confirmed enlarged left axillary lymph nodes (*thin white arrow*), and contrast-enhanced VIBRANT MP MR image (*bottom*) showed a suspicious irregular central left breast asymmetric enhancement (*thick white arrow*). MRI-guided biopsy revealed invasive lobular carcinoma

The low specificity of MRI (68 %) and high false-positive rates (32–45 %) lead to additional testing and biopsies, which can increase patient anxiety and medical costs and can delay treatment [47, 48]. If future MR technology could improve the specificity and positive predictive value of this examination, then the role of breast MRI in preoperative staging of breast cancer may become more accepted in the surgical community. The suggestion to combine MRI with functional imaging such as PET remains at a research level. The challenge for wide use in the community is the high cost of both imaging modalities and affordability for the general population in the current economy.

PET

Tumor cells may spread to distant sites via the lymphatic or circulatory system; the four major sites of distant metastasis for breast cancer are the bone, lung, brain, and liver. The bone is the most common site of metastasis from most subtypes of breast cancer, and the presence of tumor cells in the bone marrow is a strong predictor for distant metastases [6]. Cutaneous metastasis is not common, but breast carcinoma is the most common primary malignancy to spread to the skin and accounts for 24 % of all cutaneous metastases [49].

At the initial breast cancer diagnosis, it is important to determine the presence of any pathological nodal disease and distant metastases. Survival of patients with stage IV disease or metastases at presentation is poor despite new drugs and therapy, compared with patients with stage I or early breast cancer. It is estimated that about 10 % of patients with newly diagnosed breast cancer have distant metastases and 30 % of patients with early-stage breast cancer will develop recurrent disease [50].

FDG-PET/CT has been suggested to be more accurate for staging breast cancer than conventional imaging modalities such as plain chest radiography, bone scintigraphy, and axillary and liver ultrasound [51]. Riegger and colleagues reported on 106 breast cancer patients who received FDG-PET/CT and conventional imaging [51]. In 13 % of the cases, PET/CT detected synchronous tumors, nodal metastasis, or distant metastases not seen with conventional imaging (Fig. 15.11a–c) [51]. Many small-sample, single-institutional studies have confirmed that PET/CT is superior to conventional imaging in detecting unexpected distant metastases in patients with stage II to III breast cancer while maintaining a low false-positive rate [52–58]. Patients with inflammatory breast carcinoma or large noninflammatory breast carcinoma have a high risk of distant metastasis; PET/CT at the time of initial presentation is useful for detecting occult metastasis [56–58]. Most bone metastases from primary breast carcinoma are lytic or mixed. However, bone scan is still recommended for detecting sclerotic bony metastases due to the lower sensitivity of PET/CT in detecting these bony lesions [59, 60].

The role of PET/CT in the staging of early breast cancer or T1 lesion remains controversial, partially due to the limited spatial resolution of PET/CT. Small single-institu-

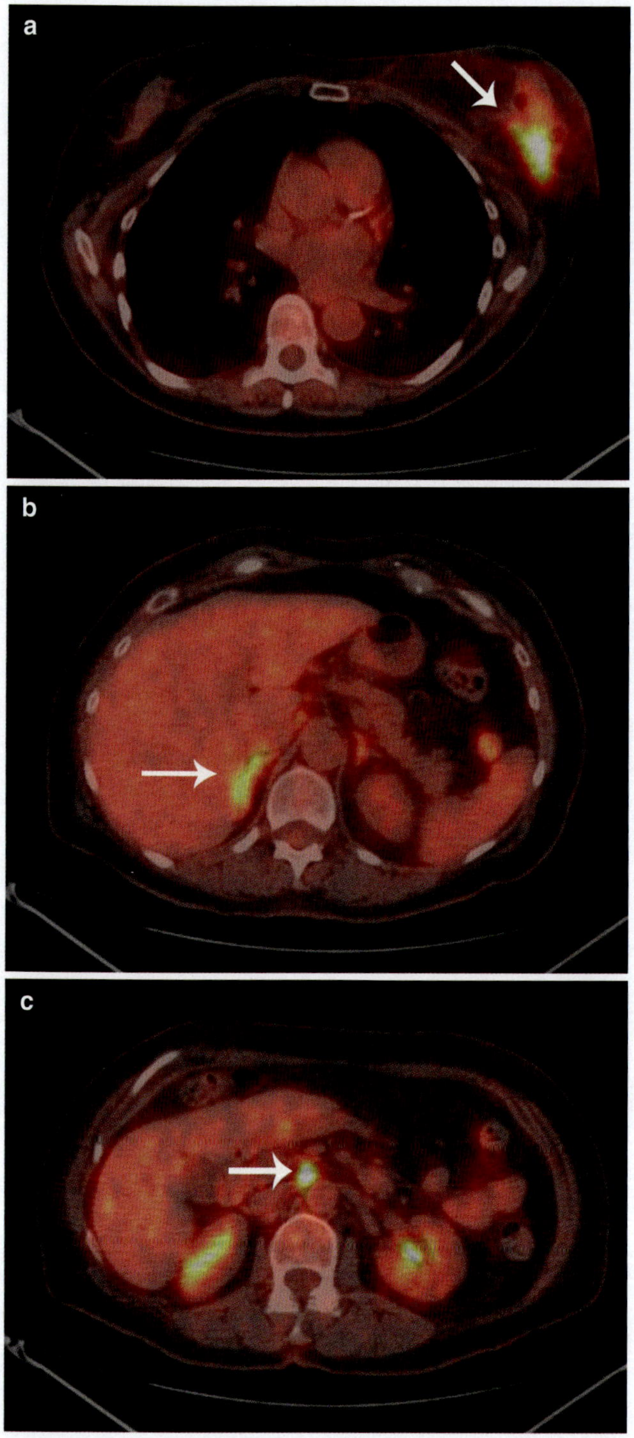

Fig. 15.11 PET/CT. Staging of a patient with newly diagnosed left breast carcinoma (**a**) with PET/CT shows right adrenal metastases (**b**) and nodal metastases (**c**) in the fused images

tional studies have confirmed that the primary lesion can be detected with PET/CT in the majority of cases, but breast MRI was superior in assessing the size of the primary breast lesion, ruling out multifocal multicentric disease, and more accurate in determining the need for mastectomy [61–64].

CT

Breast cancer commonly metastasizes to the bone, liver, lung, brain, and (less commonly) other organ systems. In patients with symptoms suspicious for pulmonary or liver metastasis from breast cancer, chest or abdominal CT is recommended. However, not all patients with newly diagnosed breast cancer receive intense surveillance with CT because it has not been shown to be useful in preoperative staging [25]. Abdominal CT is recommended in the 2013 NCCN guidelines for the staging assessment of stage I to III breast cancer cases if there are abnormal results for liver function tests, elevated alkaline phosphatase, abdominal symptoms, or abnormal results from the physical examination of the abdomen. Initial evaluation for metastatic breast cancer is important not only to determine the extent of the disease for treatment planning but also as a baseline study that can be used for future assessment of treatment effect. Even though PET/CT is becoming popular as a single test to evaluate both the visceral organs and bone, details and further characterization of the metastasis are needed for biopsy planning.

When there is a suspicion of lung metastasis, chest x-ray and CT of the chest are recommended. In newly diagnosed breast cancer cases, approximately 3 % of the women will have a solitary pulmonary nodule detected by chest x-ray, with approximately 33–40 % of those cases being pulmonary metastases from a primary breast cancer [65, 66]. Surgical resection of the solitary pulmonary metastasis has improved survival rate, with reported 5-year survival rates between 35 and 80 % [67]. The liver is the second most common site of metastasis, with hepatic metastases being found at autopsy in approximately 55–75 % of patients with breast cancer [68]. In such patients, prognosis is poor with an estimated survival of 6 months if not treated or 24 months if treated with chemotherapy [69, 70]. Therefore, abdominal CT is commonly used to evaluate hepatic metastases as well as to assess the response of these metastases to chemotherapy. Most hepatic metastases from breast cancer present on CT imaging as single or multiple vascular lesion(s) with indistinct margins, best appreciated on the portal venous phase of the test (Fig. 15.12). Some investigators have suggested that precontrast images are superior to post-contrast images in detecting these metastases [71]. In one series, 26 % of the liver metastases presented as hypervascular lesions on the arterial phase of the test [72]. Tamoxifen can result in severe fatty liver or massive hepatic steatosis as a complication of therapy [73]. Liver metastases can be more difficult to detect on abdominal CT when there is a background of hepatic steatosis. In these cases, our institution prefers abdominal MRI over CT. Some unusual patterns of liver metastases from breast cancer include cirrhotic-like appearance, lobar atrophy secondary to carcinoma involving the vascular or biliary system, and capsular retraction (Fig. 15.13) [74].

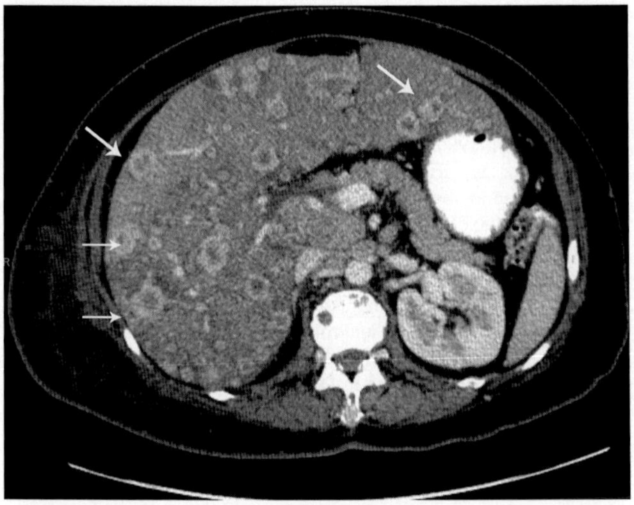

Fig. 15.12 CT of liver metastases. Contrast-enhanced computed tomography of the liver in a 52-year-old female with newly diagnosed inflammatory breast carcinoma. Staging evaluation revealed multiple vascular liver metastases (*white arrows*) and biopsy confirmed metastatic disease from breast carcinoma

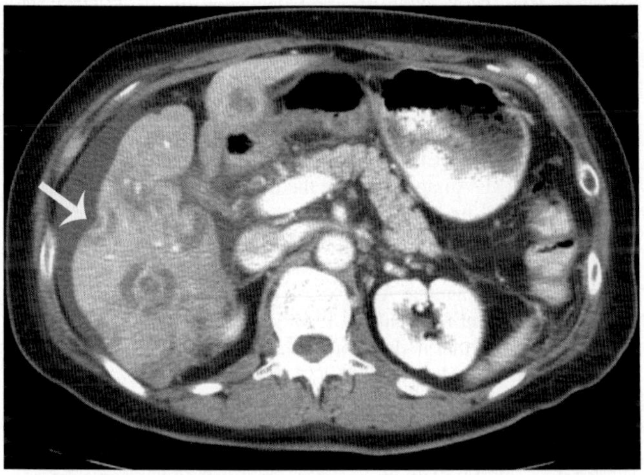

Fig. 15.13 CT of liver metastases. Contrast-enhanced computed tomography in a 63-year-old female with invasive ductal carcinoma and DCIS of the breast who developed liver metastases and associated hepatic capsular retraction (*white arrow*) from some of the metastatic lesions. Malignant ascites is also present

Restaging After Neoadjuvant Chemotherapy

SLND in Patients Undergoing NCT

Neoadjuvant chemotherapy is increasingly used in breast cancer patients because it allows for in situ assessment of tumor response as well as downsizing of the tumor, which may facilitate breast-conservation therapy. Another benefit of NCT is that 40–75 % of patients presenting with clinically involved lymph nodes will convert to pathological lymph node-negative status. Thus, SLND can lead to different results (and resulting adjuvant therapies) depending on whether it is performed before or after NCT [30, 31, 75]. Some clinicians have advocated for upfront SLND before initiating chemotherapy, arguing that SLN identification is more successful before chemotherapy and this knowledge of nodal status is important to treatment planning. However, this approach commits all women, even if the SLN is negative, to two surgical procedures. It also commits women with small-volume nodal disease that would have been easily eradicated with chemotherapy to ALND. At MD Anderson Cancer Center, we perform SLND in clinically negative women after they complete NCT during the same surgery as their breast procedure. This approach prioritizes the nodal status after NCT, which is a better prognostic indicator than the identification of occult nodal metastases pre-NCT [76]. Results from our institution have demonstrated that the SLN identification rate is not altered by NCT (98.7 % if surgery first vs. 97.4 % if SLN is performed after NCT) with similar false-negative rates (4.1 % in the surgery-first cohort vs. 5.8 % in NCT). After stratification for tumor size, the number of positive SLNs was lower if performed after NCT as opposed to before chemotherapy, and this resulted in fewer ALNDs [77].

The role of SLND in patients who present with clinically involved lymph nodes and have a clinical response to NCT is currently under review. Because a large proportion of patients have eradication of their nodal disease, there is considerable interest in finding reliable methods to restage the axilla in the hope of sparing these patients the morbidity of ALND. There have been concerns, however, that SLND may not be accurate in this setting, because tumor blockage of lymphatics may alter the lymphatic patterns and there may be discontinuous response to chemotherapy in the nodal regions. The ACOSOG Z1071 trial enrolled 689 women with clinically positive lymph nodes who then underwent NCT [78]. At surgery, participants had an SLND followed by completion ALND, and the results of the SLND were then compared with the pathological assessment of all lymph nodes. The primary endpoint of the study was to determine the false-negative rate (or number of patients with residual nodal disease who had no disease seen in the SLN). The study showed a false-negative rate of 12.6 %, slightly higher than the 10 % established before the trial began as the clinically relevant threshold. In subgroup analysis, the use of multiple mapping agents and retrieval of an increased number of SLN were associated with lower false-negative rates. The results of this trial have not yet been widely incorporated into clinical practice, although changes are expected.

Conclusion

Breast cancer remains the most common cancer for women in the developed countries despite the technical advances in the screening practice and diagnosis of this disease. Even though breast cancer mortality has declined in the United States, the survival rate of patients with a diagnosis of stage IV breast cancer has only marginally improved despite the advances in diagnosis and therapy, with a median breast cancer-specific survival of 23 months [79]. Early detection with mammography in conjunction with ultrasound or MRI and the accurate staging of newly diagnosed breast cancer are critical in the goal towards improving survival for this disease. Mammography remains the primary imaging modality for screening breast cancer in the general population. The addition of ultrasound and MRI has been shown to be beneficial in only the high-risk population. The utilization of ultrasound in the staging evaluation of newly diagnosed breast cancer cases is beneficial not only to better determine the disease extent within the breast but also to evaluate the locoregional nodal basins. MRI allows better visualization of the disease extent within the breast, while PET/CT enables detection of distant disease at the initial staging evaluation. Each imaging modalities have limitations, and finding the ideal combination of modalities remain a challenge for the medical communities while balancing the high costs of the new technology in comparison to the more traditional imaging modalities such as mammography and ultrasound.

References

1. American Cancer Society. Cancer facts & figures. Atlanta: American Cancer Society; 2014.
2. Budzar AU, Buchholz TA, Taylor SH, Hortobagyi GN, Hunt KK. Chapter 4: breast cancer. In: Rodriguez MA, Walters RS, Burke TW, editors. 60 years of survival outcomes at the University of Texas MD Anderson Cancer Center. New York: Springer; 2013. p. 19–34.
3. Edge SB, Byrd DR, Compton CC, Fritz AG, Greene FL, Trotti A. Part VII. Breast. In: American Joint Committee on Cancer, editor. Cancer staging manual. 7th ed. New York: Springer; 2010.
4. Anderson B, Yip CH, Smith RA, Shyyan R, Sener SF, Eniu A, et al. Guideline implementation for breast healthcare in low-income and middle-income countries: overview of the Breast Health Global Initiative Global Summit 2007. Cancer. 2008;113 suppl 8:2221–43.
5. Paganelli G, Galimberti V, Trifirò G, Travaini L, De Cicco C, Mazzarol G, et al. Internal mammary node lymphoscintigraphy and biopsy in breast cancer. Q J Nucl Med. 2002;46:138–44.
6. Theriault RL, Carlson RW, Allred C, Anderson BO, Burstein HJ, Edge SB, et al. National comprehensive cancer network (NCCN) clinical practice guidelines in oncology: breast, Version 3.2013. NCCN [internet]. 2013:1–176. Available from: http://www.nccn.org/professionals/physician_gls/pdf/breast.pdf.
7. Diekmann F, Bick U. Breast tomosynthesis. Semin Ultrasound CT MR. 2011;32:281–7.
8. Jakub JW, Gray RJ, Degnim AC, Boughey JC, Gardner M, Cox CE. Current status of radioactive seed for localization of non-palpable breast lesions. Am J Surg. 2010;199:522–8.
9. American College of Radiology (ACR). ACR BI-RADS® – ultrasound. In: ACR breast imaging reporting and data system, breast imaging atlas. Reston: American College of Radiology; 2003.
10. Harvey JA, Fechner RE, Moore MM. Apparent ipsilateral decrease in breast size at mammography: a sign of infiltrating lobular carcinoma. Radiology. 2000;214:883–9.
11. Le Gal M, Ollivier L, Asselain B, Meunier M, Laurent M, Vielh P, et al. Mammographic features of 455 invasive lobular carcinomas. Radiology. 1992;185:705–8.
12. Butler RS, Venta LA, Wiley EL, Ellis RL, Dempsey PJ, Rubin E. Sonographic evaluation of infiltrating lobular carcinoma. Am J Roentgenol. 1999;172(2):325–30.
13. Rissanen T, Tikkakoski T, Autio AL, Apaja-Sarkkinen M. Ultrasonography of invasive lobular breast carcinoma. Acta Radiol. 1998;39(3):285–91.
14. Skaane P, Skjorten F. Ultrasonographic evaluation of invasive lobular carcinoma. Acta Radiol. 1999;40:369–75.
15. Paramagul CP, Helvie MA, Adler DD. Invasive lobular carcinoma: sonographic appearance and role of sonography in improving diagnostic sensitivity. Radiology. 1995;195(1):231–4.
16. Selinko VL, Middleton LP, Dempsey PJ. Role of sonography in diagnosing and staging invasive lobular carcinoma. J Clin Ultrasound. 2004;32(7):323–32.
17. Yang WT, Tse GM. Sonographic, mammographic, and histopathologic correlation of symptomatic ductal carcinoma in situ. Am J Roentgenol. 2004;182(1):101–10.
18. Stavros AT. Malignant solid breast nodules: specific types. In: Stavros AT, editor. Breast ultrasound. Philadelphia: Lippincott Williams &Wilkins; 2004. p. 597–688.
19. Moon HJ, Kim MJ, Kim EK, Park BW, Youk JH, Kwak JY, et al. US surveillance of regional lymph node recurrence after breast cancer surgery. Radiology. 2009;252(3):673–81.
20. Bedi DG, Kirshnamurthy R, Krishnamurthy S, Edeiken BS, Le-Petross H, Fornage BD, et al. Cortical morphologic features of axillary lymph nodes as a predictor of metastasis in breast cancer: in vitro sonographic study. Am J Roentgenol. 2008;191:646–52.
21. Alvarez S, Anorbe E, Alcorta P, Lopez F, Alonso I, Cortes J. Role of ultrasound in the diagnosis of axillary lymph node metastases in breast cancer: a systematic review. Am J Roentgenol. 2006;186:1342–8.
22. Cabanas RM. An approach for the treatment of penile carcinoma. Cancer. 1977;39(2):456–66.
23. Morton DL, Wen DR, Wong JH, Economou JS, Cagle LA, Storm FK, et al. Technical details of intraoperative lymphatic mapping for early stage melanoma. Arch Surg. 1992;127(4):392–9.
24. Krag D, Weaver D, Ashikaga T, Moffat F, Klimberg VS, Shriver C, et al. The sentinel node in breast cancer–a multicenter validation study. N Engl J Med. 1998;339(14):941–6.
25. Veronesi U, Paganelli G, Viale G, Luini A, Zurrida S, Galimberti V, et al. A randomized comparison of sentinel-node biopsy with routine axillary dissection in breast cancer. N Engl J Med. 2003;349(6):546–53.
26. Giuliano AE, Dale PS, Turner RR, Morton DL, Evans SW, Krasne DL. Improved axillary staging of breast cancer with sentinel lymphadenectomy. Ann Surg. 1995;222(3):394–9; discussion 399–401.
27. Lucci A, McCall LM, Beitsch PD, Whitworth PW, Reintgen DS, Blumencranz PW, et al. Surgical complications associated with sentinel lymph node dissection (SLND) plus axillary lymph node dissection compared with SLND alone in the American College of Surgeons Oncology Group Trial Z0011. J Clin Oncol. 2007;25(24):3657–63.
28. Caudle AS, Hunt KK, Kuerer HM, Meric-Bernstam F, Lucci A, Bedrosian I, et al. Multidisciplinary considerations in the implementation of the findings from the American College of Surgeons Oncology Group (ACOSOG) Z0011 study: a practice-changing trial. Ann Surg Oncol. 2011;18(9):2407–12.
29. Giuliano A, Hunt K, Ballman K, Beitsch P, Whitworth P, Blumencraz P, Leitch A, Saha S, McCall L, Morrow M. Axillary dissection vs. no axillary dissection in women with invasive breast cancer and sentinel node metastasis. JAMA. 2011;305(6):569–75.
30. Dominici L, Negron Gonzalez V, Buzdar A, Lucci A, Mittendorf E, Le-Petross H, Babiera G, Meric-Bernstam F, Hunt K, Kuerer H. Cytologically proven axillary lymph node metastases are eradicated in patients receiving preoperative chemotherapy with concurrent trastuzumab for HER2-positive breast cancer. Cancer. 2010;116(12):2884–9.

31. Fisher B, Redmond C, Fisher ER, Bauer M, Wolmark N, Wickerham DL, et al. Ten-year results of a randomized clinical trial comparing radical mastectomy and total mastectomy with or without radiation. N Engl J Med. 1985;312(11):674–81.
32. Rourke LL, Hunt KK, Cormier JN. Breast cancer and lymphedema: a current overview for the healthcare provider. Womens Health (Lond Engl). 2010;6(3):399–406.
33. American College of Radiology. Breast magnetic resonance imaging (MRI) accreditation program requirements. Reston: American College of Radiology; 2008. Available at: http://www.acr.org/~/media/ACR/Documents/Accreditation/BreastMRI/Requirements.pdf.
34. American College of Radiology (ACR). ACR BI-RADS® – magnetic resonance imaging. In: ACR breast imaging reporting and data system, breast imaging atlas. Reston: American College of Radiology; 2003.
35. Houssami N, Ciatto S, Macaskill P, Lord SJ, Warren RM, Dixon JM, et al. Accuracy and surgical impact of magnetic resonance imaging in breast cancer staging: systematic review and meta-analysis in detection of multifocal and multicentric cancer. J Clin Oncol. 2008;26(19):3248–58.
36. Brennan ME, Houssami N, Lord S, Macaskill P, Irwig L, Dixon JM, et al. Accuracy and surgical impact of magnetic resonance imaging in breast cancer staging: systematic review and meta-analysis in detection of multifocal and multicentric cancer. J Clin Oncol. 2009;27:5640–9.
37. Turnbull L, Brown S, Harvey I, Olivier C, Drew P, Napp V, et al. Comparative effectiveness of MRI in breast cancer (COMICE) trial: a randomised controlled trial. Lancet. 2010;375(9714):563–71.
38. Solin LJ, Orel SG, Hwang WT, Harris EE, Schnall MD. Relationship of breast magnetic resonance imaging to outcome after breast-conservation treatment with radiation for women with early-stage invasive breast carcinoma or ductal carcinoma in situ. J Clin Oncol. 2008;26(3):386–91.
39. Lehman CD, Gatsonis C, Kuhl CK, Hendrick RE, Pisano ED, Hanna L, et al. MRI evaluation of the contralateral breast in women with recently diagnosed breast cancer. N Engl J Med. 2007;356(13):1295–303.
40. Mann RM. The effectiveness of MR imaging in the assessment of invasive lobular carcinoma of the breast. Magn Reson Imaging Clin N Am. 2010;18(2):259–76.
41. Le-Petross CH, Bidaut L, Yang WT. Evolving role of imaging modalities in inflammatory breast cancer. Semin Oncol. 2008;35(1):51–63. Review.
42. Kuhl C. The current status of breast MR imaging. Part I. Choice of technique, image interpretation, diagnostic accuracy, and transfer to clinical practice. Radiology. 2007;244:356–78.
43. Newstead GM. MR imaging of ductal carcinoma in situ. Magn Reson Imaging Clin N Am. 2010;18(2):225–40.
44. Kuhl C, Schrading S, Bieling H, et al. MRI for diagnosis of pure ductal carcinoma in situ: a prospective observational study. Lancet. 2007;370:485–92.
45. Morris E, Liberman L. Ductal carcinoma in situ. In: Morris E, Liberman L, editors. Breast MRI: diagnosis and intervention. Philadelphia: Springer; 2004. p. 164–72.
46. Kumar AJ, Chen DF, Au A, Chen YY, Leung J, Garwood ER, et al. Biologic significance of false-positive magnetic resonance imaging enhancement in the setting of ductal carcinoma in situ. Am J Surg. 2006;192(4):520–4.
47. Hillman BJ, Harms SE, Stevens G, Stough RG, Hollingsworth AB, Kozlowski KF, et al. Diagnostic performance of a dedicated 1.5-T breast MR imaging system. Radiology. 2012;265(1):51–8.
48. Bleicher RJ, Ciocca RM, Egleston BL, Sesa L, Evers K, Sigurdson ER, et al. Association of routine pretreatment magnetic resonance imaging with time to surgery, mastectomy rate, and margin status. J Am Coll Surg. 2009;209(2):180–7.
49. Sittart JA, Senise M. Cutaneous metastasis from internal carcinomas: a review of 45 years. An Bras Dermatol. 2013;88(4):541–4.
50. Harris JR, Morrow M, Bonnadonna G. Cancer of the breast. In: De Vitta Jr VT, Hellman S, Rosenberg SA, editors. Cancer: principles and practice of oncology. 4th ed. Philadelphia: JB Lippincott; 1993. p. 1264–332.
51. Riegger C, Herrmann J, Nagarajah J, Hecktor J, Kuemmel S, Otterbach F, et al. Whole-body FDG PET/CT is more accurate than conventional imaging for staging primary breast cancer patients. Eur J Nucl Med Mol Imaging. 2012;39(5):852–63.
52. Groheux D, Giacchetti S, Espie M, Vercellino L, Hamy AS, Delord M, et al. The yield of 18F-FDG PET/CT in patients with clinical stage IIA, IIB, or IIIA breast cancer: a prospective study. J Nucl Med. 2011;52(10):1526–34.
53. Koolen BB, Peeters MJTFDV, Aukema TS, Vogel WV, Oldenburg HSA, van der Hage JA, et al. 18F-FDG PET/CT as a staging procedure in primary stage II and III breast cancer: comparison with conventional imaging techniques. Breast Cancer Res Treat. 2012;131(1):117–26.
54. Aukema TS, Straver ME, Peeters MJ, Russell NS, Gilhuijs KG, Vogel WV, et al. Detection of extra-axillary lymph node involvement with FDG PET/CT in patients with stage II-III breast cancer. Eur J Cancer. 2010;46(18):3205–10.
55. Segaert I, Mottaghy F, Ceyssens S, De Wever W, Stroobants S, Van Ongeval C, et al. Additional value of PET-CT in staging of clinical stage IIB and III breast cancer. Breast J. 2010;16(6):617–24.
56. Alberini JL, Lerebours F, Wartski M, Fourme E, Le Stanc E, Gontier E, et al. 18F-fluorodeoxyglucose positron emission tomography/computed tomography (FDG-PET/CT) imaging in the staging and prognosis of inflammatory breast cancer. Cancer. 2009;115(21):5038–47.
57. Carkaci S, Macapinlac HA, Cristofanilli M, Mawlawi O, Rohren E, Gonzalez Angulo AM, et al. Retrospective study of ^{18}F-FDG PET/CT in the diagnosis of inflammatory breast cancer: preliminary data. J Nucl Med. 2009;50(2):231–8.
58. Yang WT, Le-Petross HT, Macapinlac H, Carkaci S, Gonzalez-Angulo AM, Dawood S, et al. Inflammatory breast cancer: PET/CT, MRI, mammography, and sonography findings. Breast Cancer Res Treat. 2008;109(3):417–26.
59. Schirrmeister H. Detection of bone metastases in breast cancer by positron emission tomography. Radiol Clin North Am. 2007;45(4):669–76.
60. Nakai T, Okuyama C, Kubota T, Yamada K, Ushijima Y, Taniike K, et al. Pitfalls of FDG-PET for the diagnosis of osteoblastic bone metastases in patients with breast cancer. Eur J Nucl Med Mol Imaging. 2005;32(11):1253–8.
61. Groves AM, Shastry M, Ben-Haim S, Kayani I, Malhotra A, Davidson T, et al. Defining the role of PET-CT in staging early breast cancer. Oncologist. 2012;17(5):613–9.
62. Koolen BB, van der Leij F, Vogel WV, Rutgers EJ, Vrancken Peeters MJ, Elkhuizen PH, et al. Accuracy of 18F-FDG PET/CT for primary tumor visualization and staging in T1 breast cancer. Acta Oncol. 2014;53:50–7.
63. Heusner TA, Kuemmel S, Umutlu L, Koeninger A, Freudenberg LS, Hauth EA, et al. Breast cancer staging in a single session: whole-body PET/CT mammography. J Nucl Med. 2008;49(8):1215–22.
64. Berg WA, Madsen KS, Schilling K, Tartar M, Pisano ED, Larsen LH, et al. Breast cancer: comparative effectiveness of positron emission mammography and MR imaging in presurgical planning for the ipsilateral breast. Radiology. 2011;258(1):59–72.
65. Casey JJ, Stempel BG, Scanlon EF, Fry WA. The solitary pulmonary nodule in the patient with breast cancer. Surgery. 1984;96(4):801–5.
66. McDonald ML, Deschamps C, Ilstrup DM, Allen MS, Trastek VF, Pairolero PC. Pulmonary resection for metastatic breast cancer. Ann Thorac Surg. 1994;58(6):1599–602.

67. Singletary SE, Walsh G, Vauthey JN, Curley S, Sawaya R, Weber KL, et al. A role for curative surgery in the treatment of selected patients with metastatic breast cancer. Oncologist. 2003;8(3): 241–51.
68. Hoe AL, Royle GT, Taylor I. Breast liver metastases–incidence, diagnosis and outcome. J R Soc Med. 1991;84(12):714–6.
69. Caudle A, Babiera GV. Primary tumor extirpation in stage IV disease: surgical considerations. In: Babiera GV, Skoracki RJ, Esteva FJ, editors. Advanced therapy of breast disease. Shelton: People's Medical Publishing House; 2012. p. 1001–8.
70. Dubrow RA, David CL, Libshitz HI, Lorigan JG. Detection of hepatic metastases in breast cancer: the role of nonenhanced and enhanced CT scanning. J Comput Assist Tomogr. 1990;14(3): 366–9.
71. Kim H, Han W, Moon HG, et al. The value of preoperative staging chest computed tomography to detect asymptomatic lung and liver metastasis in patients with primary breast carcinoma. Breast Cancer Res Treat. 2011;126(3):637–41.
72. Sheafor DH, Frederick MG, Paulson EK, et al. Comparison of unenhanced, hepatic arterial-dominant, and portal venous dominant phase helical CT for the detection of liver metastases in women with breast carcinoma. Am J Roentgenol. 1999;4:961–8.
73. Nishino M, Hayakawa K, Nakamura Y, Morimoto T, Mukaihara S. Effects of tamoxifen on hepatic fat content and the development of hepatic steatosis in patients with breast cancer: high frequency of involvement and rapid reversal after completion of tamoxifen therapy. Am J Roentgenol. 2003;1:129–34.
74. Roach H, Whipp E, Virjee J, et al. A Pictorial Review of the varied appearance of atypical liver metastasis from carcinoma of the breast. Br J Radiol. 2005;78:1098–103.
75. Kuerer H, Sahin A, Hunt K, Newman L, Breslin T, Ames F, Ross M, Buzdar A, Hortobagyi G. Incidence and impact of documented eradication of breast cancer axillary lymph node metastases before surgery in patients treated with neoadjuvant chemotherapy. Ann Surg. 1999;230(1):72–8.
76. Rouzier R, Extra JM, Klijanienko J, Falcou MC, Asselain B, Vincent-Salomon A, et al. Incidence and prognostic significance of complete axillary downstaging after primary chemotherapy in breast cancer patients with T1 to T3 tumors and cytologically proven axillary metastatic lymph nodes. J Clin Oncol. 2002;20(5):1304–10.
77. Hunt K, Yi M, Mittendorf E, Guerrero C, Babiera G, Bedrosian I, Hwang R, Kuerer H, Ross M, Meric-Bernstam F. Sentinel lymph node surgery after neoadjuvant chemotherapy is accurate and reduces the need for axillary dissection in breast cancer patients. Ann Surg. 2009;250(4):558–66.
78. Boughey JC, Suman VJ, Mittendorf EA, Ahrendt GM, Wilke LG, Taback B, et al. Sentinel lymph node surgery after neoadjuvant chemotherapy in patients with node-positive breast cancer: the American College of Surgeons Oncology Group (ACOSOG) Z1071 clinical trial. JAMA. 2013;310(14):1455–61.
79. Dawood S, Broglio K, Gonzalez-Angulo AM, Buzdar AU, Hortobagyi GN, Giordano SH. Trends in survival over the past two decades among white and black patients with newly diagnosed stage IV breast cancer. J Clin Oncol. 2008;26:4891–8.

The Postoperative Breast

16

Karla Arabela Sepulveda and Lilian O. Ebuoma

Introduction

Surgical interventions in the breast include excisional biopsy, lumpectomy, mastectomy, reduction, and augmentation. There are expected benign postsurgical changes following these interventions. These benign imaging findings may overlap with radiographic features of malignancy or obscure tumor recurrence. Awareness of normal postoperative imaging changes correlated with prior procedural history and time that has elapsed since those procedures is important for increasing accurate early detection of breast cancer or tumor recurrence in patients with history of breast cancer. This chapter will describe expected benign postsurgical findings and abnormal findings concerning for recurrence.

Terminology

The terms excisional biopsy, wide excision, tumorectomy, lumpectomy, and segmental mastectomy are interchanged in the literature. For the purposes of this chapter, excisional biopsy will refer to surgical excision of a benign finding, biopsy-proven atypia, or lobular neoplasia. Lumpectomy will refer to the surgical removal of malignancy. Mastectomy will refer to the surgical removal of the entire breast tissue. Excisional biopsies involve a skin incision and dissection through breast parenchyma to remove a volume of tissue containing an abnormality that is usually localized preoperatively with a wire. A lumpectomy involves the removal of a malignancy with a rim of sufficient adjacent normal tissue so that there is no cancer at the margin of the surgical specimen. Lumpectomies usually involve a larger volume of tissue than excisional biopsy.

K.A. Sepulveda, MD (✉) • L.O. Ebuoma, MD
Department of Radiology, Baylor College of Medicine, 6620 Main Street, Suite 1350, Houston, TX 77030, USA
e-mail: kasepulv@bcm.edu; ebuoma@bcm.edu

Post-excisional Biopsy

Although becoming less frequent with the increased use of minimally invasive image-guided biopsy, many patients used to undergo surgical excisional biopsy for further evaluation of indeterminate or suspicious findings on breast imaging. Currently, in the rare instances when a target cannot be accessed by image guidance or when the patient is unable to tolerate image-guided biopsy, excisional biopsy remains an alternative. In addition, excisional biopsies are performed on patients who have a history of biopsy yielding atypia or lobular neoplasia to evaluate for possible upgrade to in situ or invasive carcinoma.

Mammograms are rarely performed in the weeks following excisional biopsy. Usually a mammogram would only be performed if there is concern that a targeted lesion was not actually removed. The use of specimen radiography and accurate preoperative wire localizations limits the need for early postoperative mammogram. Typically a patient will undergo their first mammogram 6 months to 1 year after surgery. The imaging findings on the first postexcisional biopsy mammogram range from imperceptible to moderate architectural distortion. Precise preoperative wire localizations with the wire placed no more than 5–10 mm from an abnormality allow for minimal volume of tissue to be removed at the time of biopsy which minimizes the long-term changes to the breast. Immediately following biopsy, seromas and hematomas are common within the biopsy cavity. Over the following months, the fluid collections are reabsorbed and replaced with fibrosis and scarring. By the time the patient undergoes a 12-month postsurgery mammogram, it is estimated that 50–55 % of patients will heal with no scar or architectural distortion in the underlying breast parenchyma [1].

Sometimes, the only sign of intervention will be a subtle decrease in breast volume when compared with the prior mammogram or slight asymmetry in the breast parenchyma pattern compared to the contralateral breast (Fig. 16.1). In the remaining cases, excisional biopsy sites may demonstrate skin thickening, parenchymal distortion, spiculation, and,

M.K. Shetty (ed.), *Breast Cancer Screening and Diagnosis: A Synopsis*,
DOI 10.1007/978-1-4939-1267-4_16,

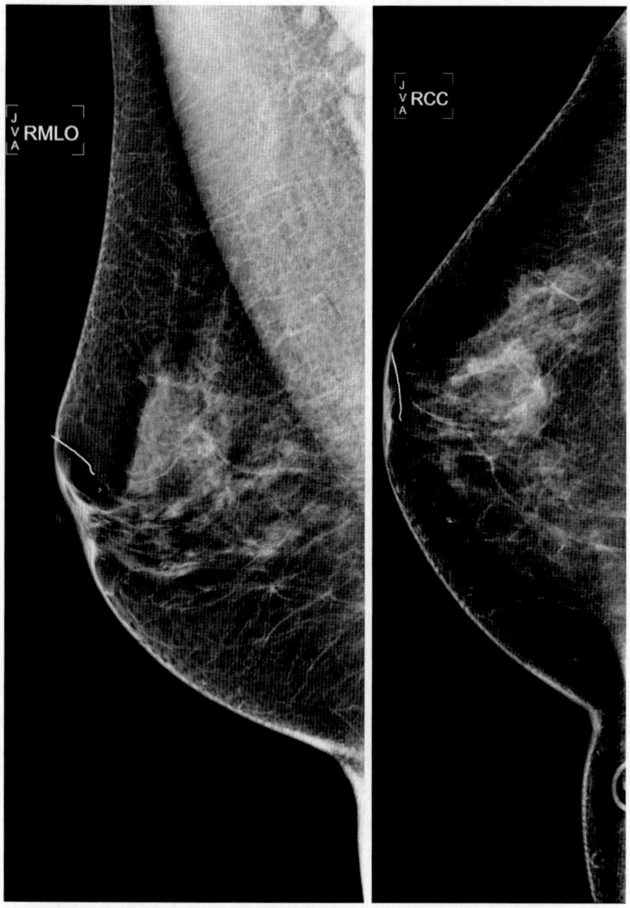

Fig. 16.1 Status post-excisional biopsy for ADH. Minimal postsurgical changes are present in the anterior upper central right breast

rarely, a persistent seroma cavity that presents as a round or oval mass (Figs. 16.2a, b, 16.3a, b, and 16.4). These findings may remain stable or slowly evolve over time gradually becoming less prominent (Fig. 16.5a–f). Coarse fat necrosis calcifications may develop gradually on follow-up exams. Variation in the amount of persistent change following biopsy is secondary to varying amount of tissue removed at the time of surgery and varying postoperative course that may include hematoma formation or infection that can produce longer term changes. A pitfall to be mindful of in the follow-up imaging of a postsurgical mammogram is the potential for parenchymal asymmetry in the breast that has not had surgery to be mistaken for disease in the contralateral breast. The apparent asymmetry is the result of the absence of tissue that has been surgically removed on the side of surgery.

Given that both scarring and carcinoma can present as spiculated masses on imaging, clinical history, physical exam, and comparison with prior studies are essential for appropriate management. When there are no prior mammograms available for comparison and when a history of biopsy is not provided, the differential diagnosis should include malignancy, radial scar, and prior trauma in addition to post-biopsy changes. Since there is a possibility for malignancy, if no prior studies are available, additional evaluation with diagnostic imaging is warranted. Technologists should obtain a thorough history of dates of prior surgical biopsies before performing imaging and marking scars in the skin to help avoid confusion. Applying a linear metallic scar marker on the skin can assist in explaining nearby architectural distortion. Some facilities place scar markers routinely while others only place them if there is uncertainty of postsurgical change correlating with a biopsy site. The skin incision can be distant from the postsurgical change, and sometimes it is more helpful to correlate with a preoperative mammogram, if available, as the mammogram will demonstrate the site of original mammographic abnormality where the postsurgical changes would be expected. Architectural distortion distant from a skin marker should be considered suspicious, particularly if the finding is new from prior exams. Review of the patient's pertinent history and symptoms will assist in increasing accuracy.

While post-biopsy imaging findings require careful evaluation, the challenge of distinguishing post-biopsy change from malignancy is usually more limited than in the post-lumpectomy mammogram given that the risk for malignancy at a site of recent benign biopsy is lower than that of a biopsy performed in a patient with known history of malignancy, particularly in the first few years following biopsy. In a prospective study by Slanetz, mammograms of 1,997 patients presenting for screening were reviewed. One hundred and seventy-three patients reported a prior history of benign biopsy. Fourteen percent (24) of the 173 patients had mammographic evidence of biopsy on the mammogram. Although 5 % (9) of the 173 post-biopsy patients were recalled for additional imaging, none of the recalls were due to confusion or diagnostic concern at the biopsy site. The rate of recall was similar to that of the group without prior history of biopsy. The study concluded that changes from previous excisional biopsy for benign breast problems are uncommon and rarely pose a diagnostic dilemma in interpretation of routine screening mammograms [2]. If there is any concern on the first exam after benign biopsy, a short-term follow up mammogram can be performed in 6 months. Any increase in calcifications, architectural distortion, or increasing asymmetries on follow-up should prompt biopsy (Fig. 16.6a–d).

In some cases, surgical excisional biopsy of an indeterminate or suspicious clinical or imaging finding is performed, rather than image-guided biopsy, and cancer is found at the time of surgery. The margins of the surgical sample are often positive and the patient needs to return to surgery for re-excision and possible axillary evaluation. In these cases, a pre-lumpectomy diagnostic mammogram with spot magnification views of the lumpectomy bed is recommended to evaluate for incompletely resected tumor. Comparison with pre-biopsy mammogram is essential to assess extent of the original disease. Correlation with the pathology report describing what aspect of the biopsy cavity has positive mar-

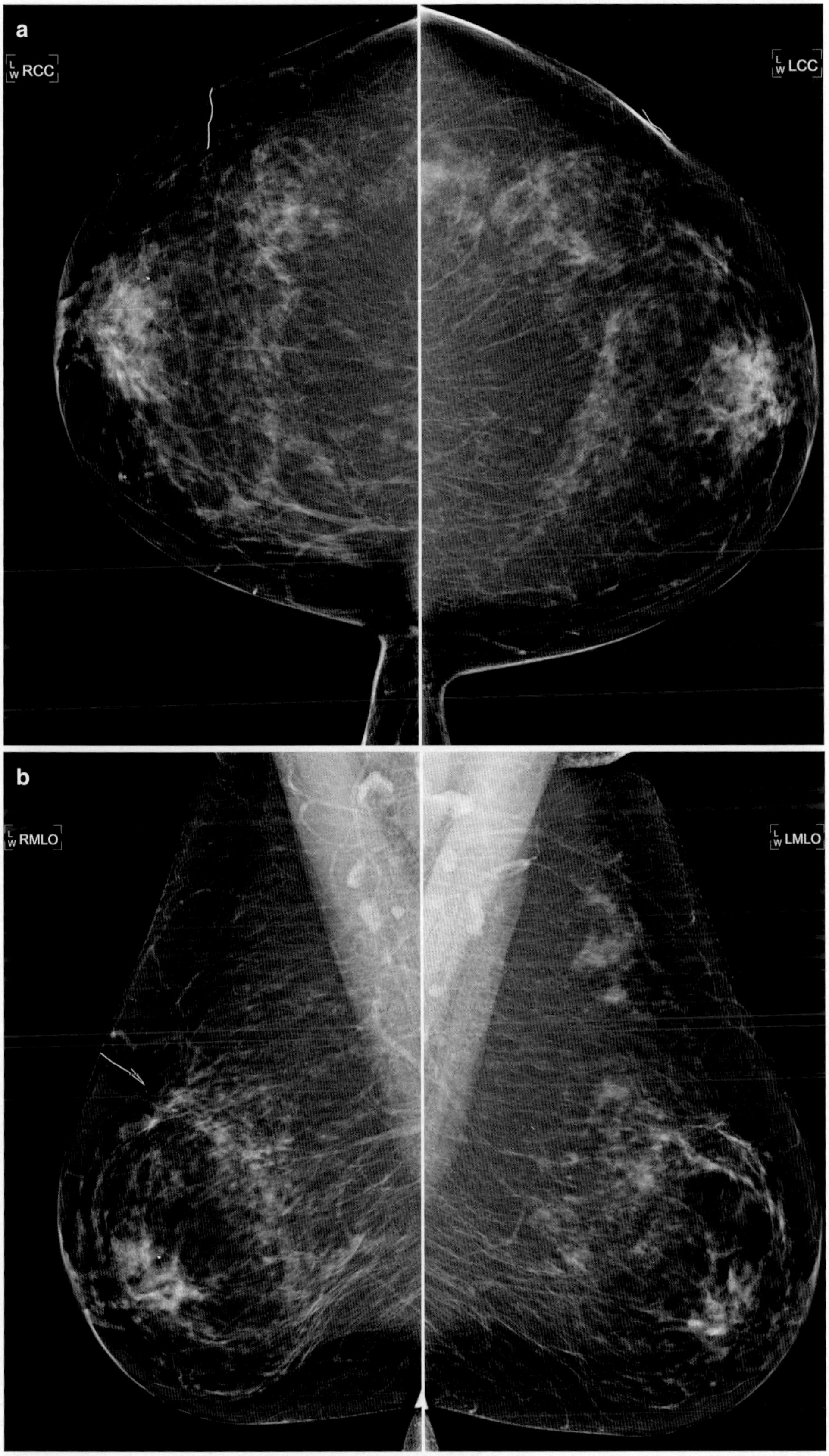

Fig. 16.2 (**a**) Prior bilateral benign excisional biopsies. Skin scar markers overlie the areas of prior biopsy and correlate to underlying subtle architectural distortion. (**b**) Note the apparent asymmetry in the posterior upper left breast due to excision of tissue on the right

Fig. 16.3 (**a**) A 73-year-old female status post benign excisional biopsy in the upper outer left breast. Architectural distortion is present in the biopsy bed. (**b**) Note the apparent asymmetry in the posterior outer right breast due to asymmetric glandular tissue after tissue was removed from the outer left breast

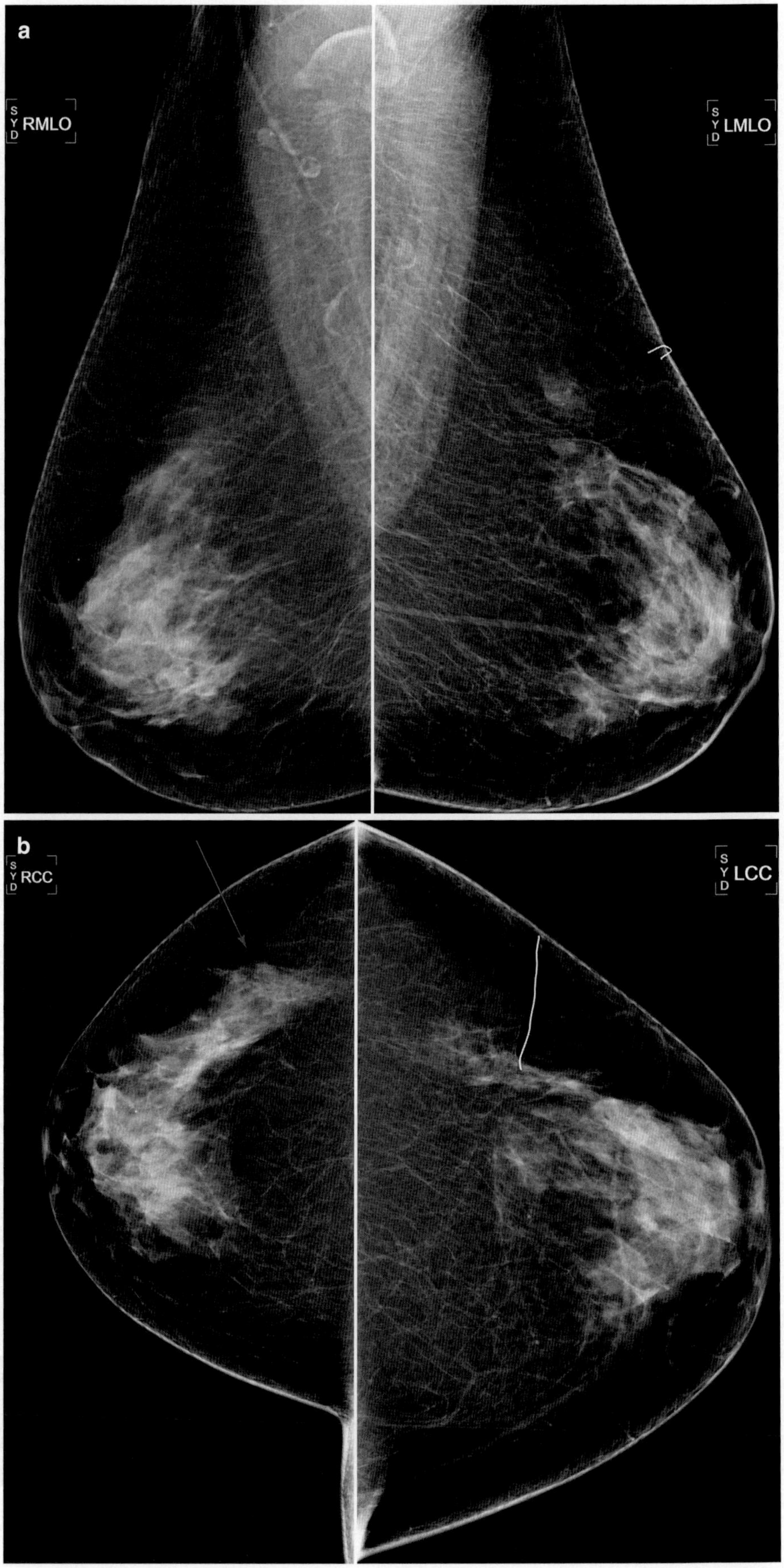

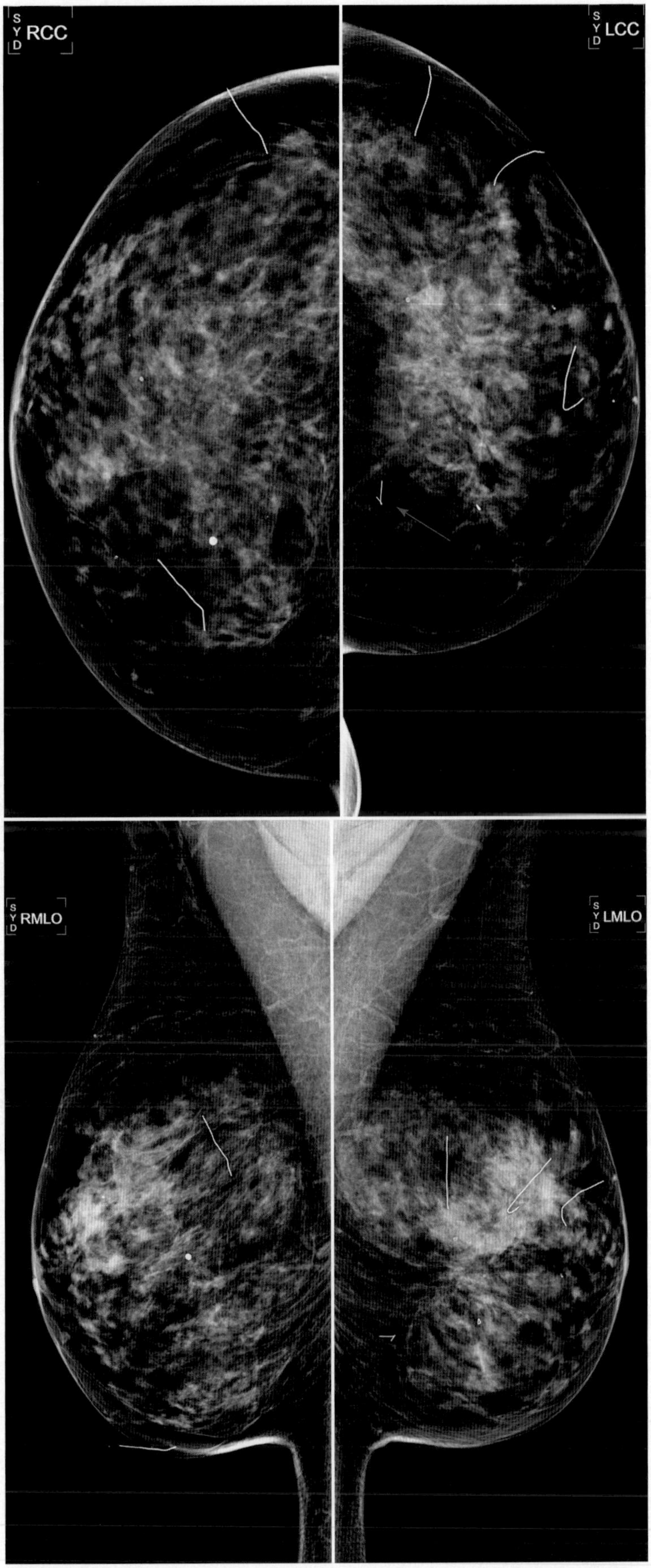

Fig. 16.4 A 59-year-old female status post multiple bilateral benign excisional biopsies. Note mild asymmetry in breast size from more biopsies being performed on the left breast and architectural distortion in the central left breast. A portion of a retained hookwire is present in the posterior medial left breast

Fig. 16.5 (**a**) A 65-year-old female with mass in the retroareolar position. (**b**) Ultrasound demonstrated a corresponding 6 mm intraductal mass. (**c**) 1 year after surgical excision of benign papilloma. Nodularity in the area of surgery is less conspicuous with spot compression. (**d**) Ultrasound demonstrated benign scar tissue. No residual or recurrent mass visualized. (**e**) Follow-up ultrasound performed 6 months (*left*) and 12 months (*right*) later shows resolving postoperative findings. (**f**) Mammogram 2 years (*left*) and 3 years (*right*) after surgery demonstrate progressively resolving postoperative changes

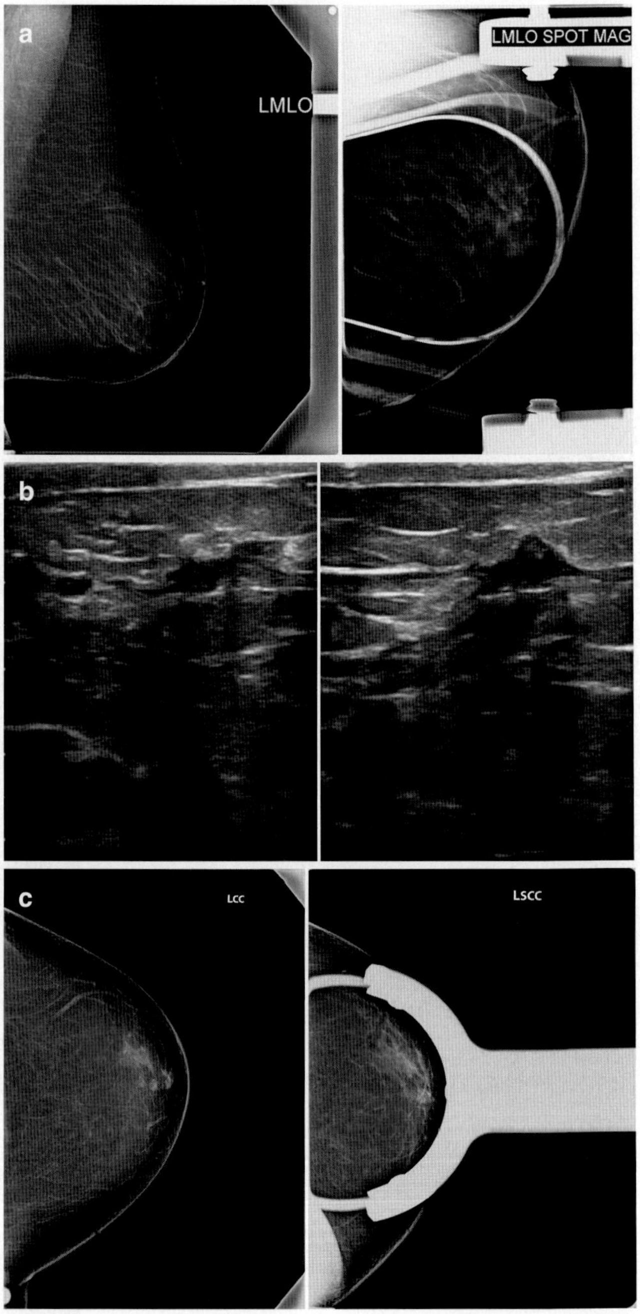

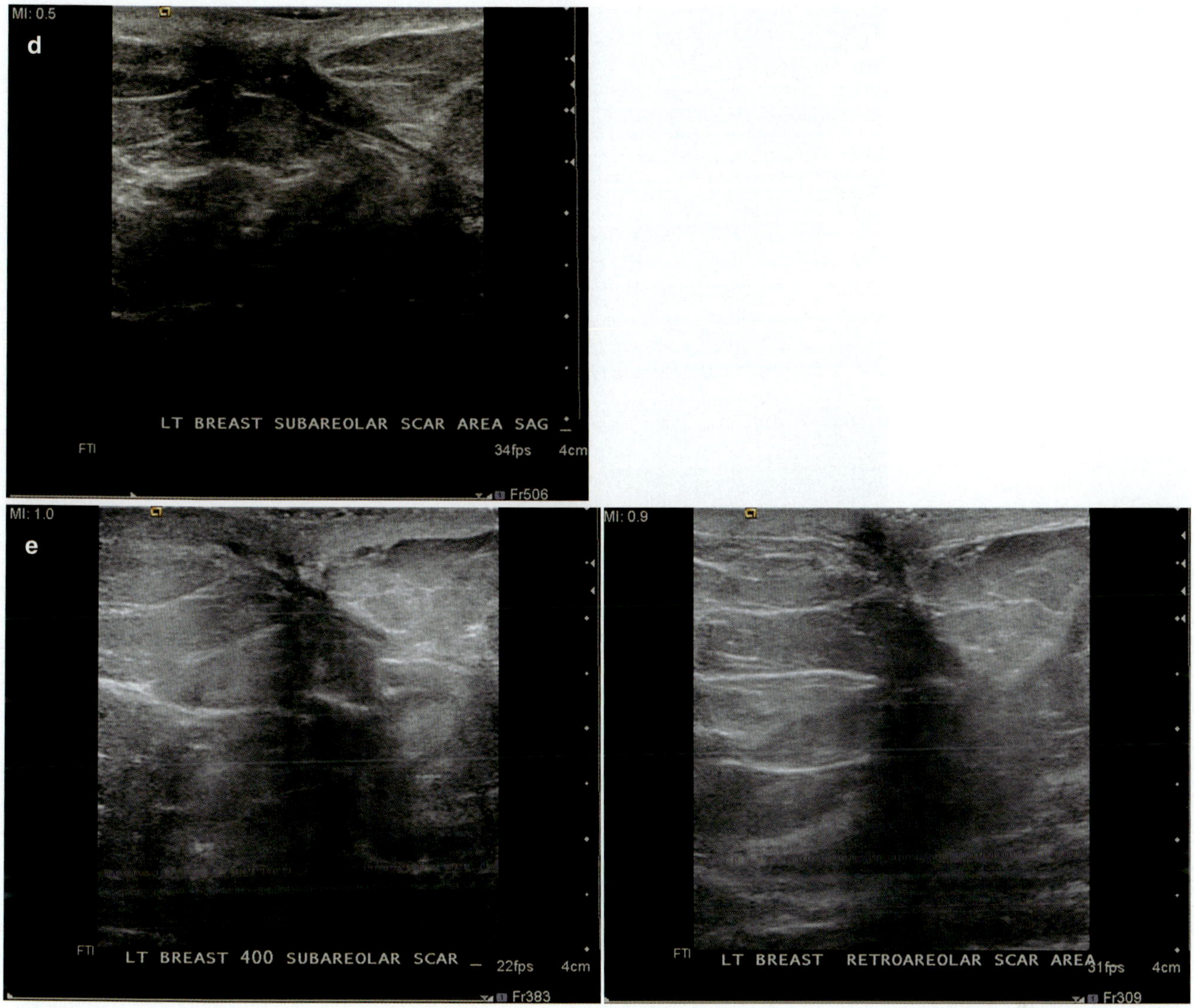

Fig. 16.5 (continued)

Fig. 16.5 (continued)

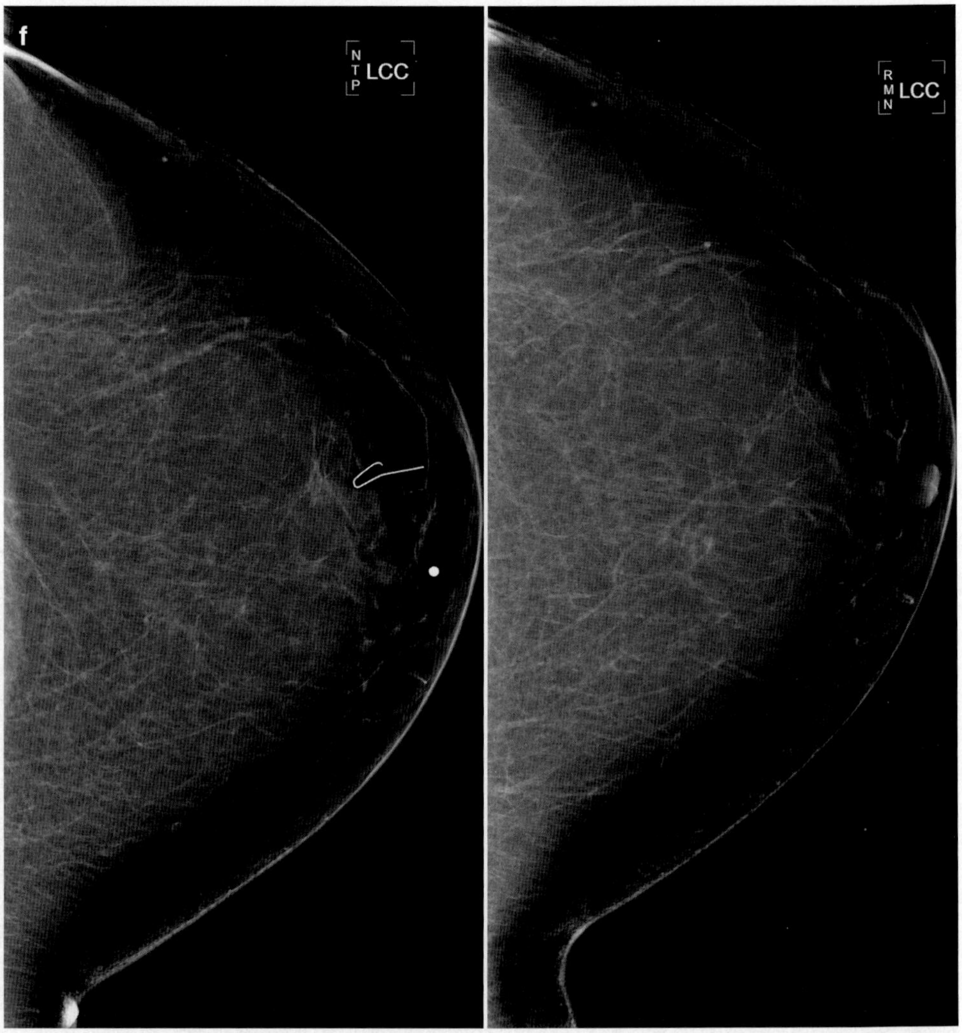

gins is also helpful to direct the imager to give additional attention to these areas. The pre-lumpectomy mammogram is particularly useful in the cases of ductal carcinoma in situ to evaluate for residual calcifications. It is important to recognize that the absence of mammographic findings does not exclude residual disease and lumpectomy is still required despite a negative mammogram. Preoperative breast MRI is also valuable to evaluate for residual disease and to assess for multicentric or contralateral disease in these patients [3–5].

Post-lumpectomy

As the use of mammography and MRI for screening has become more widespread, the detection of early-stage (I or II) breast cancer has increased. Given equivalent survival rates for breast conservation therapy and mastectomy [6, 7] in prospective, randomized trials, lumpectomy with radiation therapy has become the treatment of choice for early-stage breast cancer. Breast conservation therapy achieves local tumor control by surgical removal of the cancer with a margin of normal breast tissue followed by whole breast radiation to try to eliminate any residual microscopic disease that was not evident by radiology, surgery, or pathology.

Imaging plays an important role in evaluating breast cancer patients in both preoperative and postoperative periods. Before surgery, imaging is used to evaluate extent of disease for treatment planning. Following surgery, imaging is used to detect residual or recurrent disease on the affected side and screen the contralateral breast. The imaging challenge in evaluating these patients postsurgery is distinguishing normal benign postoperative and postradiation alterations from tumor recurrence, the imaging findings of which can overlap. The ability to differentiate between the two is usually accomplished by an understanding of expected postoperative findings in correlation with timing since surgery and with evaluation of studies in a temporal context to detect interval changes, sometimes quite subtle.

Presurgical Evaluation

Once a diagnosis of cancer is established by biopsy, review of the mammogram to reevaluate for any possible multifocal or multicentric disease can be performed prior to surgery. Spot

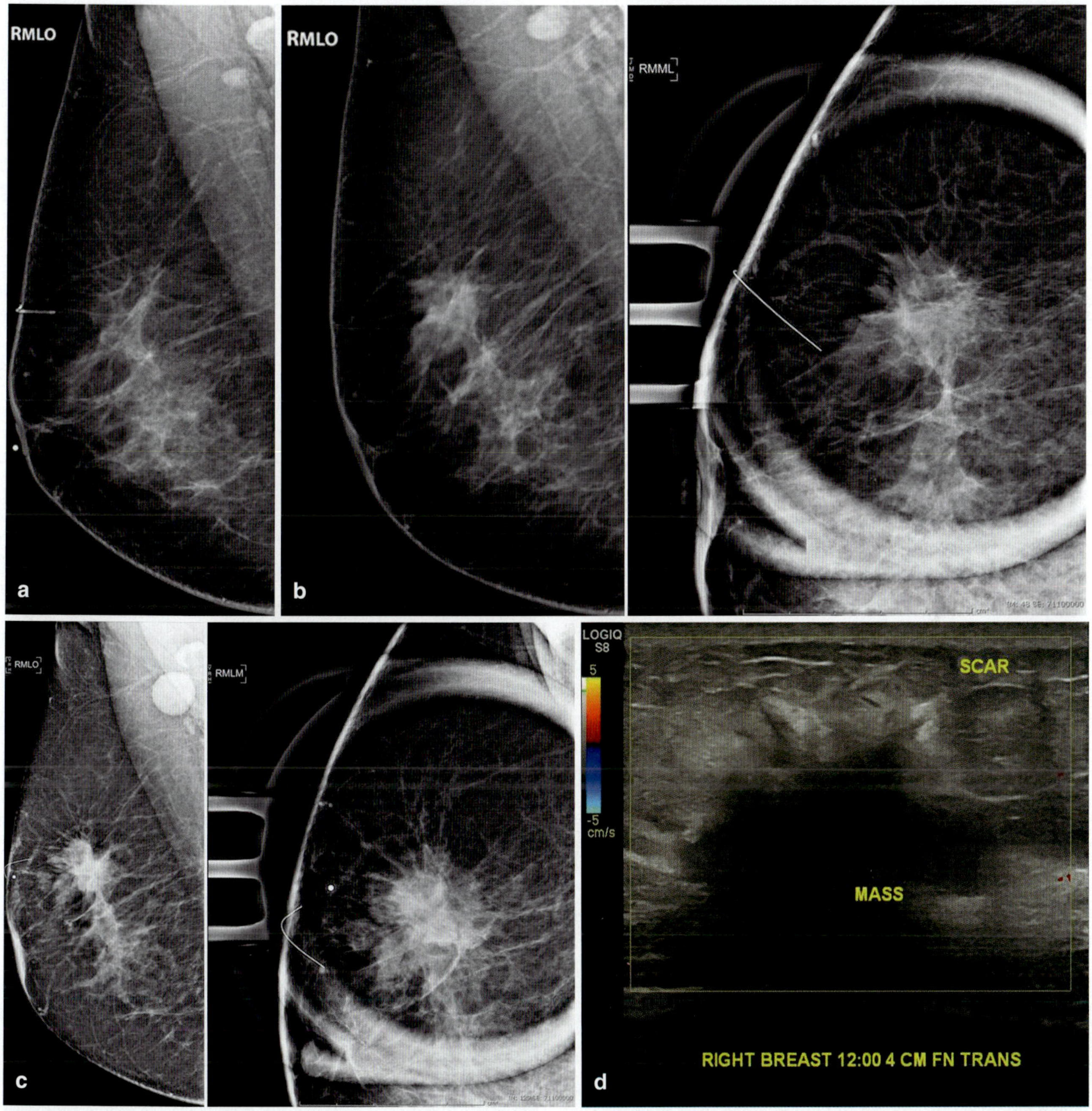

Fig. 16.6 (**a**) Right mammogram 9 months following excisional biopsy of calcifications. Pathology was benign. Mild architectural distortion is present in the mid upper breast. (**b**) The patient returns 2 years later. Increased prominence of the glandular tissue in the region of the scar prompted diagnostic mammogram which was interpreted as benign postsurgical change. (**c**) 7 months later, the patient returned complaining of a palpable abnormality. A high-density mass with irregular margins is visualized. Note enlarged right axillary lymph node. (**d**) US demonstrates a corresponding 4.2 cm hypoechoic mass superimposed on an area of architectural distortion related to a previous surgical excision site. Biopsy yielded invasive carcinoma

magnification view of indeterminate calcifications separate from the cancer and spot compression views of potential satellite nodules adjacent to the cancer or indeterminate masses in distant quadrants can be helpful to exclude additional disease.

As discussed in greater detail elsewhere in this book, breast MRI is also an important tool in the presurgical evaluation of newly diagnosed breast cancer. Multiple studies have demonstrated that MRI detects additional cancer in both the ipsilateral and contralateral breast [8–12]. Use of preoperative breast MRI varies by institution, although by the ACS guidelines breast MRI is recommended in all new diagnoses. A greater extent of the disease is often visualized on these exams.

Post-lumpectomy Evaluation

When postlumpectomy patients return for annual diagnostic imaging, it is helpful to have information on characteristics of the patient's initial cancer in order to have a better understanding of the features that may increase probability for recurrence. Important tumor features to know include tumor size and grade, proximity of tumor to margins, presence of extensive intraductal component, lymphovascular invasion, and biomarkers. It is also helpful to know if the patient was able to complete radiation and chemotherapy or antiestrogen therapy. Obtaining any prior imaging before reading the mammogram is helpful for comparing the current study to the earliest available postoperative study as detection of subtle progressive changes may not be readily apparent when comparing to exams performed 1–2 years prior. Given that 65 % of tumor recurrences are within a few centimeters of the excision site [13], dedicated attention to the lumpectomy cavity is warranted. One way of providing a more thorough examination of the lumpectomy bed is to perform spot magnification views of the surgical site. At our institution, we routinely perform these additional views for the first 5 years following surgery, although there is no published consensus on this practice.

Accurate interpretation of the postlumpectomy mammogram involves detection of potential recurrence as early as possible while limiting misinterpretation of postsurgical change as tumor recurrence. Diagnostic accuracy will be increased by familiarity of timing of tumor recurrence and expected chronological posttreatment changes. These changes include edema and skin thickening, masses and fluid collections, scarring and architectural distortion, and calcifications. These are the post-biopsy changes at the surgical site (previously discussed) with added diffuse skin thickening and breast edema associated with breast radiation. The changes seen after lumpectomy are usually more profound and prolonged than those seen after benign excision (Fig. 16.7). In comparison to the changes seen in the postlumpectomy breast, the changes following excisional biopsy usually resolve more quickly and, on occasion, completely.

Mammography performed 6–12 months after lumpectomy will demonstrate the greatest post-procedural changes [14]. The appearance of expected post-lumpectomy findings is dependent on the size of the lumpectomy and the time that has elapsed since the surgery (Figs. 16.8a–f and 16.9). Mendelson summarizes the expected time course for changes in the conservatively treated breast in the following chart (Fig. 16.10).

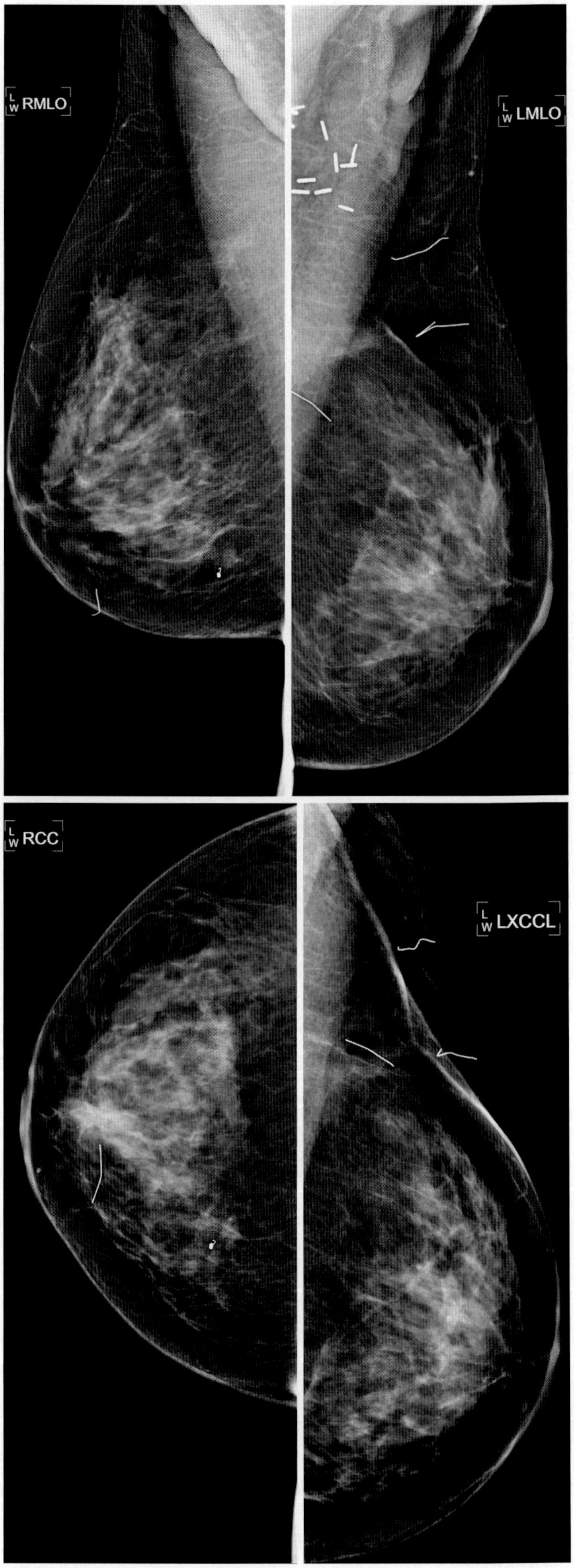

Fig. 16.7 Routine annual exam in a patient who underwent left lumpectomy and right breast excisional biopsy at the same time, 8 years prior to the exam. Note greater volume loss and postsurgical clips at the site of lumpectomy

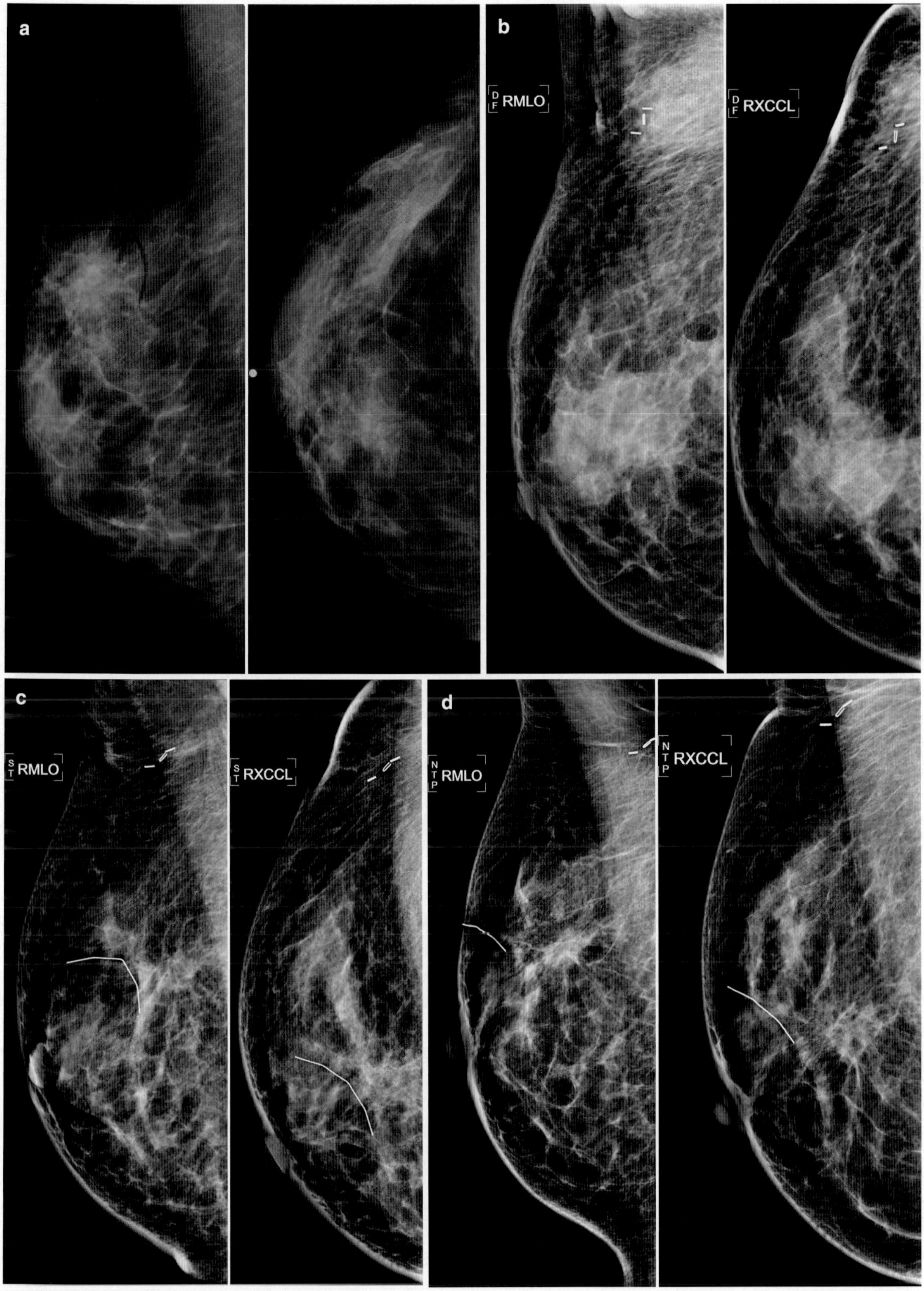

Fig. 16.8 (**a**–**f**) Progressive chronological changes in the lumpectomy cavity. (**a**) A 58-year-old with new spiculated mass in the upper inner right breast. Biopsy yielded invasive carcinoma. (**b**) The patient presented to our clinic 12 months following lumpectomy. (**c**) 18 months following lumpectomy. (**d**) 24 months post lumpectomy. (**e**) 36 months post lumpectomy. (**f**) 5 years post lumpectomy with continued decrease in edema and scarring

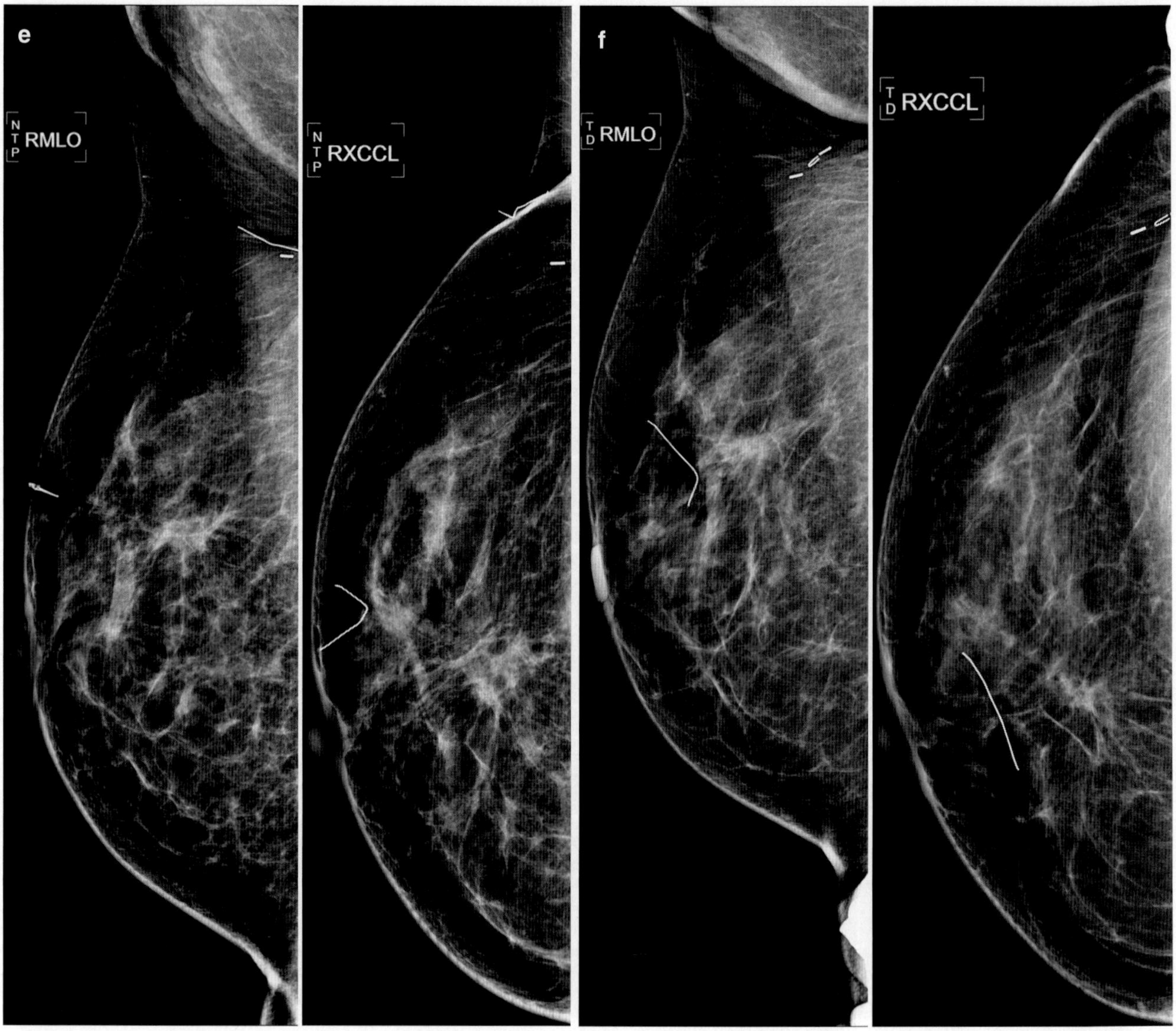

Fig. 16.8 (continued)

As demonstrated in the chart, breast edema and skin thickening are post-treatment changes with similar time courses after surgery. Breast edema manifests as skin and stromal thickening, trabecular thickening (engorgement of intramammary lymphatics) and diffusely increased breast parenchymal density [15]. The increased parenchymal density may be due to attenuation of the x-ray by edematous tissues and fibrosis and perhaps in part due to less compression secondary to patient discomfort. Initially the breast may appear enlarged due to edema. These changes are most prominent in the periareolar and dependent areas of the breast and will make the breast less compressible. Breast edema and skin thickening are particularly apparent when comparison is made with pretreatment mammograms by doing direct comparison with the contralateral breast. As the edema resolves, usually within the first 2 years after treatment, the breast will progressively decrease in size and the breast parenchyma will retain an increased density due to loss of volume and radiation fibrosis. If breast edema recurs or increases after stabilization, differential considerations include lymphatic spread of cancer, obstructed venous drainage, congestive heart failure, and infection [14].

Architectural distortion in the lumpectomy bed may be due to parenchymal scarring, fat necrosis, or recurrent cancer (Fig. 16.11a, b). The best way to discriminate scarring and recurrence on mammography is careful temporal evaluation. Scars contract and decrease in size as they mature and stabilize [14]. Radiolucent fat can be seen interspersed within the spiculated soft tissue of the scar. Mammographic findings suggestive of recurrence include lack of central radiolucent areas, new skin retraction, and increase in size, density, or nodularity of the scar [16].

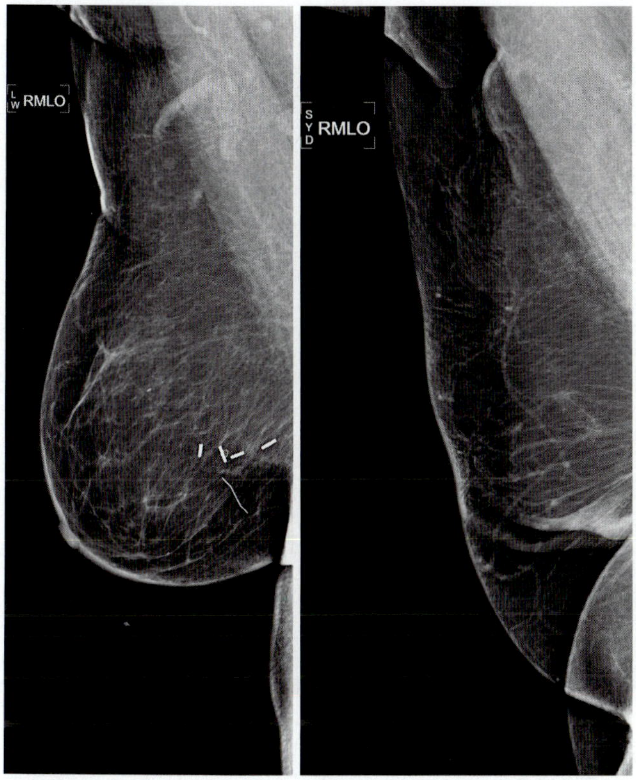

Fig. 16.9 Minimal postsurgical change (*left*) 3 years after lumpectomy for a small area of DCIS. Note the absence of findings in the axilla as no axillary dissection was performed. Compare with more significant distortion (*right*) in another patient 3 years following a more extensive lumpectomy

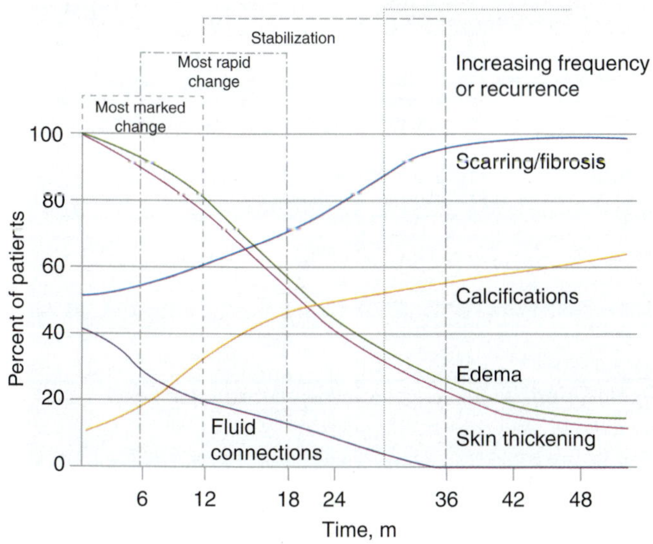

Fig. 16.10 Chronological change in appearance of the breast following lumpectomy (Used with permission from Mendelson [18])

Various fluid collections can develop following surgery including hematomas, seromas, and less commonly abscesses (Fig. 16.12a–c). These fluid collections may present as palpable or mammographically detected radiodense masses in the first year after breast conservation therapy [17]. Mammography will demonstrate postoperative fluid collections in 50 % of patients at 4 weeks and in 25 % of patients at 6 months after surgery [18]. Fluid collections are better evaluated with ultrasound and will be discussed in greater detail in the section on sonographic evaluation post lumpectomy. Most postoperative fluid collections resolve by 12 months.

Evaluation of newly developing calcifications in the postlumpectomy mammogram is of particular importance because often recurrences that present this way are not clinically detectable and provide an opportunity for early detection [13]. From a temporal standpoint, it is common for new calcifications to form in the lumpectomy bed within the first year after surgery in up to 28 % of cases [18]. Given that the risk of recurrence is greatest starting 2–3 years after surgery, most studies assign a low probability of malignancy in calcifications that occur within the first 18 months after surgery and radiation. Although most newly occurring calcifications in the postsurgical breast are benign, calcifications in post-treatment mammograms in patients with history of invasive carcinoma with extensive intraductal component or large areas of comedonecrosis should be approached with a higher level of suspicion as these tumors have higher risk of recurrence [18].

Calcifications at the lumpectomy site should be assessed in the same manner calcifications on routine screening mammograms are evaluated: calcifications with suspicious morphology or distribution increase the probability of malignancy and should prompt biopsy. The majority of calcifications that develop after surgery will be benign fat necrosis, dystrophic calcifications, or calcifying suture material (Figs. 16.13, 16.14, and 16.15). Magnification views are required to distinguish these benign calcifications from suspicious pleomorphic calcifications of cancer recurrence. Benign oil cysts present as thin rims of calcifications around a radiolucent center.

Fat necrosis calcifications typically demonstrate coarse curvilinear morphology and usually form around the periphery of a radiolucent center of fat (Figs. 16.16a, b, 16.17a, b, 16.18, 16.19a–c, and 16.20a–c). The time of development of fat necrosis is variable ranging from months to years. Although there is a classic appearance of benign calcifications, these calcifications do not always present in their classic form, making assigning benign etiology difficult, particularly when they are more faint in their early stages. When calcifications are indeterminate, careful inspection of prior mammograms may show regression of the calcifications over time or formation of the calcifications around a radiolucent center of fat, suggesting benign etiology [19]. If there is low suspicion based on morphology, monitoring with 6-month follow-up is a reasonable approach. Otherwise,

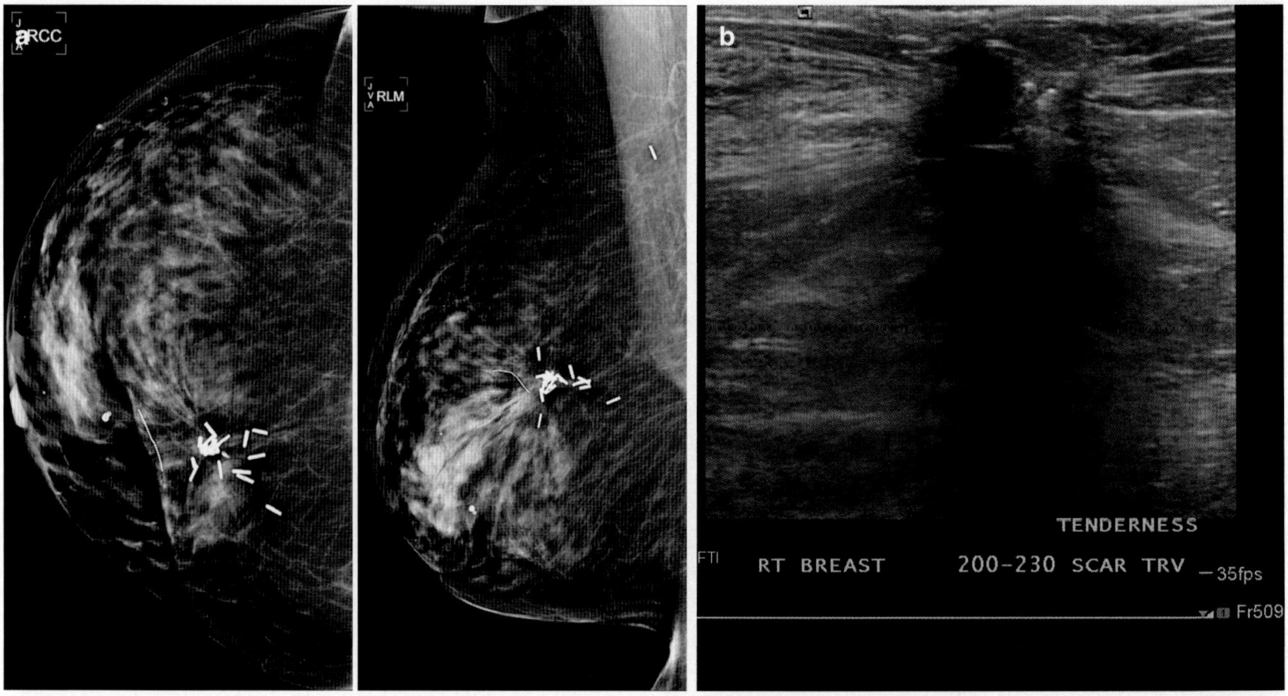

Fig. 16.11 (**a**) A 69-year-old female status post lumpectomy 12 years prior to exam. Post-lumpectomy changes are present in the upper inner right breast including surgical clips deployed at the margins of the lumpectomy site to focus follow-up mammography and to guide radiation planning. (**b**) Ultrasound of the area of prior lumpectomy shows expected sonographic findings of scar tissue

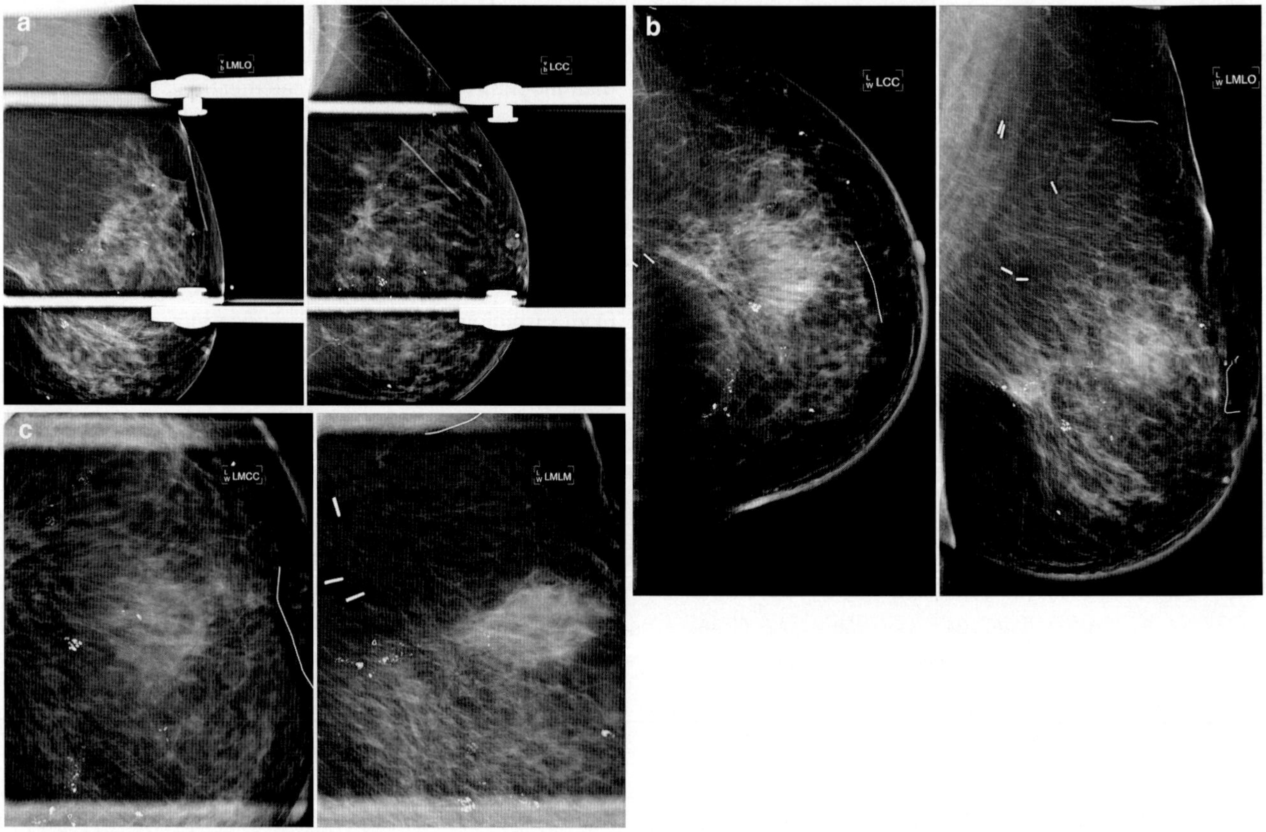

Fig. 16.12 (**a**) An 80-year-old female with new 7 mm irregular mass in the posterior upper central left breast. Biopsy yielded invasive carcinoma. (**b**) 6-month follow-up after lumpectomy. (**c**) Spot magnification views of the lumpectomy bed. Focal increased density likely represents a resolving postoperative fluid collection. Scattered benign-appearing coarse calcifications are present

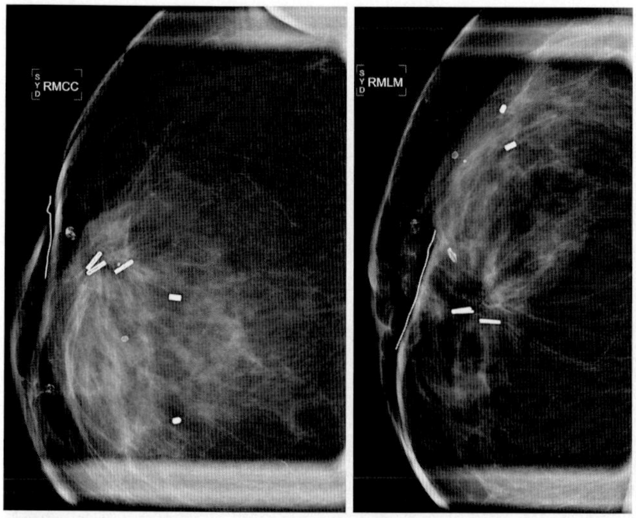

Fig. 16.13 Stable architectural distortion and benign calcifications 5 years post lumpectomy

biopsy should be performed for definitive diagnosis of benignity.

Most changes after lumpectomy diminish and regress over time and then remain stable. Stability is defined as the lack of interval change on two successive studies and occurs on average 2–3 years after breast conservation therapy is completed [18]. Fortunately for the breast imager, stability occurs around the time that tumor recurrences begin to appear [14]. Once stability is established, any increase in changes or new findings should be evaluated for tumor recurrence (Fig. 16.21a, b).

Imaging Schedule Post-lumpectomy

Currently there is no widely accepted protocol for appropriate post-lumpectomy surveillance. Although there is consensus on annual mammography of the contralateral breast, recommendations for follow-up mammography on the side of lumpectomy vary by institution and demonstrate considerable geographic variation. At some facilities, a unilateral postsurgical mammogram is performed immediately after lumpectomy but prior to initiation of radiation therapy to evaluate for residual disease at the tumor site. This is particularly recommended in patients who initially presented with extensive area of calcifications on their mammogram or may be helpful for surgical planning if positive margins were present on pathology at the time of lumpectomy. Other institutions obtain a baseline unilateral mammogram immediately following completion of radiation therapy. Some facilities will wait to perform a unilateral mammogram on the side of lumpectomy until 6 months after surgery. Thorough preoperative evaluation of the mammogram and preoperative breast MRI limit the risk for finding unexpected

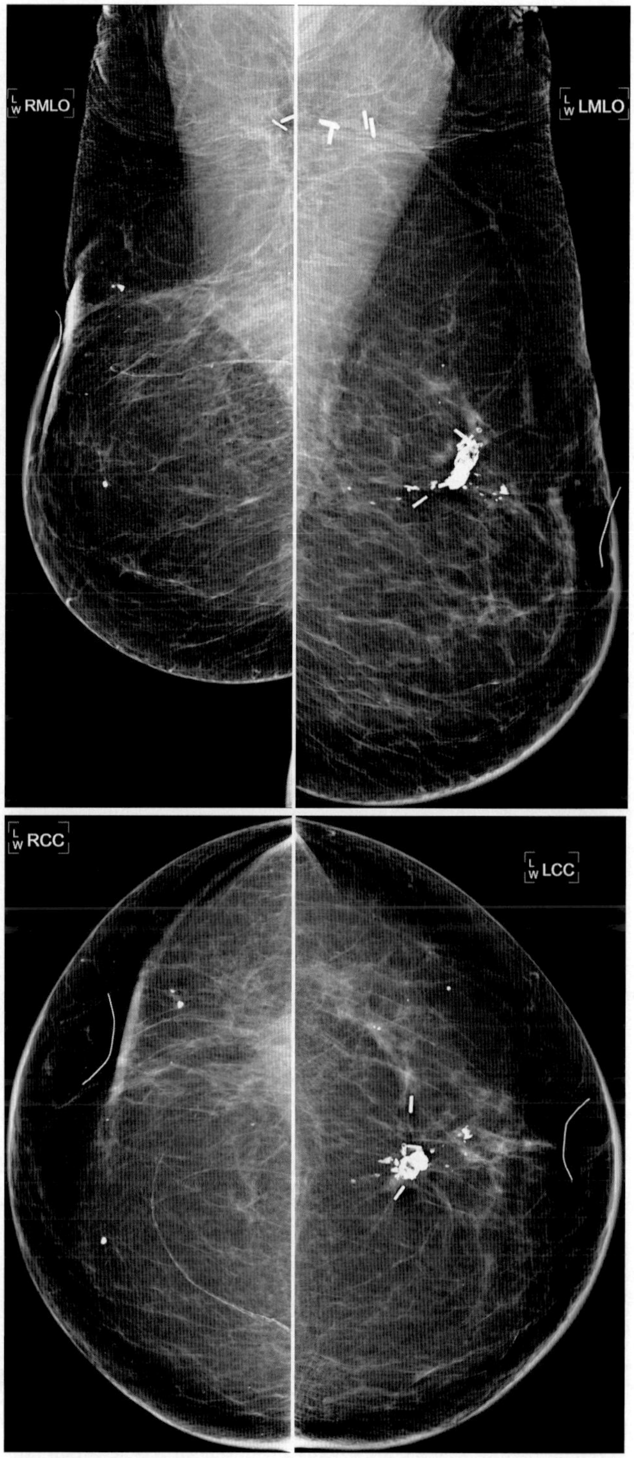

Fig. 16.14 Bilateral lumpectomies 9 years prior. The left breast shows benign fat necrosis, while the right breast has greater volume loss and architectural distortion

additional disease at the time of surgery and decrease the utility of a mammogram immediately after lumpectomy when it is often painful for the patient. In addition, an irradiated breast can be difficult to position for imaging and may

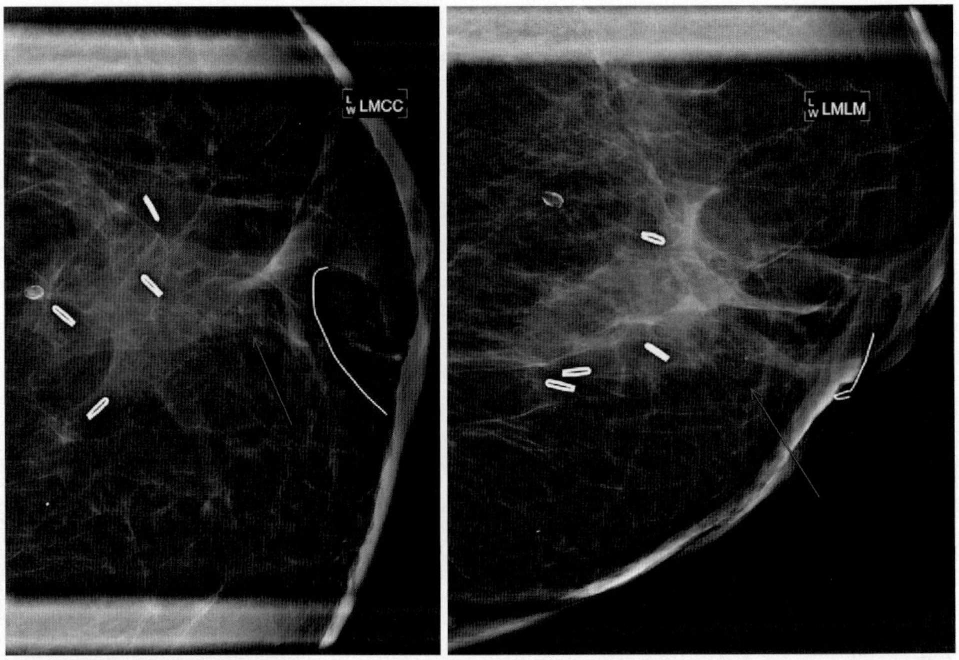

Fig. 16.15 Patient had left lumpectomy 3 years prior to exam. A new 5 mm cluster of heterogenous calcifications is visualized in the lumpectomy bed. Stereotactic biopsy was performed with pathology of dense fibrous connective tissue consistent with lumpectomy bed, histiocytic inflammatory response associated with microcalcifications and fat necrosis

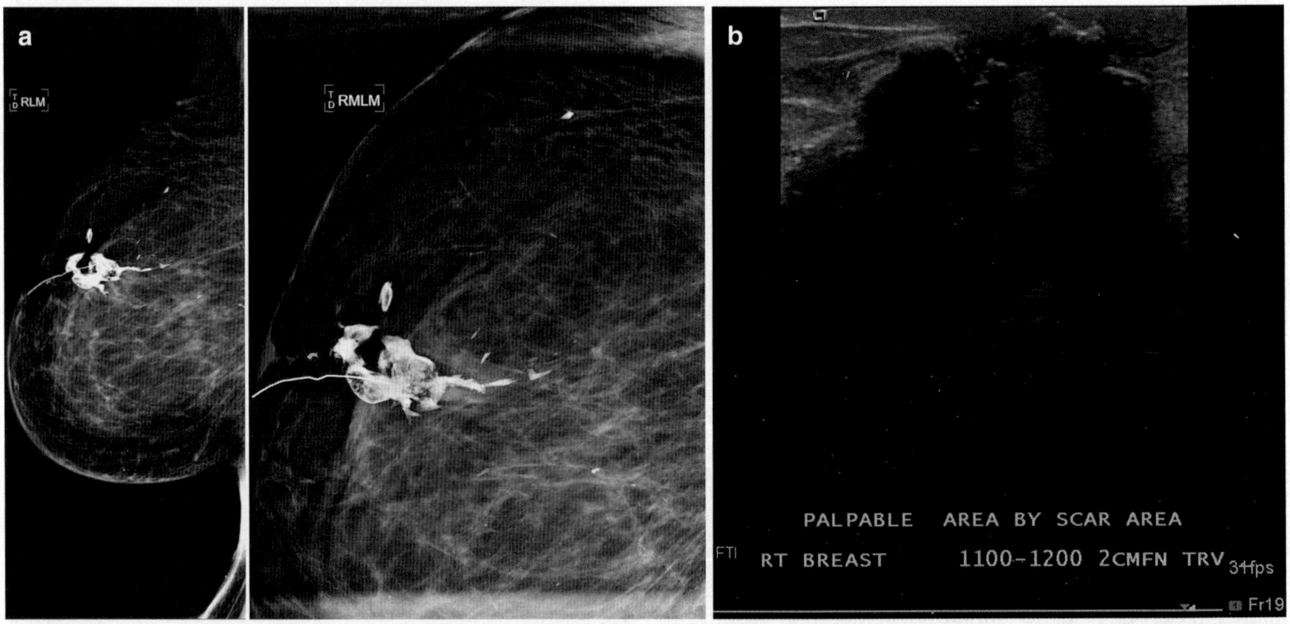

Fig. 16.16 (**a**) An 80-year-old female with history of right breast CA post lumpectomy 20 years prior to the exam. Recent 100 lb weight loss and new palpable abnormality in the right breast. The coarse fat necrosis calcifications were not significantly changed from a prior mammogram 2 years prior but was now better felt by the patient due to her weight loss. (**b**) Ultrasound of the area of palpable complaint demonstrates expected coarse calcifications and associated posterior acoustic shadowing consistent with fat necrosis

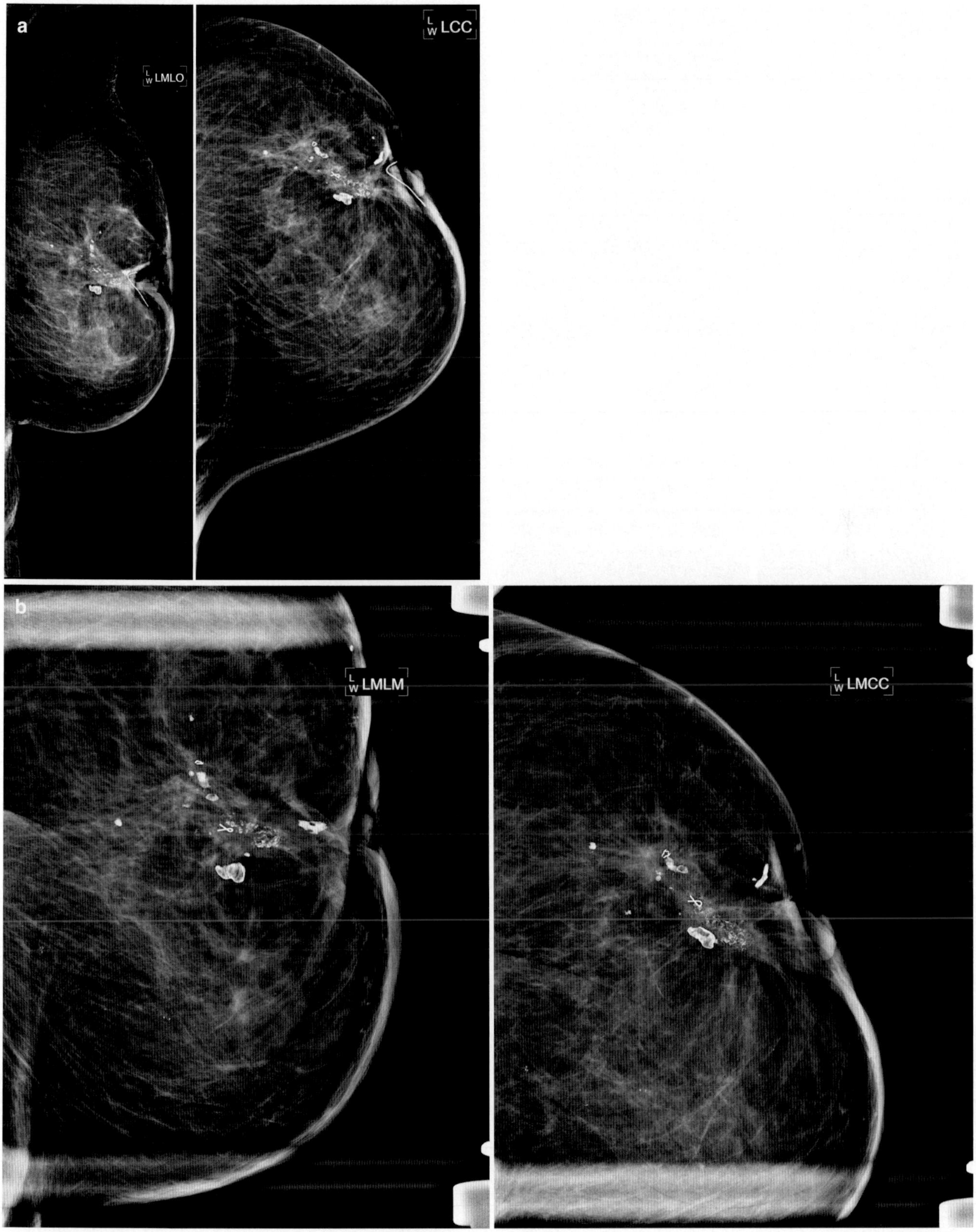

Fig. 16.17 (**a**) A 72-year-old female with history of lumpectomy 12 years prior. The patient lost 50 lb in the time since her prior mammogram and the patient and physician perceive "hardening" in the lumpectomy bed. (**b**) Spot magnification views demonstrate coarse, heterogenous fat necrosis calcifications that had been stable over several years. Note multiple biopsy clips localizing prior benign biopsies yielding fat necrosis

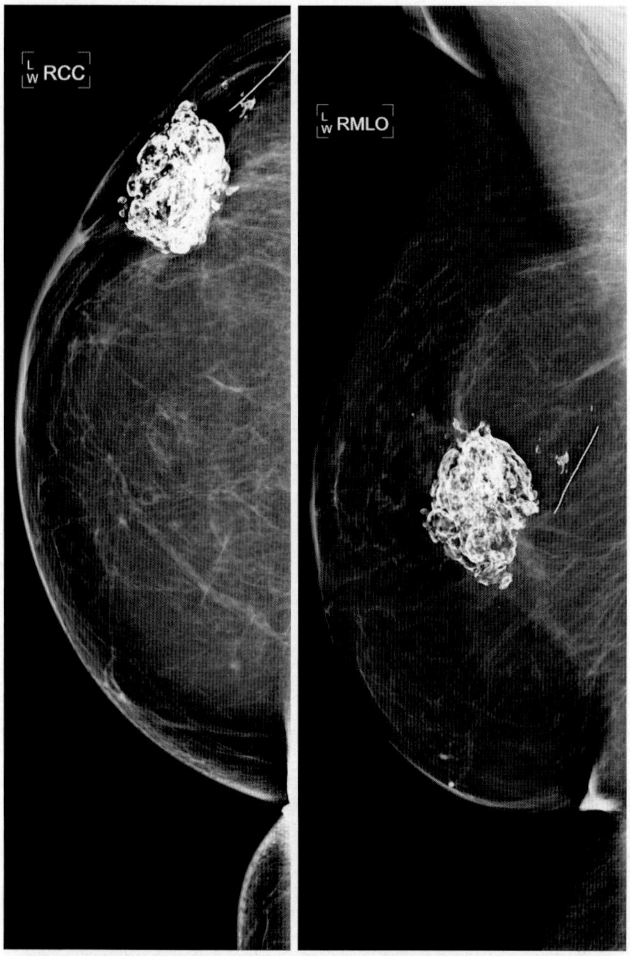

Fig. 16.18 Status post right lumpectomy with benign fat necrosis calcifications in the lumpectomy bed. Note the proximity of the calcified mass to the lateral skin making the mass palpable and leading the patient to call it "the rock" in her breast

be difficult to compress sufficiently due to patient discomfort.

After the initial unilateral mammogram 6 months post lumpectomy, bilateral mammography is performed at our facility 1 year following lumpectomy and on an annual basis thereafter, unless new imaging findings arise that require closer surveillance. However, various schedules have been proposed for follow-up mammograms after the 12-month study. Some facilities prefer to follow the post-lumpectomy breast at 6 month intervals for up to 3 years. Proponents of this schedule argue that this approach provides the optimum coverage through the "stabilization" period described in the chart. Proponents of extending 6-month follow-up out to 5 years believe that it provides better coverage when the breast transitions from the stabilization phase into the time when there is increasing frequency for recurrence. Some places will modify their schedule to perform more frequent follow-up in the patients that are at higher risk for recurrence based on the characteristics of that individual patient's cancer. We perform routine magnification views of the lumpectomy for 5 years following lumpectomy, another practice that varies by institution.

Ultrasound

There are also typical post-lumpectomy changes on sonography. Similar to mammography, familiarity with the expected sonographic appearance after surgery and radiation therapy is useful to avoid misinterpretation. Ultrasound of the lumpectomy bed within the first year after surgery usually demonstrates skin thickening and a fluid collection at the site of surgery, the size of which is variable by patient. Skin thickening after radiation therapy may reach 1 cm or greater [20]. Sonography is helpful in establishing fluid content with a mass seen in the lumpectomy cavity on mammography. The margin of the mass may be well circumscribed, ill defined, or spiculated due to the fibrotic reaction associated with healing (Fig. 16.22a, b). The fluid collection may be round or oval with varying margins (circumscribed, ill defined, or spiculated) and may appear simple or look like a complex cystic mass with septations or echogenic nodules [21] (Fig. 16.23). Aspiration of the postoperative seroma is not recommended and usually reserved for patients that have severe pain at the site or if there is suspected infection due to a tender, tense mass in a patient with fever. Ultrasound can be used for guidance if drainage is indicated. Reaccumulation of fluid following aspiration is common and there is a risk for the development of chronic draining sinuses.

Postoperative masses should remain stable, improve, or resolve. As the fluid is gradually reabsorbed, the residual fibrosis and scarring will be a hypoechoic mass with irregular margins and posterior acoustic shadowing. Identifying this finding beneath the skin scar or identifying a tract between the surgical bed and the skin is helpful in confidently identifying the mass as scar tissue. Sonography is useful in further evaluating mammographic masses as cystic or solid and can also help in further evaluating palpable masses

Fig. 16.19 (**a–c**) Evolution of fat necrosis. (**a**) The patient presented to our clinic 1 year following lumpectomy with faint, curvilinear calcifications visualized in the lumpectomy bed. Six months later, the calcifications are coarsening. (**b**) 24 and 36 months post lumpectomy. Stabilization of calcifications 3 years following surgery. (**c**) 48 months post lumpectomy

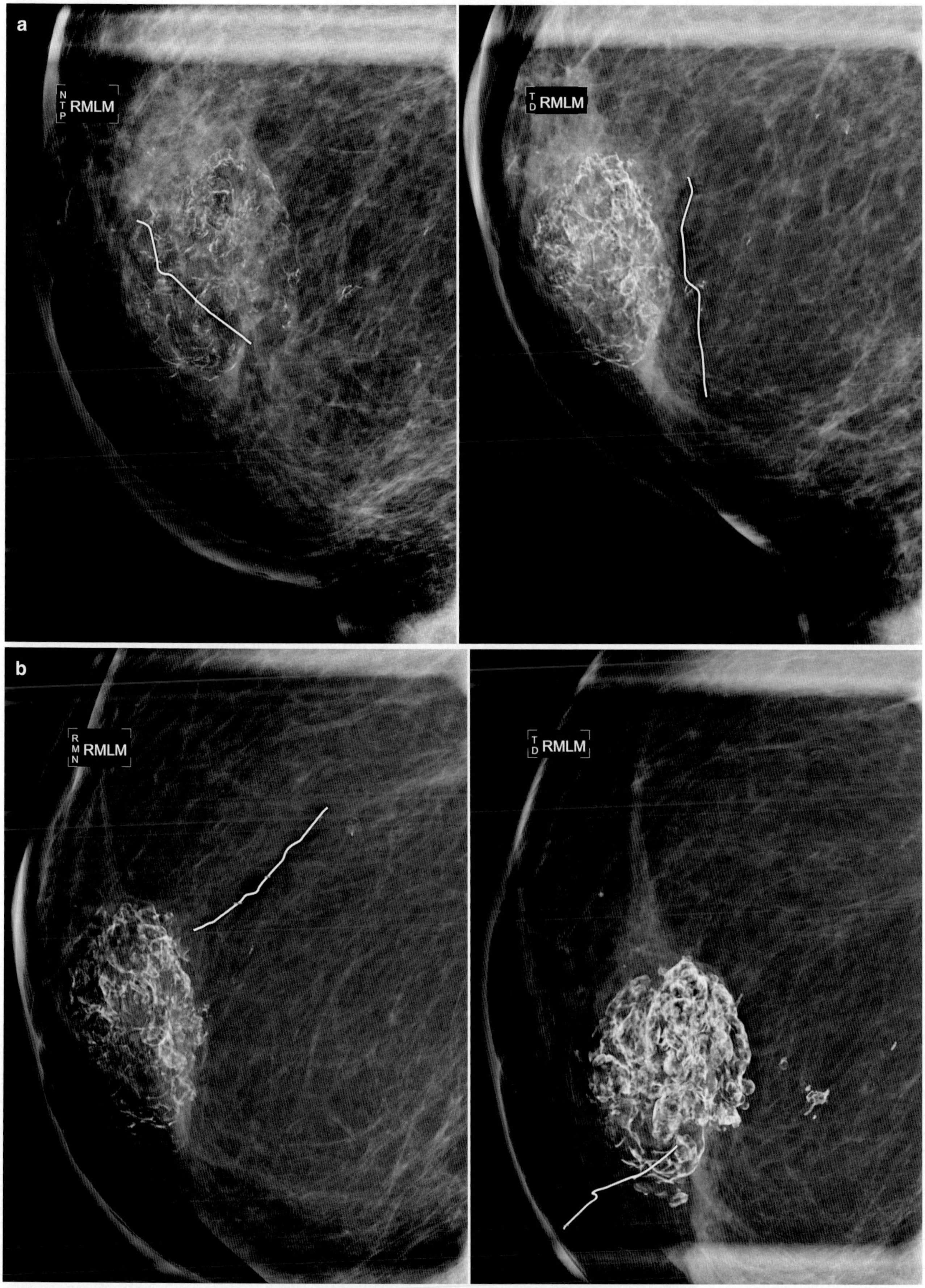
a
N T P RMLM
T D RMLM
b
R M N RMLM
T D RMLM

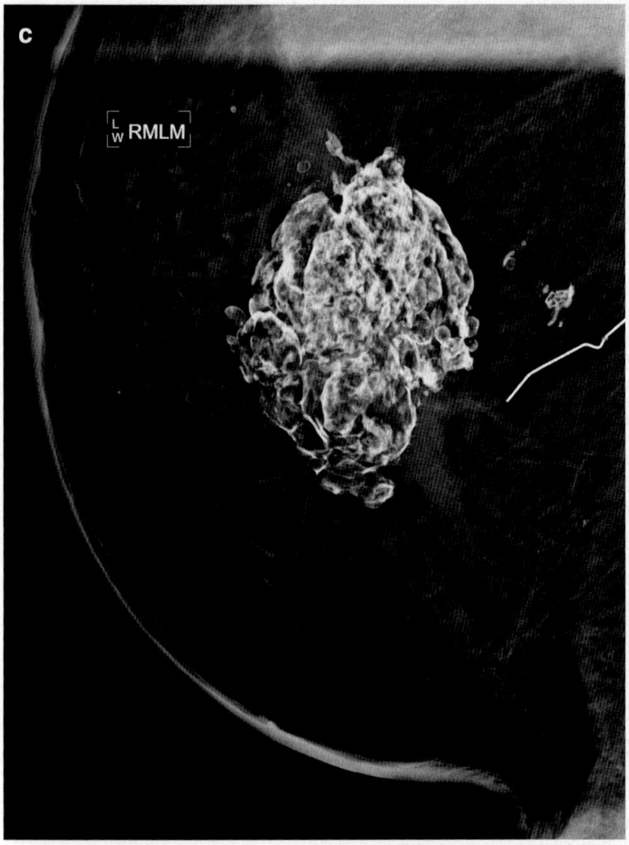

Fig. 16.19 (continued)

that are obscured by postsurgical changes or dense breast tissue. If a suspicious solid mass is identified, ultrasound can then be used to guide for biopsy. Residual skin thickening is seen in about 20 % of women 2 years after radiation therapy. Most fluid collections resolve within 2 years from the time of surgery. If a mass increases in size, further evaluation with ultrasound and possible biopsy is indicated.

MRI

Screening with breast MRI has high sensitivity, moderate specificity, and high cost when compared with mammography. In published recommendations from the Society of Breast Imaging and American College of Radiology, breast MRI may be considered in women with between 15 and 20 % lifetime risk for breast cancer on the basis of personal history of breast or ovarian cancer or biopsy-proven lobular neoplasia or ADH [4]. The American Cancer Society guidelines for breast screening with breast MRI published in 2007 stated there was insufficient evidence to recommend for or against screening women with a personal history of breast cancer [22]. A study by Morris et al. evaluated breast MRI screening in women with elevated risk of developing breast cancer and negative mammograms. The study included 245 women with personal history of breast cancer. In this group, breast MRI detected mammographically occult cancer in 4 % of the patients [23]. Consultation with referring clinicians can be helpful in selecting a subset of patients with history of breast cancer that is at

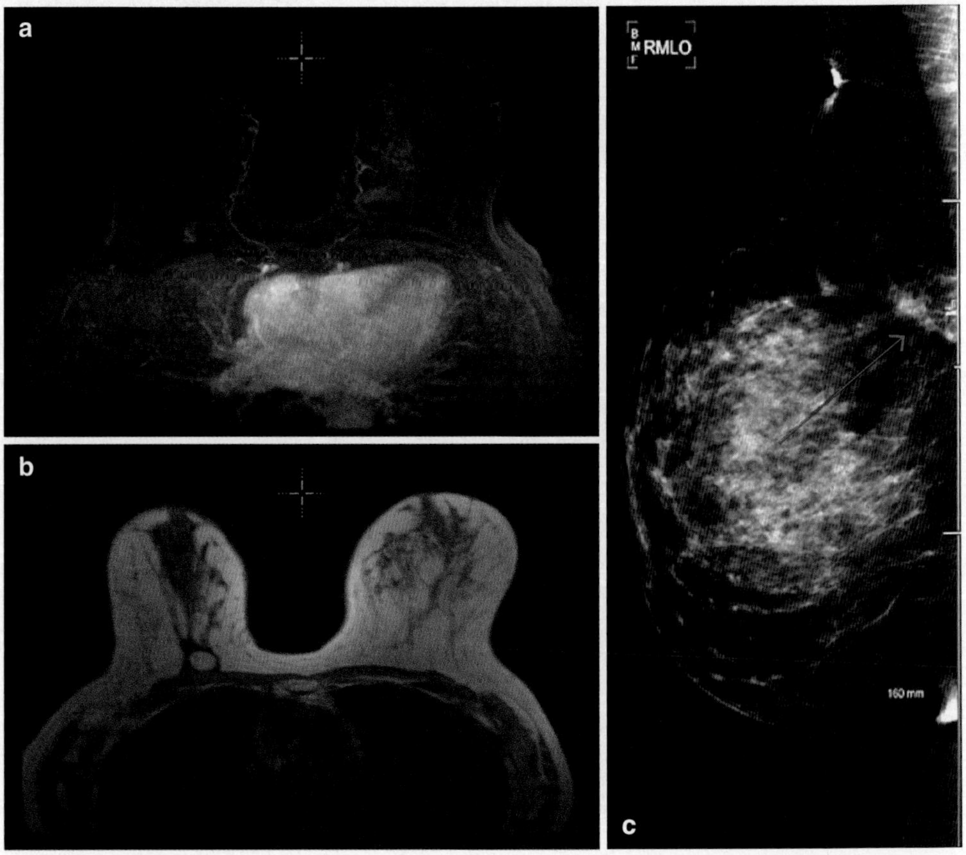

Fig. 16.20 (**a**) A 73-year-old female with history of right breast cancer status post lumpectomy 2 years prior. Patient is reporting new palpable complaint in the left breast with no mammographic or sonographic correlate. MIP image demonstrates non-mass-like enhancement in the area of palpable complaint. Biopsy was performed and yielded fat necrosis. Nodular enhancement is present in the right lumpectomy cavity. (**b**) T1 axial non-contrast image demonstrates central fat within the area of enhancement consistent with benign fat necrosis. (**c**) Right breast mammogram confirms the presence of fat necrosis

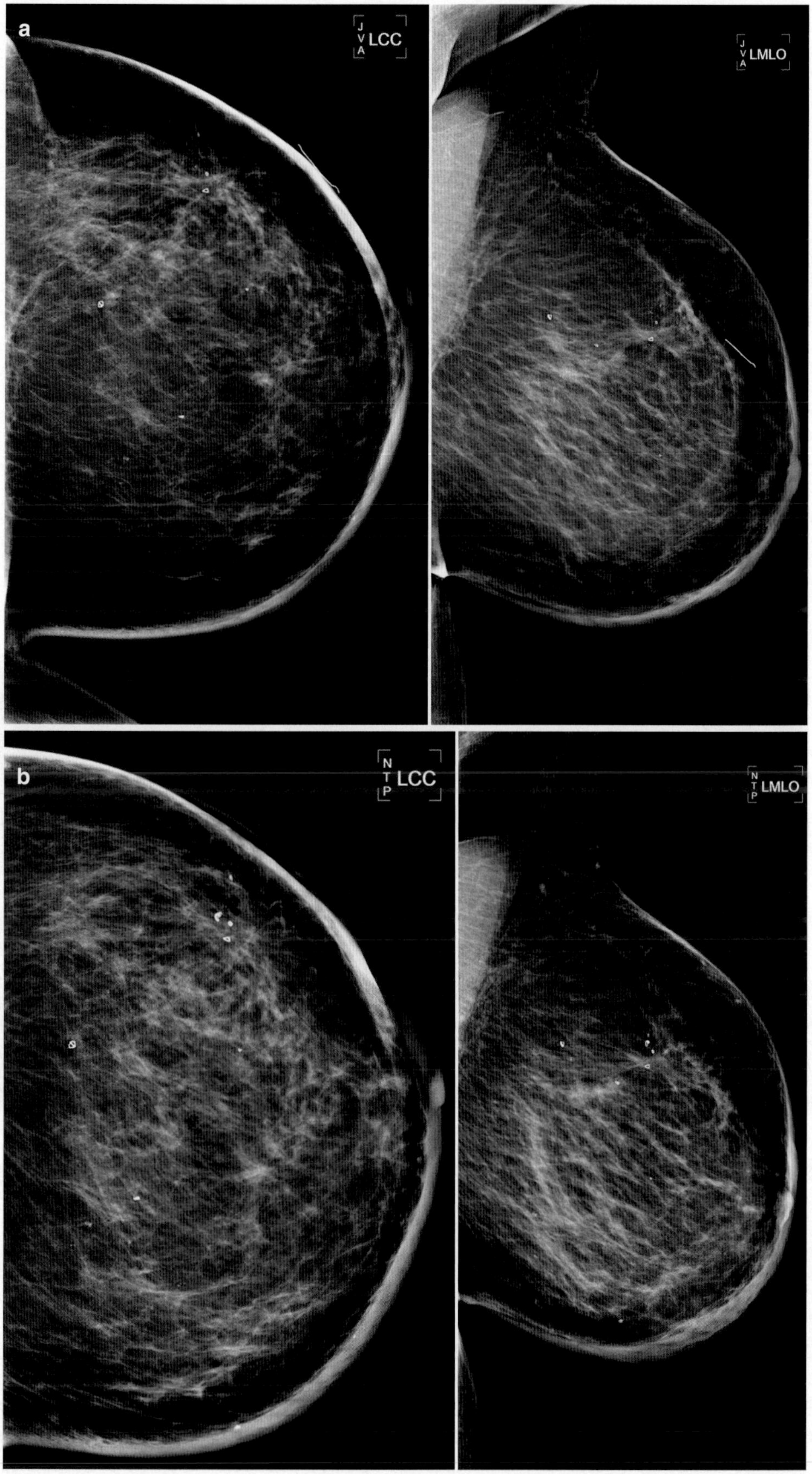

Fig. 16.21 (**a**) 10 years post lumpectomy and radiation therapy with residual skin thickening. (**b**) Over the following 3 years, the patient developed progressive increase in skin thickening. The patient reported increased breast heaviness. The interval change prompted skin biopsy which revealed dermal fibrosis consistent with scar. Following the biopsy, the patient's symptoms improved and on the subsequent mammogram the skin thickening returned to postsurgery baseline

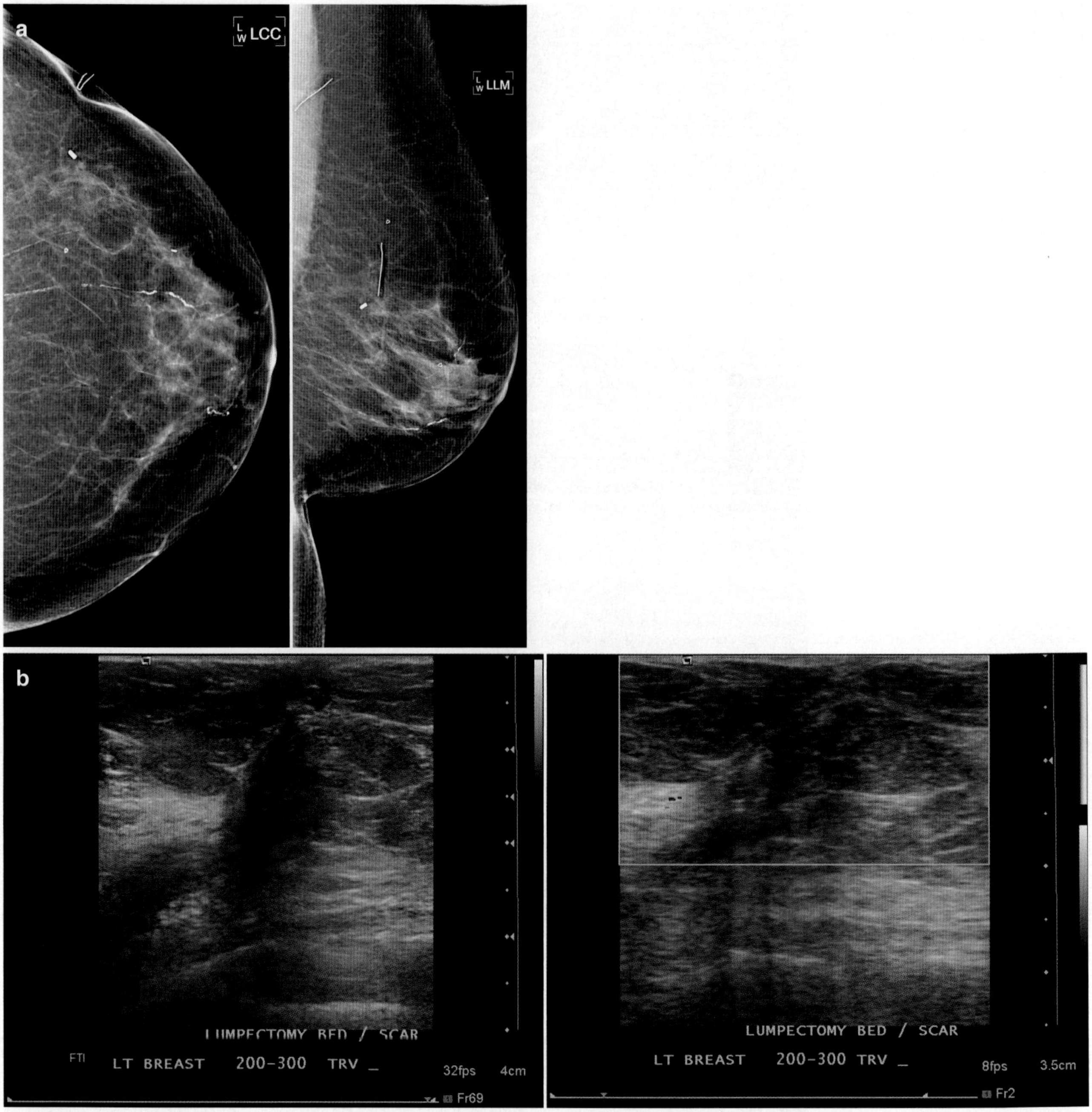

Fig. 16.22 (**a**) Left lumpectomy 8 years prior. Post-lumpectomy changes in the upper outer breast. (**b**) Ultrasound appearance of the post-lumpectomy scar area. An irregular hypoechoic area is present with changes extending to the skin. Doppler US does not demonstrate vascularity in the fibrotic scar tissue

particularly high risk for recurrence for supplemental screening with breast MRI. Importantly, the impact of breast MRI screening on breast cancer mortality has not been established by randomized clinical trials. As with its use in screening of the high risk for breast cancer population, breast MRI used in screening patients with a personal history of breast cancer should always be performed as an adjunct to mammography as some recurrences, particularly of DCIS, are detected by mammography only.

Recurrence

As therapy for breast cancer continues to improve, the number of long-term survivors is increasing and the population of patients being screened for recurrent disease is increasing. Although there are no randomized trials establishing mortality benefit of screening mammography after breast conservation therapy, the use of screening mammography has been demonstrated to decrease breast cancer mortality and

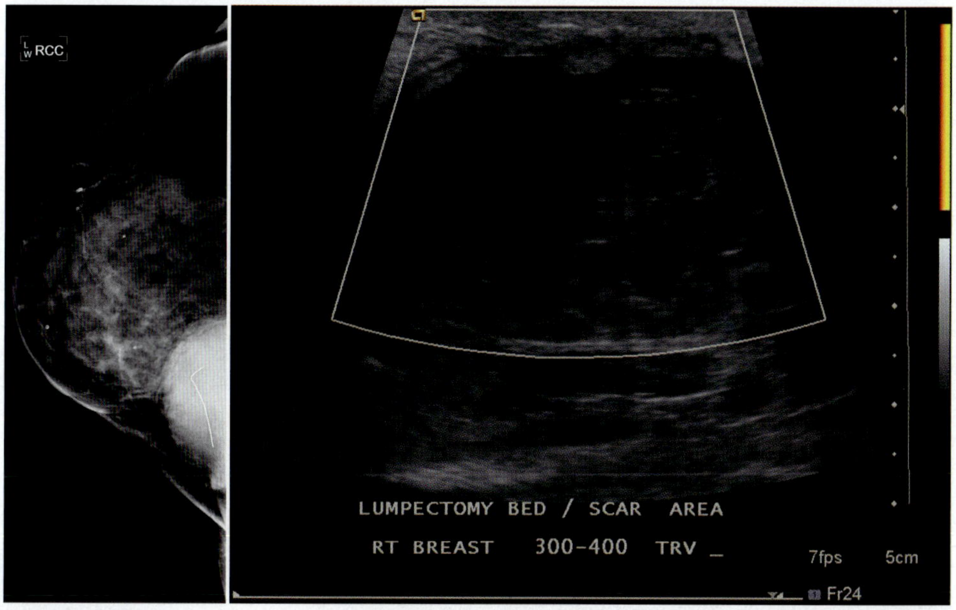

Fig. 16.23 Persistent complex postoperative seroma 2 years after lumpectomy. Hyperdense mass in the posterior inner right breast corresponds to a complex fluid collection visualized in the area of the lumpectomy scar on ultrasound. The fluid collection is decreased in size from prior exams but will likely persist on future mammograms

therefore is likely to decrease breast cancer mortality from a second primary tumor. Imaging plays a fundamental role in monitoring breast conservation patients for recurrence and, in combination with clinical history and physical exam, is an important part in optimal surveillance for breast cancer recurrence. It is estimated that 35–50 % of local recurrences will be detected with mammography in the absence of physical findings [24]. Evaluating mammograms in sequence and comparing the current mammogram to not only the prior year but also to mammograms going back several years is critical for detecting subtle findings of recurrence. The goal of surveillance is to detect recurrences at an early time point in order to initiate therapy to improve survival and to maintain a high quality of life.

Tumor recurrence can occur locally (ipsilateral treated breast), regionally (ipsilateral lymph nodes), or as a distant metastatic disease. Local tumor recurrence in the ipsilateral breast 5 years after breast-conserving therapy occurs in approximately 7 % of patients with whole breast irradiation and 26 % of patients without whole breast irradiation [25]. Most recurrences occur in the lumpectomy bed, and positive pathologic margins, younger age, higher grade tumor, larger tumor size, negative estrogen receptor status, and involvement of axillary lymph nodes have all been reported to increase the risk of ipsilateral breast tumor recurrence [25–28]. The development of pleomorphic, heterogenous, or linear calcifications, new masses, or skin thickening or increases in size or density of architectural distortion on mammography may indicate breast cancer recurrence and should prompt biopsy (Figs. 16.24a–c, 16.25a, b, 16.26a, b, 16.27a–c, 16.28a, b, 16.29a, b, 16.30a–c, 16.31a, b, and 16.32a, b).

Tumor recurrence rarely occurs in the first 2 years following treatment [18]. Changes in the mammogram in that time are more likely alterations from benign processes. Tumor recurrence in the postoperative site or quadrant peaks at a rate of 2.5 % between 2 and 6 years after breast conservation therapy. Recurrent cancers at the original tumor site usually result from failure to eradicate the original cancer and usually occur sooner than tumor developing elsewhere in the breast. Recurrence more than 10 years after therapy will more likely occur outside the treated area and likely represent new malignancies. Recurrent tumor is usually treated with salvage mastectomy. However, if the patient did not undergo radiation therapy in their initial therapy, surgical re-excision with subsequent radiation is a possible alternative.

Breast cancer in the contralateral breast of women with known history of breast cancer may represent a new primary or a metastasis from the original breast cancer (Figs. 16.33a–d, 16.34a–d, and 16.35a–c). Cancer with different pathology from the original cancer or a cancer with an associated in situ component is classified as new primaries. The risk for a metachronous, contralateral second primary breast cancer is estimated at 0.5–1.0 % per year [29]. Factors that increase the risk include a known BRCA1 or BRCA2 mutation, young age at first primary, family history of breast cancer, lobular histology for first primary breast cancer, and prior radiation exposure [30–32]. Treatment of estrogen-positive primary cancers with tamoxifen can decrease risk for contralateral breast cancer by 50 % [25]. Adjuvant endocrine therapy trials incorporating an aromatase inhibitor document an even greater reduction in the occurrence of contralateral breast cancer [33]. Knowledge of the receptor status of the patient's original tumor and possible subsequent endocrine therapy can be helpful to breast imagers in the pretest probability assessment for risk for recurrent disease.

Calcifications are an important marker for new or recurrent cancer following lumpectomy. Up to 43 % of mammographically detected cases of recurrent cancer manifest as microcalcifications [34]. The presence of pleomorphic calcifications is concerning for recurrent or residual malignancy and biopsy should be performed. In general, increasing microcalcifications in the lumpectomy bed are worrisome for breast cancer recurrence, unless the calcifications are increasing in coarseness as would be seen in fat necrosis or dystrophic calcifications. Ultrasound is limited in the evaluation of calcifications and therefore is not recommended as the primary imaging method to evaluate for recurrence. Although sonography alone is not recommended as the primary means of evaluation for recurrence, sonography can be a useful adjunctive study for supplemental screening [35].

Some patient present with perceived changes in their lumpectomy bed. The patient may describe the scar becoming more firm or larger. Usually these subjective changes are due to scar tissue or fat necrosis. If evaluation with mammography and ultrasound fails to demonstrate interval change, evaluation with breast MRI may be helpful in discriminating postsurgical scarring from recurrent tumor at the lumpectomy site [36].

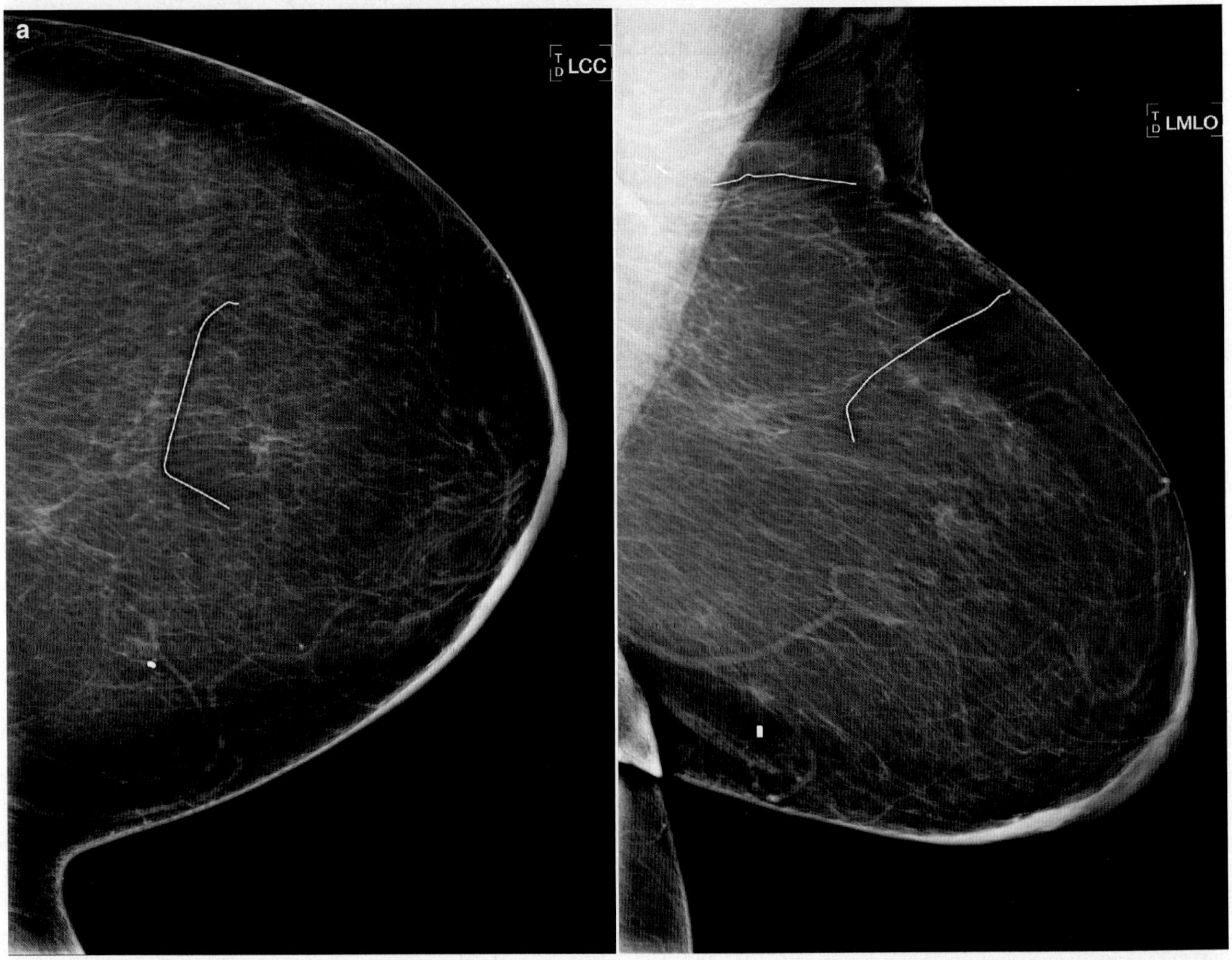

Fig. 16.24 (**a**) 8 years post left lumpectomy for a 5 mm invasive lobular carcinoma and no positive axillary lymph nodes. Following surgery and XRT, the patient took 5 years of tamoxifen. Stable postsurgical changes in the upper central breast. A small asymmetry in the mid upper central breast was unchanged from multiple prior exams. (**b**) Nine years post lumpectomy. Interval development of a high-density spiculated mass in the upper central breast. (**c**) 3 cm anterior to the lumpectomy scar, a 1.1 cm irregular hypoechoic mass with spiculated margins corresponds to the mass seen on mammography. US-guided biopsy yielded infiltrating lobular carcinoma with focal pleomorphic features. The patient underwent left mastectomy

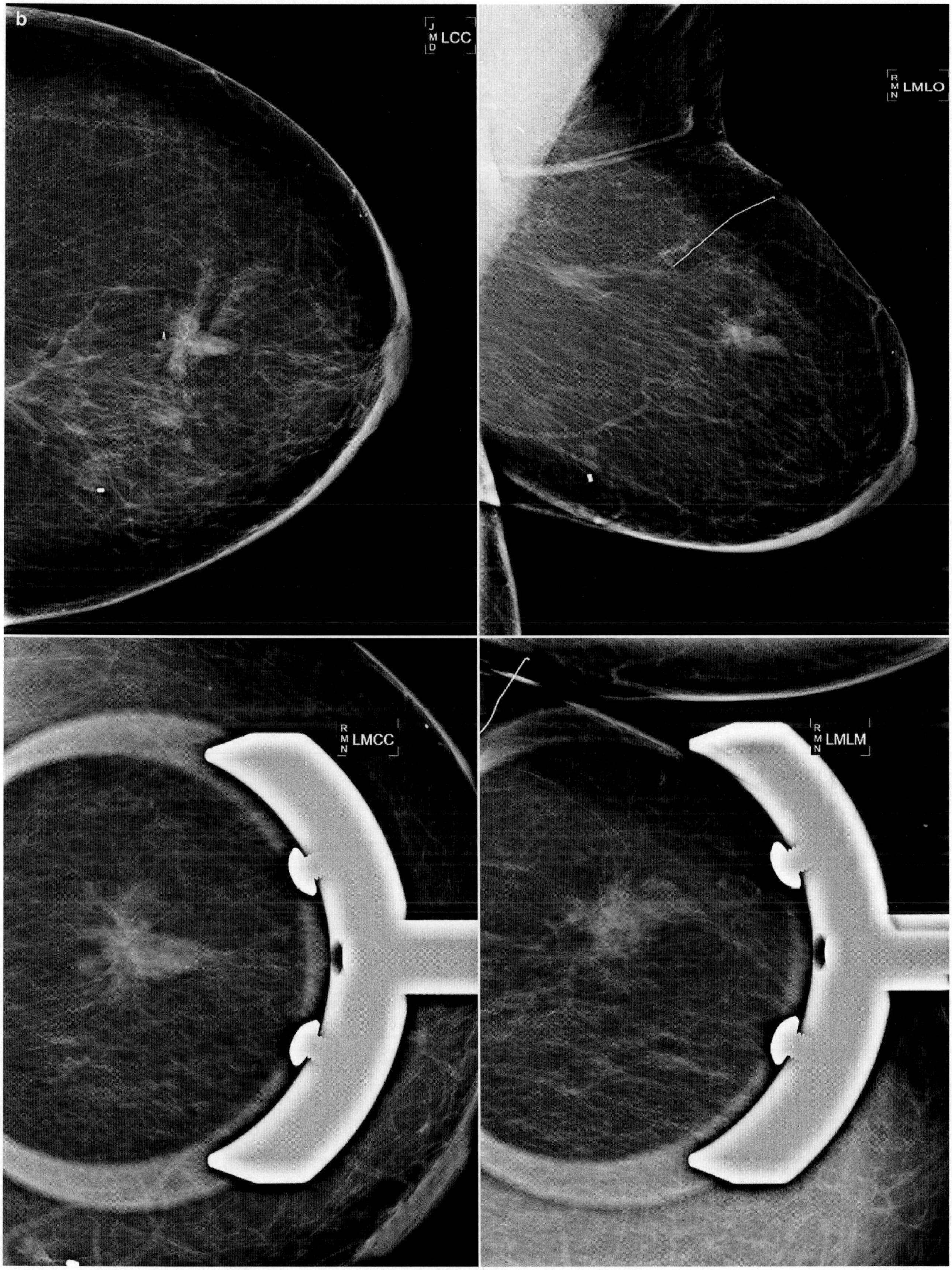

Fig. 16.24 (continued)

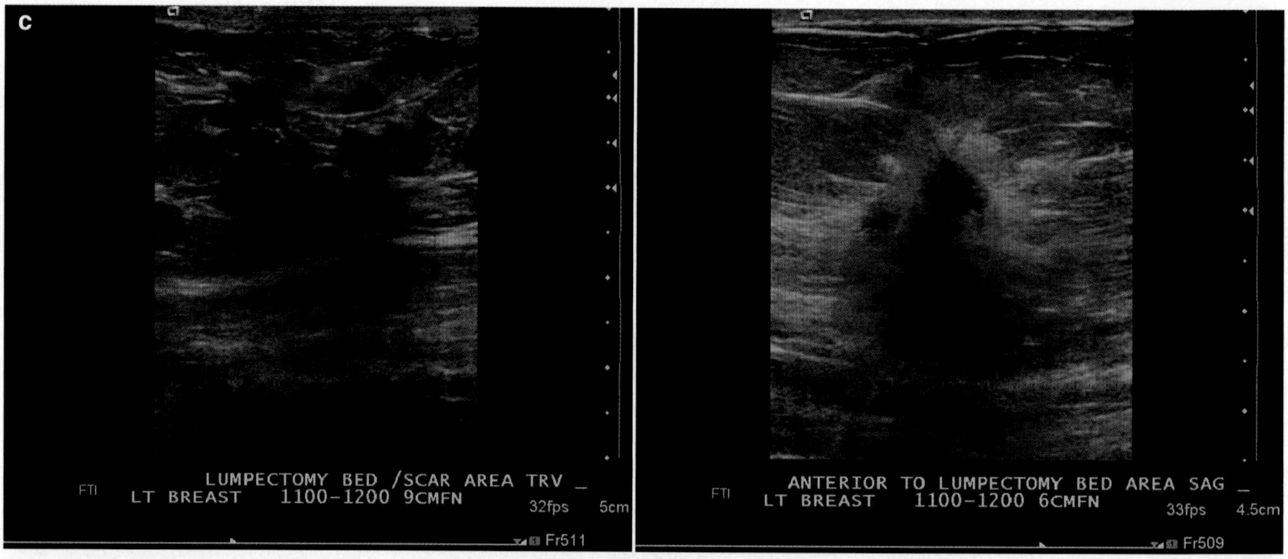

Fig. 16.24 (continued)

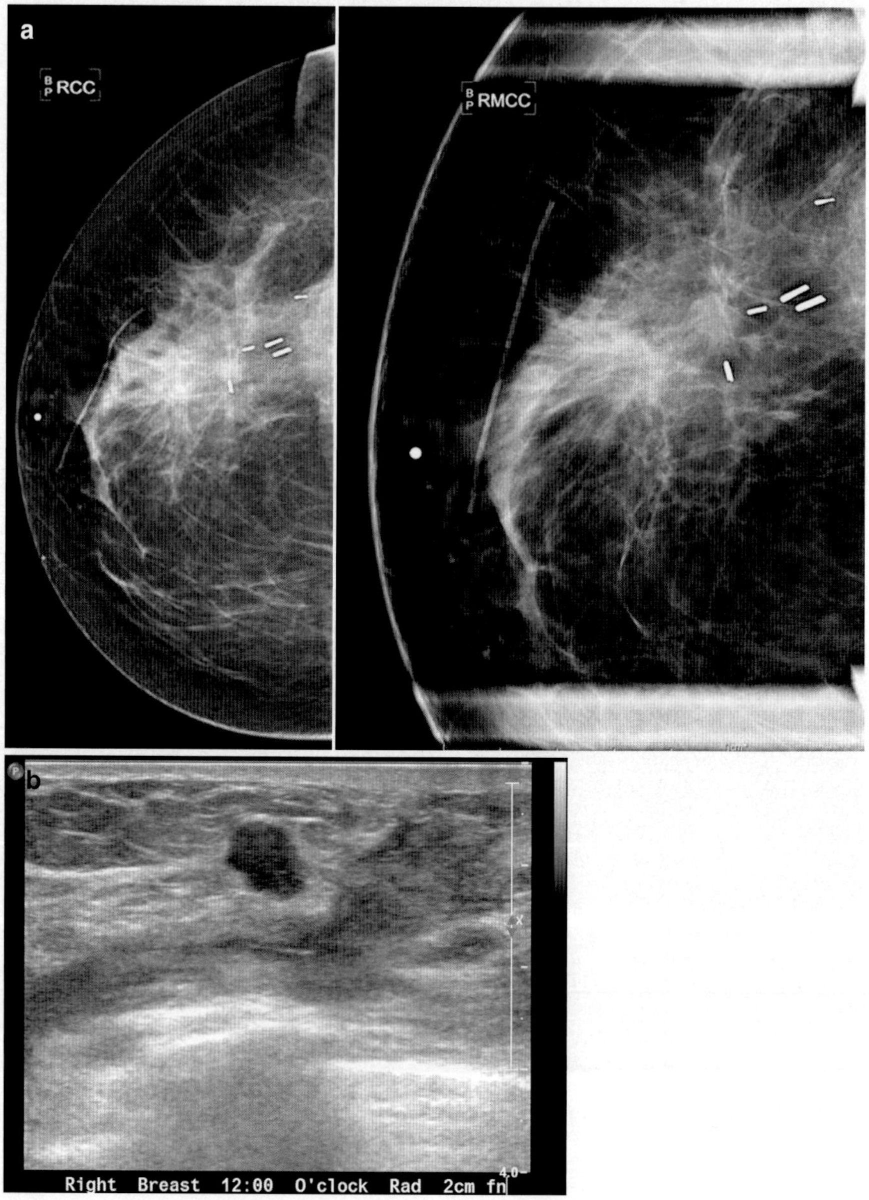

Fig. 16.25 (**a**) 6 months post lumpectomy. An 8 mm mass is visualized in the lumpectomy bed. (**b**) US demonstrates a corresponding irregular solid mass. Biopsy yielded invasive carcinoma. Biopsy yielded invasive carcinoma

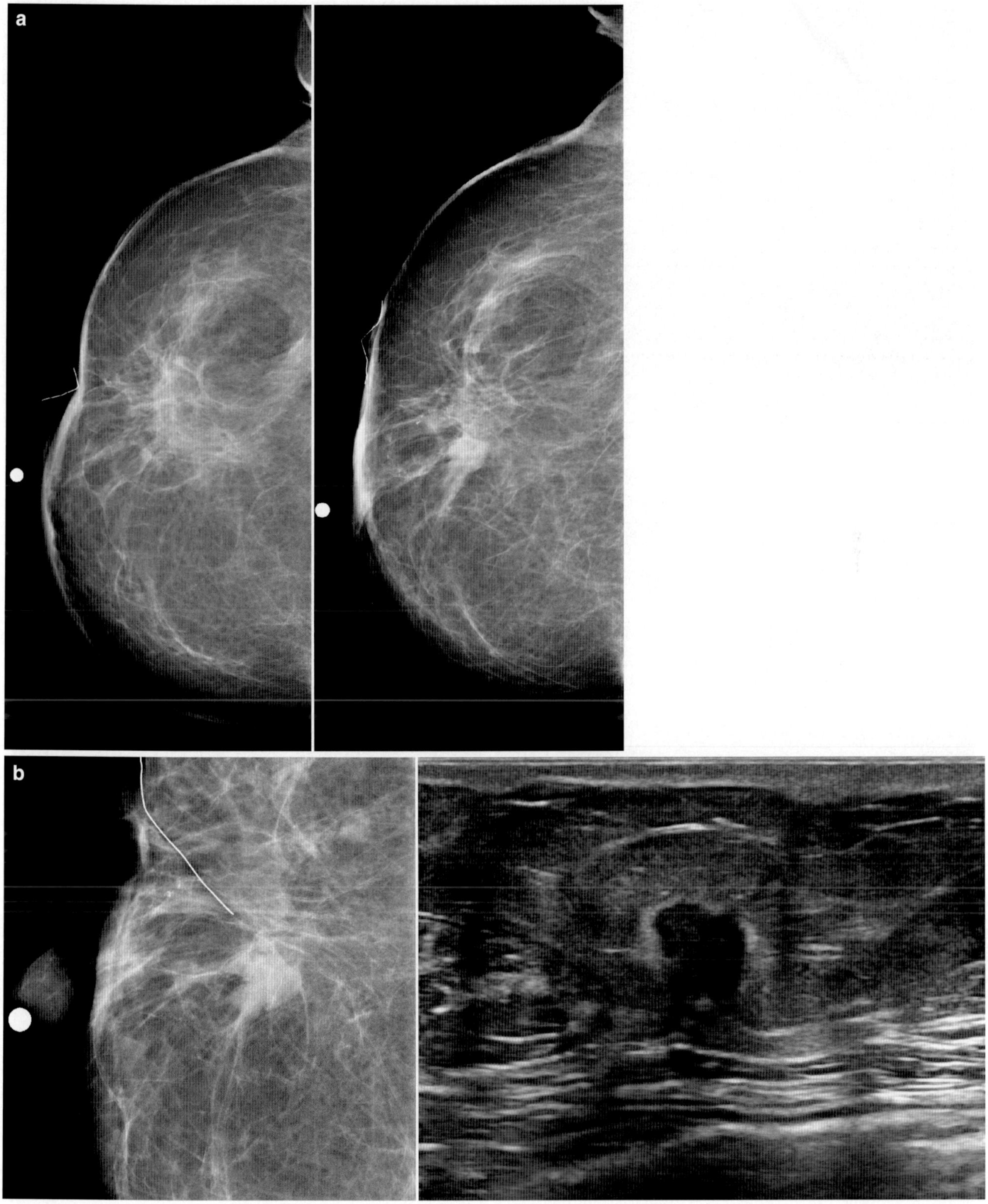

Fig. 16.26 (**a**) Right breast recurrence: Mammogram on the left was performed 3 years after lumpectomy. Mammogram on the right was performed 5 years after lumpectomy and demonstrates a new 1 cm spiculated mass in the central breast. (**b**) Spot magnification views and ultrasound demonstrate suspicious spiculated margins to the mass. US-guided core needle biopsy was performed with pathology of invasive carcinoma. The patient declined radiation therapy at the time of her lumpectomy and thus was a candidate for lumpectomy and radiation therapy for the recurrence

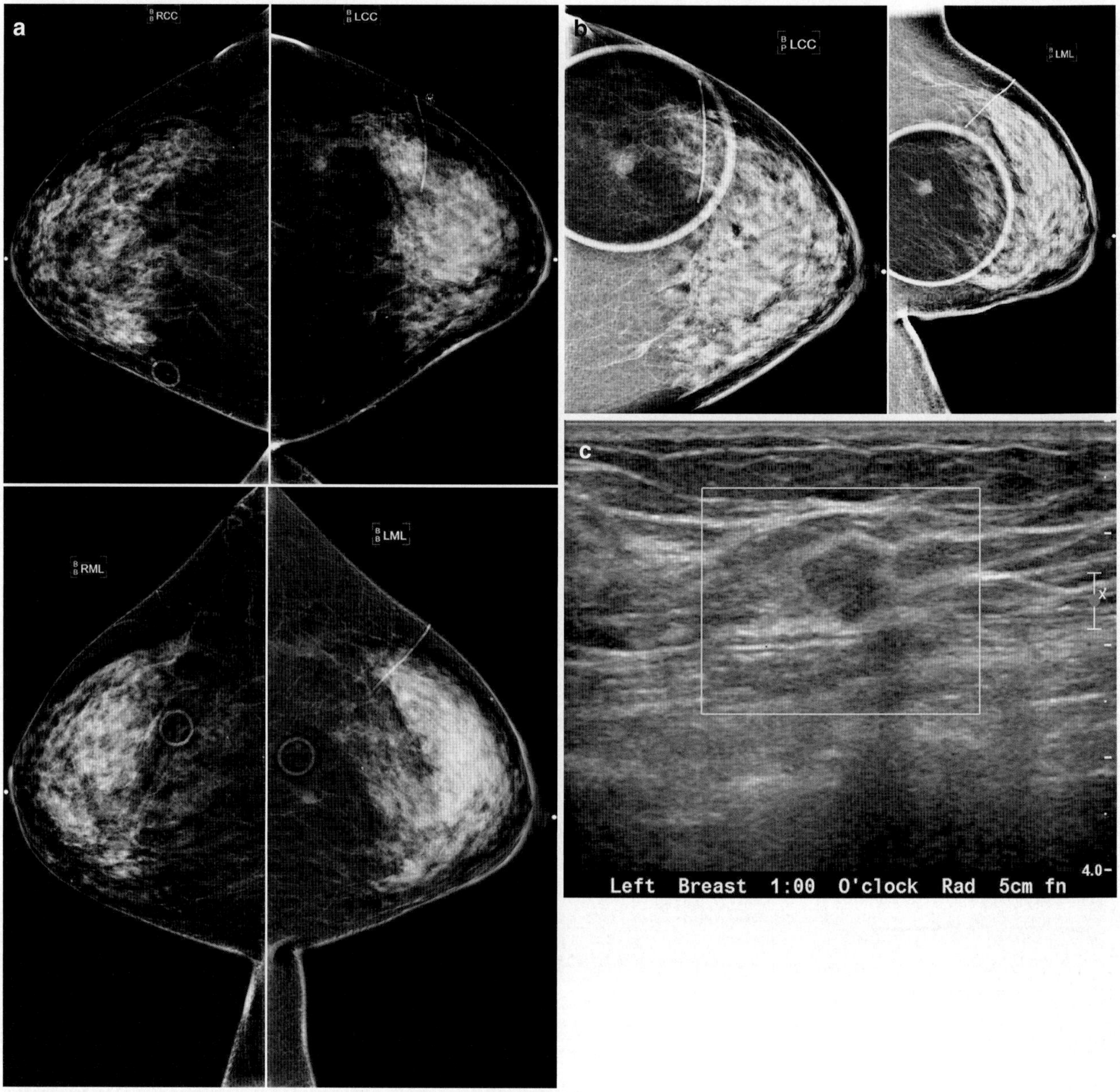

Fig. 16.27 (**a**) A 72-year-old female status post left lumpectomy for DCIS 1 year prior. (**b**) Spot magnification views confirm a new mass in the posterior upper outer left breast. (**c**) A corresponding 8 mm solid mass is seen on ultrasound. Biopsy yielded invasive carcinoma

Postmastectomy

Mastectomy is the surgical removal of the entire breast tissue. This is performed in women with breast cancer who cannot be adequately treated with breast conservation therapy or in women who prefer this method for treatment of their cancer. Also, women who have a high risk for developing breast cancer such as BRCA 1 and BRCA 2 carriers can opt to have prophylactic mastectomies. The risk of developing a breast malignancy is significantly reduced but not entirely eliminated in patients who undergo prophylactic mastectomy or any mastectomy for that matter, because a small amount of residual breast tissue remains. The lack of a distinct boundary between the breast and adjacent adipose tissue makes the removal of all breast tissue difficult [37].

Mastectomy Without Reconstruction

The type of mastectomy performed depends on the clinical scenario. A simple or total mastectomy involves the removal of only breast tissue including the nipple–areolar complex.

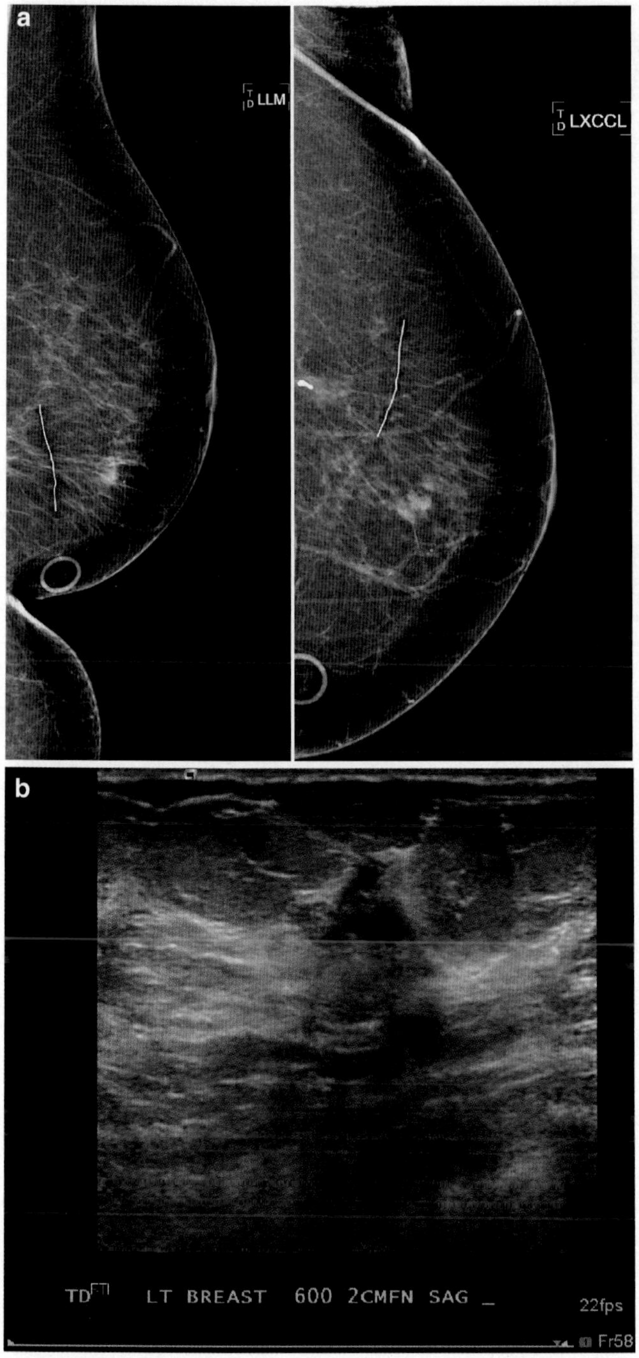

Fig. 16.28 (**a**) 10 years post lumpectomy. New 1 cm mass in the mid lower central left breast. (**b**) 1.1 cm corresponding hypoechoic mass on US. Biopsy yielded infiltrating mammary carcinoma

No removal of lymph nodes or pectoralis muscle occurs (Fig. 16.36a–d). A modified radical mastectomy involves the removal of breast tissue and nipple–areolar complex and an axillary dissection involving the removal of level I and II axillary lymph nodes (Fig. 16.37). A similar but more extensive rarely performed procedure due to its deforming nature and lack of impact on survival is the radical or extended mastectomy. Here, level I, II, and III lymph nodes and the pectoralis muscle are removed. A portion of the pectoralis muscle may be resected in a simple or modified mastectomy, if there is evidence of tumor invasion [38].

Mastectomy with Reconstruction

A woman who undergoes a mastectomy not only has to deal with the emotional and physical consequences of treatment but also the psychological impact of losing her breast. Patients who have had a mastectomy can choose to use an external prosthesis or have a reconstruction [39]. Continued improvement and advancement in the field of microsurgery provides women with choices when it comes to having a mastectomy with reconstruction. A woman can now have a mastectomy with reconstruction using her own tissue (autologous) to create a neobreast similar in appearance and even touch to her native breast. A woman can also choose to have a reconstruction with a breast prosthesis such as with a silicone or saline implant or with both autologous tissue and implants [38]. Studies have shown that having a mastectomy with breast reconstruction does not change survival compared with a simple mastectomy [40, 41].

Types of Autologous Reconstruction

For women who prefer to use their own tissue, the most standard method is through the transplantation of a transverse rectus abdominis myocutaneous (TRAM) flap into the mastectomy bed. This method provides a neobreast which is similar to the native breast in texture and appearance and is often referred to as the "tummy tuck" reconstruction. In this procedure, an autologous myocutaneous flap consisting of abdominal skin, subcutaneous fat, the rectus abdominis muscle (dual blood supply via the superior and inferior epigastric arteries), and adjoining vasculature is used for reconstruction following mastectomy. Since its introduction by Hartrampf et al. in 1982, refinements have been made to the basic technique including the pedicled, free, and delayed flap reconstruction [42, 43]. The two major technical variants of the TRAM flap include the pedicled flap which uses the superior epigastric vessels and the microsurgical free flap which uses the more robust inferior epigastric vessels. The pedicle TRAM flap requires the full length of the rectus abdominis muscle. The muscle along with its overlying lower abdominal skin and subcutaneous tissue are elevated and tunneled subcutaneously into the mastectomy defect. A portion of the skin overlying the mastectomy defect will then become the surface of the newly created neobreast. In a unilateral breast reconstruction, the contralateral muscle is used, and in cases of bilateral reconstructions, the ipsilateral rectus abdominis muscle is used to prevent vascular compromise due to crossing of the pedicles [43].

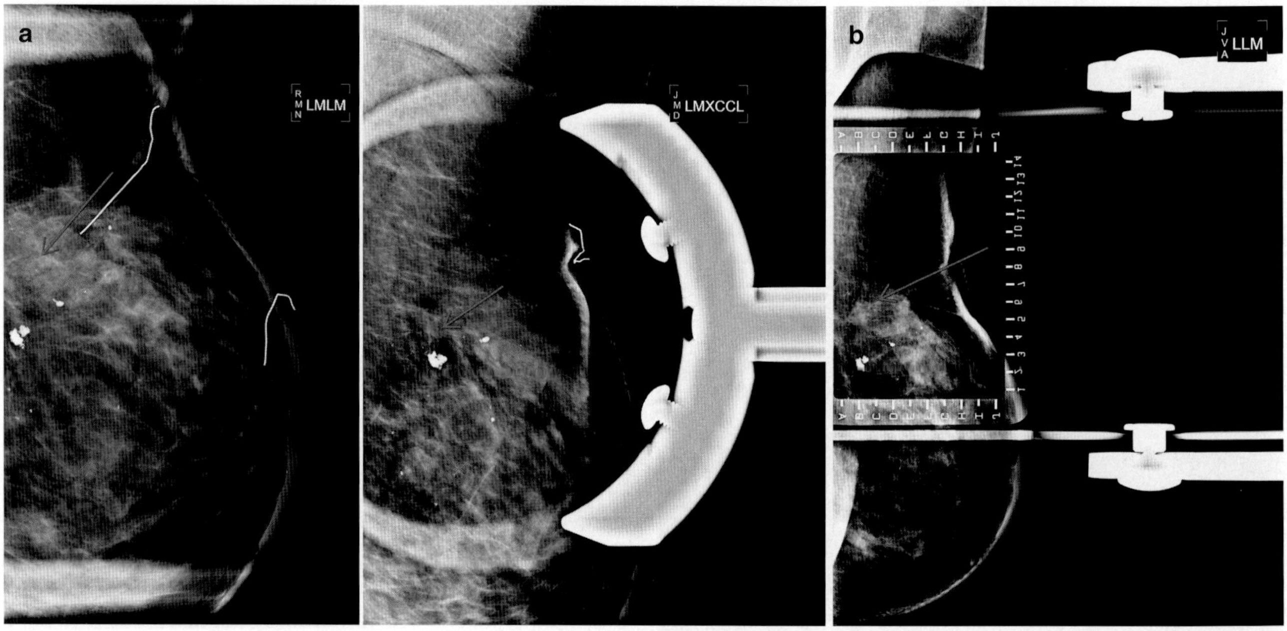

Fig. 16.29 (**a**) Left lumpectomy 3 years prior. New heterogenous calcifications are seen in the posterior aspect of the lumpectomy bed on the spot magnification views. (**b**) Localization picture for stereotactic biopsy. Pathology demonstrated ductal carcinoma in situ, atypical ductal hyperplasia

Continued improvement in microsurgical techniques led to the development of the free TRAM flap technique. This procedure utilizes the more robust inferior epigastric vasculature which is reanastomosed to the internal mammary, thoracodorsal, or subscapular vasculature. The establishment of a direct anastomosis offers a better and more predictable perfusion. Also, since only a small portion of the rectus abdominis muscle is utilized, the risk of abdominal wall hernias is decreased [43–45].

Expansion of the free tissue concept led to the development of additional flap options for autologous breast reconstruction, namely, the latissimus dorsi myocutaneous flap, based on the thoracodorsal vasculature. This reconstruction is often performed with an implant. Other flaps include the gluteal free flap, based on the inferior gluteal or superior gluteal vessels, and the lateral thigh flap which overlies the tensor fascia lata muscle with blood supply from the lateral femoral circumflex, which is long enough to be anastomosed with the axillary vessels. This flap has a low incidence of fat necrosis. The Rubens flap overlies the peri-iliac region and is supplied by the deep circumflex vessels [45, 46].

The development of perforator flap techniques added even more to the armamentarium of options for autologous breast reconstruction. The main idea here is to eliminate the harvesting of muscle entirely by establishing perfusion to a skin paddle from a single dominant perforating vessel. Although, donor site morbidity is minimized, procedure time is prolonged; therefore, appropriate patient selection matters. The deep inferior epigastric (DIEP) technique is a perforator flap technique applied to a TRAM flap. This procedure uses the lower abdominal skin and subcutaneous tissues with complete sparing of the rectus abdominis muscle. The internal mammary vessels are the preferred site of anastomosis. The DIEP flap is of tremendous benefit when a bilateral reconstruction is performed due to minimal disruption of the abdominal wall which precludes the use of an abdominal mesh and a lower incidence of abdominal wall bulges and hernias [45, 47]. The superior gluteal artery perforator (SGAP) is an additional surgical application or the perforator flap principle. The long length of the vascular pedicle and low incidence of donor site morbidity make this a good choice for autologous breast reconstruction. The superficial inferior epigastric artery (SIEP) flap is another perforator flap technique which is supplied by the superficial system. The idea behind this technique is to eliminate the need to harvest not only muscle but also the deeper vasculature. However, the unpredictable perfusion secondary to size and length of the pedicle makes this "idyllic" technique not a commonly utilized one [45].

Reconstruction with Prosthesis

If a woman does not wish to undergo autologous reconstruction, the use of breast prosthesis with a silicone or saline breast implant is an option. The benefits of this option are no additional sites of scars elsewhere in the body and no flap or donor-site complications. There is greater flexibility in determining breast size and postoperative recovery is often shorter. Reconstruction with prosthesis is often a better choice for a patient requesting reconstruction, but not having sufficient

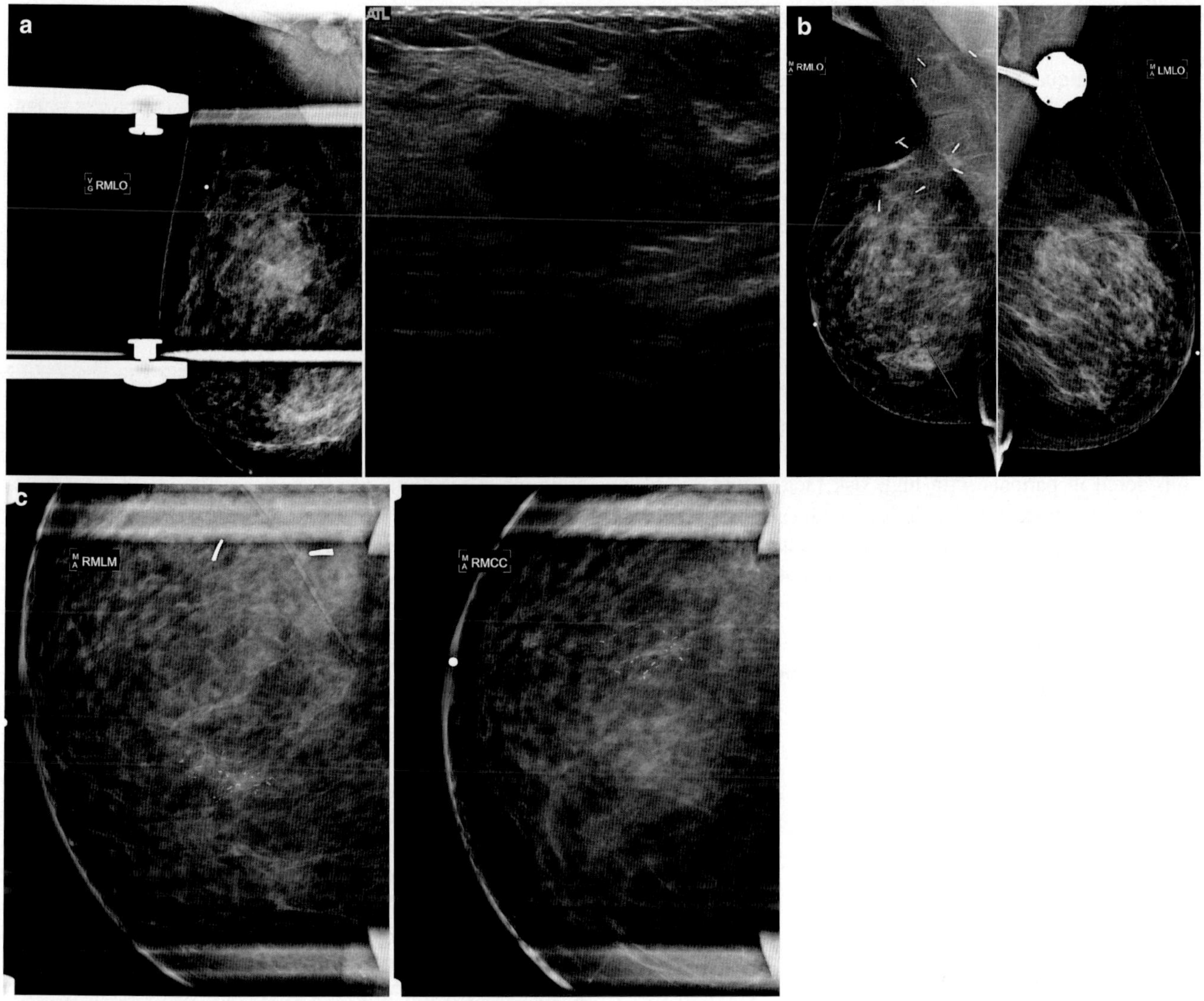

Fig. 16.30 (**a**) A 42-year-old female present with palpable abnormality in the right breast. Note prominent right axillary lymph node. US demonstrates a corresponding suspicious 1.5 cm mass. Biopsy demonstrated IDC. The patient underwent right lumpectomy and XRT. (**b**) 6 months following lumpectomy: post-lumpectomy changes are seen in the mid-posterior upper outer right breast. In the central right breast, pleomorphic calcifications span 6 cm. A scar marker overlies the upper outer left breast at the site of prior excision of a fibroadenoma. A left-sided Port-A-Cath is present. (**c**) Spot magnification views: linear branching calcifications are now seen in the mid central breast. DCIS was found at biopsy

autologous tissue for reconstruction or with comorbid medical conditions (Figs. 16.38 and 16.39). The surgery can be performed in one stage or as a two-stage operation. A two-stage surgery is often performed if there is a concern of skin viability or if the patient is requesting an increase in breast size. If performed in two stages, a tissue expander is first placed into a musculofascial pocket which consists of the pectoralis major and serratus anterior muscles. Expansion with saline is then performed periodically in an outpatient setting as the patient tolerates until the desired breast size is achieved. The tissue expander is then exchanged and replaced with an implant. With the increase use of nipple-sparing mastectomies, the one-stage approach is becoming more common [38, 44].

During breast reconstruction, the nipple–areolar complex (NAC) is sacrificed, and reconstruction of the NAC is the last stage of reconstruction. This can be performed with local flaps (contralateral nipple, inner thigh) or a tattoo [38]. With any reconstruction, the contralateral breast may require a reduction mammoplasty, a mastopexy, or an augmentation mammoplasty to achieve symmetry.

Multidisciplinary input is necessary when considering breast reconstruction regarding appropriate timing and sequencing of intervention. Factors such as delays in therapy in the setting of locally advanced breast cancer and effects of radiation on the reconstructed breast must be considered.

Nipple- and Skin-Sparing Mastectomy

A new technique which precludes the native nipple–areolar complex (NAC) reduces the prominent scars and the unnatural skin paddle on the breast mound is the skin-sparing mastectomy. A smaller periareolar incision is made, thereby requiring a smaller skin paddle to replace the areolar defect. The natural contour of the breast is preserved once the transfer of the flap takes place. The results are a more aesthetically pleasing appearance which often reduces the need for contralateral asymmetry procedures such as a reduction or a mastopexy. The skin-sparing method has garnered increased popularity due to several studies reporting local recurrence rates equivalent to traditional methods (simple mastectomy without reconstruction). Nipple-sparing mastectomy can be considered in patients with high risk factors undergoing a prophylactic mastectomy or in breast cancer patients with a low risk of nipple involvement and smaller tumor burden away from the nipple. Preoperative imaging is helpful in excluding nipple involvement [45, 48–54].

Complications associated with breast reconstruction include total or partial flap necrosis secondary to vascular compromise, fat necrosis, and donor site complications (abdominal wall hernias and umbilical necrosis). Similar to other patients with implants, there is a risk of implant rupture in patients who undergo reconstruction with implant prosthesis (Fig. 16.40). As with all surgical procedures, bleeding, infection, hematoma, seroma formation, and wound dehiscence can also occur. These risks are increased in patients who smoke, are obese, or have had previous radiation therapy [44]. Therefore, appropriate patient selection is crucial when performing breast reconstructive surgery to improve outcome.

Follow-Up Imaging

A simple mastectomy can be performed without reconstruction and surveillance is not routinely performed. Controversy exists regarding surveillance of a reconstructed breast with some advocating routine screening for early detection of non-palpable recurrent cancer in the reconstructed breast and others patients with TRAM flaps, so as to detect non-palpable lesions early [40]. While others believe that routine screening

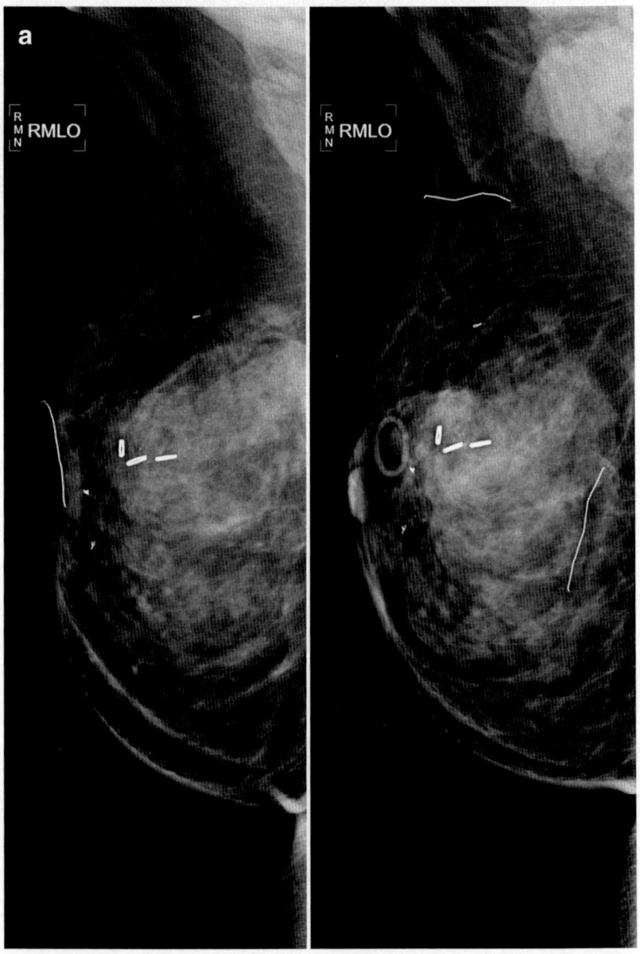

Fig. 16.31 (**a**) 2 years post right lumpectomy (*left*), there was no evidence for recurrent disease. 6 months later, the patient felt a new lump in her right axilla (*right*). (**b**) Spot magnification views of the lumpectomy bed demonstrate pleomorphic calcifications. An ill-defined hypoechoic mass with echogenic foci (calcifications) in the right 12:00 position measures approximately 3.4 cm. In the right axilla, an abnormal lymph node measures 4.4 cm. Biopsy was performed on both masses with pathology of IDC in the breast and metastatic carcinoma in the axilla

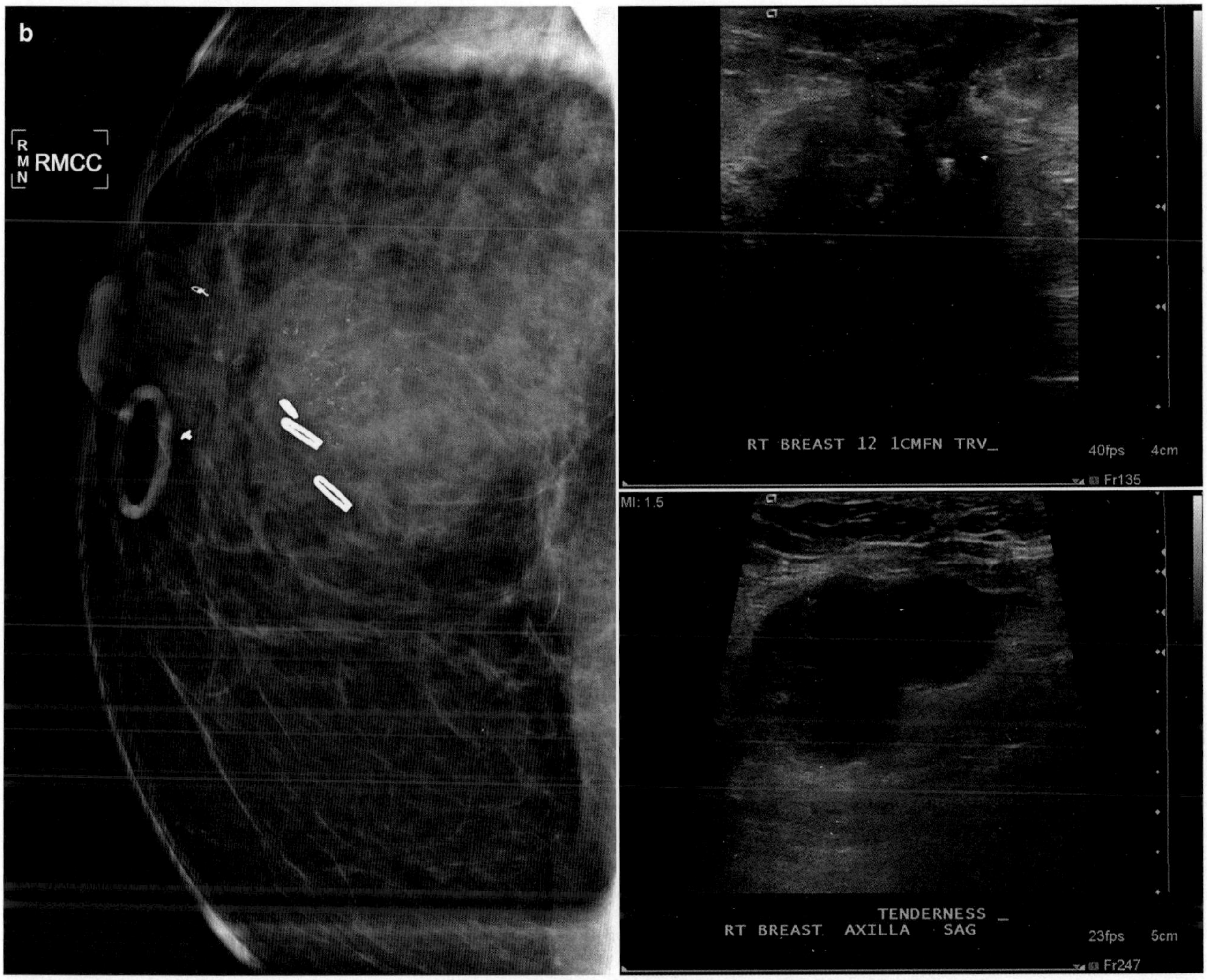

Fig. 16.31 (continued)

is not warranted due to the low incidence of recurrence in the reconstructed breast and low detection rates on mammography and MRI [55, 56]. However, given the increase in the screening of the contralateral breast with MRI in patients with a personal history of breast cancer, an opportunity exists to evaluate the reconstructed breast, chest wall, subcutaneous tissues, and overlying skin regardless of the type of mastectomy since these areas will be in the field of view if a bilateral MRI is performed.

Autologous myocutaneous flaps have a predominantly radiolucent fatty appearance on mammography and the normal fibroglandular tissue and architecture is absent. The nipple–areolar complex is also absent. The muscle pedicle has a varying appearance and can be visible posteriorly on mammography. The transplanted muscle is best seen on the mediolateral oblique view, anterior to the pectoralis muscle (Fig. 16.41). The muscle flap will be absent if a DIEP flap was used. If an LDM flap with partial mastectomy was performed, there might be residual glandular tissue. Common postoperative findings that can be noted on mammography include fat necrosis which may be seen as a lucent mass with surrounding density or curvilinear and dystrophic calcifications typically in the upper outer quadrant of the flap away from the vascular pedicle. Skin thickening, scarring, and surgical clips may also be noted. Recurrent disease will typically be noted on the chest wall and will have suspicious findings similar to the primary malignancy or masses and calcifications with suspicious features requiring further investigation, typically with ultrasound [46, 57].

Ultrasound is a useful modality in the investigation of a palpable area of concern. In a patient with an autologous reconstructed breast, diffuse fatty tissue is noted with absence of fibroglandular tissue. The vascular pedicle may be demonstrated on color Doppler. If close to the postoperative period, fluid collections representing hematomas or seromas may be demonstrated.

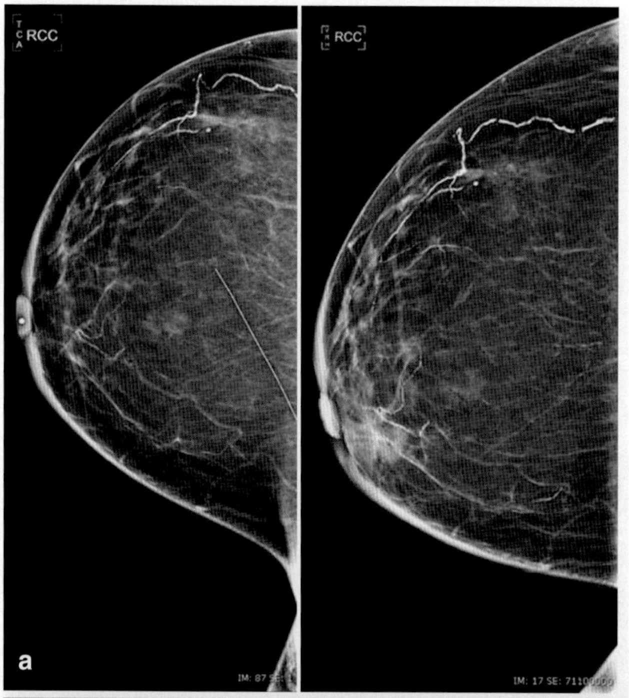

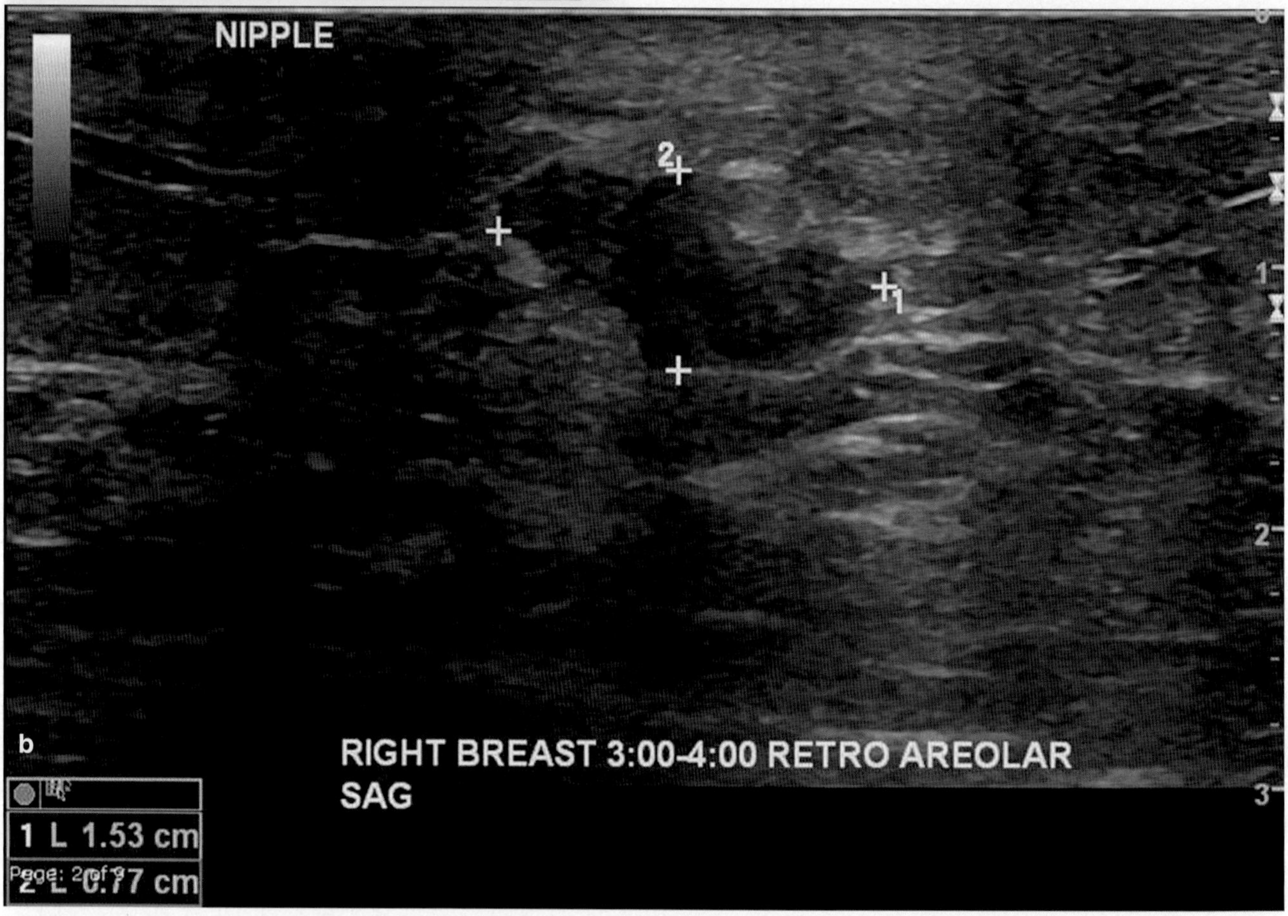

Fig. 16.32 (**a**) Patient is 17 years post lumpectomy. In a 1-year interval, the patient developed increased density and skin thickening in the retroareolar position. (**b**) US demonstrates a 1.5 cm mass with angular margins and skin thickening. Biopsy yielded invasive carcinoma

Fig. 16.33 (**a**) Left lumpectomy 11 years prior. Post-lumpectomy changes in the upper outer left breast. A new 1 cm asymmetry is visualized in the posterior upper outer right breast. (**b**) Spot magnification views of the asymmetry in the far posterior breast. (**c**) A corresponding 1.1 cm hypoechoic mass is identified in the right posterior breast on US. Note is also made of residual fluid in the left lumpectomy bed. Biopsy of the right breast mass had pathology of invasive ductal carcinoma. The patient opted for bilateral mastectomies. (**d**) 1 year following surgery, the patient presented with a new palpable abnormality in the far lateral right chest wall. A corresponding 1.4 cm hypoechoic mass was visualized with similar pathology and biomarkers as the prior right breast cancer

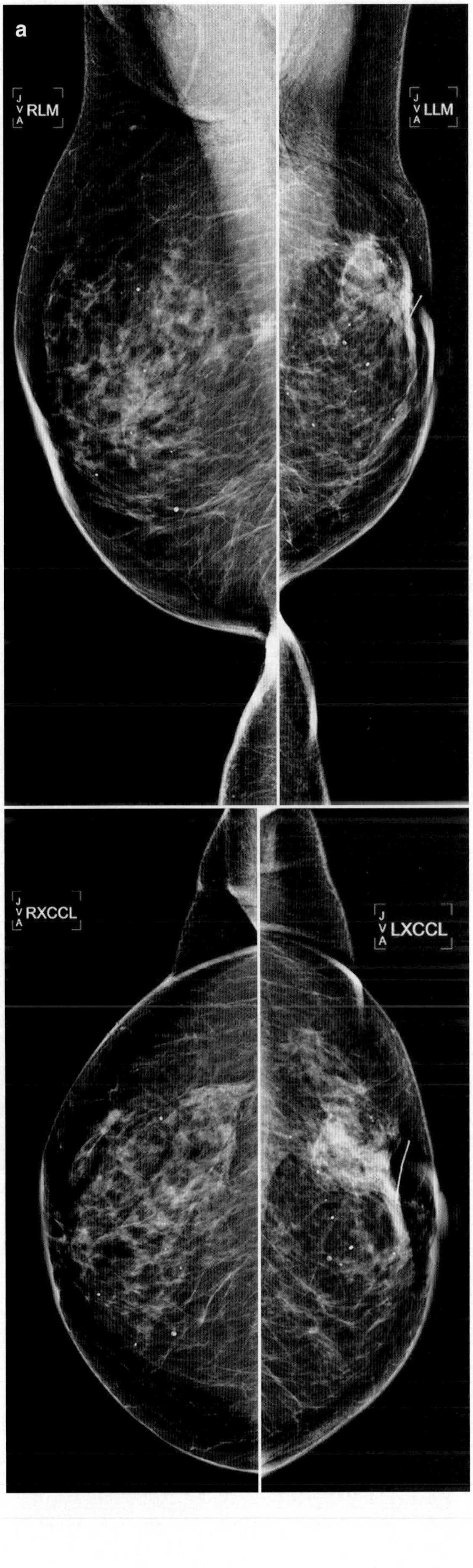

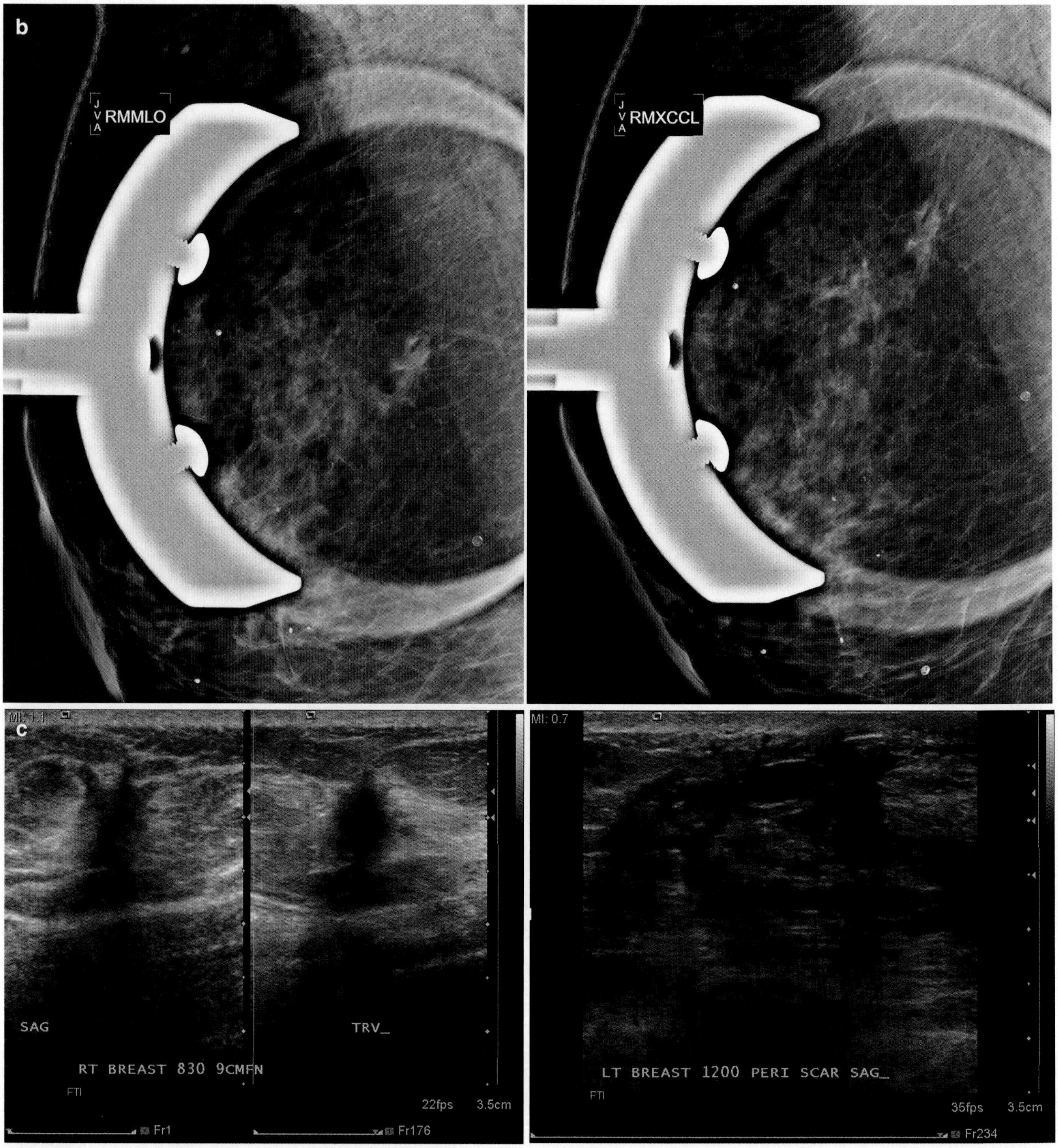

Fig. 16.33 (continued)

Fig. 16.33 (continued)

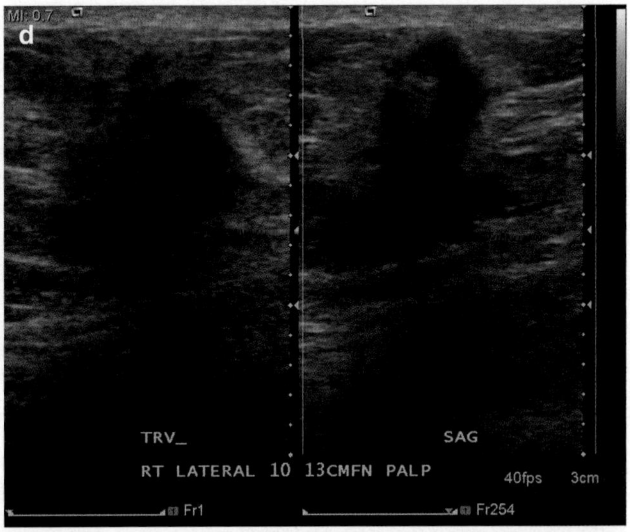

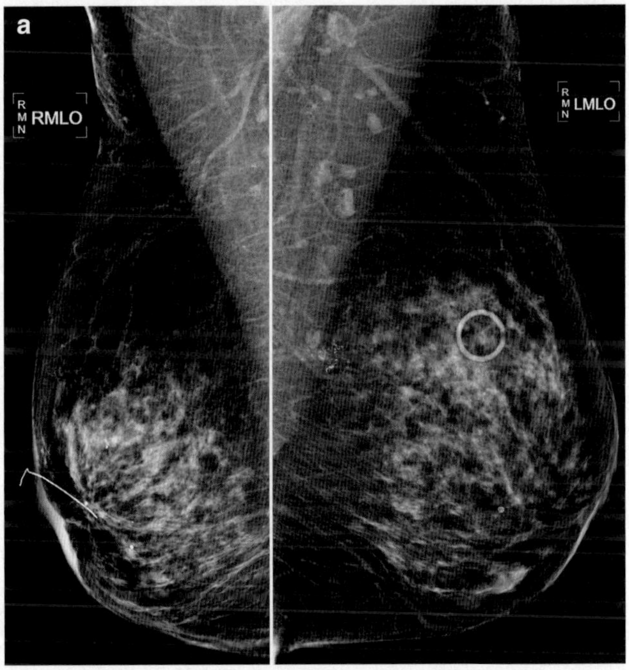

Fig. 16.34 (**a**) 7 years post right lumpectomy. New heterogenous calcifications are visualized in the posterior upper left breast. (**b**) Spot magnification views. Stereotactic biopsy demonstrated in situ carcinoma. (**c**) 6-month follow-up after lumpectomy demonstrates no residual suspicious calcifications in the lumpectomy bed. (**d**) 1 year post left lumpectectomy. Expected post surgical changes are present in the posterior upper outer left breast and right retroareolar position (8 years following surgery). *Note*: Asymmetric glandular tissue in the anterior inferior left breast is stable from prior mammogram

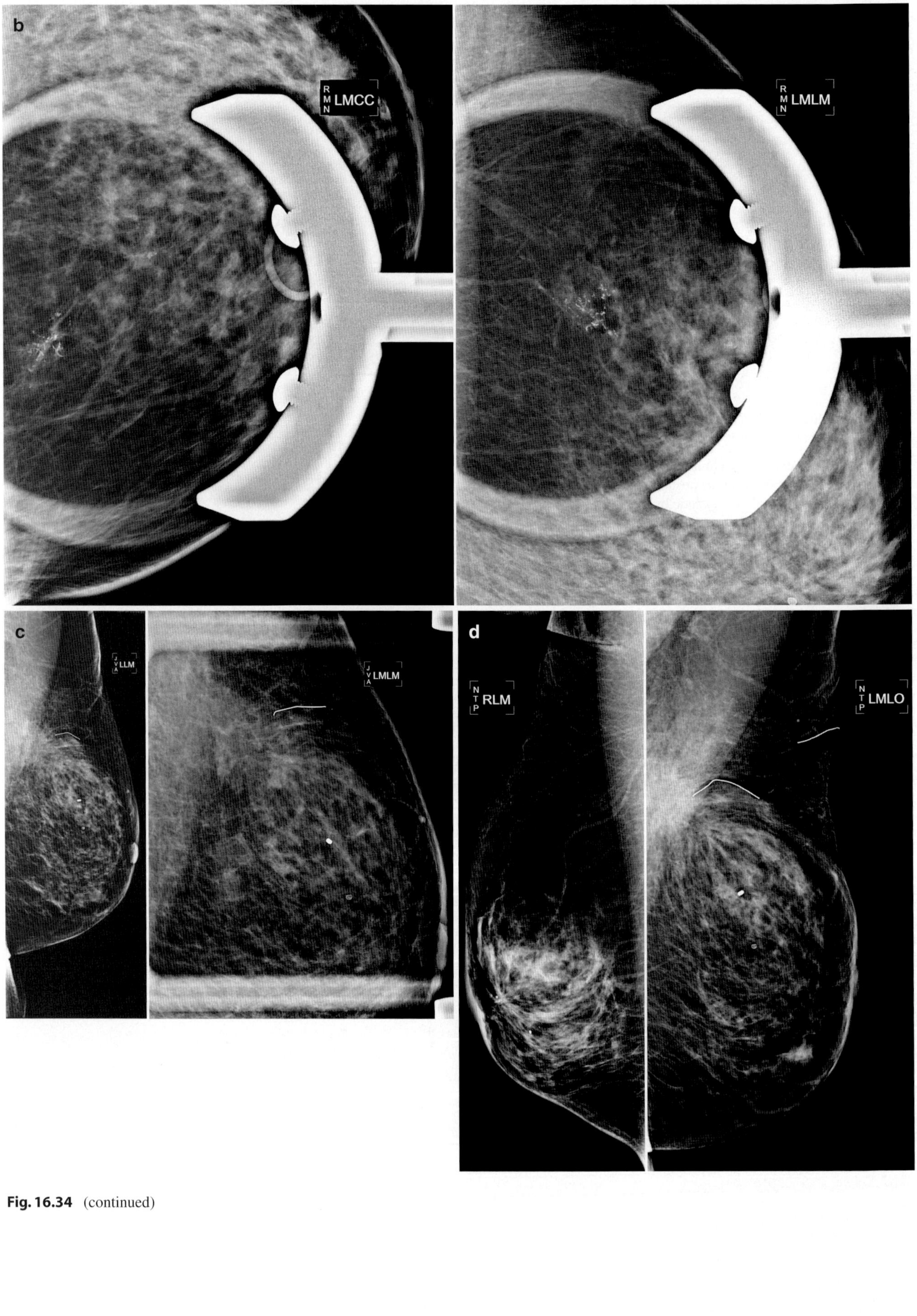

Fig. 16.34 (continued)

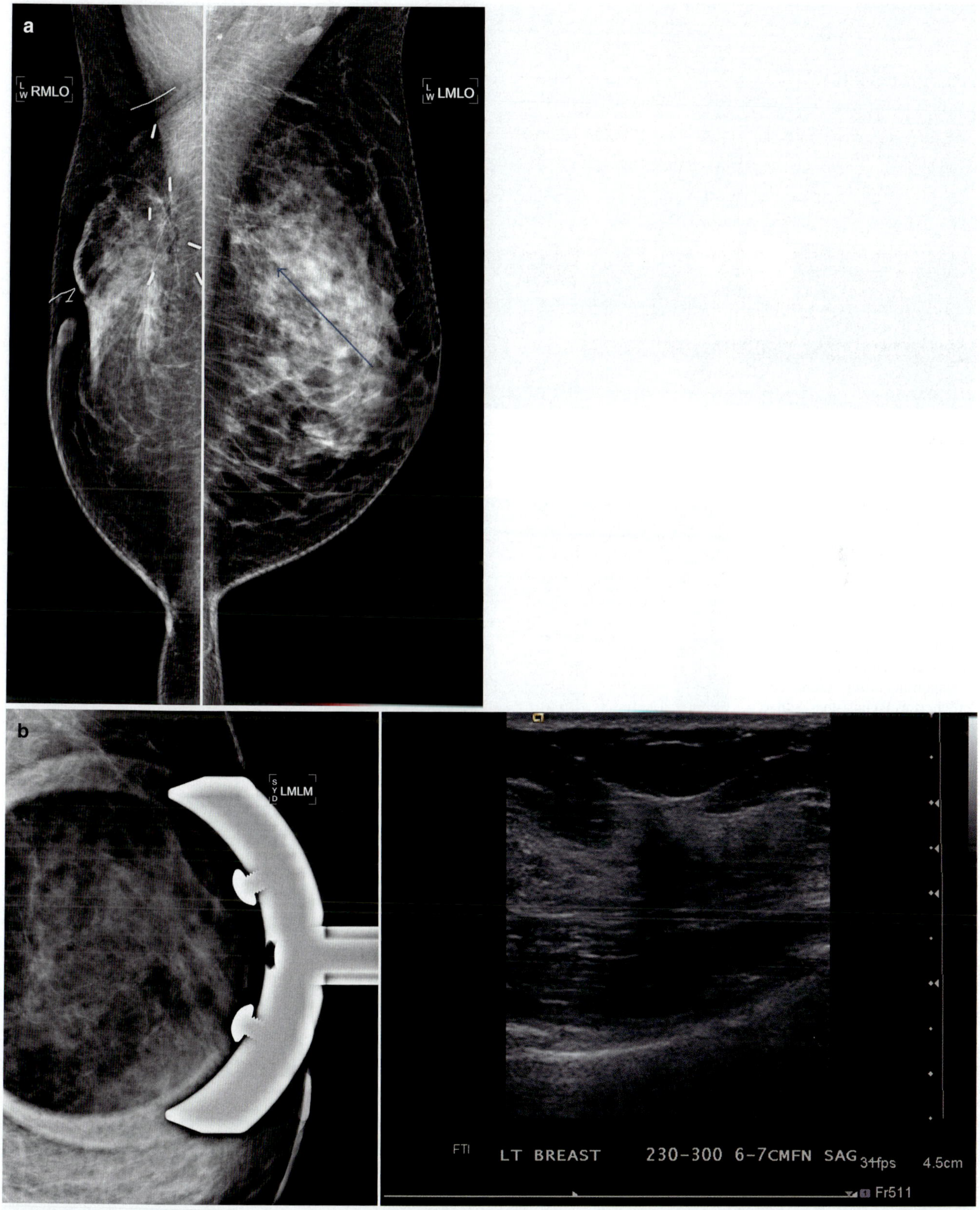

Fig. 16.35 (**a**) 6 years post right lumpectomy for 1.5 cm tubular carcinoma. Stable post-lumpectomy changes on the right. New subtle architectural distortion is seen in the posterior upper left breast. (**b**) The area is less prominent on spot compression views. However, a 1.2 cm suspicious mass is identified with ultrasound. Pathology was IDC with focal lobular growth pattern. (**c**) Post-contrast subtraction MRI images: in addition to the cancer in the posterior upper left breast, multiple additional abnormal enhancing masses extending anterior from the known cancer are seen on MRI. The total area of abnormal enhancement measures 6.2 cm. There was no evidence for recurrent disease in the right breast

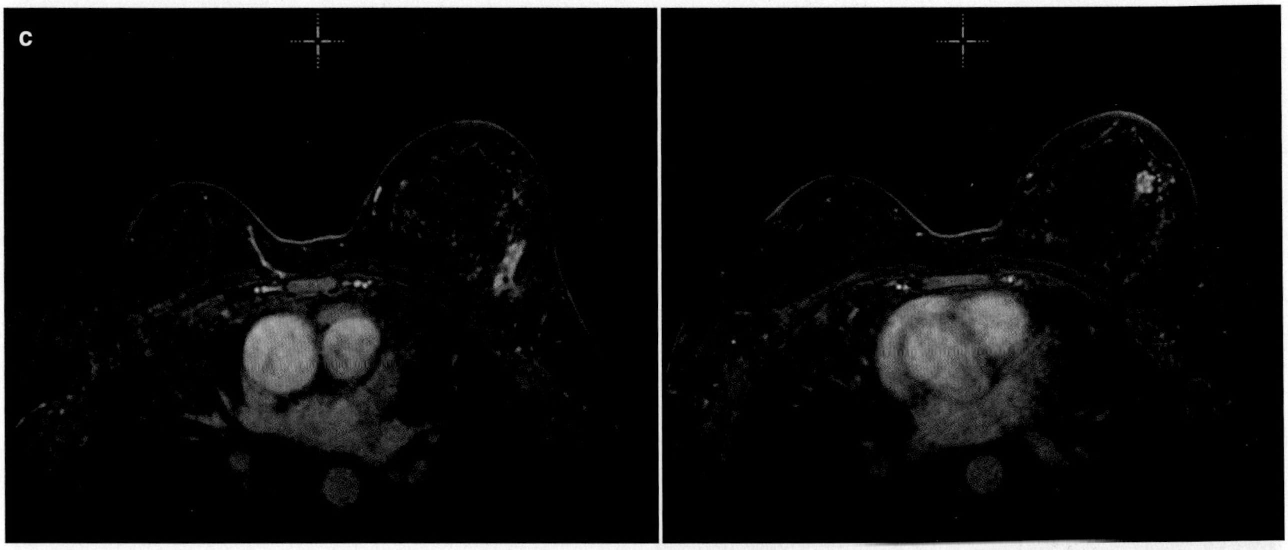

Fig. 16.35 (continued)

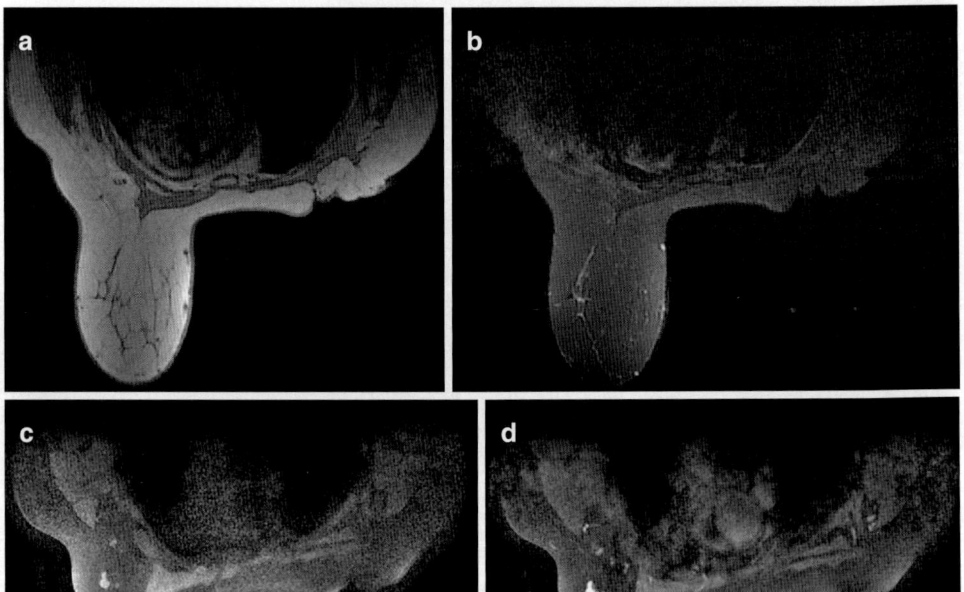

Fig. 16.36 (**a–d**) Simple mastectomy. Axial images from a bilateral breast MRI T1 weighted (**a**), T2 weighted (**b**), TI with fat saturation (**c**), and T1 with fat saturation and contrast enhancement (**d**) demonstrate evidence of an absent left breast with susceptibility artifact along the left chest wall consistent with a history of a simple (total) mastectomy

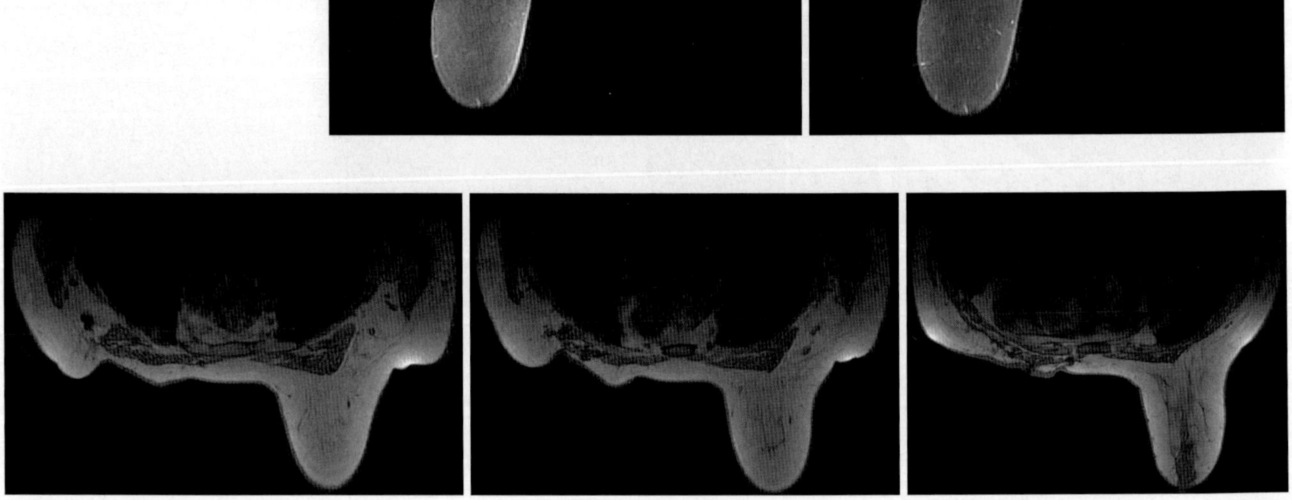

Fig. 16.37 Simple mastectomy with dissection. T1-weighted axial images from a bilateral breast MRI demonstrate evidence of an absent right with susceptibility artifact along the right chest wall and right axilla consistent with a history of a modified radical mastectomy

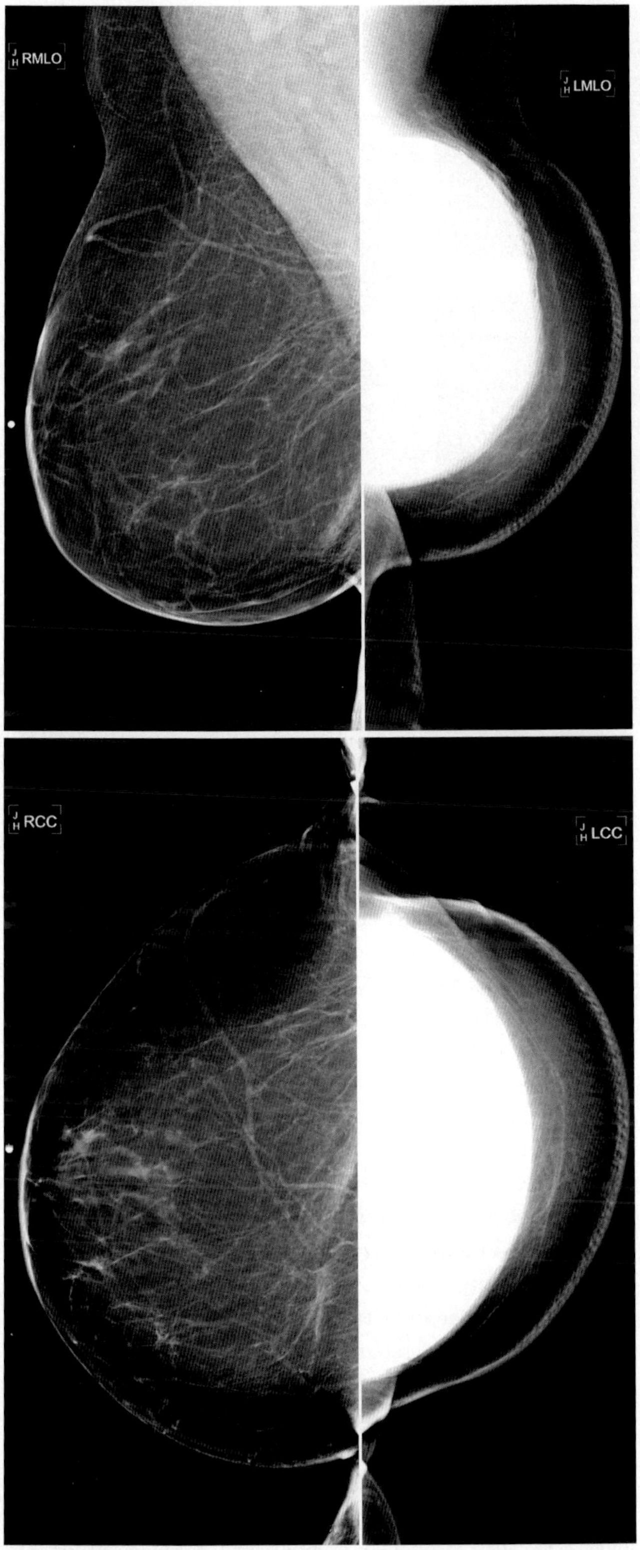

Fig. 16.38 Silicone implant reconstruction. Normal appearance of mastectomy with silicone implant reconstruction. Bilateral craniocaudal (*top*) and mediolateral oblique (*bottom*) images demonstrate evidence of a left mastectomy with silicone implant reconstruction. There is paucity of normal fibroglandular tissue in the reconstructed breast (*)

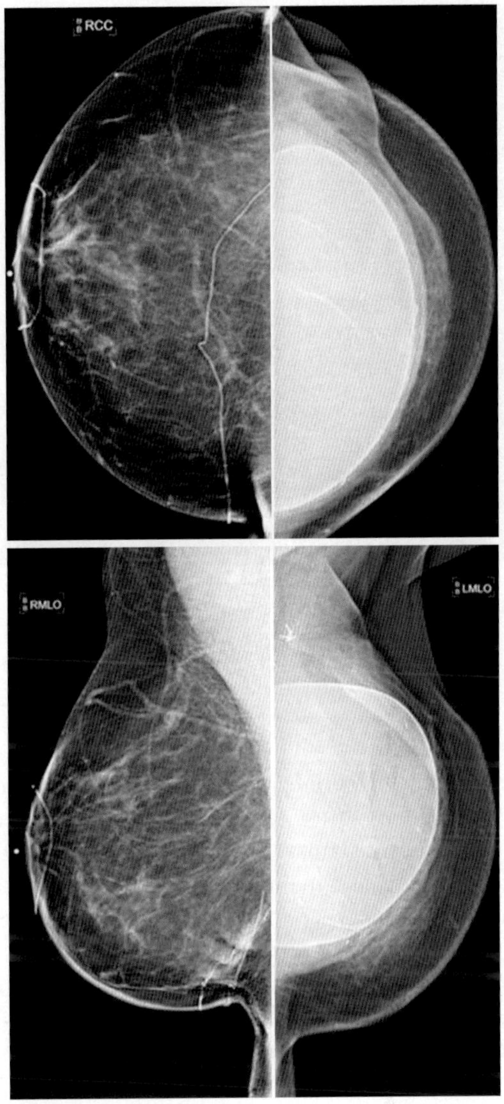

Fig. 16.39 Saline implant reconstruction. Normal appearance of mastectomy with saline implant reconstruction. Bilateral craniocaudal (*top*) and mediolateral oblique (*bottom*) images demonstrate evidence of a left mastectomy with saline implant reconstruction. There is paucity of normal fibroglandular tissue in the reconstructed breast (*). Sequelae of a breast reduction for symmetry are noted on the right breast with scar marker noted on the periareolar and inferior right breast

On MRI, the neobreast is hyperintense on T1-weighted (T1WI) consistent with fat. A thin line of hypointense signal intensity which represents de-epithelialized portion of the abdominal tissue may be seen parallel to the skin surface. The muscle pedicle is hypointense on T1WI and may be visualized inferoposterior location (Fig. 16.42a–f). On contrast-enhanced T1WI images, the vascular pedicle may be visualized. Susceptibility artifact from surgical clips may be seen in the axilla and posterior aspect of the surgical bed. In the immediate postoperative period, there might

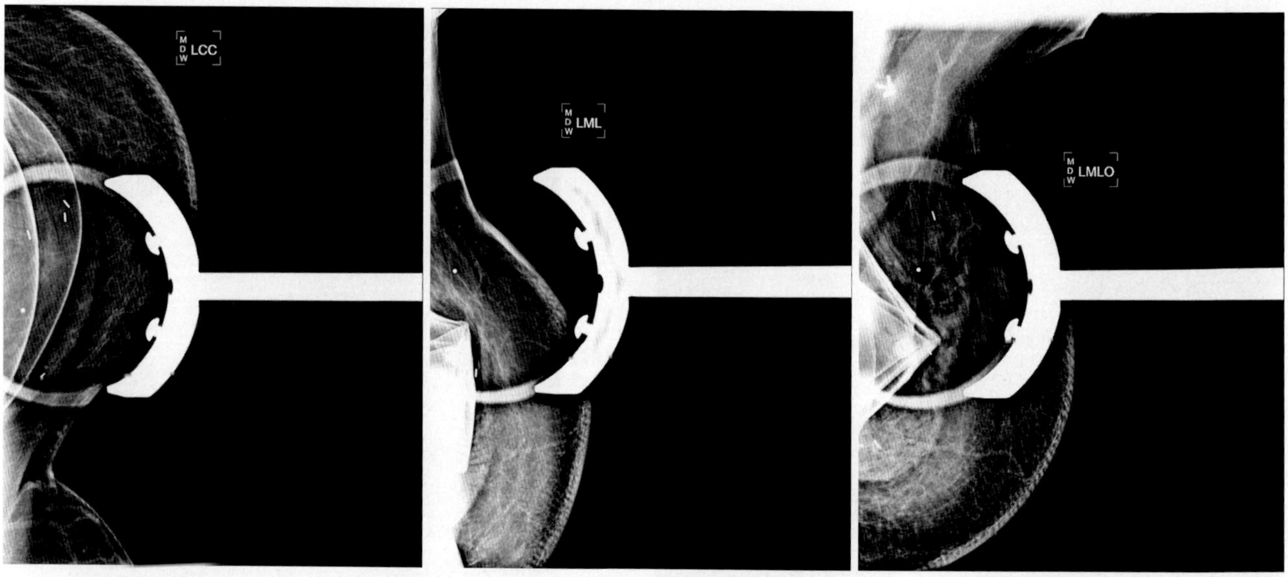

Fig. 16.40 Implant rupture: spot mammographic images in a patient with a left reconstructed breast with saline implants. The patient presented for diagnostic evaluation of a palpable area of concern denoted by a metallic BB. Review of the mammographic images shows the area of palpable concern to correspond with the port of her collapsed saline implant

be increased T2 hyperintensity noted within the skin secondary to edema. Diffuse skin thickening can be seen as a diffuse band of tissue that is hyperintense on T2-weighted images (T2WI) and hypointense on T1W1. If the patient has radiation therapy, uniform enhancement may be seen [43, 46].

Benign findings such as a hematoma, seroma, fibrosis, and fat necrosis can be noted and at times difficult to differentiate from recurrent disease. Early in the postoperative course, a hematoma is hyperintense on both T1WI and T2WI images with a hypointense hemosiderin rim later in the postoperative course. A seroma is hyperintense on T2WI with a smooth rim of enhancement on contrast-enhanced images (Fig. 16.43a–d). Fibrosis, a common sequela of radiation therapy, is often associated with architectural distortion and at times a spiculated mass which mimics malignancy. Postradiation fibrosis has none to very little enhancement on contrast-enhanced images and is hypointense on T2WI. Fat necrosis, a great mimicker on imaging, is reported to have a 25 % incidence in TRAM flap reconstructions. It can have a variable appearance on MRI with slow, gradual, rapid, or washout enhancement kinetics typically at its periphery. In general, it will be hyperintense on T1WI and follow the appearance of fat on T1 fat-saturated (T1FS) images and demonstrate persistent enhancement. A key differentiator of fat necrosis from a malignancy is the presence of central fat signal intensity within a mass (Figs. 16.44a–c and 16.45a, b). Signal void from dystorphic calcifications or findings suspicious for recurrent disease such as irregular and spiculated morphology with rapid enhancement or rim enhancement may also be noted. Given the overlap that exists between benign and malignancy findings, mammographic correlation is often helpful in establishing a diagnosis, but tissue sampling is sometimes still needed to exclude recurrent disease [43, 46, 58].

Recurrence

The incidence of recurrent local disease after a reconstruction is similar to reconstruction with simple mastectomy without reconstruction. Although uncommon, local recurrence can occur in the regional lymph nodes, chest wall, and reconstructed breast itself at sites where residual breast tissue remains (Fig. 16.46a, b). The reported ranges of recurrence in a reconstructed breast range from 2 to 11 % over a 5-year period. Most recurrent tumors occur in the skin or subcutaneous tissue of the flap and are often detected clinically. Recurrence can also occur posteriorly in the chest wall. The incidence of chest wall recurrence has been reported to be 0.2–1 % per year and these patients are more likely to have metastatic disease, a poorer prognosis, and a lower survival rate. The proposed mechanisms for recurrence are residual cancer, tumor seeding at the time of mastectomy, sequestration of tumor cells within the lymphatic system, and unspecified host factors. Benign residual tissue could also be the site of a de novo malignancy at a later time [40, 41, 54, 59–61].

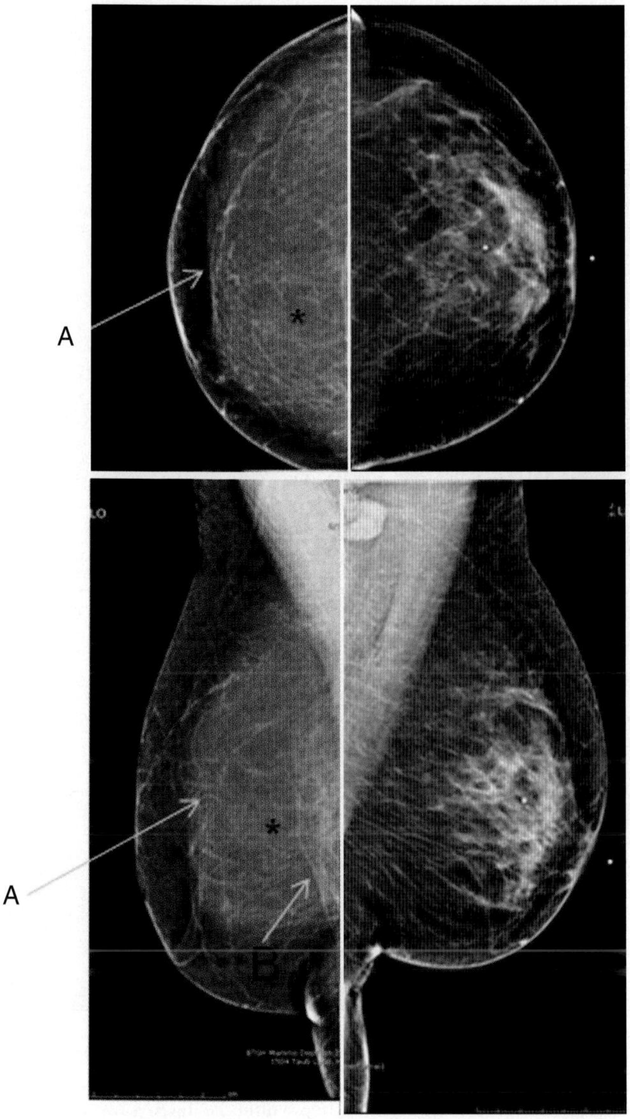

Fig. 16.41 TRAM reconstruction. Normal mammographic appearance of a TRAM flap reconstruction. Craniocaudal (*top*) and mediolateral oblique (*bottom*) views of a patient how has had a right TRAM flap reconstruction. Compared with the left heterogenously dense breast tissue, the right neobreast is entirely composed of fatty tissues (*). A thin line noted at anterior depth of both the CC and MLO views (A) represents superior edge of TRAM flap. The soft tissue in the rectus abdominis muscle can be noted at the posterior aspect of the flap (B)

When there is a clinical suspicion for recurrence, a diagnostic evaluation is performed to interrogate the area of focal complaint such as a palpable mass or pain. If the area of interest is amenable to it, a diagnostic mammogram with spot compression views can be performed. Oftentimes, a targeted ultrasound is the preferred modality of choice especially in the setting of a simple mastectomy without reconstruction where the yield of mammography is low due to lack of compressible breast tissue, hence suboptimal patient positioning and poor patient tolerance as one can imagine [43, 44]. Imaging is helpful to evaluate for fat necrosis which is a common cause for a new palpable abnormality after mastectomy (Fig. 16.47a, b). If suspicious findings are noted, a core needle or surgical excisional biopsy should be performed. Before the performance of an invasive procedure in a patient with a reconstructed breast, it is prudent to be aware of the major vascular supply of the pedicle prior to the procedure. For instance, the vasculature from a pedicle flap from the inferior epigastric vasculature would be located in the lower inner quadrant or the upper outer quadrant if a free flap with anastomosis to the thoracodorsal vasculature is present. MRI is a useful problem-solving tool for recurrent disease when there is a high suspicion for recurrence but findings on mammography or ultrasound are low yield or equivocal or in cases where the site of recurrent disease is located posteriorly and thus less likely to be clinically detectable.

Reduction Mammoplasty

A reduction mammoplasty is a type of plastic surgery performed to reduce the size and volume of the breast through the surgical removal of excess breast tissue. The indications for a breast reduction include macromastia causing physical symptoms such as upper back, chest, neck, and shoulder pain. Patients with macromastia may complain of submammary intertrigo during the summer months and skin pigmentation or grooving from the use of support bras with large shoulder straps. Not-so-common complaints are upper extremity paresthesias from compression of the brachial plexus and chronic headaches [62, 63]. Breast reduction can also be performed in a patient with macromastia for cosmesis to improve self-image and confidence, particularly in younger patients. In patients with breast cancer treated with mastectomy and reconstruction or breast conservation therapy, breast reduction may be performed on the contralateral breast for symmetry. Congenital asymmetry and gigantomastia of pregnancy are rare instances where a breast reduction may be indicated [46].

Incidence

According to the American Society for Aesthetic Plastic Surgery, over 112,000 breast reductions were performed in the United States in 2007, a 539 % increase from 1997. Thus, it is likely that a radiologist would encounter mammographic imaging on patients who have had a breast reduction. In

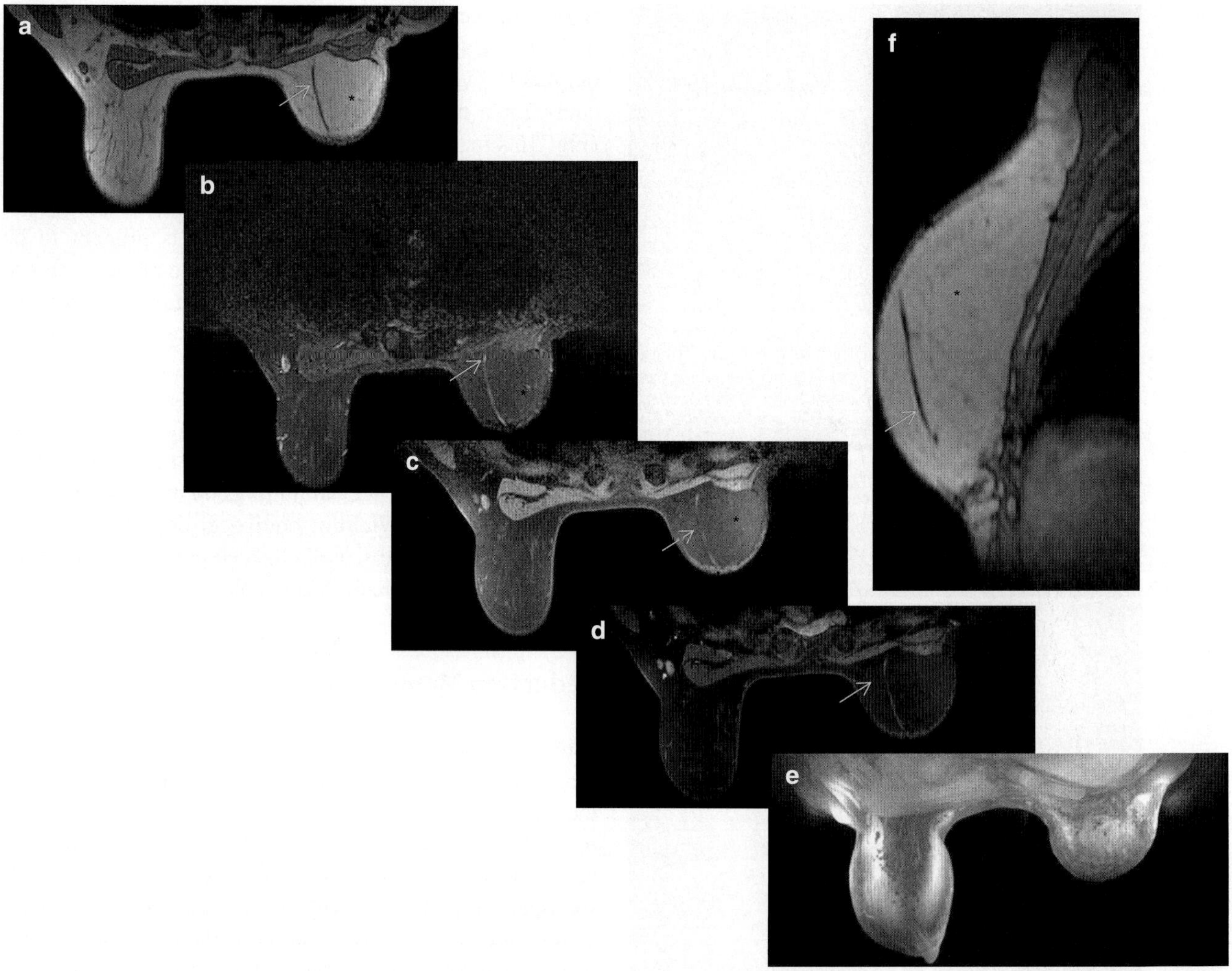

Fig. 16.42 (**a**–**f**) TRAM reconstruction. Normal MRI appearance of a TRAM flap reconstruction. Axial T1-weighted (**a**), T2-weighted (**b**), T1-weighted with fat saturation (**c**), T1-weighted with fat saturation and contrast enhancement (**d**), MIP reconstruction (**e**), and sagittal T1-weighted (**f**) images demonstrate evidence of left mastectomy with TRAM flap reconstruction. The reconstructed breast is composed entirely of fatty tissue. The thin line within the TRAM reconstruction (*arrow*) represents de-epithelialized skin from the abdominal wall

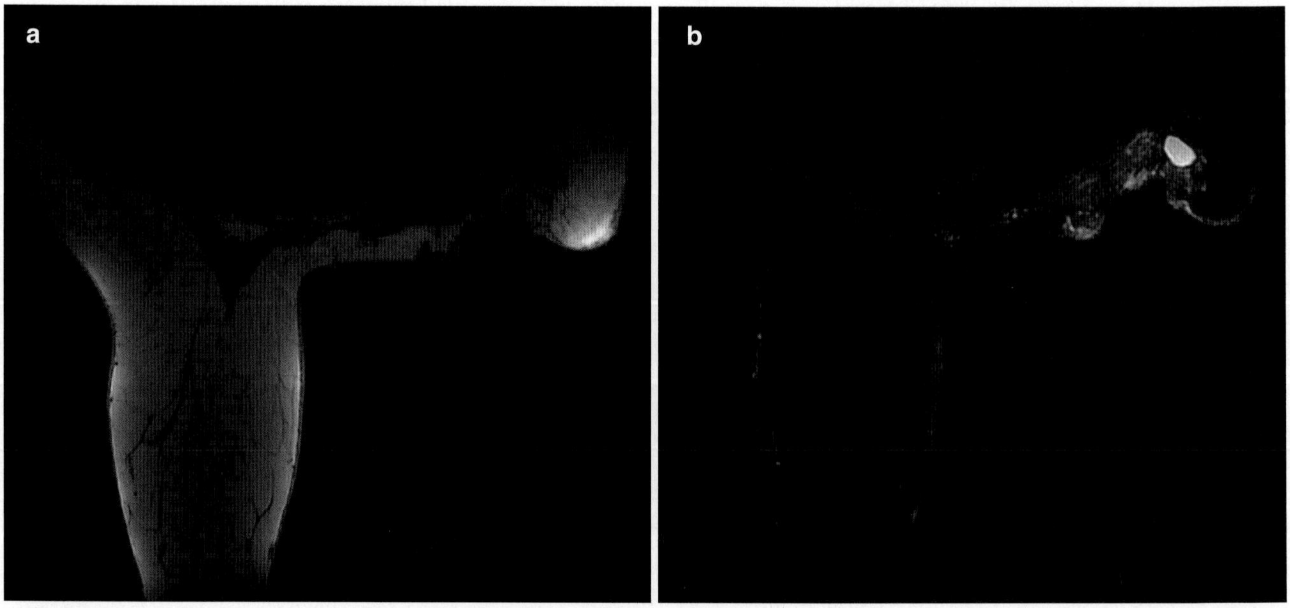

Fig. 16.43 (**a**–**d**) Seroma. Axial images from a patient who has had a left simple mastectomy. A mass is noted in the left mastectomy bed which is hypointense on T1WI (**a**, **c**) and hyperintense in T2 (**b**). No enhancement is present on T1-weighted fat-saturated contrast-enhanced images (**d**)

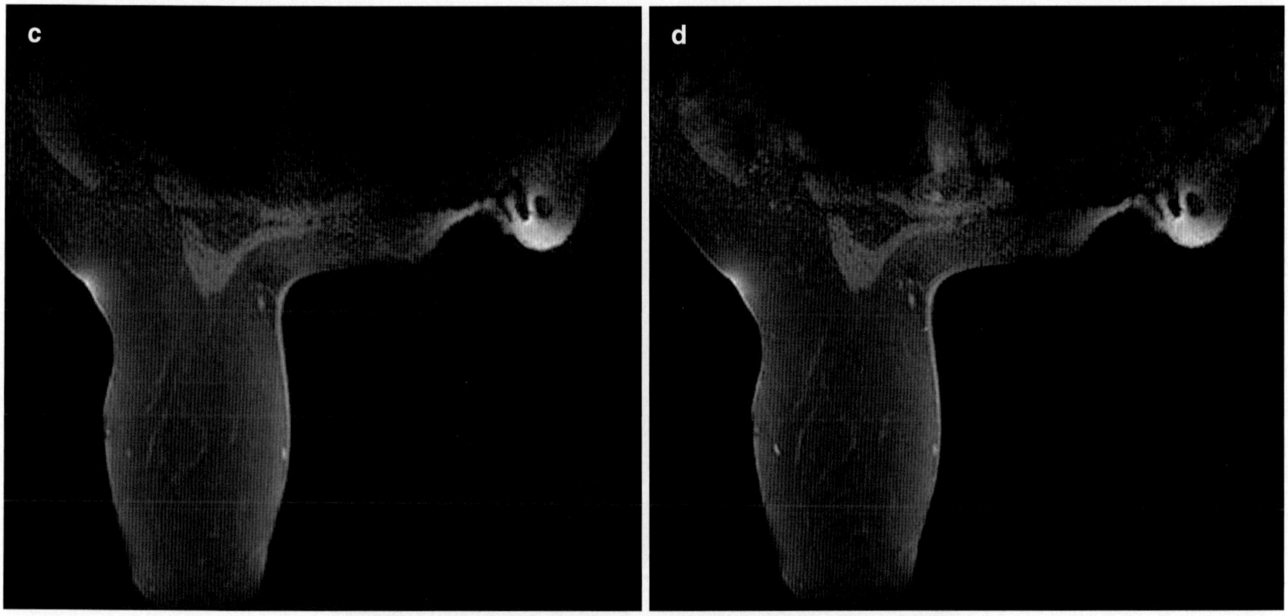

Fig. 16.43 (continued)

order not to perform unnecessary biopsies or miss subtle cancers, the recognition of the postoperative findings associated with this procedure is important [64].

Preoperative Imaging

Although rare, incidental cases of breast cancer have been reported in reduction mammoplasty specimens. This inadvertently complicates and limits treatment options [65]. Therefore, imaging clearance with mammography is recommended in women over the age of 35 presenting for breast reduction surgery. This threshold can be lowered based on risk factors such as family history, genetic disposition, previous biopsy, etc. [46, 63, 65]. Mammographic preoperative imaging can also help identify potential lesions that may need to be addressed at the time of surgery.

Surgical Technique

The general methods used to accomplish breast reduction are a transposition method, where the nipple–areolar complex remains attached to the subareolar ducts and the whole complex is transposed upwards, or a transplantation method, where a full-thickness nipple–areolar graft is severed from its ducts and transplanted upwards [66]. The free nipple graft transplantation method is often preferred when a large volume of breast tissue needs to be removed or in older patients, to decrease the risk of nipple avascular necrosis [46, 62, 66].

Two important components of the breast reduction procedure include selection of a pedicle which provides innervation and vascularity to the nipple-areolar complex and removal of selected quadrants of breast tissue. There are various surgical alternatives for a breast reduction technique. Most described techniques have both a specific pedicle and an incision pattern. The pedicle can be a monopedicle or bipedicle, e.g., McKissock vertical bipedicle technique. The pedicle and skin excision pattern are independent variables. For example, the inverted-T inferior pedicle or Wise pattern, one of the most common reduction techniques, involves an inferior pedicle and reduction of the breast volume from the superior, medial, and lateral quadrants. Other techniques include the short scar (T, vertical, horizontal, or periareolar) technique [63, 67, 68].

Postoperative Imaging

After a woman has undergone a breast reduction, postoperative imaging to establish a new baseline is often performed 6 months after the surgery. Women who have undergone a reduction mammoplasty do not have an increased risk of breast cancer when compared to the general population of women with the same risk factors; thus, the screening guidelines are the same (Fig. 16.48a, b).

Predictable changes occur within the post-reductive breast regardless of the reduction technique. These changes are well demonstrated on mammography, and their identification is essential for the prevention of unnecessary biopsies. Danikas et al. in their retrospective review of 113 patients over the age of 35 found parenchymal distribution 102 (90.2 %) and elevation of the nipple 96 (84.9 %) to be the most common findings on imaging after a breast reduction. A retroareolar fibrotic band from the transposed flap was noted in 23 patients (20.3 %). Calcifications and oil cysts

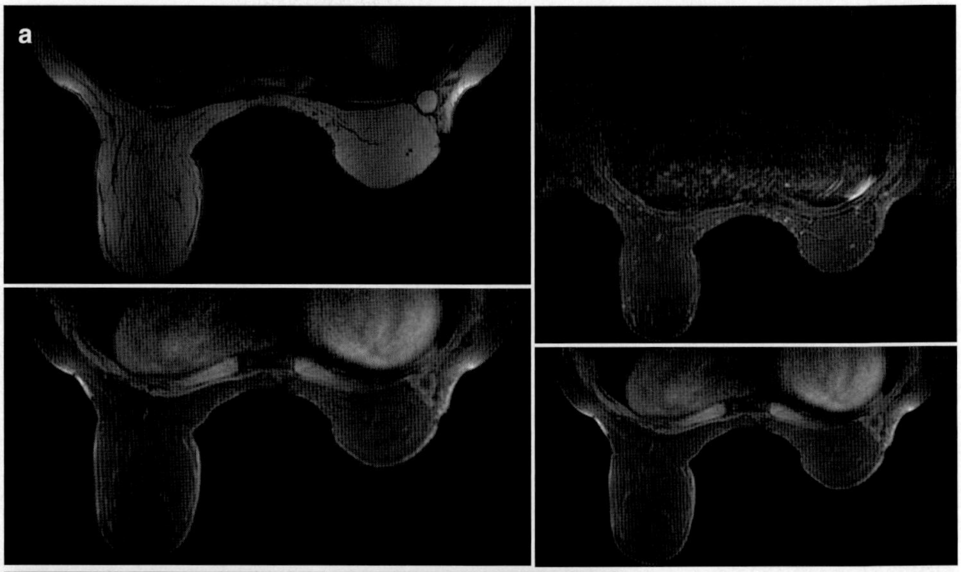

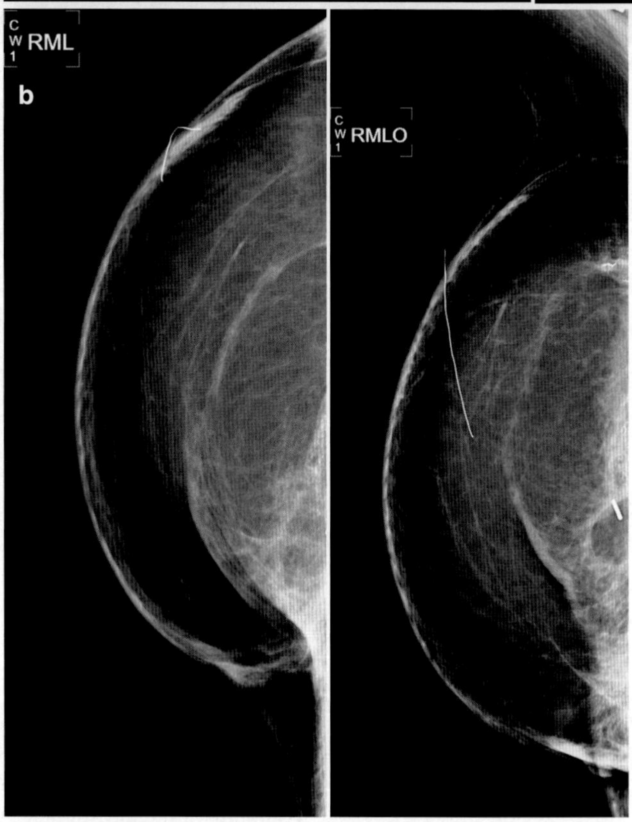

Fig. 16.44 (**a**–**c**) Fat necrosis. Multiple axial and images with T1- and T2-weighted images with and without contrast (**a**, **c**) demonstrate a mass in the lateral aspect of a left TRAM reconstruction which follows fat signal on T1-weighted images. A smooth surrounding rim of enhancement is noted on contrast-enhanced images. Correlation with mediolateral and mediolateral oblique mammographic views (**b**) confirms the MRI findings of fat necrosis

Fig. 16.45 (**a**, **b**) Fat necrosis in TRAM reconstruction. Mammographic and sonographic images (**a**) in a patient with a TRAM reconstruction who presented with an area of palpable concern. The mammogram demonstrates calcified mass with central lucency in the superior quadrant of the mass consistent with fat necrosis. Subsequent imaging (**b**) shows evidence of evolving fat necrosis with curvilinear more coarse calcifications with surrounding lucency

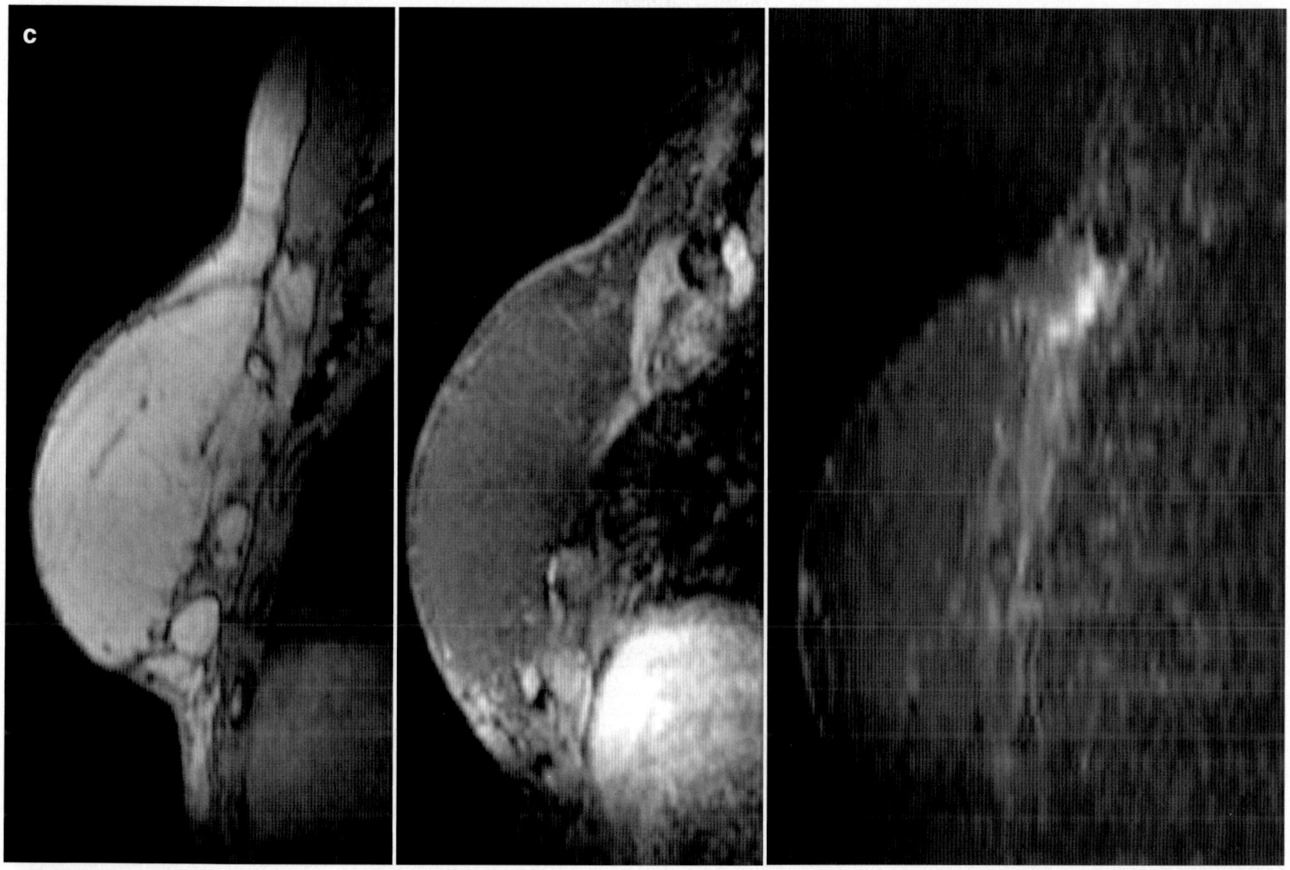

Fig. 16.44 (continued)

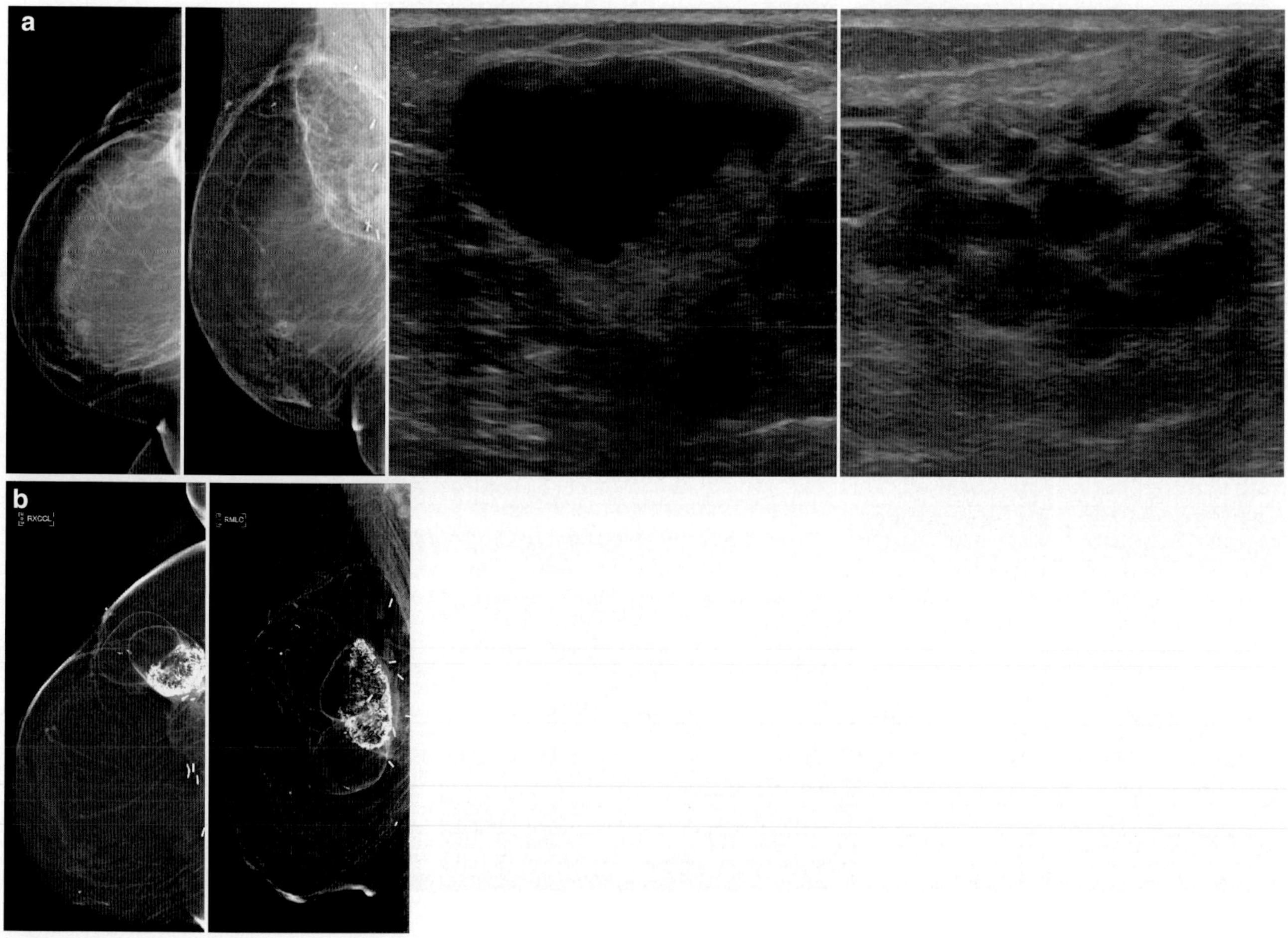

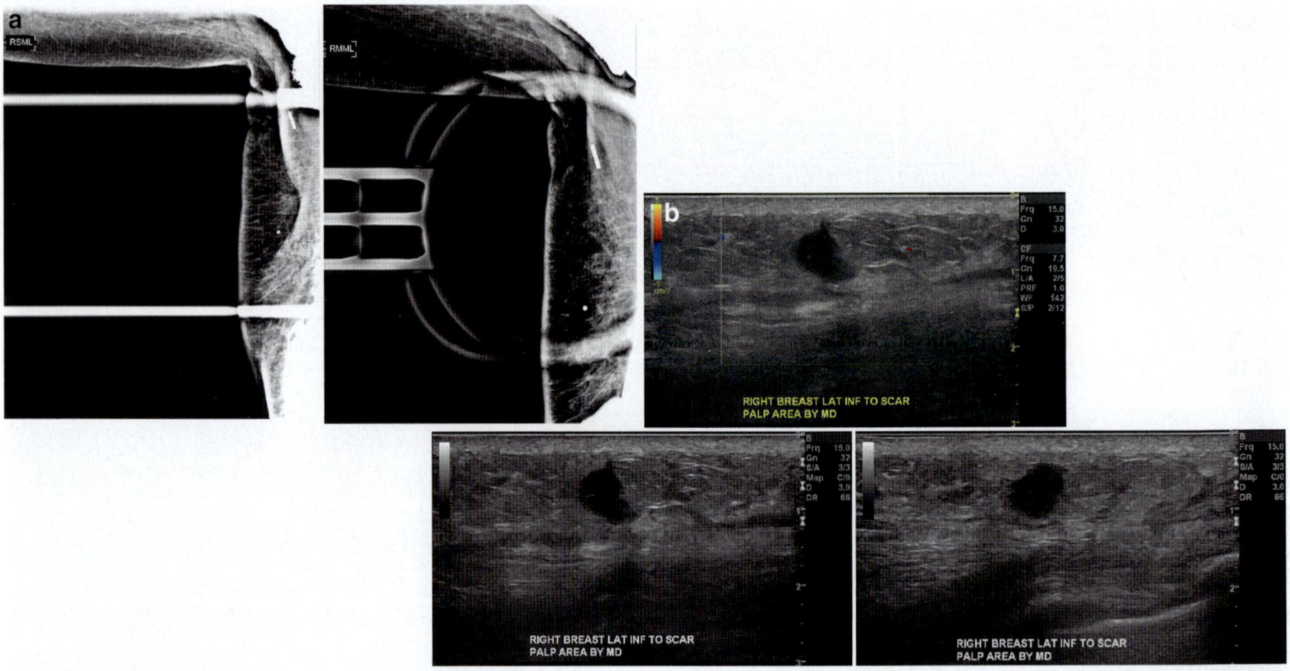

Fig. 16.46 (**a**, **b**) Recurrent malignancy. Spot mammographic images (**a**) demonstrate a focal asymmetry in the area of palpable concern denoted by a metallic BB inferior to the mastectomy scar site. Sonographic images (**b**) in the area of palpable concern show an irregular hypoechoic wider than tall mass. An ultrasound-guided core biopsy of this mass revealed recurrent malignancy

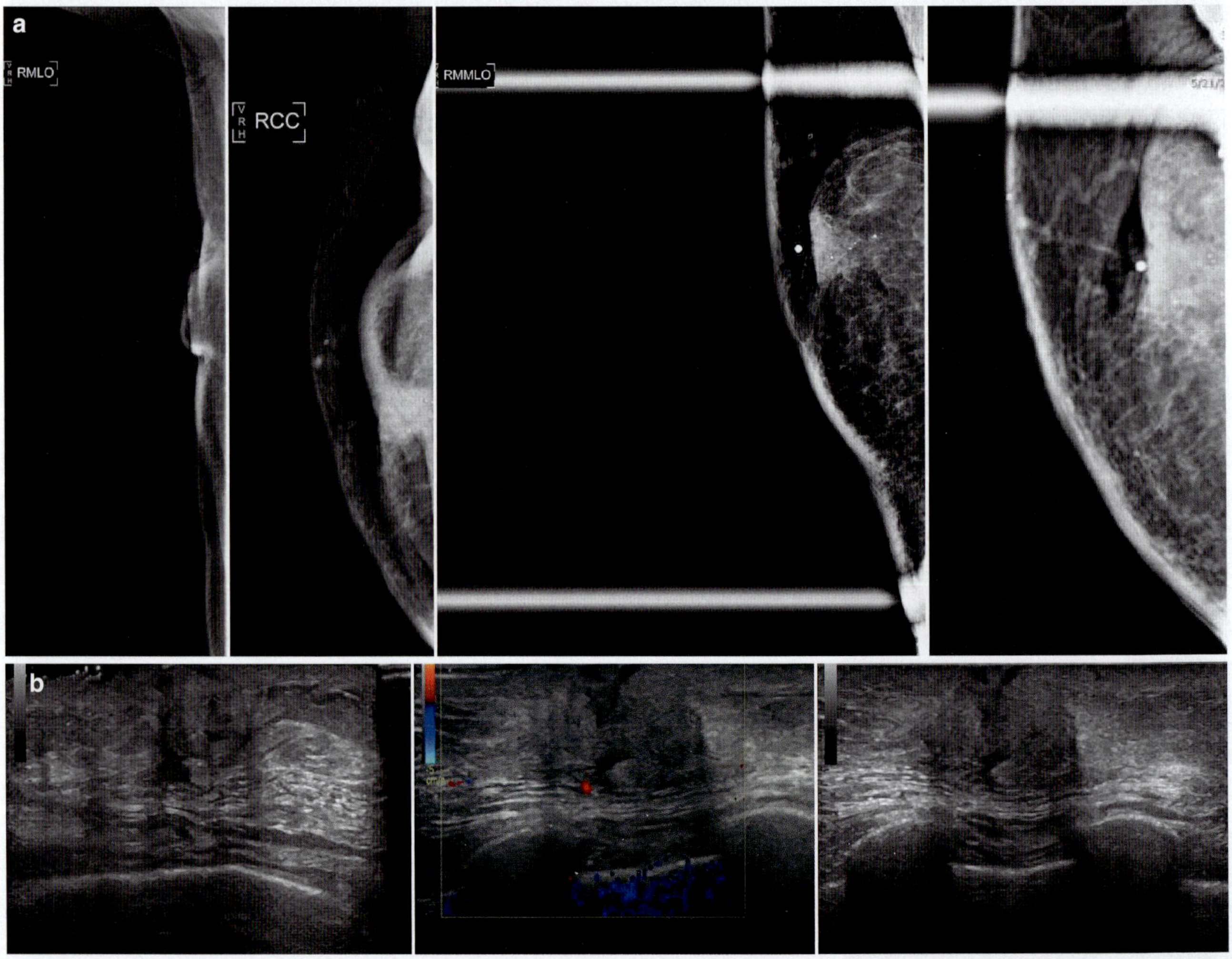

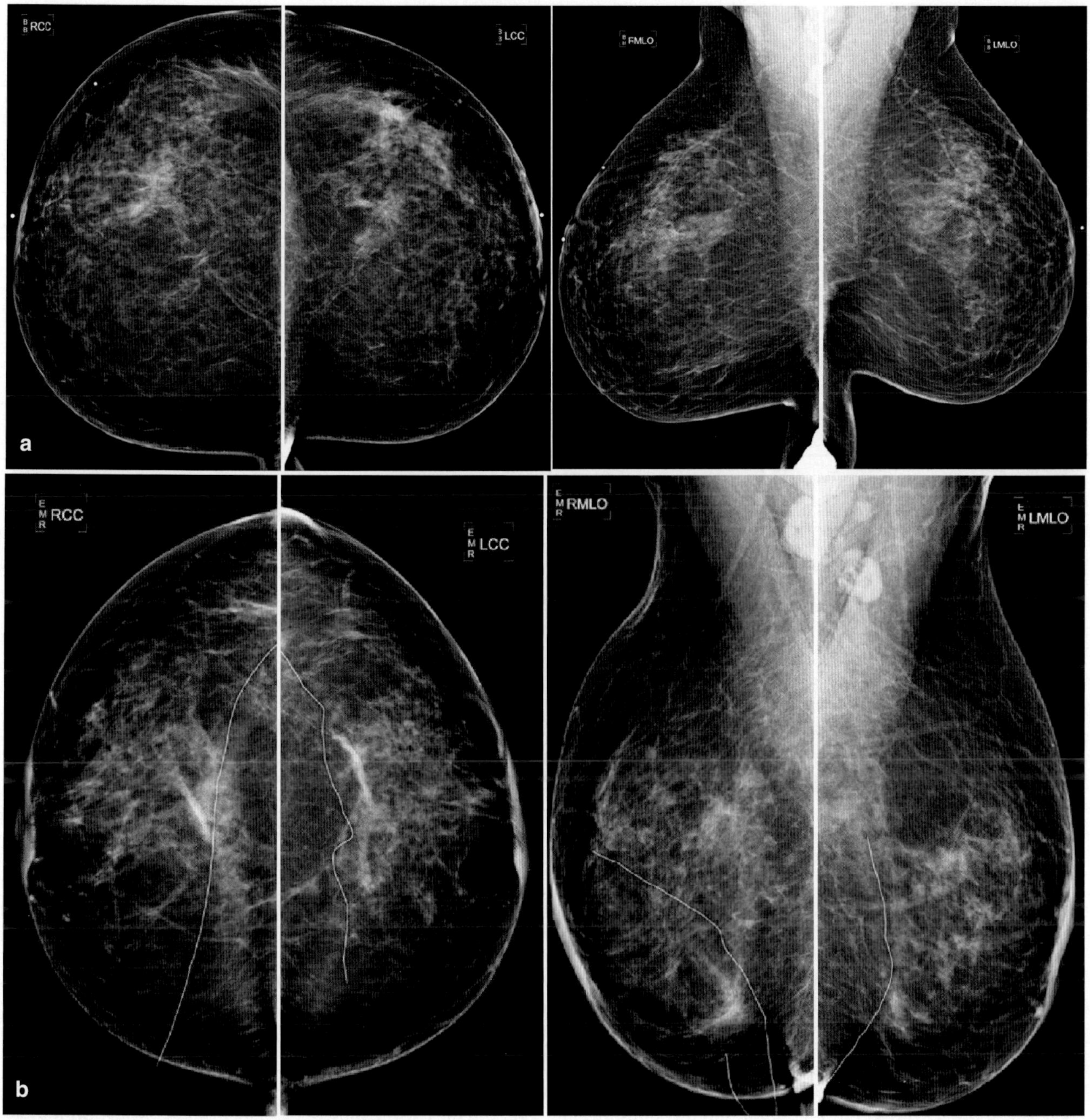

Fig. 16.48 (**a**, **b**) Pre- and postreduction mammographic findings. (**a**) Bilateral mammograms were obtained preoperatively prior to bilateral breast reduction. (**b**) Postreduction mammographic images demonstrate scar markers in the inferior and periareolar regions of both breasts. There is interval reduction in breast size. Parenchymal redistribution is noted with swirling of the breast parenchyma best demonstrated in the inferior breast on the MLO images. Note is also made of an elevated nipple-areolar complex

Fig. 16.47 (**a**, **b**) Fat necrosis. Mammographic (**a**) and sonographic (**b**) images from a patient with history of right breast malignancy treated with a total mastectomy. Clinical exam demonstrated a mass 1 cm below the mastectomy scar denoted by a metallic BB on the mammographic images. A targeted ultrasound of the area of palpable concern showed an isoechoic mass which was suspicious for malignancy. Subsequent ultrasound-guided core biopsy yielded fat necrosis

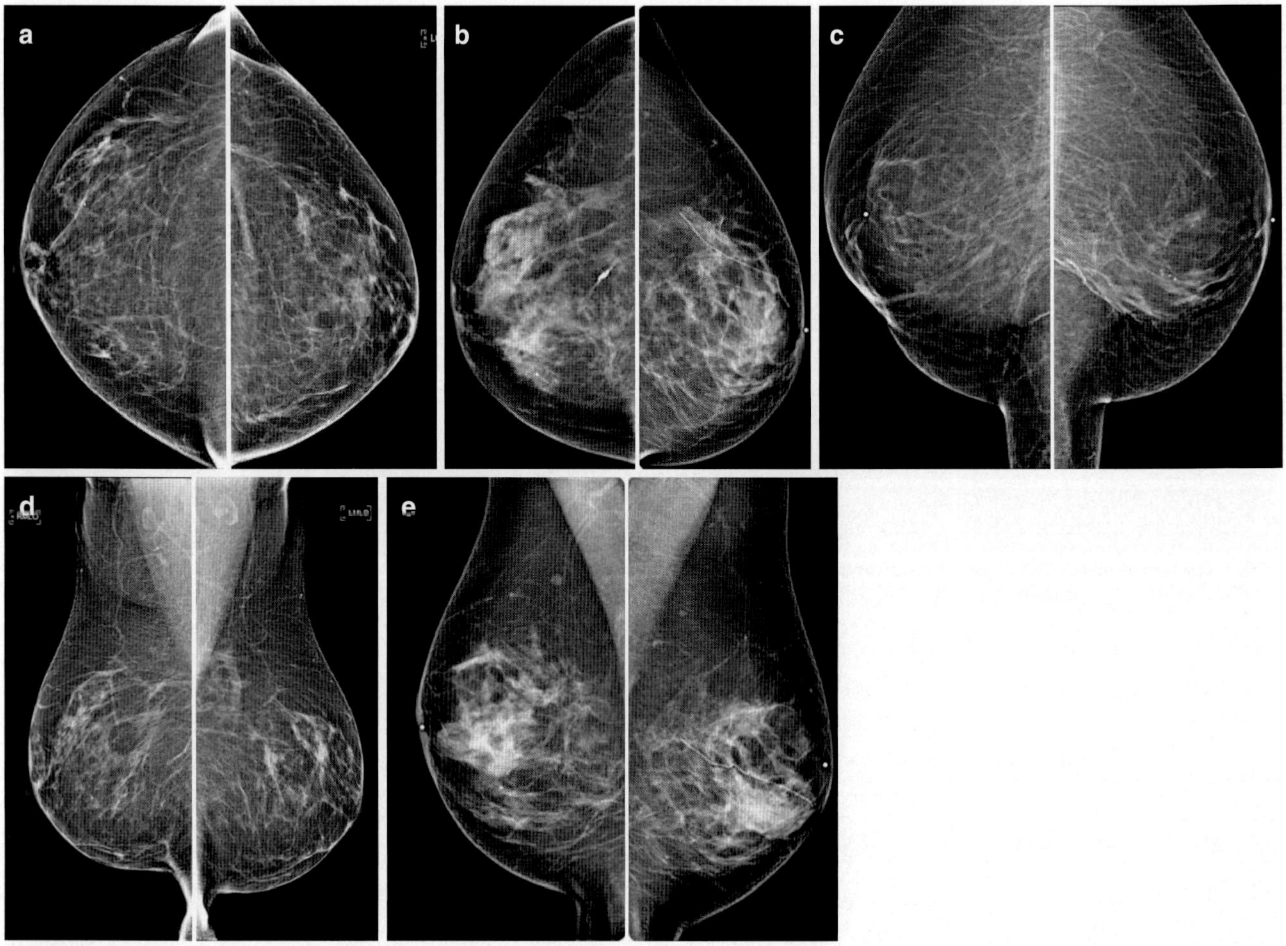

Fig. 16.49 (a–e) Distortion of breast parenchyma. Bilateral CC and MLO images from annual screening mammograms in multiple patients with history of prior bilateral reductive mammoplasty. There is diffuse distortion and a "swirling" pattern of the breast parenchyma. The nipple-areolar complex (NAC) is also in an elevated position in both breasts. These are two of the most common findings noted mammographically after a breast reduction

caused by fat necrosis were noted in 29 (25.6 %) and 22 (19.4 %) patients, respectively [69].

On imaging, the parenchymal redistribution and architectural distortion presents in a "swirling pattern" most pronounced in the inferior breast. Both of these findings are best demonstrated on the mediolateral oblique or mediolateral views. Elevation of the nipple produced by a shift of the fibroglandular tissue inferiorly will also be noted (Fig. 16.49a–e). The subareolar ducts may be disrupted or not discernible if free nipple graft transplantation was performed [66]. A retroareolar fibrotic bands which parallels the contour of the skin may be seen. Skin thickening at the incision sites in the periareolar, inferior breast, and inframammary fold (Fig. 16.50a, b) can also be seen [46, 66, 70].

Benign findings such as dermal calcifications with lucent centers may be seen at the sutural anastomosis in the periareolar and inferior regions of the breasts (Figs. 16.51 and 16.52). Sequelae of postsurgical hematomas may enhance the formation of dystrophic calcifications (Fig. 16.53) [69].

Fat necrosis, a nonsuppurative inflammatory process where local destruction of fat cells results in the development of variable-sized intracellular vacuoles filled with necrotic lipid material, can have a dramatic imaging appearance which, similar to other iatrogenic procedures and trauma, can also be seen in the setting of breast reductive surgery. Fibroblasts, multinucleated giant cells, and lipid-laden macrophages proliferate between cyst-like areas. The initial necrosis is followed by a fibrotic process where fibroblasts form a dense zone of tissue which encases the central lipid-filled cavities. As the fibrotic reaction progresses, calcifications may form characteristically at the margins of the lipid cysts. This evolving process can have a varied appearance on imaging ranging from single or multiple smooth round masses such as benign "oil cysts," coarse eggshell calcifications, and clustered pleomorphic calcifications, to spiculated masses suspicious for malignancy depending on the

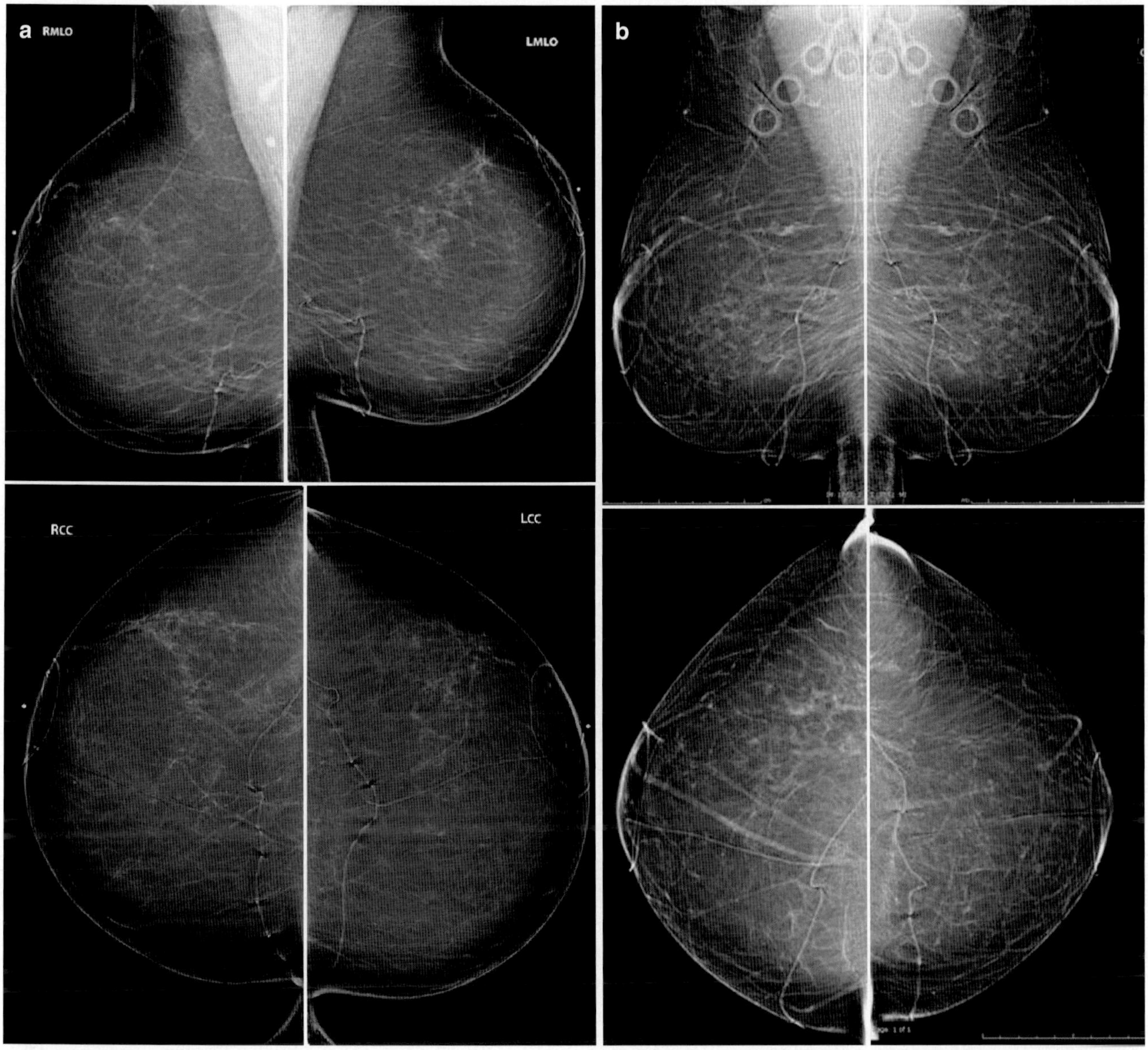

Fig. 16.50 (**a**, **b**) Scar markers. Bilateral annual screening mammogram with CC and MLO projections in two different patients who have had a bilateral reduction mammoplasty. Scar markers are noted in the distribution of the incisions made during the procedure in the periareolar and inferior regions of both breasts. Note is also made of an elevated nipple-areolar complex in both patients

underlying histopathologic changes present [71]. After a breast reduction, fat necrosis will be commonly noted around the areola and at the vertical inferior incision line (Fig. 16.54a–c).

A patient who has a prior breast reduction could present for diagnostic evaluation with an area of palpable concern at a site of developing fat necrosis. It is therefore important for the radiologist to be aware of the expected appearance and distribution of calcifications associated with breast reduction, in order to not perform unnecessary biopsies or attribute truly suspicious findings to expected postoperative changes.

Post-augmentation

There are a variety of commercially available saline and silicone breast implants that are placed surgically for breast augmentation. Less commonly in the United States, some patients will have direct injection of paraffin or liquid silicone into the breast. Although the procedure is not approved in the United States, breast imagers can see these limited mammograms on patients who had the procedure performed abroad (Fig. 16.55). A newer procedure for breast

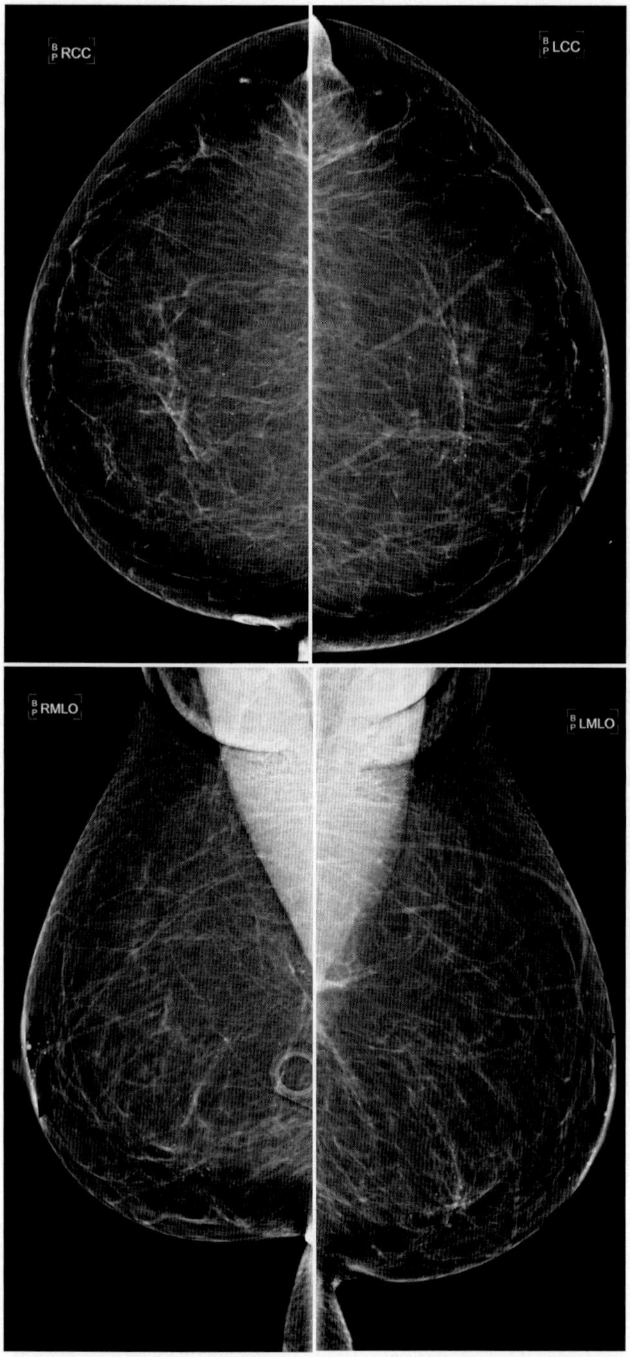

Fig. 16.51 Sutural calcifications. Bilateral CC and MLO mammogram in a patient with a history of bilateral mammoplasty. Sutural calcifications are noted at the periareolar incision site. These can also be seen in the inferior breast and inframammary fold

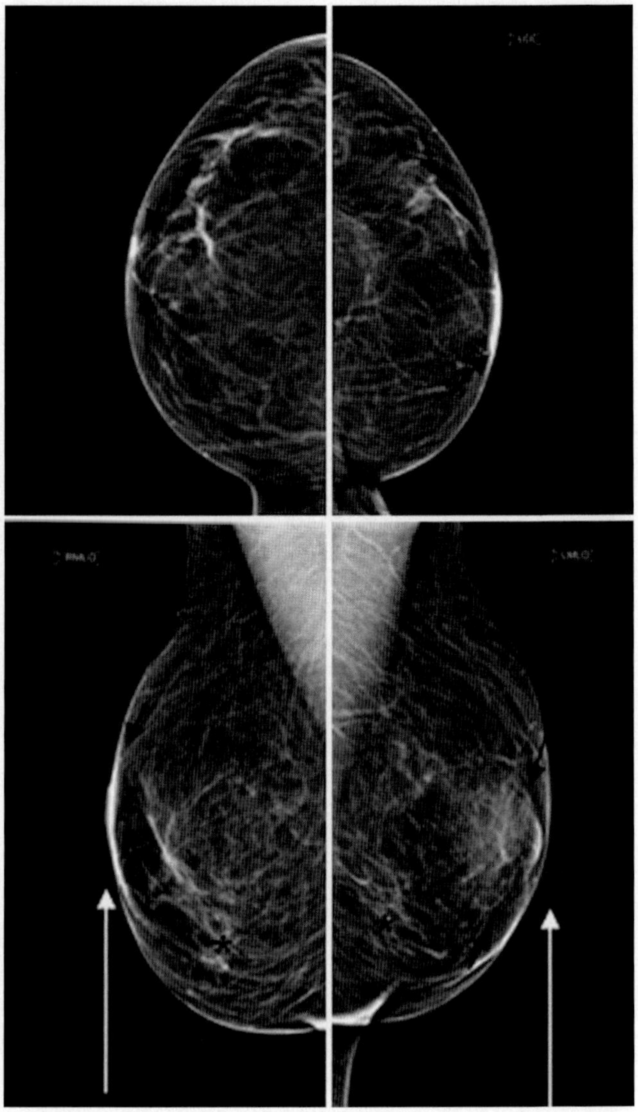

Fig. 16.52 Sutural calcifications (*black arrows*), swirling configuration in lower breast, and elevation of nipple (*white arrows*). CC and MLO views from a bilateral annual screening mammogram in a patient who has had a bilateral reduction mammoplasty. Predictable changes that occur after a reductive mammoplasty are evident. The most common is redistribution of the breast parenchyma in a swirling pattern most notable in the inferior breast (*); another very common finding is the elevation of the nipple to a more high-riding position (*white arrows*). Sutural calcifications can also be noted at the incisional anastomosis sites, namely, the periareolar (*black arrows*) and inferior and inframammary fold regions. *White arrow*, high-riding nipple; *black arrows*, calcifications at the periareolar incision site

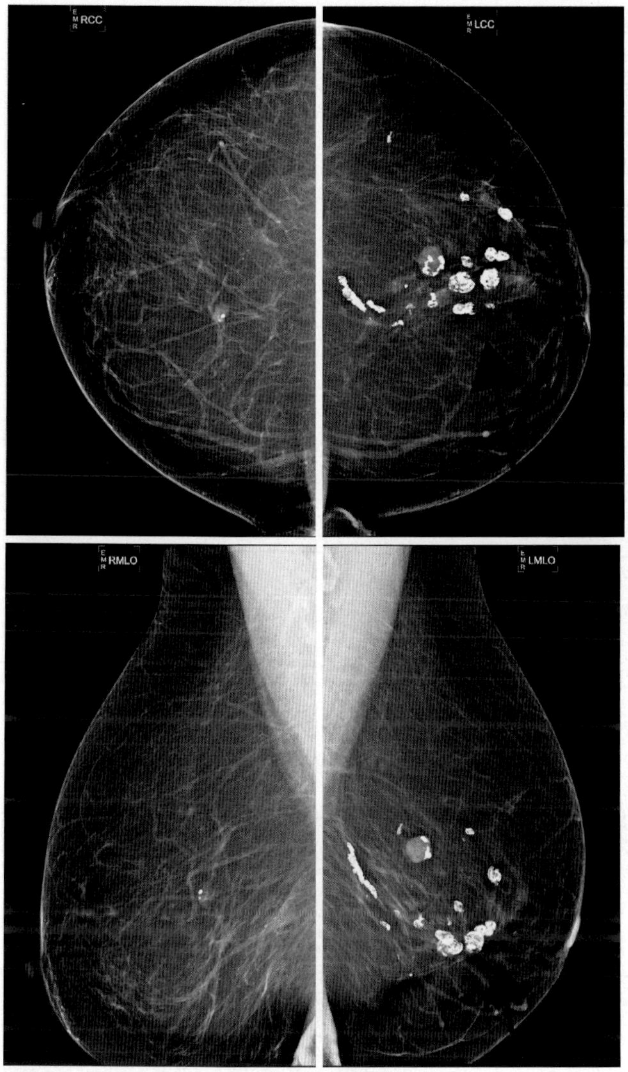

Fig. 16.53 Dystrophic calcifications. Bilateral screening mammogram with standard craniocaudal (CC) and mediolateral oblique (MLO) views. This patient has a bilateral reduction mammoplasty. Dystrophic calcifications (*black arrow*) are noted in the inferior aspects of both breasts, left greater than right. These can be seen in the setting of evolving hematomas or fat necrosis

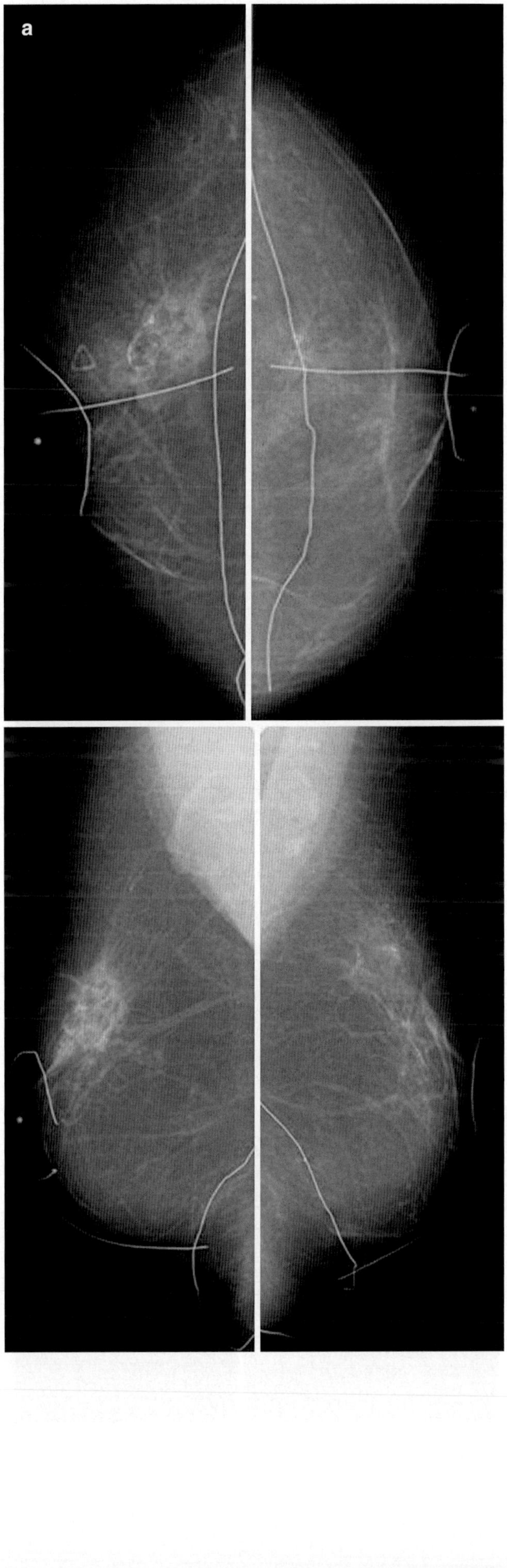

Fig. 16.54 (**a**–**c**) Fat necrosis. (**a**) Patient presents with a palpable area of concern in the upper outer quadrant of the right breast at anterior depth. CC and MLO images from a diagnostic mammogram demonstrate course curvilinear calcifications in both breasts with cystic lucencies, right greater than left. The findings are consistent with benign fat necrosis and correspond to the area of palpable concern. Note is also made of the scar markers in the inferior and periareolar region of both breasts in the typical distribution of incisions used during breast reduction surgery. On subsequent screening mammograms (**b**), the calcifications become more coarse and dystrophic in appearance. (**c**) CC and MLO images from a screening mammogram show a mass with cystic lucencies and few interspersed calcifications in the inferior right breast corresponding to the incisional pattern often used for breast reduction

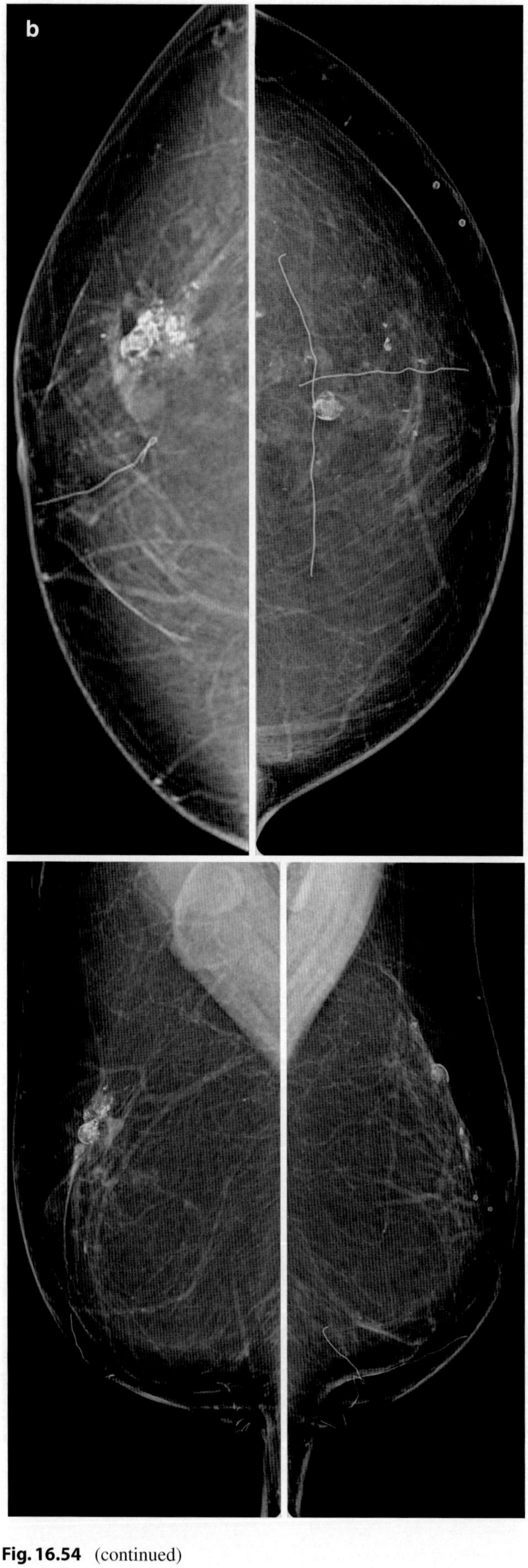

Fig. 16.54 (continued)

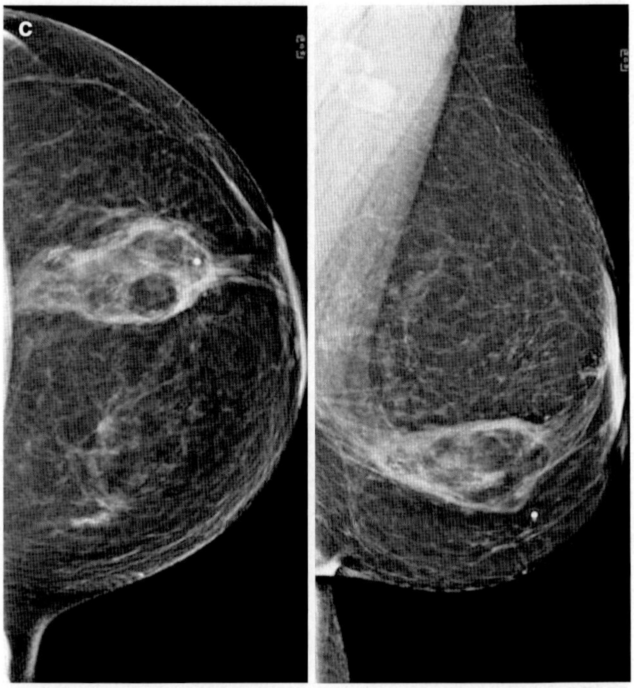

Fig. 16.54 (continued)

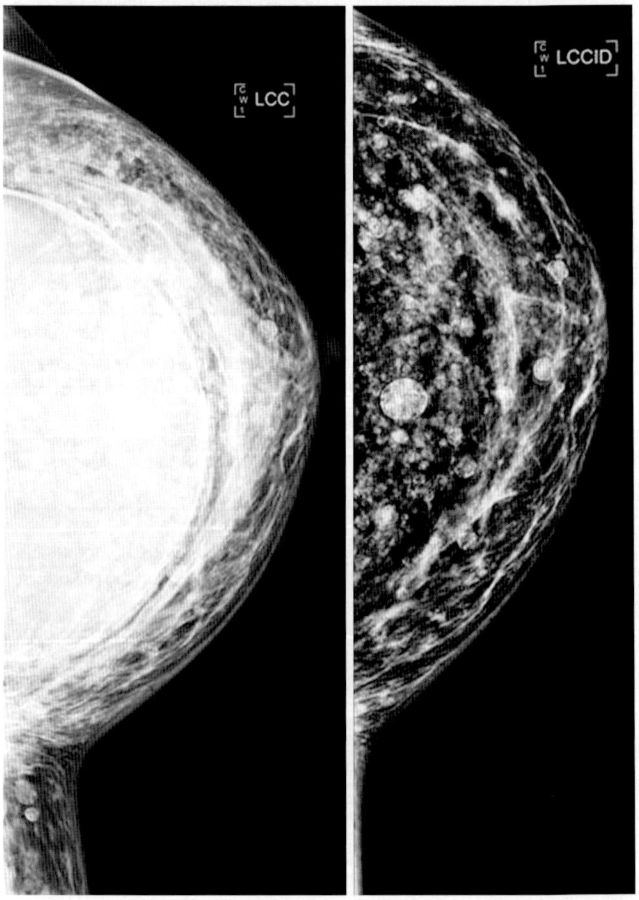

Fig. 16.55 Silicone granulomas on standard and implant-displaced CC views. Granulomas obscure the majority of the breast parenchyma making evaluation for carcinoma suboptimal

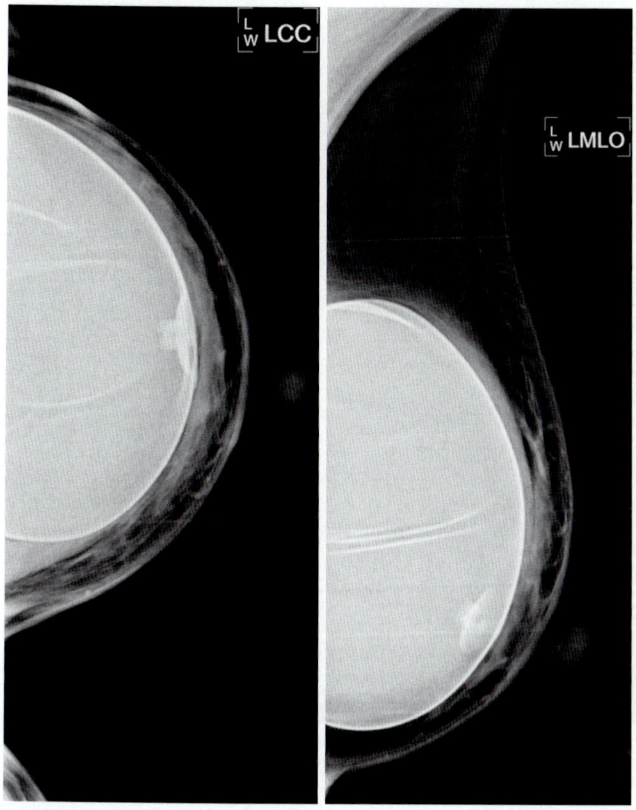

Fig. 16.56 Retropectoral saline implant is less dense than a silicone implant and demonstrates folds of the implant envelope and a valve

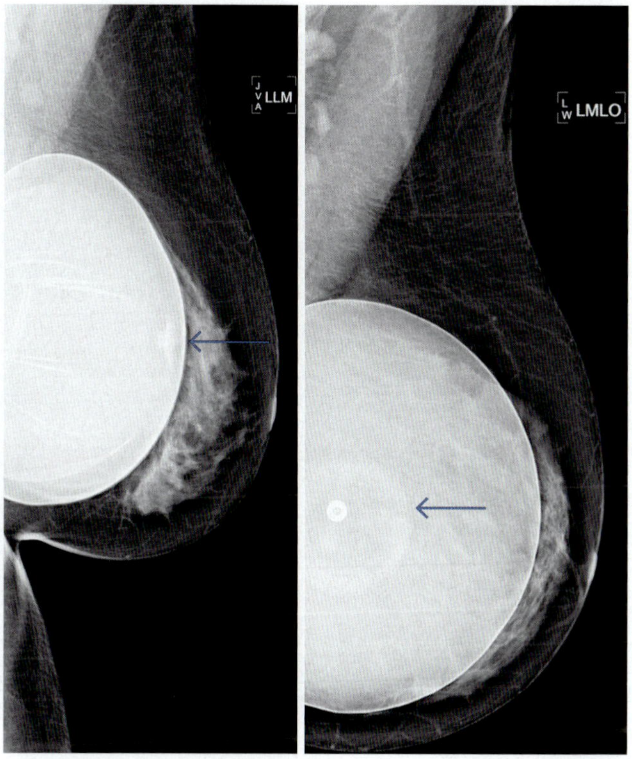

Fig. 16.57 A 67-year-old female underwent exchange of prepectoral saline implants. Images demonstrate the different types of valves that can be seen with saline implants

augmentation is autologous fat injection. This section will focus primarily on the postsurgical appearance after augmentation with implants.

The first use of silicone implants was reported in 1963. In the midst of controversy of possible association with autoimmune disorders, the US Food and Drug Administration (FDA) imposed a ban on the use of silicone implants in 1992. No definitive proof of a cause-effect relationship between implants and autoimmune disorders was ever scientifically established, and silicone implants were again made widely commercially available in 2006. Although cleared from potential harmful autoimmune diseases, implants are associated with other complications including capsular contracture and silicone gel bleed and rupture.

On mammography, saline implants are centrally radiolucent surrounded by a dense silicone outer envelope (Fig. 16.56). Saline implants are less radiodense than silicone implants and sometimes small wrinkles in the envelope and/or the implant valve can be seen (Fig. 16.57). In contrast, silicone implants are mammographically very dense and appear opaque. The presence of radiopaque implants obscures a significant amount of breast tissue on the standard views obtained for screening and decrease cancer detection. The standard CC and MLO views include both the breast tissue and the implant in the same field of view. In order to decrease the compromise in visualization of tissue by the implant, implant-displaced views are performed (Figs. 16.58 and 16.59a–c). The implant-displaced views pull the breast tissue over and in front of the implant while flattening the implant against the chest wall. By moving the implant out of the field of compression as much as possible, the breast tissue can be better compressed.

The ACR Practice Guideline for the Performance of Screening and Diagnostic Mammography recommends that the standard mammographic screening evaluation of the post-augmented breast includes four views of each breast: CC and MLO with the implant and CC and MLO views with the implant displaced. Spot magnification and compression can be performed as needed. Implant-displaced views are important to obtain better compression and visualization of the tissue surrounding the implant as compression is limited on the views with the implant. Implant integrity can be evaluated on the views with the implant. The standard views also provide better visualization of the posterior tissue that is not well seen on implant-displaced views, particularly in patients where the implant is encapsulated. Inspection of both the tissue adjacent to the implant on the nonimplant-displaced views and the tissue separated from the implant on the implant-displaced views should be performed for the most thorough screening for breast cancer.

Fig. 16.58 Patient prior to and after augmentation with a retropectoral silicone implant. Implant and implant-displaced views following augmentation demonstrated decreased visualization of breast tissue following implant placement

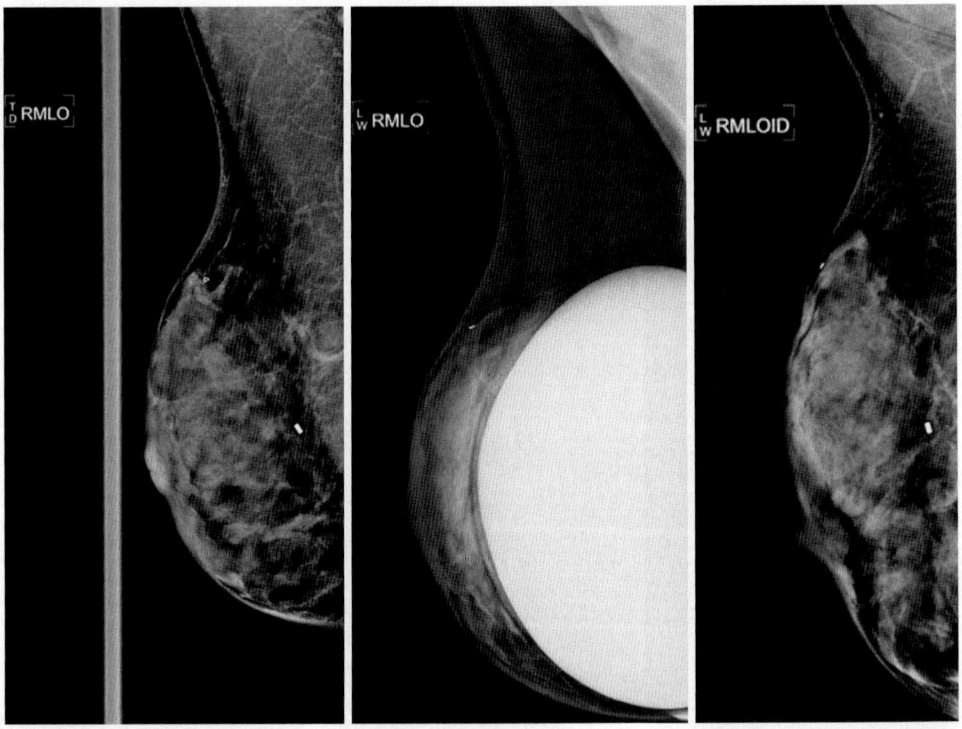

Implants can be placed in front of or behind the pectoralis muscle (Figs. 16.60 and 16.61). In prepectoral implants, the pectoralis muscle can be seen coursing posterior to the implant. A strip of pectoralis muscle will overlie the upper position of the implant in retropectoral implants. In either position, the implant incites a foreign body reaction in the body that leads to the formation of a fibrous capsule around the implant. Initially the fibrous capsule is soft and nonpalpable but with time can undergo contraction and become hard, immobile, and noncompressible. This process is reported to be more common in prepectoral implants compared to retropectoral placement. Lobulation of the silicone implant contour or in the envelope of the saline implant is a mammographic sign of contracture. Usually a capsule is not visualized on the mammogram unless it becomes calcified which can contribute to the hardness. A calcified fibrous capsule usually demonstrates dystrophic calcifications along the implant surface (Figs. 16.62, 16.63, and 16.64).

Implant rupture usually results from aging and decomposition of the implant shell. Direct trauma can also cause rupture. When a saline implant ruptures, the saline diffuses into the breast tissue and the envelope collapses against the chest wall (Fig. 16.65a, b). Not only is the rupture evident clinically, but there is also clear change in the appearance of the implant on mammography. Silicone implant rupture can be more subtle mammographically and is classified as intracapsular rupture, extracapsular rupture, or intact implant with gel bleed. Intracapsular silicone implant rupture is defined as implant envelope rupture with silicone gel contained within the fibrous capsule. Extracapsular silicone implant rupture is defined as implant envelope rupture with silicone gel extruded outside the fibrous capsule. Gel bleed is defined as a process where silicone gel leaks through an intact semipermeable elastomer shell of the implant, although some believe that this actually represents leakage of gel through small, undetected implant ruptures. This process explains why silicone can be seen within the breast parenchyma or in the axilla, despite a radiographically intact implant on MRI. This should be differentiated from extracapsular silicone gel which can only be seen outside the implant or capsule if there is rupture.

The clinical diagnosis of silicone implant rupture is more clinically challenging than saline implants, creating a more important role for imaging in diagnosis. While there can be subtle signs of silicone implant rupture on mammography, such as small collections of extravasated radiodense silicone adjacent to the implant, within the breast parenchyma, or in the axillary lymph nodes (Figs. 16.66, 16.67, and 16.68), the most useful tool for evaluation of silicone implant integrity is MRI. Mammography is particularly limited in evaluation of posterior implant rupture near the chest wall or intracapsular rupture.

Ultrasound evaluation of breasts with extravasated silicone can be very difficult. The free silicone will produce a classic "snowstorm" appearance where a hyperechoic line with posterior acoustic shadowing will be seen

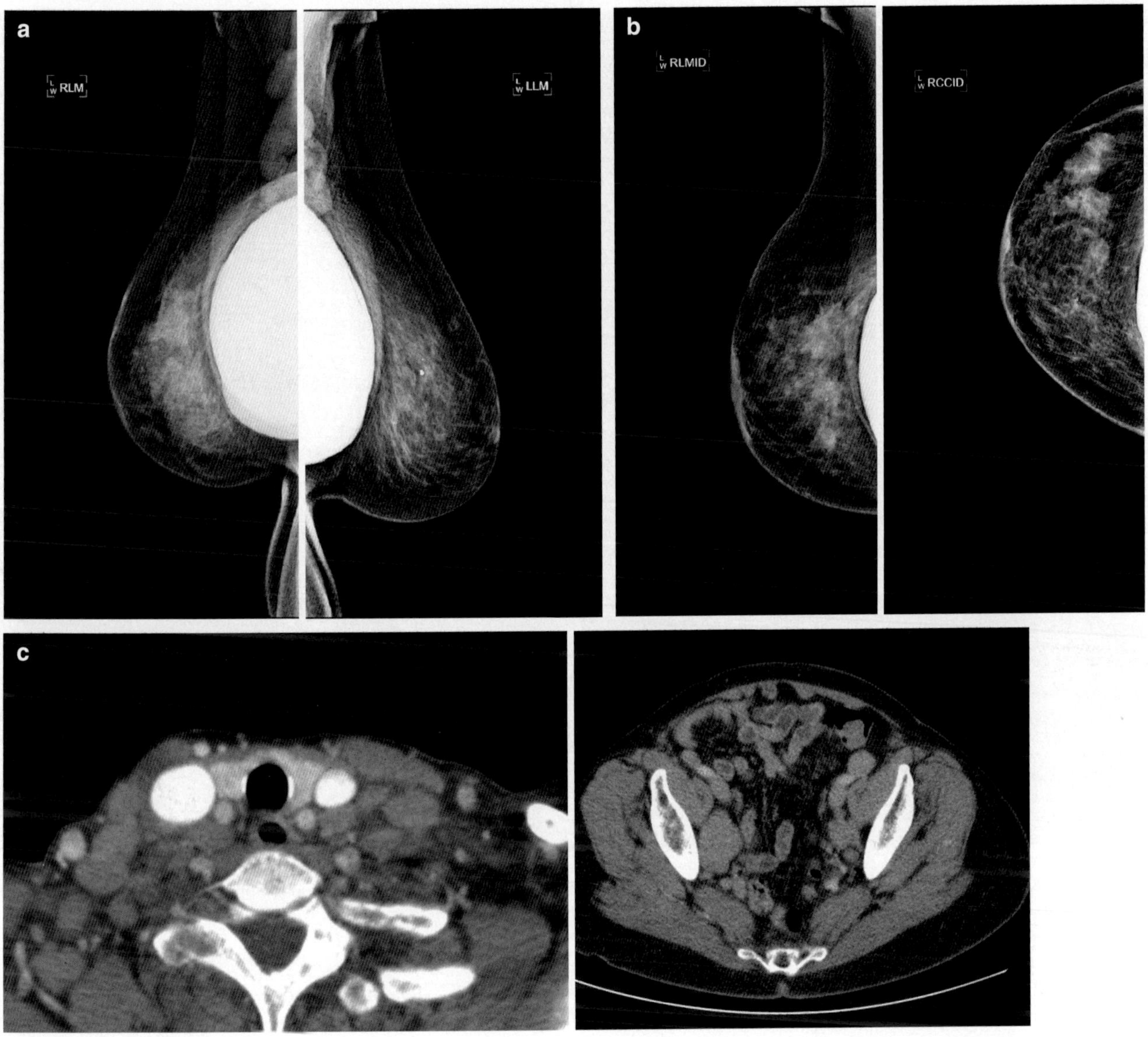

Fig. 16.59 (**a**) A 77-year-old female presents for screening. Bilateral retropectoral silicone implants are present. Multiple obscured masses are seen in the right breast. Bilateral enlarged axillary lymph nodes are seen. (**b**) Multiple masses in the upper right breast are better visualized on the implant-displaced views. Ultrasound-guided core needle biopsy of right breast masses had pathology of invasive ductal carcinoma with metaplastic features. (**c**) In addition to bilateral axillary lymphadenopathy, staging CT demonstrates extensive cervical and abdominal/pelvis lymphadenopathy. Surgical biopsy of an axillary lymph node yielded pathology of follicular lymphoma

(Fig. 16.69a–f). This appearance is secondary to the slow velocity of sound in silicone versus surrounding breast parenchyma. The shadowing produced by the silicone obscures the majority of the surrounding breast tissue and makes evaluation for possible malignancy limited. It can be helpful to place a skin marker in the region of the sonographic abnormality with subsequent mammogram performed for direct sonographic-mammographic correlation. If the patient is presenting with a new palpable abnormality, and the mammogram and ultrasound do not clearly define free silicone as the etiology, breast MRI is recommended to exclude underlying malignancy.

Breast MRI

Breast MRI is not used in the evaluation of saline implants as this is usually clinically evident and seen on mammography, as discussed previously. While contour deformities, implant bulges or herniations, capsular calcifications, and some extracapsular silicone can all be seen mammographically, intracapsular rupture and silicone gel bleed can only be visualized on MRI. Evaluation of integrity of silicone implants with MRI is the only instance when breast MRI is performed without contrast. Since gadolinium contrast is required for evaluation of malignancy, implant studies are nondiagnostic

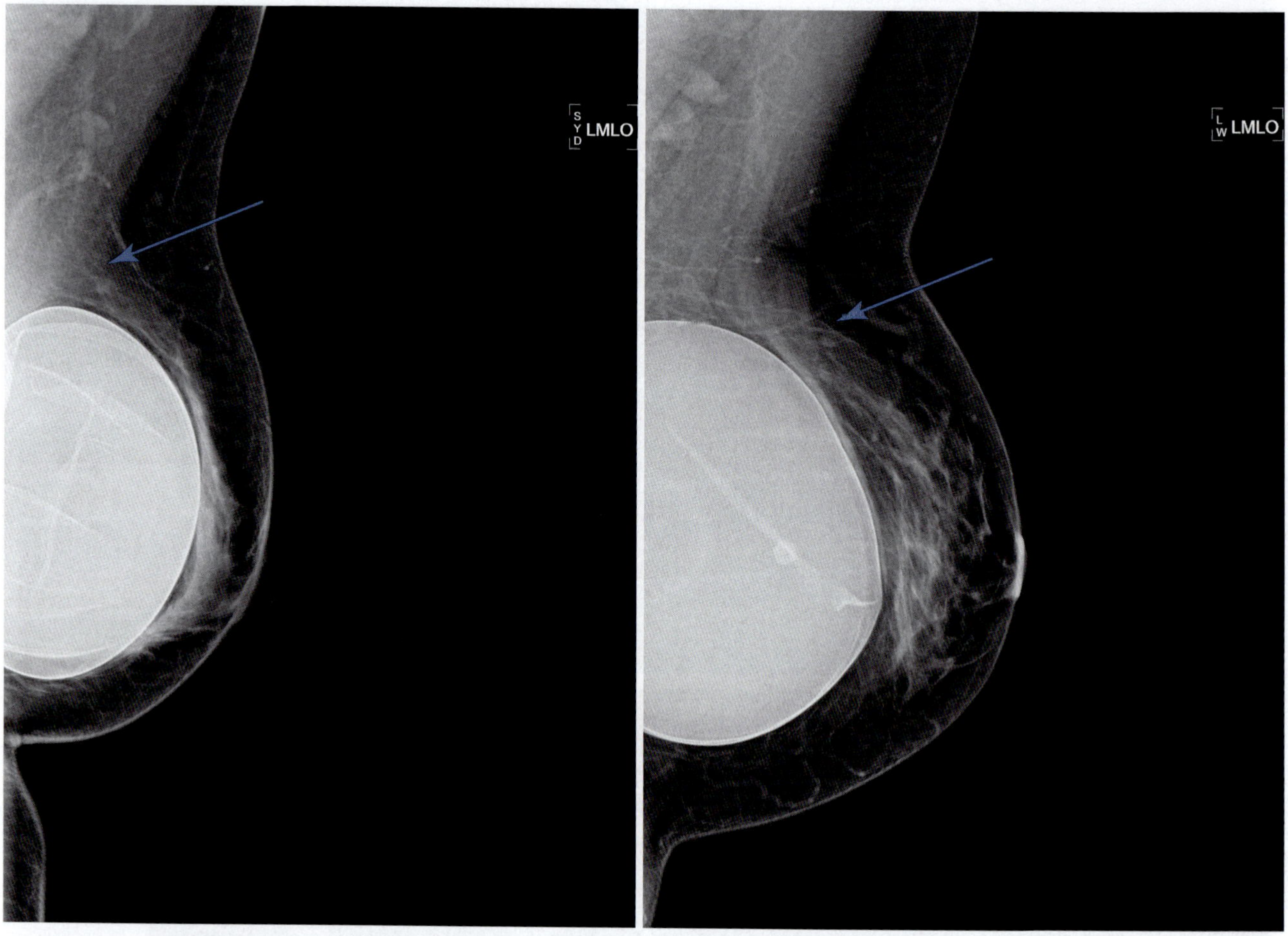

Fig. 16.60 Prepectoral versus retropectoral saline implant. Note the saline implant is less dense than silicone implants, and wrinkles and valves are seen within the saline implant

for cancer detection. In our patients with implants that undergo MRI for high-risk screening or for extent of disease in new cancer diagnosis, we perform silicone-sensitive sequences prior to the contrast portion of the study to assist in problem solving if abnormalities are seen on the contrast study that could be attributed to free silicone. This also helps to provide information on the implant integrity for preoperative planning.

Silicone-sensitive MRI sequences are utilized to differentiate silicone from water and fat. These sequences are usually T2 weighted with water suppression. Intact silicone implants will be bright on silicone-sensitive MRI sequences and may demonstrate small peripheral folds, without internal alterations (Fig. 16.70). Intracapsular rupture is diagnosed by the presence of the "linguine sign" which is created by the shell of the implant collapsing within the capsule. The fibrous capsule will be dark, as will the wavy lines of the collapsed ruptured implant which will be surrounded by the bright signal of silicone. The "keyhole" sign (or teardrop sign) is also useful in diagnosing intracapsular rupture. In this finding, silicone intersperses between dark folds in the collapsing implant shell (Figs. 16.71a, b and 16.72a–d). Extracapsular rupture is diagnosed by detecting silicone outside the capsule, within the breast parenchyma, or in the axilla. High T2 signal material will be seen surrounding the implant, within the breast parenchyma, or extending to axillary lymph nodes. It should be noted that there are double-lumen implants that can mimic rupture and knowing the implant type prior to image interpretation is essential to avoid false positives. It is also helpful to obtain a history of whether there is known prior rupture and removal/replacement for accurate assessment.

Explantation

Some women choose to remove breast implants. If the woman elects to not have another set of implants placed, typically, minimal architectural distortion will be seen in the posterior central aspect of the breast on mammography, where the implants once resided. In rare cases, the implant cavity can fill with fluid and produce a small residual mass posteriorly. If the fibrous capsule is not removed, portions of the capsule may be seen as curvilinear densities in the site previously occupied by the implant. If the capsule is calci-

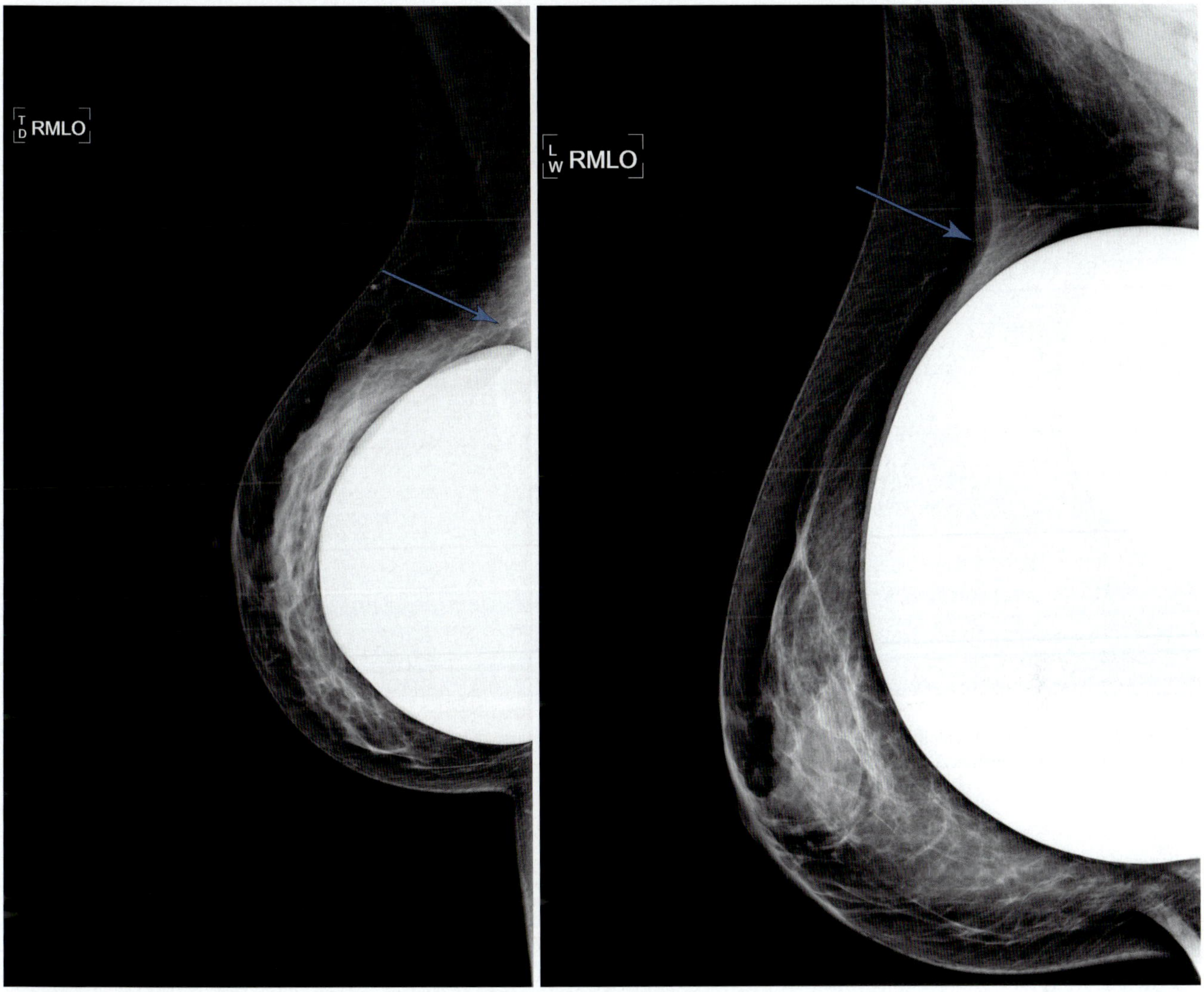

Fig. 16.61 Appearance of prepectoral versus retropectoral silicone implants. Note the pectoralis muscle coursing over the silicone implant in retropectoral implants rather than behind as seen in prepectoral implants. These findings are best visualized on the MLO view

fied, residual dystrophic calcifications in the retained fibrous capsule will be seen on mammography (Figs. 16.73, 16.74, and 16.75a, b). If the removed implants were silicone and there was prior extracapsular rupture, extravasated silicone is often left in the breast parenchyma as it is very difficult to completely remove surgically without removing a large amount of breast tissue. If the patient chooses to have another set of silicone implants placed, the residual free silicone can make diagnosing rupture of the new implants difficult.

Summary

Mammographic interpretation of the postprocedure breast requires familiarity with the various procedures and temporal changes expected following surgery. Surgical breast interventions include excisional biopsy, lumpectomy, mastectomy, reduction, and augmentation. Postsurgical imaging findings including masses, fluid collections, increased breast density, skin thickening, architectural distortion, and calcifications have characteristic sequences of evolution toward stability. Although there is overlap between post-treatment changes and breast carcinoma on imaging, recognizing characteristic post-treatment sequela and comparing interval findings on serial studies will assist in discriminating the two. Breast imagers should be informed of the spectrum of expected postoperative imaging findings, and any changes in the imaging findings after stabilization should raise concern for recurrent carcinoma and prompt biopsy. Awareness of expected findings will minimize unnecessary recall and permits early detection of recurrent breast cancer.

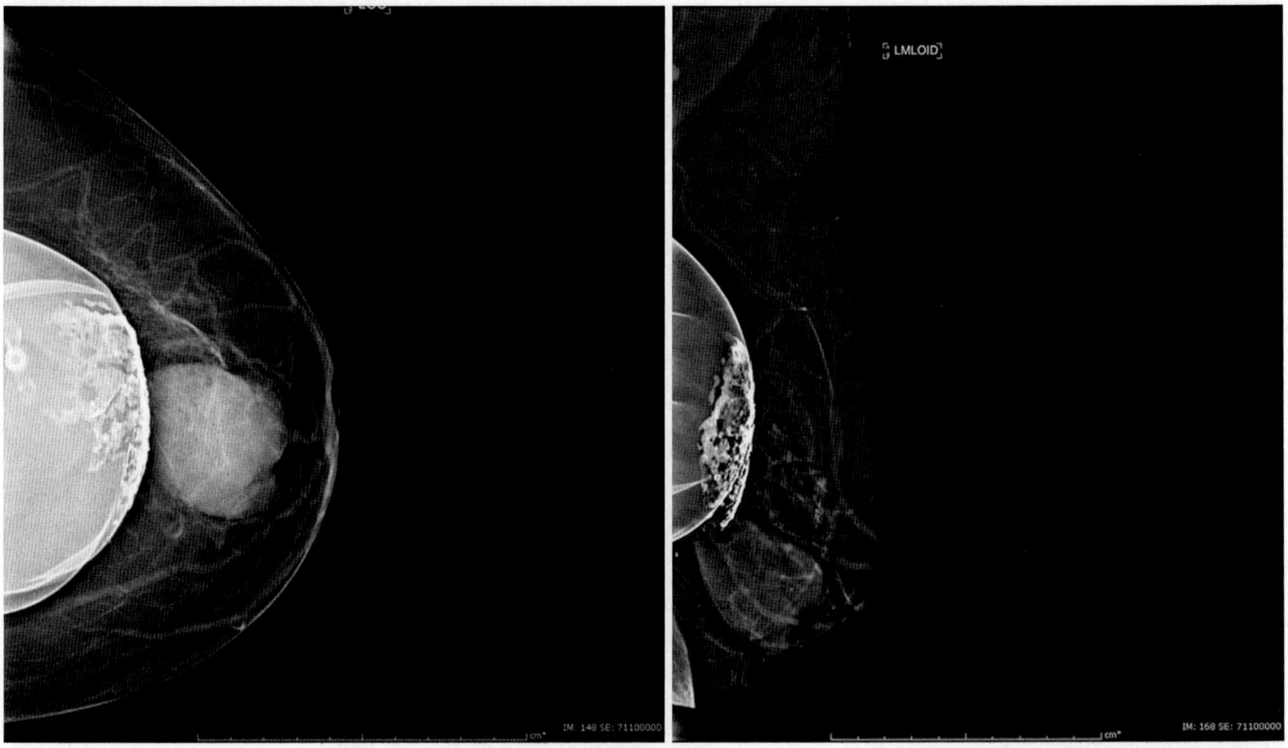

Fig. 16.62 Coarse capsular calcifications on a prepectoral saline implant. The coarse calcifications are best seen along the anterior aspect of the implant on the implant-displaced view. The mass in the lower central breast was stable over several years

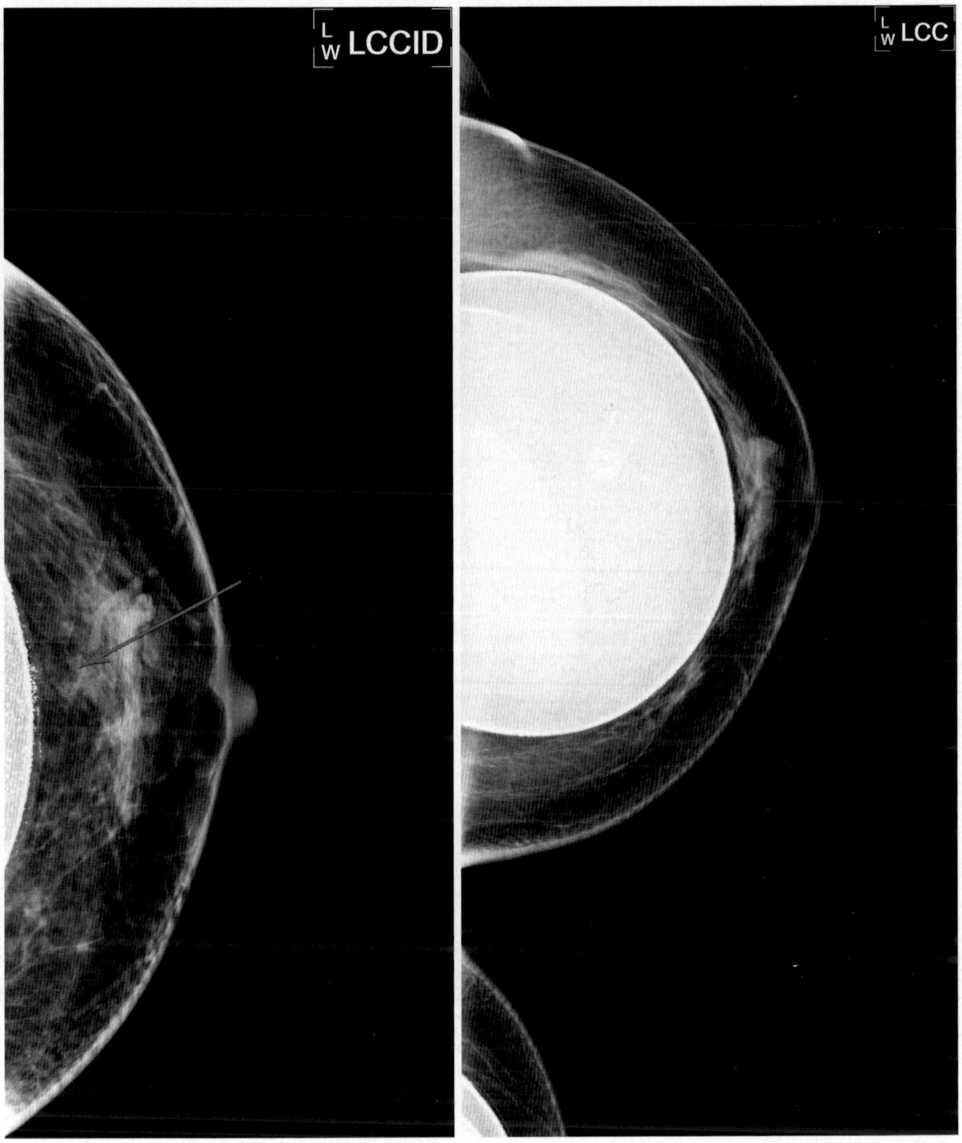

Fig. 16.63 Tiny capsular calcifications seen along the anterior aspect of a prepectoral saline implant in the implant-displaced view

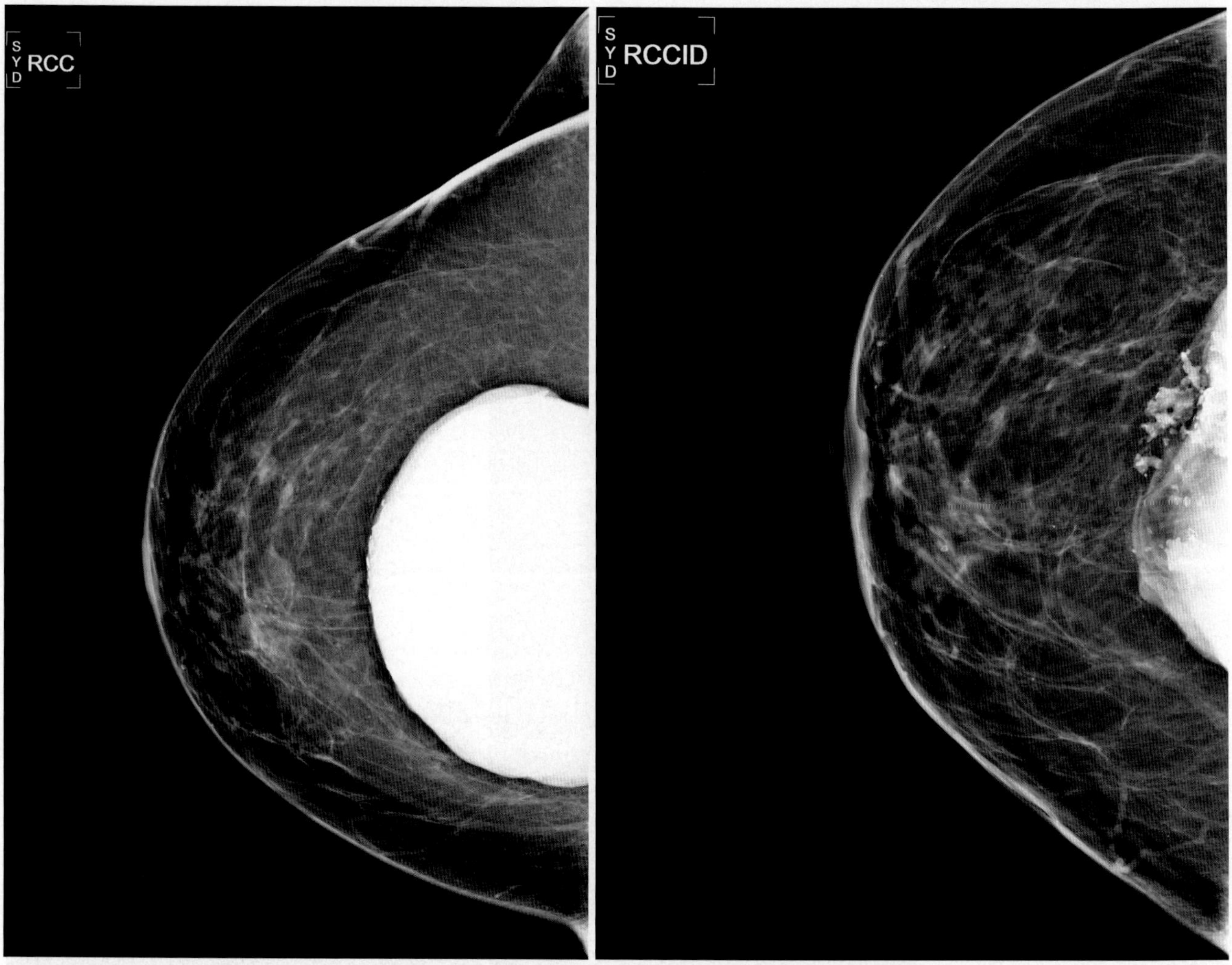

Fig. 16.64 A 77-year-old female with prepectoral silicone implant placed 25 years prior. The implant has a lobulated contour and is firm on the chest, suggesting encapsulation. Implant-displaced view demonstrates coarse capsular calcifications

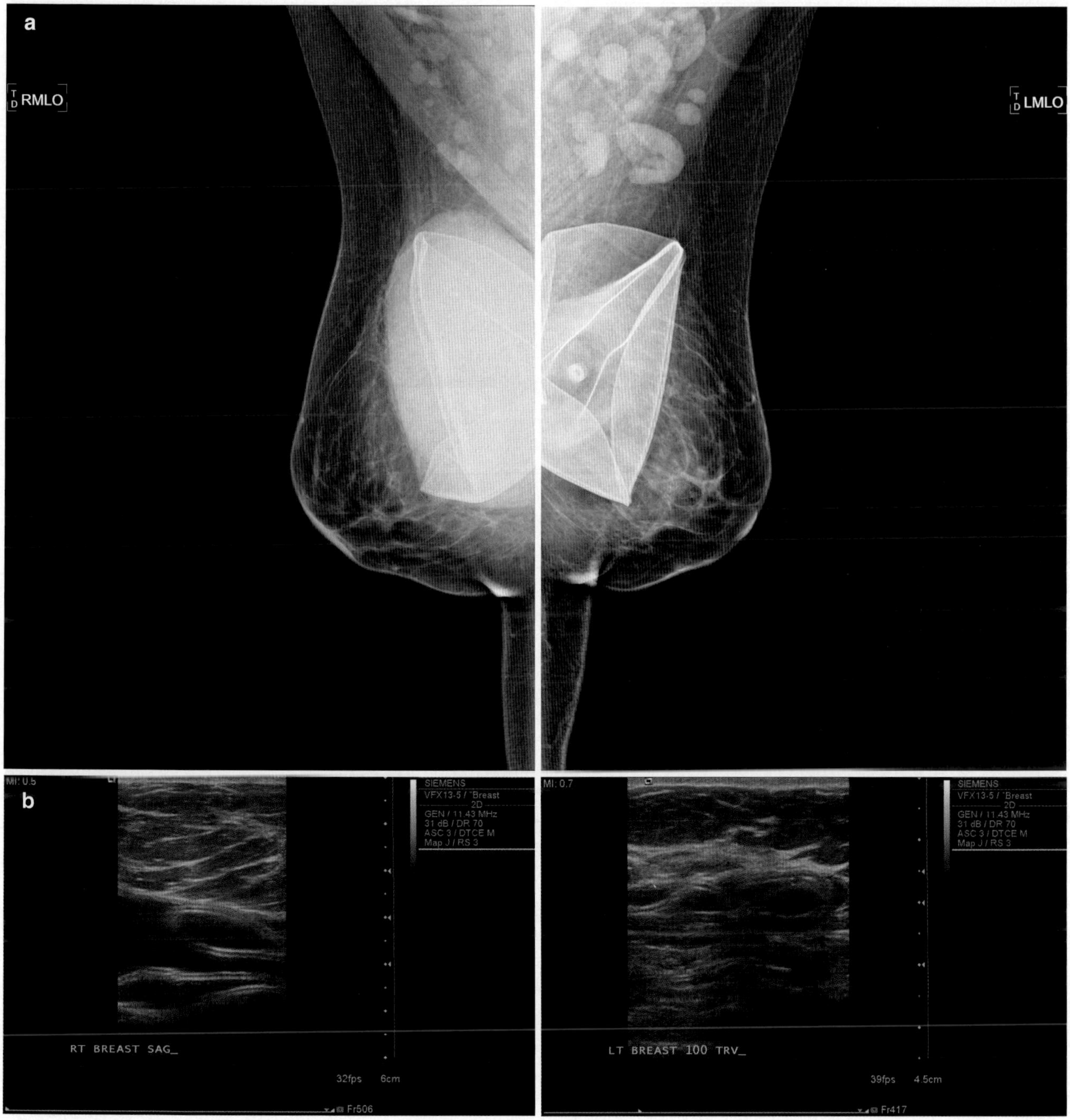

Fig. 16.65 (**a**) A 44-year-old female presents for evaluation of right breast lump. Bilateral prepectoral saline implants are ruptured. The implants were placed 17 years prior to the exam. (**b**) Residual fluid is present within the capsule on the right making the collapsed envelope more visible sonographically. The left implant is completely collapsed

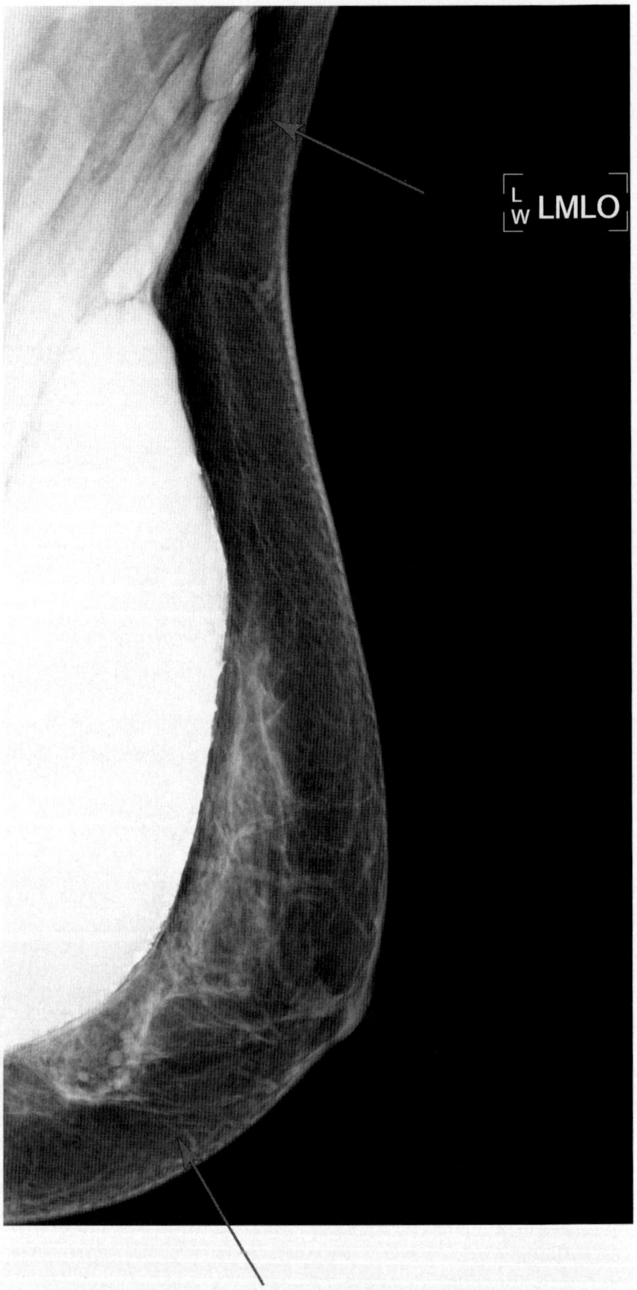

Fig. 16.66 Small collections of free silicone inferior to a prepectoral silicone implant. Dense axillary lymph nodes suggest probable silicone within the axillary lymph nodes

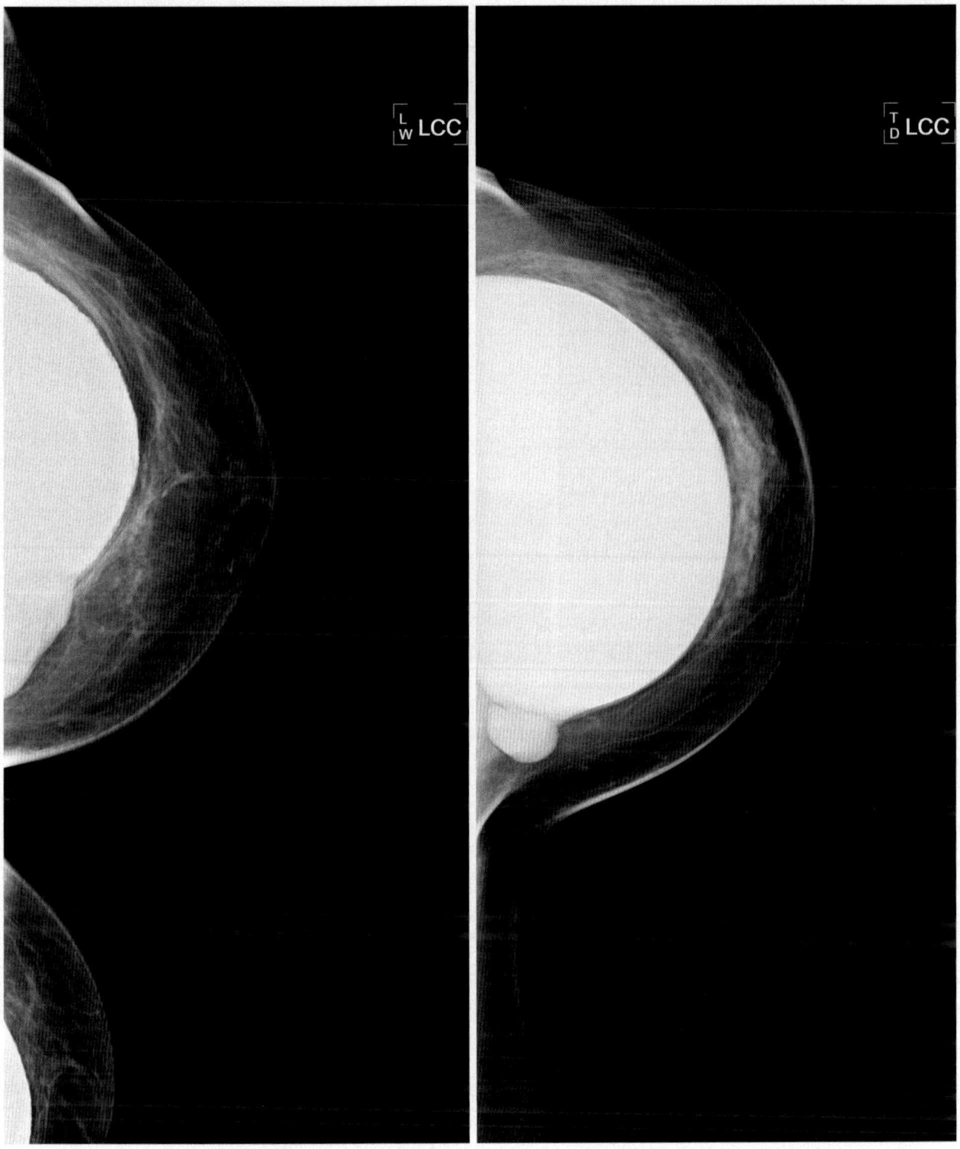

Fig. 16.67 Mammographic evidence of extracapsular rupture with free silicone within the breast parenchyma medial to the implant in two different patients

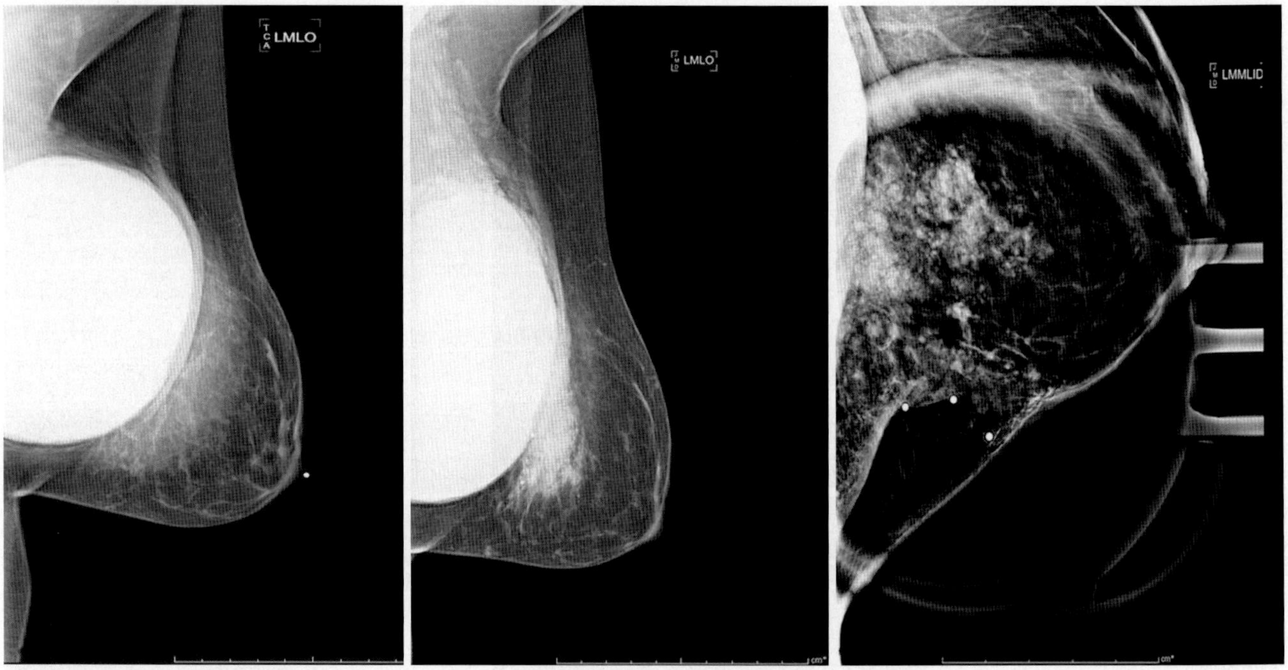

Fig. 16.68 Initial mammogram demonstrates retropectoral silicone implant. The patient returns 2.5 years later with new palpable abnormality in the lower breast. High-density material anterior to the implant in the area of complaint is consistent with extracapsular silicone

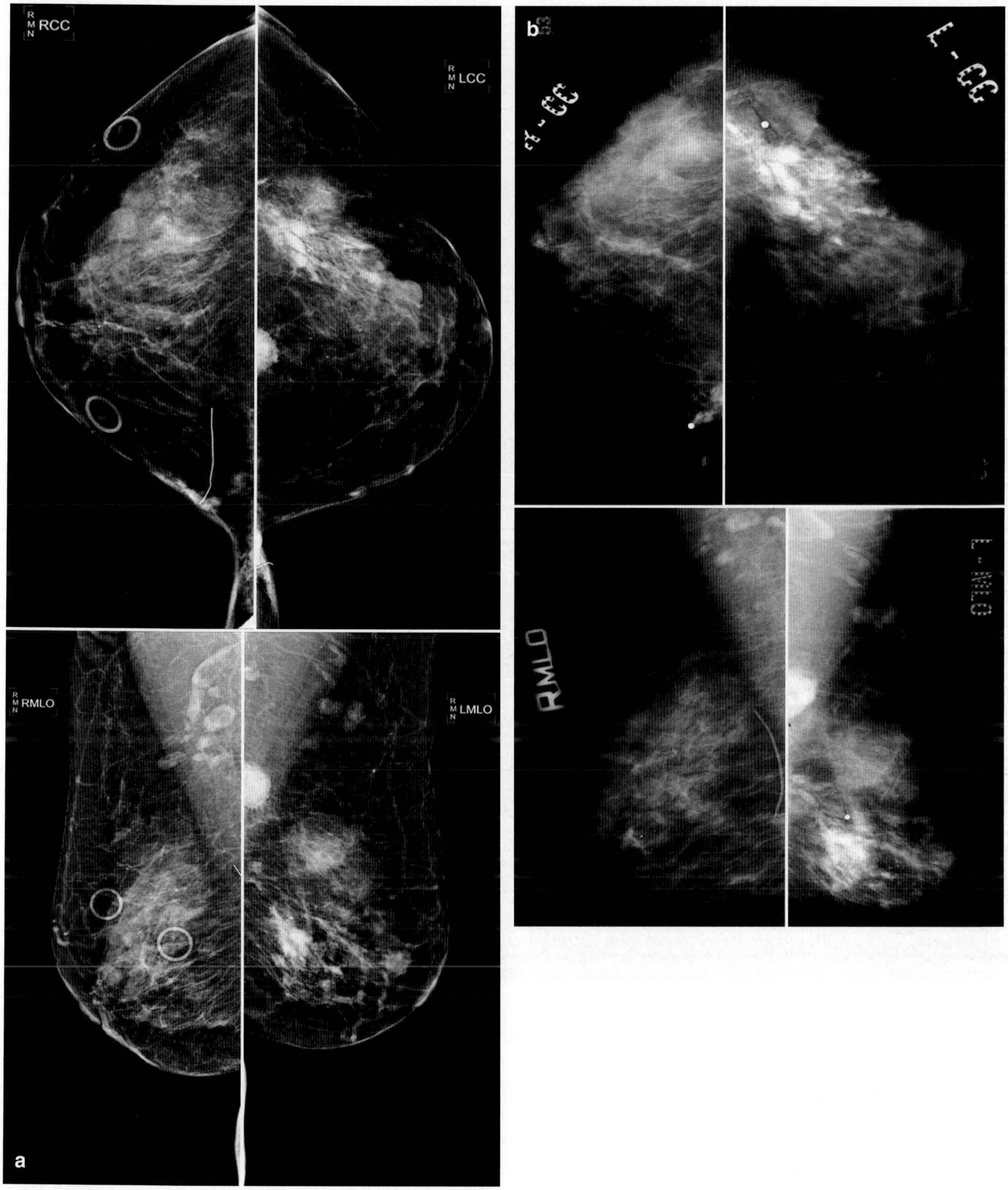

Fig. 16.69 (**a**) A 50-year-old female with history of ruptured silicone implants. Physician detects palpable abnormalities in the upper outer and lower outer left breast and upper inner right breast. (**b**) An outside mammogram from 2 years prior shows no significant change in high-density masses in area of free silicone. (**c**) Multiple silicone granulomas documented in both breasts on ultrasound. (**d**) However, ultrasound of the area of palpable complaint documents a 1.6 cm hypoechoic mass that is different in appearance from the silicone granulomas and has sonographic features of malignancy. Ultrasound-guided core needle biopsy was performed with pathology yielding invasive ductal carcinoma. (**e**) Post-procedure mammogram documents a clip in the mass in the upper outer breast. Note the higher density of the silicone granulomas. (**f**) Axial MRI silicone-sensitive sequence demonstrating high signal in one of the silicone granulomas. Note the absence of increased signal in the area of known cancer in the posterior outer breast. Post-contrast T1 images with fat saturation show enhancement in the known cancer and no enhancement in the area of the silicone granuloma

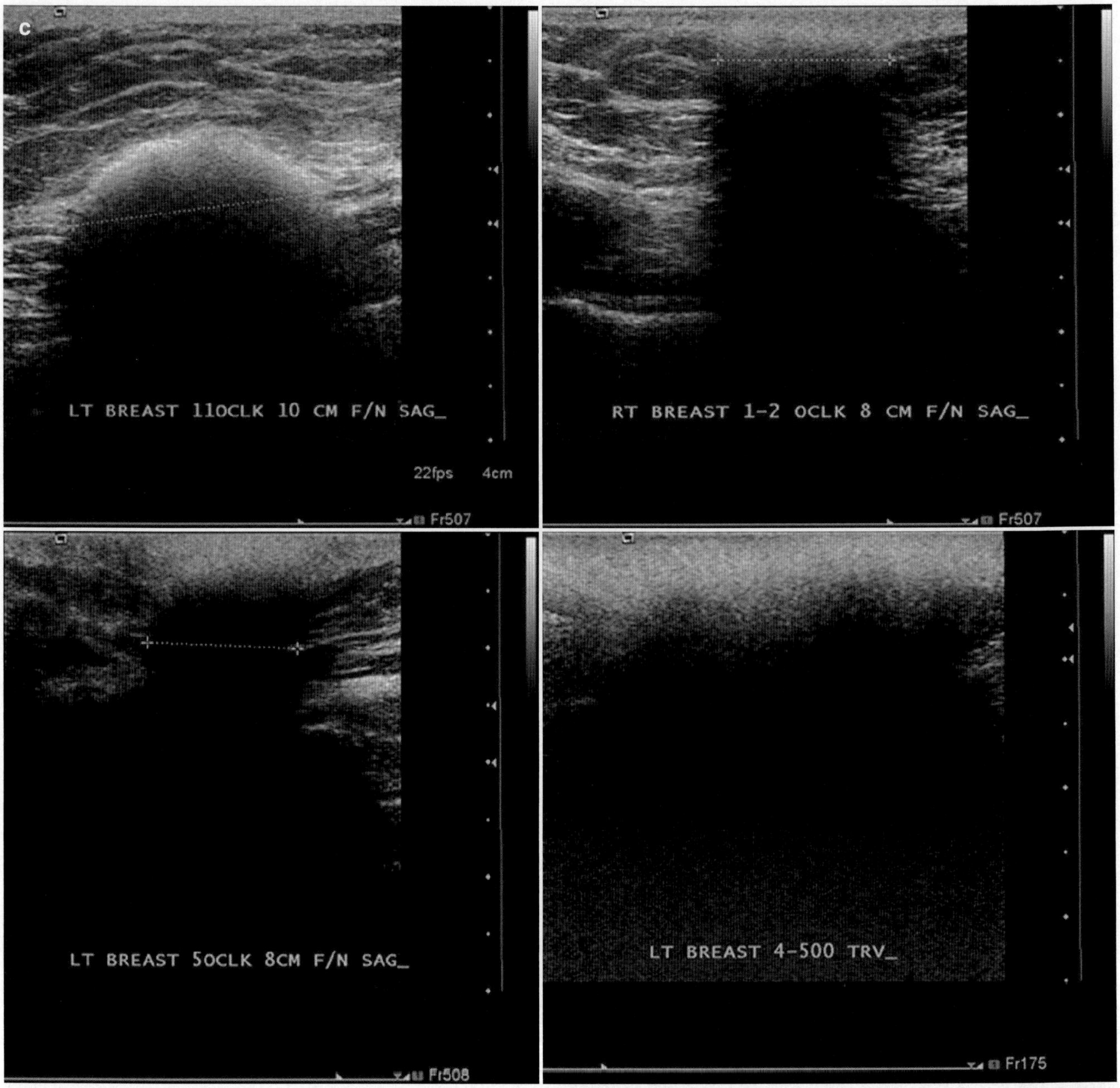

Fig. 16.69 (continued)

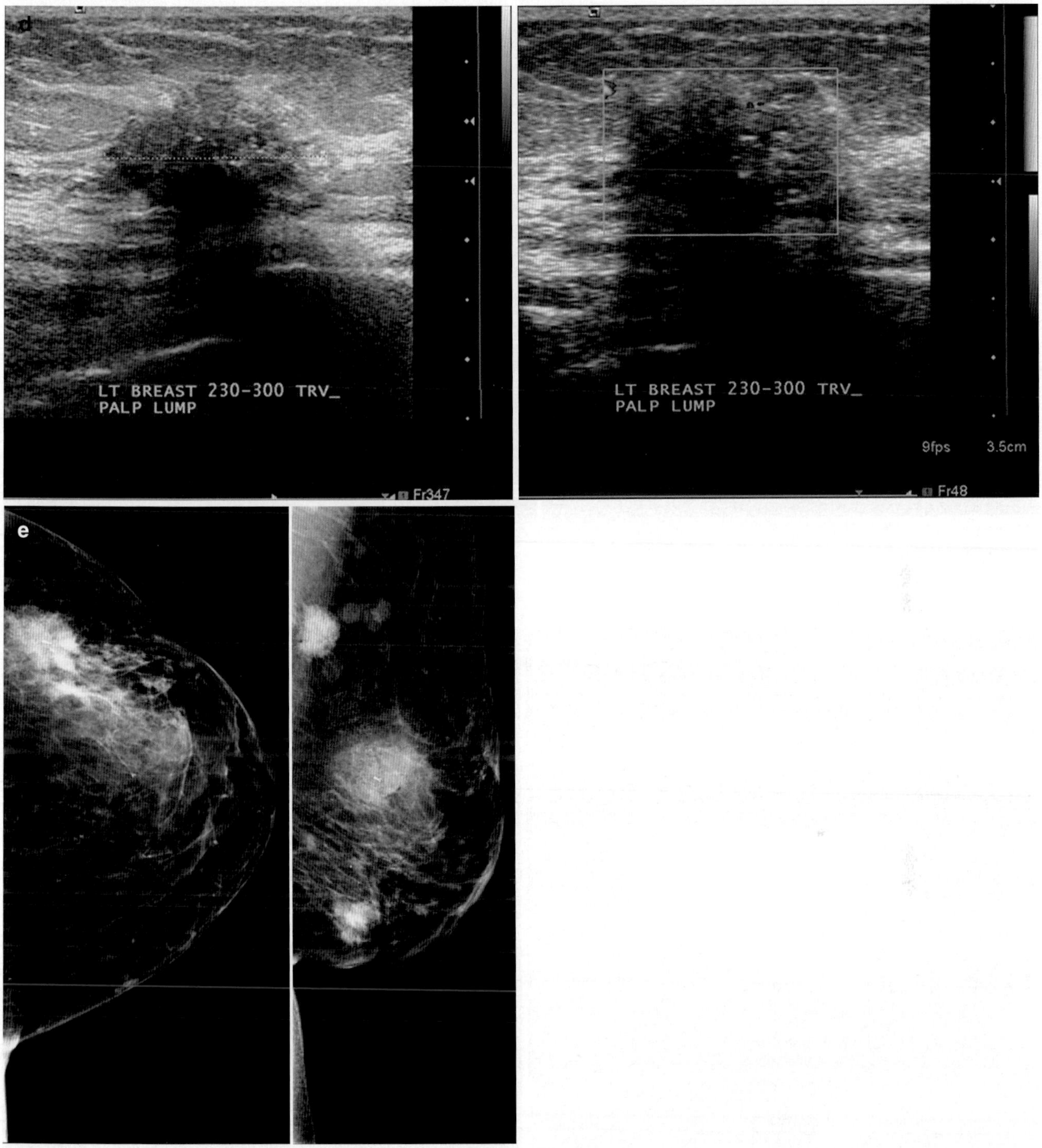

Fig. 16.69 (continued)

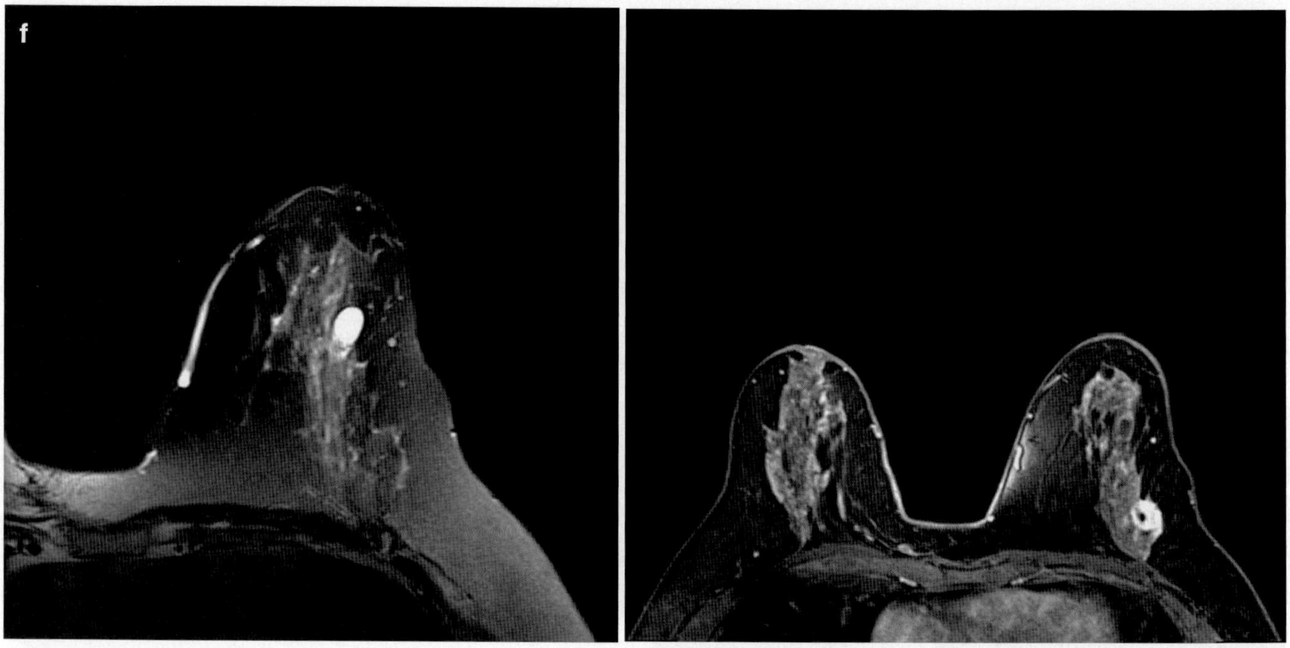

Fig. 16.69 (continued)

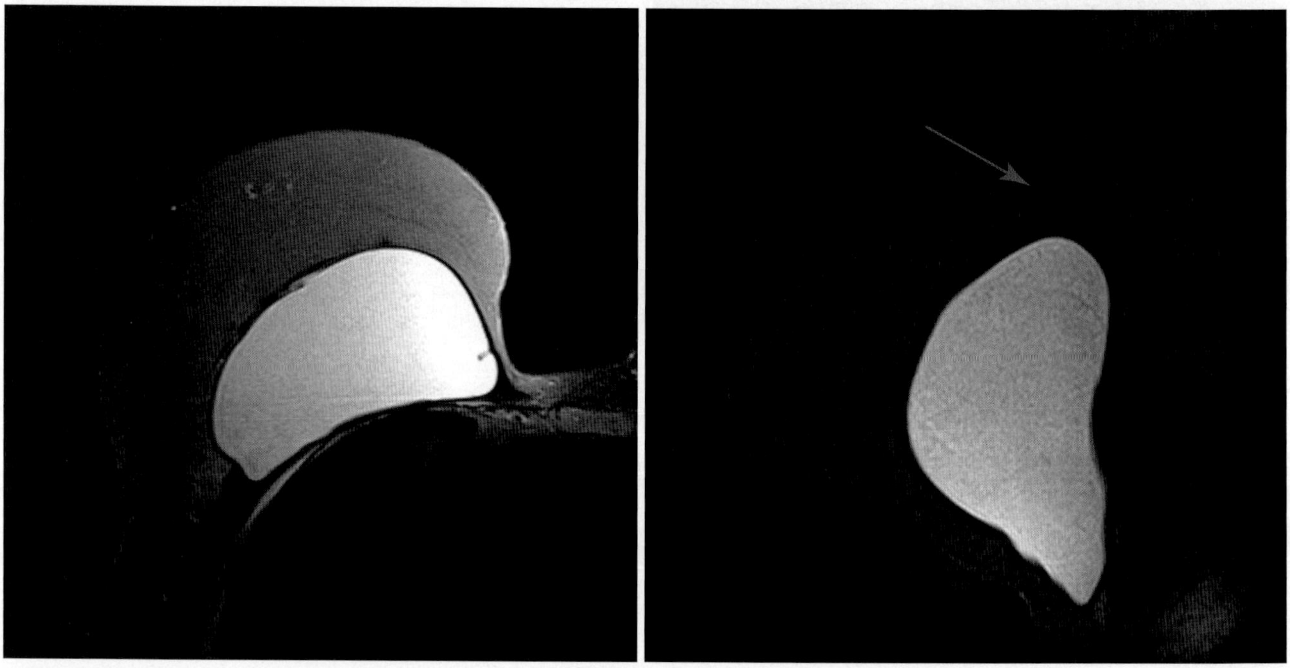

Fig. 16.70 Breast MRI with silicone-sensitive sequences demonstrates an intact retropectoral implant without evidence of intracapsular or extracapsular rupture. The pectoralis muscle (*arrow*) is visualized as a dark structure overlying the implant on the sagittal view

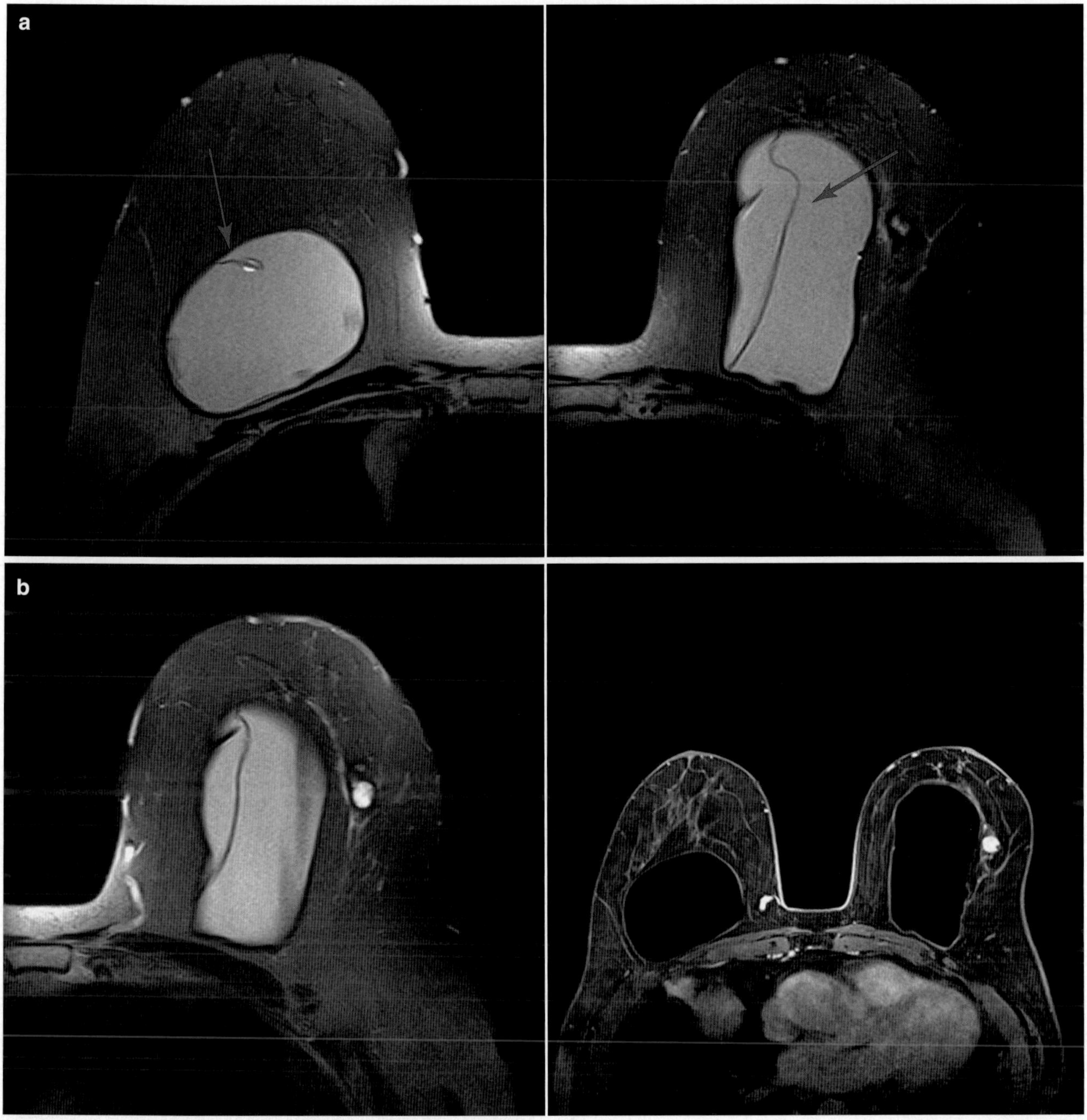

Fig. 16.71 (**a**) Bilateral prepectoral silicone implants with intracapsular rupture. The right implant demonstrates the "keyhole sign" (*arrow*) with silicone seen within a portion of free-floating envelope. The right implant demonstrates the classic "linguini" sign (*thick arrow*). Increased T2 signal lateral to the left implant raised the question of possible extracapsular silicone. (**b**) Correlation with the post-contrast study provided clarification. A 1 cm known cancer in the central outer left breast had increased T2 on a silicone-sensitive sequence. However, enhancement is present on the T1 post-contrast image with fat saturation. Free silicone should not enhance confirming the presence of malignancy rather than extracapsular silicone

Fig. 16.72 (**a**) A 60-year-old female with prepectoral silicone implants and new palpable abnormality in the medial left breast. Mammography demonstrates a focal bulge in the medial aspect of the left implant. High-density material is visualized within the breast parenchyma along the inferior aspect of the left implant. (**b**) Silicone-sensitive MRI sequences demonstrate both intracapsular and extracapsular implant rupture. A focal bulge of the implant is visualized in the medial left breast corresponding to the palpable complaint. Extracapsular silicone is also visualized anterior to the implant on the sagittal view. (**c**) Axial T2 images demonstrate intracapsular rupture bilaterally. (**d**) The patient subsequently elected for implant explantation with postsurgical changes in the posterior central breast. Note coarse capsular calcifications and nodular silicone granulomas

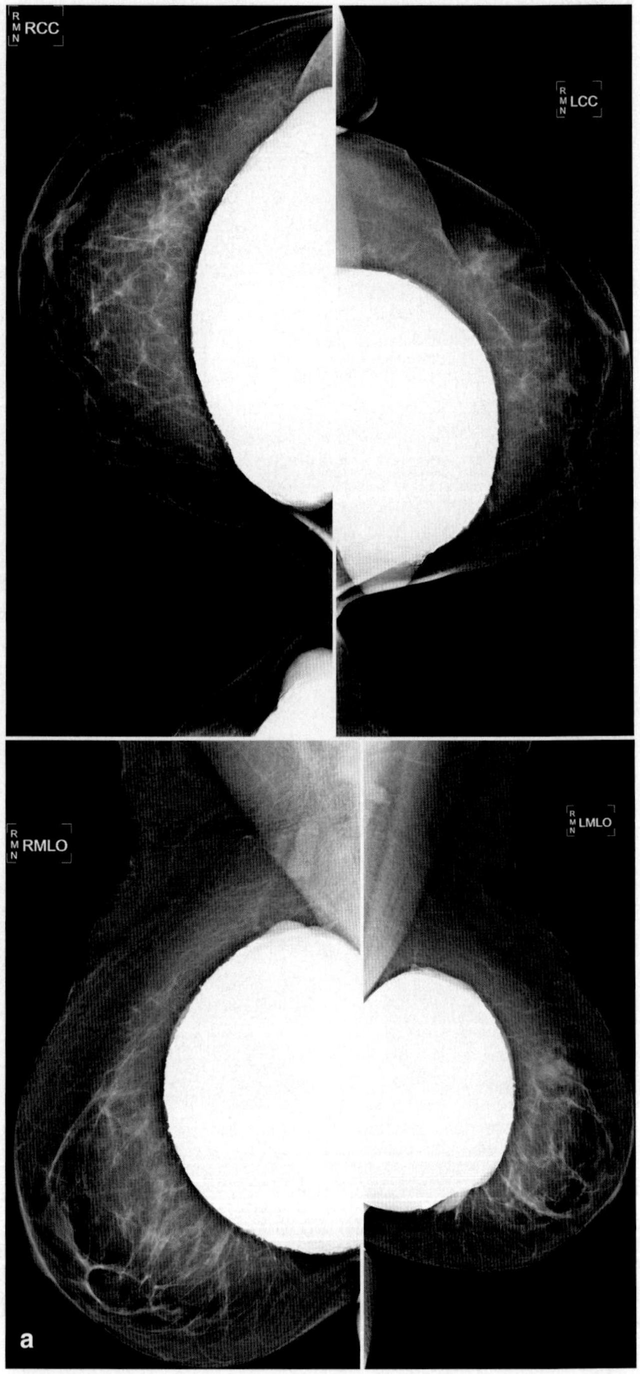

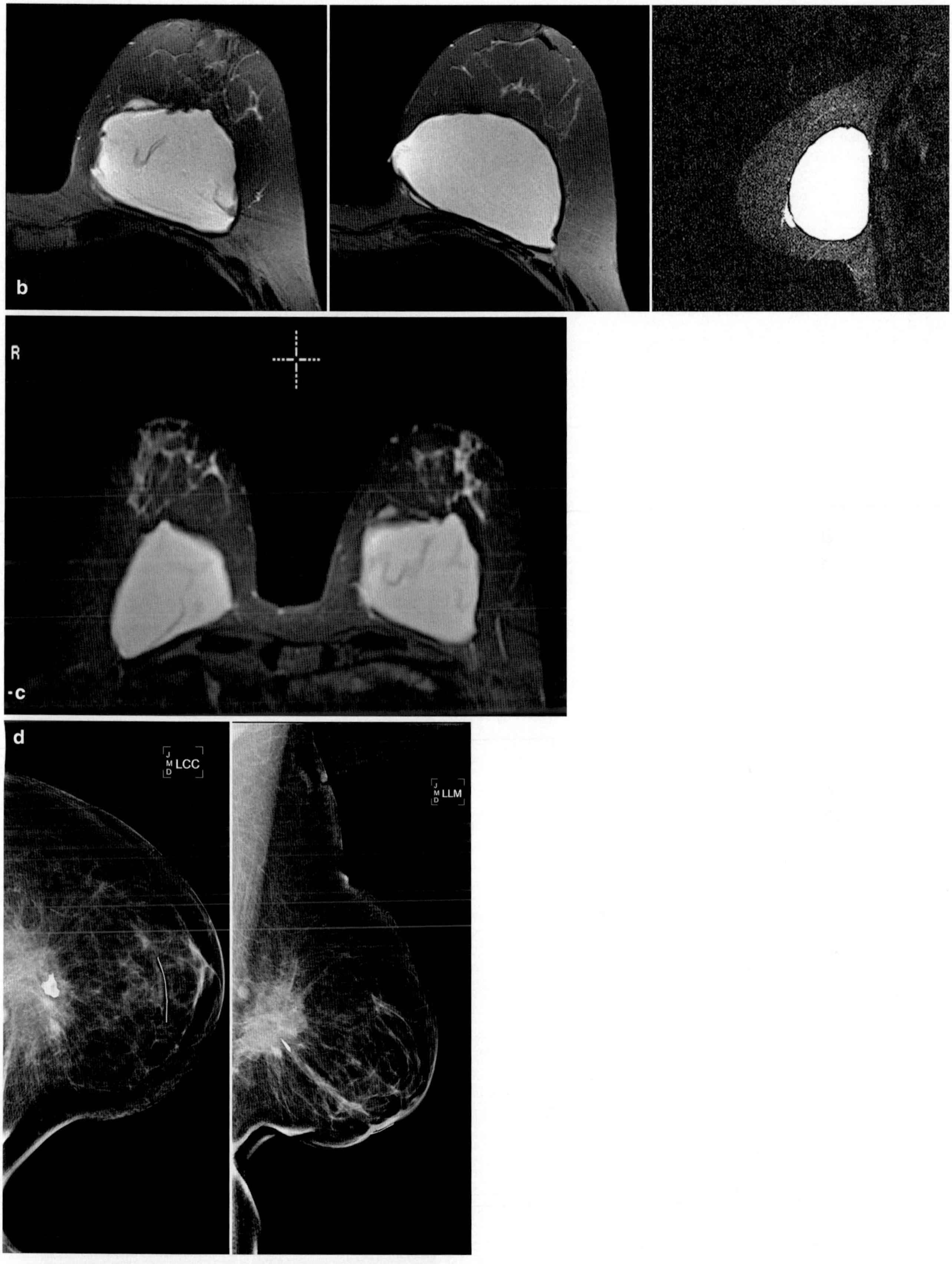

Fig. 16.72 (continued)

Fig. 16.73 A 57-year-old woman status post left lumpectomy. History of bilateral breast implant explantation 10 years prior to cancer diagnosis. Post-lumpectomy changes are present in the anterior left breast. Postsurgical calcifications and coarse capsular calcifications are visualized in the posterior central left breast. No significations that residual changes are present in the right breast

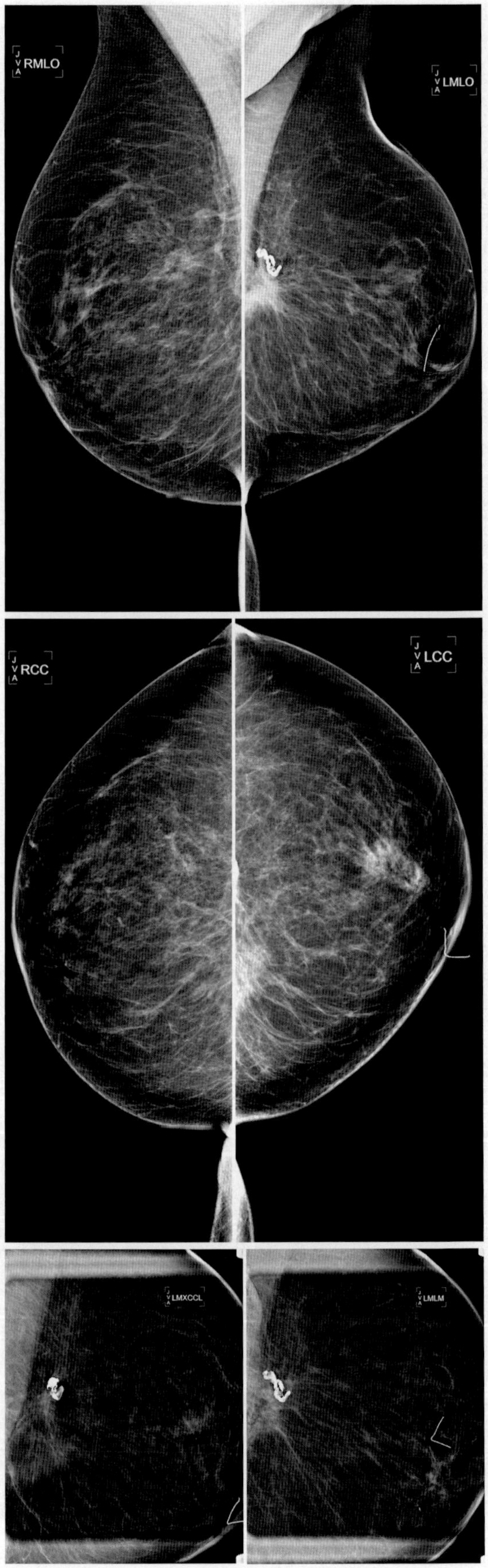

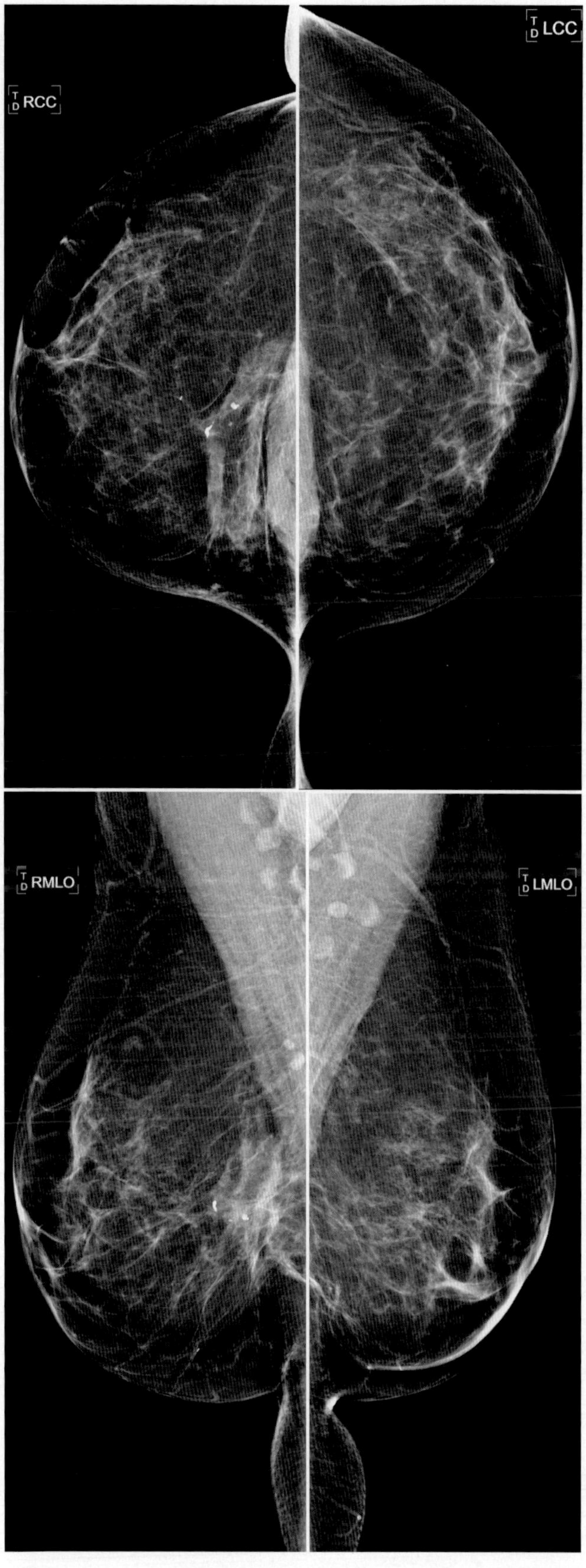

Fig. 16.74 Screening exam in a 50-year-old female with history of implant explantation. The patient had a strong family history of breast cancer in a premenopausal sister. The posterior central right breast is obscured by postsurgical changes

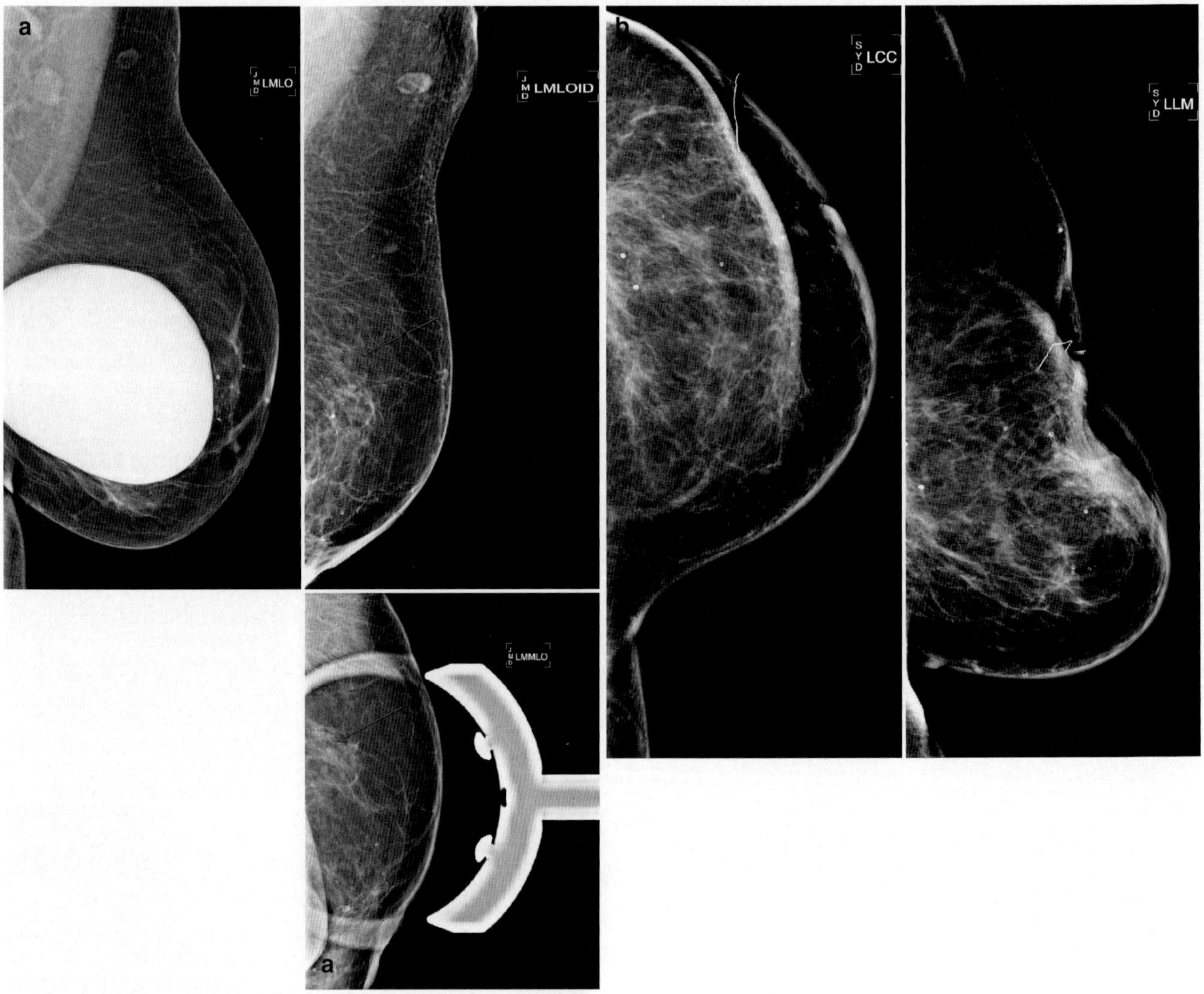

Fig. 16.75 (**a**) A 70-year-old female with faint calcifications barely perceptible on MLO implant displaced view (*arrow*) prompted spot magnification views. Spot magnification view demonstrates 8 mm of very faint heterogenous calcifications (*arrow*) just anterior to the implant. Stereotactic biopsy was performed with pathology yielding DCIS. (**b**). Six-month follow-up mammogram following lumpectomy demonstrates significant distortion of the upper outer breast at the site of lumpectomy. The silicone implant was ruptured on MRI and was removed at the time of surgery with minimal post-explantation change also noted in the posterior central breast

References

1. Brenner RJ, Pfaff JM. Mammographic changes after excisional breast biopsy for benign disease. AJR Am J Roentgenol. 1996;167(4):1047–52.
2. Slanetz PJ, et al. Previous breast biopsy for benign disease rarely complicates or alters interpretation on screening mammography. AJR Am J Roentgenol. 1998;170(6):1539–41.
3. Frei KA, et al. MR imaging of the breast in patients with positive margins after lumpectomy: influence of the time interval between lumpectomy and MR imaging. AJR Am J Roentgenol. 2000;175(6):1577–84.
4. Lee CH, et al. Breast cancer screening with imaging: recommendations from the Society of Breast Imaging and the ACR on the use of mammography, breast MRI, breast ultrasound, and other technologies for the detection of clinically occult breast cancer. J Am Coll Radiol. 2010;7(1):18–27.
5. Orel SG, et al. Breast carcinoma: MR imaging before re-excisional biopsy. Radiology. 1997;205(2):429–36.
6. Fisher B, et al. Reanalysis and results after 12 years of follow-up in a randomized clinical trial comparing total mastectomy with lumpectomy with or without irradiation in the treatment of breast cancer. N Engl J Med. 1995;333(22):1456–61.
7. Veronesi U, et al. Breast conservation is a safe method in patients with small cancer of the breast. Long-term results of three randomised trials on 1,973 patients. Eur J Cancer. 1995;31A(10):1574–9.
8. Kriege M, et al. Efficacy of MRI and mammography for breast-cancer screening in women with a familial or genetic predisposition. N Engl J Med. 2004;351(5):427–37.
9. Lee SG, et al. MR imaging screening of the contralateral breast in patients with newly diagnosed breast cancer: preliminary results. Radiology. 2003;226(3):773–8.
10. Liberman L, et al. MR imaging of the ipsilateral breast in women with percutaneously proven breast cancer. AJR Am J Roentgenol. 2003;180(4):901–10.
11. Liberman L, et al. MR imaging findings in the contralateral breast of women with recently diagnosed breast cancer. AJR Am J Roentgenol. 2003;180(2):333–41.
12. Lehman CD, et al. MRI evaluation of the contralateral breast in women with recently diagnosed breast cancer. N Engl J Med. 2007;356(13):1295–303.
13. Fowble B, et al. Breast recurrence following conservative surgery and radiation: patterns of failure, prognosis, and pathologic findings from mastectomy specimens with implications for treatment. Int J Radiat Oncol Biol Phys. 1990;19(4):833–42.
14. Krishnamurthy R, et al. Mammographic findings after breast conservation therapy. Radiographics. 1999;19:S53–62; quiz S262–3.
15. Buckley JH, Roebuck EJ. Mammographic changes following radiotherapy. Br J Radiol. 1986;59(700):337–44.
16. Mitnick J, Roses DF, Harris MN. Differentiation of postsurgical changes from carcinoma of the breast. Surg Gynecol Obstet. 1988;166(6):549–50.
17. Mendelson EB. Imaging the post-surgical breast. Semin Ultrasound CT MR. 1989;10(2):154–70.
18. Mendelson EB. Evaluation of the postoperative breast. Radiol Clin North Am. 1992;30(1):107–38.
19. Chansakul T, Lai KC, Slanetz J. The postconservation breast: part 1, Expected imaging findings. AJR Am J Roentgenol. 2012;198(2):321–30.
20. Libshitz HI, Montague ED, Paulus Jr DD. Skin thickness in the therapeutically irradiated breast. AJR Am J Roentgenol. 1978;130(2):345–7.
21. Paulus DD. Conservative treatment of breast cancer: mammography in patient selection and follow-up. AJR Am J Roentgenol. 1984;143(3):483–7.
22. Saslow D, et al. American Cancer Society guidelines for breast screening with MRI as an adjunct to mammography. CA Cancer J Clin. 2007;57(2):75–89.
23. Morris EA, et al. MRI of occult breast carcinoma in a high-risk population. AJR Am J Roentgenol. 2003;181(3):619–26.
24. Dershaw DD. Mammography in patients with breast cancer treated by breast conservation (lumpectomy with or without radiation). AJR Am J Roentgenol. 1995;164(2):309–16.
25. Early Breast Cancer Trialists' Collaborative, Group. Effects of chemotherapy and hormonal therapy for early breast cancer on recurrence and 15-year survival: an overview of the randomised trials. Lancet. 2005;365(9472):1687–717.
26. Wapnir IL, et al. Prognosis after ipsilateral breast tumor recurrence and locoregional recurrences in five National Surgical Adjuvant Breast and Bowel Project node-positive adjuvant breast cancer trials. J Clin Oncol. 2006;24(13):2028–37.
27. Komoike Y, et al. Ipsilateral breast tumor recurrence (IBTR) after breast-conserving treatment for early breast cancer: risk factors and impact on distant metastases. Cancer. 2006;106(1):35–41.
28. Horst KC, et al. Predictors of local recurrence after breast-conservation therapy. Clin Breast Cancer. 2005;5(6):425–38.
29. Samant RS, et al. Diagnosis of metachronous contralateral breast cancer. Breast J. 2001;7(6):405–10.
30. Broet P, et al. Contralateral breast cancer: annual incidence and risk parameters. J Clin Oncol. 1995;13(7):1578–83.
31. Bernstein JL, et al. Risk factors predicting the incidence of second primary breast cancer among women diagnosed with a first primary breast cancer. Am J Epidemiol. 1992;136(8):925–36.
32. Horn PL, Thompson WD. Risk of contralateral breast cancer: associations with factors related to initial breast cancer. Am J Epidemiol. 1988;128(2):309–23.
33. Howell A, et al. Results of the ATAC (Arimidex, Tamoxifen, Alone or in Combination) trial after completion of 5 years' adjuvant treatment for breast cancer. Lancet. 2005;365(9453):60–2.
34. Stomper PC, et al. Mammographic detection of recurrent cancer in the irradiated breast. AJR Am J Roentgenol. 1987;148(1):39–43.
35. Berg WA, et al. Combined screening with ultrasound and mammography vs mammography alone in women at elevated risk of breast cancer. JAMA. 2008;299(18):2151–63.
36. Belli P, et al. Magnetic resonance imaging in breast cancer recurrence. Breast Cancer Res Treat. 2002;73(3):223–35.
37. Hartmann LC, et al. Efficacy of bilateral prophylactic mastectomy in women with a family history of breast cancer. N Engl J Med. 1999;340(2):77–84.
38. Taghian AG, Smith BL, Erban JK. Breast cancer: a multidisciplinary approach to diagnosis and management. Current multidisciplinary oncology. New York: Demos Medical Pub; 2010, xviii, 335 p.
39. Glaus SW, Carlson GW. Long-term role of external breast prostheses after total mastectomy. Breast J. 2009;15(4):385–93.
40. Helvie MA, et al. Mammographic screening of TRAM flap breast reconstructions for detection of nonpalpable recurrent cancer. Radiology. 2002;224(1):211–6.
41. Noone RB, et al. Recurrence of breast carcinoma following immediate reconstruction: a 13-year review. Plast Reconstr Surg. 1994;93(1):96–106; discussion 107–8.
42. Hartrampf CR, Scheflan M, Black PW. Breast reconstruction with a transverse abdominal island flap. Plast Reconstr Surg. 1982;69(2):216–25.
43. Devon RK, et al. Breast reconstruction with a transverse rectus abdominis myocutaneous flap: spectrum of normal and abnormal MR imaging findings. Radiographics. 2004;24(5):1287–99.
44. Antoniuk PM. Breast reconstruction. Obstet Gynecol Clin North Am. 2002;29(1):209–23, ix.
45. Grotting JC, Beckenstein MS, Arkoulakis NS. The art and science of autologous breast reconstruction. Breast J. 2003;9(5):350–60.

46. Berg WA. Diagnostic imaging. Breast. 1st ed. Salt Lake City: Amirsys; 2006.
47. Blondeel N, et al. The donor site morbidity of free DIEP flaps and free TRAM flaps for breast reconstruction. Br J Plast Surg. 1997;50(5):322–30.
48. Kroll SS, et al. Local recurrence risk after skin-sparing and conventional mastectomy: a 6-year follow-up. Plast Reconstr Surg. 1999;104(2):421–5.
49. Simmons RM, et al. Local and distant recurrence rates in skin-sparing mastectomies compared with non-skin-sparing mastectomies. Ann Surg Oncol. 1999;6(7):676–81.
50. Ho CM, et al. Skin involvement in invasive breast carcinoma: safety of skin-sparing mastectomy. Ann Surg Oncol. 2003;10(2):102–7.
51. Carlson GW, et al. Local recurrence after skin-sparing mastectomy: tumor biology or surgical conservatism? Ann Surg Oncol. 2003;10(2):108–12.
52. Gerber B, et al. Skin-sparing mastectomy with conservation of the nipple-areola complex and autologous reconstruction is an oncologically safe procedure. Ann Surg. 2003;238(1):120–7.
53. Greenway RM, Schlossberg L, Dooley WC. Fifteen-year series of skin-sparing mastectomy for stage 0 to 2 breast cancer. Am J Surg. 2005;190(6):918–22.
54. Kroll SS, et al. Risk of recurrence after treatment of early breast cancer with skin-sparing mastectomy. Ann Surg Oncol. 1997;4(3):193–7.
55. Lee JM, et al. Detecting nonpalpable recurrent breast cancer: the role of routine mammographic screening of transverse rectus abdominis myocutaneous flap reconstructions. Radiology. 2008;248(2):398–405.
56. Rieber A, et al. Breast-conserving surgery and autogenous tissue reconstruction in patients with breast cancer: efficacy of MRI of the breast in the detection of recurrent disease. Eur Radiol. 2003;13(4):780–7.
57. Hogge JP, Zuurbier RA, de Paredes ES. Mammography of autologous myocutaneous flaps. Radiographics. 1999;19:S63–72.
58. Peng C, et al. MRI appearance of tumor recurrence in myocutaneous flap reconstruction after mastectomy. AJR Am J Roentgenol. 2011;196(4):W471–5.
59. Langstein HN, et al. Breast cancer recurrence after immediate reconstruction: patterns and significance. Plast Reconstr Surg. 2003;111(2):712–20; discussion 721–2.
60. Howard MA, et al. Breast cancer local recurrence after mastectomy and TRAM flap reconstruction: incidence and treatment options. Plast Reconstr Surg. 2006;117(5):1381–6.
61. Slavin SA, Love SM, Goldwyn RM. Recurrent breast cancer following immediate reconstruction with myocutaneous flaps. Plast Reconstr Surg. 1994;93(6):1191–204; discussion 1205–7.
62. Antoniuk PM. Breast augmentation and breast reduction. Obstet Gynecol Clin North Am. 2002;29(1):103–15.
63. Hammond DC, Loffredo M. Breast reduction. Plast Reconstr Surg. 2012;129(5):829e–39.
64. The American Society for Aesthetic Plastic Surgery. 15th Annual Cosmetic Surgery National Data Bank Statistics. 2011 [cited 2013 June 1]; Available from: http://www.surgery.org/sites/default/files/ASAPS-2011-Stats.pdf.
65. Keleher AJ, et al. Breast cancer in reduction mammaplasty specimens: case reports and guidelines. Breast J. 2003;9(2):120–5.
66. Miller CL, Feig SA, Fox JW. Mammographic changes after reduction mammoplasty. AJR Am J Roentgenol. 1987;149(1):35–8.
67. Andrades P, Prado A. Understanding modern breast reduction techniques with a simplified approach. J Plast Reconstr Aesthet Surg. 2008;61(11):1284–93.
68. Spear SL, Howard MA. Evolution of the vertical reduction mammaplasty. Plast Reconstr Surg. 2003;112(3):855–68; quiz 869.
69. Danikas D, et al. Mammographic findings following reduction mammoplasty. Aesthetic Plast Surg. 2001;25(4):283–5.
70. Yalin CT, et al. Breast changes after reduction mammaplasty: a case report with mammographic and ultrasonographic findings and a literature review. Breast J. 2003;9(2):133–7.
71. Hogge JP, et al. The mammographic spectrum of fat necrosis of the breast. Radiographics. 1995;15(6):1347–56.

The Multidisciplinary Approach to Breast Cancer Management

17

Sarah M. DeSnyder and Kelly K. Hunt

Introduction

Breast cancer remains the second leading cause of cancer mortality among women in the United States. The field of breast cancer treatment is rapidly changing, and as the treatment evolves, it is more important than ever for physicians involved in the diagnosis and treatment of breast cancer to work as a collaborative team. It is through multidisciplinary treatment planning that breast cancer patients are able to achieve the best possible outcomes.

Management of Ductal Carcinoma In Situ

Significant changes have occurred in the past 30 years with respect to the detection, understanding, and management of ductal carcinoma in situ (DCIS). Prior to the utilization of screening mammography, DCIS accounted for less than 1 % of all breast cancer cases and was identified most often as a palpable mass, bloody nipple discharge, or the development of Paget's disease [1]. The routine use of screening mammography has resulted in a dramatic increase in the number of women diagnosed with DCIS. In 2011, the American Cancer Society estimated that DCIS accounted for 20 % of newly diagnosed breast cancers in the United States [2].

The natural history of DCIS has been reported by several groups who followed patients with a diagnosis of DCIS without any specific therapy other than diagnostic biopsy. Approximately 25–35 % of women with DCIS experience progression to invasive carcinoma within 10 years [3–5]. Those with low-grade lesions were noted to have a longer interval without disease progression compared to those with higher-grade lesions.

S.M. DeSnyder, MD • K.K. Hunt, MD (✉)
Department of Surgical Oncology, University of Texas MD Anderson Cancer Center, 1400 Pressler Street, Unit 1484, Houston, TX 77030, USA
e-mail: sdesnyder@mdanderson.org; khunt@mdanderson.org

Although DCIS lesions are in situ or noninvasive carcinomas, they have traditionally been treated largely the same as invasive carcinomas. Initially, patients with DCIS were treated with mastectomy. However, randomized trials demonstrating equivalent overall survival (OS) in patients with invasive carcinoma treated with mastectomy and those treated with breast-conserving surgery followed by radiation therapy (breast-conserving therapy; BCT) raised questions about the necessity of mastectomy to treat all breast cancers. This led to clinical trials of breast conservation in patients with DCIS. As a result, selected patients with DCIS now have a wide variety of treatment options, including mastectomy either with or without reconstruction; BCT; and, in some highly selected patients, breast-conserving surgery alone.

Key Clinical Trials

In the 1970s and 1980s, the National Surgical Adjuvant Breast and Bowel Project (NSABP) B-06 trial and five other randomized trials were conducted in women with early-stage invasive carcinoma and demonstrated the OS equivalence of mastectomy and BCT [6–11]. Although the NSABP B-06 trial was designed to compare total mastectomy, BCT, and breast-conserving surgery alone in women with invasive carcinoma, central pathology review revealed that 78 patients actually had pure DCIS [6, 12]. Despite significant differences in local-regional recurrence rates, no OS difference was noted between patients with DCIS who underwent mastectomy and those who underwent BCT. Thus, the NSABP B-06 trial helped to establish the equivalence of mastectomy and BCT in women with DCIS.

The NSABP conducted the B-17 trial in order to assess the need for radiation following breast-conserving surgery in the management of DCIS. Patients with localized DCIS were randomly assigned to BCT or breast-conserving surgery alone [13]. After a mean follow-up time of 90 months, rates of both ipsilateral noninvasive and invasive recurrences were significantly lower in the group who received radiation. This study demonstrated the importance of postoperative radiation following surgical excision of DCIS.

M.K. Shetty (ed.), *Breast Cancer Screening and Diagnosis: A Synopsis*,
DOI 10.1007/978-1-4939-1267-4_17, © Springer Science+Business Media New York 2015

The benefit of BCT over breast-conserving surgery alone for DCIS was also demonstrated in several other randomized trials including the European Organization for Research and Treatment of Cancer (EORTC) protocol 10853; the United Kingdom, Australia, New Zealand DCIS Trial (the "UK Trial"); and the Swedish Trial [14–17]. However, it is important to recognize the current standards for specimen examination and processing—including correlation with imaging, inking of margins, and detailed pathologic examination with reporting of margin width—were not standard at the time these randomized trials were conducted.

A retrospective study by Silverstein and colleagues demonstrated that highly selected patients with DCIS may safely undergo breast-conserving surgery alone. This study examined the relationship between margin status and local control for women with DCIS [18]. The authors showed that women with margins greater than 10 mm did not benefit from radiation therapy. Women with margins between 1- and 10-mm had a relative risk of local recurrence of 1.49, compared to 2.54 for women with margins less than 1 mm. Although this was a single institution retrospective analysis, it suggested that appropriately selected patients with DCIS might not require postoperative radiation therapy.

The Radiation Therapy Oncology Group (RTOG) sought to define those patients with "good risk" DCIS who could be identified to safely undergo breast-conserving surgery alone. Eligible patients included those with unicentric, low- or intermediate-grade DCIS measuring 2.5 cm or less with a margin of 3 mm or more obtained at the time of breast-conserving surgery. Patients were randomized to whole-breast irradiation (WBI) versus no radiation. Although the trial was closed due to failure to meet required accrual numbers, the results for the 585 analyzable patients have been reported at a median follow-up was 6.46 years [19]. The local failure rate at 5 years was 0.4 % for those patients randomized to receive WBI and 3.2 % for those randomized to no radiation. This trial demonstrated a significant reduction in the local failure rate with WBI. Continued follow-up for enrolled patients is planned.

Similar to the RTOG, the Eastern Cooperative Oncology Group also prospectively evaluated patients to identify those who could safely undergo breast-conserving surgery alone [20]. Eligible patients included those with low- or intermediate-grade DCIS measuring 2.5 cm or less excised with a margin of at least 3 mm and those with high-grade DCIS measuring 1 cm or less excised with a margin of at least 3 mm. At a median follow-up of 6.2 years, those with low- or intermediate-grade DCIS had an ipsilateral breast event rate of 6.1 %, while those with high-grade DCIS had an ipsilateral breast event rate of 15.3 %. This study identified an acceptable ipsilateral breast event rate for those with low- or intermediate-grade DCIS who underwent excision alone with a margin width of at least 3 mm. In contrast, those with high-grade DCIS were not deemed to be acceptable candidates for breast-conserving surgery alone.

Selection of Surgical Therapy

Selection of therapy for patients with DCIS depends on clinical and pathologic factors, including tumor size, tumor grade, mammographic appearance, and patient preference. For most women with DCIS, the choice is between breast-conserving therapy and mastectomy. There is no single correct surgical treatment and many patients will require extensive counseling to make a decision regarding surgical therapy.

Breast-Conserving Surgery or Mastectomy

Careful selection of patients for breast-conserving surgery alone is critical to optimizing outcomes. At The University of Texas MD Anderson Cancer Center, patients with small (less than 1 cm) low-grade lesions excised with a margin of 5 mm or greater are considered candidates for breast-conserving surgery without radiation therapy [21]. The majority of patients with DCIS are candidates for BCT. However, if potential contraindications to radiation therapy exist, such as prior irradiation or the presence of collagen vascular disease, preoperative evaluation by a radiation oncologist may be indicated.

Patients with extensive suspicious calcifications identified on mammography, multicentric DCIS, close or positive margins after multiple re-excisions, prior WBI, or active collagen vascular disease should be considered candidates for mastectomy. Patients with DCIS who require mastectomy are typically candidates for skin-sparing mastectomy with immediate breast reconstruction. Certain patients are eligible for mastectomy that spares the nipple-areolar complex: patients with tumors located more than 2.5 cm from the border of the areola with smaller breast size, minimal ptosis, no prior breast surgeries requiring periareolar incisions, body mass index less than 40 kg/m^2, no active tobacco use, no prior breast irradiation, and no evidence of collagen vascular disease.

In patients eligible for BCT, the surgeon must extensively counsel the patient about the risks and benefits of BCT. It is important that patients understand that BCT is associated with a slightly higher risk of local recurrence than mastectomy, but that despite this, there is no OS difference between BCT and mastectomy.

Patient factors that may drive the decision for BCT include desire to preserve native breast tissue, desire to maintain breast and nipple sensation, and desire to minimize surgical intervention. Patient factors that may drive the decision for mastectomy include anxiety regarding recurrence, desire to minimize the need for continued imaging surveillance, concern about breast symmetry, and desire to avoid radiation therapy.

Axillary Staging

The role of axillary staging in patients with DCIS is limited. Since DCIS is a noninvasive carcinoma, it does not have the propensity to spread, and thus lymph node involvement is not expected. Despite this, for patients undergoing mastectomy as well as those with large, high-grade, or palpable tumors, axillary staging with sentinel lymph node biopsy (SLNB) may be recommended. Since most lesions are diagnosed with needle core biopsy, there is about a 20 % incidence of finding invasive breast cancer on final pathology. As it is not feasible to perform lymphatic mapping and SLNB after mastectomy, most surgeons will recommend that patients undergo SLNB at the time of mastectomy for DCIS. The technique for SLNB is described later in this chapter.

Surgical Technique

Breast-Conserving Surgery

Patients undergoing breast-conserving surgery for nonpalpable DCIS require image-guided localization of the tumor. The lesion is excised with the goal of achieving optimal cosmesis (Fig. 17.1). Incision placement is of the utmost importance to achieving this goal. For tumors located in the superior pole of the breast, creation of an incision following Langer's lines is best, while for tumors located in the inferior pole of the breast, a radial incision may be best [22]. The tumor is excised with a rim of normal breast tissue. Following excision, the specimen is oriented and sent to the pathology department, where it is imaged with specimen radiography, inked (Fig. 17.2a), sectioned (Fig. 17.2b), and reimaged. If close margins are identified on specimen radiography, re-excision is performed, and the excised tissue is sent to the pathology department for permanent-section examination. The border of the surgical cavity should be marked with radiopaque clips to facilitate radiation therapy planning. This intraoperative assessment of margins helps to achieve negative margins at the initial surgery and reduce the need for reoperation for margin control.

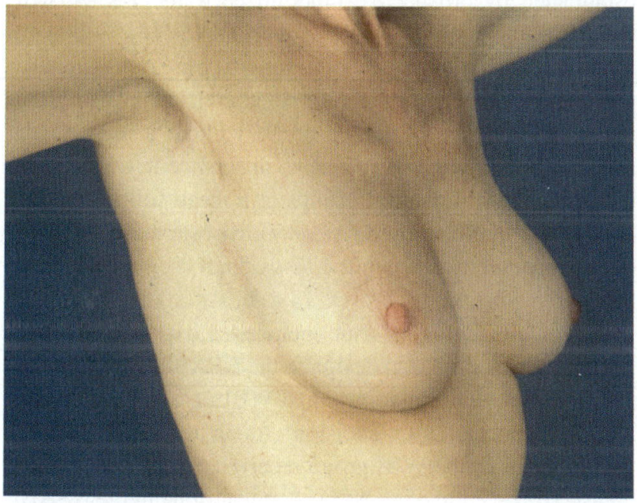

Fig. 17.1 Long-term cosmetic outcome after breast-conserving surgery performed using a periareolar incision

Various techniques may be utilized to minimize contour defects following breast-conserving surgery. For larger defects, the deep parenchyma may be re-approximated. However, if a large cosmetic defect is anticipated preoperatively, it may be beneficial to involve a plastic surgeon to perform local tissue rearrangement and possibly a procedure on the contralateral breast to achieve symmetry.

The findings on the final pathology review dictate whether additional surgical therapy will be needed. At MD Anderson, margins are re-excised if the tumor is less than 2 mm from the inked margin. As discussed previously, inability to obtain negative margins after multiple re-excisions is an indication for mastectomy.

Mastectomy

Patients undergoing mastectomy for DCIS may be considered for total mastectomy, skin-sparing mastectomy with immediate reconstruction (Fig. 17.3a), or nipple-areolar-complex-sparing mastectomy with immediate reconstruction (Fig. 17.3b).

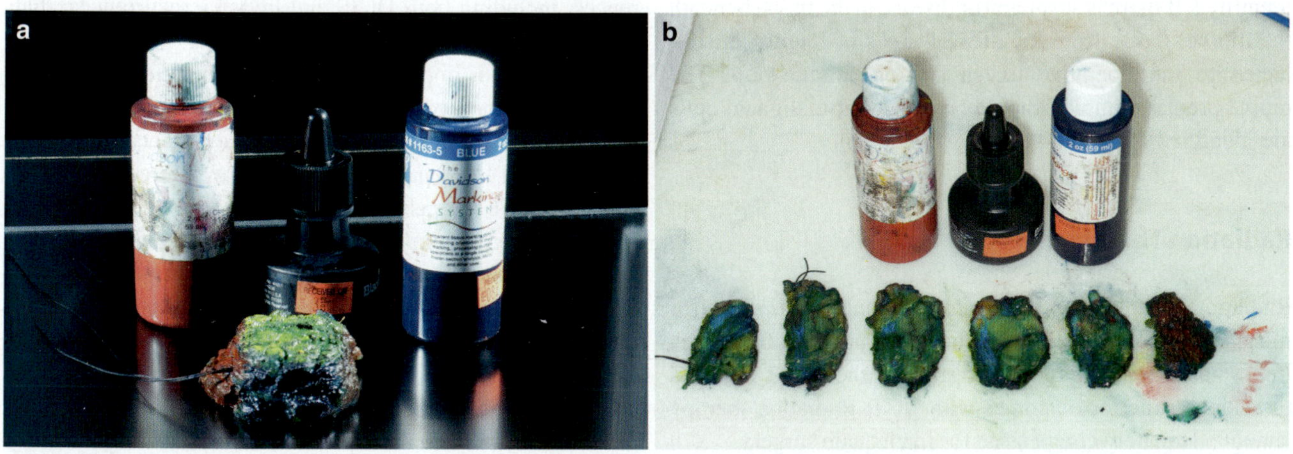

Fig. 17.2 (**a**) Segmental mastectomy specimen shown after different colors of ink have been applied to designate the anatomic margins. (**b**) Segmental mastectomy specimen shown following inking and sectioning. Both the whole specimen and the sectioned specimen are radiographed, and careful examination is performed by the pathologist and the radiologist

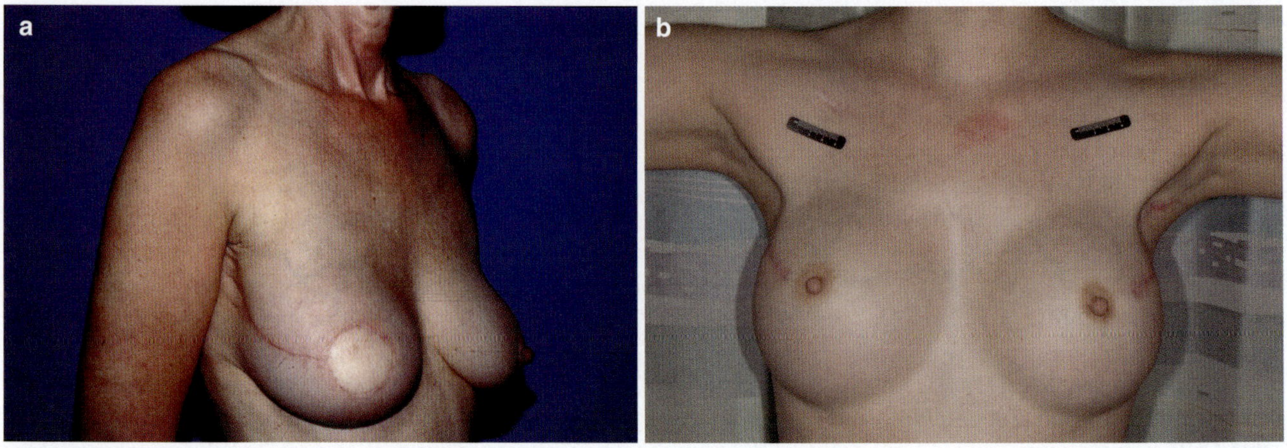

Fig. 17.3 (**a**) Skin-sparing mastectomy with TRAM flap reconstruction prior to nipple reconstruction. (**b**) Bilateral nipple-areolar-complex-sparing mastectomy with implant reconstruction

Although extensive DCIS is not a contraindication to skin-sparing mastectomy, patients with DCIS close to the skin may require excision of additional skin to achieve negative margins. Intraoperative specimen radiography is performed to determine the adequacy of margins. Excision of additional skin may be necessary if superficial disease is identified.

As discussed previously, careful selection of patients for nipple-areolar-complex-sparing mastectomy is crucial to optimize outcomes. A variety of incisions may be chosen for this type of mastectomy, including a radial incision, a lateral incision, or an inframammary incision. Incision placement may be dictated by the location of the tumor, prior biopsy scars, or patient or surgeon preference. Following excision of the breast tissue, the specimen is oriented, and clips are placed at the circumference of the areolar margin at the 3, 6, 9, and 12 o'clock positions as well as directly underneath the nipple to focus the pathologic examination. As with skin-sparing mastectomy, intraoperative specimen radiography is performed to determine the adequacy of margins. Excision of additional skin may be necessary if superficial disease is identified. If there is suspicion of disease in the tissue beneath the nipple, tissue from the area or areas of interest is subjected to intraoperative frozen section examination. The nipple-areolar complex should be excised if malignant cells are identified on frozen section examination.

Radiation Therapy

Radiation therapy is an important component of therapy for most women with DCIS who choose to undergo BCT. It is important to note that adequate surgical therapy is required to achieve superior outcomes with BCT. Radiation therapy cannot adequately compensate for inadequate surgery.

The benefit of radiation therapy for patients with DCIS undergoing breast-conserving surgery has been well established by prospective randomized trials. The NSABP B-17 trial included 814 patients with DCIS [13]. Following margin-negative tumor excision, patients were randomized to two groups, WBI and observation. Patients in the WBI group received 50 Gy to the whole breast without a boost to the tumor bed. Although there was no difference in OS between the WBI and observation groups at a mean follow-up time of 8 years, significant reductions were observed in the rates of both ipsilateral DCIS (12.1 % vs. 26.8 %, $P=0.007$) and invasive recurrence (3.9 % vs. 13.4 %, $P<0.000005$).

The EORTC 10853 trial included 1,010 patients with DCIS and was similar in design to the NSABP B-17 trial [14, 15]. Patients were randomized to WBI or observation after margin-negative tumor excision. As in the NSABP B-17 trial, patients in the WBI group received 50 Gy to the whole breast. However, in contrast to what was done in the NSABP B-17 trial, 5 % of patients in the WBI group received a boost to the tumor bed. At a median follow-up time of 10.5 years, no OS difference was seen between the two groups. However, patients randomized to postoperative WBI had fewer recurrences, including both DCIS and invasive recurrences, than patients randomized to observation (74 % vs. 85 %, $P<0.0001$). It is important to note that all patient subgroups in this trial benefited from postoperative WBI.

The UK Coordinating Committee on Cancer Research trial included 1,030 patients with DCIS or microinvasive disease (invasive disease measuring less than 1 mm) [16]. Patients were randomized to postoperative radiation therapy or observation following margin-negative tumor excision. Some patients in each group received adjuvant tamoxifen therapy. Patients randomized to postoperative radiation therapy received 50 Gy to the whole breast without a boost to the tumor bed. At a median follow-up time of 4.8 years, the incidence of recurrence in the ipsilateral breast was significantly reduced in the patients randomized to postoperative radiation therapy (6 % vs. 14 %, $P<0.001$). Although tamoxifen use was not associated with a reduced risk of ipsilateral invasive disease, it was associated with a reduced risk of ipsilateral DCIS recurrence.

In the SweDCIS trial, 1,046 women were randomized to postoperative radiation therapy or observation [17]. Patients randomized to postoperative irradiation had a 5-year incidence of ipsilateral recurrence of 7 %, compared to 22 % in the observation group ($P<0.0001$). No difference was seen in OS.

Despite these data from prospective, randomized trials supporting the benefit of postoperative radiation therapy following margin-negative tumor excision, some investigators have supported excision alone for DCIS because of the lack of OS benefit from postoperative radiation therapy. Thus, patients who are unlikely to benefit from postoperative radiation therapy may be selected for breast-conserving surgery only. The MD Anderson Cancer Center selection criteria for breast-conserving surgery alone have been discussed earlier in this chapter.

Limited data exist to support the use of accelerated partial breast irradiation (APBI) for patients with DCIS. APBI is administered two times daily over 5 days. A variety of methods exist for administration of APBI, including the use of balloon catheters or interstitial multicatheter brachytherapy devices and 3-dimensional conformal external beam radiation therapy. The published consensus statement from the American Society for Radiation Oncology (ASTRO) categorizes patients aged 50 years or older with DCIS measuring 3 cm or less in the "cautionary" group for APBI use; patients younger than 50 years of age and those with DCIS larger than 3 cm are considered to be "unsuitable" for APBI [23]. The ASTRO task force asserted that the paucity of data on the use of APBI in patients with DCIS has resulted in uncertainty regarding its use. The ASTRO guidelines encouraged enrollment of patients with DCIS measuring less than 3 cm in the RTOG 04-13/NSABP B-39 clinical trial. This clinical trial was opened in March 2005 and has recently completed accrual. The goal of this trial is to examine the efficacy of APBI modalities compared to each other as well as to WBI.

Adjuvant Tamoxifen

Results from studies to date indicate that following counseling regarding the risks and benefits of tamoxifen therapy, women with estrogen receptor (ER)-positive DCIS without contraindications to tamoxifen therapy should be offered adjuvant tamoxifen for a duration of 5 years.

The NSABP B-24 trial demonstrated a significant reduction in ipsilateral tumor events with adjuvant tamoxifen therapy for patients with DCIS [24]. This trial included 1,804 women with DCIS regardless of ER status. Women were randomized to BCT with tamoxifen or BCT without tamoxifen. At a median follow-up time of 74 months, the rate of breast cancer events was lower in the tamoxifen group (8.2 % vs. 13.4 %, $P=0.0009$).

Allred and colleagues retrospectively evaluated 41 % of patients with DCIS in the NSABP B-24 trial to determine the relationship between DCIS ER status and the effects of tamoxifen [25]. In this study, 76 % of women had DCIS that was ER positive. Patients with ER-positive DCIS had a greater reduction in ipsilateral breast tumor recurrence with tamoxifen than patients with ER-negative DCIS (11 % vs. 5.2 %, $P<0.001$).

Management of Early-Stage Breast Cancer

Early-stage (stage I and II) breast cancer may be managed successfully with either BCT or mastectomy.

Key Clinical Trials

Trials Comparing BCT and Mastectomy

The NSABP B-06 trial established the survival equivalence of BCT and mastectomy for patients with early-stage breast cancer [6]. This trial compared lumpectomy and axillary lymph node dissection (ALND) either with or without WBI to modified radical mastectomy in patients with a tumor size of 4 cm or less and either N0 or N1 nodal status. A total of 2,163 patients were randomized. No difference was noted between the treatment groups in disease-free survival (DFS) or OS. This was maintained at 20 years of follow-up [26]. Notably, there were significant differences in the local control rates. Patients treated with lumpectomy without WBI had an in-breast recurrence rate of 39.2 %, those treated with lumpectomy with WBI had an in-breast recurrence rate of 14.3 %, and those treated with mastectomy had a chest wall recurrence rate of 10.2 %. In addition to the NSABP B-06 trial, five other randomized trials have demonstrated no difference in DFS and OS between BCT and mastectomy for patients with early-stage disease [7–11].

Axillary Staging

Axillary lymph node status remains the most important prognostic factor for women with operable breast cancer. Much like the treatment of the primary breast tumor, staging and treatment of the axilla has become less invasive over the past several decades. Historically, ALND was required for axillary staging. However, randomized trials evaluating less invasive techniques for operable breast cancer demonstrated that elective ALND had no survival benefit over ALND performed in a delayed fashion once clinically palpable axillary disease became evident [26, 27]. The routine use of ALND for staging of the axilla overtreats the 75 % percent of women with operable breast cancer in whom the axillary lymph nodes are histologically negative. These findings prompted the development of lymphatic mapping and SLNB for breast cancer patients with a clinically negative axilla [28].

In 1991, Giuliano and colleagues initiated a pilot study to examine the use of SLNB for patients with breast cancer. Of the 174 patients enrolled, 114 (65.5 %) had a SLN successfully identified. In 109 of these 114 patients (95.6 %), the status of the SLN accurately predicted the status of the axilla. The results of this pilot study, reported in 1994, revolutionized axillary surgery. Today, SLNB is recognized as a minimally invasive and accurate technique to stage the axilla with the advantage of decreased morbidity [28, 29].

The NSABP B-32 trial compared clinically node-negative patients undergoing SLNB followed by ALND with patients undergoing SLNB with ALND only if a SLN was positive for metastatic disease [30]. A total of 5,611 patients were randomized. The SLN identification rate was 97 %, and the false-negative rate was 9.7 %. Twenty-six percent of patients in the trial had positive SLNs. Over 60 % of patients with metastatic disease in the SLNs had no further positive lymph nodes within the ALND specimen. The NSABP B-32 clinical trial and other randomized trials demonstrated no difference in DFS, OS, and local-regional control rates between patients with negative SLNs who underwent SLNB alone and those who underwent ALND [31, 32]. In addition, patients who undergo SLNB alone have been noted to have decreased morbidity and improved quality of life compared to patients who undergo ALND [32, 33].

The American College of Surgeons Oncology Group (ACOSOG) Z0011 trial evaluated the utility of ALND in patients with clinical T1-2, N0 breast cancer with one or two positive SLNs for whom BCT with WBI was planned [34]. Patients were not eligible if they received neoadjuvant chemotherapy or neoadjuvant hormonal therapy or if their treatment plan included mastectomy, lumpectomy without radiation, or lumpectomy with alternative forms of radiation delivery such as APBI. WBI was administered using standard tangential fields without additional fields. Patients with one or two positive SLNs were randomized to completion ALND or no further surgery. Decisions regarding adjuvant therapy were left to the treating clinicians. The primary endpoint was OS, and the secondary endpoint was local-regional recurrence. After a median follow-up time of over 6 years, no difference was noted between patients randomized to completion ALND and those randomized to no further surgery in terms of OS (91.9 and 92.5 %, respectively; $P=0.25$) or DFS (82.2 and 83.8 %, respectively; $P=0.14$).

Data from the ACOSOG Z0011 trial also demonstrated that patients randomized to SLNB alone were less likely to have adverse effects than were patients randomized to completion ALND (25 % vs. 70 %, $P \leq 0.001$) [35]. Patients in the SLNB-alone group were less likely to have wound infections (3 % vs. 8 %, $P \leq 0.0016$), seromas (6 % vs. 14 %, $P \leq 0.0001$), paresthesias (9 % vs. 39 %, $P < 0.0001$), and subjectively reported lymphedema (2 % vs. 13 %, $P < 0.0001$).

Prior to the reporting of the ACOSOG Z0011 data, completion ALND was the standard of care for patients with metastatic disease identified within SLNs. Following publication of the ACOSOG Z0011 trial, the National Comprehensive Cancer Network (NCCN) added a footnote to its published breast cancer guidelines stating that there was no OS difference for patients with one or two positive SLNs treated with BCT who underwent completion ALND and those who underwent no further surgery [36]. In addition, the American Society of Breast Surgeons issued a consensus statement that supported the omission of completion ALND for patients who meet the ACOSOG Z0011 criteria [37]. The results of the ACOSOG Z0011 trial have revolutionized treatment of the axilla in selected patients with axillary metastasis.

The International Breast Cancer Study Group (IBCSG) 23-01 trial had a design similar to that of the ACOSOG Z0011 trial [38]. In the IBCSG 23-01 trial, patients with micrometastatic disease within the SLN were randomized to ALND versus no further surgery. Unlike the ACOSOG Z0011 trial, the IBCSG 23-01 trial did not exclude patients undergoing mastectomy. Approximately 9 % of patients in each arm of the trial were treated with mastectomy. The investigators recently published the results and showed no differences in OS or local-regional recurrence between the study arms [39].

Recently, the ACOSOG Z1071 trial examined the role of SLNB in patients who presented with N1-2 nodal disease and received neoadjuvant chemotherapy [40]. This trial included patients with clinical T1-4, N1-2 breast cancer who received neoadjuvant chemotherapy. All patients underwent SLNB followed by completion ALND. Complete resolution of axillary disease was noted in 40 % of patients. SLNB identified the nodal status correctly in 84 % of patients; the false-negative rate was 12.4 %. Although this false-negative rate was higher than the predefined acceptable rate of 10 %, removal of two or more SLNs at the time of SLNB reduced the false-negative rate. The results of this trial were recently published in the Journal of the American Medical Association. This trial may significantly impact treatment of the axilla in patients with axillary nodal disease at presentation in whom axillary disease resolves following neoadjuvant chemotherapy.

Selection of Surgical Therapy

BCT or Mastectomy

Selection of therapy for patients with early-stage breast cancer depends on a variety of tumor and patient factors, including the ratio of tumor size to breast size, the presence of multicentric disease, whether the patient can tolerate radiation therapy, and patient preference. Patients with a large tumor in relation to the size of the breast may not achieve an adequate cosmetic outcome after BCT and may be better served by mastectomy. BCT is typically reserved for patients with a tumor size of 4 cm or less. However, BCT with a good cosmetic outcome may also be achievable in women with larger tumors and relatively large breasts. Patients with larger tumors who wish to pursue BCT may be candidates for either neoadjuvant chemotherapy or neoadjuvant hormonal therapy to decrease the tumor size and thus permit BCT. In addition, patients with larger tumors who opt for BCT may be candidates for local tissue rearrangement or placement of myocutaneous tissue flaps to repair the defect resulting from BCT. Patients with multicentric disease are better served by mastectomy as they are considered to have an increased risk of recurrence after BCT.

It is also important to recognize that BCT requires adjuvant radiation therapy. Thus, patients for whom BCT is planned should be evaluated by a radiation oncologist if they have undergone prior irradiation of the breast or a region close to the breast or have a collagen vascular disease. In addition, patients for whom BCT is planned must be willing and able to attend all planned radiation therapy appointments.

Breast Reconstruction After Mastectomy

Mastectomy for early-stage breast cancer may be performed either with or without breast reconstruction. Many patients with early-stage breast cancer who undergo mastectomy are candidates for breast reconstruction.

For many patients, reconstruction can be performed immediately at the time of mastectomy. Immediate reconstruction allows for skin-sparing mastectomy which preserves the patient's own skin, thus optimizing cosmetic outcomes. Highly selected women with early-stage breast cancer may be candidates for immediate reconstruction with preservation of the nipple-areolar complex. Eligibility for this procedure has been described previously in this chapter. Patients for whom adjuvant radiation therapy is planned are not ideal candidates for nipple-areolar-complex-sparing mastectomy because of the effects of radiation on the preserved nipple. In addition to providing improved cosmesis resulting from preservation of the skin and/or the nipple-areolar complex, immediate reconstruction provides a psychological benefit for the patient. Patients undergoing immediate reconstruction also benefit from completing therapy and reconstruction in one surgery.

If no postoperative radiation therapy is planned, patients may have immediate reconstruction performed using implants or autologous tissue; tissue flaps that can be used include the transverse rectus abdominis myocutaneous flap, deep inferior epigastric perforator flap, latissimus dorsi flap with an implant, and other tissue flaps. However, if adjuvant radiation therapy may be required, a tissue expander should be placed. A tissue expander allows for preservation of the skin at the time of mastectomy, and the expander can be deflated at the time of radiation therapy to permit adequate irradiation of the chest wall and regional nodal basins. Removal of the tissue expander and reconstruction with either an implant or autologous tissue takes place approximately 1 year after completion of radiation therapy.

Axillary Staging

Axillary staging is required for all patients with early-stage breast cancer. Information about the axillary nodal status is valuable prognostic information and assists in tailoring adjuvant therapies. For example, for patients with small tumors without lymph node involvement, adjuvant chemotherapy may not be recommended; however, detection of lymph node involvement in a patient with a small tumor would prompt a recommendation for chemotherapy. In addition, detection of axillary lymph node involvement in a patient younger than 40 years or more than four involved axillary lymph nodes in any patient would prompt a recommendation for adjuvant radiation therapy in patients treated with mastectomy, whereas in the absence of nodal metastases, postmastectomy radiation therapy (PMRT) would not be recommended.

Thus, patients with clinically node-negative breast cancer should undergo SLNB for staging of the axilla. Patients with a positive SLN should be appropriately selected for completion ALND versus no further surgery according to the principles outlined previously.

At MD Anderson, patients for whom BCT with WBI is planned and who meet the eligibility criteria used in the ACOSOG Z0011 trial undergo intraoperative lymphatic mapping with SLNB at the time of segmental mastectomy. At the time of SLNB, the SLNs are sent to the pathology department for permanent-section examination. Patients with one or two positive SLNs who have negative tumor margins proceed to adjuvant systemic therapy and WBI with no further surgery.

The current MD Anderson practice regarding completion ALND was established during a multidisciplinary conference held to discuss the results of the ACOSOG Z0011 trial and apply these results safely to patients [41]. This conference included clinicians from the Departments of Surgical Oncology, Radiation Oncology, Breast Medical Oncology, Diagnostic Radiology, and Pathology. The participants reached a consensus that omission of completion ALND was appropriate for patients with clinical T1-2, N0 breast cancer and one or two positive SLNs expected to undergo BCT with WBI but not for patients expected to undergo mastectomy or APBI or for patients who underwent neoadjuvant chemotherapy or neoadjuvant hormonal therapy. Special consideration was given to patients with lobular histology as patients with lobular carcinoma were underrepresented in the ACOSOG Z0011 trial and small-volume axillary disease may be of clinical relevance in patients with lobular histology. Both of these factors should be taken into consideration when patients with lobular histology are counseled about completion ALND. Hormone receptor status is also an important consideration as 83 % of ACOSOG Z0011 participants had ER-positive disease. Although ER status was not significantly associated with local-regional recurrence on multivariable analysis, at MD Anderson, hormone receptor status is considered within a broad context of factors when patients are counseled about completion ALND. Age is another important factor to consider. More than 62 % of patients in each arm of the ACOSOG Z0011 trial were older than 50 years. In addition, age younger than 50 years was a significant predictor of local-regional recurrence on multivariable analysis. Thus, patients younger than 50 years should be carefully counseled regarding completion ALND. Nodal burden may also play an important role in risk determination. At MD Anderson, a nomogram that incorporates the size of SLN metastases and the ratio of positive to negative nodes harvested at SLNB may be used to counsel patients regarding the need for completion ALND [42]. At MD Anderson, patients with a positive SLNB expected to undergo mastectomy and those expected to undergo BCT with alternative forms of radiation therapy undergo completion ALND.

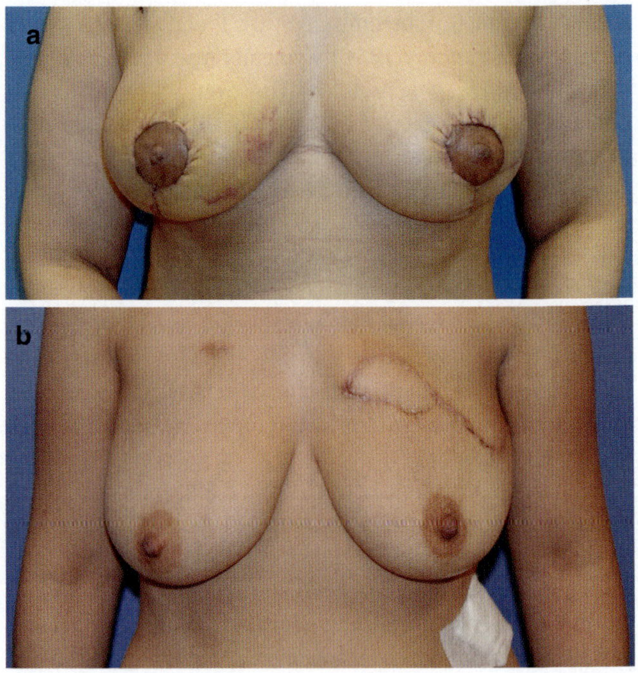

Fig. 17.4 (**a**) Cosmetic outcome in a patient requiring re-excision for margin control with local tissue rearrangement and contralateral symmetry procedure. (**b**) Breast-conserving surgery with repair of the partial mastectomy defect using a latissimus dorsi flap for volume replacement (Photos courtesy of Dr. David M. Adelman)

Surgical Techniques

Breast-Conserving Surgery

Patients undergoing breast-conserving surgery for nonpalpable early-stage breast cancer require image-guided localization of the tumor.

Incision placement is key to achieving optimal cosmetic outcomes. The tumor is excised with a rim of normal breast tissue. The specimen is then oriented and sent to the pathology department, where it is imaged with specimen radiography, inked, sectioned, and reimaged. If close margins are identified on specimen radiography, re-excision is performed, and the excised tissue is sent to the pathology department for permanent-section examination. The border of the surgical cavity is marked with radiopaque clips to facilitate radiation therapy planning.

Patients with larger defects after tumor excision may benefit from involvement of a plastic surgeon for local tissue rearrangement (Fig. 17.4a) or reconstruction using a latissimus dorsi flap (Fig. 17.4b). If necessary, a procedure may be performed on the contralateral breast to achieve symmetry, either during the same surgery when the tumor is excised or following completion of radiation therapy at a second surgery.

The findings on the final pathology review dictate whether additional surgical therapy will be needed. As described previously, at MD Anderson, a margin of less than 2 mm prompts consideration for a return to the operating room for re-excision. If negative margins cannot be achieved after multiple re-excisions, mastectomy is indicated.

Mastectomy

Surgical options for patients undergoing mastectomy for early-stage breast cancer include total mastectomy, skin-sparing mastectomy, and, for some highly selected patients, nipple-areolar-complex-sparing mastectomy.

Regardless of the type of mastectomy, intraoperative specimen radiography is performed to determine the adequacy of margins. Excision of additional skin may be necessary if superficial disease is identified.

As discussed previously, careful selection of patients for nipple-areolar-complex-sparing mastectomy is crucial to optimize outcomes. If there is suspicion of disease beneath the nipple or areola, intraoperative assessment of the tissue underlying the circumference of the areolar margin at 3, 6, 9, and 12 o'clock as well as directly underlying the nipple may be performed by the pathologist using frozen section examination. The nipple-areolar complex should be excised if malignant cells are identified on frozen section examination.

Patients undergoing skin-sparing mastectomy or nipple-areolar-complex-sparing mastectomy undergo initiation of reconstruction with placement of a tissue expander. If the likelihood of adjuvant radiation therapy is very small, immediate reconstruction can be performed using an implant or a myocutaneous flap.

Axillary Lymph Node Staging

In patients with a clinically negative axilla, axillary staging should be performed with SLNB. SLNB requires lymphatic mapping, which can be accomplished with blue dye or a radioactive tracer, and SLN dissection. Some surgeons choose to have patients undergo preoperative lymphoscintigraphy as well to identify patterns of lymphatic drainage.

For patients undergoing preoperative lymphoscintigraphy, lymphoscintigraphy is most often performed with injection of high-dose technetium-labeled sulfur colloid (2.5 mCi) on the day prior to surgery. The technetium-labeled sulfur colloid can be injected peritumorally or under the areola. Patients with nonpalpable tumors require imaging guidance for peritumoral injection. Peritumoral injection has the advantage of identifying drainage patterns of the tumor outside of the axilla, such as drainage to the internal mammary lymph nodes. Lymphoscintigraphy is performed 15–30 min following radiocolloid injection and then at 30- to 60-min intervals thereafter until drainage to the SLN is identified. The inability of lymphoscintigraphy to identify a SLN on the day before surgery does not necessarily indicate failure of mapping; in some patients, drainage to SLNs will occur, and a SLN will be identified with a handheld gamma probe at the time of surgery. However, if drainage is not identified on lymphoscintigraphy performed the day before surgery, consideration should be given to reinjection of low-dose technetium-labeled sulfur colloid on the day of surgery.

On the day of surgery, patients injected the day before surgery with high-dose technetium-labeled sulfur colloid are taken directly to the operating room. Patients who did not undergo injection of high-dose technetium-labeled sulfur colloid the day before surgery should be injected with a low dose (0.5–1 mCi) of technetium-labeled sulfur colloid 1–4 h before they are taken to the operating room. If dual-modality SLN mapping is planned (i.e., use of both blue dye and radiotracer), prophylaxis for allergic reactions to the blue dye solution should be administered intravenously in the operating room. This prophylaxis includes diphenhydramine, steroids, and famotidine. Five milliliters of lymphazurin blue dye should be injected peritumorally for patients undergoing breast-conserving surgery or either peritumorally or under the areola for patients undergoing mastectomy. The breast should be massaged for 5 min to facilitate lymphatic drainage. A handheld gamma probe is used to transcutaneously localize the SLN within the axilla. A transverse incision is made close to the transcutaneously identified node along the standard ALND incision line below the axillary hairline. The gamma probe may be utilized to guide the dissection. Alternatively, blue-stained lymphatics may be used to guide the dissection. SLNs are defined as blue-stained lymph nodes and lymph nodes containing radioactivity as identified by the gamma probe.

Patients in whom mapping is more likely to fail to identify a SLN include patients who have undergone prior breast surgery, patients over 70 years of age, and obese patients. Patients who do not have a SLN identified should undergo ALND. The technique for ALND is described later in this chapter.

Radiation Therapy

The Early Breast Cancer Trialists' Collaborative Group (EBCTCG) has examined all of the randomized trials where breast conservation was performed with or without radiation therapy [43]. At 15 years of follow-up, the absolute reduction in mortality with radiation therapy after breast-conserving surgery was 5.1 % in node-negative patients and 7.1 % in node-positive patients. These data suggest that the addition of radiation not only improves local control but also improves survival.

Two randomized trials have suggested that in selected older patients with small, low-grade tumors, breast-conserving surgery without radiation therapy may be appropriate [44, 45]. The Cancer and Leukemia Group B (CALGB) C9343 trial included women over 70 years of age with T1N0 breast cancer and randomized them to breast-conserving surgery with or without radiation therapy. All women, 97 % of whom had ER-positive tumors, were treated with adjuvant tamoxifen. No differences in DFS and OS were seen although the local recurrence rate was lower in patients randomized to radiation (1 % vs. 4 %, $P<0.001$). The Canadian trial was similar to the CALGB C9343 trial. Although the Canadian trial was open to women 50 years of age and older, the mean age was 68 years, and 80 % of women had ER-positive tumors. At a median follow-up time of 5.6 years, no difference was seen in DFS or OS although the local recurrence rate was lower in patients randomized to radiation (0.6 % vs. 7.7 %, $P<0.001$). Generally, patients with early-stage breast cancer selected for breast-conserving surgery without radiation include women 70 years of age or older with an expected survival of less than 10 years with T1, N0, ER-positive breast cancer.

APBI is an option for carefully selected patients with early-stage breast cancer. A variety of methods exists for administration of APBI as have been described previously in this chapter. Proponents of APBI argue that the majority of breast cancer recurrences occur in or adjacent to the tumor bed; the abbreviated course of treatment may increase the feasibility of BCT for many women; and the abbreviated course of treatment may improve radiation therapy compliance. The previously discussed RTOG 04-13/NSABP B-39 trial, which directly compares WBI to APBI in early-stage breast cancer, will provide data on local recurrence and survival and assess differences in outcomes between the two radiation treatment strategies.

While the results of this trial are awaited, a consensus statement from ASTRO was developed to guide the use of APBI outside of the context of a clinical trial [23]. According to the consensus statement, patients suitable for APBI include patients 60 years of age or older with a unifocal, T1, ER-positive tumor with no lymphovascular invasion and resection margins of at least 2 mm. Patients for whom ASTRO was not certain about the appropriateness of APBI include patients with invasive lobular histology, a tumor size of 2.1 cm to 3 cm, ER-negative disease, focal lymphovascular invasion, or margins less than 2 mm. Patients considered unsuitable for APBI include those with T3 or T4 disease, ER-negative disease, multifocality, multicentricity, extensive LVI, or positive margins.

Adjuvant Systemic Therapy

Adjuvant chemotherapy, biologic therapy, and hormonal therapy have all contributed to improved outcomes for breast cancer patients. The timing of systemic therapy may alter surgical therapy options and provide valuable prognostic information. Thus, it is important that the timing of therapies be determined using a multidisciplinary approach.

Chemotherapy may be administered as either neoadjuvant or adjuvant treatment. The NSABP B-18 trial demonstrated that neoadjuvant and adjuvant chemotherapy are equivalent with respect to DFS and OS [46]. However, in that trial, 12 % of patients who were initially not candidates for BCT were candidates for BCT at the conclusion of their neoadjuvant chemotherapy. In addition, administering chemotherapy in the neoadjuvant setting allows clinicians to assess the tumor's sensitivity to the regimen, which in turn allows clinicians to alter regimens for tumors that appear resistant, limiting the administration of ineffective chemotherapeutics.

The NCCN guidelines on breast cancer treatment, available at www.nccn.org, provide expert opinion based on synthesis of the available evidence. For patients with early-stage breast cancer, the most current NCCN guidelines, published in 2013, recommend neoadjuvant chemotherapy for patients with stage IIA (T2N0) and IIB (T2N1, T3N0) disease who are not initially candidates for BCT but desire to undergo BCT [47]. For patients with stage II disease who desire mastectomy, chemotherapy may be administered as adjuvant therapy or as neoadjuvant therapy.

Adjuvant chemotherapy has the potential to benefit all patients with early-stage breast cancer. However, most patients with stage I disease have a small risk of local recurrence, metastasis, and death due to breast cancer and thus a smaller potential benefit from adjuvant chemotherapy. Chemotherapy may be appropriate for some patients with stage I disease. However, when patients with stage I disease are counseled about adjuvant therapy options, it is important to consider tumor characteristics such as ER status, tumor size, and other prognostic factors.

Patients with ER-positive disease and a tumor smaller than 1 cm are unlikely to derive significant benefit from chemotherapy. In contrast, patients with ER-positive disease and a tumor size of 1–2 cm should be considered for adjuvant systemic therapy. Patients with ER-positive disease should be administered endocrine therapy for 5 years. Premenopausal patients should be recommended tamoxifen, while postmenopausal patients should be considered for an aromatase inhibitor.

Patients with ER-negative disease smaller than 0.5 cm are not usually recommended to receive adjuvant therapy. Those with ER-negative disease measuring 0.6–1 cm and unfavorable features such as young age, high tumor grade, and LVI should be considered for adjuvant chemotherapy. Patients with ER-negative disease larger than 1 cm should also be considered for adjuvant chemotherapy.

The NCCN guidelines recommend trastuzumab-based therapy for all patients with node-positive HER2-positive disease and patients with node-negative HER2-positive tumors larger than 1 cm. The guidelines also recommend that trastuzumab-based therapy be considered for patients with HER2-positive disease measuring 0.6–1 cm.

To individualize therapy decisions, it is important to consider the anticipated benefit for each patient. For patients for whom the NCCN guidelines recommend consideration of chemotherapy, tools to assist with decision making about systemic therapy may be helpful. These tools include Adjuvant! Online (Adjuvant! Inc.), Oncotype DX® (Genomic Health, Inc.), and MammaPrint® (Agendia). Adjuvant! Online is a computer model based on the Surveillance, Epidemiology, and End Results registry that estimates the 10-year risk of recurrence and death due to breast cancer according to age, comorbidities, ER status, tumor size, tumor grade, and nodal status. The Adjuvant! Online website creates easy to understand charts to assist with patient counseling. Adjuvant! Online does have limitations, however. Because it is based on registry data, inaccuracies may exist with respect to the data captured. In addition, information on women younger than 35 years and information on HER2 status was not captured, and thus, the use of Adjuvant! Online does not provide the best outcome information for these patients. Oncotype DX is a 21-gene assay developed to quantify the risk of recurrence and predict the benefit from chemotherapy for patients with ER-positive, node-negative disease [48, 49]. Oncotype DX also provides easy-to-understand graphics to assist in patient counseling. The MammaPrint assay, another tool used to predict both prognosis and the benefit of adjuvant therapy, is a 70-gene assay that categorizes patients as being at either low or high risk for recurrence, regardless of ER status.

Management of Locally Advanced Breast Cancer

Patients with locally advanced breast cancer must undergo multimodality treatment including systemic therapy, surgery, and radiation therapy to optimize outcomes. This patient group includes patients without clinically detected metastatic disease with tumors larger than 5 cm, tumors that invade the chest wall, tumors that involve the overlying breast skin, fixed or matted axillary lymph nodes, internal mammary involvement, or supraclavicular lymph node involvement.

Selection of Surgical Therapy

Traditionally, patients with locally advanced breast cancer required modified radical mastectomy; however, in a select group of patients, neoadjuvant chemotherapy may shrink the primary tumor enough to render patients candidates for BCT. Neoadjuvant chemotherapy is now the standard of care for patients with locally advanced disease.

In patients with internal mammary lymph node involvement, supraclavicular lymph node involvement, or chest wall invasion, neoadjuvant chemotherapy may render the disease resectable. In patients with locally advanced breast cancer considered operable at initial evaluation, neoadjuvant chemotherapy may make surgical intervention technically less difficult. In patients with large primary tumors who desire BCT, neoadjuvant chemotherapy may shrink the primary tumor enough to render patients candidates for this therapy. Patients who experience a decrease in the size of the primary tumor but still have a contour defect at the time of surgery may benefit from involvement of a plastic surgeon at the time of breast-conserving surgery to perform local tissue rearrangement or myocutaneous flap placement to restore volume and minimize the defect.

In a study to assess the feasibility of BCT for patients with locally advanced disease, patients who received neoadjuvant chemotherapy for locally advanced disease underwent pathologic examination of their mastectomy specimens [50]. Mastectomy specimens from 143 patients were examined, and 33 patients (23 %) were found to be appropriate candidates for BCT with ALND following completion of neoadjuvant chemotherapy. Requirements for BCT with ALND in this study included resolution of skin edema, residual tumor size less than 5 cm, lack of multicentricity, lack of extensive lymphovascular invasion, and lack of extensive suspicious microcalcifications.

More recently, an assessment of patients undergoing BCT following neoadjuvant chemotherapy, including patients with locally advanced disease, demonstrated that appropriately selected patients with locally advanced breast cancer can undergo BCT with an acceptable rate of local recurrence [51]. The 5-year ipsilateral breast tumor recurrence-free survival rate did not differ significantly between patients with T1, T2, T3, and T4 tumors. However, it is important to note that patients with T3 and T4 tumors were offered BCT according to their response to neoadjuvant chemotherapy. In addition, patients with multifocal T3 and T4 disease had a worse 5-year ipsilateral breast tumor recurrence-free survival rate than patients without multifocal disease (80 % vs. 97 %, $P=0.0008$).

The administration of neoadjuvant chemotherapy to patients with chest wall involvement or extensive skin involvement may result in resolution of this involvement, thus permitting resection with modified radical mastectomy. However, if chest wall or extensive skin involvement does not resolve following neoadjuvant chemotherapy, chest wall resection or extensive skin resection may be required. Chest wall or extensive skin resection necessitates a multidisciplinary surgical team including a surgical oncologist, a plastic surgeon, and a thoracic surgeon. If skeletal resection is required, complex planning is necessary to achieve optimal outcomes, as resection of the chest wall may result in instability, exposure of underlying vital structures, and respiratory difficulty.

Chest wall reconstruction stabilizes the chest wall, protects underlying structures, and prevents paradoxical chest wall movement. A variety of mesh products and even metal plates may be considered for repair of chest wall defects. In addition, consideration of various soft tissue reconstruction options is important. These are necessary to provide coverage after chest wall resection as well as to provide closure after extended skin resection. Options for soft tissue closure range from skin graft placement to local tissue transfer to use of a myocutaneous flap.

Surgical Techniques

Breast-Conserving Surgery

It is of the utmost importance for patients with locally advanced breast cancer to undergo placement of a marker prior to initiation of neoadjuvant chemotherapy. This marker ensures that it will be possible to localize the tumor if a complete imaging response occurs. Patients with a nonpalpable tumor following neoadjuvant chemotherapy require image-guided localization of the tumor at the time of surgery. The technique for BCT has been described earlier in this chapter.

Mastectomy

Surgical options for patients who undergo mastectomy for locally advanced breast cancer include total mastectomy and, for a highly selected group of patients, skin-sparing mastectomy. The decision to proceed with skin-sparing mastectomy should be a joint decision of the breast surgeon, the plastic surgeon, and the radiation oncologist. Continued skin involvement after neoadjuvant chemotherapy, including edema, chest wall involvement, or diffuse, suspicious-appearing calcifications close to the overlying skin, indicates the need for total mastectomy. Intraoperative specimen radiography is performed to determine the adequacy of margins. Excision of additional skin may be necessary if superficial disease is identified.

Patients undergoing skin-sparing mastectomy have initiation of reconstruction with placement of a tissue expander. The use of a tissue expander allows for administration of PMRT as deflation of the expander permits adequate targeting of the chest wall and regional nodal basins. Patients should not have immediate reconstruction with either an implant or a myocutaneous flap as patients with locally advanced breast cancer will require PMRT.

Axillary Lymph Node Dissection

In patients who undergo a total mastectomy, ALND is performed through the lateral portion of the elliptical incision. In patients who undergo BCT or a skin-sparing mastectomy, ALND is performed through a separate axillary incision. Skin flaps are raised superiorly, medially, laterally, and inferiorly within the axilla. Posterolaterally, the anterior border of the latissimus muscle is identified. Anteromedially, the lateral border of the pectoralis major muscle is identified. The axillary vein is then identified cephalad. Using these landmarks as the anatomic boundaries, a level I and II ALND is performed. Dissection proceeds from cephalad to caudad along the latissimus muscle up to the axillary vein. Dissection then proceeds from lateral to medial along the axillary vein. The thoracodorsal nerve and vessels are identified and protected from injury. Branches of the axillary vein are ligated with either ties or clips. The long thoracic nerve is identified as it travels within the investing fascia of the serratus anterior muscle and protected from injury. The fascia along the lateral border of the pectoralis muscle is then incised, and the fatty lymphatic contents are swept off the posterior axilla and chest wall, with care taken to leave the serratus fascia intact (Fig. 17.5).

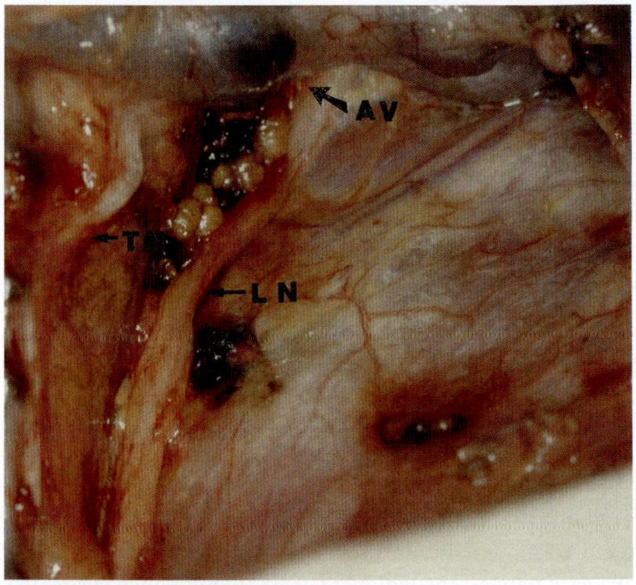

Fig. 17.5 Vital structures identified during axillary lymph node dissection including the axillary vein (*AV*), thoracodorsal nerve (*TN*), and long thoracic nerve (*LN*)

Standard ALND does not include the level III axillary lymph nodes. Routine excision of level III axillary nodes provides little benefit and increases the risk of lymphedema. However, if palpable lymphadenopathy exists at the axillary apex, the tendinous portion of the pectoralis minor muscle may be divided at its insertion to allow excision of level III lymph nodes.

Radiation Therapy

The administration of WBI in patients with locally advanced breast cancer requires a skilled radiation oncologist. The use of multiple adjacent fields is complex, and incorrect planning of such treatment may result in either inadequate coverage of the chest wall and regional lymphatics or administration of elevated doses with burning of the tissue. However, in the hands of an experienced radiation oncologist, BCT is feasible for patients with locally advanced breast cancer with a good response to neoadjuvant chemotherapy and successful breast-conserving surgery.

In patients treated with mastectomy, PMRT is well known to effectively reduce the burden of residual local-regional disease. The Danish Breast Cancer Cooperative Group's protocol 82b randomized premenopausal women with high-risk breast cancer who underwent modified radical mastectomy to either chemotherapy or chemotherapy with radiation therapy [52]. Patients with a primary tumor larger than 5 cm, positive lymph nodes, skin invasion, or pectoralis fascia invasion were considered high risk. Radiation was delivered to the chest wall and regional nodal basins. At a median follow-up time of 114 months, patients who received PMRT had a significantly lower local-regional recurrence rate (9 % vs. 32 %) and higher DFS (48 % vs. 35 %) and OS rates (54 % vs. 45 %) compared to patients who did not receive PMRT.

The Danish Breast Cancer Cooperative Group's protocol 82c examined postmenopausal women with high-risk breast cancer who underwent modified radical mastectomy and randomized them to either tamoxifen or tamoxifen with PMRT [53]. At a median follow-up time of 10 years, patients in the PMRT group had a significantly lower local-regional recurrence rate (8 % vs. 35 %) and significantly higher DFS (36 % vs. 24 %) and OS rates (45 % vs. 36 %).

The British Columbia trial randomized premenopausal node-positive breast cancer patients who had undergone modified radical mastectomy to adjuvant chemotherapy alone versus adjuvant chemotherapy with PMRT [54]. At a median follow-up time of 20 years, patients randomized to receive adjuvant chemotherapy with PMRT had a significantly lower local-regional recurrence rate (13 % vs. 39 %) and significantly higher DFS (48 % vs. 31 %) and OS rates (47 % vs. 37 %).

The Danish and British Columbia trials demonstrate that patients at high risk for local-regional recurrence have disease that cannot be addressed solely by systemic therapy and surgery. These patients clearly benefit from PMRT, which reduces the local-regional recurrence rate, thereby improving both DFS and OS.

The EBCTCG examined the effect of radiation versus no radiation on local recurrence and 15-year survival in patients treated on randomized trials [43]. Among patients with node-positive disease, those who underwent PMRT had significantly decreased rates of local-regional recurrence at 15 years (8 % vs. 29 %). Not surprisingly, larger reductions in the local-regional recurrence rate were seen in subgroups of patients with higher-risk disease. The EBCTCG concluded that treatments that significantly lower the risk of local-regional recurrence would over the course of 15 years prevent one breast cancer death for every four local recurrences prevented, thus resulting in an improved 15-year OS rate.

It is important that PMRT be applied appropriately to avoid toxic effects for patients at low risk of local-regional recurrence. Katz and colleagues examined patients treated with systemic therapy without PMRT to better define patients at intermediate and high risk of local-regional recurrence, who would benefit from PMRT [55, 56]. Patients with metastases in more than three axillary lymph nodes had a greater than 20 % risk of local-regional recurrence. Patients with one to three positive axillary lymph nodes with a tumor larger than 4 cm, gross extranodal extension, inadequate ALND, skin or nipple invasion, or inadequate margins also had rates of local-regional recurrence that warranted PMRT. These studies helped to define the patients for whom the benefit of PMRT outweighs the risk of toxic effects.

Patients undergoing neoadjuvant chemotherapy and modified radical mastectomy should be carefully evaluated for PMRT after mastectomy is complete and final pathology is available. In general, all patients who present with stage III disease will receive PMRT regardless of response to chemotherapy. Patients who present with stage II disease may not require PMRT, depending on the response to chemotherapy and the amount of residual disease in the breast and regional lymph nodes. Buchholz and colleagues demonstrated that patients who met criteria for PMRT prior to neoadjuvant chemotherapy and patients with more than three axillary lymph nodes positive for disease on final pathology benefit from PMRT [57]. It is important to note that even patients who met the criteria for PMRT at diagnosis but experienced a pathologic complete response to neoadjuvant chemotherapy were at high risk of local–regional recurrence and benefited from PMRT.

Systemic Therapy

Many patients with locally advanced breast cancer have inoperable disease at diagnosis. Delivering neoadjuvant systemic therapy may allow patients with disease initially deemed inoperable to become candidates for surgical resection. In addition, administration of neoadjuvant systemic therapy allows direct observation of tumor response, which provides valuable prognostic information and allows for alterations in ineffective chemotherapy regimens, limiting exposure to ineffective agents. Patients who experience a pathologic complete response to neoadjuvant chemotherapy have survival outcomes superior to those of patients who experience a partial response or no response; patients who experience progression of disease during neoadjuvant chemotherapy have the worst survival outcomes [58].

The effectiveness of chemotherapy regimens in the management of breast cancer are usually tested first in the metastatic setting. Once an agent has been shown to be effective in the metastatic setting, it is tested in adjuvant therapy trials to determine the impact on OS and DFS. Similar chemotherapy regimens will be utilized for neoadjuvant therapy in locally advanced breast cancer as are utilized in the adjuvant setting for patients with earlier stage disease. An EBCTCG update published in 2005 reviewed the results of all the randomized trials with different regimens to provide the evidence for adjuvant treatment decisions [59]. The EBCTCG concluded that polychemotherapy regimens such as CMF (cyclophosphamide, methotrexate, and 5-fluorouracil), FEC (5-fluorouracil, epirubicin, and cyclophosphamide), and FAC (5-fluorouracil, doxorubicin, and cyclophosphamide) along with some polychemotherapy regimens containing taxanes were more effective than single-agent chemotherapy in reducing breast cancer recurrence and mortality. It is important to note that HER2 status was not considered in this analysis. The use of trastuzumab to treat HER2-positive breast cancer has been demonstrated to significantly improve both DFS and OS. Currently, the NCCN guidelines include several regimens containing trastuzumab for both neoadjuvant and adjuvant chemotherapy [47].

Endocrine therapy also may be administered as neoadjuvant therapy in patients with hormone-receptor-positive breast cancer, particularly for elderly women who are deemed to be poor candidates for chemotherapy. Review of the NSABP B-14 and B-20 data demonstrated that less benefit was derived from chemotherapy with increasing age [60]. ER concentration, nuclear grade, histologic grade, tumor type, and proliferation markers should be considered in the decision between chemotherapy and endocrine therapy. Patients who may benefit from neoadjuvant endocrine therapy include those with locally advanced breast cancer that may become operable, those with large tumors who with a good response to neoadjuvant therapy may become eligible for BCT, and those with a short life expectancy for whom neoadjuvant endocrine therapy can provide long-term disease control.

All patients with hormone-receptor-positive disease should be offered adjuvant endocrine therapy as part of their multidisciplinary treatment. The EBCTCG analysis demonstrated benefit with the use of adjuvant tamoxifen therapy in patients with hormone-receptor-positive disease but not hormone-receptor-negative disease [59]. The recommended duration of therapy is 5 years. Although American Society of Clinical Oncology (ASCO) guidelines support using an aromatase inhibitor in postmenopausal women, as aromatase inhibitors are superior to tamoxifen in postmenopausal women with respect to DFS and toxic effects, it is important to note that tamoxifen is effective in both premenopausal and postmenopausal women with hormone-receptor-positive tumors [61].

Surveillance for Breast Cancer Patients Who Have Completed Curative Treatment

The American Cancer Society estimated that 230,480 new cases of invasive breast cancer and 57,650 new cases of in situ breast cancer were diagnosed in US women in 2011 [2]. Because of continued improvements in the detection and treatment of breast cancer together with the increasing population of the United States, the number of breast cancer survivors continues to increase. As a result, surveillance for breast cancer patients who have completed curative treatment and survivorship programs to address the physical and emotional needs of breast cancer survivors have become more important than ever before.

In 1994, a multicenter randomized controlled trial was published that examined the impact of two follow-up protocols on breast cancer survival and health-related quality of life in patients treated for breast cancer with curative intent [62]. The study enrolled 1,420 women with stage I, II, and III breast cancer. Women were randomized to an intensive surveillance group or a control group. Patients in the intensive surveillance group had routine visits with imaging including bone scan, liver echography, chest radiography, and laboratory studies at predefined intervals, while patients in the control group had follow-up visits at the same intervals with additional testing only if clinically indicated. No significant differences were seen in survival or time to detection of recurrence between the two groups at 71 months. In addition, no difference in quality of life was noted between these two groups. As a result, the investigators concluded that routine testing during breast cancer surveillance should be discouraged.

The National Research Council Project on Breast Cancer conducted a similar study that addressed the question of surveillance intensity for survivors [63]. A total of 1,243 patients were randomized to either clinical follow-up with physical examination and mammography or intensive follow-up with additional chest radiography and bone scan every 6 months. Although patients in the intensive follow-up group had earlier detection of recurrence, no difference in overall survival was noted. As a result, clinical follow-up was recommended over intensive follow-up.

Guidelines for Follow-up After Breast Cancer Treatment

The NCCN guidelines recommend that patients treated for DCIS have a history and physical examination every 6–12 months for the first 5 years after the completion of treatment and then annually, along with annual mammography [47]. Patients treated with BCT should have their initial follow-up mammogram 6–12 months after the completion of radiation therapy. The NCCN recommends that patients treated for invasive breast cancer be followed up by members of the treatment team. Clinical follow-up with history and physical examination should be performed every 4–6 months for the first 5 years and then annually. Mammograms should be performed annually. These guidelines clearly state that routine laboratory studies and imaging are not recommended for asymptomatic patients.

Women taking tamoxifen who have not undergone hysterectomy should have an annual gynecologic evaluation, and any vaginal spotting in a postmenopausal woman on tamoxifen therapy should be investigated promptly because of the risk of endometrial carcinoma.

Women with ovarian failure taking aromatase inhibitors should undergo baseline bone mineral density testing followed by testing at regular intervals. If bisphosphonate treatment is initiated, baseline dental examination and preventive dental care should be done prior to initiation of treatment. Patients treated with bisphosphonates should take calcium and vitamin D supplements.

Updated guidelines from ASCO are similar to those of the NCCN [64]. ASCO recommends a history and physical examination every 3–6 months for the first 3 years, every 6–12 months for the next 2 years, and then annually. Mammography is recommended annually. Patients who underwent BCT should have their first posttreatment mammogram 6 months after the completion of radiation therapy and then annually. ASCO specifies that laboratory studies and imaging are not recommended for asymptomatic patients. Routine gynecologic follow-up is recommended for all women. The ASCO guidelines state that surveillance care may take place under the direction of a primary care physician beginning 1 year after diagnosis for women with a tumor size less than 5 cm and less than four positive axillary lymph nodes. If a primary care physician takes over surveillance care, the primary care physician as well as the patient should be informed of recommended surveillance guidelines.

Actual Practice Patterns

Although clear guidelines have been established for surveillance in breast cancer patients who have undergone therapy with curative intent, actual practice patterns vary markedly. This has been illustrated by Margenthaler and colleagues, who surveyed ASCO members to determine how they perform breast cancer surveillance [65]. The results of this survey demonstrated wide deviation from the guidelines. The surveillance strategy most commonly recommended by the respondents was history and physical examination, mammography, and laboratory studies, although the frequency with which these various elements of surveillance were performed varied considerably. Over 80 % of ASCO members surveyed recommended laboratory studies at least annually even though the ASCO recommendations oppose the use of such tests. In addition, 7–15 % of those surveyed recommended various imaging studies at least annually even though the guidelines specifically oppose the use of imaging surveillance.

As the number of breast cancer survivors increases, the need to educate those performing surveillance for these patients has become increasingly important. The use of imaging studies only for patients who are symptomatic is the most appropriate and cost-effective strategy. With the economics of healthcare attracting increased attention, providers who fail to perform surveillance according to the NCCN and ASCO guidelines may experience decreasing reimbursement for unnecessary tests.

NCCN Guidelines for Breast Cancer Survivors

The 2013 version of the NCCN practice guidelines for breast cancer included new guidelines for addressing survivorship issues [47]. The NCCN defines a survivor as "an individual… from the time of diagnosis, through the balance of his or her life." As screening improves, treatment modalities become more effective, and as the population ages, the population of breast cancer survivors grows. Breast cancer survivors have many special needs besides cancer surveillance. The NCCN survivorship guidelines focus on "the potential impact on health, physical and mental states, health behaviors, professional and personal identity, sexuality, and financial standing." For survivors, the NCCN recommends performing healthcare assessments at regular intervals to screen for and provide interventions to address survivorship issues.

Acknowledgments The authors are grateful to Stephanie Deming for editorial assistance with the manuscript.

References

1. Nemoto T, Vana J, Bedwani RN, Baker HW, McGregor FH, Murphy GP. Management and survival of female breast cancer: results of a national survey by the American College of Surgeons. Cancer. 1980;45(12):2917–24.
2. Breast cancer facts & figures 2011–2012. Atlanta: American Cancer Society, Inc. www.cancer.org/acm/graips/content/eepideriologysurverlance/document/acspc-030975.pdf.
3. Page D, Rogers L, Schuyler P, et al. The natural history of ductal carcinoma in situ of the breast. In: Silverstein MS, Recht A, Lagios MD, eds. Ductal carcinoma in situ of the breast. 2nd ed. Philadelphia: Lippincott Williams & Wilkins; 2002. p. 17–21.
4. Sanders ME, Schuyler PA, Dupont WD, Page DL. The natural history of low-grade ductal carcinoma in situ of the breast in women treated by biopsy only revealed over 30 years of long-term follow-up. Cancer. 2005;103(12):2481–4.
5. Rosen PP, Senie R, Schottenfeld D, Ashikari R. Noninvasive breast carcinoma: frequency of unsuspected invasion and implications for treatment. Ann Surg. 1979;189(3):377–82.
6. Fisher B, Redmond C, Poisson R, Margolese R, Wolmark N, Wickerham L, et al. Eight-year results of a randomized clinical trial comparing total mastectomy and lumpectomy with or without irradiation in the treatment of breast cancer. N Engl J Med. 1989;320(13):822–8.
7. Veronesi U, Cascinelli N, Mariani L, Greco M, Saccozzi R, Luini A, et al. Twenty-year follow-up of a randomized study comparing breast-conserving surgery with radical mastectomy for early breast cancer. N Engl J Med. 2002;347(16):1227–32.
8. Blichert-Toft M, Nielsen M, During M, Moller S, Rank F, Overgaard M, et al. Long-term results of breast conserving surgery vs. mastectomy for early stage invasive breast cancer: 20-year follow-up of the Danish randomized DBCG-82TM protocol. Acta Oncol. 2008; 47(4):672–81.
9. Jacobson JA, Danforth DN, Cowan KH, D'Angelo T, Steinberg SM, Pierce L, et al. Ten-year results of a comparison of conservation with mastectomy in the treatment of stage I and II breast cancer. N Engl J Med. 1995;332(14):907–11.
10. Sarrazin D, Le MG, Arriagada R, Contesso G, Fontaine F, Spielmann M, et al. Ten-year results of a randomized trial comparing a conservative treatment to mastectomy in early breast cancer. Radiother Oncol. 1989;14(3):177–84.
11. van Dongen JA, Bartelink H, Fentiman IS, Lerut T, Mignolet F, Olthuis G, et al. Randomized clinical trial to assess the value of breast-conserving therapy in stage I and II breast cancer, EORTC 10801 trial. J Natl Cancer Inst Monogr. 1992;11:15–8.
12. Fisher B, Bauer M, Margolese R, Poisson R, Pilch Y, Redmond C, et al. Five-year results of a randomized clinical trial comparing total mastectomy and segmental mastectomy with or without radiation in the treatment of breast cancer. N Engl J Med. 1985;312(11):665–73.
13. Fisher B, Dignam J, Wolmark N, Mamounas E, Costantino J, Poller W, et al. Lumpectomy and radiation therapy for the treatment of intraductal breast cancer: findings from National Surgical Adjuvant Breast and Bowel Project B-17. J Clin Oncol. 1998;16(2):441–52.
14. Julien JP, Bijker N, Fentiman IS, Peterse JL, Delledonne V, Rouanet P, et al. Radiotherapy in breast-conserving treatment for ductal carcinoma in situ: first results of the EORTC randomised phase III trial 10853. EORTC Breast Cancer Cooperative Group and EORTC Radiotherapy Group. Lancet. 2000;355(9203):528–33.
15. Bijker N, Meijnen P, Peterse JL, Bogaerts J, Van Hoorebeeck I, Julien JP, et al. Breast-conserving treatment with or without radiotherapy in ductal carcinoma-in-situ: ten-year results of European Organisation for Research and Treatment of Cancer randomized phase III trial 10853–a study by the EORTC Breast Cancer Cooperative Group and EORTC Radiotherapy Group. J Clin Oncol. 2006;24(21):3381–7.

16. Houghton J, George WD, Cuzick J, Duggan C, Fentiman IS, Spittle M. Radiotherapy and tamoxifen in women with completely excised ductal carcinoma in situ of the breast in the UK, Australia, and New Zealand: randomised controlled trial. Lancet. 2003;362(9378):95–102.
17. Emdin SO, Granstrand B, Ringberg A, Sandelin K, Arnesson LG, Nordgren H, et al. SweDCIS: radiotherapy after sector resection for ductal carcinoma in situ of the breast. Results of a randomised trial in a population offered mammography screening. Acta Oncol. 2006;45(5):536–43.
18. Silverstein MJ, Lagios MD, Groshen S, Waisman JR, Lewinsky BS, Martino S, et al. The influence of margin width on local control of ductal carcinoma in situ of the breast. N Engl J Med. 1999; 340(19):1455–61.
19. McCormick B. RTOG 9804: a prospective randomized trial for "good risk" ductal carcinoma in situ (DCIS), comparing radiation (RT) to observation (OBS). J Clin Oncol. 30(suppl);abstr 1004.
20. Hughes LL, Wang M, Page DL, Gray R, Solin LJ, Davidson NE, et al. Local excision alone without irradiation for ductal carcinoma in situ of the breast: a trial of the Eastern Cooperative Oncology Group. J Clin Oncol. 2009;27(32):5319–24.
21. Hunt K, Meric-Bernstam F. Surgical options for breast cancer. In: Hunt KK, Robb GL. Strom EA, Ueno NT, editors. Breast cancer. 2nd ed. New York: Springer; 2008. p. 198–232.
22. Brunnert K. The Osnabrueck experience with reconstruction of the partial mastectomy defect. In: Spear S, editor. Surgery of the breast: principles and art. Philadelphia: Lippincott-Raven; 1998. p. 197–220.
23. Smith BD, Arthur DW, Buchholz TA, Haffty BG, Hahn CA, Hardenbergh PH, et al. Accelerated partial breast irradiation consensus statement from the American Society for Radiation Oncology (ASTRO). J Am Coll Surg. 2009;209(2):269–77.
24. Fisher B, Dignam J, Wolmark N, Wickerham DL, Fisher ER, Mamounas E, et al. Tamoxifen in treatment of intraductal breast cancer: National Surgical Adjuvant Breast and Bowel Project B-24 randomised controlled trial. Lancet. 1999;353(9169):1993–2000.
25. Allred DC, Anderson SJ, Paik S, Wickerham DL, Nagtegaal ID, Swain SM, et al. Adjuvant tamoxifen reduces subsequent breast cancer in women with estrogen receptor-positive ductal carcinoma in situ: a study based on NSABP protocol B-24. J Clin Oncol. 2012;30(12):1268–73.
26. Fisher B, Jeong JH, Anderson S, Bryant J, Fisher ER, Wolmark N. Twenty-five-year follow-up of a randomized trial comparing radical mastectomy, total mastectomy, and total mastectomy followed by irradiation. N Engl J Med. 2002;347(8):567–75.
27. Fisher B, Redmond C, Fisher ER, Bauer M, Wolmark N, Wickerham DL, et al. Ten-year results of a randomized clinical trial comparing radical mastectomy and total mastectomy with or without radiation. N Engl J Med. 1985;312(11):674–81.
28. Giuliano AE, Kirgan DM, Guenther JM, Morton DL. Lymphatic mapping and sentinel lymphadenectomy for breast cancer. Ann Surg. 1994;220(3):391–8; discussion 398–401.
29. Giuliano AE, Dale PS, Turner RR, Morton DL, Evans SW, Krasne DL. Improved axillary staging of breast cancer with sentinel lymphadenectomy. Ann Surg. 1995;222(3):394–9; discussion 399–401.
30. Krag DN, Anderson SJ, Julian TB, Brown AM, Harlow SP, Ashikaga T, et al. Technical outcomes of sentinel-lymph-node resection and conventional axillary-lymph-node dissection in patients with clinically node-negative breast cancer: results from the NSABP B-32 randomised phase III trial. Lancet Oncol. 2007;8(10):881–8.
31. Veronesi U, Paganelli G, Viale G, Luini A, Zurrida S, Galimberti V, et al. A randomized comparison of sentinel-node biopsy with routine axillary dissection in breast cancer. N Engl J Med. 2003; 349(6):546–53.
32. Veronesi U, Viale G, Paganelli G, Zurrida S, Luini A, Galimberti V, et al. Sentinel lymph node biopsy in breast cancer: ten-year results of a randomized controlled study. Ann Surg. 2010;251(4):595–600.
33. Ashikaga T, Krag DN, Land SR, Julian TB, Anderson SJ, Brown AM, et al. Morbidity results from the NSABP B-32 trial comparing sentinel lymph node dissection versus axillary dissection. J Surg Oncol. 2010;102(2):111–8.
34. Giuliano AE, Hunt KK, Ballman KV, Beitsch PD, Whitworth PW, Blumencranz PW, et al. Axillary dissection vs no axillary dissection in women with invasive breast cancer and sentinel node metastasis: a randomized clinical trial. JAMA. 2011;305(6):569–75.
35. Lucci A, McCall LM, Beitsch PD, Whitworth PW, Reintgen DS, Blumencranz PW, et al. Surgical complications associated with sentinel lymph node dissection (SLND) plus axillary lymph node dissection compared with SLND alone in the American College of Surgeons Oncology Group Trial Z0011. J Clin Oncol. 2007;25(24):3657–63.
36. National Comprehensive Cancer Center (NCCN) Clinical practice guidelines in oncology: Breast, version 1.2012. Available from: www.nccn.org/professionals/physician_/gls/pdf/breast.pdf.
37. The American Society of Breast Surgeons position statement on management of the axilla in patients with invasive breast cancer. Available from: http://www.breastsurgeons.org/statements/PDF_Statements/Axillary_Management.pdf.
38. Galimberti V, Cole BF, Zurrida S, et al. S3-1: update of International Breast Cancer Study Group trial 23-01 to compare axillary dissection versus no axillary dissection in patients with clinically node negative breast cancer and micrometastases in the sentinel node. Cancer Res. 2011;71(24 Supplement):S3–1.
39. Galimberti V, Cole BF, Zurrida S, Viale G, Luini A, Veronesi P, et al. Axillary dissection versus no axillary dissection in patients with sentinel-node micrometastases (IBCSG 23-01): a phase 3 randomised controlled trial. Lancet Oncol. 2013;14(4):297–305.
40. Boughey JC, Suman VJ, Mittendorf EA, et al. The role of sentinel lymph node surgery in patients presenting with node positive breast cancer (T0-4, N1-2) who receive neoadjuvant chemotherapy – results from the ACOSOG Z1071 trial. Cancer Res. 2012;72 (24 Supplement):S2–1.
41. Caudle AS, Hunt KK, Kuerer HM, Meric-Bernstam F, Lucci A, Bedrosian I, et al. Multidisciplinary considerations in the implementation of the findings from the American College of Surgeons Oncology Group (ACOSOG) Z0011 study: a practice-changing trial. Ann Surg Oncol. 2011;18(9):2407–12.
42. Mittendorf EA, Hunt KK, Boughey JC, Bassett R, Degnim AC, Harrell R, et al. Incorporation of sentinel lymph node metastasis size into a nomogram predicting nonsentinel lymph node involvement in breast cancer patients with a positive sentinel lymph node. Ann Surg. 2012;255(1):109–15.
43. Clarke M, Collins R, Darby S, Davies C, Elphinstone P, Evans E, et al. Effects of radiotherapy and of differences in the extent of surgery for early breast cancer on local recurrence and 15-year survival: an overview of the randomised trials. Lancet. 2005; 366(9503):2087–106.
44. Fyles AW, McCready DR, Manchul LA, Trudeau ME, Merante P, Pintilie M, et al. Tamoxifen with or without breast irradiation in women 50 years of age or older with early breast cancer. N Engl J Med. 2004;351(10):963–70.
45. Hughes KSSL, Berry D, Cirrincione C, McCormick B, Shank B, Wheeler J, Champion LA, Smith TJ, Smith BL, Shapiro C, Muss HB, Winer E, Hudis C, Wood W, Sugarbaker D, Henderson IC, Norton L, Cancer and Leukemia Group B, Radiation Therapy Oncology Group, Eastern Cooperative Oncology Group. Lumpectomy plus tamoxifen with or without irradiation in women 70 years of age or older with early breast cancer. N Engl J Med. 2004;351:971–7.
46. Fisher B, Brown A, Mamounas E, Wieand S, Robidoux A, Margolese RG, et al. Effect of preoperative chemotherapy on local-regional disease in women with operable breast cancer: findings from National Surgical Adjuvant Breast and Bowel Project B-18. J Clin Oncol. 1997;15(7):2483–93.

47. National Comprehensive Cancer Center (NCCN) Clinical Practice Guidelines in Oncology: Breast Cancer Version 2.2013. nccn.org. Available from: www.nccn.org/professionals/physician_/gls/pdf/breast.pdf.
48. Paik S, Shak S, Tang G, Kim C, Baker J, Cronin M, et al. A multigene assay to predict recurrence of tamoxifen-treated, node-negative breast cancer. N Engl J Med. 2004;351(27):2817–26.
49. Paik S, Tang G, Shak S, Kim C, Baker J, Kim W, et al. Gene expression and benefit of chemotherapy in women with node-negative, estrogen receptor-positive breast cancer. J Clin Oncol. 2006; 24(23):3726–34.
50. Singletary SE, McNeese MD, Hortobagyi GN. Feasibility of breast-conservation surgery after induction chemotherapy for locally advanced breast carcinoma. Cancer. 1992;69(11):2849–52.
51. Chen AM, Meric-Bernstam F, Hunt KK, Thames HD, Oswald MJ, Outlaw ED, et al. Breast conservation after neoadjuvant chemotherapy: the MD Anderson cancer center experience. J Clin Oncol. 2004;22(12):2303–12.
52. Overgaard M, Hansen PS, Overgaard J, Rose C, Andersson M, Bach F, et al. Postoperative radiotherapy in high-risk premenopausal women with breast cancer who receive adjuvant chemotherapy. Danish Breast Cancer Cooperative Group 82b Trial. N Engl J Med. 1997;337(14):949–55.
53. Overgaard M, Jensen MB, Overgaard J, Hansen PS, Rose C, Andersson M, et al. Postoperative radiotherapy in high-risk postmenopausal breast-cancer patients given adjuvant tamoxifen: Danish Breast Cancer Cooperative Group DBCG 82c randomised trial. Lancet. 1999;353(9165):1641–8.
54. Ragaz J, Olivotto IA, Spinelli JJ, Phillips N, Jackson SM, Wilson KS, et al. Locoregional radiation therapy in patients with high-risk breast cancer receiving adjuvant chemotherapy: 20-year results of the British Columbia randomized trial. J Natl Cancer Inst. 2005;97(2):116–26.
55. Katz A, Strom EA, Buchholz TA, Theriault R, Singletary SE, McNeese MD. The influence of pathologic tumor characteristics on locoregional recurrence rates following mastectomy. Int J Radiat Oncol Biol Phys. 2001;50(3):735–42.
56. Katz A, Strom EA, Buchholz TA, Thames HD, Smith CD, Jhingran A, et al. Locoregional recurrence patterns after mastectomy and doxorubicin-based chemotherapy: implications for postoperative irradiation. J Clin Oncol. 2000;18(15):2817–27.
57. Buchholz TA, Tucker SL, Masullo L, Kuerer HM, Erwin J, Salas J, et al. Predictors of local-regional recurrence after neoadjuvant chemotherapy and mastectomy without radiation. J Clin Oncol. 2002; 20(1):17–23.
58. Kuerer HM, Newman LA, Smith TL, Ames FC, Hunt KK, Dhingra K, et al. Clinical course of breast cancer patients with complete pathologic primary tumor and axillary lymph node response to doxorubicin-based neoadjuvant chemotherapy. J Clin Oncol. 1999; 17(2):460–9.
59. Early Breast Cancer Trialists' Collaborative Group (EBCTCG). Effects of chemotherapy and hormonal therapy for early breast cancer on recurrence and 15-year survival: an overview of the randomised trials. Lancet. 2005;365(9472):1687–717.
60. Fisher B, Jeong JH, Bryant J, Anderson S, Dignam J, Fisher ER, et al. Treatment of lymph-node-negative, oestrogen-receptor-positive breast cancer: long-term findings from National Surgical Adjuvant Breast and Bowel Project randomised clinical trials. Lancet. 2004;364(9437):858–68.
61. Burstein HJ, Griggs JJ, Prestrud AA, Temin S. American society of clinical oncology clinical practice guideline update on adjuvant endocrine therapy for women with hormone receptor-positive breast cancer. J Oncol Pract. 2010;6(5):243–6.
62. Impact of follow-up testing on survival and health-related quality of life in breast cancer patients. A multicenter randomized controlled trial. The GIVIO Investigators. JAMA. 1994;271(20):1587–92.
63. Rosselli Del Turco M, Palli D, Cariddi A, Ciatto S, Pacini P, Distante V. Intensive diagnostic follow-up after treatment of primary breast cancer. A randomized trial. National Research Council Project on Breast Cancer follow-up. JAMA. 1994;271(20):1593–7.
64. Khatcheressian JL, Hurley P, Bantug E, Esserman LJ, Grunfeld E, Halberg F, et al. Breast cancer follow-up and management after primary treatment: American Society of Clinical Oncology clinical practice guideline update. J Clin Oncol. 2013;31(7):961–5.
65. Margenthaler JA, Allam E, Chen L, Virgo KS, Kulkarni UM, Patel AP, et al. Surveillance of patients with breast cancer after curative-intent primary treatment: current practice patterns. J Oncol Pract. 2012;8(2):79–83.

Design and Operation of a Comprehensive Breast Care Center

18

Stamatia Destounis, Renee Morgan, and Andrea Arieno

Introduction

In 2014, an estimated 235,080 new cases of invasive breast cancer were expected to be diagnosed in men and women in the United States [1]. The disease continues to be a leading cause of death in women, second only to lung cancer. Early detection and diagnosis is crucial to reduce mortality, and screening mammography has been the gold standard for breast cancer diagnosis. A comprehensive and efficiently operating breast care facility is vital to provide the best environment for breast cancer screening and diagnosis.

This chapter will discuss the background of our breast imaging center, the current status, and the required setup. Throughout the chapter, an overview of current practices that allow for optimal patient care will be provided.

An Overview of Elizabeth Wende Breast Care, LLC

Our facility, Elizabeth Wende Breast Care, LLC (EWBC), is located in Rochester, New York, and was established in 1976 [2]. From its inception, EWBC's mission has been to provide patients with the highest quality breast imaging and excellent care that considers each patient's physical and emotional well-being. EWBC has grown to be the largest freestanding breast imaging center in the United States, seeing approximately 80,000 patients annually. Figures 18.1 and 18.2 demonstrate the distribution of our patients from across the state and country.

Our practice has expanded over the years and currently includes a main office which is approximately 33,500 square feet (Fig. 18.3) and three satellite offices: 1,200 square feet (a rural location southeast of the main office), 2,000 square feet (northwest of the main office), and 2,300 square feet (east of the main office). Combined, we serve approximately 420 patients daily: 340 screening, 60 diagnostic, 20 screening ultrasound, eight magnetic resonance imaging (MRI) examinations, and six genetic appointments.

The first floor of the main office is designated for patient care, and the second floor is designated for medical record storage, administrative offices, and the genetics department. The main office, on a bus line and with ample free parking, sees an average of 265 screening appointments and an average of 60 diagnostic appointments daily. The office includes six radiologists, four full-time and two part-time, in addition to a staff of 134 employees, 97 full-time and 37 part-time. The majority of our work is done online (patients have the option to wait for results) from 6:45 a.m. to 5:00 p.m., which can make for a long day for staff and radiologists.

Screening services available include digital mammography, digital breast tomosynthesis, ultrasound, and breast MRI. All examinations are interpreted at the main office, as the satellite office studies are transferred via our extended network circuits to the main office. Each screening mammography examination is read with the use of computer-aided detection (CAD), and same-day results are offered to those patients who choose to wait. For those who do wait for results (approximately 62 % of our population), additional views, ultrasound, and needle biopsy can all be performed during the same visit, if necessary. Whether our patients travel a distance for their appointment, make special

S. Destounis, MD, FACR (✉) • R. Morgan, RT • A. Arieno, BS
Elizabeth Wende Breast Care LLC, 170 Sawgrass Drive, Rochester, NY 14620, USA
e-mail: sdestounis@ewbc.com; rmorgan@ewbc.com; aarieno@ewbc.com

M.K. Shetty (ed.), *Breast Cancer Screening and Diagnosis: A Synopsis*,
DOI 10.1007/978-1-4939-1267-4_18, © Springer Science+Business Media New York 2015

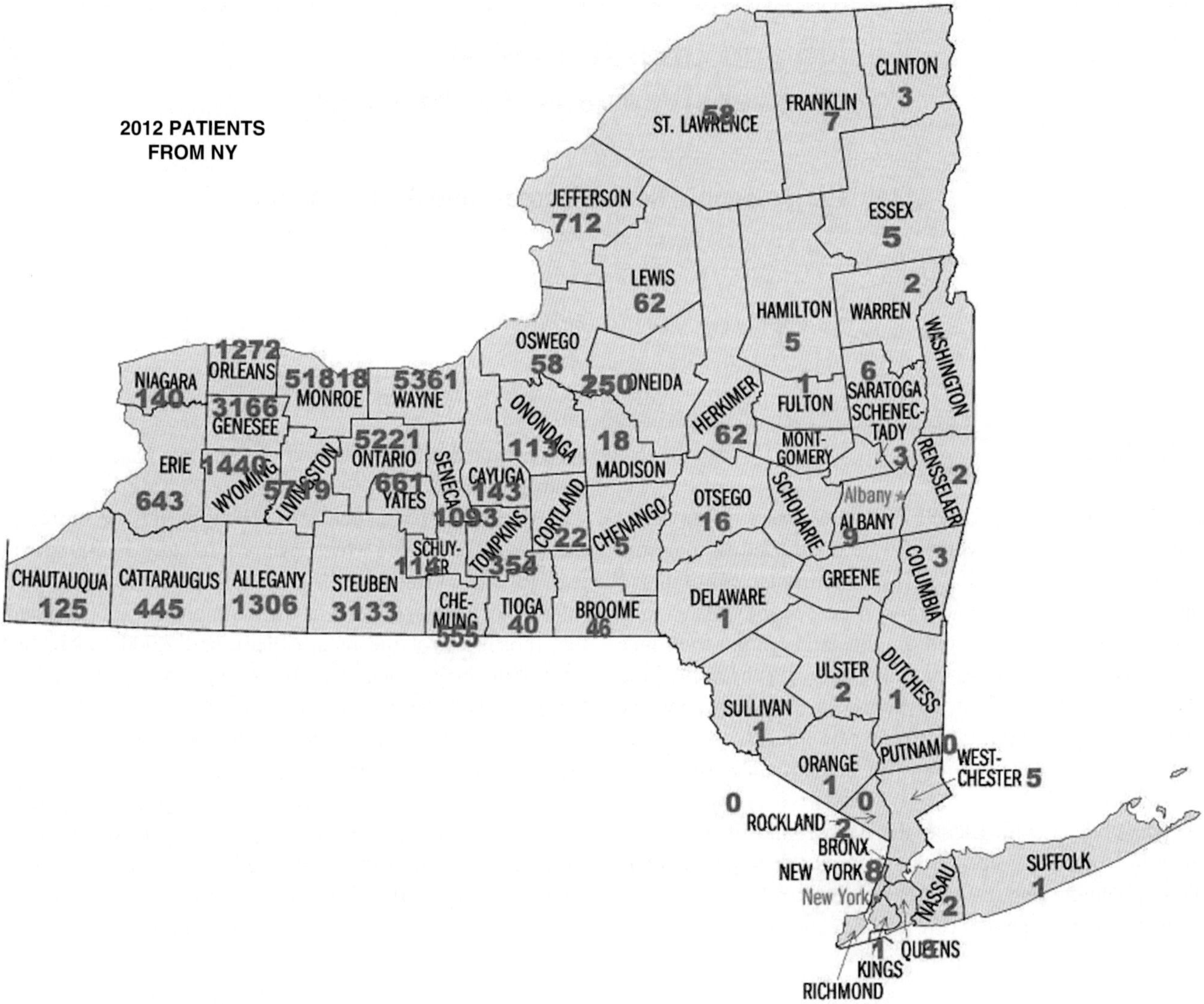

Fig. 18.1 Map of New York State displays the distribution of patients that we serve

transportation arrangements, or are anxious for their results, the option to have the mammogram and additional work-up, if necessary, during the same visit is very important. For those fitting the appointment into a busy life schedule, the option to not wait for results is appreciated.

In addition to the screening services mentioned previously, we also offer diagnostic services which include diagnostic ultrasound, breast MRI, ductography, fine-needle aspiration cytology (FNAC), and needle core biopsy for all imaging modalities (stereotactic, ultrasound, and MRI).

Breast MRI was a modality that was added to our practice in 2003. We began with MRI 1 day per week with a mobile lease and eventually, due to the high patient demand, built an addition to house a permanent unit to be utilized daily. Having access to an extensive range of diagnostic services has allowed our facility to provide care to a wide array of patients, whether recently diagnosed with breast cancer or those considered at high lifetime breast cancer risk.

As of 2010, we implemented a risk assessment/genetics program and have had a certified genetic counselor on staff since 2011. The process began when we realized patients with multiple risk factors for breast or ovarian cancer had many questions and needed counseling at a level that our current staff could not provide. This program has allowed us to reach out to our high-risk population and ultimately provide additional and potentially lifesaving services, such as screening MRI.

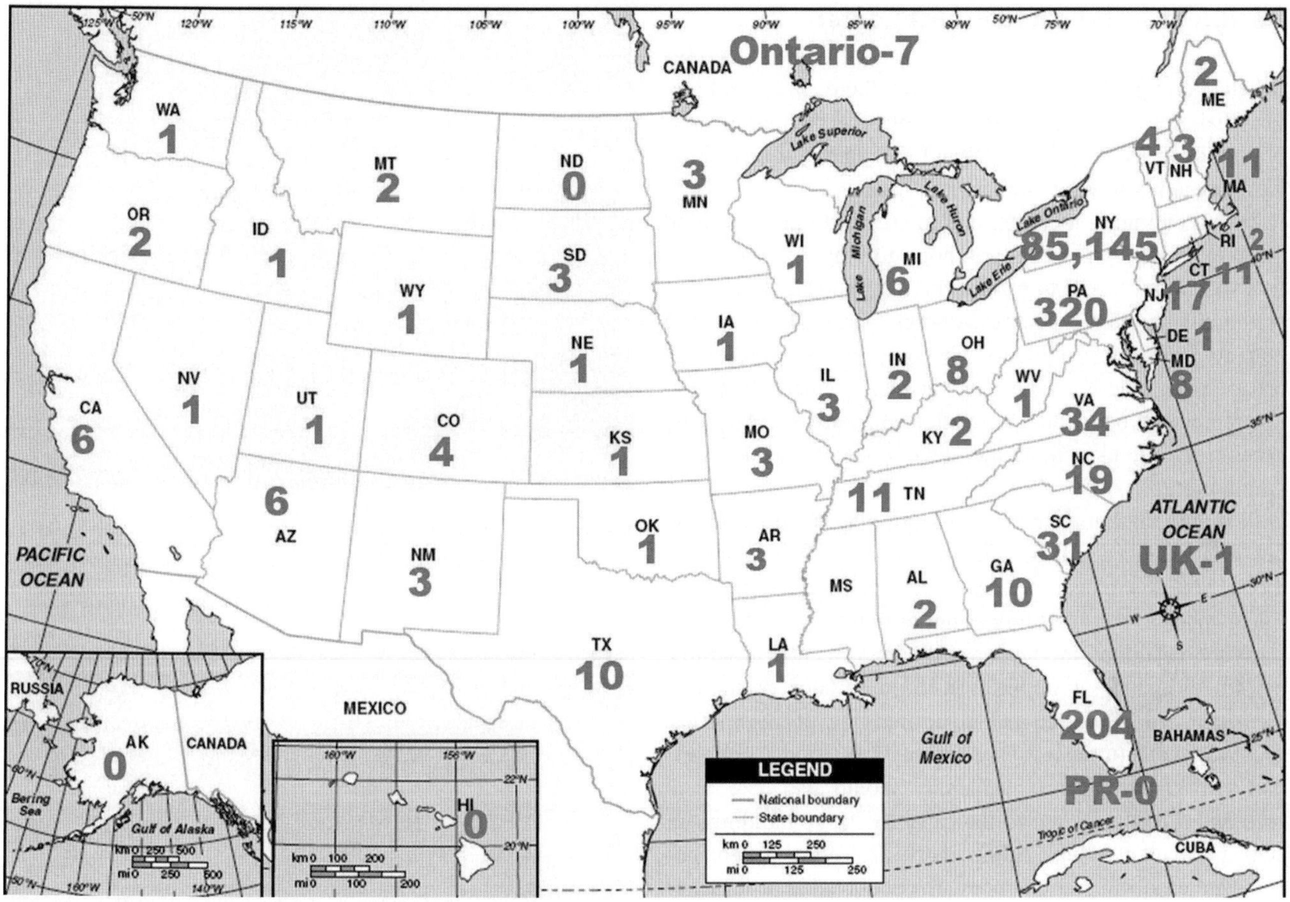

Fig. 18.2 Map of the United States and Canada showing the distribution of patients that travel to our facility

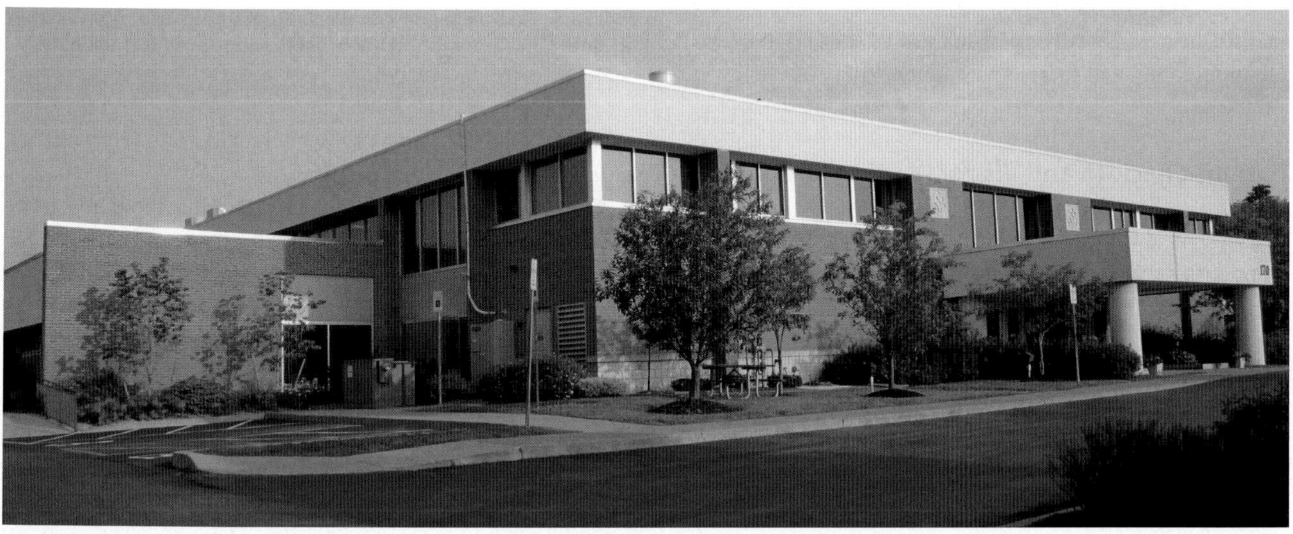

Fig. 18.3 Elizabeth Wende Breast Care, LLC, located in Rochester, New York

Design of a Dedicated Breast Center

When opening a breast imaging center, there are several factors that need to be considered. From the beginning, it is important to know and understand the state and local laws that may apply in your area.

When picking a location, it is important to keep in mind the population of patients you hope to reach. A city location will allow access to patients in many surrounding areas, as the city is often a central location. A rural location will help to reach those patients who may not have access to urban areas. Another aspect to consider is where the imaging center will be located in relation to a bus line. Allowing access for patients without their own mode of transportation is important.

It is optimal that from the very beginning stages, you plan out what services will be offered to patients, but even with the best plans in place, a practice may grow and require additional space to include services not initially anticipated.

When designing the layout of the breast center, it will be helpful to include an architect in the discussion on the services that will be offered and the desired flow of the practice. This will help to design an efficient layout for a seamless daily workflow. Parking availability should also be considered and directly related to the capacity of the building, for staff and patients alike. Additionally, protecting patient privacy and ensuring that practices are conducted in accordance with Health Insurance Privacy and Accountability Act (HIPAA) will need to be considered when designing the center. This needs to be considered from the time the patient checks in and continued throughout the office visit. Most of the health and human services (hhs.gov) [3] sites are an excellent resource to assure proper protection for patient privacy.

The following subsections will discuss the layout of our facility, from patient check-in and visitor waiting room to the mammography and radiologists' suites.

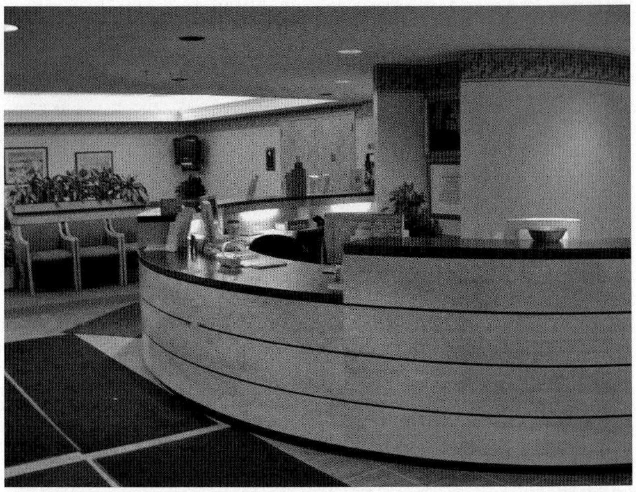

Fig. 18.4 The original reception area was an open design which did not allow for much privacy while a patient checked in with reception staff

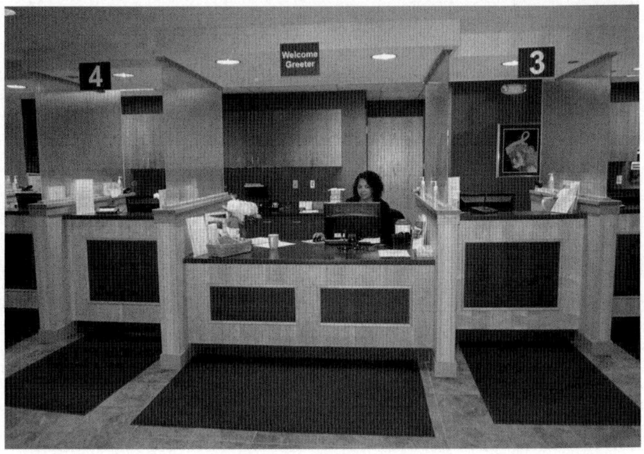

Fig. 18.5 Remodeling of the reception area was performed to ensure adequate privacy for the patient while checking in at the front desk

Patient Check-In and Visitor Waiting Room

When a patient first enters the facility, she approaches the front desk staff in the main waiting room. The outside waiting room should include varying-sized chairs or benches to accommodate patients and visitors of all sizes. Armchairs are important for patients with limited mobility who may need assistance when getting to a standing position, while bench-style seating (armless) is important as it provides comfort for the overweight patient who may require slightly more room than the standard chair. A waiting room bathroom should be incorporated, as family members tend to accompany and wait for the patient's visit to be complete. Building codes and specifications will need to be adhered to, to ensure requirements for handicap accessibility are met, for example, a large doorway for wheelchairs, scooters, walkers, or those requiring extra assistance.

Our front reception area went through remodeling to be designed in accordance with HIPAA. It is essential that the check-in process is as private as possible to protect the patients' protected health information (PHI). Figures 18.4 and 18.5 show the transition of the reception area as the facility adapted to HIPAA regulations. Each receptionist has her own computer and desk, separated from the next receptionist by a glass partition. The partition provides the privacy needed for review of PHI that takes place at check-in (Fig. 18.6).

Aside from the physical design of the outside waiting area, we offer a wide selection of reading materials, as well as herbal teas and decaffeinated coffee, television, and wireless internet for both patients and those who may be accompanying them for the appointment.

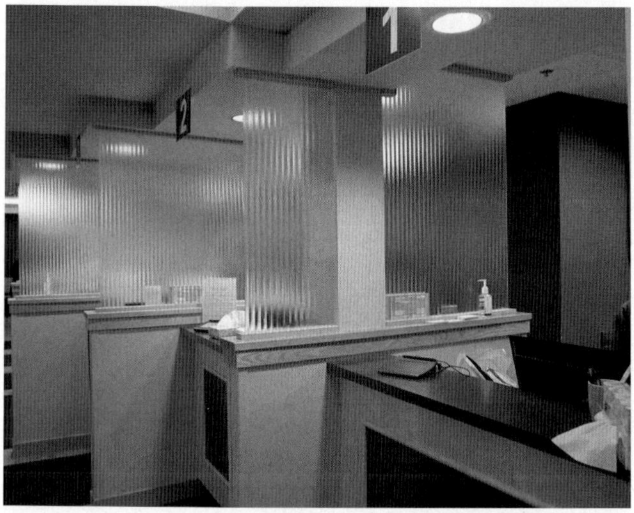

Fig. 18.6 Glass partitions divide the reception desk to protect the patients' health information

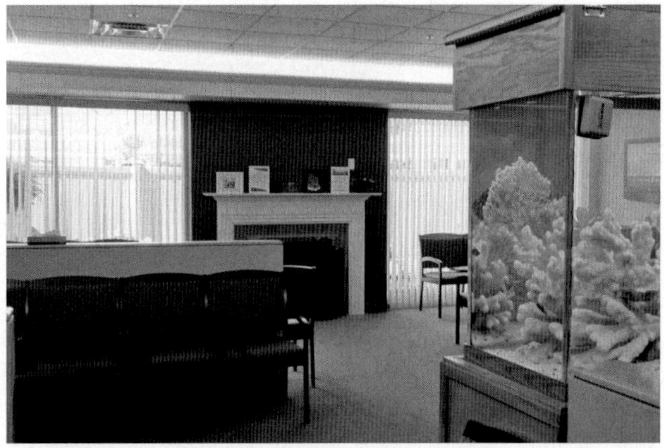

Fig. 18.7 The waiting room for patients attending screening mammography contains aquariums and a fireplace as it was designed to be a tranquil and serene environment

Patient Waiting Room Design

Due to the volume of patients we service and the fact that some patients may experience a lengthy visit, the office was designed with two inside patient waiting areas. The asymptomatic screening patients, whether waiting for results or not, have a shorter appointment time, approximately 1 h from check-in to checkout. However, the symptomatic diagnostic patient may be with us for several hours for a complete work-up. The decision of designing two separate waiting areas came from past experience; when all patients shared one waiting area, regardless of appointment type, we found that patients were noticing others would arrive after them and leave before them, and this added additional anxiety to an already stressful appointment. At the earliest opportunity (when further space became available), the decision was made to separate the diagnostic patients and the screening patients. Incorporating the two waiting rooms has turned out to be an excellent decision, as the dynamics of each scenario fit the respective waiting room.

The screening changing area contains 10 changing booths and 72 lockers; the screening waiting room allows seating for 51. A smaller waiting room is adjacent to the large screening waiting room; this room is utilized if a patient requires a smaller setting. The diagnostic changing area has five changing booths and 36 lockers; the diagnostic waiting room is smaller allowing for seating for 34. Both waiting rooms have a fireplace and fish tank to promote a tranquil environment. Decaffeinated coffee and herbal teas are offered for patients, along with reading material (Figs. 18.7 and 18.8).

As with the visitor waiting room, it is important to have comfortable chairs for patients of all sizes. It has been reported that patients with weight issues often do not adhere to screening tests, but if the environment is accommodating, these patients may be more inclined to keep their appointments [4]. Research has shown that obese women have higher mortality rates for breast and cervical cancer [5], and one bad experience may turn a patient away from a lifesaving screening exam.

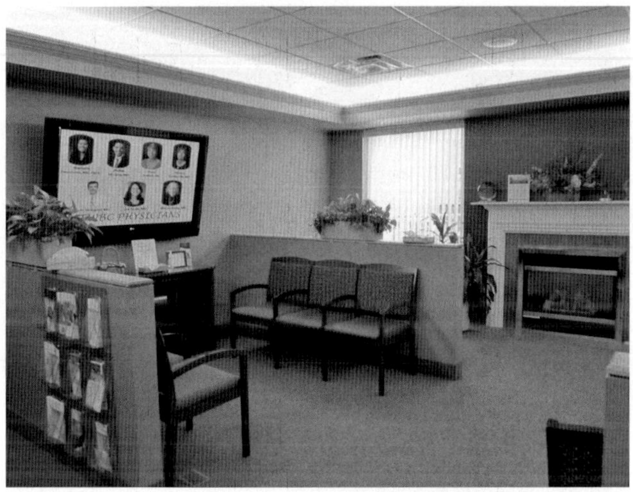

Fig. 18.8 The waiting room for patients presenting for a diagnostic appointment is a smaller version of the screening waiting room, also housing a fireplace as well as a flat-screen television

Mammography Suites

The main office has ten mammography suites that are centrally located from the two patient waiting rooms. Each room is equipped with a direct ray full field digital mammography (FFDM) unit with attachments and all supplies necessary for the study (Fig. 18.9).

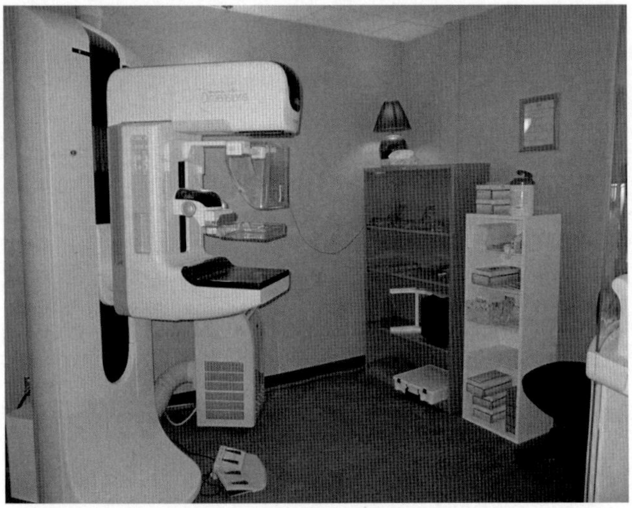

Fig. 18.9 A typical mammography room at our facility

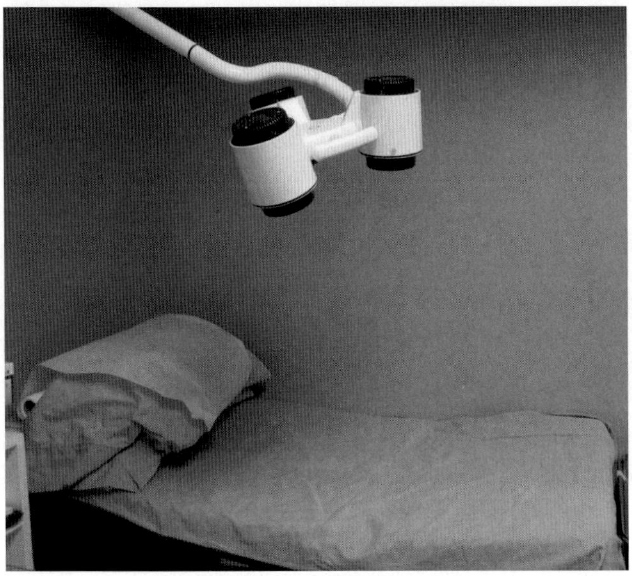

Fig. 18.10 The largest mammography room is utilized for procedures such as ductography and contains a bed to aid with the procedure so that the patient does not need to be transferred to another room for imaging

The largest mammography suite has been designated for localization procedures and is also equipped with an examination table used for ductography cannulation (Fig. 18.10).

Utilizing this larger room for interventional procedures is a benefit, as added staff may be needed during the procedure, such as a nurse, in cases where the patient needs extra assistance. Additionally, in each room, a thin client computer is provided for access to the radiology information system (RIS) and picture archiving and communication system (PACS) (Fig. 18.11). The technologist has the ability to review prior reports and images as well as update electronic health information that may be provided during the patient interview portion of the examination.

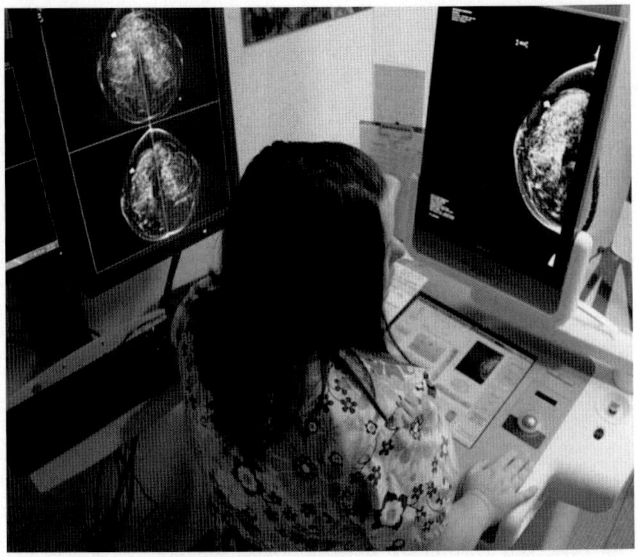

Fig. 18.11 The technologists have access to prior imaging while preparing for the patient in the mammography suite

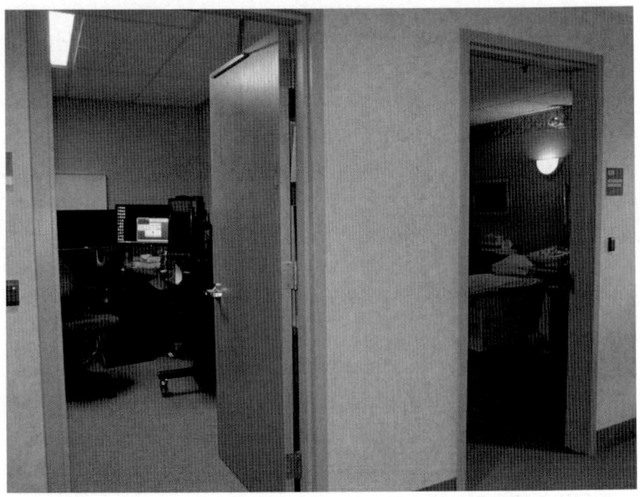

Fig. 18.12 The radiologists' reading room and examination room can both be accessed from the hallway, as well as by a doorway between the two rooms

Radiologist Suite

Each radiologist at our facility has a two-room suite consisting of a reading room and an attached examination and ultrasound room (Fig. 18.12). There is hallway access to both rooms, as well as an inside doorway connecting the two rooms. This allows the patient to be escorted in from the outer hallway and allows the radiologist to enter the examination room from their reading room (Fig. 18.13). Daily, each radiologist has a medical assistant scheduled with them to assist with patient flow.

The radiologist reading room reflects the current modern, ergonomic design for the digital era. Due to the sedentary nature of the digital reading room, it is crucial that ergonomics

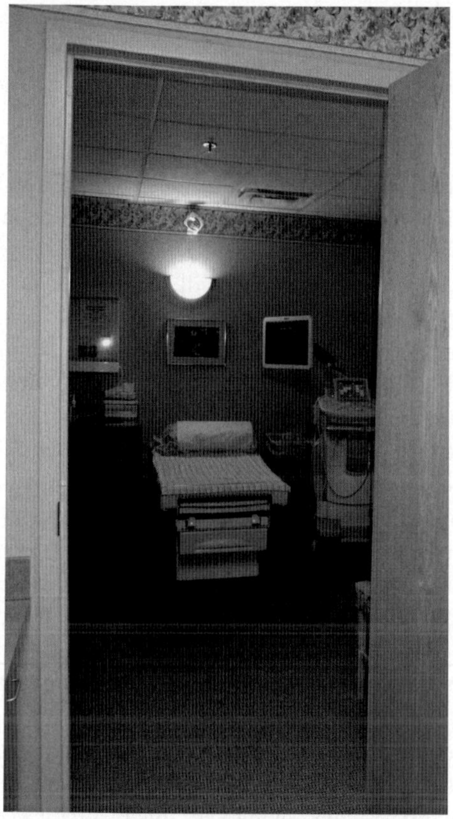

Fig. 18.13 A view into the examination room from the reading room demonstrates the convenience for the radiologist when preparing to examine a patient

be addressed to minimize eyestrain, lower back strain, carpel tunnel syndrome, and fatigue [6]. Each radiologist's office is equipped with a lumbar-supportive chair and a height adjustable desk that can be used for seated or standing reading (Figs. 18.14 and 18.15).

Two 5 megapixel monitors can be height adjusted and tilted for optimal viewing to minimize neck strain. Each room has overhead fluorescent lighting, but when interpreting digital mammograms, it is not used due to the reflective glare on the monitors. Instead, ambient lighting (with a low-wattage bulb) that is located behind the monitors is used. Each radiologist has an ergonomic keyboard and mouse allowing for their hand and wrist to be neutrally positioned. A programmable gaming mouse is used and programmed so that with slight hand movement, the reading protocol can be advanced and CAD can be applied.

The ultrasound room attached to the reading room allows for an efficient workflow for the radiologist. This room is used for clinical breast examination, handheld ultrasound, and clinically guided procedures such as cyst aspirations, antegrade ductography injection, FNAC, and core biopsy. In addition to this attached room, there is an overflow ultrasound/examination room that is shared amongst the radiologists if needed on a busy day. This allows the radiologist to see their next patient without waiting for the turnover and cleaning of the room just used. The combination of having an individual suite and a medical assistant assigned to help maintain adequate patient flow is an important aspect in the design of our facility.

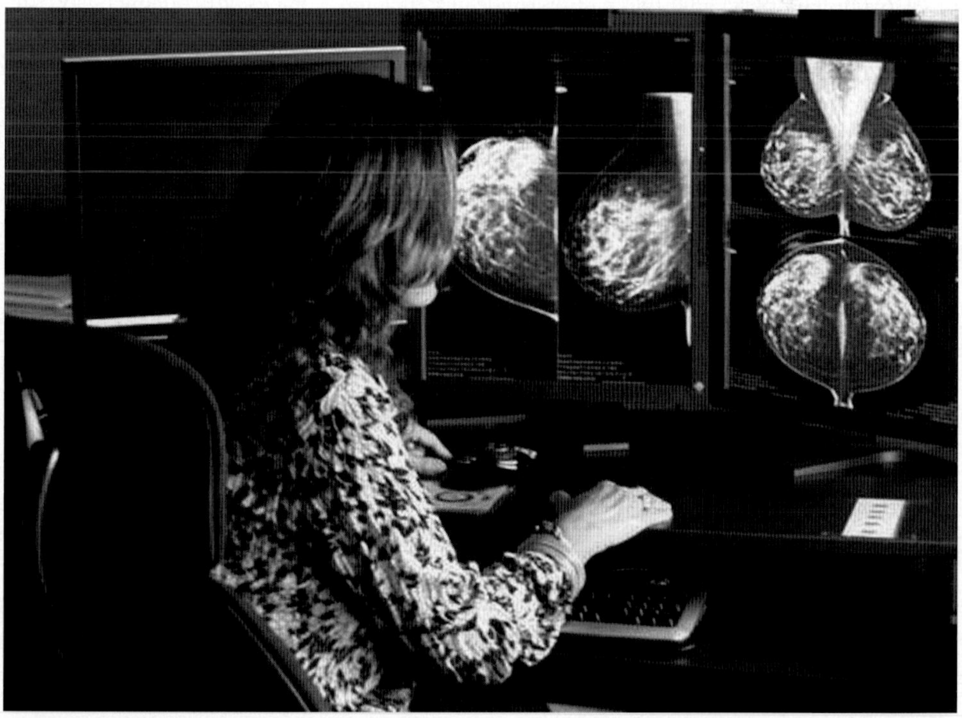

Fig. 18.14 With the new ergonomically designed workstations, the radiologists can read while remaining seated in a lumbar-supportive chair

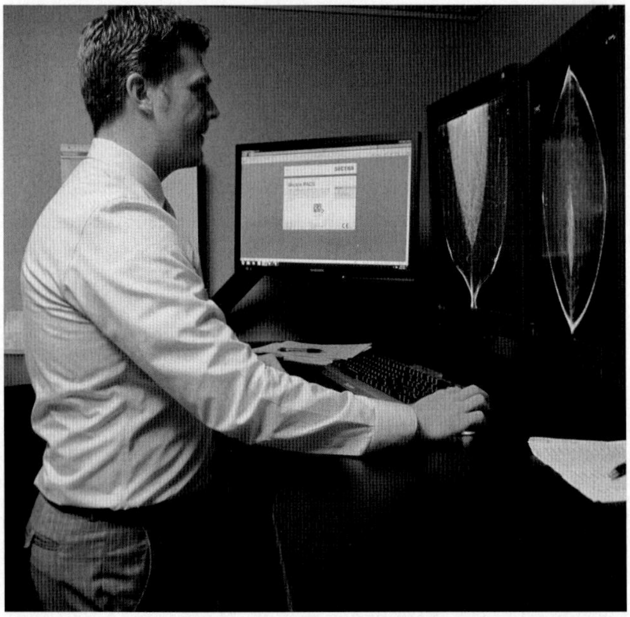

Fig. 18.15 The ergonomically designed workstations can also be adjusted to allow the radiologist to stand while interpreting examinations

Running the Office

This section will review how our systems are integrated to provide a seamless daily clinical workflow.

RIS and PACS

In 2008, our facility became 100 % digital and since then has been converting to a paperless, chartless environment. Our facility uses an electronic proprietary RIS (Avairis). This system is closely integrated with our PACS system (Sectra). The two systems, using bidirectional Health Level 7 (HL7) messaging, have allowed us to follow and manage all aspects of our patients' visits electronically, as well as maintain an electronic chart for each patient.

Our operation has gone through many changes over the years, and it is important to describe the progression that has brought us to the present functionality. Originally, during the time of film-screen mammography, PACS was solely used to view the new digital images as we began to implement FFDM. As the years progressed, our Information Technology (IT) department and PACS administrators have integrated PACS closely with the RIS. Prior patient information has been added into the patients' record on PACS to ensure that all information on a patient is directly available to the radiologist. In the transition from film screen to digital, film images have been digitized into PACS. Additionally, all radiology reports have been tied into the exams in PACS and can be viewed directly alongside the images. Personal and family history and prior needle or surgical biopsy information are also now included in PACS and can easily be viewed by the radiologist while reviewing a case. Changes such as these have allowed the radiologists to read all examinations from their own workstations within their own offices.

Today, when a patient schedules an appointment, a message (made possible with HL7) containing appointment information is sent to PACS. PACS performs an automatic "pre-fetch" of prior images from archive the night before the appointment. All prior images will be available for the radiologist to review and compare with the current examination.

During the appointment, PACS will send an HL7 message to the RIS when the radiologist has completed reading the examination. Immediately after screening examinations are interpreted and marked by the radiologists as normal, a message is sent to the RIS, the patient result letter is automatically printed, and the date of the next appointment is set for the patient. Once the letter is printed, the medical assistant knows that the patient's visit is complete and can then give the patient her results. At the same time, the report is also automatically sent to the patient's referring physicians, and the name of the reading radiologist is sent to the billing program in the RIS and charges are posted.

When a radiologist needs additional imaging, they will mark either "finding" or "assessment" on the exam in PACS. If "assessment" is marked, this is a request for extra mammographic images to be performed. A message is automatically sent to the RIS where an extra view/exam is created on the "dashboard" (which will be explained in the next section) and is available for the technologist. The process will repeat itself until the patient is marked as normal. If "finding" is marked, which means the additional mammographic views are obtained and the radiologist is still concerned about the area of investigation, a message is automatically sent to the RIS to create a new exam for an ultrasound, and the patient will present on the ultrasound "dashboard" for the sonographers or the radiologist, converting the exam to a diagnostic appointment.

Dashboard

The "dashboard" that has been mentioned previously is a feature of Avairis that is used to electronically track patients during their appointment at our facility. The dashboard is used by staff members and departments that have direct patient care (Fig. 18.16).

At the start of the day, all patient names are pre-populated to the dashboard through appointment scheduling. Once the patient enters the office, a staff member at the front desk, who is logged into the "greeter view," will begin the movement of the patient as she/he proceeds through the stages of the appointment. This is done electronically by dragging the patient icon on the dashboard to the next step in the visit. The movement of the patient on the dashboard immediately

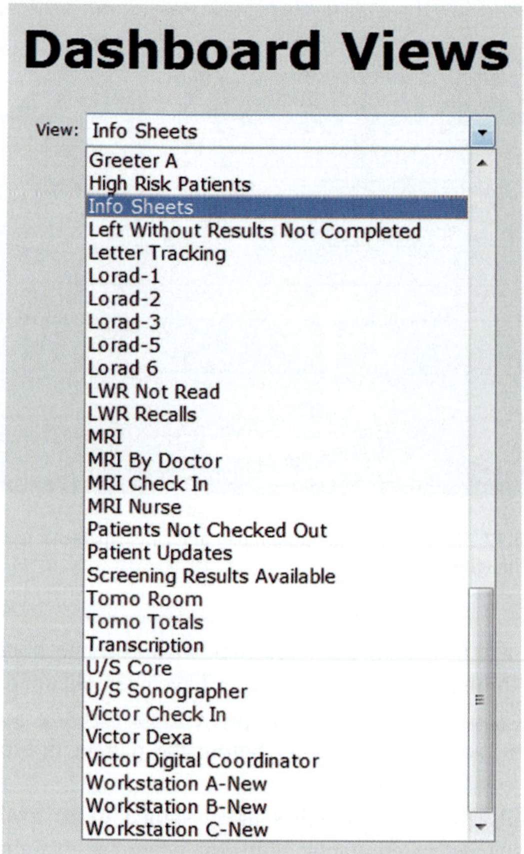

Fig. 18.16 The dashboard is used by all departments within our facility and was created with many different views depending on the needs of the department or individual staff member

notifies the next staff member who will interact with the patient that she/he is ready. For example, once Mrs. Smith has completed check-in and is ready to be brought back to change for the examination, her name will appear on the "bring back" dashboard. This alerts the designated staff member to bring her to the inside waiting room. The patient will then show on the digital coordinator's dashboard, and the coordinator will move the patient into one of the available mammography rooms. The technologist assigned to that room will then see she/he has a patient and will begin the exam. When she/he begins and ends the exam on the dashboard, HL7 messages will be sent to PACS to change the status of the patient. This process continues throughout the patient's appointment at the office and messages are sent between the RIS, PACS, and our Dolbey reporting system as well.

Department Functionality

The ability to have a highly efficient breast center requires having all the necessary departments with specific expertise interact with one another. The following will discuss the important roles of each department in our facility.

Call Center/Front Desk (Reception)

The front desk (reception) and the call center share a group of 25 employees that rotate between the two departments. The call center is the first impression of the office, and it is essential to have knowledgeable staff answering the calls in a timely fashion. This department answers approximately 850 calls daily.

After an automatic triage the patient is directed to screening, diagnostic, bone densitometry, or MRI scheduling. These calls average 1 min in length. A select group of employees (medical assistants and select call center staff) rotate through diagnostic scheduling. It is important that these individuals are well trained and very familiar with breast problems and the urgency of particular symptoms. In addition, the diagnostic schedulers need to have a complete understanding of the office workflow and the doctor's schedules in order to properly inform the patient of the time that should be allotted for the diagnostic appointment. This knowledge base helps minimize diagnostic scheduling errors which ultimately results in high patient satisfaction.

The call center staff is also responsible for managing patients who were auto-scheduled for their next screening visit. This is automatically generated at the end of their last routine screening appointment. The call center staff will mail out a health history form 45 days prior to the appointment. An automated phone message is also in place to remind patients of the upcoming appointment 2 days prior to the appointment date.

Front Desk (Reception)

Upon entering the building, the patient encounters the front desk employees for check-in in the outside waiting room. A receptionist will greet the patient, confirm the appointment is scheduled correctly, and ensure that the health history form is completed (which is sent by mail prior to the appointment date). Once these requirements have been satisfied, the greeter will send the patient on to check in. The check-in receptionist will confirm patient identification (ID) by photo ID. Patients are asked to electronically sign two consent statements: one confirms that the patient has read our facility privacy statement and authorizes us to obtain their medical information as well as use their medical information for education and research purposes; the other confirms the patient has read and understands our facility policy regarding insurance. Insurance information is verified and the current insurance card is scanned to ensure we have the most up-to-date subscriber number. Two full-time employees verify all insurance information in advance, but if any questions arise, the receptionist has the ability to check insurance eligibility through the internet right at the front desk. As part of our genetics program, the receptionists also verify with the patient that we have the correct personal and family history of breast cancer information in the electronic record.

If the patient presents for a diagnostic appointment and has brought outside films or digital images with her, a reception staff member will sort through the films and reports. The films will be provided to the medical records department for digitization into PACS, or with digital images; the medical records department will upload into PACS. For a diagnostic appointment, the patient is also asked to bring in outside radiology and pathology reports for the radiologist at our facility to review. Based on the type of diagnostic appointment (e.g., second opinion, check-up, new problem), the chart is brought either to the radiologists' reading room to order specific mammographic views or directly to the technologist to perform routine mammographic imaging.

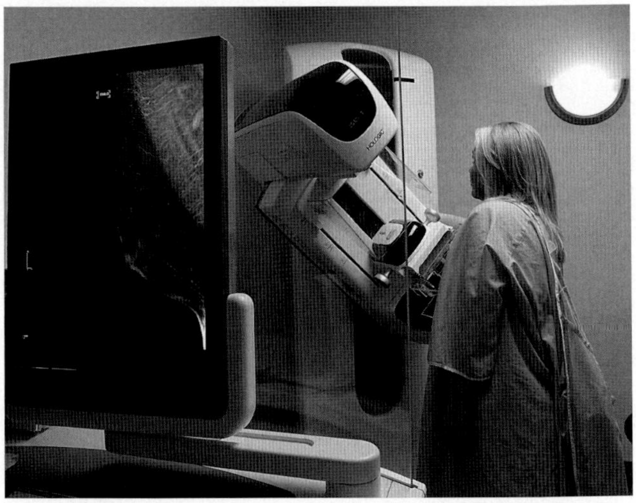

Fig. 18.17 Three of our mammography units are capable of tomosynthesis imaging

Technologist Department

The technical staff consists of 35 mammography technologists and three sonographers, 19 full-time and 24 part-time (part-time hours range from 25 to 38 h weekly). The technologists cover the main office as well as the three satellite offices. One technologist has an additional certification in MRI. Years of experience in breast imaging range from 1 to 30 years, with some spending their entire career at our breast center. Eleven technologists assist through a rotational schedule with stereotactic core biopsies, and three rotate through the MRI department. Seven technologists perform quality control of the units with two specifically supervising the compliance aspect of quality control. Each day, two technologists are scheduled late; these two stay until all imaging and interventional procedures for the day have been completed.

Technologist training is crucial for the success of the facility. It is important that newly hired technologists undergo training by those most familiar and knowledgeable with breast imaging and particularly with the philosophy of the breast center. The four most senior technologists at our facility are assigned with training the newly hired technologist. They follow a training curriculum that begins with screening examinations, leading up to diagnostic imaging. Training may take upward of a year to complete.

The main office has ten FFDM rooms, three of which have tomosynthesis capabilities (Fig. 18.17). Each mammography room is scheduled with two technologists per day. The technologists scheduled to a particular room will see their patient's name come up on the dashboard and will place the patient to an "in progress" designation when she/he is ready to begin the exam. The technologist goes to the waiting room (either the screening or diagnostic room, which is indicated by a color code on the dashboard) and escorts the patient into the mammography room. The patient's name, date of birth, and reason for exam are confirmed by the technologist prior to imaging. After the images have been obtained, they are checked for proper technique, correct labeling, subject motion, and general quality before the patient is escorted back to the waiting room.

Daily, four technologists are assigned to be available to assist with stereotactic biopsies, when the examination is ordered. When not assisting with stereotactic biopsies, these technologists are performing diagnostic or screening mammograms. Our facility has two stereotactic prone biopsy tables and performs an average of five (range 6–22) stereotactic biopsies daily. Generally two technologists, or a technologist and a medical assistant, will be responsible for each biopsy performed. Their duties include retrieving (printing) the necessary images for review, room and biopsy equipment preparation, escorting the patient to the biopsy room, patient preparation (pre- and post biopsy), and positioning the patient so the radiologist can be called upon for a "biopsy-ready" patient [7]. Post biopsy, the technologist will hold pressure and bandage the biopsy site as well as review printed post biopsy instructions with the patient. The patient will be called by the radiologist in the next 24–48 h with the results of the biopsy. Any imaging, such as post biopsy clip placement views, will be performed by the same set of technologists who assisted with the biopsy. The technologists will then clean the room in preparation for the next pending biopsy.

Managing the patient flow via the dashboard in the technologist area is an integral part of assuring that the patients are imaged in a timely fashion. This duty is performed by the digital coordinator (typically the control technologist), who will route patients to prospective mammography rooms. This allows for the most efficient use of the mammography rooms and technical staff. In addition, the digital coordinator will review any comments regarding special needs or concerns, the patient's breast density, and history or risk of breast cancer, as these factors play a role in the decision of which room the patient will be assigned to. The digital coordinator is able to see the progression of the exam in the mammography room through a web-based PACS and assigns the next patient to be imaged accordingly. The technologists in the mammography rooms and the digital coordinator have the ability to communicate with each other through instant messaging; this is useful in that communication between the technologist and coordinator remains open, as occasionally a patient may need additional time or the technologist requires additional help with positioning a difficult patient. This allows the coordinator to route the next patient to another room. Throughout the day, patients requiring additional views after screening mammography will reappear at the top of the dashboard list, and the color will change to red (a visual). The digital coordinator will expedite such an exam to the next available mammography room due to fact that the patient has already been waiting after routine imaging.

Medical Assistants

Our facility has 17 medical assistants who work closely with the radiologists daily. Their duties include examination room preparation, escorting the patient back and forth from the waiting room, patient preparation in the ultrasound room, ultrasound assistance, biopsy preparation and assistance, billing assistance, and follow-up visit scheduling. In addition to direct patient care, the assistants rotate through the following positions:

- Digital hanger: Each mammography examination is individually confirmed to be in the correct hanging protocol prior to the radiologist read. Once confirmed, these images are then sent to the radiologists' workstation for interpretation.
- Diagnostic recall scheduler: Phone calls are made to those patients who have been recalled from a screening mammogram to schedule further imaging evaluation.
- Screening results: Normal results from screening examinations are given by a medical assistant. The patient is also informed of her breast density (per the new 2013 New York State law). The assistant will answer any questions the patient may have regarding the visit after discussing with the radiologist.
- Lab coordinator: Paperwork (laboratory requests and labels for specimens) is prepared for patients having a biopsy procedure.

Ideally, the most efficient daily workflow is to consistently have five radiologists each scheduled to see 15 diagnostic patients; true diagnostics (those presenting with a new concern), second opinions, checkups, and recalled patients from screening. In addition to the diagnostic schedule, each radiologist will read a portion of the daily MRIs. If there is a cancellation and enough time allows, the call center staff will try to fill the opening with another diagnostic patient from the waiting list. This scheduling works best for assistant staffing, imaging capabilities, and overall capacity of the building and parking lot.

In addition to the radiologists' diagnostic schedule, each will be assigned to read screening examinations throughout the day. Reader assignment is an automatic process that occurs as the patients are imaged. The screening examinations of patients waiting for their results are put in the correct work-list to be read by the radiologists. These patients, if requiring further work-up, will also be added to the radiologist's diagnostic schedule. The medical assistants help to ensure the radiologists continuously read the screening examinations of the patients waiting in the office for results [2]. The assistant will notify the radiologist specifically when there is a patient who has been waiting longer than usual as well as inform the radiologist when additional imaging that was requested is ready to be reviewed.

When the patient is ready to be seen by the radiologist, the assistant will escort the patient to the ultrasound suite. After reviewing the current study and any priors, the radiologist along with the assistant will join the patient in the examination room and go over medical history and existing problems. Physical examination and ultrasound are performed by the radiologist, with support of the assistant, and the results are then discussed with the patient. If a biopsy is determined to be necessary due to a suspicious finding, the radiologist will discuss this with the patient. The patient is most often told the biopsy can be performed right away, unless medically discouraged for reasons such as Coumadin or aspirin use. Most patients are thankful to be able to have the biopsy performed at the time of the appointment, but a few may choose to reschedule. The assistant will prepare the necessary paperwork as well as prepare the biopsy tray. If an ultrasound-guided biopsy is to be performed, the assistant will provide support with the procedure. After the biopsy and after post biopsy care is provided, the patient is given written aftercare instructions and the cell phone number of the radiologist, should any concerns arise after the procedure. Specimens are sent out to local laboratories for results which are usually available within 24 h, unless it is late in the day, Friday, or before a holiday. Each patient is called with the results personally by the radiologist who performed the biopsy whether the results are benign or malignant.

MRI Department

A brief history of incorporating breast MRI into our practice was provided earlier. The MRI addition to the building has

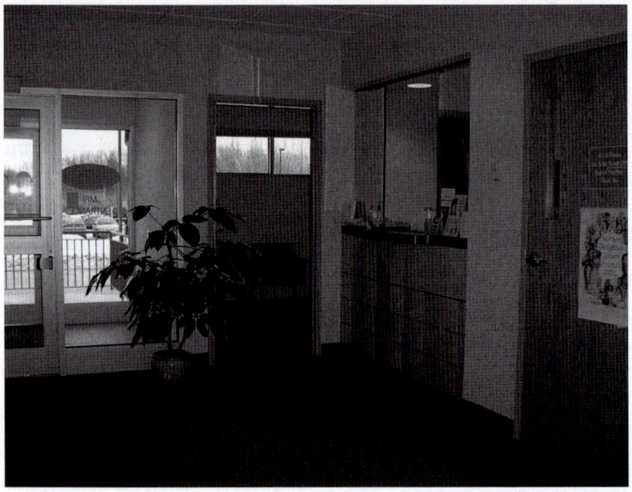

Fig. 18.18 The MRI department has a separate entrance, creating a quiet and calm environment

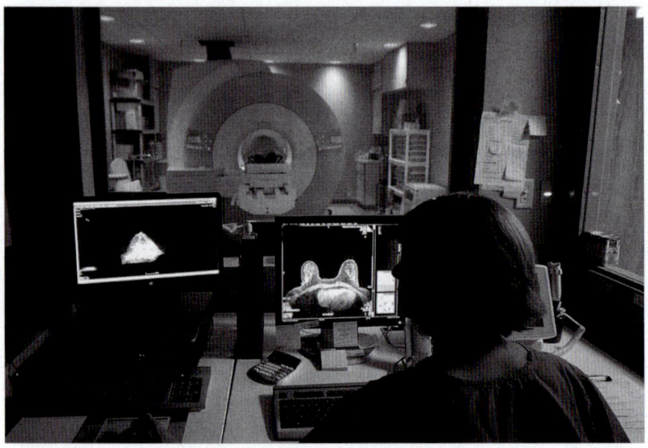

Fig. 18.19 View from the MRI technologist's workstation while scanning a patient

its own entrance and reception area, which adds a quiet, less congested atmosphere (Fig. 18.18).

The MRI department staff consists of two full-time office employees that assist with insurance pre-authorization, scheduling, and MRI contraindication screening. A nurse is on staff for intravenous access, for contrast injection, and for any emergencies or reactions that may arise. Three MRI trained technologists (one with MRI certification) rotate between the mammography department and MRI department, assisting with scanning and MRI-guided biopsies (Fig. 18.19).

Interestingly, in 2003 when first incorporating breast MRI, the majority of the examinations performed were for presurgical extent of disease evaluation; today the majority of the breast MRI examinations performed are for high-risk screening, reflecting the transition within our MRI practice and the implementation of our high-risk and genetics program (Fig. 18.20).

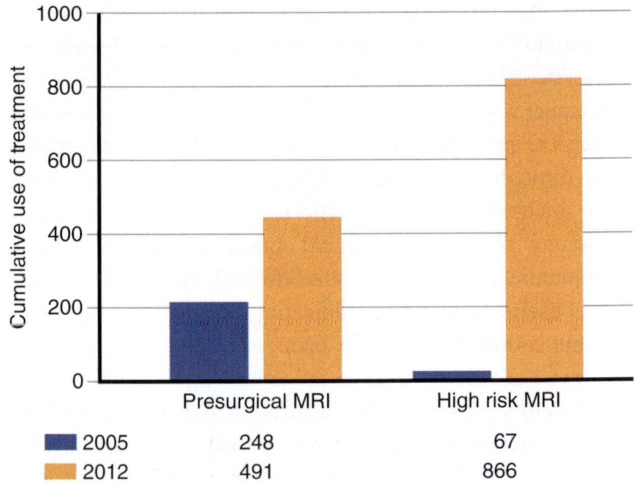

Fig. 18.20 Over the years, we have seen a change in the distribution of indications for breast MRI. In 2005, examinations performed for presurgical assessment were the most common; however, as of 2012, examinations performed for evaluation of high-risk patients had become more frequent than any other indication

Genetics Department

The need for a genetics program was based on several factors for us; the number of high-risk MRIs we were performing steadily increased over the last several years; our physicians found themselves spending a larger amount of time counseling patients regarding their risk of breast cancer, and patients were increasingly initiating the discussion with staff during visits at our facility. It has been estimated that approximately 1.4 million women in the United States have family history of breast cancer that, based on criteria established by the US Preventive Services Task Force (USPSTF), permits referral for genetic counseling and potentially genetic testing [8, 9]. Yet fewer than 2 % of respondents who would be candidates for genetic counseling report having been tested [8]. We began to understand that there was a need in our community for genetic counseling and testing, and being a comprehensive breast center, we felt it would be an important service we could provide to our patients.

We began to implement the program by utilizing the health history forms completed by patients. When a patient checks in at the front desk, the medical history information is entered by reception staff into the electronic dashboard. Patients are flagged if the responses on the health history form meet specified NCCN (National Comprehensive Cancer Network) guidelines [10]; high-risk flagging is based on two points (Table 18.1).

Letters are generated based on the high-risk flagging through the dashboard. Initially when we first began to implement this program, our nurse and a trained medical assistant called those patients who were flagged as potential

Table 18.1 High-risk flagging is based on a two-point assessment

Risk factor	Point assessment
Any family history of ovarian/cancer	Each occurrence, 1 point
Personal history of cancer age 50 and over	Each occurrence, 1 point
Personal history of cancer age 50 and under	Each occurrence, 2 points
Ashkenazi Jewish ancestry	1 point

high risk. We have found that approximately 17 % of our patient population is flagged as high risk. As the program progressed, we found that the demand was too high for our staff to keep up with, so we made the decision to hire a certified genetic counselor part-time. The need continued to grow and the position is now staffed full-time. The counselor now works with a trained medical assistant who fields an average of 30 calls daily. The assistant screens patients over the phone to determine if the patient is eligible to continue on to genetic counseling and/or testing. When a patient is determined to be eligible for counseling, the counselor performs a detailed interview. This helps to determine if the patient is eligible for testing. The primary model utilized is Tyrer-Cuzick risk assessment. Gail model or BRCAPRO may be used when Tyrer-Cuzick is not all inclusive for the particular patient; for example, if the patient has male family history, Tyrer-Cuzick cannot be used as it is not incorporated in the risk assessment with that model. All patients who undergo testing are asked to return when the results are available to have a discussion with the counselor as there is much to be discussed that can be quite detailed and complicated. The results are discussed, as well as the implications for the patient's family, and recommendations for medical management are provided. To date we have had 34 positive test results. By identifying patients with genetic mutations, we can review recommended medical management strategies for these patients, including breast MRI, preventative surgery, and/or chemoprevention. Patients can discuss results with their primary physician and establish a customized medical management plan. This helps us to provide the most comprehensive care we can to our patients.

Patient Advocates

Three patient advocates are utilized in our main office to help ensure that we meet the needs of our patients (Fig. 18.21). These staff members provide our patients with personal support and often provide immediate answers to questions a patient may have during the visit. These individuals check in with each inside waiting room at 30 min intervals to determine if there are any patient needs and questions they can address. In some instances, a patient advocate will become involved when a patient will require additional

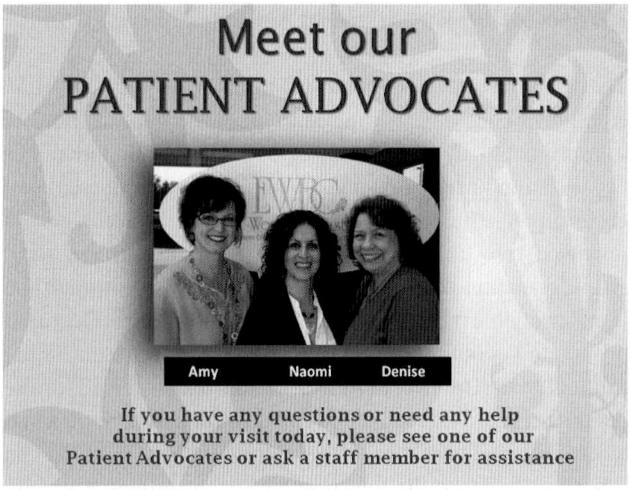
Meet our
PATIENT ADVOCATES
Amy
Naomi
Denise
If you have any questions or need any help
during your visit today, please see one of our
Patient Advocates or ask a staff member for assistance

Fig. 18.21 The patient advocates are always available to ensure that all patients' needs are met throughout their visit at our facility

imaging by talking to the patient about the fees associated with the additional views. This interaction is beneficial as it will allow the patient to become aware of the additional billing involved.

The advocates also serve as a liaison between the radiologist and the patient to assist with, for example, a newly diagnosed cancer patient who may ask about support services. In such an instance, our advocates can supply information about support groups and provide the patient with contact phone numbers.

Additionally, these staff members are often called upon to assist with a patient who has special needs or a patient who is anxious. For example, if a diabetic patient is in need of something to eat, the advocate will provide a light snack and juice. For a nervous patient, it is not out of the ordinary for an advocate to sit by her side through the whole appointment. The advocates also assist with patients who are underinsured or not insured at all. Our facility works closely with a government-run organization in our region that helps provide funding for uninsured patients. If a patient comes in with no insurance, a patient advocate will call this organization (Cancer Services) and help to qualify the patient for coverage. Over the last couple years, due to the high volume of patients currently under- or uninsured, we have opened up our schedule on several Saturdays throughout the year to screen these patients. Our patient advocates help coordinate this in association with Cancer Services, and on average, 65 patients will be scheduled. In addition to imaging, radiologists are present to perform physical examination and complete the breast care for these patients. This program is very important to our community as it provides care that may otherwise be unobtainable.

Transcription Department

The transcription department is staffed with four full-time employees and one part-time employee. The transcriptionists transcribe and edit approximately 140 diagnostic letters per day utilizing Fusion Text and Fusion Speech through Dolbey & Company, Inc. The text dictated by the radiologist is reviewed for clarity and accuracy by the department staff. All information contained in the text is verified through the use of available programs such as PACS and the RIS. Required billing and coding information is added if not present in the original text. Upon completion of the necessary edits, the document is provided to the radiologist for a final review and electronic signature. Once the radiologist signs off on the report, it is sent to the referring physician through a variety of methods as requested by the referring physicians, including faxing, mailing, or electronic delivery. There is also a built-in electronic delay in transmitting the reports to the referring physicians to allow time for our auditing staff to communicate any additional changes required to transcription staff. The majority of the reports are sent out within 24 h. Any additional changes that are required after the report has been signed and transmitted to referring physicians are made and sent as an amended document.

Billing Department

Our billing department is staffed with five full-time employees. Four are Certified Medical Coders and one is a Certified Professional Coder (CPC) with a Certified Evaluation and Management Coder (CEMC) specialty. In a private practice it is important to collect all reimbursement assigned per service performed. The overhead is very high, and in order to maintain the building, the equipment, and the staff, we have hired billing specialists to help us achieve the highest possible collection rate. After a patient has completed her visit, a billing sheet is generated to reflect the services provided, which is sent to the billing department for auditing. Before being processed to the insurance company, all billing sheets are audited for clarity; this is done by matching up the procedure and diagnosis codes to the examination report that will be sent to the referring physician. Once payment has been issued from the insurance company, it will be applied to the patient account. Our billing department will work with patients who have large out-of-pocket expenses due to high deductible insurance plans. These patients are given the ability to pay a monthly installment. The billing staff also offers large discounts to patients who cannot afford our services.

In addition to submitting to the insurance companies, every 2 weeks staff members are assigned to investigate claims for payments that are overdue (over 30 days). It is necessary to follow through to determine why the payers have not issued payment. This process is an important check to assure that "timely filing" (a rule in place by insurance companies to guarantee proper payment) is in place, so the center will not lose out on the claim. Periodically our CEMC specialist will check insurance websites to ensure the office is working in accordance with billing procedures and coding procedures. Additionally, this employee will run internal audits once a quarter to periodically check for accuracy. The results of this audit will be discussed with staff members; this allows us to determine where improvements can be made, with the hope of increased reimbursement rates.

Medical Records and Record Retention

The medical records department is staffed with five full-time employees. These employees oversee all aspects of maintaining the physical medical record, as well as burning compact discs at the request of the patient or referring physician. As our center is working toward an electronic chart, we still utilize a physical chart for all diagnostic and MRI appointments. Because of this, film requests and chart preparation are conducted several days ahead of the appointment. The medical records department staff also downloads patient studies from outside facilities into PACS and digitizes outside analog films so that the exams are available to the interpreting radiologist for comparison at the time of the appointment. Additionally, patients can drop off films or request images 5 days a week after the proper paperwork has been obtained.

Approximately 235,000 patient charts are stored on-site in a 3,470 square feet area with an additional 40,000 stored off-site at a secure location. Our policy is that a chart will stay on-site and never be destroyed if a patient has had a diagnosis of breast cancer. If the patient is deceased, the chart will be sent to off-site storage, but will never be destroyed. If a patient has not returned to our center in 10 years, the chart will be destroyed. All charts of deceased patients will be stored at the off-site location for 10 years and then destroyed.

IT and PACS Department

The IT and PACS department is made up of five full-time employees and one part-time employee. One staff member oversees all aspects of the dashboard, working on development and maintenance with the programmer. Two staff members manage PACS and are available to troubleshoot on a daily basis with staff members throughout the office. The PACS managers ensure that all exams are pre-fetched for the day. The PACS managers were integral to the transition of our facility to digital. The remaining members of the department serve as Windows Systems Administrator, Linux and Network Systems Administrator, and IT support. These staff members oversee the network and all system programs. Due to the electronic nature of our practice, the IT and PACS department is extremely vital to our daily operation. As we continue to make improvements within our facility, whether it be to establish a more efficient workflow or to integrate a new imaging modality, our PACS and IT department continue to play a major role. They address issues as they arise and work to ensure workflow is minimally interrupted when there is a problem. The department has helped to give us the ability to transition to a chartless environment.

Medical Outcomes

One full-time employee and two part-time employees electronically track all biopsy patients and collect all surgical information. This department is crucial for regulatory reporting, such as for Mammography Quality Standards Act (MQSA). This department also updates the electronic chart of every patient that is seen for an abnormality or is recalled from screening.

Human Resources

Our center has a dedicated human resource manager whose primary job functions are to hire new staff, research and implement benefit packages, assist with disability claims, manage payroll, and protect the rights of the employees while adhering to the rules and regulations set in place by the office and the government. The human resource manager has an open-door policy in place for grievances as well as suggestions.

Office Management and Marketing

Management

With any service-oriented business, it is crucial to maintain positive office morale and retain good employees. The office philosophy regarding staff has been to provide good benefits, competitive wages, and flexible work schedules in a safe environment. We cross-train the office staff to minimize job burnout and post new job openings to allow staff to migrate to jobs within the facility [2]. Having 134 employees and acknowledging the specialties of each department as well as maintaining open communication has been the key to maintain office morale.

Staff suggestions are welcome and often changes are made based on these suggestions. Each department has at least one team leader who is the supervisor. The team leaders are responsible for training new staff, updating department policy, maintaining the department schedule, and coordinating the department vacation schedule. The team leaders from all departments, along with the office manager, facilities manager, and human resource manager, hold weekly meetings during which time policy changes and office issues are discussed. This open flow of information between departments enables us to provide accurate and efficient services for our patients. The meeting notes are transcribed into a weekly office memo and are provided for the entire staff to ensure continued education for all.

With the costs of medical services increasing every year while reimbursement continues to decline or remain flat, radiologists are forced to be both a medical doctor and business manager. Practices are forced to make adjustments in all areas of their business. It is important to periodically evaluate contracts and renegotiate with insurance providers. When doing so, it is important to report on expenses. Our facility uses the relative value unit (RVU) cost analysis for this, as this will provide information on the cost of a procedure in comparison to provider reimbursement [11]. Being aware of your clinical outcomes and reporting on this information will provide the biggest advantage when negotiating with payers, proving that your service is providing excellent patient care.

Marketing

A facility will need to expend time and energy into retaining existing patients and recruiting new ones. The marketing plan should be revised yearly to adapt to the constantly changing medical climate [11]. Marketing your practice can be done by a number of methods. One method that we continually use is to solicit feedback through surveys from our patients and referring physicians. These surveys help us measure our patient and referring physician satisfaction level and provide us the knowledge that allows us to make changes that have a substantial impact. Patient and referring physician satisfaction will be the best source of marketing. If a patient receives exceptional care, it will be spread through word of mouth, as will a negative opinion if a patient is unhappy with the care received. The same goes for the referring physicians. It is crucial that a center maintains and exceeds the expectations of the patients and the referring physician base. During the office visit, we strive to satisfy the patient by prompt and courteous appointment scheduling, a respectful and pleasant check-in at the front desk, and a knowledgeable and efficient technologist interaction during imaging.

Outside of the office, a complete interactive website that is easily searchable is used to educate and inform new patients and returning patients. Educating the community is important; this can be done through fundraising events (American Cancer Society's Making Strides Walk) and support groups (Gilda's Club and American Cancer Society). Participation with local organizations is a good way to market the center with a visual presence. It is important that a successful center continues to lead the market with clinical and operational excellence as well as constant improvements to stay on the cutting edge.

New Technologies

A comprehensive breast center not only will need to stay informed of new technologies entering the field but will need to embrace and incorporate these technologies into practice. Our facility has a research department staffed with four full-time employees who coordinate clinical trials involving new breast imaging modalities. Over the years we have continued to add and also modify our daily workflow for research projects. The radiologists' role in research is conducted, for the most part, after hours. This has been as important as it allows our facility to stay current with technology and new modalities coming into the market. Digital breast tomosynthesis, breast computed tomography, automated breast ultrasound, ultrasound elastography, and CAD are examples of projects, both past and present, that we have participated in at our facility. Our patients have a very positive attitude toward research; they are willing to participate in studies that evaluate these new technologies. Our patients drive us to continue research as they question and demand better breast care and improved diagnostic techniques.

Conclusion

The design and operation of a comprehensive breast imaging center is critical to ensure effective workflow and daily operation. Seamless workflow is acquired through departments interacting and working in tandem. The support of the staff such as medical assistants and technologists helps to lighten the workload for the radiologists, allowing them to have the time necessary to evaluate a greater number of patients. Interoffice planning, communication, and education foster this proficient environment. This philosophy has proven beneficial as shown by a recorded patient return rate of 90 % from 2011 to 2012. It is always important to remember that breast cancer screening can be an emotional experience for a patient; having highly trained staff that are in tune to the needs of the patient is imperative for the success of the facility as well as patient satisfaction. Our mission has been, and always will be, to provide quality breast imaging and excellent patient care, considering the patients' physical and emotional well-being.

Acknowledgments The authors would like to thank Annette Wiebeld, MS, CPC; Diana Kissel, MS; and Anne Horan for their invaluable input.

References

1. American Cancer Society. Cancer facts and figures 2014. Atlanta: American Cancer Society.
2. Logan-Young W. The breast imaging center: successful management in today's environment. Radiol Clin North Am. 2000;38(4): 853–60.
3. Understanding Health Information Privacy. www.hhs.gov/ocr/privacy/hipaa/understanding/index.html.
4. Destounis S, Newell M, Pinsky R. Breast imaging and intervention in the overweight and obese patient. AJR Am J Roentgenol. 2011; 196:296–302.
5. Wee CC, McCarthy EP, Davis RB, Phillips RS. Screening for cervical and breast cancer: is obesity an unrecognized barrier to preventive care? Ann Intern Med. 2000;132:699–704.
6. Harisinghani MG, Blake MA, Saksena M, Hahn PF, Gervais D, Zalis M, et al. Importance and effects of altered workplace ergonomics in modern radiology suites. Radiographics. 2004;24: 615–27.
7. Somerville P. A Day at Elizabeth Wende Breast Care, LLC: Work and Patient Flow. Semin Breast Dis. 2008;11(4):169–79.
8. Hall IJ, Middlebrooks A, Coughlin SS. Population prevalence of first-degree family history of breast and ovarian cancer in the United States: implications for genetic testing. Open Health Serv Policy J. 2008;1:34–47.
9. US Preventive Services Task Force. Genetic risk assessment and BRCA mutation testing for breast and ovarian cancer susceptibility: recommendation statement. Ann Intern Med. 2005;143:355–61.
10. National Comprehensive Cancer Network clinical practice guidelines in oncology. Breast cancer screening and diagnosis. NCCN Version 1. 2012.
11. Wade T, Seifert P. Marketing the practice. Semin Breast Dis. 2008;11(4):187–94.

Emerging Technologies in Breast Imaging

19

Mary S. Newell and Anna I. Holbrook

Introduction

Mammographic screening has been validated as an effective way to decrease breast cancer deaths, responsible for a 30–40 % mortality reduction in participating populations. However, despite its success, it remains an imperfect tool, especially in certain subsegments of patients. Some cohorts for which mammographic evaluation proves less sensitive include women with dense breasts, women with genetic predisposition to breast cancers, and women with prior history of breast cancer. As a result, there is impetus to develop and refine new screening and diagnostic technologies that address the limitations of mammography. These include advanced mammographic applications such as digital tomosynthesis, stereoscopic mammography and contrast-enhanced digital mammography; dedicated breast computed tomography (CT); advanced applications of breast ultrasound and MRI; dedicated breast molecular imaging; and optical imaging. We describe these evolving technologies and outline their strengths and weaknesses.

Tomosynthesis

Tomosynthesis is thought to improve detection of cancers and reduce false-positive exams by eliminating the overlap of normal fibroglandular tissue (Fig. 19.1a, b). In tomosynthesis, an x-ray tube is moved in an arc above the breast and detector, and multiple images are obtained as the tube moves. These images are then reconstructed, creating a series of individual in-plane images through the entire breast [1]. Tomosynthesis has showed promising results and in 2011 was approved by the FDA [2]. Waldherr et al. found that one-view tomosynthesis had better sensitivity and negative predictive value than did full-field digital mammography (FFDM). This was true not only in dense breasts but also in fatty breasts. While 23 % of FFDMs required additional imaging to further evaluate a suspected abnormality, only 11 % of tomosynthesis exams did so [3]. Svahn et al. also found an improved sensitivity of one-view tomosynthesis when compared to FFDM (90 % vs. 79 %), but with no difference in false-positive exams [4]. However, data are conflicting when tomosynthesis is compared to FFDM, as some studies showed no difference in the diagnostic performance [5, 6].

In contrast, many studies have found optimistic results when examining tomosynthesis in combination with FFDM. Skaane et al. found that tomosynthesis in combination with mammography versus mammography alone resulted in a 27 % increase in the cancer detection rate ($p=0.001$), with a 15 % decrease in false positives ($p<0.001$). Also encouraging is that they found that adding tomosynthesis allowed for a 40 % increase in detection of invasive cancers [7]. Rafferty et al. had similar results, with a significantly increased area under the receiver operation characteristic (ROC) curve when tomosynthesis was combined with mammography compared to mammography alone. Recall rates for non-cancer cases significantly decreased for all readers. They also found that the increased sensitivity was greatest for invasive cancers [8]. Poplack and colleagues found a reduction of 40 % in the screening recall rate when tomosynthesis was used in addition to mammography [9], while Gur et al. found a decrease of 30 % [10]. A recent study by Rose and associates [11] found that after addition of tomosynthesis to FFDM in routine clinical practice, recall rates decreased from 8.7 to 5.5 % ($p<0.001$), and the positive predictive value for recalls increased from 4.7 to 10.1 % ($p<0.001$). Several studies have evaluated the use of tomosynthesis in lieu of additional mammographic views in characterizing noncalcified lesions. Some have found the two techniques to be comparable [12, 13], while Zuley et al. found that the area under the ROC curve (AUC) was significantly greater for

M.S. Newell, MD (✉) • A.I. Holbrook, MD
Department of Radiology and Imaging Sciences, Emory University, Atlanta, GA 30345, USA
e-mail: mary.newell@emoryhealthcare.org; anna.holbrook@emoryhealthcare.org

M.K. Shetty (ed.), *Breast Cancer Screening and Diagnosis: A Synopsis*,
DOI 10.1007/978-1-4939-1267-4_19, © Springer Science+Business Media New York 2015

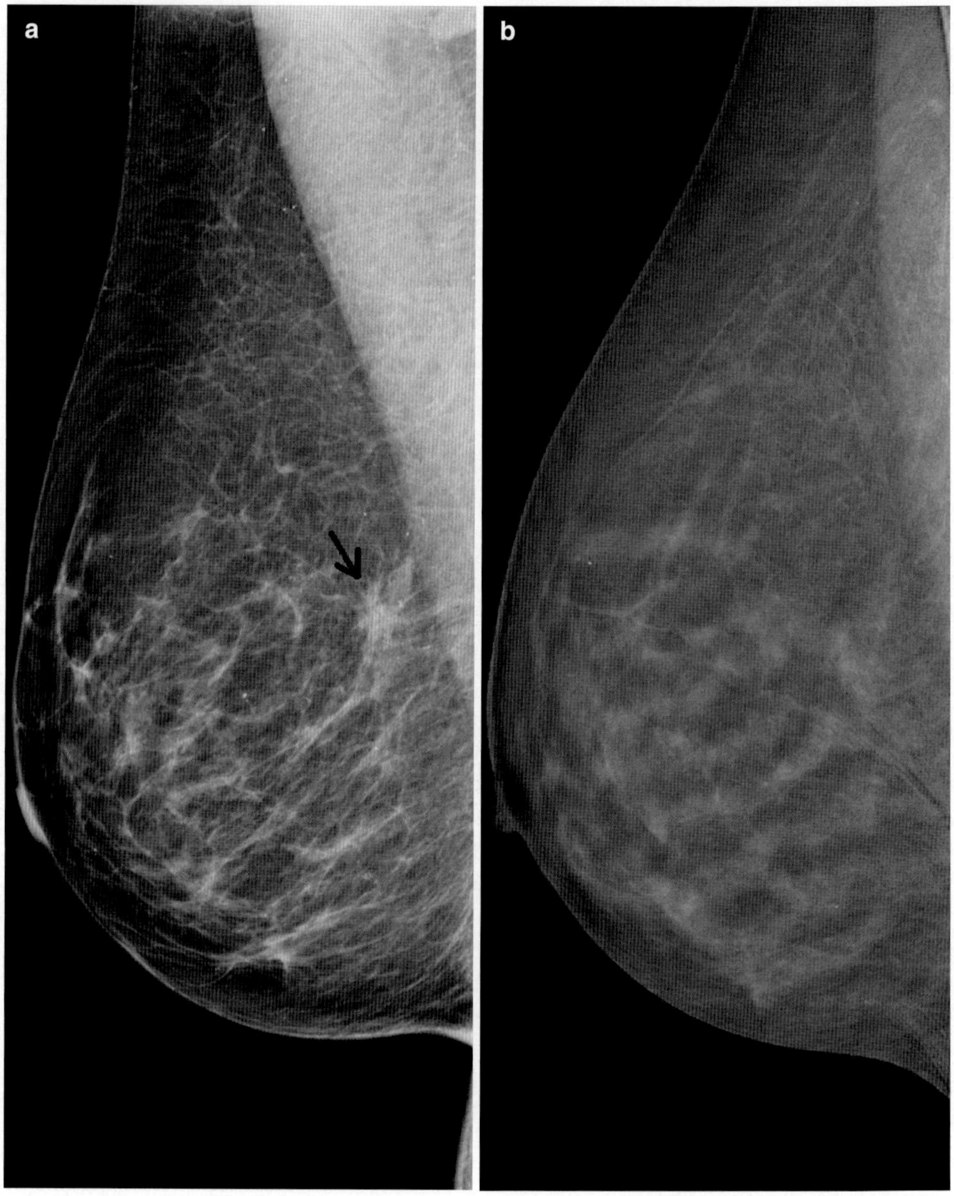

Fig. 19.1 (**a**) Mammogram (MLO view) demonstrates an area of possible architectural distortion (*arrow*). (**b**) Corresponding image from tomosynthesis examination shows no suspicious abnormality. The distortion was due to overlap of normal fibroglandular tissue (Images courtesy of Hologic® and Carl J. D'Orsi, MD)

tomosynthesis versus supplemental mammographic views (0.87 vs. 0.83) [14].

In order to decrease radiation dose and interpretation time, single-view as opposed to two-view tomosynthesis imaging has been explored. Wallis et al. found single-view tomosynthesis examinations to have equivalent diagnostic accuracy to a standard FFDM exam, while two-view tomosynthesis offered an improved accuracy, but only for readers with less than 10 years of experience [15].

Tomosynthesis is thought to be less sensitive than mammography for the detection of calcifications. This is due to images being reviewed as slabs of user-defined thickness. There is an inherent trade-off with the thickness of slabs: thicker slabs allow for the perception of 3D clusters of calcifications, but also lead to decreased spatial resolution of each individual calcification [16]. Poplack et al. found that in general, the image quality of calcifications was better with mammography than with tomosynthesis [9]. However, another study found that though FFDM was slightly more sensitive than tomosynthesis for the detection of calcifications, the diagnostic performance as measured by AUR between the two modalities was not significantly different [16]. Further improvements in image acquisition and display may lead to improvement in calcification detection. An additional drawback of tomosynthesis is an approximate doubling of interpretation time when compared to mammography alone [7, 15]. However, it is anticipated that this will be balanced by reduction in recalled screening examinations, follow-up studies, and biopsies [14]. Another limitation is increased radiation dose. Using tomosynthesis in combination with FFDM results in a doubling of radiation dose, though in many cases, this is still less than the FDA limit for a single standard mammogram exam [1, 8]. However, it is desirable to keep radiation doses as low as reasonably achievable. One solution to this is in the use of synthetically reconstructed two-dimensional images, created from the tomosynthesis data, in lieu of the additional corresponding full-field view. This technology has recently been approved by the FDA [17].

Stereoscopic Mammography

Similar to the idea behind tomosynthesis is that of stereoscopic mammography, which attempts to overcome 2D mammography's limitation of overlying normal tissue obscuring and mimicking lesions. Stereoscopic imaging uses two images of the breast acquired above and below the 0° axis. These images are viewed with cross-polarized glasses on a display consisting of two cross-polarized monitors at 110° from one another, each displaying one of the images, and a silver-coated glass plate bisecting the 110° angle (Fig. 19.2). In this setup, each eye sees only one of the two images, and the reader's visual system fuses the images into a single in-depth image. One study that evaluated stereoscopy clinically found that it had significantly higher specificity and accuracy and a lower recall rate when compared to standard mammography, with a similar sensitivity [18]. Further research will need to be done to confirm these results and to see if good results can be obtained at a lower radiation dose.

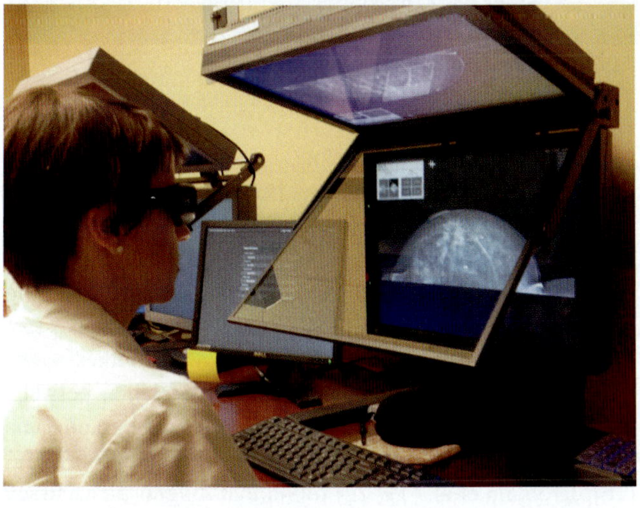

Fig. 19.2 Stereoscopic mammographic dedicated viewing station

Contrast-Enhanced Mammography (CEM)

Another modification that has been developed to overcome the limitations of conventional mammography is the addition of intravenous contrast. This is postulated to improve lesion detection due to the preferential uptake of contrast material within cancers, as seen in contrast-enhanced MRI (magnetic resonance imaging). Contrast-enhanced mammography could theoretically be an alternative for those unable to have an MRI.

There are two methods of obtaining contrast-enhanced mammographic images. One is to use temporal subtraction, in which a pre-contrast mask image is obtained followed by the injection of contrast and a series of additional exposures [19]. The mask image is then subtracted from those taken after contrast injection to show the distribution of contrast. This method is limited by the requirement for compression, motion artifacts due to long imaging times, and the ability to only image one breast in one view per injection. Another method uses dual-energy acquisition, in which, after iodinated contrast injection, two images are performed in rapid succession—a low-energy image below the k edge of iodine (33.2 keV) and a high-energy image above the k edge. The high-energy image preferentially demonstrates the contrast distribution, as photons just above the k edge are more likely to be attenuated by iodine than those below or far above it [20]. The images are then processed to suppress background breast tissue and highlight iodine-enhanced areas [21] (Fig. 19.3a, b). This dual-energy technique allows both breasts to be imaged in multiple views with only one injection [22]. It also permits shorter acquisition times, minimizing motion artifact and the duration of breast compression [22]. A disadvantage of this method is that as contrast is present on both acquisitions, some of the iodine is subtracted out of the processed image [20].

An initial study by Jong et al. showed that with the temporal subtraction method, 8/10 (80 %) cancers enhanced and 7/12 (58 %) benign lesions did not [23]. Another preliminary investigation by Diekmann and associates found that by using temporal subtraction, contrast could be seen within known tumors in all seven participating patients [24]. A subsequent study showed that adding temporal subtraction CEM to conventional mammography increased sensitivity for detecting cancer from 43 to 62 %. The improvement in sensitivity was even greater in patients with dense breasts [25]. Another study of temporal subtraction CEM found that its sensitivity for known cancers was 80 % [26]. Interestingly, in 2 of 20 patients, the cancers were in the posterior part of the breast and moved out of the field of view between the mask and contrast-enhanced images. This highlights one of the limitations of the temporal subtraction technique: prolonged acquisition times resulting in patient motion.

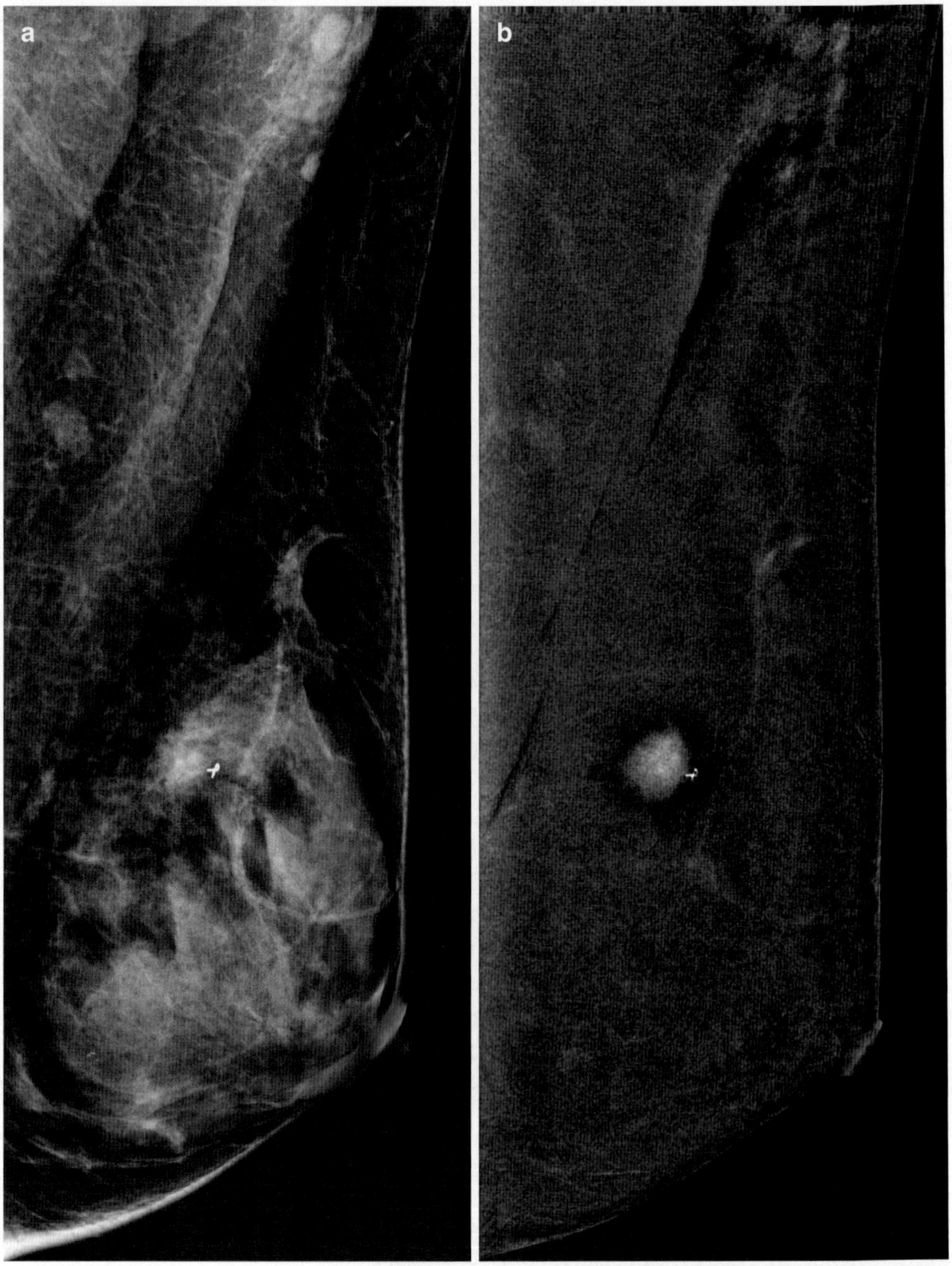

Fig. 19.3 A 48-year-old with grade 1 invasive ductal carcinoma, post biopsy. (**a**) Standard MLO view mammogram. (**b**) Dual-energy contrast-enhanced digital mammogram (CEDM). The cancer is not readily apparent on standard mammography (**a**) but is well demonstrated on CEDM (**b**) (Images courtesy of John Lewin, MD)

A preliminary study of the feasibility of duel-energy contrast-enhanced (DE CE) mammography was done by Lewin et al. [27]. They demonstrated that all 14/14 cases of cancer enhanced, while out of 12 patients with benign lesion, only 4 enhanced. Jochelson and associates compared DE CE mammography with conventional mammography and with MRI in 52 patients with known cancer [21]. They found that DE CE mammography and MRI both had a sensitivity of 96 % for index tumors, more than conventional mammography, which had a sensitivity of 81 %. Sixteen of the 52 patients had multifocal or multicentric cancers, and MRI was better at detecting these additional ipsilateral cancers than was DE CE mammography (88 % vs. 56 %). However, MRI had more false-positive findings (13/52 or 25 %) than did DE CE mammography (2/52 or 4 %). The Jochelson study found that the size of lesions as measured on DE CE mammography accurately represented the pathologic size in all but two patients, in which it overestimated the size by 1 and 1.7 cm. MRI accurately depicted the size in both. Another study, however, found that there was a good correlation between the size of lesions as measured on CE mammography and histological specimens (coefficient of correlation of 95 %) [26]. Dromain et al. [19, 22] found that diagnostic accuracy was improved when DE CE mammography was performed in addition to conventional mammography with or without ultrasound when compared to conventional mammography with or without ultrasound alone. The area under the ROC curve increased for each reader when DE CE mammography was added to conventional mammography +/– ultrasound.

Interestingly, unlike the rapid washout of contrast seen in malignancies during MRI imaging, enhancement with CE mammography remains present for at least 10 min. This may be due to differences between gadolinium and iodine [21] or as a consequence of breast compression [26]. Because of this lack of washout, kinetic enhancement information is not a helpful discriminator in CE mammography as it is in MRI [25].

Limitations of contrast-enhanced mammography include a decreased ability to evaluate the breast periphery due to a rind of increased density from radiation scatter [19, 21]. Additionally, there is a small increase in radiation exposure compared to conventional mammography. Several authors have calculated that the total additional radiation dose was equivalent to approximately one additional mammographic view [21, 22]. Lastly, there is a possibility of allergic reaction to the iodinated contrast, which can be life-threatening [22]. More studies will need to be done to verify that the risks are justified by a significant improvement in the detection of cancer.

Breast Ultrasound

Background

The appeal of using breast ultrasound (US) as a diagnostic adjunct to mammography was first noted in the 1960s–1970s, related to its "nondestructive technique" [28]. Kobayashi and colleagues reported early success using ultrasound to differentiate between benign and malignant breast lesions, employing a 5 MHz transducer and an automated system. They reported 84 % accuracy in predicting benign pathology and 90 % accuracy with malignant lesions, using only two sonographic criteria, which roughly correlate in today's terminology to (1) the echo pattern of the lesion itself and surrounding tissue (the latter actually concentrating on the posterior lesion margin) and (2) lesion posterior acoustic features [29]. Their cohort consisted only of palpable lesions that were suspicious enough to warrant excision/mastectomy, however. In addition, the smallest mass they were able to find was 5 mm, even when they were directed to the site in question by clinical findings. Dodd and associates concluded that US lacked the spatial resolution to detect and characterize subclinical cancers [28]. As a result, breast US was largely relegated to differentiating cystic from solid masses detected clinically or mammographically, at which it proved skillful. As sonographic equipment became more sophisticated, with resolution improved by the introduction of higher-frequency transducers of at least 10 MHz, US became an increasingly sought-after tool to supplement mammography in the evaluation of breast problems. Multiple studies have confirmed its utility in determining which mammographically detected solid masses might undergo short-term surveillance rather than requiring biopsy (negative predictive value in the region of 99.5 %), assuming strict morphologic criteria were followed [30, 31] (Fig. 19.4).

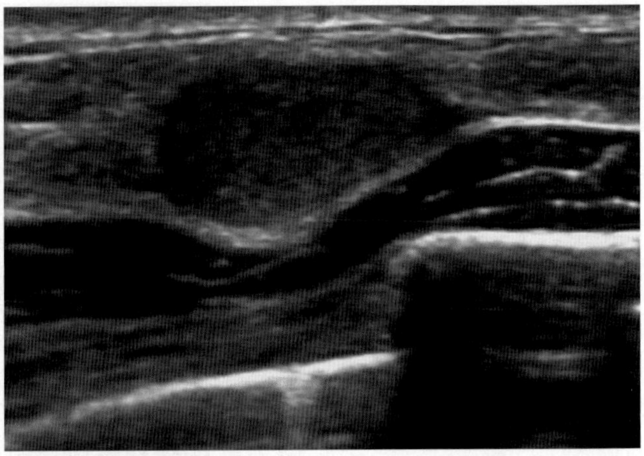

Fig. 19.4 This mass shows multiple features (gently lobulated margins, oval shape, parallel orientation, homogeneously mild hypoechogenicity, absence of suspicious features) that allow surveillance rather than biopsy, despite its solid nature

As the ability of breast US to find and characterize mammographically occult lesions became validated, the possibility of using US as an adjunct screening tool, at least for women at increased risk and/or with dense tissue, has gained momentum. ACRIN (American College of Radiology Investigational Network) 6666, a prospective multicenter study, was designed to compare mammography alone to mammography plus ultrasound in a screening setting, using a cohort of patients at elevated risk for breast cancer and heterogeneously or extremely dense breast tissue in at least one quadrant as determined by mammogram. Among their 2,637 patients, 12 cancers were seen on ultrasound alone, representing a supplemental yield of 4.2 cancers per 1,000 over mammography alone. The cancers found with US alone tended to be smaller and more often node negative [32]. Two additional multicenter studies have confirmed the results noted in ACRIN 6666 [33, 34], showing additional cancer detection yield of 4.2–4.4 per 1,000.

However, breast US has limitations, including imperfect specificity and, at least in the screening setting, many false positives. ACRIN 6666 revealed a near doubling of false-positive rate (8.1 % vs. 4.4 %), a lower positive predictive value for biopsy (PPV_2) (8.9 % vs. 22.6 %), and a higher rate of short-term follow-up recommendation (8.6 % vs. 2.2 %) with US alone compared to mammography. Thus, the additionally detected cancers came with a "price," including unnecessary biopsies and added work-up. Another limitation includes its

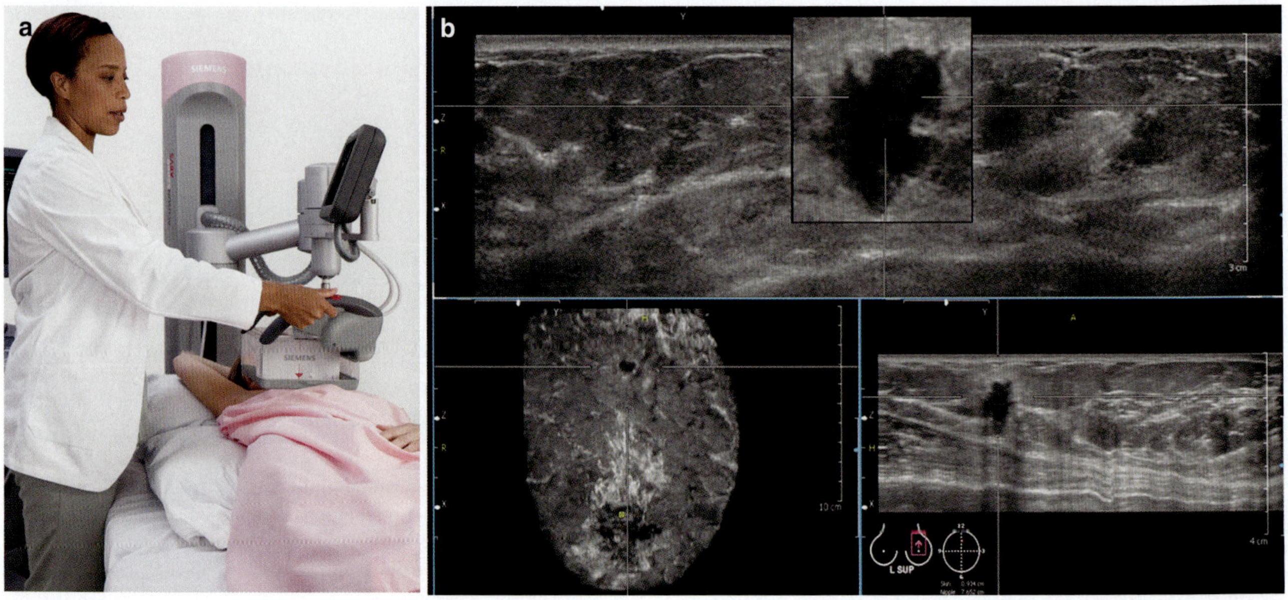

Fig. 19.5 (**a**) Automated whole-breast ultrasound unit with large footprint transducer covering breast. (**b**) Breast cancer outlined in three orthogonal views (Images courtesy of Siemens Healthcare)

diminished sensitivity for in situ cancers compared to mammography [32]. Handheld technique is also highly operator dependent: given its real-time nature, if a lesion is not detected and recorded during active scanning, it will be missed. In a screening setting, it is time and labor intensive, especially of concern when requiring physician scanning involvement during times of decreasing technical and professional reimbursement. In ACRIN 6666, the reported average scan time per patient was 19 min for a bilateral exam (often much longer in patient with large breasts or multiple findings), excluding time spent talking to the patient, reviewing and reporting the exam, and comparing to prior exams [32]. Evolving ultrasound technology is primed to address many of these limitations.

New Technologies

Automated whole-breast ultrasound (AWBU) is being revisited, improved, and refined after its introduction in the 1960s–1970s. AWBU has the potential to standardize and expedite study acquisition. It theoretically can be performed by a technologist without requiring physician involvement during scanning. A variety of prototypes are under development and clinical evaluation. Each uses unique acquisition and presentation methods and employs high-frequency probes. One vendor uses a robotically guided but standard transducer to scan the entirety of both breasts, with presentation of the images in a cine loop in 2D axial projection. Another employs a large footprint transducer placed over the central part of each breast with patient supine, with presentation of the reconstructed images in the coronal plane, as well as the orthogonal source images (Fig. 19.5a, b). A third prototype makes use of a custom transducer to scan a pendant, immersed breast, with presentation of 3D reconstructed images [35]. Wang and colleagues showed that the diagnostic accuracy of AWBU in differentiating benign from malignant lesions is comparable to handheld US [36]. A 2010 multicenter prospective screening study comparing mammography to automated whole-breast screening showed that automated US screening resulted in an increase in cancer yield by 3.6 per 1,000 compared to mammography alone [37]. These authors also found an improved PPV (30.7 % vs. 8.9 %) and a higher detection rate of subcentimeter US-only cancers (14.3 % vs. 6.2 %) when their automated technique was compared to the handheld technique used in ACRIN 6666. These results require validation by other large studies, but suggest the potential efficacy of AWBU for increasing throughput in a screening setting, while retaining accuracy. Some potential limitations of AWBU included its limited field of evaluation (the axillae and, with some systems, the periphery of the breasts are excluded) and diminished effectiveness with large breasts (deep lesions may not be well visualized/characterized). As specialized add-on equipment or complete replacement systems will be required to carry out AWBU, cost will rise.

Ultrasound elastography (USE) is another exciting emerging technology that may improve specificity for lesions detected with ultrasound, aiding in more cost-effective but equally safe management of these lesions. USE essentially evaluates the stiffness of tissue, as is done more grossly and subjectively during physical examination of the breast. Two types of USE are currently being evaluated: compressive (strain) elastography and shear-wave elastography (SWE). In each, one can ascertain the stiffness of a mass and its adjacent environment by observing its reaction to the application of an external stressor. With compressive elastography, gentle transducer pressure is used to apply external force (stress) to the surface of the breast over the

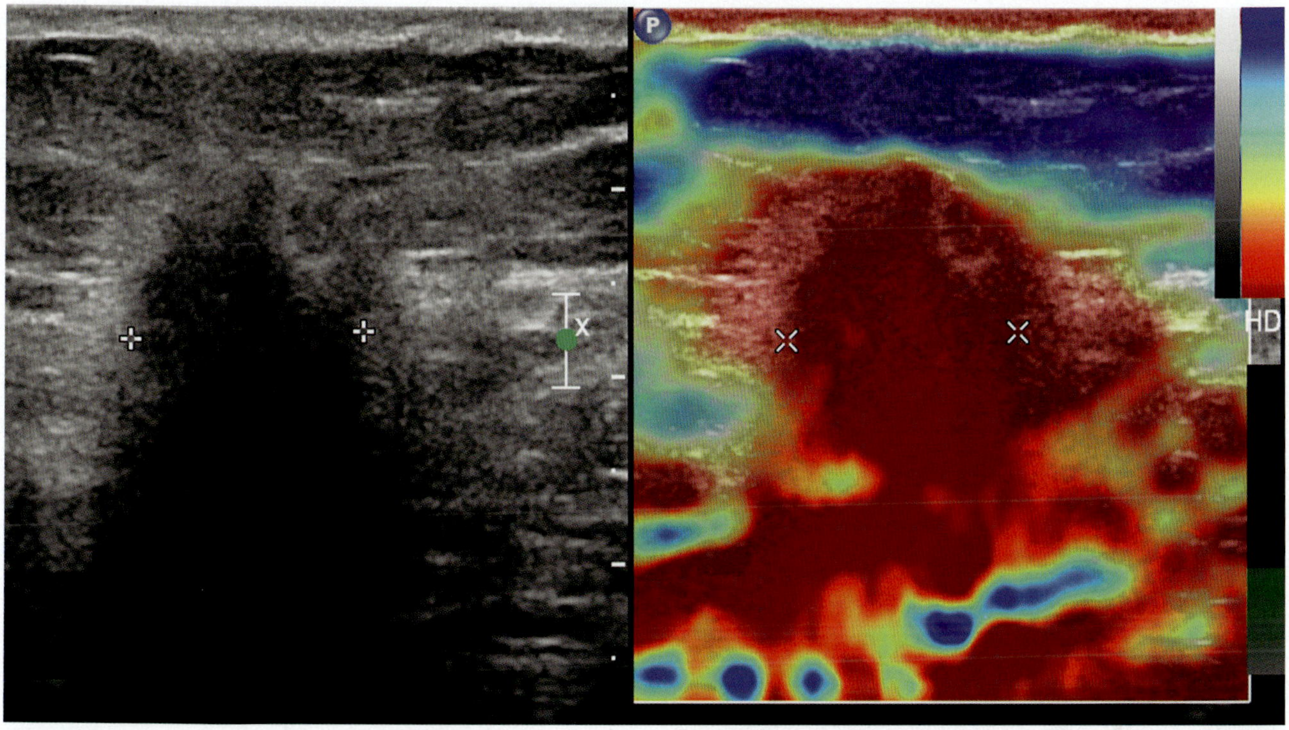

Fig. 19.6 Compression elastography. A mass is seen on standard US image (*left*). The corresponding elastogram (*right*) shows the mass to display low strain (assigned *red* here), indicating a firm consistency compared to other breast tissue. Note that the red coloration extends beyond the margins of the mass as outlined by cursor placement, indicating an Itoh score of 5

lesion in question; the resultant "strain" (the degree to which the tissue changes in shape, size, and position when the stress is applied) has implications about likelihood of malignancy. Upon detection of an equivocal lesion during real-time scanning, elastography software allows side-by-side display of the B-mode image and the corresponding "elastogram" (a color-coded visual display of the semiquantitative strain data generated automatically and behind the scenes) (Fig. 19.6). This elastogram is then qualitatively evaluated and/or assigned a score, as described by Itoh and associates [38]. They described a spectrum of elastogram patterns: a lesion displaying uniform high strain (diffusely soft and malleable) would receive a score of 1; at the other extreme, a lesion and its surrounding tissue showing low strain (firm and immobile) would receive a score of 5. A meta-analytic comparison of USE to conventional B-mode (N=5,511 lesions) showed an improvement in specificity from 70 % (B-mode) to 88 % (USE) [39]. However, USE alone was far less sensitive than conventional US (79 % vs. 96 % for B-mode), demonstrating that this technique cannot serve as a replacement for conventional US, but rather as a triage tool that may allow safe deferral of biopsy of borderline suspicious (i.e., BIRADS (Breast Imaging and Reporting System) 4a) lesions which have a low elastography score, thereby decreasing the unacceptably high false-positive rate of screening US. This method of USE has some intrinsic limitations. It is operator dependent (related to subjective application of "light" transducer pressure as the source of mechanical stress) and semiquantitative in nature and therefore may lack reproducibility [40].

Shear-wave elastography (SWE) represents another method of interrogating the stiffness of tissue. Instead of relying on transducer pressure to stress tissue, SWE measures tissue stiffness by calculating the speed at which that tissue variably propagates shear waves. These shear waves are generated as a result of a transducer-produced acoustic radiation force impulse (ARFI), which perturbs the tissue (Fig. 19.7). Ultrafast scanning is required to record the minute degrees of tissue displacement that occurs as the transversely oriented shear waves travel through tissue at varying speeds, depending on tissue stiffness. As the stress imparted by this pulse wave is known, the resultant strain of the interrogated tissue can be quantified. SWE requires no active participation by the technologist over and above scanning and therefore is operator independent and highly reproducible. Therefore, SWE mitigates many of the limitations of strain elastography. This technology is coupled with B-mode imaging. Research is ongoing to determine which single or combination of elastographic features (e.g., quantitative features such as maximum, median, or minimum elasticity value; elastographic lesion homogeneity; elastographic shape; elastographic lesion size vs. B-mode size) serve best to improve specificity and even sensitivity. Results of the BE1 Multinational Study [41] comparing conventional US to US plus SWE confirmed that by considering certain elastographic features, some BIRADS 4a lesions could be safely downgraded. In addition, some BIRADS 3 (and even BIRADS 2) lesions were accurately upgraded: 4 of 4 BIRADS 3 lesions that were morphologically benign appearing but showed suspicious elastographic

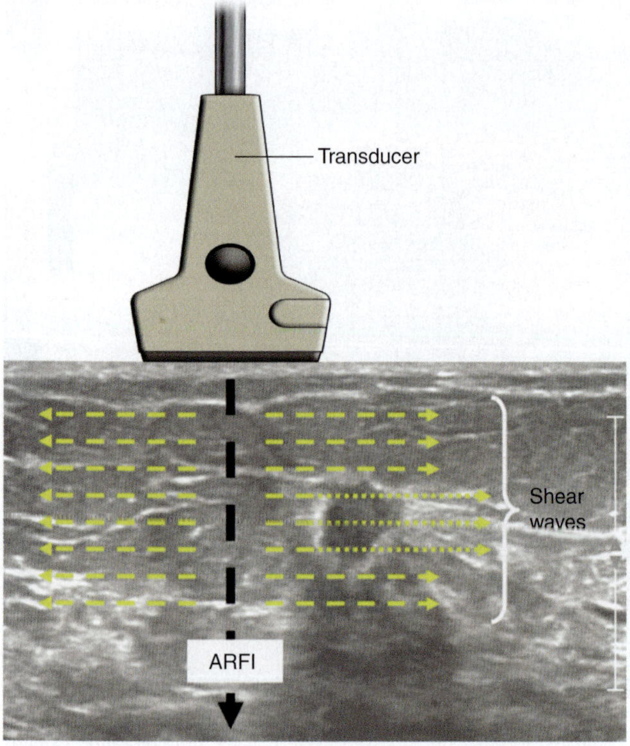

Fig. 19.7 Schematic of shear-wave propagation. An acoustic wave force impulse (*ARFI*) is sent from transducer into breast, resulting in propagation of transverse shear waves. These waves traverse the mass present here faster than normal tissue and can be quantified and visually displayed

features proved to be cancer. By adding SWE, specificity was increased from 61.1 to 78.5 %. Both SWE and strain elastography allow accurate differentiation of complicated cysts from solid masses, a situation encountered frequently when using US in both the screening and diagnostic arenas, allowing improvement in specificity and diminishment in false positive biopsy and short-term follow-up rates.

The use of computer-assisted diagnosis (CADx) for US is another way that improved performance can likely be realized. As opposed to computer-assisted detection technology used in mammography, US CADx is used not to detect lesions but to help predict their likelihood of malignancy once detected, based on combined morphologic features. Kashikura and associates showed that reader accuracy (as measured by AUC) on the average improved from 0.716 to 0.864 ($p = .006$) when CADx was used by three experienced imagers to help evaluate a series of 390 US masses [42].

Dedicated Breast Computed Tomography

Dedicated breast computed tomography (DBCT) represents an additional investigational modality that seeks to address the 2D limitations imposed by standard mammography. Its theoretical appeal includes the ability to image and display the breast in isotropic three-dimensionality, as has been exquisitely demonstrated when imaging other organs, and the lack of need for breast compression.

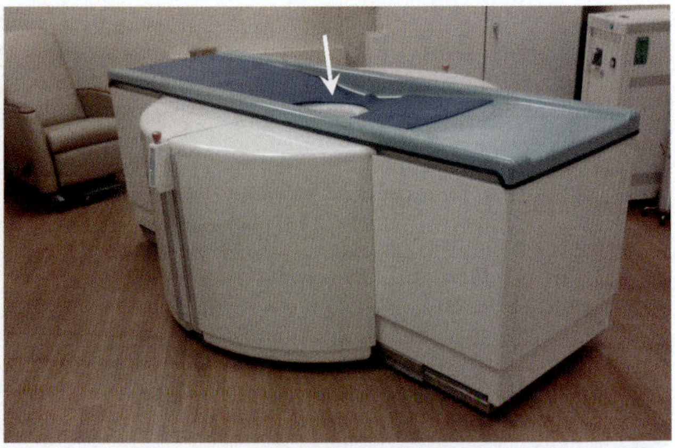

Fig. 19.8 Dedicated breast CT scanner. The patient lies prone and hangs breast in vertical gantry (*arrow*) (Courtesy of Ioannis Sechopoulos, PhD)

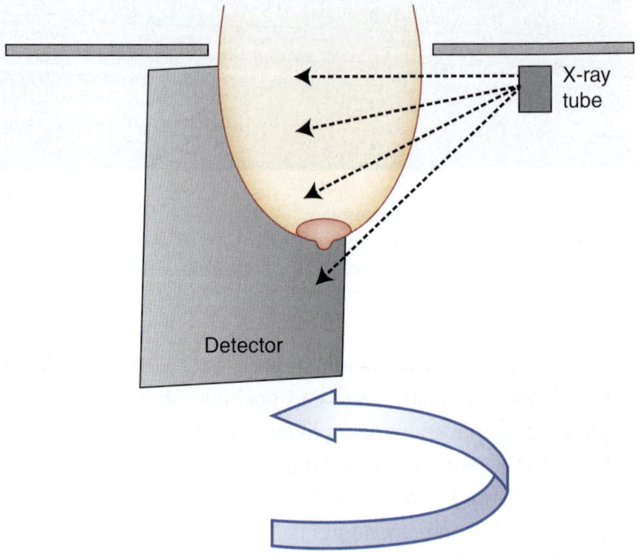

Fig. 19.9 Schematic of dedicated breast CT scanner. The X-ray source consists of a half cone beam (collimated to target only breast) and detector, both of which rotate in synchronized opposition around the pendant breast

Several prototype models are undergoing evaluation. They are configured such that the patient lies prone on a table with her breast placed pendant into a dedicated gantry (Fig. 19.8). Rather than traditional cone beam geometry used for whole-body CT, a half cone beam is used, dictated by the need for the X-ray tube and the detector to rotate as closely opposed to the undersurface of the table as possible to allow visualization of posterior breast tissue and, optimally, a portion of chest wall (Fig. 19.9). Flat panel detectors are used, with a 40×30 cm field of view (PAXSCAN™ detector, Varian Imaging Systems®, Salt Lake City, UT, USA). A variety

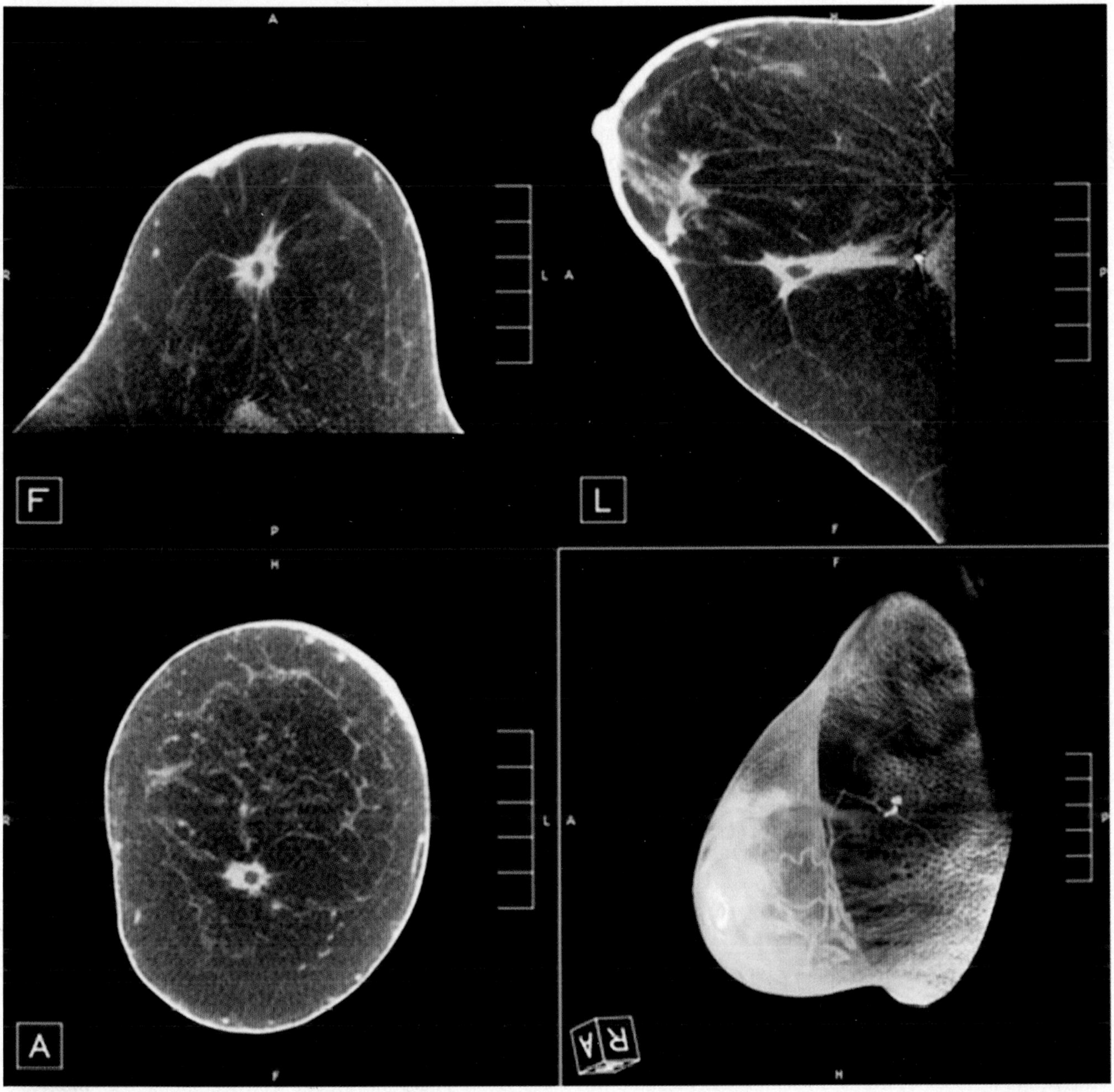

Fig. 19.10 Non-contrast breast CT. A mass (showing spiculated margins but central fat: fat necrosis) is displayed in three orthogonal views. A maximum intensity projection (*lower right*) is also displayed, which can be rotated in any projection (Courtesy of Hologic® and Carl J. D'Orsi, MD)

of X-ray source types has been employed, operating at kVps from 49 to 80, with resultant scan times ranging from 10 to 16.6 s, allowing single breath hold [43]. These original prototypes allow spatial resolution in the range of 150–400 μm, less than is achieved with standard digital mammography [44]. The images are reconstructed in three orthogonal planes and evaluated by scrolling through an imaging volume. 3D and maximum intensity projection (MIP) can be created as well (Fig. 19.10). Using this general technique, radiation dose per breast per series is comparable to a two-view mammogram [45].

Adequacy of breast coverage was evaluated by O'Connell and associates. They found that greater tissue inclusion was demonstrated medially, laterally, inferiorly, and posteriorly, with equivalent coverage noted superiorly. However, by using axillary nodes as a marker for comparison, they noted that mammography allowed better coverage of axillary tail. Patient acceptance must be considered in evaluating this modality, since avoidance of breast compression is touted as a potential advantage. O'Connell's group also assessed patient acceptance and comfort. A minority of patients (13 %) found DBCT to be less comfortable than mammography, with most finding it more (43.5 %) or equally (43.5 %) comfortable compared to mammography [45].

The clinical data regarding DBCT are relatively sparse. Initially, work was done without the use of intravenous contrast. Lindfors and colleagues scanned a cohort of 69 women with BIRADS 4 or 5 lesions, as well as 10 healthy volunteers. They compared DBCT images to the patients' mammograms in a nonblinded fashion for lesion conspicuity. Overall, there was no difference in lesion detectability between modalities; however, masses were better seen with DBCT, and calcifications were better detected with mammography, reaching significance in both scenarios [46]. These data were confirmed on follow-up studies by the same group [43] and suggest that the lack of comparable spatial resolution achieved with the original DBCT prototypes limits the clinical efficacy of DBCT, at least in the non-contrast setting, when evaluating calcifications. O'Connell et al., using a different prototype scanner, also found, in comparing mammography to non-contrast DBCT, that CT was inferior in detecting calcifications when compared to mammography. In their study, 13.5 % of calcifications seen on mammography were not detectable on DBCT [45].

Non-contrast DBCT is dependent on morphology and differences in intrinsic soft tissue contrast to allow lesion detection. More recent work has looked at leveraging the physiological differences between normal parenchyma, benign tumors, and malignant lesions by using intravenous contrast material, as has been done with breast MRI. In a study of similar design to that described previously, Prionas and associates compared mammography and non-contrast DBCT to contrast-enhanced DBCT (CE-DBCT) in 46 women with BIRADS 4 or 5 lesion who underwent all three imaging studies prior to biopsy. They found that all malignant lesions ($N=29$) were better seen on CE-DBCT than on mammography, especially masses. Interestingly, malignant calcifications ($N=7$; 5 of 7 were pure DCIS) were also better seen on CE-DBCT, albeit only slightly and not reaching statistical significance. Conversely, benign calcification was seen with greater conspicuity on mammography, raising the possibility that CE-DBCT might allow for greater specificity in calcium evaluation by essentially "missing" benign calcifications. Since degree of enhancement is quantifiable, these investigators were able to show that differential enhancement may allow prediction of malignancy, with an area under the ROC curve of 0.876 [47].

The logistics of CE-DBCT deserve consideration. One of the benefits of dynamic contrast-enhanced (DCE) MRI is that robust temporal and spatial information is obtained with technology that allows parallel imaging of both breasts synchronously. With DBCT, however, only one breast is imaged at a time. It has not been established how best to combine the imaging of both breasts with the timing of contrast administration. Prionas' group [47] used the following scan sequence: pre-contrast unaffected breast, pre-contrast affected breast, post-contrast affected breast, and post-contrast unaffected breast. Therefore, two patient position changes were required. Obviously, some kinetic data are lost in this situation when compared to DCE MRI, where multiple sequential and bilaterally parallel postcontrast time points are acquired. This group, however, noted that morphology is likely more important than kinetics when evaluating lesions, and DBCT with its superior resolution, may make this logistical point relatively moot. Further study is needed to validate that observation. Prionas' group also reported that decisions regarding contrast dose and delay after injection were derived empirically. Again, ongoing work will help determine optimal scanning protocols.

The early work regarding DBCT appears promising. In an interesting discussion of what the "perfect" replacement for mammography would look like, Kalender et al. noted that that tool must meet the following specifications: 3D capabilities, good soft tissue contrast, dynamic/kinetic proficiency, high spatial resolution (100 μm), dose comparable to two-view mammography, patient comfort without need for significant compression, biopsy capabilities, and low cost [48]. It appears from these studies that DBCT comes close to meeting this challenge. However, a few concerns remain. The original prototype models, on which the available clinical studies have been performed, offer spatial resolution in the range of 300–400 μm, inferior to that demanded by Kalender. However, several groups are working on new prototypes that achieve improved resolution while maintaining acceptable dose, using spiral technique and other modifications [48, 49]. Additionally, a "clinic-ready" fully shielded model has been developed that employs an open geometry which will allow integration of a (yet-to-be-developed) biopsy system. Its developers indicate that a clinical throughput of 11 min/patient can be expected and a cost comparable to a tomosynthesis unit [49]. Even the original prototypes achieve a rapid per-sequence scan time of 10–16 s. Thus, the kinetic considerations will likely be addressed. These new prototypes await clinical validation. Although it appears that the theoretically "perfect" breast imaging machine has nearly been built, it remains to be seen if DBCT can garner the excitement that DCE breast MRI and tomosynthesis have.

Magnetic Resonance Imaging

Magnetic resonance imaging (MRI) has been validated as a robust breast imaging tool, largely related to its high sensitivity for detection of breast cancer, in the range of 94–99 %. Its many indications include high-risk screening, determination of the extent of disease in newly diagnosed breast cancer patients, assessment of treatment response in patients undergoing neoadjuvant hormonal or chemotherapy, problem-solving in selected cases where a suspected imaging finding can be neither dismissed safely nor validated/localized by standard imaging, and further evaluation of suspicious clinical symptoms where a biopsy target or cause cannot be identified by routine imaging. However, it suffers from some drawbacks, including reported relative low specificity (range 37–86 %) [50] and high cost, when compared to mammography. Newer technologies, which explore parameters other than lesion morphology and kinetic enhancement characteristics, are being developed to address these limitations.

Magnetic Resonance Spectroscopy (MRS)

Magnetic resonance spectroscopy interrogates the chemical composition of tissue in vivo in a noninvasive manner. This technique has been applied to the brain and prostate with success and continues to undergo investigation for use in breast cancer evaluation. The bulk of chemical material in the breast consists of water and fat. However, other molecules can be detected via MRS, including some relatively specific for breast neoplasia, namely, choline-containing compounds (grouped together and referred to as total choline). These molecules have a role in membrane synthesis and metabolism and therefore may serve as signature molecules for the presence of breast cancer, where such metabolism is elevated. This total choline is present in high enough concentrations that its presence can be detected by the small magnetic field alterations its protons create (Fig. 19.11a, b). Choline can be present in normal breast tissue and benign breast lesions, indicating that quantification and not just identification of its presence is paramount [51]. One appealing potential use for MRS would be to increase the specificity of MRI. Bartella and associates found that by incorporating MRS into the MR protocol, the positive predictive value of biopsy could be increased from 35 to 82 %, with MRS showing specificity of 88 %, while maintaining 100 % sensitivity [52]. Dorrius and colleagues showed that BIRADS 3 lesions could be accurately reassigned based on choline concentrations. In their study, the use of MRS would have allowed proper identification of the two of eight malignant lesions initially called BIRADS 3 on routine MRI as well six of eight benign lesions that could have been safely reassigned to the BIRADS 2 category. There was no overlap between the choline concentrations of benign and malignant lesions, and their AUC was 1.00, compared to 0.0964 for standard MRI [53]. However, both studies only interrogated lesions 1 cm or greater in size. Tozaki's results were less compelling, showing overall sensitivity and specificity of 44 and 85 %, respectively. When only lesions >1.5 cm were considered, sensitivity increased to 82 % but specificity fell to 69 % [50].

Another area where MRS may be useful is in the early prediction of treatment response to neoadjuvant chemotherapy (NAC). An optimal tool would allow prediction as early in treatment as possible, to allow midcourse regimen change in nonresponders. Mammography, ultrasound, and physical exam rely on decrease in tumor size as a marker of response, but this has been shown to be unreliable in some cases and may lag behind real response. MRI is a more accurate tool, as it can show physiologic changes that may precede size change [54]. However, as MRS is measuring tumor metabolites in the form of choline compounds, it could provide even more specific information about treatment response and cell death. Meisamy showed that using a 4 T unit, changes in tumor choline concentrations could be detected within 24 h after treatment initiation [55]. Tozaki used a 1.5 T unit to show that this indication was feasible with current clinically available hardware and found that tumor choline was reduced after two treatment cycles in eventual responders compared to nonresponders, despite no significant change in tumor size at that point between the two groups. Positive and negative predictive values were 89 and 100 %, respectively [56].

MRS is hampered by several limitations. Lesion size is one. Most studies have narrowed inclusion criteria to lesions ≥1 cm, as partial volume averaging makes specific detection of choline difficult in smaller lesions. This decreases its utility for lesion characterization/management, especially in non-mass enhancements. However, Razek and colleagues were able to show improved sensitivity and specificity over MRI for lesion characterization even for lesions as small as 0.5 cm with MRS, when using a 3 T system. They attribute their favorable results to higher field strength [57]. Other limitations of MRS include low sensitivity for detection of DCIS, as choline is often absent in in situ lesions; the capability of examining only a single lesion when single-voxel technique (most common) is used; and false-negative exams, especially when inadequate fat suppression allows the spectroscopic peak of fat to broaden and obscure the relatively small choline peak. Additionally, no commercial analytic software has been developed specific to breast MRS [58]. Therefore, for several reasons, MRS remains outside of routine clinical practice at this point, but holds promise.

Diffusion-Weighted Imaging (DWI)

Diffusion-weighted imaging is another emerging MRI technique that probes lesion physiology and local architecture rather than just morphology and kinetic characteristics. It assesses the ability of water to move freely and randomly in tissue (Brownian motion). This motion may be relatively restricted under certain circumstances, such as in the presence of increased cellular density, cellular swelling, changes in membrane permeability, and the presence of cell lysis.

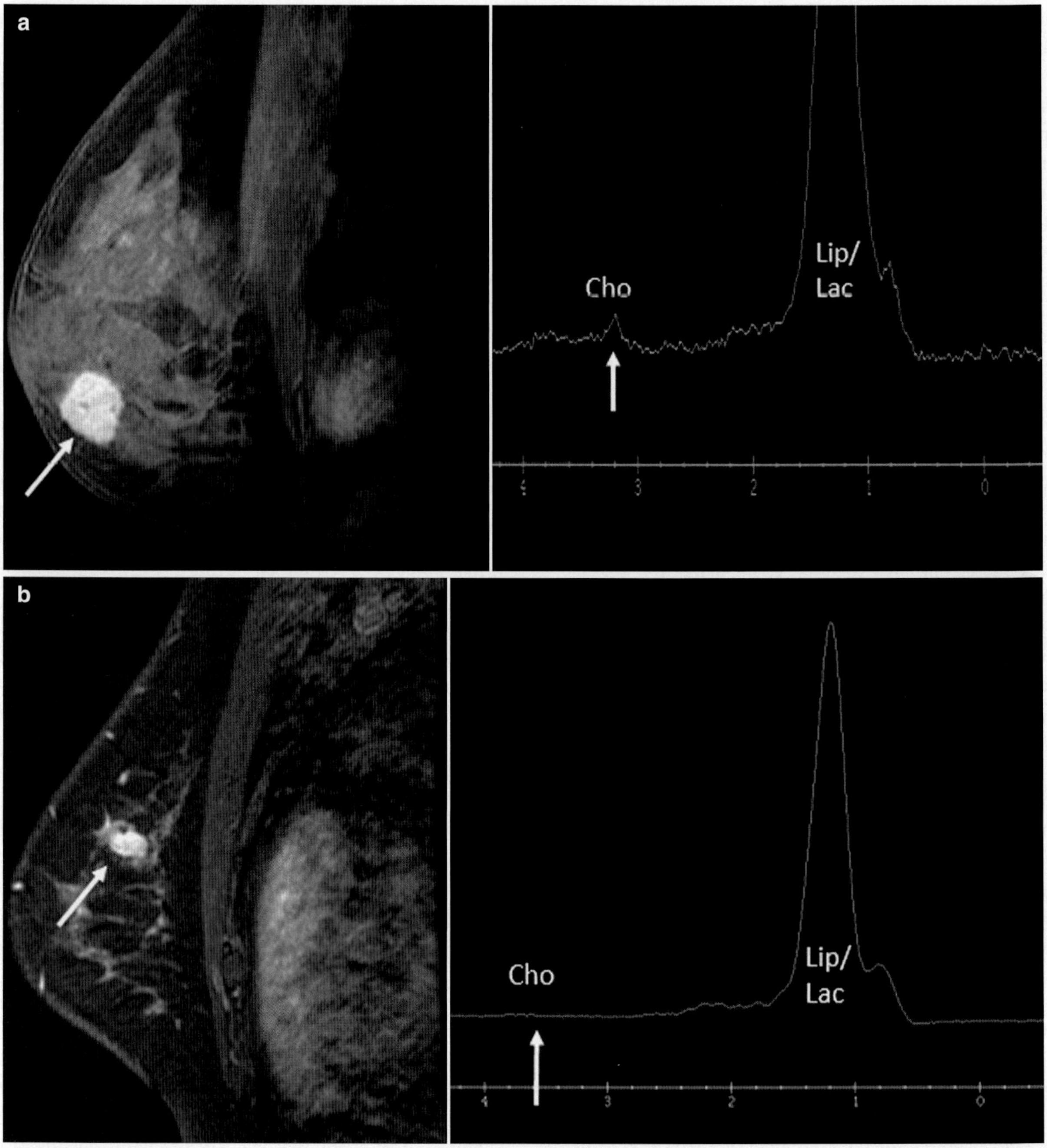

Fig. 19.11 Examples of MR spectroscopy (MRS). (**a**) The malignant mass shown on conventional post-contrast MR image on *left* (*arrow*) displays an elevated choline peak (*right*, *arrow*) when interrogated by MRS. (**b**) The fibroadenoma outlined on post-contrast MR image (*left*, *arrow*) shows no elevation in choline spectral peak (*right*, *arrow*), in keeping with its benign nature. *Lip/Lac* lipid/lactate (Images courtesy of Sunitha B. Thakur, PhD)

Each of these may occur in cancer. As a result, the free motion of water is restricted compared to adjacent normal tissue. This process can be quantified, referred to as the apparent diffusion coefficient (ADC), and can be mapped to allow correlation to standard images of the breast (Fig. 19.12). Many studies have confirmed that the ADC values differ between malignant and benign lesion, with ADCs tending to be lower in cancers (likely related mainly to dense cellularity) [59, 60]. Partridge and associates showed that low ADC was a significant predictor of malignancy and that even when a relatively high discriminating ADC threshold was set so as to allow 100 % sensitivity, biopsy could have been avoided in 33 % of benign cases. Very importantly, that group demonstrated that the improved PPV was realized for non-mass

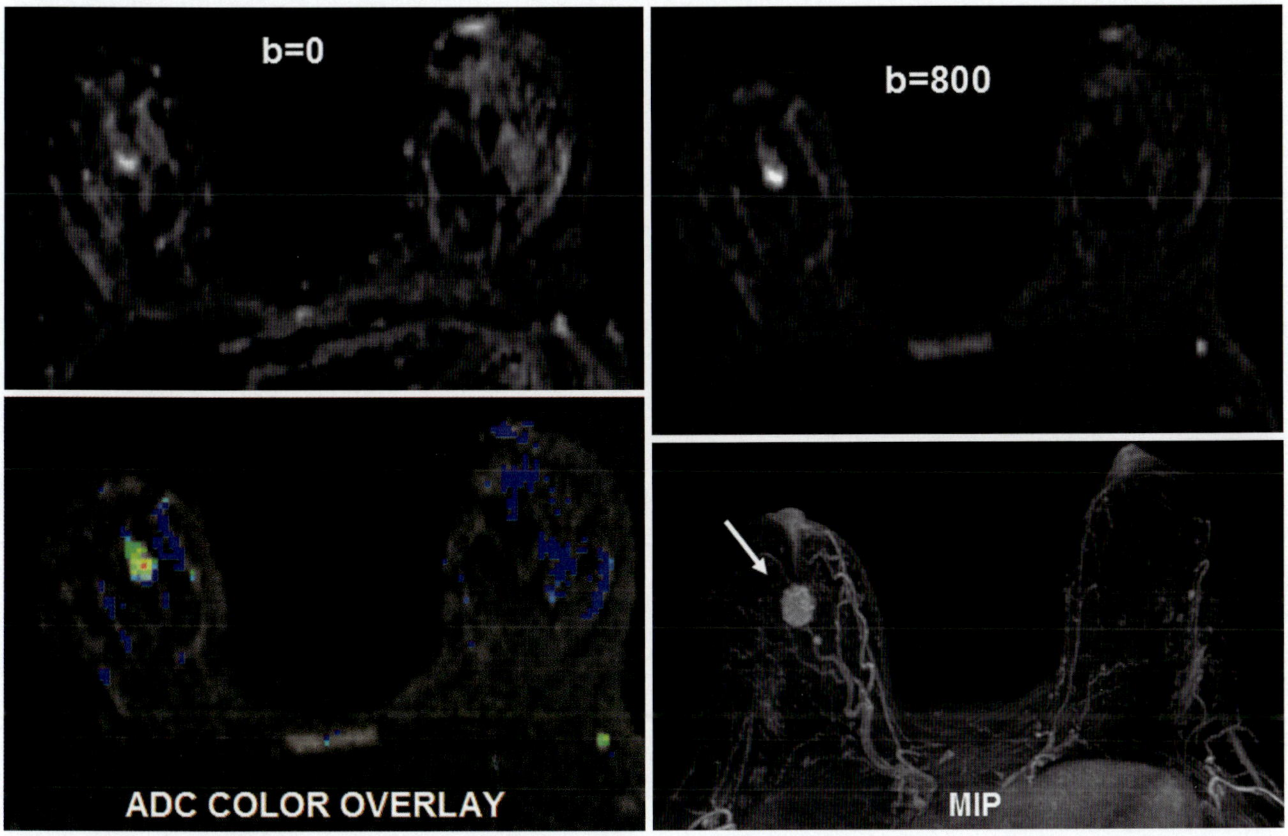

Fig. 19.12 Diffusion-weighted imaging. The cancer seen on the MIP imaged (*lower right, arrow*) can be visualized on the DWIs (*top images*) obtained at b values of 0 and 800. Average ADC (1.0 in this case, *low*) is calculated for area of interest, and values are qualitatively displayed by color map (*lower left*) (*red* low ADC) (Courtesy of Hologic®)

lesions and lesions <1 cm, a weakness for MRS [61]. Pinker and associates developed an interpretation system that combined BIRADS features with ADC values. They set ADC discriminator thresholds and used those to potentially modify BIRADS final assessments. For example, if a mass was assigned BIRADS 4 assessment based on morphology and kinetics, but had and ADC >1.39, it was reassigned as a BIRADS 2 lesion. Conversely, a BIRADS 3 lesion could be upgraded if it had an ADC less than the threshold value. Using this system, the group maintained the high sensitivity of standard MRI but improved specificity to 89.4 % [62].

DWI may allow early detection of treatment response to NAC. Several studies have shown that ADC values rise as tumors respond to treatment, often before a change in tumor size is noted and as early as 3 weeks after the start of therapy [63–65]. This likely reflects a change in cell density as tumor dies. DWI may also be able to predict the presence of an invasive component when DCIS is evaluated with MRI. Mori and colleagues showed a statistical difference between the ADC of invasive disease and surrounding DCIS, outlining an invasive nest as small as 1.5 mm [66]. Other exciting work suggests that axillary nodal metastasis detection may eventually become noninvasive. Two groups have found that ADC values between normal nodes and malignant nodes differ significantly [67, 68]. Unfortunately, the groups differed regarding whether involved nodes displayed an increased or decreased ADC compared to normal nodes. This brings to light some important limitations regarding DWI. There is overlap in ADC values between benign and malignant lesions. No absolute discriminatory ADC values have been identified; values identified in the literature appear investigator specific. Additionally, due to poor spatial resolution (related in part to slice thickness), tumor conspicuity as on DWI images suffers compared to standard MRI. These issues will likely be solved, especially with increasing penetration of 3 T units in the market, and DWI is expected to become a routine component of breast MRI evaluation in the near future, with software analytic tools currently available on several dedicated breast MRI interpretation systems.

Other potential technical advances related to MRI are undergoing current evaluation. Tumor micro-vascularity, qualitatively (lesion enhancement morphology) and semiquantitatively (kinetic curves) assessed during routine MR imaging, can be examined more quantitatively, by measuring parameters such as vascular permeability (k^{trans}), the capacity of tissue to absorb contrast (v_e), and flux of contrast within tissue (k_{ep}). Each of these perfusion parameters reflects the presence of tumor neoangiogenesis, the new, abnormal vessels that form with cancers. There is much interest in using this information to predict the presence of invasion in lesions thought to be pure DCIS, tumor grade and subtype, and prognostic information noninvasively. For example, Koo and associates found that these parameters could predict tumors with poor prognostic features as defined by tumor markers (estrogen receptor and her-2-neu) [69]. This perfusion work is ongoing and currently the results have not reached consensus, but one can see the progressive refinement of noninvasive measures that will allow increasing personalized tumor detection, prognosis, and treatment assessment. While some of this work is possible at 1.5 T, it is likely that use of 3 T units will allow more robust advancement in these technologies, related to improved temporal and spatial resolution and improved signal-to-noise ratio [70].

Breast-Specific Gamma Imaging

Breast-specific gamma imaging (BSGI), also known as molecular breast imaging (MBI) or breast scintigraphy, is an imaging modality which capitalizes on physiologic differences between breast cancer and normal tissue in order to allow for the detection of neoplasm (Fig. 19.13). The most widely used radiotracer is Tc-99 m sestamibi, which localizes within mitochondria. It is thought that both the higher concentration of mitochondria within cancer cells and the increased delivery of the radiotracer to the tumors because of neovascularity lead to greater uptake of Tc-99 m sestamibi within the cancers relative to the surrounding normal breast tissue. As physiologic, rather than anatomic, characteristics of the breast are imaged, BSGI is postulated to overcome several limitations confounding the interpretation of mammograms including high breast density, postoperative scarring, and breast implants [71].

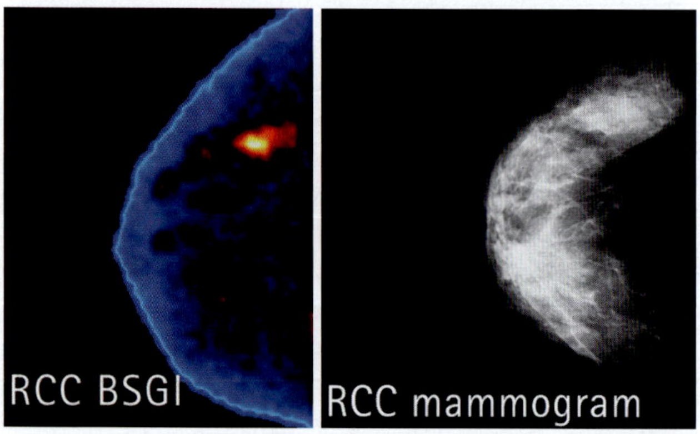

Fig. 19.13 BSGI image demonstrates multiple areas of uptake in the right breast, representing multicentric lobular carcinoma. Mammogram (CC view) demonstrates dense tissue, without abnormality (Images courtesy of Dilon Technologies)

BSGI has its origins in what is known as scintimammography, which used a traditional gamma camera and imaged the patient prone in the lateral and AP positions. This technique was limited in its ability to detect subcentimeter lesions due to the poor resolution of the cameras as well as the inability to position the detector close to the breast [72]. Current gamma imaging employs a high-resolution gamma camera which images the slightly compressed breast in the craniocaudal and mediolateral oblique positions, as is done in mammography. 15–25 mCi of Tc-99 m sestamibi (or, less frequently, Tc-99 m tetrofosmin) are injected, and each image is obtained to 100,000 counts, for a total of approximately 45 min per exam. With the high-resolution camera, the sensitivity for the detection of subcentimeter lesions has improved [73]. Another benefit of the breast-specific gamma camera is that the breast can be imaged in positions comparable to those used in mammography, so that direct correlation between the two imaging modalities can be made [74]. In the past, if a suspicious abnormality was identified on a BSGI examination, second review of the mammogram, directed ultrasound, or MRI were used to attempt to identify the abnormality for targeting for biopsy. Today, a gamma-guided stereotactic localization device is available [71].

BSGI has shown promising results. Brem et al. [75] found that BSGI had a high sensitivity (96.4 %) and a moderate specificity (59.5 %) in a study of 146 patients. This result was echoed in a larger, multicenter trial by Weigert et al. [76] of 1,042 patients which found that gamma imaging had an overall sensitivity of 91 % and a specificity of 77 %. A recent meta-analysis of studies investigating BSGI again concluded that it has a high sensitivity (95 %) and moderate specificity (80 %) [77].

Many believe that BSGI can be a useful imaging modality in patients with dense breasts in whom mammography is known to be of decreased sensitivity. In a study of BSGI as an adjunct to mammography in 936 women with dense breasts, the sensitivity of both modalities combined was significantly higher than that of mammography alone (91 % vs. 27 %), and most detected cancers were node negative [78]. Kim et al. found that gamma imaging was able to detect more additional sites of cancer than mammography in 28/121 women with dense breasts and cancer (83.1 % vs. 44.1 % sensitivity) [79]. Studies suggest that BSGI can be useful in detecting ductal carcinoma in situ (DCIS). In a study of 22 cases, BSGI demonstrated statistically equivalent sensitivity (91 %) for the detection of DCIS when compared to mammography (82 %) and MRI (88 %) [73]. Another study of 33 women demonstrated that BSGI had an equal sensitivity to mammography for the detection of DCIS (93.9 % vs. 90.9 %), but better assessed the extent of disease when correlation with histopathology was done [80]. BSGI has also been shown to be at least as effective in the detection of invasive lobular carcinoma (ILC) as mammography, ultrasound, and MRI. Brem et al. [74] found in a study of 28 lesions that the sensitivity of BSGI for detecting ILC was 93 %, as compared to 83 % with MRI, 79 % with mammography, and 68 % with ultrasound, though the differences were not statistically significant.

Several studies have compared the utility of BSGI and MRI as adjuncts to mammography. In a study of 33 mammographically indeterminate lesions evaluated both by BSGI and MRI, BSGI was found to have an equal sensitivity to MRI (89 % vs. 100 %, not statistically significant), but a higher specificity (71 % vs. 25 %) [81]. The results of a study of 66 patients with known cancer comparing BSGI to MRI echo these findings of equal sensitivity (88.8 % vs. 92.3 %) and higher specificity (90.1 % vs. 39 %) [82]. One advantage of BSGI over MRI is that it can be used in patients with contraindications to MRI, such as pacemakers, defibrillators, or aneurysm clips, and in patients with claustrophobia who cannot tolerate MRI. Additionally, the potentially hazardous use of gadolinium in patients with renal disease can be avoided. Another advantage is that the number of images generated by BSGI, generally 4–16, is much less than the sometimes thousands of images produced by an MRI, thus not placing such a high burden on storage space and potentially decreasing image interpretation time [71].

Thus, there are many studies that support the use of BSGI as a tool for the detection of breast cancer. However, a limitation of these data is that most of the studies that have been published to date have small sample sizes and are retrospective. More prospective studies with large sample sizes showing the effectiveness of BSGI must be performed before this modality is accepted into mainstream practice. In the end, however, the most critical limitation of BSGI that must be considered is its very high radiation exposure when compared to mammography. Not only is the radiation exposure of BSGI much higher, but the effects are not limited to the breasts as in the case of mammography, as the biodistribution of the tracer throughout the body exposes many organs and tissues to the radiation [83]. It is estimated that at current typical doses, a single BSGI study is associated with a fatal radiation-induced cancer risk comparable to that of a lifetime of annual screening mammography in women starting at age 40 [84]. Therefore, at current doses, it is difficult to support the widespread use of BSGI.

Positron Emission Tomography/Positron Emission Mammography

As mammography, ultrasound and MRI are not without limitations, there has been interest in the use of alternative modalities for the detection and staging of breast cancer. Fluorine-18 (^{18}F) fluorodeoxyglucose (FDG) positron emission tomography (PET) is one such modality. ^{18}F-FDG is a structural glucose analogue that is taken up by and trapped within cells. The more metabolically active the cell, the greater the glucose requirement, and therefore the greater the accumulation of FDG within. Labeling with the positron emitter fluorine-18 allows detection, localization, and quantification of FDG accumulation by PET instrumentation [85]. PEt allows for visualization of tumors based on physiologic, and not anatomic, factors. Therefore, it is not limited by breast density, as in the case of mammography. It also overcomes several limitations imposed by MRI, as it can be performed in patients with claustrophobia, poor renal function, and implanted metal devices and is not affected by hormonal status [86]. Additionally, it allows for whole-body imaging, facilitating staging of malignancy. Its combination with CT permits specific anatomic localization of FDG accumulation [87].

However, PET is not without significant limitations. Most studies have found whole-body PET with or without CT to be of lower utility than MRI in the detection of primary breast tumors. Though in a study by Heusner et al., PET/CT had a statistically equivalent sensitivity for the detection of primary cancers when compared to MRI, MRI was better able to classify the T stage [87]. Most other studies have found a poor performance of whole-body PET in the detection of primary tumor. Choi and colleagues calculated a sensitivity of 89.6 % for PET/CT in detecting the primary lesion, compared to 99.4 % for ultrasound and 98.5 % for MRI [88]. They found that this low sensitivity of PET/CT in detecting the primary tumor was dependent on size—though it was able to detect all T2 or larger cancers, it detected only 81 % of T1 lesions and only 70.8 % of 1 cm or smaller cancers. Avril et al. [89] found that whole-body PET was unable to detect any tumor smaller than 0.5 cm. Sensitivity only increased to 12.5 % for lesions 0.5–1.0 cm in size. For stage T2 tumors, sensitivity increased to 80.6–91.9 %.

Several studies also demonstrate the limitations of whole-body PET in determining the extent of disease in the breast. Though the Heusner et al. study [87] found that PET/CT was better able to correctly classify the focality pattern of lesions when compared to MRI, another study [88] found PET/CT to be a poor detector of multifocality, with a sensitivity of 12.5 % compared to 80.0 % (US) and 81.1 % (MRI). Uematsu et al. [90] also found that PET was significantly less accurate in evaluating tumor extent when compared to MRI (43.5 % vs. 91 %). PET/CT has also been found to be of relatively low utility for staging the axilla, with a mean sensitivity of 63 % [87, 88, 90–93]. This is comparable to the sensitivity of clinical exam, ultrasound, and MRI [87, 88, 92, 93]. As the sensitivity is lower than that of sentinel node biopsy, it cannot be used as a substitute [93].

Many groups have attempted to determine whether the degree of FDG uptake in tumors can be used as a prognostic indicator, but results are conflicting. Several studies [94–98] agree that tumors expressing more Ki-67 have a greater FDG

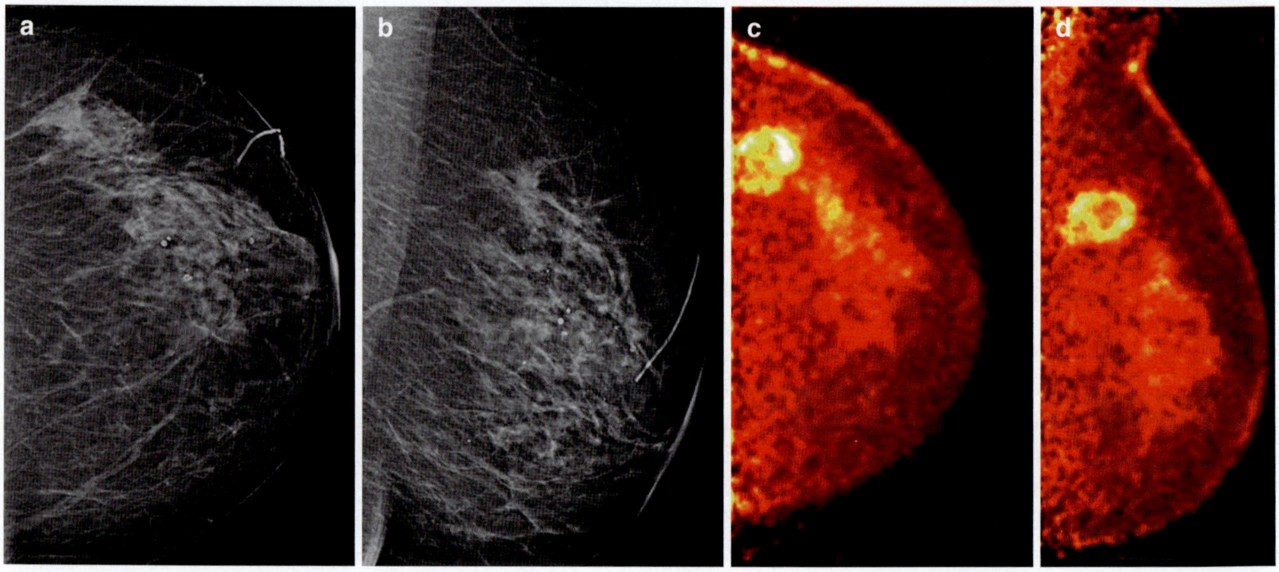

Fig. 19.14 CC (**a**) and MLO mammographic (**b**) views demonstrate no abnormality. Corresponding PEM images (**c, d**) show uptake in the upper outer quadrant, representing invasive lobular carcinoma (Images courtesy of Kathy Schilling, MD)

uptake. Some studies have found that tumors with ductal histology have a higher FDG uptake than those with lobular [94–96, 99] though others [97, 98] have found no correlation between FDG uptake and histology. Similarly, there are conflicting data regarding the association between FDG uptake and tumor size, histological grade, axillary lymph node status, and hormone receptor positivity [94–101]. At least two investigators have found an association between triple negativity and increased FDG uptake [99, 102]. Another found that patients with tumors that had high FDG uptake had a significantly poorer prognosis than those whose tumors had low uptake [101]. One study attempted to determine what tumor characteristics were associated with a false-negative PET [103]. It found that tumor size (less than or equal to 10 mm) and low tumor grade were associated with a false-negative result.

The utility of whole-body PET in breast cancer diagnosis appears to be not in the evaluation of the breast and axilla, but rather, in combination with CT, for the detection of distant metastatic disease. The sensitivity and specificity of PET/CT for detecting distant metastases is much higher than that of conventional imaging (100 and 96.4–98 % vs. 60–61.5 and 83–99.2 %) [88, 91]. This detection of unexpected sites of metastatic disease by PET/CT led to a change in the initial staging in 8–42 % of patients in multiple studies [91, 92, 104]. Whether the detection of these additional sites of disease leads to improved patient survival is yet to be seen. Current recommendations are to use PET in combination with CT [85] in those with clinically suspected metastatic disease. PET/CT has also been found to be useful in the evaluation of patients with recurrent breast cancer. Aukema et al. found that PET/CT changed the clinical management in almost half the patients with tumor recurrence when compared to evaluation with conventional staging procedures (physical examination, MRI, chest radiograph, liver US or CT, and bone scan) [105]. Only one metastasis detected by conventional imaging was missed by PET/CT and was determined to have no clinical consequence for the patient. The authors suggest that PET/CT may replace conventional staging procedures in the future.

Positron emission mammography (PEM), or breast PET, was developed in order to take advantage of PET's benefits in detecting breast cancer (e.g. not being dependent on breast density or hormonal status) while overcoming its limitations, specifically its low sensitivity for small cancers [106]. This is thought to be possible because the dedicated PEM cameras are small and are able to be positioned closer to the breast, and also use compression, which reduces the effects of motion [107]. PEM uses two parallel photon detectors that are positioned on the breast similar to a mammography unit [108]. Initial studies showed that PEM could be effective in identifying breast cancers (Fig. 19.14a–d). One study of 18 lesions demonstrated that PEM had a sensitivity of 86 %, specificity of 91 %, and overall diagnostic accuracy of 89 % [109]. Another pilot study of 23 patients also demonstrated a sensitivity of 86 % and demonstrated that PEM can be effective in finding cancers as small as 4 mm [110]. A third preliminary study of 44 women with known breast cancer found that most index cancers (39/44 or 89 %) could be seen with PEM, while PEM was also able to detect three incidental cancers not seen by any other modality. This study also found that PEM could be effective in predicting margin status, as out of 19 patients who underwent breast-conserving surgery, PEM correctly predicted 6/8 (75 %) with positive margins and 11/11 (100 %) of those with negative margins [111].

Larger studies confirm these results. A study of 94 patients with known or suspected cancers found that PEM had a sensitivity of 90 % and specificity of 86 % [112].

Compared to whole-body PET, PEM is able to see smaller cancers. PEM was found to be more sensitive than PET/CT in the detection of cancer, and the difference in sensitivity was accentuated in small tumors [108]. A pilot study found a cancer as small as 4 cm [110]. Berg et al. found that PEM had a sensitivity of 63 % for cancers smaller than 1 cm [106]. In a large series of 472 patients with newly diagnosed breast cancer, Berg et al. [112, 113] compared the performance of PEM with that of MRI in detecting cancer in the ipsilateral and contralateral breasts. When evaluating the ipsilateral breast, MRI was found to have greater lesion-level sensitivity for additional malignant lesions (53 % vs. 47 %) and to more accurately predict the need for mastectomy, though breast-level sensitivity was comparable. PEM was found to have greater specificity (79.9 % vs. 65.6 %). In the contralateral breast, sensitivity of PEM for cancer detection was lower than that of MRI (73 % vs. 93 %). Another study [86] comparing PEM with MRI found that they had the same index lesion depiction sensitivity (92.8 %), greater than whole-body PET (67.9 %). Similarly, there was no significant difference between PEM and MRI in the detection of additional unsuspected lesions.

One limitation of PEM is that the far posterior portion of the breast may not be adequately imaged due to limited coincidence-count sampling at the edge, as well as detector plates excluding the far posterior breast from the field of view. One study found that all three false-negative cases (out of 20 total cases) were of cancers located in the posterior breast [110]. Another significant limitation of PEM is that it employs ionizing radiation. It is estimated that at current typical doses, a single PEM study is associated with a fatal radiation-induced cancer risk comparable to that of a lifetime of annual screening mammography in women starting at age 40 [84]. Therefore, given the evidence that it is, at best, comparable to MRI in detecting breast cancer, PEM is unlikely to be widely accepted as the preferred study in patients able to undergo MRI examinations.

Optical Imaging

The use of light for the detection and characterization of breast cancer is appealing on many levels. It uses no ionizing radiation, does not require significant breast compression and can provide functional information. Max Cutler used optical imaging (OI) in its most basic form in the 1920s when he transilluminated the breast in an attempt to outline and characterize pathology [114]. Dr. Cutler applied a narrow-beam light source to the undersurface of the flattened breast of a seated patient and observed from above. He noted that the various tissues encountered in the breast differentially transmitted or absorbed light. Fatty tissue and cysts were translucent, while solid masses and anything containing hemorrhagic material were "intensely opaque." He evaluated palpable masses and felt he could differentiate simple cysts (which he recognized as clinically unimportant) from hemorrhagic cysts and solid masses (clinically important). Additionally, he used transillumination technique to evaluate bloody nipple discharge and was able to identify and localize papillomas in some cases, thereby precluding the need for mastectomy, which was sometimes the treatment for suspicious nipple discharge in that period. However, despite Dr. Cutler's enthusiasm, the technique did not gain a foothold. In the 1970s and 1980s, interest was revived, using improved technology consisting of a near-infrared (NIR) light source and dedicated detectors, as the human eye is insensitive to NIR light. The literature surrounding this technique was largely anecdotal but claimed some success. When scrutinized in a more methodological manner, it was found wanting, detecting only 53 % of cancers present in a study population of 1,239 women compared to 96 % found with mammography and only 19 % of subclinical and small (<1 cm) cancers [115].

Given its theoretical appeal, however, experimentation with the technology continued, with resultant emergence of more sophisticated methods of transmitting and receiving NIR light as well as interrogation of more physiologic and functional tissue attributes, over and above simple light transmission versus absorption. Some of these improvements included development of diffuse optical tomography (DOT), which sends laser-generated NIR light into the breast in multiple projections and, using mathematical reconstruction, can create a 3D map of the breast. Traditional tissue absorption information is obtained. However, additionally, when light of varying frequencies is delivered, spectroscopic data can be ascertained. Some of the main "chromophores" (tissue absorbers) in the breast include oxyhemoglobin, deoxyhemoglobin, water, and lipid, and via their unique and quantifiable spectroscopic footprint, they can be mapped within the breast. Each of these chromophores has an implication in tissue metabolism, neoangiogenesis, necrosis, and extracellular water content and thus the presence, etiology, and status of a breast tumor.

A comprehensive review of the clinical data surrounding breast optical imaging was performed by Leff and colleagues [116]. They concluded that the technique allows lesion detection in 85 % of cases, due mainly to increased concentrations of tissue oxyhemoglobin (reflecting neovascularity) and deoxyhemoglobin (indicative of tissue metabolism). It underperforms in detecting small cancers (due to poor spatial resolution). Importantly, they observed that the data do not convincingly demonstrate the ability of optical imaging to differentiate between benign and malignant lesions. Given these data, when combined with non-superior sensitivity, they concluded that in its current form optical

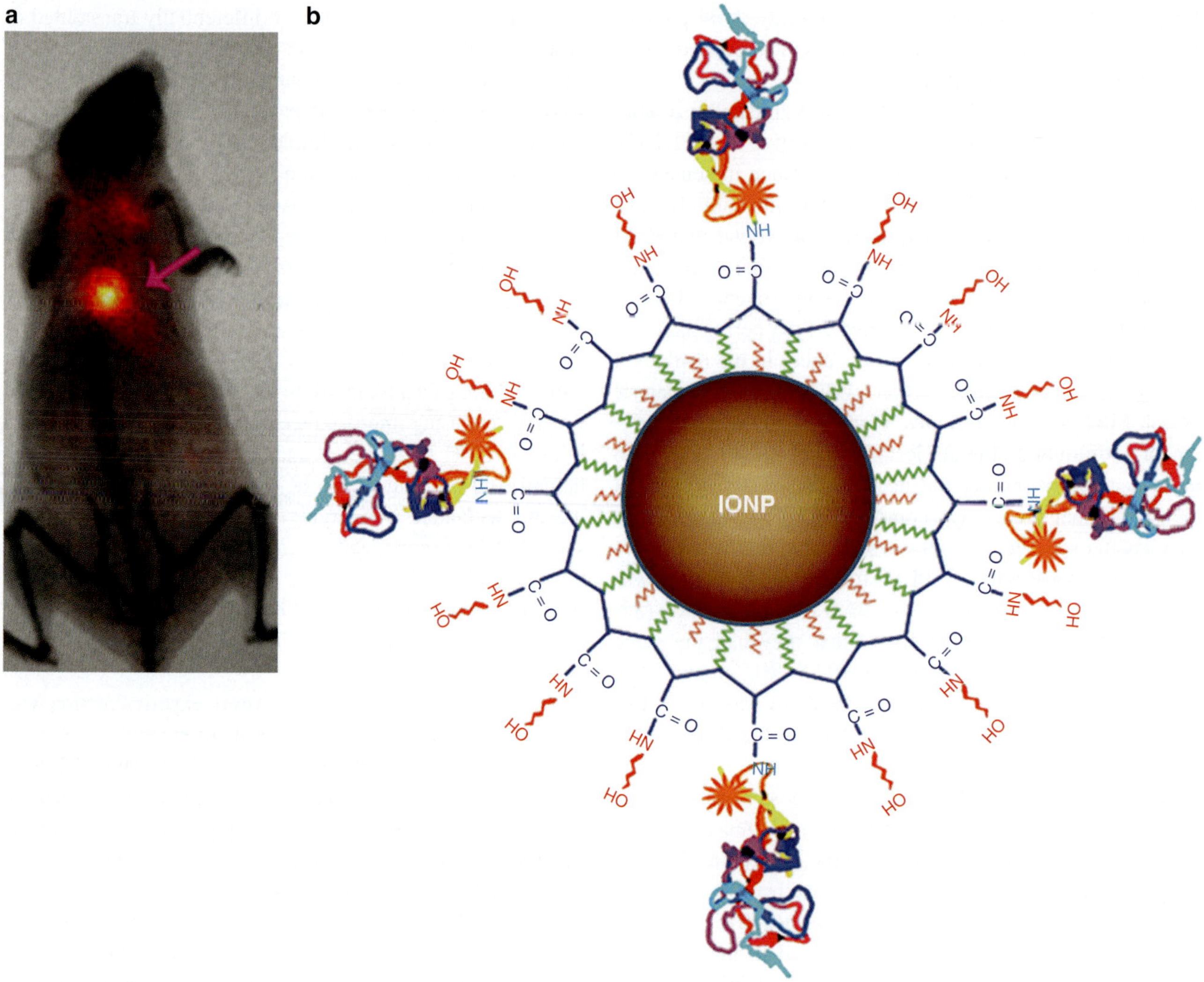

Fig. 19.15 (**a**) NIR optical imaging. 4T1 mouse mammary tumor model. Fluorescent dye attached to a nanoparticle is injected intravenously and concentrates selectively (*outlined by arrow*) in a mammary tumor in this mouse. It is activated by near-infrared light and can be imaged. The nanoparticle, displayed schematically (**b**), can be made tumor specific and may also be bound to chemotherapeutic agents, creating a "theranostic" particle [122]. *IONP* Iron oxide nanoparticles (Images courtesy of Lily Yang, MD, PhD)

imaging cannot supplant mammography, but with further refinement, may play a part in multimodality breast imaging in certain scenarios. For example, Soliman et al. showed that optical imaging may be a useful, noninvasive, relatively inexpensive way to determine response to neoadjuvant chemotherapy in patients with locally advanced breast cancer as early as 4 weeks into treatment [117].

Exciting new refinements are currently being evaluated. Fluorescent dyes are being explored as way to improve sensitivity and specificity. These cyanine-based dyes are administered intravenously and collect in neoplastic tissue, related to leaky tumor vascularity, similar to MRI and CT contrast material. Not only do they act as NIR light absorbers when concentrated within tumors (just as oxy- and deoxyhemoglobin, lipid, and water do), but they also fluoresce when excited by external application of NIR light, allowing detection and localization by an optical imaging tomographic unit. In a multicenter clinical trial, Poellinger and associates [118] confirmed potential clinical utility for this technology, noting 100 % sensitivity for cancer detection at certain administered doses of this dye in a dose-escalating design study. However, they also noted that sensitivity was related to dose, lesion size, breast size, and lesion depth, with overall sensitivity of 60.9 % for invasive cancers. Additionally, the optimal imaging dose they defined was far different from that determined by other authors [119], suggesting that this work is still in its developmental stages. Other related, potentially "game-changing" work is undergoing in vivo evaluation on an animal level. In this work, fluorescent dyes are being made tumor specific by attaching estrogen [120] or Her2-targeted Affibody molecules [121] (Fig. 19.15a, b). Since these molecules/nanoparticles (the number and type of which will likely be expanded rapidly as more is discovered about tumor-specific surface and intracellular markers) would be expected to attach specifically to primary cancers and metastases, and not to normal cells, the specter of tailored detection and tumor monitoring is easily imagined. With the addition of a chemotherapeutic agent to the nanoparticle (rendering it "theranostic"), as has been developed by Shalviri and colleagues [122], highly tailored therapy is added to the mix, potentially markedly diminishing the debilitating systemic effects of treatment, as only the cancer is being targeted and not healthy tissue.

Conclusion

The exciting new technologies outlined previously will likely allow for improved sensitivity and specificity in breast cancer detection and lesions characterization. However, the field of breast imaging finds itself at an unusual crossroads. On one hand, there is pressure, even from politicians and the public, to image more, especially in populations deemed to be at elevated risk. On the other hand, many of our tools have been accused of leading to overdiagnosis, mental anguish in patients, unnecessary added interventions, and cost run-ups. It seems prudent to move forward with technological developments and research, rather than retreat, with the goal of further refining our tools so that they can be applied appropriately, even if sometimes selectively, to maximize outcomes benefit.

References

1. Niklason LT, Christian BT, Niklason LE, Kopans DB, Castleberry DE, Opsahl-Ong BH, et al. Digital tomosynthesis in breast imaging. Radiology. 1997;205(2):399–406.
2. FDA. Selenia Dimensions 3D System- P080003. 2011 [updated 20 May 2013; cited 05 Jun 2013]. Available from: http://www.fda.gov/MedicalDevices/ProductsandMedicalProcedures/DeviceApprovalsandClearances/Recently-ApprovedDevices/ucm246400.htm.
3. Waldherr C, Cerny P, Altermatt HJ, Berclaz G, Ciriolo M, Buser K, et al. Value of one-view breast tomosynthesis versus two-view mammography in diagnostic workup of women with clinical signs and symptoms and in women recalled from screening. AJR Am J Roentgenol. 2013;200(1):226–31.
4. Svahn TM, Chakraborty DP, Ikeda D, Zackrisson S, Do Y, Mattsson S, et al. Breast tomosynthesis and digital mammography: a comparison of diagnostic accuracy. Br J Radiol. 2012;85(1019):e1074–82.
5. Teertstra HJ, Loo CE, van den Bosch MA, van Tinteren H, Rutgers EJ, Muller SH, et al. Breast tomosynthesis in clinical practice: initial results. Eur Radiol. 2010;20(1):16–24.
6. Gennaro G, Toledano A, di Maggio C, Baldan E, Bezzon E, La Grassa M, et al. Digital breast tomosynthesis versus digital mammography: a clinical performance study. Eur Radiol. 2010;20(7):1545–53.
7. Skaane P, Bandos AI, Gullien R, Eben EB, Ekseth U, Haakenaasen U, et al. Comparison of digital mammography alone and digital mammography plus tomosynthesis in a population-based screening program. Radiology. 2013;267(1):47–56.
8. Rafferty EA, Park JM, Philpotts LE, Poplack SP, Sumkin JH, Halpern EF, et al. Assessing radiologist performance using combined digital mammography and breast tomosynthesis compared with digital mammography alone: results of a multicenter, multireader trial. Radiology. 2013;266(1):104–13.
9. Poplack SP, Tosteson TD, Kogel CA, Nagy HM. Digital breast tomosynthesis: initial experience in 98 women with abnormal digital screening mammography. AJR Am J Roentgenol. 2007;189(3):616–23.
10. Gur D, Abrams GS, Chough DM, Ganott MA, Hakim CM, Perrin RL, et al. Digital breast tomosynthesis: observer performance study. AJR Am J Roentgenol. 2009;193(2):586–91.
11. Rose SL, Tidwell AL, Bujnoch LJ, Kushwaha AC, Nordmann AS, Sexton Jr R. Implementation of breast tomosynthesis in a routine screening practice: an observational study. AJR Am J Roentgenol. 2013;200(6):1401–8.
12. Brandt KR, Craig DA, Hoskins TL, Henrichsen TL, Bendel EC, Brandt SR, et al. Can digital breast tomosynthesis replace conventional diagnostic mammography views for screening recalls without calcifications? A comparison study in a simulated clinical setting. AJR Am J Roentgenol. 2013;200(2):291–8.
13. Noroozian M, Hadjiiski L, Rahnama-Moghadam S, Klein KA, Jeffries DO, Pinsky RW, et al. Digital breast tomosynthesis is comparable to mammographic spot views for mass characterization. Radiology. 2012;262(1):61–8.
14. Zuley ML, Bandos AI, Ganott MA, Sumkin JH, Kelly AE, Catullo VJ, et al. Digital breast tomosynthesis versus supplemental diagnostic mammographic views for evaluation of noncalcified breast lesions. Radiology. 2013;266(1):89–95.
15. Wallis MG, Moa E, Zanca F, Leifland K, Danielsson M. Two-view and single-view tomosynthesis versus full-field digital mammography: high-resolution X-ray imaging observer study. Radiology. 2012;262(3):788–96.
16. Spangler ML, Zuley ML, Sumkin JH, Abrams G, Ganott MA, Hakim C, et al. Detection and classification of calcifications on digital breast tomosynthesis and 2D digital mammography: a comparison. AJR Am J Roentgenol. 2011;196(2):320–4.
17. FDA. Selenia Dimensions 3D System – P080003/S001 2013 [updated 23 May 2013; cited 20 Jun 2013]. Available from: http://www.fda.gov/MedicalDevices/ProductsandMedicalProcedures/DeviceApprovalsandClearances/Recently-ApprovedDevices/ucm353734.htm.
18. D'Orsi CJ, Getty DJ, Pickett RM, Sechopoulos I, Newell MS, Gundry KR, et al. Stereoscopic digital mammography: improved specificity and reduced rate of recall in a prospective clinical trial. Radiology. 2013;266(1):81–8.
19. Dromain C, Thibault F, Muller S, Rimareix F, Delaloge S, Tardivon A, et al. Dual-energy contrast-enhanced digital mammography: initial clinical results. Eur Radiol. 2011;21(3):565–74.
20. Lewin JM, Niklason L. Advanced applications of digital mammography: tomosynthesis and contrast-enhanced digital mammography. Semin Roentgenol. 2007;42(4):243–52.
21. Jochelson MS, Dershaw DD, Sung JS, Heerdt AS, Thornton C, Moskowitz CS, et al. Bilateral contrast-enhanced dual-energy digital mammography: feasibility and comparison with conventional digital mammography and MR imaging in women with known breast carcinoma. Radiology. 2013;266(3):743–51.
22. Dromain C, Thibault F, Diekmann F, Fallenberg EM, Jong RA, Koomen M, et al. Dual-energy contrast-enhanced digital mammography: initial clinical results of a multireader, multicase study. Breast Cancer Res. 2012;14(3):R94.
23. Jong RA, Yaffe MJ, Skarpathiotakis M, Shumak RS, Danjoux NM, Gunesekara A, et al. Contrast-enhanced digital mammography: initial clinical experience. Radiology. 2003;228(3):842–50.
24. Diekmann F, Diekmann S, Taupitz M, Bick U, Winzer KJ, Huttner C, et al. Use of iodine-based contrast media in digital full-field mammography–initial experience. Rofo. 2003;175(3):342–5.

25. Diekmann F, Freyer M, Diekmann S, Fallenberg EM, Fischer T, Bick U, et al. Evaluation of contrast-enhanced digital mammography. Eur J Radiol. 2011;78(1):112–21.
26. Dromain C, Balleyguier C, Muller S, Mathieu MC, Rochard F, Opolon P, et al. Evaluation of tumor angiogenesis of breast carcinoma using contrast-enhanced digital mammography. AJR Am J Roentgenol. 2006;187(5):W528–37.
27. Lewin JM, Isaacs PK, Vance V, Larke FJ. Dual-energy contrast-enhanced digital subtraction mammography: feasibility. Radiology. 2003;229(1):261–8.
28. Dodd GD. Present status of thermography, ultrasound and mammography in breast cancer detection. Cancer. 1977;39(6 Suppl):2796–805.
29. Kobayashi T, Takatani O, Hattori N, Kimura K. Differential diagnosis of breast tumors. The sensitivity graded method ultrasonotomography and clinical evaluation of its diagnostic accuracy. Cancer. 1974;33(4):940–51.
30. Graf O, Helbich TH, Hopf G, Graf C, Sickles EA. Probably benign breast masses at US: is follow-up an acceptable alternative to biopsy? Radiology. 2007;244(1):87–93.
31. Stavros AT. Breast ultrasound. Philadelphia: Lippincott Williams & Williams; 2004.
32. Berg WA, Blume JD, Cormack JB, Mendelson EB, Lehrer D, Bohm-Velez M, et al. Combined screening with ultrasound and mammography vs mammography alone in women at elevated risk of breast cancer. JAMA. 2008;299(18):2151–63.
33. Tohno E, Ueno E, Watanabe H. Ultrasound screening of breast cancer. Breast Cancer. 2009;16(1):18–22.
34. Corsetti V, Ferrari A, Ghirardi M, Bergonzini R, Bellarosa S, Angelini O, et al. Role of ultrasonography in detecting mammographically occult breast carcinoma in women with dense breasts. Radiol Med. 2006;111(3):440–8.
35. Kelly KM, Richwald GA. Automated whole-breast ultrasound: advancing the performance of breast cancer screening. Semin Ultrasound CT MR. 2011;32(4):273–80.
36. Wang HY, Jiang YX, Zhu QL, Zhang J, Dai Q, Liu H, et al. Differentiation of benign and malignant breast lesions: a comparison between automatically generated breast volume scans and handheld ultrasound examinations. Eur J Radiol. 2012;81(11):3190–200.
37. Kelly KM, Dean J, Comulada WS, Lee SJ. Breast cancer detection using automated whole breast ultrasound and mammography in radiographically dense breasts. Eur Radiol. 2010;20(3):734–42.
38. Itoh A, Ueno E, Tohno E, Kamma H, Takahashi H, Shiina T, et al. Breast disease: clinical application of US elastography for diagnosis. Radiology. 2006;239(2):341–50.
39. Sadigh G, Carlos RC, Neal CH, Dwamena BA. Ultrasonographic differentiation of malignant from benign breast lesions: a meta-analytic comparison of elasticity and BIRADS scoring. Breast Cancer Res Treat. 2012;133(1):23–35.
40. Regner DM, Hesley GK, Hangiandreou NJ, Morton MJ, Nordland MR, Meixner DD, et al. Breast lesions: evaluation with US strain imaging–clinical experience of multiple observers. Radiology. 2006;238(2):425–37.
41. Berg WA, Cosgrove DO, Dore CJ, Schafer FK, Svensson WE, Hooley RJ, et al. Shear-wave elastography improves the specificity of breast US: the BE1 multinational study of 939 masses. Radiology. 2012;262(2):435–49.
42. Kashikura Y, Nakayama R, Hizukuri A, Noro A, Nohara Y, Nakamura T, et al. Improved differential diagnosis of breast masses on ultrasonographic images with a computer-aided diagnosis scheme for determining histological classifications. Acad Radiol. 2013;20(4):471–7.
43. Lindfors KK, Boone JM, Newell MS, D'Orsi CJ. Dedicated breast computed tomography: the optimal cross-sectional imaging solution? Radiol Clin North Am. 2010;48(5):1043–54.
44. Kalender WA. Concepts for high-resolution CT of the breast. In: Digital mammography. Berlin/Heidelberg: Springer; 2010. p. 421–7.
45. O'Connell A, Conover DL, Zhang Y, Seifert P, Logan-Young W, Lin CF, et al. Cone-beam CT for breast imaging: radiation dose, breast coverage, and image quality. AJR Am J Roentgenol. 2010;195(2):496–509.
46. Lindfors KK, Boone JM, Nelson TR, Yang K, Kwan AL, Miller DF. Dedicated breast CT: initial clinical experience. Radiology. 2008;246(3):725–33.
47. Prionas ND, Lindfors KK, Ray S, Huang SY, Beckett LA, Monsky WL, et al. Contrast-enhanced dedicated breast CT: initial clinical experience. Radiology. 2010;256(3):714–23.
48. Kalender WA, Beister M, Boone JM, Kolditz D, Vollmar SV, Weigel MC. High-resolution spiral CT of the breast at very low dose: concept and feasibility considerations. Eur Radiol. 2012;22(1):1–8.
49. McKinley RL, Tornai MP, Tuttle LA, et al. Development and initial demonstration of a low-dose dedicated fully 3-D CT system. In: Maidment ADA, Bakic P, Gavenonis D, editors. Breast imaging. Berlin/Heidelberg: Springer; 2012. p. 442–9.
50. Tozaki M, Fukuma E. 1H MR spectroscopy and diffusion-weighted imaging of the breast: are they useful tools for characterizing breast lesions before biopsy? AJR Am J Roentgenol. 2009;193(3):840–9.
51. Bolan PJ, Meisamy S, Baker EH, Lin J, Emory T, Nelson M, et al. In vivo quantification of choline compounds in the breast with 1H MR spectroscopy. Magn Reson Med. 2003;50(6):1134–43.
52. Bartella L, Morris EA, Dershaw DD, Liberman L, Thakur SB, Moskowitz C, et al. Proton MR spectroscopy with choline peak as malignancy marker improves positive predictive value for breast cancer diagnosis: preliminary study. Radiology. 2006;239(3):686–92.
53. Dorrius MD, Pijnappel RM, van der Weide Jansen MC, Jansen L, Kappert P, Oudkerk M, et al. The added value of quantitative multi-voxel MR spectroscopy in breast magnetic resonance imaging. Eur Radiol. 2012;22(4):915–22.
54. Mann RM, Kuhl CK, Kinkel K, Boetes C. Breast MRI: guidelines from the European Society of Breast Imaging. Eur Radiol. 2008;18(7):1307–18.
55. Meisamy S, Bolan PJ, Baker EH, Bliss RL, Gulbahce E, Everson LI, et al. Neoadjuvant chemotherapy of locally advanced breast cancer: predicting response with in vivo (1)H MR spectroscopy–a pilot study at 4 T. Radiology. 2004;233(2):424–31.
56. Tozaki M, Sakamoto M, Oyama Y, Maruyama K, Fukuma E. Predicting pathological response to neoadjuvant chemotherapy in breast cancer with quantitative 1H MR spectroscopy using the external standard method. J Magn Reson Imaging. 2010;31(4):895–902.
57. Razek NMA. Role of proton MR spectroscopy in high field magnet (3T) in diagnosis of indeterminate breast masses (BIRDS 3 & 4). Egypt J Radiol Nucl Med. 2012;43(4):657–62.
58. McLaughlin R, Hylton N. MRI in breast cancer therapy monitoring. NMR Biomed. 2011;24(6):712–20.
59. Partridge SC, Mullins CD, Kurland BF, Allain MD, DeMartini WB, Eby PR, et al. Apparent diffusion coefficient values for discriminating benign and malignant breast MRI lesions: effects of lesion type and size. AJR Am J Roentgenol. 2010;194(6):1664–73.
60. Marini C, Iacconi C, Giannelli M, Cilotti A, Moretti M, Bartolozzi C. Quantitative diffusion-weighted MR imaging in the differential diagnosis of breast lesion. Eur Radiol. 2007;17(10):2646–55.
61. Partridge SC, DeMartini WB, Kurland BF, Eby PR, White SW, Lehman CD. Quantitative diffusion-weighted imaging as an adjunct to conventional breast MRI for improved positive predictive value. AJR Am J Roentgenol. 2009;193(6):1716–22.

62. Pinker K, Bickel H, Helbich TH, Gruber S, Dubsky P, Pluschnig U, et al. Combined contrast-enhanced magnetic resonance and diffusion-weighted imaging reading adapted to the "Breast Imaging Reporting and Data System" for multiparametric 3-T imaging of breast lesions. Eur Radiol. 2013;23(7):1791–802.
63. Tozaki M, Oyama Y, Fukuma E. Preliminary study of early response to neoadjuvant chemotherapy after the first cycle in breast cancer: comparison of 1H magnetic resonance spectroscopy with diffusion magnetic resonance imaging. Jpn J Radiol. 2010;28(2):101–9.
64. Manton DJ, Chaturvedi A, Hubbard A, Lind MJ, Lowry M, Maraveyas A, et al. Neoadjuvant chemotherapy in breast cancer: early response prediction with quantitative MR imaging and spectroscopy. Br J Cancer. 2006;94(3):427–35.
65. Nilsen L, Fangberget A, Geier O, Olsen DR, Seierstad T. Diffusion-weighted magnetic resonance imaging for pretreatment prediction and monitoring of treatment response of patients with locally advanced breast cancer undergoing neoadjuvant chemotherapy. Acta Oncol. 2010;49(3):354–60.
66. Mori N, Ota H, Mugikura S, Takasawa C, Tominaga J, Ishida T, et al. Detection of invasive components in cases of breast ductal carcinoma in situ on biopsy by using apparent diffusion coefficient MR parameters. Eur Radiol. 2013;23(10):2705–12.
67. Kamitani T, Hatakenaka M, Yabuuchi H, Matsuo Y, Fujita N, Jinnouchi M, et al. Detection of axillary node metastasis using diffusion-weighted MRI in breast cancer. Clin Imaging. 2013; 37(1):56–61.
68. Luo N, Su D, Jin G, Liu L, Zhu X, Xie D, et al. Apparent diffusion coefficient ratio between axillary lymph node with primary tumor to detect nodal metastasis in breast cancer patients. J Magn Reson Imaging. 2013;38(4):824–8.
69. Koo HR, Cho N, Song IC, Kim H, Chang JM, Yi A, et al. Correlation of perfusion parameters on dynamic contrast-enhanced MRI with prognostic factors and subtypes of breast cancers. J Magn Reson Imaging. 2012;36(1):145–51.
70. Rahbar H, Partridge SC, DeMartini WB, Thursten B, Lehman CD. Clinical and technical considerations for high quality breast MRI at 3 Tesla. J Magn Reson Imaging. 2013;37(4):778–90.
71. Brem RF, Rechtman LR. Nuclear medicine imaging of the breast: a novel, physiologic approach to breast cancer detection and diagnosis. Radiol Clin North Am. 2010;48(5):1055–74.
72. Taillefer R. Clinical applications of 99mTc-sestamibi scintimammography. Semin Nucl Med. 2005;35(2):100–15.
73. Brem RF, Fishman M, Rapelyea JA. Detection of ductal carcinoma in situ with mammography, breast specific gamma imaging, and magnetic resonance imaging: a comparative study. Acad Radiol. 2007;14(8):945–50.
74. Brem RF, Ioffe M, Rapelyea JA, Yost KG, Weigert JM, Bertrand ML, et al. Invasive lobular carcinoma: detection with mammography, sonography, MRI, and breast-specific gamma imaging. AJR Am J Roentgenol. 2009;192(2):379–83.
75. Brem RF, Floerke AC, Rapelyea JA, Teal C, Kelly T, Mathur V. Breast-specific gamma imaging as an adjunct imaging modality for the diagnosis of breast cancer. Radiology. 2008;247(3): 651–7.
76. Weigert JM, Bertrand ML, Lanzkowsky L, Stern LH, Kieper DA. Results of a multicenter patient registry to determine the clinical impact of breast-specific gamma imaging, a molecular breast imaging technique. AJR Am J Roentgenol. 2012;198(1): W69–75.
77. Sun Y, Wei W, Yang HW, Liu JL. Clinical usefulness of breast-specific gamma imaging as an adjunct modality to mammography for diagnosis of breast cancer: a systemic review and meta-analysis. Eur J Nucl Med Mol Imaging. 2013;40(3):450–63.
78. Rhodes DJ, Hruska CB, Phillips SW, Whaley DH, O'Connor MK. Dedicated dual-head gamma imaging for breast cancer screening in women with mammographically dense breasts. Radiology. 2011;258(1):106–18.
79. Kim BS, Moon BI, Cha ES. A comparative study of breast-specific gamma imaging with the conventional imaging modality in breast cancer patients with dense breasts. Ann Nucl Med. 2012;26(10):823–9.
80. Spanu A, Sanna D, Chessa F, Cottu P, Manca A, Madeddu G. Breast scintigraphy with breast-specific gamma-camera in the detection of ductal carcinoma in situ: a correlation with mammography and histologic subtype. J Nucl Med. 2012;53(10):1528–33.
81. Brem RF, Petrovitch I, Rapelyea JA, Young H, Teal C, Kelly T. Breast-specific gamma imaging with 99mTc-Sestamibi and magnetic resonance imaging in the diagnosis of breast cancer–a comparative study. Breast J. 2007;13(5):465–9.
82. Kim BS. Usefulness of breast-specific gamma imaging as an adjunct modality in breast cancer patients with dense breast: a comparative study with MRI. Ann Nucl Med. 2012;26(2):131–7.
83. O'Connor MK, Li H, Rhodes DJ, Hruska CB, Clancy CB, Vetter RJ. Comparison of radiation exposure and associated radiation-induced cancer risks from mammography and molecular imaging of the breast. Med Phys. 2010;37(12):6187–98.
84. Hendrick RE. Radiation doses and cancer risks from breast imaging studies. Radiology. 2010;257(1):246–53.
85. Fletcher JW, Djulbegovic B, Soares HP, Siegel BA, Lowe VJ, Lyman GH, et al. Recommendations on the use of 18F-FDG PET in oncology. J Nucl Med. 2008;49(3):480–508.
86. Schilling K, Narayanan D, Kalinyak JE, The J, Velasquez MV, Kahn S, et al. Positron emission mammography in breast cancer presurgical planning: comparisons with magnetic resonance imaging. Eur J Nucl Med Mol Imaging. 2011;38(1):23–36.
87. Heusner TA, Kuemmel S, Umutlu L, Koeninger A, Freudenberg LS, Hauth EA, et al. Breast cancer staging in a single session: whole-body PET/CT mammography. J Nucl Med. 2008;49(8):1215–22.
88. Choi YJ, Shin YD, Kang YH, Lee MS, Lee MK, Cho BS, et al. The effects of preoperative (18)F-FDG PET/CT in breast cancer patients in comparison to the conventional imaging study. J Breast Cancer. 2012;15(4):441–8.
89. Avril N, Rose CA, Schelling M, Dose J, Kuhn W, Bense S, et al. Breast imaging with positron emission tomography and fluorine-18 fluorodeoxyglucose: use and limitations. J Clin Oncol. 2000;18(20):3495–502.
90. Uematsu T, Kasami M, Yuen S. Comparison of FDG PET and MRI for evaluating the tumor extent of breast cancer and the impact of FDG PET on the systemic staging and prognosis of patients who are candidates for breast-conserving therapy. Breast Cancer. 2009;16(2):97–104.
91. Fuster D, Duch J, Paredes P, Velasco M, Munoz M, Santamaria G, et al. Preoperative staging of large primary breast cancer with [18F]fluorodeoxyglucose positron emission tomography/computed tomography compared with conventional imaging procedures. J Clin Oncol. 2008;26(29):4746–51.
92. Segaert I, Mottaghy F, Ceyssens S, De Wever W, Stroobants S, Van Ongeval C, et al. Additional value of PET-CT in staging of clinical stage IIB and III breast cancer. Breast J. 2010;16(6):617–24.
93. Cooper KL, Harnan S, Meng Y, Ward SE, Fitzgerald P, Papaioannou D, et al. Positron emission tomography (PET) for assessment of axillary lymph node status in early breast cancer: a systematic review and meta-analysis. EurJ Surg Oncol. 2011;37(3):187–98.
94. Gil-Rendo A, Martinez-Regueira F, Zornoza G, Garcia-Velloso MJ, Beorlegui C, Rodriguez-Spiteri N. Association between [18F] fluorodeoxyglucose uptake and prognostic parameters in breast cancer. Br J Surg. 2009;96(2):166–70.
95. Buck A, Schirrmeister H, Kuhn T, Shen C, Kalker T, Kotzerke J, et al. FDG uptake in breast cancer: correlation with biological and clinical prognostic parameters. Eur J Nucl Med Mol Imaging. 2002;29(10):1317–23.

96. Avril N, Menzel M, Dose J, Schelling M, Weber W, Janicke F, et al. Glucose metabolism of breast cancer assessed by 18F-FDG PET: histologic and immunohistochemical tissue analysis. J Nucl Med. 2001;42(1):9–16.
97. Shimoda W, Hayashi M, Murakami K, Oyama T, Sunagawa M. The relationship between FDG uptake in PET scans and biological behavior in breast cancer. Breast Cancer. 2007;14(3): 260–8.
98. Ikenaga N, Otomo N, Toyofuku A, Ueda Y, Toyoda K, Hayashi T, et al. Standardized uptake values for breast carcinomas assessed by fluorodeoxyglucose-positron emission tomography correlate with prognostic factors. Am Surg. 2007;73(11):1151–7.
99. Groheux D, Giacchetti S, Moretti JL, Porcher R, Espie M, Lehmann-Che J, et al. Correlation of high 18F-FDG uptake to clinical, pathological and biological prognostic factors in breast cancer. Eur J Nucl Med Mol Imaging. 2011;38(3):426–35.
100. Mavi A, Cermik TF, Urhan M, Puskulcu H, Basu S, Yu JQ, et al. The effects of estrogen, progesterone, and C-erbB-2 receptor states on 18F-FDG uptake of primary breast cancer lesions. J Nucl Med. 2007;48(8):1266–72.
101. Inoue T, Yutani K, Taguchi T, Tamaki Y, Shiba E, Noguchi S. Preoperative evaluation of prognosis in breast cancer patients by [(18)F]2-Deoxy-2-fluoro-D-glucose-positron emission tomography. J Cancer Res Clin Oncol. 2004;130(5):273–8.
102. Basu S, Chen W, Tchou J, Mavi A, Cermik T, Czerniecki B, et al. Comparison of triple-negative and estrogen receptor-positive/progesterone receptor-positive/HER2-negative breast carcinoma using quantitative fluorine-18 fluorodeoxyglucose/positron emission tomography imaging parameters: a potentially useful method for disease characterization. Cancer. 2008;112(5):995–1000.
103. Kumar R, Chauhan A, Zhuang H, Chandra P, Schnall M, Alavi A. Clinicopathologic factors associated with false negative FDG-PET in primary breast cancer. Breast Cancer Res Treat. 2006; 98(3):267–74.
104. van der Hoeven JJ, Krak NC, Hoekstra OS, Comans EF, Boom RP, van Geldere D, et al. 18F-2-fluoro-2-deoxy-d-glucose positron emission tomography in staging of locally advanced breast cancer. J Clin Oncol. 2004;22(7):1253–9.
105. Aukema TS, Rutgers EJ, Vogel WV, Teertstra HJ, Oldenburg HS, Vrancken Peeters MT, et al. The role of FDG PET/CT in patients with locoregional breast cancer recurrence: a comparison to conventional imaging techniques. Eur J Surg Oncol. 2010;36(4): 387–92.
106. Berg WA, Weinberg IN, Narayanan D, Lobrano ME, Ross E, Amodei L, et al. High-resolution fluorodeoxyglucose positron emission tomography with compression ("positron emission mammography") is highly accurate in depicting primary breast cancer. Breast J. 2006;12(4):309–23.
107. MacDonald L, Edwards J, Lewellen T, Haseley D, Rogers J, Kinahan P. Clinical imaging characteristics of the positron emission mammography camera: PEM Flex Solo II. J Nucl Med. 2009;50(10):1666–75.
108. Eo JS, Chun IK, Paeng JC, Kang KW, Lee SM, Han W, et al. Imaging sensitivity of dedicated positron emission mammography in relation to tumor size. Breast. 2012;21(1):66–71.
109. Levine EA, Freimanis RI, Perrier ND, Morton K, Lesko NM, Bergman S, et al. Positron emission mammography: initial clinical results. Ann Surg Oncol. 2003;10(1):86–91.
110. Rosen EL, Turkington TG, Soo MS, Baker JA, Coleman RE. Detection of primary breast carcinoma with a dedicated, large-field-of-view FDG PET mammography device: initial experience. Radiology. 2005;234(2):527–34.
111. Tafra L, Cheng Z, Uddo J, Lobrano MB, Stein W, Berg WA, et al. Pilot clinical trial of 18F-fluorodeoxyglucose positron-emission mammography in the surgical management of breast cancer. Am J Surg. 2005;190(4):628–32.
112. Berg WA, Madsen KS, Schilling K, Tartar M, Pisano ED, Larsen LH, et al. Breast cancer: comparative effectiveness of positron emission mammography and MR imaging in presurgical planning for the ipsilateral breast. Radiology. 2011;258(1):59–72.
113. Berg WA, Madsen KS, Schilling K, Tartar M, Pisano ED, Larsen LH, et al. Comparative effectiveness of positron emission mammography and MRI in the contralateral breast of women with newly diagnosed breast cancer. AJR Am J Roentgenol. 2012;198(1):219–32.
114. Cutler M. Transillumination of the breast. Ann Surg. 1931;93(1): 223–34.
115. Sickles EA. Breast cancer detection with transillumination and mammography. AJR Am J Roentgenol. 1984;142(4):841–4.
116. Leff DR, Warren OJ, Enfield LC, Gibson A, Athanasiou T, Patten DK, et al. Diffuse optical imaging of the healthy and diseased breast: a systematic review. Breast Cancer Res Treat. 2008;108(1):9–22.
117. Soliman H, Gunasekara A, Rycroft M, Zubovits J, Dent R, Spayne J, et al. Functional imaging using diffuse optical spectroscopy of neoadjuvant chemotherapy response in women with locally advanced breast cancer. Clin Cancer Res. 2010;16(9):2605–14.
118. Poellinger A, Persigehl T, Mahler M, Bahner M, Ponder SL, Diekmann F, et al. Near-infrared imaging of the breast using omocianine as a fluorescent dye: results of a placebo-controlled, clinical, multicenter trial. Invest Radiol. 2011;46(11):697–704.
119. van de Ven S, Wiethoff A, Nielsen T, Brendel B, van der Voort M, Nachabe R, et al. A novel fluorescent imaging agent for diffuse optical tomography of the breast: first clinical experience in patients. Mol Imaging Biol. 2010;12(3):343–8.
120. Jose I, Deodhar KD, Desai UB, Bhattacharjee S. Early detection of breast cancer: synthesis and characterization of novel target specific NIR-fluorescent estrogen conjugate for molecular optical imaging. J Fluoresc. 2011;21(3):1171–7.
121. van de Ven SM, Elias SG, Chan CT, Miao Z, Cheng Z, De A, et al. Optical imaging with her2-targeted affibody molecules can monitor hsp90 treatment response in a breast cancer xenograft mouse model. Clin Cancer Res. 2012;18(4):1073–81.
122. Shalviri A. Evaluation of new bi-functional terpolymeric nanoparticles for simultaneous in vivo optical imaging and chemotherapy of breast cancer. Drug Deliv Transl Res. 2012;2(6):437–53.

Index

M.K. Shetty (ed.), *Breast Cancer Screening and Diagnosis: A Synopsis*,
DOI 10.1007/978-1-4939-1267-4, © Springer Science+Business Media New York 2015

C

Printed in the United States of America